Nutritional On

Nutritional Oncology
Nutrition in Cancer Prevention, Treatment, and Survivorship

Edited by

David Heber, MD, PHD
UCLA Center for Human Nutrition
David Geffen School of Medicine at UCLA
Los Angeles, California

Zhaoping Li, MD, PHD
UCLA Center for Human Nutrition
David Geffen School of Medicine at UCLA
Los Angeles, California

Vay Liang W. Go, MD
UCLA Center for Human Nutrition
David Geffen School of Medicine at UCLA
Los Angeles, California

Foreword by
Michael Milken

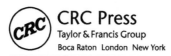

CRC Press
Taylor & Francis Group
Boca Raton London New York

CRC Press is an imprint of the
Taylor & Francis Group, an **informa** business

First edition published 2022
by CRC Press
6000 Broken Sound Parkway NW, Suite 300, Boca Raton, FL 33487-2742

and by CRC Press
2 Park Square, Milton Park, Abingdon, Oxon, OX14 4RN

Library of Congress Cataloging-in-Publication Data
Names: Heber, David, editor. | Li, Zhaoping, 1962- editor. | Go, Vay Liang W., editor.
Title: Nutritional oncology : nutrition in cancer prevention, treatment,
and survivorship / edited by David Heber, Zhaoping Li, Vay Liang W. Go.
Other titles: Nutritional oncology (Heber)
Description: First edition. | Boca Raton : CRC Press, 2021. | Includes
bibliographical references and index. | Summary: "Nutritional Oncology:
Nutrition in Cancer Prevention, Treatment, and Survivorship presents
evidence-based approaches to the study and application of nutrition in
all phases of cancer including prevention, treatment, and survivorship.
There is a long history of interest in the role of nutrition in cancer
but only in the last 50 years has this interdisciplinary field developed
scientific evidence from a combination of population studies, basic
research, and clinical studies. Precision oncology, targeted therapies
and immunonutrition have led to advances in cancer treatment and
prevention. Highlighting insights from Precision Oncology and Precision
Nutrition to improve cancer prevention, treatment and survival is the
core mission of this book. The editors have over 40 years of clinical
and research experience integrating science with practical advice based
on available evidence for healthcare professionals while highlighting
research vistas for the scientific community"— Provided by publisher.
Identifiers: LCCN 2021011033 | ISBN 9780367272494 (hardback) |
ISBN 9781032002613 (paperback) | ISBN 9780429317385 (ebook)
Subjects: MESH: Neoplasms—diet therapy | Neoplasms—etiology |
Neoplasms—prevention & control | Nutritional Physiological Phenomena |
Diet—adverse effects
Classification: LCC RC271.D52 | NLM QZ 266 | DDC 616.99/40654–dc23
LC record available at https://lccn.loc.gov/2021011033

ISBN: 9780367272494 (hbk)
ISBN: 9781032002613 (pbk)
ISBN: 9780429317385 (ebk)

Typeset in Times
by codeMantra

Printed and bound by CPI Group (UK) Ltd, Croydon, CR0 4YY

We dedicate this textbook on Nutritional Oncology to the scientists listed below who contributed so much during their long careers to the field of nutrition and cancer research. We stand on the shoulders of these giants whom we remember as we hope to inspire a future generation of researchers and clinicians.

Dr. George Blackburn

Dr. Donald S. Coffey

Dr. Robert Elashoff

Dr. Norman Farnsworth

Dr. Sydney Finegold

Dr. Judah Folkman

Dr. David Golde

Dr. David Kritchevsky

Dr. John Milner

Dr. Paul Talalay

Dr. Vernon R. Young

Dr. Ernst Wynder

Contents

Preface

Advances in molecular and cellular biology have led to Precision Oncology and the emerging fields of Personalized and Precision Nutrition. Increasingly cancer is seen as a systemic and not an organ-confined disease which can increasingly be controlled and converted into a chronic disease rather than an acute fatal disease. Millions of cancer survivors around the world are seeking information on how they got this disease and what can be done to reduce the risk of relapse or second cancers. Scientific advances in cancer, molecular signal networks in tumor cells, angiogenesis and the tumor microenvironment, targeted molecular cancer therapies and immunotherapies as well as the discovery of the gut microbiome, immunonutrition, and personalization of nutrient requirements combine to create the knowledge base of Nutritional Oncology. Nutrition has long been associated with cancer through population studies defining associations of diet and cancer. Basic studies have demonstrated the potential of nutrition to modulate gene expression and cellular signals. The recent observation that the gut microbiome and immune system may be involved in the response of patients to immunotherapy has opened new avenues for research on the role of nutrition in cancer therapy. Nutrition plays a key role in risk factor reduction for cancer prevention, response to cancer treatment, and in the prevention of relapse and promotion of quality of life for the increasing population of cancer survivors.

As cancer is evolving to become more treatable as a chronic disease, the impact of Nutritional Oncology joining together advances in Precision Oncology and Personalized and Precision Nutrition will be an increasingly important part of the care of the growing global cancer patient and cancer survivor populations as well as an area ripe with research opportunities.

This book fulfills a growing need for cancer patients and their physicians who are puzzled about the role of nutrition in cancer and need more information. Unlike many texts and popular books on nutrition and cancer where alternative, integrative, and unproven nutritional therapies for cancer are presented as facts with little more than testimonial evidence, this text on Nutritional Oncology supports its assertions with scientific references, identifies future hypotheses for testing, and presents an overview of the evolution of the science of nutrition in cancer from editors with over 40 years of clinical and research experience in the field of Nutritional Oncology.

Foreword

On hearing the words "You have prostate cancer" in 1993, my first thought was about my family—the impact it would have on my wife and children. The next thought was of the many relatives, including my father and mother-in-law, who had received cancer diagnoses. Every one of them had died, and my prognosis was for a life expectancy of only 12–18 months. What could I do that they had not done? One realization was that none of them had made any significant changes in their diets.

Over the next year, we expanded the Milken Family Foundation's previous medical philanthropy by founding CaP CURE (now the Prostate Cancer Foundation). At the same time, even while undergoing extensive tests, androgen deprivation therapy and radiation, I studied the full range of treatment options. CaP CURE published epidemiological studies showing the negative health effects of Western diets on Asians who moved to America. This led me to Dr. David Heber, co-editor of this book and a respected nutritional oncologist. I knew Dr. Heber from our previous support of programs at University of California, Los Angeles (UCLA) but now sought his advice as an expert on nutrition and cancer.

Throughout my life to that point, I'd been a junk food enthusiast, even winning college fraternity eating contests that involved consuming shocking numbers of hot dogs. But now I decided that no hot dog was worth dying for. With David's encouragement, I changed 180 degrees to a plant-based diet. By this time, I was in remission, felt great, became a nutrition evangelist and eventually hired chef Beth Ginsberg, who joined me in writing two cookbooks of cancer-fighting recipes. We served delicious plant-based substitutes for high-fat foods in such locations as the U.S. Senate dining room and the ABC Television commissary. We even held competitions to show that most people couldn't tell the difference between junk food and the healthier versions Beth created.

At CaP CURE's 1994 Scientific Retreat, the agenda was filled with highly technical presentations on developments in cancer, especially the biology of prostate cancer. I had personally invited Dr. Heber to speak and that, it turned out, was a problem. No one questioned his qualifications as an experienced physician and author of many widely cited professional papers. It was the *subject* of his proposed lecture that bothered the program committee. "This conference is about hard science," one of the committee members said. "It's not about unproven theories of nutrition."

When I protested that there was widespread evidence of links between nutrition and the prevention or progression of disease", he was dismissive. "Mike, we appreciate your help in supporting our research, but now you're telling us crazy stuff. If you think eating vegetables or anything else can prevent or treat cancer, prove it." Eventually, we reached a compromise. We'd leave Dr. Heber off the formal agenda, but allow him to speak to the group at lunch.

In 1994, anecdotal evidence suggested associations between diet and cancer; but no one could prove a clear causal effect because cancer is a disease that begins at the cellular level. At the time, technology didn't exist to study the cellular interactions of food metabolites and incipient tumors. Today, thanks to revolutionary advances in genomic sequencing, proteomics and imaging, we can *prove* the link as documented in this important book.

The very concept of nutritional oncology that had been resisted at our 1994 conference dominated the agenda a quarter century later: at the 2019 Scientific Retreat, 20 percent of the program dealt with some aspect of the microbiome, diet and its effect on gene expression. Fringe ideas had become mainstream.

Hypotheses that were poorly understood three decades ago—the impact of obesity, the lipids-cancer link, and activation of a chronic immune response—are now widely accepted by clinicians. Dietary interventions have transformed the standard of care for cancer patients. Earlier work demonstrated that those patients who reduced caloric intake experienced less toxicity from radiation, decreased tumor size and fewer metastases. More recent studies using microbiome sequencing go further by marrying precision medicine with precision nutrition. This involves creating personalized diets that match the vulnerabilities of specific tumors.

Many other studies have buttressed the idea that food is medicine. There's no doubt in my mind it is that medicine which allows me to be here writing these words 28 years after a terminal diagnosis. It also strengthens my belief that our healthcare system should put greater emphasis on prevention. It makes no sense to allocate more than 90 percent of spending to treatment and less than 10 percent to the preventive strategies that can often reduce the need for treatment.

These kinds of advances add to 200 years of medical progress that economic historians credit for as much as half of all economic gains since the nineteenth century. After thousands of years of nearly imperceptible growth, the world's wealth began doubling every few decades starting about 1820. The largest stimulus for this growth was increased worker productivity made possible by improved health and extended lifespans—the result of better disease prevention and the cures produced by research.

The importance of research is especially appreciated by those of us who have seen the lives of close friends and relatives tragically cut short by cancer and other serious illnesses. Our time with them was precious. Not a day goes by that I don't think about loved ones who have passed away. So even as we focus on access to healthcare and its costs, let's never forget that each life saved by preventing disease and developing improved treatments is priceless. In that sense, this is a book not only about science, but also about hope. The hope of longer lives, of course, but also something greater—healthier, more meaningful lives for people everywhere.

Michael Milken
Founder, Prostate Cancer Foundation

Editors

Dr. David Heber is Professor Emeritus of Medicine and Public Health at the David Geffen School of Medicine at UCLA and is internationally prominent in the field nutrition and cancer as well as in obesity, and age-related chronic diseases and the application of nutrition in common forms of cancer including prostate and breast cancer. He is also the Founding Director of the UCLA Center for Human Nutrition and founding Chief of the Division of Clinical Nutrition in the UCLA Department of Medicine where he directed multiple NIH-funded research programs including the National Cancer Institute-funded UCLA Clinical Nutrition Research Unit, The NIH-funded UCLA Dietary Supplements Research Center: Botanicals and the NIH-National Institutes of Diabetes, Digestive, and Kidney Diseases UCLA Nutrition and Obesity Training Program where he oversaw the training of research fellows many of whom are currently in academic or industry positions. He has published over 250 research papers and numerous professional texts internationally. In 2014, he co-wrote a textbook with Dr. Bharat Aggarwal entitled *Immunonutrition* (CRC Press). Dr. Heber is board-certified in Internal Medicine, and Endocrinology and Metabolism by the American Board of Internal Medicine. He earned his MD at Harvard Medical School and his PhD in Physiology at the University of California, Los Angeles. In 2014, he was elected a Fellow of the American Society for Nutrition, the highest honor of the society. In 2017, he co-wrote a textbook for doctors together with Dr. Zhaoping Li, entitled *Primary Care Nutrition: Writing the Nutrition Prescription* (CRC Press, 2017).

Zhaoping Li, MD, PhD, is the Lynda and Stewart Resnick Endowed Chair in Human Nutrition, Professor and Chief of the Division of Clinical Nutrition in the Department of Medicine at the David Geffen School of Medicine at UCLA. She is also the Vice Chair of Medicine at the Greater Los Angeles VA Health System and is the Director of the multidisciplinary UCLA Center for Human Nutrition which includes the renowned UCLA Weight Management Program, the Nutritional Medicine Consultation Service, and a Nutritional Oncology Consultation Program serving cancer patients in over 80 practices within the UCLA Health Care System. She has been working with Dr. Heber in the Division of Clinical Nutrition since 1997. Dr. Li is board-certified in internal medicine, physician nutrition specialists, a fellow of American College of Physicians, and is a former President of the National Board of Physician Nutrition Specialists and a member of the Board of Directors of the American Society for Nutrition. Her research interests span both basic and clinical research in obesity, cancer, and other age-related chronic diseases and she supervises a faculty of MD clinical physician scientists and PhD laboratory scientists investigating gene–nutrient interaction, nutritional modulation of the microbiome, and health impacts of phytonutrients. Dr. Li has been a principal investigator for over 100 investigator-initiated National Institutes of Health and industry-sponsored clinical trials and published over 200 peer-reviewed scientific papers. In addition to the present volume she co-wrote *Primary Care Nutrition: Writing the Nutrition Prescription* with Dr. David Heber, published by CRC Press in 2017.

Vay Liang W. Go, MD, is a distinguished professor and co-director of the UCLA Agi Hirshberg Center for Pancreatic Diseases at the David Geffen School of Medicine at UCLA, Editor-in-Chief of *Pancreas*, and co-founder of the American Pancreatic Association. Over a five-decade academic career, his research has focused on the regulation of the human exocrine and endocrine pancreas and gut-brain axis in health and disease. He expanded to nutrition and cancer prevention and the mechanism of action of phytochemicals on pancreatic diseases utilizing metabolomics technologies. He received his internal medicine and gastroenterology training and subsequently became a professor of medicine at the Mayo Clinic. From 1985 to 1988, Dr. Go served in three related capacities at the National Institutes of Health, all involving digestive diseases and nutrition. He became the Executive Chairman, UCLA Department of Medicine from 1988 to 1992. In 1994, he co-founded the UCLA Center for Human Nutrition with Dr. David Heber. He was the Associate Director of the NCI-funded UCLA Clinical Nutrition Research Unit, Director of the Nutrition Education program, and co-principal investigator of the NIH funded nutrition curriculum development grants and the cancer prevention curriculum program. Dr. Go has authored and coauthored more than 400 peer reviewed manuscripts and mentored and trained more than 80 fellows in the field of gastroenterology, nutrition, endocrinology, and pancreatology, many of whom have attained leadership roles in their respective fields.

Contributors

Sidharth R. Anand
Division of Medical Oncology
Department of Medicine
David Geffen School of Medicine at UCLA
Los Angeles, California

Michael D. Bastasch
Department of Radiation Oncology
University of Texas East Health
Athens, Texas

Bettina M. Beech
Departments of Medicine and Surgery
Vanderbilt University School of Medicine
Nashville, Tennessee

Catherine L. Carpenter
UCLA Center for Human Nutrition
School of Nursing, Medicine and Public Health
Los Angeles, California

Bridget A. Cassady
Abbott Nutrition Research & Development
Columbus, Ohio

Mohamed El-Gamal
Toxicology Department
Faculty of Medicine
Mansoura University
Mansoura, Egypt

Stephen F. Freedland
Department of Surgery
Samuel Oschin Comprehensive Cancer Center
Cedars-Sinai Medical Center
Los Angeles, California
and
Section of Urology
Durham VA Medical Center
Durham, North Carolina

Michael R. Freeman
Department of Surgery
Samuel Oschin Comprehensive Cancer Center
Cedars-Sinai Medical Center
Los Angeles, California

Michael Garcia
UCLA Center for Human Nutrition
Department of Medicine
David Geffen School of Medicine at UCLA
Los Angeles, California

John A. Glaspy
Division of Medical Oncology
Department of Medicine
David Geffen School of Medicine at UCLA
Los Angeles, California

Refaat Hegazi
Abbott Nutrition Research & Development
Columbus, Ohio
and
Faculty of Medicine
Mansoura University
Mansoura, Egypt

Susanne Henning
UCLA Center for Human Nutrition
Department of Medicine
David Geffen School of Medicine at UCLA
Los Angeles, California

Shafiq A. Khan
Center for Cancer Research and Therapeutic
    Development
Clark Atlanta University
Atlanta, Georgia

Lauren Lemieux
UCLA Center for Human Nutrition
Department of Medicine
David Geffen School of Medicine at UCLA
Los Angeles, California

William W. Li
The Angiogenesis Foundation
Cambridge, Massachusetts

Berkeley N. Limketkai
Division of Gastroenterology
Department of Medicine
David Geffen School of Medicine at UCLA
Los Angeles, California

Qing-Yi Lu
UCLA Center for Human Nutrition
Department of Medicine
David Geffen School of Medicine at UCLA
Los Angeles, California

Elad Mashiach
The Angiogenesis Foundation
Cambridge, Massachusetts

William J. McCarthy
Department of Health Policy and Management
UCLA Fielding School of Public Health
Los Angeles, California

Steven D. Mittelman
Division of Endocrinology
Department of Pediatrics
David Geffen School of Medicine at UCLA
Los Angeles, California

Keith C. Norris
Division of General Internal Medicine and
    Health Services Research
Department of Medicine
David Geffen School of Medicine at UCLA
Los Angeles, California

Rebecca L. Paszkiewicz
Division of Endocrinology
Department of Pediatrics
David Geffen School of Medicine at UCLA
Los Angeles, California

Gail S. Prins
Departments of Urology, Physiology,
    Biophysics, and Pathology
University of Illinois at Chicago
Chicago, Illinois

Katie N. Robinson
Abbott Nutrition Research & Development
Columbus, Ohio

Navindra Seeram
College of Pharmacy
University of Rhode Island
Kingston, Rhode Island

Vijaya Surampudi
UCLA Center for Human Nutrition
Department of Medicine
David Geffen School of Medicine at UCLA
Los Angeles, California

Sara Thomas
Abbott Nutrition Research & Development
Columbus, Ohio

Emily Truong
Division of Gastroenterology
Department of Medicine
David Geffen School of Medicine at UCLA,
Los Angeles, California

Smrruthi V. Venugopal
Department of Surgery
Samuel Oschin Comprehensive Cancer Center
Cedars-Sinai Medical Center
Los Angeles California

David G.A. Williams
Duke Clinical Research Institute
Duke University
Durham, North Carolina

Lishi Xie
Departments of Urology, Physiology,
    Biophysics, and Pathology,
University of Illinois at Chicago
Chicago, Illinois

Zuo-Feng Zhang
Center for Environmental Genomics
Department of Epidemiology
UCLA Fielding School of Public Health
Los Angeles, California

1 Historical Evolution of the Role of Nutrition in Cancer

David Heber and Vay Liang W. Go
UCLA Center for Human Nutrition

CONTENTS

INTRODUCTION

The role nutrition plays in cancer causation, treatment, and survivorship has received significant interest leading to an active area of research by scientists and physicians, but it still engenders considerable controversy in the oncology community and among many basic scientists. Within the cancer research and clinical community, nutrition has been traditionally considered a side issue. It was the interest of the cancer patient community in the potential benefits of diet, lifestyle, and supplements through lobbying of legislators that led to the formation of the American Cancer Society (ACS) and the National Cancer Institute (NCI) to attack cancer. The "War on Cancer" in the 1970s focused attention on the etiology and prevention of cancer, nutrition took its place alongside smoking cessation as a significant prevention research area at the NCI.

In 1980, the NCI commissioned the National Research Council (NRC) to conduct a comprehensive study of the scientific information pertaining to the relationship of diet and nutrition to cancer. The NCI requested that a committee "review the state of knowledge and information pertinent to diet/nutrition and the incidence of cancer" and "develop a series of recommendations related to dietary components (nutrients and toxic contaminants)". It also requested that the NRC "based on the above state-of-the-art appraisals and the identification of gap areas develop a series of research recommendations related to dietary components and nutritional factors and the incidence of cancer". The NCI then asked that two reports be prepared: the first to advise the NCI and the public whether evidence indicates that certain dietary habits may affect the risk of developing cancer and the second to inform the NCI and the scientific community about useful directions research might take to increase our knowledge in this area. This effort was organized as the Diet, Nutrition, and Cancer Program of the NCI.

The three major sources of scientifically valid data used in the report were epidemiological studies on human populations; experimental studies on animals; and in vitro tests for genetic toxicity. Special attention was given to the degree of concordance between epidemiological and experimental

1

evidence for individual components of the diet; the greater the concordance, the more useful the information obtained. Various sections of the work reviewed nutrients, nonnutrients, and the current state of knowledge concerning trends in cancer incidence, focusing on the role that diet plays in the occurrence of cancer at specific sites.

In order to pursue multidisciplinary integrated research on diet, nutrition, and cancer, the NCI participated in the National Institutes of Health Clinical Nutrition Research Units (CNRU) program by funding two of eight CNRU's nationally to concentrate on nutrition and cancer research at Sloane-Kettering Cancer Center in New York and at the University of California, Los Angeles (UCLA) in Los Angeles. The authors of this chapter (D.H. and V.L.W.G.) led the CNRU funded by the NCI at the UCLA from 1992 to 2006 involving over 100 scientists from multiple disciplines. Studies of genenutrient interaction in patients with colonic adenomatous polyps, phytonutrient effects on skin, breast, and prostate cancer effects of weight reduction on hormones and inflammation were carried out. The CNRU had a series of cores (lipid-hormone, gene-nutrient, biostatistics, molecular oncology, etc.) which served many projects in multiple divisions and departments at UCLA and other institutions nationally. The NCI also funded human intervention studies utilizing low fat diets including the Women's Health Initiative and Women's Nutrition Intervention Study, as well as many investigator-initiated research studies. The NCI also developed a public education program geared at increasing fruit and vegetable intake patterned after the "5-A-Day for Better Health" program of the California Department of Health Services reflecting the considerable population, clinical, and basic research evidence demonstrating the anticancer benefits of phytonutrients found in colorful fruits and vegetables.

Over the last 15 years, the increased use of genotyping of cancer specimens using next generation sequencing has led to the development of therapies that take advantage of the amplified metabolic pathways and surface receptors for growth factors in cancer. The discovery of imatinib and other tyrosine kinase inhibitors has revolutionized cancer therapy. Advances in immunotherapy coupled with the appreciation of the role of the gut microbiome in immunity have given new relevance to nutrition research in cancer. Genetics for precision oncology and understanding personalized nutrition based on phenotype and genotype promise a new era in the evolution of nutrition research in cancer prevention, treatment, and survivorship.

CANCER MALNUTRITION

The starvation, anorexia, and cachexia accompanying advanced cancer must have been observed in ancient times as it is today, but we have no record of such observations from either the early Egyptian observations on breast cancer or the writings on cancer from the Hippocratic school in Greece. There were scattered observations in the 1800s but it was the metabolic observations of Warburg and Corey in 1924 on tumor metabolism that were seminal in establishing major research efforts on the potential role of nutrition in cancer treatment. Today there is an increased understanding of the fuel choices of cancer cells to meet their demands for energy and for the production of biosynthetic precursors which are affected by intrinsic and extrinsic factors including oncogene mutations, nutrient and oxygen availability, and factors in the tumor microenvironment (DeNicola and Cantley 2015).

Nutrition support was provided as an afterthought in most hospitals treating advanced cancer until the 1960s when total parenteral nutrition (TPN) was developed first in dogs and then in humans by Dr. Stanley Dudrick at the Peter Bent Brigham Hospital in Boston and Harvard Medical School. TPN became available as a "high-tech" approach to nutrition supposedly superior to other methods and was used in advanced cancer patients in an attempt to improve antitumor responses (1981). Current guidelines from the European Society for Enteral and Parenteral Nutrition recognize that efforts at nutritional therapy in patients with cancer are impeded or precluded by the frequent development of metabolic derangements in induced by the tumor or by its treatment (Arends et al. 2017).

Early research in this area was motivated by the observation that many cancer patients did not gain weight despite the provision of adequate or even excess calories based on their apparent metabolic needs. While cancer patients since the 1970s have been screened for the risk or the presence of malnutrition, there have been few well-controlled trials demonstrating the benefit of nutrition on responses to therapy or survival. This area of research has receded in popularity and the pragmatic current situation is that all cancer patients with the exception of those at the end of life are provided energy and substrates as required in a stepwise manner of supportive nutrition from counseling to enteral and/or parenteral nutrition. To counter malnutrition in patients with advanced cancer there are a few pharmacological agents which produce weight gain and some nutrient approaches that improve cachexia and anorexia but these have only limited effects unless the tumor responds to treatment. General advice to cancer survivors is also limited and amounts to encouraging regular physical activity and adoption of a "prudent" diet.

VITAMINS AND CANCER

Vitamins were an exciting area of nutrition research in the early twentieth century leading to the award of several Nobel prizes for the isolation and chemical characterization of the essential vitamins we know today. It was considered from the earliest time that these substances in tiny amounts had amazing effects in vitamin-deficient animals and humans. Studying childhood leukemia in the 1940s, Dr. Sidney Farber had read about folic acid and its benefits for normal cells in malnourished individuals and thought it might be beneficial to the nutrition of children with leukemia. He gave folic acid to children with leukemia, and unexpectedly, these children had relapses and got worse not better. Dr. Farber knew Dr. Yellapragada Subbarow who was conducting research in the 1940s at Lederle Labs trying to synthesize folic acid after being denied tenure at Harvard Medical School. His experiments led to the synthesis of antifolic acid vitamin analogs. His discoveries of aminopterin and methotrexate acting as antivitamins induced remissions in some children ultimately initiating an era of chemotherapy research for decades. Through the efforts of Dr. Farber, the namesake of the Dana-Farber Center in Boston (Farber 1949) an era in which combination chemotherapy and the extensive and successful use of the randomized control trials through the NCI would set a standard that nutrition studies in cancer would rarely achieve.

However, vitamin C or ascorbic acid in large doses was touted as a cure for cancer by Dr. Linus Pauling who at the time had won Nobel Prizes in Chemistry and Peace, and many scientists were aghast at this suggestion. Nutrition science has developed a great deal of information on vitamin C, known as ascorbic acid or ascorbate. It is synthesized in animals except for humans, monkeys, guinea pigs, and several other animal species. Humans underwent a series of inactivating mutations of the gene encoding gluconolactone oxidase, a key enzyme in vitamin C biosynthesis most likely due to the abundance of vitamin C in the plants that made up the ancient human diet. Today, the human diet includes vegetables and fruits, including brussels sprout, broccoli, cauliflower, bell pepper, chili pepper, lettuce, kale, tomato, citrus fruits, strawberry, papaya, kiwifruit, pineapple, and mango.

Vitamin C supplements taken orally produce plasma concentrations that are tightly controlled so that plasma concentrations do not further increase readily at doses of 200 mg or above per day. On the other hand, intravenous injections of large doses of vitamin C can produce millimolar concentrations of plasma vitamin C (Padayatty et al. 2004). Intracellular concentrations of vitamin C are in the millimolar range in many cells as a result of transport of the oxidized form of vitamin C (dehydroascorbate) into cells where it is chemically reduced to vitamin C (Agus, Vera, and Golde 1999). Tumor and muscle cells have the highest concentrations of vitamin C but this does not imply that vitamin C promotes tumor growth as some have surmised, and there is recent evidence that high-dose vitamin C administered intravenously may improve the response to chemotherapy in some tumors (Blaszczak et al. 2019).

A hallmark of acute promyelocytic leukemia is the expression of PML/RARα fusion protein. Treatment with all-trans retinoic acid (ATRA), a metabolite of vitamin A, results in the terminal differentiation of neutrophil granulocytes (Wang et al. 2019, Wang and Chen 2008). Since the introduction of ATRA in the treatment and optimization of the ATRA-based regimens, the clinical response rate was raised up to 90%–95% and 5-year disease-free survival to 74% in this form of leukemia (Wang and Chen 2008).

A systematic review to support the European Palliative Care Research Collaboration development of clinical guidelines for cancer patients suffering from cachexia examined 4,214 publications with 21 of these included in the final evaluation (Mochamat et al. 2017). Vitamin E in combination with omega-3 fatty acids displayed an effect on survival in a single study, vitamin D showed improvement of muscle weakness in prostate cancer patients, and vitamin C supplementation led to an improvement of various quality of life aspects in a sample with a variety of cancer diagnoses. For proteins, a combination therapy of β-hydroxy-β-methylbutyrate, arginine, and glutamine led to an increase in lean body mass after 4 weeks in a study of advanced solid tumor patients, whereas the same combination did not show a benefit on lean body mass in a large sample of advanced lung and other cancer patients. After 8 weeks. L-carnitine led to an increase of body mass index and an increase in overall survival in advanced pancreatic cancer patients. Adverse effects of food supplementation were rare and were of mild intensity. At this time, the systematic review did not identify enough solid evidence to recommend the use of minerals, vitamins, proteins, or other supplements in cancer. On the other hand, no serious adverse effects have been reported with dietary supplementation.

CANCER CAUSATION

Research into cancer causation began with the observation by the British surgeon Percivall Pott in 1775 that cancer of the scrotum was a common disease among chimney sweeps (Brown and Thornton 1957). It was later noted that coal tar dyes also caused skin cancer, an observation which stimulated research to this day on chemical carcinogenesis (Moustafa et al. 2015).

By the early twentieth century the observations of Professor Frederick L. Hoffman (1885–1946) on the causes of cancer in the nineteenth century, published in 1937, documented an increase in the incidence of cancer in the early twentieth century. Between 1900 and 1916, cancer-related mortality grew by nearly 30%, and by 1926, cancer had become America's second most common lethal disease only surpassed by heart disease. The ACS was founded in 1913 by 15 physicians and businessmen in New York City under the name American Society for the Control of Cancer. The NCI was established through the National Cancer Act of 1937. The passage of this law represented the culmination of nearly three decades of efforts to formalize the U.S. government's role in cancer research.

In the US, a 1958 food additives amendment to the US Food, Drug, and Cosmetic Act, known as the Delaney Clause, stated that chemicals capable of causing cancer should not be permitted in food (Weisburger 1996). The concept that chemical carcinogens are a major cause of human cancer whether in food or in occupational and general settings is still an active area of scientific research today that is related to nutrition and cancer research.

CHEMICAL CARCINOGENESIS

The Delaney Clause created the need for an experimental animal bioassay program to identify chemicals having this property. Indeed, legislation mandated a program to determine and assess chemicals with the potential to cause human cancer (Zeiger 2017). Dr. Bruce Ames developed the Ames test for chemical mutagens in the 1970s. The test assessed the ability of chemicals to induce mutations in the bacterium *Salmonella typhimurium* (Rueff, Rodrigues, and Kranendonk 2019). Several synthetic substances including dyes, which caused mutations, were banned. The test made

Ames a hero to environmentalists. However, he later changed his position on synthetic chemicals, following the realization that smoking cessation and changes in diet and lifestyle were more important in cancer prevention (Ames and Gold 1997). As a result, during the 1990s, he came into conflict with environmentalists who had once praised him as a scientist who contributed to their cause by developing the Ames Test. Ames devoted much of his career to the study of nutrition, aging, and cancer at the University of California and later at the Children's Hospital in Oakland, California. He was active in research and advocacy for nutrition research well into his 90s.

To this day, several government agencies and laboratories participate in the effort to identify chemical carcinogens, including the Food and Drug Administration, Environmental Protection Agency, the Occupational Safety and Health Administration and the Consumer Product Safety Commission (Huff, Jacobson, and Davis 2008). The lead organization in this effort is the National Toxicology Program of the Public Health Service which summarizes evidence in reports on chemical carcinogens. Chemicals are classified into those that are "known to be human carcinogens" and those that are "reasonably anticipated to be human carcinogens" (Elmore et al. 2018).

At the international level, the International Agency for Research on Cancer (IARC) of the World Health Organization has been conducting since 1971 a relatively sophisticated program of carcinogen evaluation as part of their Monograph Program, gathering information from a variety of sources (Rousseau, Straif, and Siemiatycki 2005). IARC distinguishes five main groups or physical factors on the basis of existing scientific data to assess their carcinogenic potential:

(1) the agent may be a carcinogenic mixture for humans (proven carcinogen or certainly carcinogenic). The exposure circumstance entails exposures that are carcinogenic to humans. This category is only used when sufficient indications of carcinogenicity for humans are available. As of 2012, 108 agents were classified in Group 1 of IARC. This group is divided into subgroups: agents and groups of agents, complex mixtures, occupational exposures, and others; (2) Agents that are probably carcinogenic for human beings where there is no formal evidence of carcinogenicity in humans, but corroborating indicators of its carcinogenicity for humans and sufficient evidence of carcinogenicity in experimental animals. As of 2012, 64 agents and group of agents were included in this group called 2A; (3) a subgroup of the second group (called 2B) included as of 2012 some 272 agents judged probably carcinogenic to humans. There is limited evidence of carcinogenicity in humans for this group and evidence for animals, or insufficient evidence for human beings but sufficient evidence of carcinogenicity in experimental animals (possible carcinogens); (4) 508 agents are included in Group 3 and are not classifiable as to their carcinogenicity to humans. (Insufficient evidence for human beings and insufficient or limited for animals.); and (5) agents which are probably not carcinogenic for human beings are in a group where evidence suggesting lack of carcinogenicity in humans and in experimental animals is evident.

These research and policy communities acknowledge that conducting experimental research on putative carcinogens and assessing their risk to humans is not a very quantitative science because their activities are affected by a variety of experimental, lifestyle, and environmental factors (Guyton et al. 2018, Smith et al. 2016, Goodman and Lynch 2017).

NUTRITION AND CANCER

In 1975, under the leadership of the late Ernst Wynder (1922–1999), the American Health Foundation in conjunction with the NCI sponsored the 1975 Key Biscayne Conference on nutrition in the causation of cancer (Wynder 1975). Dr. Wynder had distinguished himself with seminal studies conducted on the relationship of tobacco and lung cancer. His research on the nutritional causes of large bowel cancer presented at the Biscayne Conference led to the following summary: "Results from epidemiological studies have provided clues as to etiological factors involved in the development of large bowel cancer. Overnutrition, especially in terms of dietary fat consumed, appears to be a key etiological variable affecting the rate of colon cancer. Epidemiologists can provide the leads for chemists and bacteriologists to pursue in population groups and for experimentalists to test in laboratory animals. Coordination of and cooperation between many disciplines is necessary in order to contribute to the prevention of this man-made disease".

Then, in 1977, the U.S. Senate Committee recommended some simple and clear dietary goals for all Americans, mostly based on diet and heart disease (1977, Lee 1978). Based on the growing implications that diet played a role in cancer, the U.S. Senate appropriated funds to the National Academy of Sciences (NAS) enabling the preparation and publication of the 1982 NAS Diet, Nutrition and Cancer report (1982). Subsequently, many more public policy reports including the Surgeon General's Report on Nutrition and Health repeated that about one-third of all cancers were caused by diet (McGinnis 1988). These estimates were based on epidemiological studies by Doll and Peto which have held true over decades of further research (Blot and Tarone 2015).

The interest of the NCI in cancer control initially focused on early detection and treatment. Less attention was focused on prevention with the exception of research on tobacco and cancer. Then, in the late 1960s and 1970s, this began to change. Researchers associated a growing number of occupational, environmental, and lifestyle factors with cancer, and Congress and advocacy groups pressured the NCI to devote more resources to studies of cancer causation and primary prevention. Research on diet, nutrition, and cancer following the 1971 Cancer Act increased at the beginning of what was known then as the War on Cancer. Federal support for diet and nutrition research was increased as part of the growing interest in prevention (Cantor 2012). Research on diet, nutrition, and cancer following the 1971 Cancer Act increased at the beginning of what was known then as the War on Cancer.

DIET AND NUTRITION

While the basic research on metabolism in cancer was proceeding, there was a parallel development of dietary assessment tools in nutritional epidemiology and these tools were applied to understanding diet, nutrition, and cancer through observational studies (Satija et al. 2015). Nutritional epidemiology studies examined the association of differences in nutrient intake, or dietary patterns with the observed incidence of cancer.

There are two major study designs used in nutritional epidemiology: (1) case–control studies which compare patients with cancer and healthy age-matched controls. These studies do not control for the changes in eating patterns of individuals that have cancer or who changed their diet before or after diagnosis as a result of the perception that diet could be a contributing factor to their cancer or precancerous condition; and (2) prospective cohort studies which identify a large group of individuals and follow their incidence of new cancers over time. The interpretation of that data often informs public policy and results in recommendations to the public which are controversial due to the biases of the public and the interests of established producers of specific food categories or products which are judged to be beneficial or harmful in these analyses. These large cohorts developed many years ago tend not to reflect the demographic changes that have occurred over the last 40 years. When contradictory "man bites dog" data are developed, they receive a lot of press and undermine the public's confidence in nutrition science. For many reasons, data derived from nutritional epidemiology have often been attacked in the popular press making it difficult to promote healthy eating habits among the general public.

For both types of studies, the food frequency questionnaire (FFQ) is often used especially in very large studies where it is the most practical alternative. FFQs consist of a structured food list and a frequency response section on which the participant indicates the usual frequency of intake of each food over a certain period of time in the past. It is the most common choice for measuring intake in large observational studies owing to its ease of use, low participant burden, and ability to capture usual long-term dietary intake. These features make possible repeated assessments over time, which can capture long-term variations in diet trends.

Systematic sources of variation in the FFQ and other dietary assessment tools include omission of occasional foods consumed by individuals, errors in estimating portion sizes, and over- or under-reporting due to desired social approval and praise or social desirability. Biological specimens can augment the food intake data obtained from questionnaires. For example, doubly labeled water can be used to assess total energy intake (Westerterp 2018); urinary urea nitrogen can be used to estimate protein intake (Okuda, Asakura, and Sasaki 2019); and blood lipid profiles or nutritional lipidomics (Smilowitz et al. 2013). Various blood levels of phytonutrients such as lycopene from tomato products can assess specific fruit and vegetable intake.

A recent meta-analysis (Grosso et al. 2017) examined 93 studies including over 85,000 cases, 100,000 controls, and 2,000,000 exposed individuals. Data were extracted from each identified study using a standardized form by two independent authors. The most convincing evidence from prospective cohort studies supported an association between healthy dietary patterns and a decreased risk of colon and breast cancer. Limited evidence was found of a relation between an unhealthy dietary pattern and risk of upper aerodigestive tract, pancreatic, ovarian, endometrial, and prostatic cancers based only on case–control studies. Unhealthy dietary patterns were associated with higher body mass index and energy intake, while healthy patterns were associated with higher education, physical activity, and less smoking. Potential differences across geographical regions require further evaluation. These results which typify the conclusions reached by nutritional epidemiologists studying nutrition and cancer suggest a potential role of diet in certain cancers, but the evidence is not conclusive and may be driven or mediated by lifestyle factors.

NUTRIGENOMICS

The sequencing of the human genome at the turn of the century stimulated the development of research into nutrigenomics (Mathers 2017) and precision medicine with a focus on cancer (Collins and Varmus 2015). Nutrigenomics is a term used to denote both the field of nutrigenetics which applies genomics in population studies which also consider dietary intake and nutrients to search for gene–nutrient interactions and the field of nutrigenomics where basic researchers examine the effects of nutrients on the genome examining RNA transcribed, proteins formed, and cellular phenotype. Much of the early hype around possible applications of this new science was the fiction that you could go to a doctor and he would tell you what to eat based on your genome which would then allow you to link to a food producer who would send customized food to your home to help you prevent age-related chronic diseases including common forms of cancer (Sikalidis 2019).

This early hype was unhelpful and led to commercial ventures that sent you some information on common genetic variants or single-nucleotide polymorphisms (Levy et al. 2007). All humans are 99.9% genetically identical, but that 0.1% difference can be studied for its impact on the contribution of genetic variation to a wide range of phenotypes including common forms of cancer (Hoppe et al. 2018).

Innovative genetic research of multiple genes at once, copy number variants, and of interactions between genotype and dietary factors in determining phenotypes are leading to some new understandings of the difference among individuals in their response to a healthy diet for cancer prevention. At the same time, stem cell-based approaches and genome editing have huge potential to transform mechanistic nutrition and cancer research for both treatment and prevention.

The application of nutrigenetics research may improve public health through the use of metabolomics approaches to identify novel biomarkers of food intake, which will lead to more objective and robust measures of dietary exposure. The discovery of the microbiome led to the concept of two metabolomes—the food metabolome and the endogenous metabolome. As food is digested and metabolized, the endogenous metabolome is formed. The microbiome also digests foods and releases metabolites into the circulation where they enter the endogenous metabolome. Therefore, the food metabolome results from both endogenous and microbiota-mediated metabolism (Scalbert et al. 2014).

Identical twins have the same 23,000 human genes, but can have up to a 20% difference in their microbiome genes. A study of 3,500 identical twins as part of the United Kingdom Biobank examined the differences in the food metabolomes of twins and found significant variations in both metabolites and metabolic pathways among identical twins (Pallister et al. 2016). With the largest nutritional metabolomics data set to date, they identified 73 novel candidate biomarkers of food intake for potential use in nutritional epidemiological studies.

Nutrigenomics may also provide new insights in the development of personalized nutrition interventions, which may facilitate larger, more appropriate and sustained changes in eating and other lifestyle behaviors. However, it is important to remember what most humans have in common including the adaptation to starvation and poor adaptation to overnutrition as well as the metabolic and epigenetic changes resulting from changes in physical activity (Heianza and Qi 2017).

Personalized nutrition in cancer is about more than diet alone. Differences in body composition, fat depots, and changes with aging that impact metabolic resilience are all important topics that go beyond genomics and are relevant to individual rather than public health interventions in cancer prevention, treatment, and survival.

PRECISION ONCOLOGY

Oncology was an obvious choice for enhancing the near-term impact of the revolution in human genomics. Precision oncology research has revealed many of the molecular lesions that drive cancer development and metastasis. Beyond its organ of origin (e.g., breast or prostate), each cancer has its own genomic signature, with some tumor-specific features and some features common to multiple types. Inherited cancers confer an increased susceptibility to damage to the genome from diet and environment to different degrees. Heritable cancers are estimated to account for 10%–15% of all cancers and even these cancers are impacted by diet and environmental factors. Precision oncology offers a new approach to oncogenic mechanisms and their interaction with environment influences for risk assessment, diagnosis, and determination of the best therapeutic strategies. With the increasing use of drugs and antibodies targeted to specific cancer genotypes, precision oncology is designed to counter the influence of specific molecular drivers of tumor growth and metastasis. Many targeted therapies are being developed, and several have been shown to confer benefits. In addition, novel immunologic approaches have recently produced some profound responses, with signs that molecular signatures may be strong predictors of benefit.

Precision nutrition is an advance beyond personalized nutrition which developed in the era of the sequencing of the human genome and mainly concerned gene–nutrient interaction. Precision nutrition is an emerging science that considers individual variability in the response to foods based on genetic and epigenetic variation (Zeisel 2019) and the microbiome (Mills et al. 2019).

Research combining the insights from precision oncology and precision nutrition holds the promise of determining the impact of bioactive nutrients in foods, herbs, and spices on cancer prevention and treatment. By modulating angiogenesis, tumor progression, metastasis, and responses to chemotherapy, nutrition may play an adjunctive role in treatment and a primary role in prevention. Bioactive phytonutrients including the large class of polyphenols may be used in future therapies targeting common forms of cancer including breast, colon, and prostate cancers (Reglero and Reglero 2019).

Quercitin has demonstrated chemopreventive effects in colon cancer on cell cycle arrest, increase in apoptosis, antioxidant replication, modulation of estrogen receptors, regulation of signaling pathways, inhibition of metastasis and angiogenesis (Darband et al. 2018, Henning et al. 2017).

The health benefits of pomegranate polyphenol consumption in juice from whole pomegranates or extracts of pomegranate are attributed to ellagitannins and their metabolites. Ellagitannins are hydrolyzed to ellagic acid which is absorbed into the circulation, but the majority of the polyphenols remain in the intestine where they stimulate growth of bacteria and the formation of urolithins. In a study of 20 healthy participants who consumed 1,000 mg of pomegranate extract capsules (POM) daily for 4 weeks, we found three different "metabotypes" based on variations in the individual urinary and fecal contents of the POM metabolite urolithin A (UA). We observed three distinct groups: (1) individuals with no baseline UA presence but induction of UA formation by POM extract consumption (n=9); (2) baseline UA formation which was enhanced by POM extract consumption (N=5); and (3) no baseline UA production, which was not inducible (N=6) (Li et al. 2015). Compared to baseline the phylum Actinobacteria was increased and Firmicutes decreased significantly in individuals forming UA (producers). Verrucomicrobia (*Akkermansia muciniphila*) was 33- and 47-fold higher in stool samples of UA producers compared to nonproducers at baseline and after 4 weeks, respectively. In UA producers, the genera Butyrivibrio, Enterobacter, Escherichia, Lactobacillus, Prevotella, Serratia, and Veillonella were increased and Collinsella decreased significantly at week 4 compared to baseline (Li et al. 2015). This study demonstrated that pomegranate polyphenols are prebiotic but also demonstrated the differences among individuals based on their ability to form UA, termed a postbiotic. The study also raised the possibility that responses to POM extract consumption in cancer patients may vary secondary to changes in the microbiota and resulting metabotype.

A diet rich in cruciferous vegetables is associated with a lower risk of developing breast, lung, prostate, and colorectal cancer (Feskanich et al. 2000, Benabdelkrim, Djeffal, and Berredjem 2018). The chemoprotective effect of cruciferous vegetables is due to their high glucosinolate content and the capacity of glucosinolate metabolites, such as isothiocyanates (ITC) and indoles, to modulate biotransformation enzyme systems (e.g., cytochromes P450 and conjugating enzymes). Data from molecular epidemiologic studies suggest that genetic and associated functional variations in biotransformation enzymes, particularly glutathione S-transferase (GST)M1 and GSTT1, which metabolize ITC, alter cancer risk in response to cruciferous vegetable exposure (Lampe and Peterson 2002).

In addition to polyphenols, curcumin (diferuloylmethane) is one of the most studied phytonutrients in recent years as a potential therapeutic product for cancer. Curcumin has been reported to modulate growth factors, enzymes, transcription factors, kinase, inflammatory cytokines, and proapoptotic (by upregulation) and antiapoptotic (by downregulation) proteins (Giordano and Tommonaro 2019).

Botanical dietary supplements including Notoginseng have been proposed as potential ingredients of precision nutritional supplements in cancer therapy (Wang, Anderson, and Yuan 2016). Notoginseng is a Chinese herbal medicine with a long history of use. It has a distinct ginsenoside profile compared to other ginseng herbs such as Asian ginseng and American ginseng. Over 80 dammarane saponins have been isolated and elucidated from different plant parts of notoginseng. The role of the microbiome in mediating notoginseng metabolism, bioavailability, and pharmacological actions is being studied. Emphasis has also been placed on the identification and isolation of enteric microbiome-generated notoginseng metabolites. Future investigations should provide key insights into notoginseng's bioactive metabolites as clinically valuable anticancer compounds.

Rapidly proliferating tumor cells consume large amounts of energy and substrates to build new cell membranes and other cellular structures. Lipids, functioning as essential structural components of membranes and serving as important energy resources, are critical macromolecules for tumor growth. Recent studies have demonstrated that both lipid synthesis and uptake are significantly elevated in malignancies to support tumor growth. Steroid regulatory element binding proteins (SREBPs) are transcription factors that regulate transcription of the genes for the low-density lipoprotein receptor and β-Hydroxy β-methylglutaryl-Coenzyme A (HMG-CoA) reductase, the rate limiting enzyme in cholesterol synthesis. One of these elements (SREBP-1) is highly expressed in glioblastoma, in prostate, endometrial, breast cancers, hepatocellular carcinoma, ovarian cancer, and pancreatic cancer (Cheng, Li, and Guo 2018). As more evidence of the relationship of lipid biosynthesis and carcinogenesis is developed, there may be a role for examining the differences in lipid metabolism among individuals which is an area where there is established variation.

Elevations in triglycerides and cholesterol in the blood are broadly classified under the heading of dyslipidemias and these are the most common abnormalities of lipid metabolism observed in Western society. Dyslipidemia is common in overweight and obesity, and is a risk factor for cardiometabolic diseases. The individual variations in lipid metabolism have been ascribed to both genetic factors and diet. Genome-wide association studies have identified over 150 loci related to elevations in lipid levels. However, genetic variation only explains about 40% of the total variation (Matey-Hernandez et al. 2018). The unexplained variance has been attributed to environmental factors including diet, physical activity, and lifestyle. The gut microbiota digestion of different dietary components including fats and polysaccharides can also cause changes in lipid metabolism. Future research on lipids and cancer will assess the contributing role of host genetics, diet, and the gut microbiome to dyslipidemia which may have therapeutic implications, the prevention and treatment of common forms of cancer including breast cancer and prostate cancer.

Finally, multitargeting profiles of food and herbal ingredients are being investigated regarding their potential roles triggering anticancer molecular mechanisms through the modulation of certain gene expressions or signaling pathways, epigenetic mechanisms, and tumor metabolism. Clearly, precision nutrition in cancer is an ambitious but potentially valuable area for basic and clinical research.

CONCLUSION

Nutrition has a clear role to play in cancer prevention, treatment, and survival, but much research remains to be done in terms of integrating the latest insights from precision nutrition and precision oncology into practical advances. The interest of the public in this approach has exceeded the development of supportive scientific evidence. What is needed in the future is a partnership of the oncology and nutrition science research communities in collaborative research. It is vital to move from cellular research to clinical trials demonstrating real differences in outcome when weight management, dietary patterns, and food ingredients within foods or supplements are included in protocols. While the randomized controlled trial and observational epidemiology have both made contributions to our understanding of nutrition and cancer, future studies must integrate approaches across different nutritional scientific approaches reviewed in subsequent chapters.

REFERENCES

Agus, D. B., J. C. Vera, and D. W. Golde. 1999. "Stromal cell oxidation: a mechanism by which tumors obtain vitamin C." *Cancer Res* 59 (18):4555–8.

Ames, B. N., and L. S. Gold. 1997. "Environmental pollution, pesticides, and the prevention of cancer: misconceptions." *FASEB J* 11 (13):1041–52. doi: 10.1096/fasebj.11.13.9367339.

Arends, J., P. Bachmann, V. Baracos, N. Barthelemy, H. Bertz, F. Bozzetti, K. Fearon, E. Hutterer, E. Isenring, S. Kaasa, Z. Krznaric, B. Laird, M. Larsson, A. Laviano, S. Muhlebach, M. Muscaritoli, L. Oldervoll, P. Ravasco, T. Solheim, F. Strasser, M. de van der Schueren, and J. C. Preiser. 2017. "ESPEN guidelines on nutrition in cancer patients." *Clin Nutr* 36 (1):11–48. doi: 10.1016/j.clnu.2016.07.015.

Benabdelkrim, M., O. Djeffal, and H. Berredjem. 2018. "GSTM1 and GSTT1 polymorphisms and susceptibility to prostate cancer: a case-control study of the Algerian population." *Asian Pac J Cancer Prev* 19 (10):2853–2858. doi: 10.22034/APJCP.2018.19.10.2853.

Blaszczak, W., W. Barczak, J. Masternak, P. Kopczynski, A. Zhitkovich, and B. Rubis. 2019. "Vitamin C as a modulator of the response to cancer therapy." *Molecules* 24 (3):453. doi: 10.3390/molecules24030453.

Blot, W. J., and R. E. Tarone. 2015. "Doll and Peto's quantitative estimates of cancer risks: holding generally true for 35 years." *J Natl Cancer Inst* 107 (4):djv044. doi: 10.1093/jnci/djv044.

Brown, J. R., and J. L. Thornton. 1957. "Percivall Pott (1714–1788) and chimney sweepers' cancer of the scrotum." *Br J Ind Med* 14 (1):68–70. doi: 10.1136/oem.14.1.68.

Cantor, D. 2012. "Between prevention and therapy: Gio Batta Gori and the National Cancer Institute's Diet, Nutrition and Cancer Programme, 1974–1978." *Med Hist* 56 (4):531–61. doi: 10.1017/mdh.2012.73.

Cheng, X., J. Li, and D. Guo. 2018. "SCAP/SREBPs are central players in lipid metabolism and novel metabolic targets in cancer therapy." *Curr Top Med Chem* 18 (6):484–493. doi: 10.2174/1568026618666180523104541.

Collins, F. S., and H. Varmus. 2015. "A new initiative on precision medicine." *N Engl J Med* 372 (9):793–5. doi: 10.1056/NEJMp1500523.

Darband, S. G., M. Kaviani, B. Yousefi, S. Sadighparvar, F. G. Pakdel, J. A. Attari, I. Mohebbi, S. Naderi, and M. Majidinia. 2018. "Quercetin: a functional dietary flavonoid with potential chemo-preventive properties in colorectal cancer." *J Cell Physiol* 233 (9):6544–6560. doi: 10.1002/jcp.26595.

DeNicola, G. M., and L. C. Cantley. 2015. "Cancer's fuel choice: new flavors for a picky eater." *Mol Cell* 60 (4):514–23. doi: 10.1016/j.molcel.2015.10.018.

"Dietary goals for the United States: statement of The American Medical Association to the Select Committee on Nutrition and Human Needs, United States Senate." 1977. *R I Med J* 60 (12):576–81.

Elmore, S. A., V. Carreira, C. S. Labriola, D. Mahapatra, S. R. McKeag, M. Rinke, C. Shackelford, B. Singh, A. Talley, S. M. Wallace, L. M. Wancket, and C. J. Willson. 2018. "Proceedings of the 2018 National Toxicology Program Satellite Symposium." *Toxicol Pathol* 46 (8):865–97. doi: 10.1177/0192623318800734.

Feskanich, D., R. G. Ziegler, D. S. Michaud, E. L. Giovannucci, F. E. Speizer, W. C. Willett, and G. A. Colditz. 2000. "Prospective study of fruit and vegetable consumption and risk of lung cancer among men and women." *J Natl Cancer Inst* 92 (22):1812–23. doi: 10.1093/jnci/92.22.1812.

Giordano, A., and G. Tommonaro. 2019. "Curcumin and cancer." *Nutrients* 11 (10):2376. doi: 10.3390/nu11102376.

Goodman, J., and H. Lynch. 2017. "Improving the International Agency for Research on Cancer's consideration of mechanistic evidence." *Toxicol Appl Pharmacol* 319:39–46. doi: 10.1016/j.taap.2017.01.020.

Grosso, G., F. Bella, J. Godos, S. Sciacca, D. Del Rio, S. Ray, F. Galvano, and E. L. Giovannucci. 2017. "Possible role of diet in cancer: systematic review and multiple meta-analyses of dietary patterns, lifestyle factors, and cancer risk." *Nutr Rev* 75 (6):405–19. doi: 10.1093/nutrit/nux012.

Guyton, K. Z., I. Rusyn, W. A. Chiu, D. E. Corpet, M. van den Berg, M. K. Ross, D. C. Christiani, F. A. Beland, and M. T. Smith. 2018. "Application of the key characteristics of carcinogens in cancer hazard identification." *Carcinogenesis* 39 (4):614–22. doi: 10.1093/carcin/bgy031.

Heianza, Y., and L. Qi. 2017. "Gene-diet interaction and precision nutrition in obesity." *Int J Mol Sci* 18 (4):787. doi: 10.3390/ijms18040787.

Henning, S. M., P. H. Summanen, R. P. Lee, J. Yang, S. M. Finegold, D. Heber, and Z. Li. 2017. "Pomegranate ellagitannins stimulate the growth of Akkermansia muciniphila in vivo." *Anaerobe* 43:56–60. doi: 10.1016/j.anaerobe.2016.12.003.

Hoppe, M. M., R. Sundar, D. S. P. Tan, and A. D. Jeyasekharan. 2018. "Biomarkers for homologous recombination deficiency in cancer." *J Natl Cancer Inst* 110 (7):704–13. doi: 10.1093/jnci/djy085.

Huff, J., M. F. Jacobson, and D. L. Davis. 2008. "The limits of two-year bioassay exposure regimens for identifying chemical carcinogens." *Environ Health Perspect* 116 (11):1439–42. doi: 10.1289/ehp.10716.

Lampe, J. W., and S. Peterson. 2002. "Brassica, biotransformation and cancer risk: genetic polymorphisms alter the preventive effects of cruciferous vegetables." *J Nutr* 132 (10):2991–4. doi: 10.1093/jn/131.10.2991.

Lee, P. R. 1978. "Nutrition policy--from neglect and uncertainty to debate and action." *J Am Diet Assoc* 72 (6):581–8.

Levy, S., G. Sutton, P. C. Ng, L. Feuk, A. L. Halpern, B. P. Walenz, N. Axelrod, J. Huang, E. F. Kirkness, G. Denisov, Y. Lin, J. R. MacDonald, A. W. Pang, M. Shago, T. B. Stockwell, A. Tsiamouri, V. Bafna, V. Bansal, S. A. Kravitz, D. A. Busam, K. Y. Beeson, T. C. McIntosh, K. A. Remington, J. F. Abril, J. Gill, J. Borman, Y. H. Rogers, M. E. Frazier, S. W. Scherer, R. L. Strausberg, and J. C. Venter. 2007. "The diploid genome sequence of an individual human." *PLoS Biol* 5 (10):e254. doi: 10.1371/journal.pbio.0050254.

Li, Z., S. M. Henning, R. P. Lee, Q. Y. Lu, P. H. Summanen, G. Thames, K. Corbett, J. Downes, C. H. Tseng, S. M. Finegold, and D. Heber. 2015. "Pomegranate extract induces ellagitannin metabolite formation and changes stool microbiota in healthy volunteers." *Food Funct* 6 (8):2487–95. doi: 10.1039/c5fo00669d.

Matey-Hernandez, M. L., F. M. K. Williams, T. Potter, A. M. Valdes, T. D. Spector, and C. Menni. 2018. "Genetic and microbiome influence on lipid metabolism and dyslipidemia." *Physiol Genomics* 50 (2):117–26. doi: 10.1152/physiolgenomics.00053.2017.

Mathers, J. C. 2017. "Nutrigenomics in the modern era." *Proc Nutr Soc* 76 (3):265–75. doi: 10.1017/S002966511600080X.

McGinnis, J. M. 1988. "The Surgeon General's report on nutrition and health." *R I Med J* 71 (10):373.

Mills, S., C. Stanton, J. A. Lane, G. J. Smith, and R. P. Ross. 2019. "Precision nutrition and the microbiome, Part I: Current state of the science." *Nutrients* 11 (4):923. doi: 10.3390/nu11040923.

Mochamat, H. Cuhls, M. Marinova, S. Kaasa, C. Stieber, R. Conrad, L. Radbruch, and M. Mucke. 2017. "A systematic review on the role of vitamins, minerals, proteins, and other supplements for the treatment of cachexia in cancer: a European Palliative Care Research Centre cachexia project." *J Cachexia Sarcopenia Muscle* 8 (1):25–39. doi: 10.1002/jcsm.12127.

Moustafa, G. A., E. Xanthopoulou, E. Riza, and A. Linos. 2015. "Skin disease after occupational dermal exposure to coal tar: a review of the scientific literature." *Int J Dermatol* 54 (8):868–79. doi: 10.1111/ijd.12903.

National Research Council (US) Committee on Diet, Nutrition, and Cancer. 1982. *Diet, Nutrition, and Cancer.* Washington (DC): National Academies Press.

"Nutrition classics. Surgery, Volume 64, 1968. Long-term total parenteral nutrition with growth, development, and positive nitrogen balance: Stanley J. Dudrick, Douglas W. Wilmore, Harry M. Vars, Jonathan E. Rhoads." 1981. *Nutr Rev* 39 (7):278–81. doi: 10.1111/j.1753–4887.1981.tb06788.x.

Okuda, M., K. Asakura, and S. Sasaki. 2019. "Protein intake estimated from brief-type self-administered diet history questionnaire and urinary urea nitrogen level in adolescents." *Nutrients* 11 (2):319. doi: 10.3390/nu11020319.

Padayatty, S. J., H. Sun, Y. Wang, H. D. Riordan, S. M. Hewitt, A. Katz, R. A. Wesley, and M. Levine. 2004. "Vitamin C pharmacokinetics: implications for oral and intravenous use." *Ann Intern Med* 140 (7):533–7. doi: 10.7326/0003-4819-140-7-200404060-00010.

Pallister, T., A. Jennings, R. P. Mohney, D. Yarand, M. Mangino, A. Cassidy, A. MacGregor, T. D. Spector, and C. Menni. 2016. "Characterizing blood metabolomics profiles associated with self-reported food intakes in female twins." *PLoS One* 11 (6):e0158568. doi: 10.1371/journal.pone.0158568.

Reglero, C., and G. Reglero. 2019. "Precision nutrition and cancer relapse prevention: a systematic literature review." *Nutrients* 11 (11):2799. doi: 10.3390/nu11112799.

Rousseau, M. C., K. Straif, and J. Siemiatycki. 2005. "IARC carcinogen update." *Environ Health Perspect* 113 (9):A580–1. doi: 10.1289/ehp.113–1280416.

Rueff, J., A. S. Rodrigues, and M. Kranendonk. 2019. "A personally guided tour on some of our data with the Ames assay-A tribute to Professor Bruce Ames." *Mutat Res* 846:503094. doi: 10.1016/j.mrgentox.2019.503094.

Satija, A., E. Yu, W. C. Willett, and F. B. Hu. 2015. "Understanding nutritional epidemiology and its role in policy." *Adv Nutr* 6 (1):5–18. doi: 10.3945/an.114.007492.

Scalbert, A., L. Brennan, C. Manach, C. Andres-Lacueva, L. O. Dragsted, J. Draper, S. M. Rappaport, J. J. van der Hooft, and D. S. Wishart. 2014. "The food metabolome: a window over dietary exposure." *Am J Clin Nutr* 99 (6):1286–308. doi: 10.3945/ajcn.113.076133.

Sikalidis, A. K. 2019. "From food for survival to food for personalized optimal health: a historical perspective of how food and nutrition gave rise to nutrigenomics." *J Am Coll Nutr* 38 (1):84–95. doi: 10.1080/07315724.2018.1481797.

Smilowitz, J. T., A. M. Zivkovic, Y. J. Wan, S. M. Watkins, M. L. Nording, B. D. Hammock, and J. B. German. 2013. "Nutritional lipidomics: molecular metabolism, analytics, and diagnostics." *Mol Nutr Food Res* 57 (8):1319–35. doi: 10.1002/mnfr.201200808.

Smith, M. T., K. Z. Guyton, C. F. Gibbons, J. M. Fritz, C. J. Portier, I. Rusyn, D. M. DeMarini, J. C. Caldwell, R. J. Kavlock, P. F. Lambert, S. S. Hecht, J. R. Bucher, B. W. Stewart, R. A. Baan, V. J. Cogliano, and K. Straif. 2016. "Key characteristics of carcinogens as a basis for organizing data on mechanisms of carcinogenesis." *Environ Health Perspect* 124 (6):713–21. doi: 10.1289/ehp.1509912.

Wang, C. Z., S. Anderson, and C. S. Yuan. 2016. "Phytochemistry and anticancer potential of notoginseng." *Am J Chin Med* 44 (1):23–34. doi: 10.1142/S0192415X16500026.

Wang, X., H. Fan, C. Xu, G. Jiang, H. Wang, and J. Zhang. 2019. "KDM3B suppresses APL progression by restricting chromatin accessibility and facilitating the ATRA-mediated degradation of PML/RARalpha." *Cancer Cell Int* 19:256. doi: 10.1186/s12935-019-0979-7.

Wang, Z. Y., and Z. Chen. 2008. "Acute promyelocytic leukemia: from highly fatal to highly curable." *Blood* 111 (5):2505–15. doi: 10.1182/blood-2007-07-102798.

Weisburger, J. H. 1996. "Human protection against non-genotoxic carcinogens in the US without the Delaney Clause." *Exp Toxicol Pathol* 48 (2–3):201–8. doi: 10.1016/S0940-2993(96)80045-5.

Westerterp, K. R. 2018. "Exercise, energy expenditure and energy balance, as measured with doubly labelled water." *Proc Nutr Soc* 77 (1):4–10. doi: 10.1017/S0029665117001148.

Wynder, E. L. 1975. "The epidemiology of large bowel cancer." *Cancer Res* 35 (11 Pt. 2):3388–94.

Zeiger, E. 2017. "Reflections on a career and on the history of genetic toxicity testing in the National Toxicology Program." *Mutat Res* 773:282–92. doi: 10.1016/j.mrrev.2017.03.002.

Zeisel, S. H. 2019. "A conceptual framework for studying and investing in precision nutrition." *Front Genet* 10:200. doi: 10.3389/fgene.2019.00200.

2 Cancer Metabolism and Nutrition

David Heber
UCLA Center for Human Nutrition

CONTENTS

INTRODUCTION

As lifespans have increased over the last few centuries, the overall incidence of cancer has increased markedly in populations around the world (Riscuta 2016). The risk of cancer increases with age as a result of a number of factors. One primary factor is increased production of reactive oxygen species produced in the course of normal metabolism during aging by mitochondria. These reactive oxygen species can damage cells at the DNA, RNA, and protein level and work in concert with chronic inflammation to increase cancer risk (Zong, Rabinowitz, and White 2016). Diet and lifestyle affect physiological aging and there are individual differences in how quickly physiological aging at the cellular level advances (Belsky et al. 2015). Many of the processes that define malignant phenotypes at the cellular level, including DNA damage responses, oxidative stress, metabolic reprogramming, and cellular senescence, are also integral to the biology of aging. Therefore, the mechanisms of aging are shared with those affecting the development of common forms of cancer (Cordani et al. 2019).

Overweight and obesity through the actions of adipocytes and stromal cells as well as the gut microbiome can stimulate increased inflammation systemically and can accelerate the process of carcinogenesis (Iyengar et al. 2018). Mitochondrial production of reactive oxygen species is accelerated by a sedentary lifestyle, obesogenic diets, and obesity. When chronic inflammation is present in association with obesity and chronic diseases, it acts as a further stimulus to increased oxidant stress and mutagenesis over time.

Seventy percent of the immune system is located in the gut-associated lymphatic tissue around the intestines, where diet and lifestyle can modulate immune function systemically (Rooks and Garrett 2016). The products produced by the gut microbiome including short-chain fatty acids (SCFA) circulate throughout the body and can affect organ function (Vander Heiden and DeBerardinis 2017).

Nutrition affects carcinogenesis beginning at the cellular level but extending throughout the body's homeostatic organ and tissue systems through the effects of diet and lifestyle. At the cellular level, the genetic changes that occur in cancer cells can transform normal metabolic pathways in ways that benefit the growth of cancer cells and also utilize substrates in perturbed normal metabolic pathways in ways that promote tumor growth (Boroughs and DeBerardinis 2015).

In considering the impact of host nutrition on cancer prevention and treatment, it is important to appreciate the metabolic resilience of cancer cells when considering nutritional approaches as either preventive or adjunctive to cancer treatment. Nutrition can clearly play a role in cancer prevention and risk reduction as well as support of the cancer patient during treatment (de Las Penas et al. 2019). There are several examples of recently discovered small molecules that target cellular proteins controlling cancer cell metabolism including cyclin-dependent kinase 4 and 6 (CDK4/6), poly (adenosine diphosphate-ribose) polymerase (PARP), and phosphoinositide 3-kinase (PI3K) in breast cancer among others (Nur Husna et al. 2018). Research on metabolic inhibitors of cancer cell growth based on genetic profiling and precision oncology are being examined in basic research and may someday yield less toxic and more cancer-specific treatments for cancer.

CELLULAR AND MOLECULAR BASIS OF CANCER

Most normal cells follow a steady cycle of cell growth and death. New normal cells replace lost cells. The cellular and molecular lesions secondary to aging that promote an increased risk of cancer can be genetic including mutations, deletions, or translocations or they can be epigenetic. Epigenetic changes over time include DNA methylation and histone modification. Among epigenetic changes, global DNA methylations accumulate with aging and directly contribute to cell transformation. Some cancers are associated with decreased methylation as well but the common link is that the normal control of gene activation is perturbed (Sapienza and Issa 2016).

It is impossible to predict whether a given individual of any age will develop cancer. Risk factors clearly affect cancer incidence and cancer risk increases with age. Tomasetti and Vogelstein (2015) proposed that a significant portion of human cancers were simply due to "bad luck" statistically driven somatic cell mutation events during DNA replication and only a few to carcinogens, pathogens, or inherited genes and that this should impact public health approaches to cancer prevention.

Albini and co-workers (2015) pointed to an alternative explanation of the association of cancer and aging called the cancer stem cell (CSC) hypothesis. This concept argues that cancers are derived from tissue stem cells and not from somatic differentiated cells, and emphasizes the importance of the tissue microenvironment in the growth of transformed cells.

The difference between these two concepts is an important distinction in messaging to the public. Since aging is inevitable, the statistical mutation model supposes that individuals cannot avoid developing common forms of cancer. The facts is that many cancer can be prevented given our extensive knowledge of known risk factors and behaviors that can lower the risk for specific cancers including smoking cessation and changes in diet and lifestyle. While some tumors will still occur due to aging and chance, prevention should still be a primary goal for public health policies.

THE ROLE OF STEM CELLS AND CANCER PROGENITOR CELLS

Stem cells can divide indefinitely and ultimately produce all the mature cell types that constitute an organ in order to provide for normal tissue growth and repair (Noguchi, Miyagi-Shiohira, and Nakashima 2018). Adult tissue-specific stem cells contain tissue-specific genetic information and the stability of DNA in these cells is preserved by normal homeostasis in protected microenvironments. On the other hand, stem cells that accumulate genetic lesions are tumor-initiating stem cells also termed cancer progenitor cell (Reya et al. 2001). Mismatched repair of DNA damage in stem and progenitor cells can promote carcinogenesis. Studies suggest that distinct "cells of origin" within an organ can give rise to different subtypes of cancer (Sutherland and Visvader 2015). Tissue-specific stem and progenitor cells are the predominant targets that evolve to tumor initiation. Various factors in the microenvironment can act on the cell of origin by causing dedifferentiation, and these cell populations can be detected for earlier diagnosis and detection of premalignant clones at the time of diagnosis and prior to relapse. Detection using circulating biomarkers of abnormal cells could conceivably be used in the design of prevention regimens for families at high genetic risk and for treatment regimens in cancer survivors who relapse. The genetic signature of the progenitor cells is transmitted to daughter cells. As these daughter stem cells accumulate more cells with genetic lesions they proliferate leading to cancer formation, but subclones may also form from the mutation of stem and progenitor cells within a tumor.

Certain aberrations in DNA that accumulate in cells eventually confer a survival advantage over normal cells allowing them to grow uncontrollably. DNA changes through mutation or epigenetic changes lead to the stimulation of metabolism that favors cancer cell growth over normal cells. These cancer cells go through an epithelial to mesenchymal transition (EMT) which enables them to cross normal cell and organ boundaries and metastasize throughout the body through the support of oncogenic metabolism and extrinsic factors in the microenvironment where they spread.

Metastasis accounts for 90% of deaths from malignant tumors. Extracellular vesicles and exosomes remodel the primary microenvironment and prepare the secondary microenvironment for spread (Liu et al. 2017). The extracellular vesicles and exosomes contain various molecules including nucleic acids, proteins, lipids, messenger RNA, micro-RNAs, and noncoding RNAs. This cargo can provide communication between neighboring and distant cells. Cancer cells release these molecules to alter the host microenvironment to favor metastases (Liu et al. 2017, O'Loghlen 2018, Becker et al. 2016, Bebelman et al. 2018, Lu et al. 2017, Lobb, Lima, and Moller 2017).

Prior to metastasizing, cancer cells undergo an EMT. The EMT is the critical first step in tumor metastasis. Epithelial cancer cells undergoing EMT lose epithelial cell polarity and gain mesenchymal proteins (Tsai and Yang 2013, Smith and Bhowmick 2016, De Craene and Berx 2013, Lin and Wu 2020, Sciacovelli and Frezza 2017, Sciacovelli et al. 2016, Lamouille, Xu, and Derynck 2014, Du and Shim 2016, Suresh et al. 2016). EMT also contributes to the acquisition of CSC phenotypes. EMT-inducing transcription factors also regulate cancer cell stemness, inhibit senescence and apoptosis defense responses, determine resistance to chemotherapy, and promote tumor angiogenesis and metabolic alterations (Puisieux, Brabletz, and Caramel 2014, Ansieau, Collin, and Hill 2014). Cancer cell metabolism has been demonstrated to regulate EMT, cell invasion, and metastasis as well as CSC phenotype by inducing metabolic enzyme genes.

Extrinsic mechanisms, such as the metabolic, stromal, and immunological microenvironments, can support metastasis (Yang and Lin 2017). According to the "seed and soil" hypothesis, cancer cells find a microenvironment which supports colonization and further metastasis since it is difficult for cancer cells to survive outside their original environment (Liu et al. 2017).

Subclones of cells in metastatic lesions can accumulate changes in their DNA that are different from the primary tumor and other metastatic cells even within the same tumor mass leading to heterogeneity of cells (San Juan et al. 2019). This heterogeneity makes it more difficult to treat advanced metastatic cancers than primary cancers or early metastatic disease. As cancers grow, they repeatedly adopt multiple metabolic pathways that are also present in normal cells. This presents a challenge for the development of targeted metabolic therapies that optimally would have a much greater effect on tumor cells than surrounding normal cells.

METABOLIC CHANGES FAVORING GROWTH IN CANCER CELLS

Warburg and Cori in the 1920s discovered that there are fundamental differences in the central metabolic pathways operating in malignant tissue (Potter, Newport, and Morten 2016). While they proposed their theory as an explanation for tumorigenesis, the identification of gene alterations including oncogenes and tumor suppressor genes in the 1970s in cancer cells, a multistep process of carcinogenesis based on genetic alterations, reduced interest in nutrition and metabolism among cancer researchers (Vogelstein et al. 2013). As proteomic and metabolomics research has progressed, there are nutrition research challenges and opportunities in the area of cancer metabolism (Romagnolo and Milner 2012).

Various subcellular signaling pathways amplified in cancer cells secondary to genetic mutations favor the growth of cancer cells in the microenvironment where these cells interact with stromal cells (Wu, Clausen, and Nielsen 2015). Some of these alterations may be susceptible to inhibition, but the general interest in treating metabolic targets as a research area is far less prevalent than precision oncology based on cancer genetics and more recently immunotherapy (Velcheti and Schalper 2016).

Metabolic reprogramming of cancer cells while promoting cancer cell growth makes them potentially susceptible to agents that selectively starve cancer cells of their metabolic substrates in order to delay or suppress tumor growth (Ward and Thompson 2012, Cheong et al. 2011, Shafaee et al. 2015). Thus, a better understanding of cancer cell metabolism may pave the way for research and development of metabolic adjunctive nutrition regimens that reduce the toxicity of therapy to normal cells (Rodriguez-Enriquez et al. 2019, Pacheco-Velazquez et al. 2018, Marin-Hernandez et al. 2014, Marin-Hernandez et al. 2011).

In both normal and cancer cells, carbohydrates, fats, and proteins are broken down to glucose, fatty acids, and amino acids which enter metabolic pathways in the mitochondria to produce adenosine triphosphate (ATP). However, there is a shift in the metabolism of cancer cells away from energy production as ATP toward the production of substrates for cancer cell growth (Schulze and Yuneva 2018). Research on nutritional adjuncts for cancer treatment being explored include targeting glycolysis, the Krebs cycle, oxidative phosphorylation, glutamine metabolism, fatty acid oxidation, nucleic acid synthesis, lipid synthesis, and amino acid metabolism (Li et al. 2016).

Normal cells do not metabolize glucose to lactate when oxygen is available, since oxidative phosphorylation through tricarboxylic acid cycle is much more efficient in producing ATP (42 molecules of ATP secondary to oxidative phosphorylation in mitochondria versus only 6 ATP through anaerobic glycolysis). As Warburg and Cori found, cancer cells metabolized glucose to lactate even in the presence of oxygen and tumor slices consumed glucose and secreted lactate at a higher rate than normal tissues (Li et al. 2016).

The observation that tumor cells import more glucose than normal cells is the basis for some forms of Positron Emission Tomography (PET) (Shin et al. 2015) as a diagnostic method for identifying tumor metastases. Increased glucose uptake is mediated through isoforms of membrane glucose transporters which are expressed by cancer cell genes and reside in the tumor cell membrane. Fluorinated deoxyglucose is not metabolized once transported into the cells by glucose transporters but when made with a specific isotope of fluoride emits positrons at the sites of metastases which can be detected and their location visualized by a PET scan.

A major advantage of the amplified glycolytic pathway in tumor cells is the generation of intermediates that are precursors to anabolic metabolism including the pentose phosphate pathway generating NADPH, ribose-6-phosphate, amino acid, lipids, and other cellular substrates supporting production and growth of new cells (Pavlova and Thompson 2016, Yoshida 2015, Guido et al. 2012).

The first step is the conversion of glucose by a hexokinase enzyme to glucose-6-phosphate (G-6P). G-6P is converted to fructose-6-phosphate by phosphoglucose isomerase. Then using the energy from ATP, fructose-6-phosphate is converted to fructose-1,6-diphosphate. Fructose-1,6-diphosphate is converted to glyceraldehyde-3-phosphate dehydrogenase (GAPDH) and dihydroxyacetone phosphate aldolase. Then in combination with NAD+, the enzyme converts GAPDH to 1,3-bisphosphoglycerate.

Branching off of the linear path of conversions from glucose to pyruvate are (1) production of ribose-5-phosphate, a precursor to nucleotide synthesis; (2) dihydroxyacetone phosphate for lipid synthesis; (3) production of serine from 3-phosphoglycerate which can be converted to cysteine and glycine amino acids for protein synthesis; and (4) lactate from pyruvate.

Mitochondrial oxidative phosphorylation is focused on ATP generation in nonproliferating cells. However, the tricarboxylic acid cycle (TCA) also has an anabolic role in that it stimulates aspartate biosynthesis in proliferating cancer cells (Birsoy et al. 2015, Sullivan et al. 2015). The functional role for the shift from energy production to substrate production in cancer cells is the biosynthesis of the nucleotides and amino acids needed for cell assembly and growth. Aspartate is required supply for nucleotide and protein biosynthesis in proliferating cells.

The aspartate in the circulation is not adequate for cell proliferation, so this must be synthesized intracellularly in cancer cells, and in study of 35 breast cancer patients compared to 35 controls circulating aspartate levels were low (Xie et al. 2015). Metabolic transformation is a means for cancer cells to sustain proliferation and resist cell death signals. The lowered aspartate level is specific to breast cancer as this was not found in a series of gastric and colorectal cancer patients. There was a higher level of aspartate in breast cancer tissues than in adjacent nontumor tissues in 20 patients. In addition, MCF-7 breast cancer cell had a higher concentration intracellularly of aspartate than immortalized normal MCF-10A cells, suggesting that the depleted level of aspartate in blood of breast cancer patients is due to increased tumor aspartate utilization. Together, these findings suggest that lowed circulating aspartate is a key metabolic feature of human breast cancer.

Cancer cells utilize pyruvate generated from the glycolytic pathway to generate a variety of substrates for cell growth. The TCA cycle intermediates are precursors to fatty acids, nucleotides, hemes, and porphyrins, which are essential building blocks for DNA, proteins, and lipids. Alpha-ketoglutarate formed from isocitrate, succinate from succinyl-CoA, fumarate and malonate, and ultimately oxaloacetate maintain the activity of the TCA cycle also called the Krebs cycle.

Cancer cells also take up and metabolize glutamine. Glutaminase catalyzes the conversion of glutamine to glutamate, which subsequently forms alpha-ketoglutarate that enters the TCA cycle. Glutamine is the most abundant circulating nonessential amino acid, and glutamate generated from glutamine is also a precursor of other nonessential amino acids (e.g., aspartate, alanine, arginine, and proline). Glutamine is the source of nitrogen for the biosynthesis of glycosylated molecules and nucleotides, and it serves as a substrate for fatty acid synthesis in hypoxic cells or cells with activation of hypoxia-inducible factor-1-alpha (Metallo et al. 2011).

The hypoxia-inducible factors, HIF-1α/2α, work together with cancer-associated mutations that deregulate hypoxia signaling and mediate a complementary metabolic shift to a glutamine-maintained TCA cycle, through the activation of reductive carboxylation of α-ketoglutarate, a metabolic reaction that is heavily used to maintain de novo lipogenesis under hypoxia (Shafaee et al. 2015). Human clear cell renal cell carcinomas are driven by HIF-2α, due to mutational inactivation of the von Hippel–Lindau tumor suppressor gene, and provide a cancer model for studying reprogramming of metabolism by hypoxia signaling (Gameiro et al. 2013, Kaelin 2008).

Nutrient-sensing mechanisms in cancer cells link cellular activities with nutrient availability. The links between metabolite pools and protein post-translational modifications include acetylation, methylation, and glycosylation (Campbell and Wellen 2018). Through these enzymatic modifications, cancer cells undergo metabolic reprogramming and exhibit metabolic plasticity that allows them to survive and proliferate within the tumor microenvironment.

Mutations of proteins in the tricarboxylic acid cycle can prevent the oxidation of pyruvate to acetyl-CoA. In that situation, the cell becomes dependent on the alpha-ketoglutarate formed from glutamate. Then alpha-ketoglutarate is converted into citrate through increased carboxylation by an isocitrate dehydrogenase-2-dependent reaction (Mullen et al. 2014, Mullen et al. 2011). Reductive carboxylation of glutamine to citrate is also an alternative pathway for lipid synthesis. Glutamine is also utilized to synthesize glutathione, an important intracellular antioxidant.

Both glycolysis and glutaminolysis metabolic pathways are active in several cancer types. Triple-negative breast cancers (TNBCs) lack progesterone and estrogen receptors and do not have amplified human epidermal growth factor receptor 2, the main therapeutic targets for managing breast cancer. However, TNBCs have altered cellular metabolism, including an increased Warburg effect and glutamine dependence, making the glutaminase inhibitors therapeutically promising for this tumor type and potentially for others.

In a nutrient-rich microenvironment, cancer cells take up glucose and amino acids through trans-membrane transport channels and these are used to support glycolysis and the tricarboxylic acid cycle which maintain production of ATP and metabolic intermediates for tumor anabolism. Pancreatic ductal adenocarcinoma cells are surrounded by dense fibrous tissue limiting nutrients needed for tumor cells including amino acids. In response, the adenocarcinoma cells develop two different mechanisms for degrading lysosomal contents including proteins and using the nutrients to support tumor cell growth. Autophagy is used to digest damaged cytoplasmic organelles. Pinocytosis is used to degrade extracellular components that were internalized by the cell. The serine biosynthesis pathway is essential in breast cancer and is associated with poor 5-year survival in breast cancer patients (Possemato et al. 2011).

TUMOR–HOST METABOLIC INTERACTION

Targeting glycolysis and/or mitochondrial metabolism in cancer cells or catabolism in neighboring stromal cells may be effective in inhibiting tumor progression and metastasis (Bailey et al. 2012). The challenge is how to target these cells specifically and utilize inhibitors that are toxic to tumor cells but do not affect normal cells.

Tumors have both aerobic and anaerobic regions depending on the vascular supply of oxygen to different parts of a solid tumor. In addition to this oxygen gradient, new blood vessel formation called angiogenesis is critically required for tumors to grow beyond a few microns. New blood vessels are formed in hypoxic areas through the activation of hypoxia-inducible factors. However, these new vessels formed through angiogenesis are not efficient at supplying oxygen to the tumor tissue. There is a metabolic interaction between the hypoxic and oxygenated areas of tumors (Pokorny et al. 2015). Lactate generated from glycolysis in hypoxic cells is secreted and taken up by aerobic cancer cells and converted to pyruvate which then enters the mitochondria to generate ATP via the TCA cycle. This has been called the "reverse Warburg effect" or the "Lactate shuttle".

The ATP produced by the well-oxygenated tumor or stromal cells leaves more glucose for hypoxic cancer cell metabolism and survival (Rawat et al. 2019). Monocarboxylate transporter 1 (MCT1) moves lactate between cancer-associated stromal cells and cancer cells. MCT4, present in fibroblasts, is responsible for exporting L-lactate out of stromal cells, and MCT1 in epithelial cancer cells mediates lactate uptake. MCT1 transporter could be inhibited to deprive hypoxic cancer cells of adequate glucose for growth.

Numerous tumor–host metabolic interactions are an important phenomenon in cancer progression through interactions of tumor cells with the surrounding stromal microenvironment (Akhtar et al. 2019, de Groot et al. 2017).

Prostate cancer cells exhibit altered cellular metabolism but, notably, not the hallmarks of Warburg metabolism. Prostate cancer cells exhibit increased de novo synthesis of fatty acids. Extracellular-derived FAs are primary building blocks for complex lipids and heterogeneity in FA metabolism in prostate cancer that can influence tumor cell behavior (Balaban et al. 2019). When implanting breast tumors in mice, the breast fat is the typical site for successful implantation (Kocaturk and Versteeg 2015).

It is possible to inhibit fatty acid oxidation by inhibiting carnitine palmitoyltransferase which is the enzyme responsible for promoting the uptake of long-chain fatty acids into the mitochondria. Inhibition of energy production as a strategy for potentiation of anticancer chemotherapy was investigated using 1 glycolysis inhibitor and 1 fatty acid beta-oxidation inhibitor-2-deoxyglucose and etomoxir, respectively, both known to be clinically well tolerated. Eighteen anticancer drugs were screened for potentiation by these inhibitors. 2-Deoxyglucose potentiated acute apoptosis over 24 hours induced mainly by some, but not all, genotoxic drugs, whereas etomoxir had effect only on cisplatin (Hernlund et al. 2008).

Glycolytic and mitochondrial metabolism can be targeted to slow cancer growth, but this is complicated by the use of these metabolic pathways in normal cells as well. Currently, there exist several inhibitors of transmembrane glucose transporters, including cytochalasin B and selected tyrosine kinase inhibitors which are somewhat less toxic to normal cells than tumor cells (Bailey et al. 2012).

CANCER CELL GENE REGULATION AND TUMOR CELL METABOLISM

The metabolic reprogramming of cancer goes beyond activation of glycolysis as originally proposed by Warburg. A recent systematic analysis of expression of metabolic genes across several cancer types showed that, besides glycolysis, other metabolic pathways, including nucleotides and protein synthesis, are activated in cancer (Hu et al. 2013). This study of the convergence of metabolic pathways in cancer analyzed 8,161 cancer and normal samples for gene expression in 20 different types of solid cancers. These cancers exhibited common metabolic signatures but maintained some features of their tissue of origin. By identifying those metabolic signatures that were tissue-specific and tissue-independent signals, investigators were led to the observation that activation of nucleotide synthesis and inhibition of mitochondrial oxidative phosphorylation are the main features of the convergent metabolic reprogramming of cancer cells.

TUMOR CELL METABOLISM AND METASTASIS

The key difference between benign and life-threatening malignant tumors is metastasis (Beans 2018, Bleau et al. 2014, Lamouille, Xu, and Derynck 2014). Malignant tumors spread to surrounding tissue and to distant metastatic sites through invasion and metastasis. Metastatic progression is promoted by both internal cellular mechanisms and external metabolic, stromal, and immunological factors in the microenvironment and circulation (Yang and Lin 2017, Boussadia et al. 2018, Yuan et al. 2016, Ren et al. 2018, Leong, Aktipis, and Maley 2018). Metastatic cancer cells seek out a favorable microenvironment that favors colonization, growth, and further metastasis (Liu and Cao 2016, Liu et al. 2017). Tumor-produced extracellular vesicles and exosomes promote the remodeling of the primary tumor microenvironment and prime the secondary microenvironment which is the "soil" where the tumor "seed" of the "seed and soil" concept of tumor spread (Liu et al. 2017). The vesicles and exosomes contain nucleic acids, proteins, lipids, messenger RNA, microRNAs, and noncoding RNAs, which alter the primary tumor microenvironment to a premetastatic microenvironment (Liu et al. 2017, Steinbichler et al. 2017, Mashouri et al. 2019, Bebelman et al. 2018, Lu et al. 2017).

Mitochondria accumulate defects with aging and in tumors as a result of defects in mitophagy, the process that normally clears defective mitochondria that can increase oxidant stress (Bernardini, Lazarou, and Dewson 2017). In turn, oxidant stress promotes metastasis through activation of SRC and protein tyrosine kinase 2 beta signaling (Bernardini, Lazarou, and Dewson 2017, Zong, Rabinowitz, and White 2016, Zielonka and Kalyanaraman 2008, Bargiela, Burr, and Chinnery 2018, Corbet and Feron 2017). Evidence of mitochondrial dysfunction is linked to cancer metastasis and patient outcomes through increased oxidant stress at a level that promotes tumorigenesis (Sciacovelli and Frezza 2017, Gill, Piskounova, and Morrison 2016, Ren et al. 2017).

EMT is an essential first step in the development of metastatic potential. Cancer cell metabolism plays an important role in the regulation of EMT via induction of metabolic enzyme genes that activate an oncogenic metabolism pattern. Tumor epithelial cells that undergo EMT undergo cellular changes including the loss of polarity and increased mesenchymal proteins (Sciacovelli and Frezza 2017, Smith and Bhowmick 2016, De Craene and Berx 2013, Liu et al. 2015, Nieto et al. 2016). Disturbance of a controlled epithelial balance is triggered by altering several layers of regulation, including the transcriptional and translational machinery, expression of noncoding RNAs, alternative splicing and protein stability (De Craene and Berx 2013). EMT also leads to resistance to chemotherapy, and promotes tumor angiogenesis and metabolic alterations (Antony, Thiery, and Huang 2019, van Staalduinen et al. 2018).

As cancer cells grow and divide they can go into a senescent state as the result of oxidative stress and the activation of oncogenes (Campisi 1997, Liu, Ding, and Meng 2018, Loaiza and Demaria 2016, Hemann and Narita 2007, Nelson et al. 2014, Coppe et al. 2008). Oncogene-induced senescence has been found in premalignant tumors. Telomere shortening in senescence causes DNA damage (Nelson et al. 2014). Oncogene-induced senescence is also associated with further DNA damage (Halazonetis, Gorgoulis, and Bartek 2008, Matt and Hofmann 2016, Barnes, Fouquerel, and Opresko 2019). Senescence suppresses cell division in preneoplastic lesions (Drullion et al. 2018, Roos, Thomas, and Kaina 2016, Halazonetis, Gorgoulis, and Bartek 2008, Basu and Nohmi 2018). Senescent cells have been found in different cancers including B cell lymphoma and lung, breast, colorectal, and thyroid cancers (Kim et al. 2017, Gayle et al. 2019, Tsolou et al. 2019). Recently, senescence has also been implicated in the promotion of tumor progression. Senescent cells secrete growth factors, chemokines, cytokines, extracellular matrix remodeling proteases including matrix metalloproteinases. Cytokines and damaged DNA trigger an immune response. At early stages of cancer development immune factors inhibit growth, while at later stages, immune factors can promote angiogenesis and tumor development. Furthermore, senescent cells exhibit increased glycolysis, which is regulated by the counterbalance of p53 and Rb. Finally, the senescent secretory phenotype induces EMT, invasion, metastasis, and angiogenesis that are crucial for tumor progression.

CONCLUSION

Nutrition can impact cancer prevention and treatment in the modern era as more is understood of the molecular and metabolic resilience of cancer cells. Cancer cells exhibit oncogenic metabolic alterations including in glutamine metabolism, the pentose phosphate pathway, and pathways for the synthesis of fatty acids and cholesterol. These cancer cell metabolic pathways produce biochemical precursors for nucleic acids, lipids, and proteins. Cancer cells achieve metabolic advantages for survival and proliferation as a result of these metabolic changes mediated by cancer-related transcription factors, including HIF1-alpha, c-Myc, and p53 linked to metabolic pathways such as PI3K and 5' adenosine monophosphate-activated protein kinase (AMPK).

There are examples of recently discovered small molecules that can target the cellular proteins that control oncogenic metabolism including cyclin-dependent kinase 4 and 6 (CDK4/6), poly (adenosine diphosphate-ribose) polymerase (PARP) and phosphoinositide 3-kinase (PI3K). Research on metabolic inhibitors of cancer cell growth based on genetic profiling and precision oncology are being examined in basic research and may someday yield less toxic and more cancer-specific treatments for cancer. The focus of cancer research and treatment has shifted from treating cancer based on type and histology to treating the specific cancer mutations of individuals through precision oncology. As the nutritional and metabolic characteristics of individual patients including genome, epigenome, proteome, metabolome, and microbiome comprise precision nutrition. In the future, research in precision oncology and precision nutrition will likely proceed in parallel to result in better prevention and treatment options for common forms of cancer.

REFERENCES

Akhtar, M., A. Haider, S. Rashid, and Admh Al-Nabet. 2019. "Paget's "Seed and Soil" theory of cancer metastasis: an idea whose time has come." *Adv Anat Pathol* 26 (1):69–74. doi: 10.1097/PAP.0000000000 000219.

Albini, A., S. Cavuto, G. Apolone, and D. M. Noonan. 2015. "Strategies to prevent "Bad Luck" in cancer." *J Natl Cancer Inst* 107 (10):djv213. doi: 10.1093/jnci/djv213.

Ansieau, S., G. Collin, and L. Hill. 2014. "EMT or EMT-promoting transcription factors, where to focus the light?" *Front Oncol* 4:353. doi: 10.3389/fonc.2014.00353.

Antony, J., J. P. Thiery, and R. Y. Huang. 2019. "Epithelial-to-mesenchymal transition: lessons from development, insights into cancer and the potential of EMT-subtype based therapeutic intervention." *Phys Biol* 16 (4):041004. doi: 10.1088/1478-3975/ab157a.

Bailey, K. M., J. W. Wojtkowiak, A. I. Hashim, and R. J. Gillies. 2012. "Targeting the metabolic microenvironment of tumors." *Adv Pharmacol* 65:63–107. doi: 10.1016/B978-0-12-397927-8.00004-X.

Balaban, S., Z. D. Nassar, A. Y. Zhang, E. Hosseini-Beheshti, M. M. Centenera, M. Schreuder, H. M. Lin, A. Aishah, B. Varney, F. Liu-Fu, L. S. Lee, S. R. Nagarajan, R. F. Shearer, R. A. Hardie, N. L. Raftopulos, M. S. Kakani, D. N. Saunders, J. Holst, L. G. Horvath, L. M. Butler, and A. J. Hoy. 2019. "Extracellular fatty acids are the major contributor to lipid synthesis in prostate cancer." *Mol Cancer Res* 17 (4):-949–962. doi: 10.1158/1541-7786.MCR-18-0347.

Bargiela, D., S. P. Burr, and P. F. Chinnery. 2018. "Mitochondria and hypoxia: metabolic crosstalk in cell-fate decisions." *Trends Endocrinol Metab* 29 (4):249–259. doi: 10.1016/j.tem.2018.02.002.

Barnes, R. P., E. Fouquerel, and P. L. Opresko. 2019. "The impact of oxidative DNA damage and stress on telomere homeostasis." *Mech Ageing Dev* 177:37–45. doi: 10.1016/j.mad.2018.03.013.

Basu, A. K., and T. Nohmi. 2018. "Chemically-induced DNA damage, mutagenesis, and cancer." *Int J Mol Sci* 19 (6):1767. doi: 10.3390/ijms19061767.

Beans, C. 2018. "News feature: targeting metastasis to halt cancer's spread." *Proc Natl Acad Sci U S A* 115 (50):12539–12543. doi: 10.1073/pnas.1818892115.

Bebelman, M. P., M. J. Smit, D. M. Pegtel, and S. R. Baglio. 2018. "Biogenesis and function of extracellular vesicles in cancer." *Pharmacol Ther* 188:1–11. doi: 10.1016/j.pharmthera.2018.02.013.

Becker, A., B. K. Thakur, J. M. Weiss, H. S. Kim, H. Peinado, and D. Lyden. 2016. "Extracellular vesicles in cancer: cell-to-cell mediators of metastasis." *Cancer Cell* 30 (6):836–848. doi: 10.1016/j.ccell.2016.10.009.

Belsky, D. W., A. Caspi, R. Houts, H. J. Cohen, D. L. Corcoran, A. Danese, H. Harrington, S. Israel, M. E. Levine, J. D. Schaefer, K. Sugden, B. Williams, A. I. Yashin, R. Poulton, and T. E. Moffitt. 2015. "Quantification of biological aging in young adults." *Proc Natl Acad Sci U S A* 112 (30):E4104–E4110. doi: 10.1073/pnas.1506264112.

Bernardini, J. P., M. Lazarou, and G. Dewson. 2017. "Parkin and mitophagy in cancer." *Oncogene* 36 (10):1315–1327. doi: 10.1038/onc.2016.302.

Birsoy, K., T. Wang, W. W. Chen, E. Freinkman, M. Abu-Remaileh, and D. M. Sabatini. 2015. "An essential role of the mitochondrial electron transport chain in cell proliferation is to enable aspartate synthesis." *Cell* 162 (3):540–551. doi: 10.1016/j.cell.2015.07.016.

Bleau, A. M., A. Agliano, L. Larzabal, A. L. de Aberasturi, and A. Calvo. 2014. "Metastatic dormancy: a complex network between cancer stem cells and their microenvironment." *Histol Histopathol* 29 (12):1499–1510. doi: 10.14670/HH-29.1499.

Boroughs, L. K., and R. J. DeBerardinis. 2015. "Metabolic pathways promoting cancer cell survival and growth." *Nat Cell Biol* 17 (4):351–359. doi: 10.1038/ncb3124.

Boussadia, Z., J. Lamberti, F. Mattei, E. Pizzi, R. Puglisi, C. Zanetti, L. Pasquini, F. Fratini, L. Fantozzi, F. Felicetti, K. Fecchi, C. Raggi, M. Sanchez, S. D'Atri, A. Care, M. Sargiacomo, and I. Parolini. 2018. "Acidic microenvironment plays a key role in human melanoma progression through a sustained exosome mediated transfer of clinically relevant metastatic molecules." *J Exp Clin Cancer Res* 37 (1):245. doi: 10.1186/s13046-018-0915-z.

Campbell, S. L., and K. E. Wellen. 2018. "Metabolic signaling to the nucleus in cancer." *Mol Cell* 71 (3):-398–408. doi: 10.1016/j.molcel.2018.07.015.

Campisi, J. 1997. "The biology of replicative senescence." *Eur J Cancer* 33 (5):703–709. doi: 10.1016/S0959-8049(96)00058-5.

Cheong, J. H., E. S. Park, J. Liang, J. B. Dennison, D. Tsavachidou, C. Nguyen-Charles, K. Wa Cheng, H. Hall, D. Zhang, Y. Lu, M. Ravoori, V. Kundra, J. Ajani, J. S. Lee, W. Ki Hong, and G. B. Mills. 2011. "Dual inhibition of tumor energy pathway by 2-deoxyglucose and metformin is effective against a broad spectrum of preclinical cancer models." *Mol Cancer Ther* 10 (12):2350–2362. doi: 10.1158/1535-7163. MCT-11-0497.

Coppe, J. P., C. K. Patil, F. Rodier, Y. Sun, D. P. Munoz, J. Goldstein, P. S. Nelson, P. Y. Desprez, and J. Campisi. 2008. "Senescence-associated secretory phenotypes reveal cell-nonautonomous functions of oncogenic RAS and the p53 tumor suppressor." *PLoS Biol* 6 (12):2853–2858. doi: 10.1371/journal. pbio.0060301.

Corbet, C., and O. Feron. 2017. "Cancer cell metabolism and mitochondria: nutrient plasticity for TCA cycle fueling." *Biochim Biophys Acta Rev Cancer* 1868 (1):7–15. doi: 10.1016/j.bbcan.2017.01.002.

Cordani, M., M. Donadelli, R. Strippoli, A. V. Bazhin, and M. Sanchez-Alvarez. 2019. "Interplay between ROS and autophagy in cancer and aging: from molecular mechanisms to novel therapeutic approaches." *Oxid Med Cell Longev* 2019:8794612. doi: 10.1155/2019/8794612.

De Craene, B., and G. Berx. 2013. "Regulatory networks defining EMT during cancer initiation and progression." *Nat Rev Cancer* 13 (2):97–110. doi: 10.1038/nrc3447.

de Groot, A. E., S. Roy, J. S. Brown, K. J. Pienta, and S. R. Amend. 2017. "Revisiting seed and soil: examining the primary tumor and cancer cell foraging in metastasis." *Mol Cancer Res* 15 (4):361–370. doi: 10.1158/1541-7786.MCR-16-0436.

de Las Penas, R., M. Majem, J. Perez-Altozano, J. A. Virizuela, E. Cancer, P. Diz, O. Donnay, A. Hurtado, P. Jimenez-Fonseca, and M. J. Ocon. 2019. "SEOM clinical guidelines on nutrition in cancer patients (2018)." *Clin Transl Oncol* 21 (1):87–93. doi: 10.1007/s12094-018-02009-3.

Drullion, C., G. Marot, N. Martin, J. Desle, L. Saas, C. Salazar-Cardozo, F. Bouali, A. Pourtier, C. Abbadie, and O. Pluquet. 2018. "Pre-malignant transformation by senescence evasion is prevented by the PERK and ATF6alpha branches of the Unfolded Protein Response." *Cancer Lett* 438:187–196. doi: 10.1016/j.canlet.2018.09.008.

Du, B., and J. S. Shim. 2016. "Targeting epithelial-mesenchymal transition (EMT) to overcome drug resistance in cancer." *Molecules* 21 (7):965. doi: 10.3390/molecules21070965.

Gameiro, P. A., J. Yang, A. M. Metelo, R. Perez-Carro, R. Baker, Z. Wang, A. Arreola, W. K. Rathmell, A. Olumi, P. Lopez-Larrubia, G. Stephanopoulos, and O. Iliopoulos. 2013. "In vivo HIF-mediated reductive carboxylation is regulated by citrate levels and sensitizes VHL-deficient cells to glutamine deprivation." *Cell Metab* 17 (3):372–385. doi: 10.1016/j.cmet.2013.02.002.

Gayle, S. S., J. M. Sahni, B. M. Webb, K. L. Weber-Bonk, M. S. Shively, R. Spina, E. E. Bar, M. K. Summers, and R. A. Keri. 2019. "Targeting BCL-xL improves the efficacy of bromodomain and extra-terminal protein inhibitors in triple-negative breast cancer by eliciting the death of senescent cells." *J Biol Chem* 294 (3):875–886. doi: 10.1074/jbc.RA118.004712.

Gill, J. G., E. Piskounova, and S. J. Morrison. 2016. "Cancer, oxidative stress, and metastasis." *Cold Spring Harb Symp Quant Biol* 81:163–175. doi: 10.1101/sqb.2016.81.030791.

Guido, C., D. Whitaker-Menezes, C. Capparelli, R. Balliet, Z. Lin, R. G. Pestell, A. Howell, S. Aquila, S. Ando, U. Martinez-Outschoorn, F. Sotgia, and M. P. Lisanti. 2012. "Metabolic reprogramming of cancer-associated fibroblasts by TGF-beta drives tumor growth: connecting TGF-beta signaling with "Warburg-like" cancer metabolism and L-lactate production." *Cell Cycle* 11 (16):3019–3035. doi: 10.4161/cc.21384.

Halazonetis, T. D., V. G. Gorgoulis, and J. Bartek. 2008. "An oncogene-induced DNA damage model for cancer development." *Science* 319 (5868):1352–1355. doi: 10.1126/science.1140735.

Hemann, M. T., and M. Narita. 2007. "Oncogenes and senescence: breaking down in the fast lane." *Genes Dev* 21 (1):1–5. doi: 10.1101/gad.1514207.

Hernlund, E., L. S. Ihrlund, O. Khan, Y. O. Ates, S. Linder, T. Panaretakis, and M. C. Shoshan. 2008. "Potentiation of chemotherapeutic drugs by energy metabolism inhibitors 2-deoxyglucose and etomoxir." *Int J Cancer* 123 (2):476–483. doi: 10.1002/ijc.23525.

Hu, J., J. W. Locasale, J. H. Bielas, J. O'Sullivan, K. Sheahan, L. C. Cantley, M. G. Vander Heiden, and D. Vitkup. 2013. "Heterogeneity of tumor-induced gene expression changes in the human metabolic network." *Nat Biotechnol* 31 (6):522–529. doi: 10.1038/nbt.2530.

Iyengar, N. M., I. C. Chen, X. K. Zhou, D. D. Giri, D. J. Falcone, L. A. Winston, H. Wang, S. Williams, Y. S. Lu, T. H. Hsueh, A. L. Cheng, C. A. Hudis, C. H. Lin, and A. J. Dannenberg. 2018. "Adiposity, inflammation, and breast cancer pathogenesis in asian women." *Cancer Prev Res (Phila)* 11 (4):227–236. doi: 10.1158/1940-6207.CAPR-17-0283.

Kaelin, W. G., Jr. 2008. "The von Hippel-Lindau tumour suppressor protein: O_2 sensing and cancer." *Nat Rev Cancer* 8 (11):865–873. doi: 10.1038/nrc2502.

Kim, Y. H., Y. W. Choi, J. Lee, E. Y. Soh, J. H. Kim, and T. J. Park. 2017. "Senescent tumor cells lead the collective invasion in thyroid cancer." *Nat Commun* 8:15208. doi: 10.1038/ncomms15208.

Kocaturk, B., and H. H. Versteeg. 2015. "Orthotopic injection of breast cancer cells into the mammary fat pad of mice to study tumor growth." *J Vis Exp* (96):51967. doi: 10.3791/51967.

Lamouille, S., J. Xu, and R. Derynck. 2014. "Molecular mechanisms of epithelial-mesenchymal transition." *Nat Rev Mol Cell Biol* 15 (3):178–196. doi: 10.1038/nrm3758.

Leong, S. P., A. Aktipis, and C. Maley. 2018. "Cancer initiation and progression within the cancer microenvironment." *Clin Exp Metastasis* 35 (5–6):361–367. doi: 10.1007/s10585-018-9921-y.

Li, C., G. Zhang, L. Zhao, Z. Ma, and H. Chen. 2016. "Metabolic reprogramming in cancer cells: glycolysis, glutaminolysis, and Bcl-2 proteins as novel therapeutic targets for cancer." *World J Surg Oncol* 14 (1):15. doi: 10.1186/s12957-016-0769-9.

Lin, Y. T., and K. J. Wu. 2020. "Epigenetic regulation of epithelial-mesenchymal transition: focusing on hypoxia and TGF-beta signaling." *J Biomed Sci* 27 (1):39. doi: 10.1186/s12929-020-00632-3.

Liu, Q., H. Zhang, X. Jiang, C. Qian, Z. Liu, and D. Luo. 2017. "Factors involved in cancer metastasis: a better understanding to "seed and soil" hypothesis." *Mol Cancer* 16 (1):176. doi: 10.1186/s12943-017-0742-4.

Liu, X. L., J. Ding, and L. H. Meng. 2018. "Oncogene-induced senescence: a double edged sword in cancer." *Acta Pharmacol Sin* 39 (10):1553–1558. doi: 10.1038/aps.2017.198.

Liu, X., F. Yun, L. Shi, Z. H. Li, N. R. Luo, and Y. F. Jia. 2015. "Roles of signaling pathways in the epithelial-mesenchymal transition in cancer." *Asian Pac J Cancer Prev* 16 (15):6201–6206. doi: 10.7314/apjcp.2015.16.15.6201.

Liu, Y., and X. Cao. 2016. "Characteristics and significance of the pre-metastatic niche." *Cancer Cell* 30 (5):668–681. doi: 10.1016/j.ccell.2016.09.011.

Loaiza, N., and M. Demaria. 2016. "Cellular senescence and tumor promotion: Is aging the key?" *Biochim Biophys Acta* 1865 (2):155–167. doi: 10.1016/j.bbcan.2016.01.007.

Lobb, R. J., L. G. Lima, and A. Moller. 2017. "Exosomes: key mediators of metastasis and pre-metastatic niche formation." *Semin Cell Dev Biol* 67:3–10. doi: 10.1016/j.semcdb.2017.01.004.

Lu, J., J. Li, S. Liu, T. Wang, A. Ianni, E. Bober, T. Braun, R. Xiang, and S. Yue. 2017. "Exosomal tetraspanins mediate cancer metastasis by altering host microenvironment." *Oncotarget* 8 (37):62803–62815. doi: 10.18632/oncotarget.19119.

Marin-Hernandez, A., J. C. Gallardo-Perez, S. Rodriguez-Enriquez, R. Encalada, R. Moreno-Sanchez, and E. Saavedra. 2011. "Modeling cancer glycolysis." *Biochim Biophys Acta* 1807 (6):755–767. doi: 10.1016/j.bbabio.2010.11.006.

Marin-Hernandez, A., S. Y. Lopez-Ramirez, I. Del Mazo-Monsalvo, J. C. Gallardo-Perez, S. Rodriguez-Enriquez, R. Moreno-Sanchez, and E. Saavedra. 2014. "Modeling cancer glycolysis under hypoglycemia, and the role played by the differential expression of glycolytic isoforms." *FEBS J* 281 (15):3325–3345. doi: 10.1111/febs.12864.

Mashouri, L., H. Yousefi, A. R. Aref, A. M. Ahadi, F. Molaei, and S. K. Alahari. 2019. "Exosomes: composition, biogenesis, and mechanisms in cancer metastasis and drug resistance." *Mol Cancer* 18 (1):75. doi: 10.1186/s12943-019-0991-5.

Matt, S., and T. G. Hofmann. 2016. "The DNA damage-induced cell death response: a roadmap to kill cancer cells." *Cell Mol Life Sci* 73 (15):2829–2850. doi: 10.1007/s00018-016-2130-4.

Metallo, C. M., P. A. Gameiro, E. L. Bell, K. R. Mattaini, J. Yang, K. Hiller, C. M. Jewell, Z. R. Johnson, D. J. Irvine, L. Guarente, J. K. Kelleher, M. G. Vander Heiden, O. Iliopoulos, and G. Stephanopoulos. 2011. "Reductive glutamine metabolism by IDH1 mediates lipogenesis under hypoxia." *Nature* 481 (7381):380–384. doi: 10.1038/nature10602.

Mullen, A. R., Z. Hu, X. Shi, L. Jiang, L. K. Boroughs, Z. Kovacs, R. Boriack, D. Rakheja, L. B. Sullivan, W. M. Linehan, N. S. Chandel, and R. J. DeBerardinis. 2014. "Oxidation of alpha-ketoglutarate is required for reductive carboxylation in cancer cells with mitochondrial defects." *Cell Rep* 7 (5):1679–1690. doi: 10.1016/j.celrep.2014.04.037.

Mullen, A. R., W. W. Wheaton, E. S. Jin, P. H. Chen, L. B. Sullivan, T. Cheng, Y. Yang, W. M. Linehan, N. S. Chandel, and R. J. DeBerardinis. 2011. "Reductive carboxylation supports growth in tumour cells with defective mitochondria." *Nature* 481 (7381):385–388. doi: 10.1038/nature10642.

Nelson, D. M., T. McBryan, J. C. Jeyapalan, J. M. Sedivy, and P. D. Adams. 2014. "A comparison of oncogene-induced senescence and replicative senescence: implications for tumor suppression and aging." *Age (Dordr)* 36 (3):9637. doi: 10.1007/s11357-014-9637-0.

Nieto, M. A., R. Y. Huang, R. A. Jackson, and J. P. Thiery. 2016. "Emt: 2016." *Cell* 166 (1):21–45. doi: 10.1016/j.cell.2016.06.028.

Noguchi, H., C. Miyagi-Shiohira, and Y. Nakashima. 2018. "Induced tissue-specific stem cells and epigenetic memory in induced pluripotent stem cells." *Int J Mol Sci* 19 (4). doi: 10.3390/ijms19040930.

Nur Husna, S. M., H. T. Tan, R. Mohamud, A. Dyhl-Polk, and K. K. Wong. 2018. "Inhibitors targeting CDK4/6, PARP and PI3K in breast cancer: a review." *Ther Adv Med Oncol* 10. doi: 10.1177/1758835918808509.

O'Loghlen, A. 2018. "Role for extracellular vesicles in the tumour microenvironment." *Philos Trans R Soc Lond B Biol Sci* 373 (1737). doi: 10.1098/rstb.2016.0488.

Pacheco-Velazquez, S. C., D. X. Robledo-Cadena, I. Hernandez-Resendiz, J. C. Gallardo-Perez, R. Moreno-Sanchez, and S. Rodriguez-Enriquez. 2018. "Energy metabolism drugs block triple negative breast metastatic cancer cell phenotype." *Mol Pharm* 15 (6):2151–2164. doi: 10.1021/acs.molpharmaceut.8b00015.

Pavlova, N. N., and C. B. Thompson. 2016. "The emerging hallmarks of cancer metabolism." *Cell Metab* 23 (1):27–47. doi: 10.1016/j.cmet.2015.12.006.

Pokorny, J., J. Pokorny, A. Foletti, J. Kobilkova, J. Vrba, and J. Vrba. 2015. "Mitochondrial dysfunction and disturbed coherence: gate to cancer." *Pharmaceuticals (Basel)* 8 (4):675–695. doi: 10.3390/ph8040675.

Possemato, R., K. M. Marks, Y. D. Shaul, M. E. Pacold, D. Kim, K. Birsoy, S. Sethumadhavan, H. K. Woo, H. G. Jang, A. K. Jha, W. W. Chen, F. G. Barrett, N. Stransky, Z. Y. Tsun, G. S. Cowley, J. Barretina, N. Y. Kalaany, P. P. Hsu, A. M. Chan, B. Yuan, L. A. Garraway, D. E. Root, M. Mino-Kenudson, E. F. Brachtel, E. M. Driggers, and D. M. Sabatini. 2011. "Functional genomics reveal that the serine synthesis pathway is essential in breast cancer." *Nature* 476 (7360):346–350. doi: 10.1038/nature10350.

Potter, M., E. Newport, and K. J. Morten. 2016. "The Warburg effect: 80 years on." *Biochem Soc Trans* 44 (5):1499–1505. doi: 10.1042/BST20160094.

Puisieux, A., T. Brabletz, and J. Caramel. 2014. "Oncogenic roles of EMT-inducing transcription factors." *Nat Cell Biol* 16 (6):488–494. doi: 10.1038/ncb2976.

Rawat, D., S. K. Chhonker, R. A. Naik, A. Mehrotra, S. K. Trigun, and R. K. Koiri. 2019. "Lactate as a signaling molecule: journey from dead end product of glycolysis to tumor survival." *Front Biosci (Landmark Ed)* 24:366–381.

Ren, B., M. Cui, G. Yang, H. Wang, M. Feng, L. You, and Y. Zhao. 2018. "Tumor microenvironment participates in metastasis of pancreatic cancer." *Mol Cancer* 17 (1):108. doi: 10.1186/s12943-018-0858-1.

Ren, T., H. Zhang, J. Wang, J. Zhu, M. Jin, Y. Wu, X. Guo, L. Ji, Q. Huang, H. Zhang, H. Yang, and J. Xing. 2017. "MCU-dependent mitochondrial Ca(2+) inhibits NAD(+)/SIRT3/SOD2 pathway to promote ROS production and metastasis of HCC cells." *Oncogene* 36 (42):5897–5909. doi: 10.1038/onc.2017.167.

Reya, T., S. J. Morrison, M. F. Clarke, and I. L. Weissman. 2001. "Stem cells, cancer, and cancer stem cells." *Nature* 414 (6859):105–111. doi: 10.1038/35102167.

Riscuta, G. 2016. "Nutrigenomics at the interface of aging, lifespan, and cancer prevention." *J Nutr* 146 (10):1931–1939. doi: 10.3945/jn.116.235119.

Rodriguez-Enriquez, S., A. Marin-Hernandez, J. C. Gallardo-Perez, S. C. Pacheco-Velazquez, J. A. Belmont-Diaz, D. X. Robledo-Cadena, J. L. Vargas-Navarro, N. A. Corona de la Pena, E. Saavedra, and R. Moreno-Sanchez. 2019. "Transcriptional regulation of energy metabolism in cancer cells." *Cells* 8 (10). doi: 10.3390/cells8101225.

Romagnolo, D. F., and J. A. Milner. 2012. "Opportunities and challenges for nutritional proteomics in cancer prevention." *J Nutr* 142 (7):1360S-1369S. doi: 10.3945/jn.111.151803.

Rooks, M. G., and W. S. Garrett. 2016. "Gut microbiota, metabolites and host immunity." *Nat Rev Immunol* 16 (6):341–352. doi: 10.1038/nri.2016.42.

Roos, W. P., A. D. Thomas, and B. Kaina. 2016. "DNA damage and the balance between survival and death in cancer biology." *Nat Rev Cancer* 16 (1):20–33. doi: 10.1038/nrc.2015.2.

San Juan, B. P., M. J. Garcia-Leon, L. Rangel, J. G. Goetz, and C. L. Chaffer. 2019. "The complexities of metastasis." *Cancers (Basel)* 11 (10):1575. doi: 10.3390/cancers11101575.

Sapienza, C., and J. P. Issa. 2016. "Diet, nutrition, and cancer epigenetics." *Annu Rev Nutr* 36:665–681. doi: 10.1146/annurev-nutr-121415-112634.

Schulze, A., and M. Yuneva. 2018. "The big picture: exploring the metabolic cross-talk in cancer." *Dis Model Mech* 11 (8). doi: 10.1242/dmm.036673.

Sciacovelli, M., and C. Frezza. 2017. "Metabolic reprogramming and epithelial-to-mesenchymal transition in cancer." *FEBS J* 284 (19):3132–3144. doi: 10.1111/febs.14090.

Sciacovelli, M., E. Goncalves, T. I. Johnson, V. R. Zecchini, A. S. da Costa, E. Gaude, A. V. Drubbel, S. J. Theobald, S. R. Abbo, M. G. Tran, V. Rajeeve, S. Cardaci, S. Foster, H. Yun, P. Cutillas, A. Warren, V. Gnanapragasam, E. Gottlieb, K. Franze, B. Huntly, E. R. Maher, P. H. Maxwell, J. Saez-Rodriguez, and C. Frezza. 2016. "Fumarate is an epigenetic modifier that elicits epithelial-to-mesenchymal transition." *Nature* 537 (7621):544–547. doi: 10.1038/nature19353.

Shafaee, A., D. Z. Dastyar, J. P. Islamian, and M. Hatamian. 2015. "Inhibition of tumor energy pathways for targeted esophagus cancer therapy." *Metabolism* 64 (10):1193–1198. doi: 10.1016/j.metabol.2015.07.005.

Shin, Y. S., J. Kim, D. Johnson, A. A. Dooraghi, W. X. Mai, L. Ta, A. F. Chatziioannou, M. E. Phelps, D. A. Nathanson, and J. R. Heath. 2015. "Quantitative assessments of glycolysis from single cells." *Technology (Singap World Sci)* 3 (4):172–178. doi: 10.1142/S2339547815200058..

Smith, B. N., and N. A. Bhowmick. 2016. "Role of EMT in metastasis and therapy resistance." *J Clin Med* 5 (2). doi: 10.3390/jcm5020017.

Steinbichler, T. B., J. Dudas, H. Riechelmann, and Skvortsova, II. 2017. "The role of exosomes in cancer metastasis." *Semin Cancer Biol* 44:170–181. doi: 10.1016/j.semcancer.2017.02.006.

Sullivan, L. B., D. Y. Gui, A. M. Hosios, L. N. Bush, E. Freinkman, and M. G. Vander Heiden. 2015. "Supporting aspartate biosynthesis is an essential function of respiration in proliferating cells." *Cell* 162 (3):552–563. doi: 10.1016/j.cell.2015.07.017.

Suresh, R., S. Ali, A. Ahmad, P. A. Philip, and F. H. Sarkar. 2016. "The role of cancer stem cells in recurrent and drug-resistant lung cancer." *Adv Exp Med Biol* 890:57–74. doi: 10.1007/978-3-319-24932-2_4.

Sutherland, K. D., and J. E. Visvader. 2015. "Cellular mechanisms underlying intertumoral heterogeneity." *Trends Cancer* 1 (1):15–23. doi: 10.1016/j.trecan.2015.07.003.

Tomasetti, C., and B. Vogelstein. 2015. "Cancer etiology. Variation in cancer risk among tissues can be explained by the number of stem cell divisions." *Science* 347 (6217):78–81. doi: 10.1126/science.1260825.

Tsai, J. H., and J. Yang. 2013. "Epithelial-mesenchymal plasticity in carcinoma metastasis." *Genes Dev* 27 (20):2192–2206. doi: 10.1101/gad.225334.113.

Tsolou, A., I. Lamprou, A. O. Fortosi, M. Liousia, A. Giatromanolaki, and M. I. Koukourakis. 2019. "'Stemness' and 'senescence' related escape pathways are dose dependent in lung cancer cells surviving post irradiation." *Life Sci* 232:116562. doi: 10.1016/j.lfs.2019.116562.

van Staalduinen, J., D. Baker, P. Ten Dijke, and H. van Dam. 2018. "Epithelial-mesenchymal-transition-inducing transcription factors: new targets for tackling chemoresistance in cancer?" *Oncogene* 37 (48):6195–6211. doi: 10.1038/s41388-018-0378-x.

Vander Heiden, M. G., and R. J. DeBerardinis. 2017. "Understanding the intersections between metabolism and cancer biology." *Cell* 168 (4):657–669. doi: 10.1016/j.cell.2016.12.039.

Velcheti, V., and K. Schalper. 2016. "Basic overview of current immunotherapy approaches in cancer." *Am Soc Clin Oncol Educ Book* 35:298–308. doi: 10.14694/EDBK_156572; doi: 10.1200/EDBK_156572.

Vogelstein, B., N. Papadopoulos, V. E. Velculescu, S. Zhou, L. A. Diaz, Jr., and K. W. Kinzler. 2013. "Cancer genome landscapes." *Science* 339 (6127):1546–1548. doi: 10.1126/science.1235122.

Ward, P. S., and C. B. Thompson. 2012. "Metabolic reprogramming: a cancer hallmark even warburg did not anticipate." *Cancer Cell* 21 (3):297–308. doi: 10.1016/j.ccr.2012.02.014.

Wu, P., M. H. Clausen, and T. E. Nielsen. 2015. "Allosteric small-molecule kinase inhibitors." *Pharmacol Ther* 156:59–68. doi: 10.1016/j.pharmthera.2015.10.002.

Xie, G., B. Zhou, A. Zhao, Y. Qiu, X. Zhao, L. Garmire, Y. B. Shvetsov, H. Yu, Y. Yen, and W. Jia. 2015. "Lowered circulating aspartate is a metabolic feature of human breast cancer." *Oncotarget* 6 (32):-33369–33381. doi: 10.18632/oncotarget.5409.

Yang, L., and P. C. Lin. 2017. "Mechanisms that drive inflammatory tumor microenvironment, tumor heterogeneity, and metastatic progression." *Semin Cancer Biol* 47:185–195. doi: 10.1016/j.semcancer.2017.08.001.

Yoshida, G. J. 2015. "Metabolic reprogramming: the emerging concept and associated therapeutic strategies." *J Exp Clin Cancer Res* 34:111. doi: 10.1186/s13046-015-0221-y.

Yuan, Y., Y. C. Jiang, C. K. Sun, and Q. M. Chen. 2016. "Role of the tumor microenvironment in tumor progression and the clinical applications (Review)." *Oncol Rep* 35 (5):2499–2515. doi: 10.3892/or.2016.4660.

Zielonka, J., and B. Kalyanaraman. 2008. ""ROS-generating mitochondrial DNA mutations can regulate tumor cell metastasis"--a critical commentary." *Free Radic Biol Med* 45 (9):1217–1219. doi: 10.1016/j.freeradbiomed.2008.07.025.

Zong, W. X., J. D. Rabinowitz, and E. White. 2016. "Mitochondria and Cancer." *Mol Cell* 61 (5):667–676. doi: 10.1016/j.molcel.2016.02.011.

3 Precision Oncology and Nutrition

John A. Glaspy and Sidharth R. Anand
David Geffen School of Medicine at UCLA

David Heber
UCLA Center for Human Nutrition

CONTENTS

INTRODUCTION

The goal of precision oncology as defined by the American Society for Clinical Oncology is simply to deliver the right cancer treatment to the right patient at the right dose and at the right time (Schwartzberg et al. 2017). Cancer comprises several hundred heterogeneous diseases, meaning that differences exist not only between cancer cells from various patients but also between cancer cells within a single patient. Tumors are constantly developing characteristics to evade cell death. No single drug has been effective in "curing" all cancers as each cancer type has its own genetic and metabolic characteristics and these evolve through the stages of carcinogenesis and metastasis. Precision oncology is based on using a combination of the unique characteristics of each patient's tumor cells to direct therapy. Government regulatory policies have paved the way for the adoption of "big data" genetic profiling techniques to guide patient therapies, such as those described by the NCI-MATCH (Molecular Analysis for Therapy Choice) or the NCI-MPACT (Molecular Profiling-based Assignment of Cancer Therapy) initiatives. In this chapter, the argument is made that new research combines precision oncology and precision nutrition by integrating information on the nutrition and metabolism of the tumor and the patient with the genomics and metabolism of cancer cells, and even the microbiome of the patient may lead to new approaches to cancer prevention and therapy and better results when molecularly targeted therapies and immunotherapy are used to treat specific forms of cancer using the precision made possible by molecular oncology and molecular nutrition.

PRECISION ONCOLOGY

Key research advances occurred over the last 50 years that led to the development of the field of precision oncology. In 1970, the independent and simultaneous discovery of reverse transcriptase in retroviruses (then RNA tumor viruses) by David Baltimore and Howard Temin was recognized through the award of the Nobel Prize in Physiology and Medicine in 1975. The discovery of reverse transcriptase revolutionized molecular biology and laid the foundations for retrovirology and cancer biology. Harold Varmus and Michael Bishop through the discovery of the cellular origin of retroviral oncogenes earned the Nobel Prize in Physiology and Medicine in 1989 (Varmus 2019). The first draft sequence of the human genome was accomplished in 2001 (Venter et al. 2001), followed by the sequencing of cancer genomes (Lin et al. 2007). These discoveries led to the deployment of assays that could detect alterations in tumor biopsy specimens which could be performed utilizing polymerase chain reaction methods quickly and inexpensively. The discovery of oncogenes led to molecular cloning that enhanced the search for human cancer viruses and oncogenes leading to the understanding of how oncogenes and tumor suppressor genes were key to the unregulated growth of cancer cells and the multistep process of carcinogenesis (Coffin and Fan 2016).

The insight that genetic changes within our own cells programmed by inherited mutations or extrinsic genotoxic factors as we age could trigger cancer sparked the idea that inhibiting the activities of oncogenes could lead to targeted therapies that would be more effective and less toxic than chemotherapy. Epigenetic alterations such as DNA methylation defects and aberrant covalent histone modifications occur within all cancers and are selected for throughout the natural history of tumor formation, with changes being detectable in early onset, progression, and ultimately recurrence and metastasis. The epigenome changes with age and numerous studies have been published documenting age-related DNA hypermethylation and acceleration of this process that suggests that age-related epigenetic changes may be a biomarker of cancer risk potentially affected by diet and lifestyle (Werner, Kelly, and Issa 2017). At the same time, the knowledge that oxidant stress affected the integrity of the genome during aging sparked the idea that factors such as smoking, environmental pollution, toxins, and unbalanced nutrition could promote carcinogenesis. In parallel with the evolution of knowledge in basic cancer biology, population studies beginning with the effects of tobacco on lung cancer expanded into studies of many environmental factors including nutrition and obesity (Giovannucci 2018).

The discovery of the human epidermal growth factor receptor 2 (HER2)/neu proto-oncogene and its role in the pathogenesis of breast cancer tumors in 1987 by Dr. Dennis Slamon at the University of California, Los Angeles led to the 2019 Lasker-DeBakey Clinical Medical Research Award as the result of the development of an effective anti-HER2 monoclonal antibody drug (trastuzumab), directed against the HER2 receptor protein. The award honored Dr. Slamon and his collaborators H. Michael Shepard and Axel Ullrich for developing and testing the first monoclonal antibody drug available for the treatment of cancer. This was a major milestone in encouraging the development of precision oncology in breast cancer and other tumors. Clinical trials in HER2-positive (Her2+) patients demonstrated that the combined use of targeted therapy with trastuzumab in conjunction with cytotoxic chemotherapy was associated with improved time to disease progression and overall survival. Patients with Her2+ breast cancer represent 20%–25% of all breast cancer patients and have high relapse rates and poorer prognosis. The combined antibody and chemotherapy treatment of Her2+ breast cancer has led to a reduction in relapse rates of up to 50% (Chung et al. 2015).

With these advances and recognition of the genetic heterogeneity of human tumor cells, it became feasible to propose using genetic biomarkers drive treatment decisions in cancer patients. This idea increased interest in molecular profiling and gave birth to the new field of precision oncology. Sequencing technology and costs improved rapidly during the early 2000s, particularly with the advent of Next Generation Sequencing on formalin-fixed, paraffin-embedded tissue whereby massive parallel sequencing allows determination of alterations in a large number of genes through a rapid and cost-effective process (Wakai et al. 2019).

MONOCLONAL ANTIBODIES

In 1975, George Kohler and Cesar Milstein developed methodologies to create hybrid monoclonal antibodies specific to different antigens, with the fusion of murine B lymphocytes and human myeloma cells. This subsequently led to the development of the first monoclonal antibody to treat cancer in murine models, and to the first attempts at human monoclonal antibody-based cancer treatments with the murine monoclonal antibody AB89 (Bernstein, Tam, and Nowinski 1980, Nadler et al. 1980).

It was not until the late 1980s and early 1990s that the first effective monoclonal antibody-based therapies became available for human use with the discovery of traztuzumab, which blocks the HER2/neu glycoprotein receptor and also leads to antibody mediated cellular toxicity, a key mechanism also used by other monoclonal antibody-based therapies.

Since then the field has exploded with the advancement of new drug discovery techniques. Multiple monoclonal antibodies, including murine, chimeric, humanized, and human monoclonal antibodies, have been tested in preclinical murine models and subsequent clinical trials to determine if there are therapeutic benefits for cancer patients.

In the mid-1990s, inspired by murine monoclonal antibodies against cell surface antigen CD-20, IDEC pharmaceuticals created a chimeric monoclonal antibody named IDEC-28, subsequently approved by the United States Food and Drug Administration (FDA) in 1997 to be used in patients affected by lymphoproliferative B lymphocyte disorders. This molecule, known as Rituxan, was subsequently studied in multiple clinical trials involving refractory Non-Hodgkins Lymphoma (NHLs) as well as indolent lymphomas and was shown to have benefits (Maloney et al. 1994, Coiffier et al. 2002, Reff et al. 1994).

The next important discovery in the evolution of monoclonal antibodies used in cancer therapy was antibodies to the epidermal growth factor receptor (EGFR) receptor. One of the earliest in this line of therapy was Cetuximab, a chimeric mouse/human monoclonal antibody which inhibits EGFR signaling transduction and blocks cell cycle progression, leading to EGFR internalization and antibody-dependent cell-mediated cytotoxicity (Vincenzi et al. 2010). Cetuximab is now used in a variety of cancer treatments including nonsmall cell lung cancer (NSCLC), head and neck cancer, and colorectal cancers. In colorectal cancer, patients who do not have an activating mutation in Kirsten rat sarcoma viral oncogene (KRAS) (KRAS "wild-type") can benefit from monoclonal antibodies to KRAS with cetuximab and newer agents targeting the KRAS pathway such as panitumumab (Lievre 2006).

Further innovations in antibody development led to the approval of Panitumumab directed to EGFR in 2006, for the treatment of metastatic colorectal cancer patients with wild-type KRAS, including in the front-line setting (Poulin-Costello et al. 2013, Modest, Pant, and Sartore-Bianchi 2019).

Monoclonal antibodies have continued to evolve, targeting the various potential avenues for neoplastic growth and survival. One of the major suspected pathways of focus has been tumor angiogenesis. In order to sustain growth, tumors need nutrients and must get rid of metabolic waste, thus requiring tumor-associated neovascularization. As described by Folkman in the 1990s, in tumor angiogenesis, an "angiogenic switch" remains active in tumor tissue, leading to constant formation of new vasculature to sustain tumor growth (Hanahan and Folkman 1996). The vascular endothelial growth factor (VEGF) pathway was identified as playing a key role in this new blood vessel growth and subsequently monoclonal antibodies were discovered to target this pathway (Ferrara and Henzel 1989). This ultimately led to the development and first clinical trials of bevacizumab in 1997, and subsequently the use of bevacizumab in combination with chemotherapy

(Gordon et al. 2001). This monoclonal antibody to VEGF is now used in metastatic colorectal carcinoma, metastatic renal cancer, metastatic ovarian and cervical cancer, metastatic lung cancer, and metastatic breast cancer.

ANTIBODY-DRUG CONJUGATES

Antibody-drug conjugates (ADCs) are intended to spare normal cells while specifically targeting and killing cancer cells. ADCs have a cytotoxic anticancer drug bound to an antibody that specifically targets a protein tumor marker found on cancer cells. The antibody attaches itself to the target protein so that the cell internalizes the antibody and the drug so that the drug is released intracellularly to kill the cancer cell while ideally sparing surrounding normal cells. Advances in molecular biology techniques led to the development of an ADC with the monoclonal antibody Herceptin chemically linked to the antimitotic agent emtansine (DM1 or mertansine). This drug shows more efficacy than Traztuzumab alone with the monoclonal antibody inhibiting cell growth through by binding the HER2 receptor, and inhibiting the mitogen-activated protein kinase (MAPK) and PI3K/AKT pathway, and emtansine entering the cell and binding tubulin to block DNA duplication. Historically used successfully in the metastatic HER2+ breast cancer setting, TDM1 is now growing in use in the adjuvant setting for patients with residual disease after HER2-directed therapy in the neoadjuvant setting (LoRusso et al. 2011, Barok, Joensuu, and Isola 2014, Hurvitz et al. 2018, von Minckwitz et al. 2019). A number of additional ADCs are under study or have received FDA designation including brentuximab vedotin, sacituzumab govitecan, and DS-8201. Brentuximab vedotin selectively targets CD30, which is highly expressed in Hodgkin's lymphoma. This ADC is now used in combination with chemotherapy as a front-line treatment of patients with advanced Hodgkin's lymphoma. The ADC sacituzumab govitecan (IMMU-132) targets trophoblast cell-surface antigen (Trop-2) and selectively delivers high doses of SN-38, the active metabolite of the topoisomerase 1 inhibitor, irinotecan in patients with metastatic triple-negative breast cancer. DS-8201 is used for the treatment of patients with HER2-positive, locally advanced or metastatic breast cancer who have received trastuzumab (Herceptin) and pertuzumab (Perjeta) treatment and have disease progression after therapy with ado-trastuzumab emtansine. Further research is needed to develop safe and effective ADCs with the promise of more specific precision oncology approaches in cells that express surface protein markers even if they are not functional proteins.

SELECTIVE TYROSINE KINASE AND SMALL MOLECULE INHIBITORS

Tyrosine kinases are enzymes that transfer a phosphate group from Adenosine Triphosphate (ATP) to a protein in a cell. Tyrosine kinases are a subclass of many protein kinases in cells that function as an "on" or "off" switch in many cellular metabolic control points including those that impact cell proliferation. The tyrosine name of this class is based on the fact that the phosphate group is attached to the amino acid tyrosine on the target protein. Other tyrosine kinases can attach phosphate groups to serine and threonine. Kinase-mediated phosphorylation is an important mechanism in communicating signals within a cell and regulating cellular activities. Protein kinases can become mutated, stuck in the "on" position, and cause unregulated growth of the cell, which is a necessary step for the development of cancer. Therefore, kinase inhibitors can be effective cancer treatments.

A stunning discovery led to the development of the tyrosine kinase inhibitor, imatinib, which radically changed the treatment paradigm and outcomes for chronic myelogenous leukemia (CML) and the less common gastrointestinal stromal tumors (GIST) by targeting mutated receptor proteins on the surface of tumor cells. C-abl is a proto-oncogene that codes for a member of the tyrosine kinase family. The human c-abl gene is located on the long arm of chromosome 9. It is activated by translocation to the breakpoint cluster region (bcr) on chromosome 22 in CML. The c-abl and breakpoint cluster genes are in a head-to-tail configuration chimeric gene (BCR-ABL1) that codes for proteins that result in upregulated tyrosine kinase activity. The BCR-ABL1 gene is necessary and sufficient to cause CML (Lambert et al. 2013).

The BCR-ABL1 rearrangement in CML was successfully targeted by the small molecule imatinib. The 2009 Lasker-DeBakey Clinical Medical Research Award honored the three scientists who developed the tyrosine kinase inhibitor treatment for CML. This discovery converted this fatal cancer into a manageable chronic condition by targeting the molecular basis of this cancer, with life expectancy now close to that of the general population (Hochhaus et al. 2017). The award was shared by Charles L. Sawyers (Memorial Sloan-Kettering Cancer Center formerly at UCLA). Brian J. Druker (Oregon Health and Science University), and Nicholas B. Lydon (formerly at Novartis), who broke new ground in cancer therapy and saved the lives of thousands of patients with CML and GIST. Second-generation and third-generation bcr abl inhibitors have subsequently been developed over the years, such as Dasatinib, Nilotinib, Bosutinib, and Ponatinib, each with its own efficacy and side-effect profile.

Multiple, nonoverlapping driver mutations and tyrosine kinase inhibitors with clinically effective inhibitory properties were discovered for the treatment of NSCLC (Sgambato et al. 2018). Erlotinib (Tarceva) and Gefitinib (Iressa) are two of these important tyrosine kinase inhibitors, specifically directed toward the EGFR ATP binding site to inhibit the activation of MAPK and PI3K/AKT pathways (Nicholson, Gee, and Harper 2001). These molecules were first approved in the early 2000s for NSCLC and have subsequently shown activity in the inhibition of EGFR (and HER2 kinases) in lung, ovarian, breast, and colon cancers.

NSCLC has emerged as the prototype disease where genomic data from at least several well-documented alterations with approved targeted agents are essential for optimal treatment from diagnosis to progression to advanced disease. Due to the development of resistance to targeted therapies, resampling and retesting of tumors, including using liquid biopsy technology after clinical progression, are used in making treatment decisions. The value of molecular profiling depends on avoiding both underutilization for well-documented variant target-drug pairs and overutilization of variant-drug therapy without proven benefit. As techniques evolve and become more cost-effective, the use of molecular testing may prove to add more specificity and improve cancer outcomes for a larger number of patients.

Many kinase-signaling pathways drive various hallmarks of tumor development such as survival, metabolism, motility, proliferation, angiogenesis, and evasion of immune surveillance. Tyrosine kinase inhibitors (e.g., lorlatinib) have been developed which target the anaplastic lymphoma kinase (ALK)/ROS1 (c-ros oncogene 1) in patients with ALK-positive metastatic NSCLC previously treated with one or more ALK inhibitors. Osimertinib (Tagrisso) is a third-generation EGFR tyrosine kinase inhibitor for the first-line treatment of patients with metastatic EGFR mutation-positive NSCLC.

A class of tyrosine kinase inhibitors with properties of VEGF inhibition evolved over time in parallel to these important advances in NSCLC. Small-molecule tyrosine kinase inhibitors (TKIs) directed to the ATP-binding pocket of the VEGF receptor (antiangiogenic) showed significant activity in a variety of malignancies. Sunitinib (Sutent) has been used in difficult-to-treat pancreatic neuroendocrine tumors (NET) , GIST, and renal cell carcinomas, and Sorefenib (Nexavar) has been a mainstay in the treatment of renal and hepatocellular carcinoma (Herrmann et al. 2008, Imbulgoda, Heng, and Kollmannsberger 2014, Hasskarl 2018).

A different class of targeted therapy small-molecule inhibitors; mammalian target of rapamycin (mTOR) inhibitors are also widely used in the treatment of multiple tumors. mTOR inhibitors are a class of drugs which inhibit the mTOR pathway, which is an intracellular serine-/threonine-specific kinase responsible for cellular signaling and metabolism, particularly cell cycle progression from G1 to S phase. As indicated in its name, this drug category was discovered through the identification of a powerful antifungal drug, Rapamycin, produced by the microorganism *Streptomyces hydroscopicus*. Everolimus and Temserolimus are two of the many mTOR medications currently in use for cancer-directed therapy, initially approved for the treatment of progressive NET tumors, hormone positive metastatic breast cancer, and advanced renal cell carcinoma (Hasskarl 2018, Lee, Ito, and Jensen 2018).

CYCLIN-DEPENDENT KINASES

Cyclin-dependent kinases (CDKs) are the families of protein kinases first discovered for their role in regulating the cell cycle. CDKs are small proteins with molecular weights ranging from 34 to 40kDa and contain primarily a kinase domain. CDKs bind a regulatory protein called a cyclin. Without cyclin, CDKs have little kinase activity; only the cyclin-CDK complex is an active kinase. CDKs phosphorylate their substrates on serines and threonines, so they are serine-threonine kinases. Most of the known cyclin-CDK complexes regulate the progression through the cell cycle. Animal cells contain at least nine CDKs, four of which, CDK1, 2, 3, and 4, are directly involved in cell cycle regulation. They are also involved in regulating transcription, mRNA processing, and cell differentiation.

CDK4 and CDK6 (CDK4/6) are commonly deregulated and overactivated in many types of cancer cells. CDK4/6 inhibitors have been developed to attenuate growth-signaling pathways and restore control of cell cycle in cancer cells. CDK4/6 interact with cyclin D, which is synthesized at the start of G1, and these cyclin/CDK complexes drive cell cycle progression from G1 to S phase. Inhibitors block these kinases to stop the cells' transition from G1 to S phase.

For estrogen receptor-positive (HR+)/HER2− advanced breast cancer patients endocrine therapies were first line therapy until recently when a CDK4/6 inhibitor in combination with endocrine therapy was shown to be effective in the treatment of premenopausal and postmenopausal women with HR+/HER2− advanced breast cancer. Three CDK4/6 inhibitors, palbociclib, ribociclib, and abemaciclib, have been approved for the treatment of HR+/HER2 advanced breast cancer (Choo and Lee 2018).

CDK4/6 have been extensively tested against breast cancer, but additional studies are underway in patients with liposarcoma, mantle cell lymphoma, NSCLC, glioblastoma (GBM), pancreatic adenocarcinoma, urothelial cancer, head and neck squamous cell carcinoma, metastatic castrate-resistant prostate cancer, ovarian cancer, and endometrial cancer (Klein et al. 2018).

IMMUNOTHERAPY

These approvals are a reflection of the plethora of ground-breaking changes in cancer treatment and the willingness of the FDA to assure that patients have faster access to these life-saving treatments.

The Nobel Prize in Physiology or Medicine in 2018 was awarded jointly to James P. Allison and Tasuku Honjo for their discovery of cancer therapy by inhibition of negative immune regulation. Immune checkpoint inhibitor drugs counter the effects of PD-1 or PD-L1 proteins made by tumor cells which blind the immune system to the presence of tumor cells. Drugs in this category enable the patient's T cells to attack tumor cells throughout the body even when cancer cells have widely metastasized.

Antiprogrammed death 1 (anti-PD-1) antibodies, pembrolizumab and nivolumab, and antiprogrammed death ligand 1 (anti-PD-L1) antibody atezolizumab have led to a significantly longer survival of lung cancer patients with a manageable safety profile. They are now approved as first- or second-line treatment options in patients with advanced NSCLC. Only the pembrolizumab approval is limited to the PD-L1-positive NSCLC; both nivolumab and atezolizumab can be currently used irrespective of tumor PD-L1 expression. Biomarkers for the response to PD-1/PD-LI checkpoint inhibitors beyond PD-L1 expression levels are being investigated in order to select patients who are most likely to benefit from antibodies targeting the PD-1 axis. Platinum-based chemotherapy remains the standard first-line treatment for advanced NSCLC when there are no genetic alterations identified, such as production of PD-L1, sensitizing mutations of EGFR, or translocations of the ALK gene.

Pembrolizumab (Keytruda) appears to be the most versatile and widely tested PD-1 inhibitor. It is approved to treat classical Hodgkin lymphoma (cHL) in adult and pediatric patients with refractory cHL or who have relapsed after three or more previous therapeutic approaches. In 2017, it was approved as first-line combination therapy with pemetrexed and carboplatin for patients with metastatic nonsquamous NSCLC, independent of PD-L1 expression and was also approved for patients with locally advanced or metastatic urothelial carcinoma that has progressed following platinum-containing chemotherapy. Pembrolizumab is also approved for patients with recurrent locally advanced or metastatic, gastric, or gastroesophageal junction adenocarcinoma that express PD-L1, and it was the first cancer treatment approved for any unresectable or metastatic tumor that expresses either the microsatellite instability-high or mismatch repair deficient biomarker. This is the first application of this therapy that was not prescribed based on tumor type, making it potentially applicable to a wide range of tumors.

The majority of melanomas have mutations associated with the MAPK pathway, an important signal transduction pathway involved in cell growth, proliferation, and survival. Oncogenic activation of the MAPK pathway can occur via multiple mechanisms, the most common of which in melanoma is constitutive activation of the Baton Rouge Area Foundation (BRAF) kinase via mutation, which occurs in ~40%–60% of cases. BRAF encodes a cytoplasmic serine–threonine kinase. More than 97% of BRAF mutations are located in codon 600 of the BRAF gene. The most common mutation (in up to 90% of cases) is the result of a transversion of T to A at nucleotide 1799, which results in a substitution of valine (V) for glutamic acid (E) at position 600.26 of the BRAF oncogene. BRAF mutations have been found in about half of all cases of melanoma with the V600E being the most common. BRAF mutations are also often found in other disorders and different types of cancer, including cancers of the colon, thyroid, and ovaries. Cancers with a BRAF mutation tend to be more serious than those without the mutation. In unresectable or metastatic advanced melanomas the V600E mutation in the BRAF gene is the most common. Targeted therapy with BRAF and MEK inhibitors is associated with significant long-term treatment benefit in patients with BRAF V600-mutated melanoma (Cheng et al. 2018).

Molecular profiling has shown that mutation load increases with melanoma tumor progression and that unique patterns of genetic changes and evolutionary trajectories for different melanoma subtypes can occur. Changes in the BRAF mutational status between primary and metastatic lesions, as well as genetic heterogeneity within tumors of different clones, are known to occur.

Despite a high initial response rate, the durability of responses to combination BRAF and MEK inhibitor therapy has been limited to durations under 6 months. Further research uncovered numerous mechanisms of therapeutic resistance to BRAF inhibitor monotherapy, with many of these contributing to MAPK reactivation. Concurrent with the clinical development of BRAF-targeted therapy was the clinical development of another type of immune checkpoint inhibitor. This class of agents blocks immunomodulatory molecules on the surface of T cells or their ligands. This results in reactivation of potentially anergic T cells. Ipilimumab and tremelimumab are monoclonal antibodies that block the cytotoxic T lymphocyte antigen 4 (CTLA-4) receptor on the surface of T lymphocytes. CTLA-4 functions to downregulate the priming phase of an immune response, and blocking this interaction results in T cell activation via engagement of antigen presenting cells. CTLA4 blockade may also function through depletion of immune-suppressive regulatory T cells or Treg via antibody-dependent cellular cytotoxicity. Patients with metastatic melanoma demonstrated a survival benefit over then standard-of-care chemotherapy, leading to FDA approval of these drugs in 2011. Though overall objective response rates were modest (10%–15%), treatment with CTLA-4 blockade is associated with long-term disease control in a subset of patients, with approximately 20% of treated patients achieving durable disease control for over 10 years after initiation of therapy. Treatment with monoclonal antibodies blocking PD-1 was associated with response rates of approximately 40% in patients with metastatic melanoma and two such drugs were FDA-approved for melanoma in 2014 (pembrolizumab and nivolumab). Combination regimens with CTLA-4 and PD-1 blockade were tested in clinical trials demonstrating a high response rate of over 60% and improvement in overall survival, though treatment with this regimen was also associated with a very high rate of toxicity.

BRAF- and MEK-targeted therapies have multiple, complex, and interrelated mechanisms of action and encourage the further investigation of combination treatment strategies with targeted therapy and immune checkpoint inhibitors, as well as other therapies that modulate the immune microenvironment. Clinical trials investigating preoperative and adjuvant BRAF-targeted therapy for high-risk, BRAF-mutated melanoma are also needed. The hope is that the genetic profile of tumors can match patients with the BRAF V600E mutation treatment regimens including combination with BRAF inhibitors. Results of next-generation sequencing have shown that most patients do not have "actionable" mutations like the BRAF V600E. In other words, we do not yet have a drug that can target every specific mutation identified in cancer patients. Also cancers can have more than one "driver" mutation. However, combination therapies seem to hold promise in overcoming some of these issues.

MOLECULAR RADIOTHERAPY

Since the time of Marie and Pierre Curie in the late 1900s, with the discovery of radium and the possible use of x-rays for the treatment of tumors, radiation therapy has evolved to become increasingly targeted in order to limit potential toxicity to surrounding tissues (Kulakowski 2011). Radiation therapy is now indicated in the treatment of a variety of malignancies in the neoadjuvant and adjuvant, definitive/curative, and palliative settings. Molecular radiotherapy uses similar principles of radioactivity to target cancer cells but in a much more precise manner. In molecular radiotherapy, radioactive compounds are taken up by particular cancer subtypes depending on the intrinsic properties of a radioactive isotope such as Iodine 131 in the thyroid gland, or through the creation of drug conjugates that incorporate radioactive isotopes.

An exciting development using the principles of molecular radiotherapy is in the treatment of metastatic neuroendocrine tumors, with the discovery of peptide receptor radionucleotide therapy. This technique works because particular tumors express increased membrane peptide receptors compared to normal tissue, particularly somatostatin receptors in neuroendocrine tumors. Analogs such as octreotide which can target tumor cells expressing somatostatin are combined with radioactive compounds such as lutetium-177, indium-111, or yttrium-90. These analogs are highly effective as a treatment and similarly can be utilized for diagnostic purposes in patients with these tumors (Strosberg et al. 2017).

ADOPTIVE CELL THERAPIES

Adoptive cell therapies are the newest precision medicine technique available for cancer treatment, involving the collection of immune cells from a patient or a donor, followed by ex vivo manipulation of these cells and reinfusion. One of the latest and most exciting developments is chimeric antigen receptor (CAR-T cell therapy). CAR-T uses gene editing technologies to insert a gene construct into T cell DNA to create chimeric T cells with a monoclonal antibody with high specificity to cancer cells. CARs (first-generation) are composed of an extracellular binding domain, hinge region, transmembrane domain, and one or more intracellular signaling domains (Makita and Tobinai 2017). CAR-T cell treatment is now approved in the treatment of relapsed/refractory diffuse large B cell lymphoma and relapsed/refractory B cell precursor ALL, namely, axicabtagene ciloleucel (Yescarta®) and tisagenlecleucel (Kymriah) which both target CD 19 (Kochenderfer and Rosenberg 2013, Kuwana et al. 1987, Choe, Williams, and Lim 2020).

There are now a number of preclinical and clinical studies to examine the role of various additional CAR-T therapies targeting other cell surface receptors such as CD 20 and CD 22, and dual targeting techniques as well as new clinical indications in hematologic malignancies such as multiple myeloma as well as solid tumors.

THE MICROBIOME

Factors beyond tumor genomics influence cancer development and responses to anticancer therapies including traditional chemotherapy and immunotherapies. A number of studies have shown that the gut microbiome may influence antitumor immune responses via innate and adaptive immunity (Gopalakrishnan et al. 2018). The human gut harbors trillions of bacteria including over 1,000 species that vary widely between individuals and are influenced by diet and lifestyle. These bacteria engage in nutrient metabolism, the production of metabolites, and communication with the gut-associated lymphatic tissue, which comprises 70% of the host immune system (Ivanov and Honda 2012).

Anti-PD-L1 and anti-CTLA4 therapies are more effective in patients who demonstrate antitumor immunity prior to treatment, consistent with the concept that these therapies promote preexisting immunity rather than induce de novo responses (Tumeh et al. 2014, Ji et al. 2012).

Recent studies demonstrated that gut bacteria are involved in tumor control using conventional therapies such as cyclophosphamide and oxaliplatin, both of which depend on activation of antitumor immunity for their therapeutic effects (Iida et al. 2013, Viaud et al. 2013). This concept is further supported by studies that illustrate an important role for gut microbes in promoting the efficacy of anti-PD-L1 and anti-CTLA-4 therapies (Sivan et al. 2015, Vetizou et al. 2015).

Bifidobacteria are widely considered to be beneficial and have shown some benefit in treating inflammatory bowel disease (Vieira, Teixeira, and Martins 2013). Oral gavage with a Bifidobacterium cocktail impaired tumor growth in mice and addition of anti-PD-L1 further enhanced tumor control. Critically, the therapeutic effect of Bifidobacterium supplementation and anti-PD-L1 therapy was strictly dependent on CD8+ T cells.

In mice and patients, T cell responses specific for Bifidobacterium (B.) thetaiotaomicron or B. fragilis were associated with the efficacy of CTLA-4 blockade. Tumors in antibiotic-treated or germ-free mice did not respond to CTLA blockade. This defect was overcome by gavage with B. fragilis, immunization with B. fragilis polysaccharides, or by adoptive transfer of B. fragilis-specific T cells. Fecal microbial transplantation from humans to mice confirmed that treatment of melanoma patients with antibodies against CTLA-4 favored the outgrowth of B. fragilis with anticancer properties. These observations support a key role for the microbiome and some Bacteroides species in the immunostimulatory effects of CTLA-4 blockade. Defining the mechanisms involved in mediating the role of the microbiome in cancer therapy could also lead to the development of specific dietary modulation of the microbiome or the use of bacteria-derived metabolites or antigens that could serve as immunotherapy adjuvants.

GLUCOSE RESTRICTION

Unlike normal cells, cancer cells often depend on glycolysis for energy generation in the presence of oxygen and produce lactate, a metabolic adaptation that favors tumor growth known as the Warburg effect. One strategy proposed to inhibit or slow tumor growth is glucose restriction by administration of a high-fat, low-carbohydrate ketogenic diet (KD). Under these conditions, ketone bodies are generated as an important energy source for most normal cells and organs while starving the tumor of glucose.

A classic 4:1 KD delivers 90% of its calories from fat, 8% from protein, and only 2% from carbohydrate. KDs in the 1920s were extremely bland and restrictive diets which were difficult to follow. KDs have evolved since then to make adherence easier and have gained some popularity in the treatment of obesity and diabetes.

In a recent review of 57 preclinical studies of KD and 30 clinical observation studies (Weber et al. 2020), 60% of preclinical studies demonstrated an antitumor effect of KDs, 17% did not detect an influence on tumor growth, and 10% reported adverse or pro-proliferative effects. In 10% of the preclinical studies, a statement on the effect on cancer cells cannot be made due to the lack of proper control groups. Three percent of the preclinical studies did not report data on tumor progression but investigated the effect of the KD on tumor microvasculature, gene expression, or glucose uptake. Most of the studies were performed in GBM models with no adverse effects observed. Most clinical studies were case reports or pilot/feasibility studies focusing on safety and tolerability of the KD. Only one randomized controlled trial is available to date (Cohen et al. 2018). Questionnaires were administered at baseline and after 12 weeks on the assigned diet to assess changes in mental and physical health, perceived energy, appetite, and food cravings. Typically, a moderate reduction of blood glucose and induction of ketosis was observed without any serious adverse events or toxicity. A majority of clinical studies that are currently underway are examining effects on patients with GBM.

AMINO ACID DEPRIVATION

The body cannot synthesize nine essential amino acids and these must be obtained from the diet to prevent loss of lean body mass and impaired immune function. The nine essential amino acids are histidine, isoleucine, leucine, lysine, methionine, phenylalanine, threonine, tryptophan, and valine. Nonessential amino acids can be made in the body and include alanine, arginine, asparagine, aspartic acid, cysteine, glutamic acid, glutamine, glycine, proline, serine, and tyrosine. Complete proteins contain all 21 common amino acids including both the essential and nonessential amino acids. Eating essential and nonessential amino acids at every meal is less important than getting a balance of them over the whole day. With the increased popularity of plant-based diets, it is important to note that a diet based on a single plant item will not be adequate. It is important that over the day, a balance of essential amino acids is obtained to prevent the body from utilizing amino acids in muscle protein for the metabolic needs of the body leading to muscle loss. Therefore, it is challenging to deplete amino acid levels in the tumor microenvironment without causing severe whole-body reduction of these amino acids with significant side effects.

In vitro and in animals, nonessential amino acids can be required in large amounts by cancer cells for various anabolic processes, and depriving cells of specific amino acids often severely compromises their viability, regardless of their ability to synthesize these amino acids.

The potential of dietary methionine restriction to enhance cancer treatment has been tested in various mouse models and types of cancer, including sarcoma, glioma, prostate cancer, colorectal cancer, breast cancer, and melanoma. Recently, it was shown that methionine restriction in humans results in similar metabolic changes to those observed in methionine-deprived tumor-bearing mice with inhibition of both one-carbon metabolism and nucleotide synthesis.

Methionine restriction influences tumor growth in animal models through controlled and reproducible changes in the folate pathway of one-carbon metabolism. This pathway metabolizes methionine and is the target of a variety of cancer interventions that involve chemotherapy and radiation. Methionine restriction produced therapeutic responses in two patient-derived xenograft models of chemotherapy-resistant RAS-driven colorectal cancer, and in a mouse model of autochthonous soft-tissue sarcoma driven by a G12D mutation in KRAS and knockout of p53 (KrasG12D/+; Trp53−/−) that is resistant to radiation. Metabolomics revealed that the therapeutic mechanisms operated via effects on flux through one-carbon metabolism that affected redox and nucleotide metabolism interacting with the antimetabolite or radiation intervention. In a controlled and tolerated feeding study in humans, methionine restriction resulted in effects on systemic metabolism that were similar to those obtained in mice (Gao et al. 2019).

Oncogenic drivers elevate lipid reactive oxygen species (ROS) production in many tumor types including pancreatic ductal adenocarcinoma (PDAC) and can be counteracted by metabolites of the amino acid cysteine. Ferroptosis is a form of cell death that is triggered by lipid ROS normally counteracted by endogenous antioxidants including glutathione and coenzyme A. The uptake by PDAC cells of oxidized cysteine (cystine) is a critical factor in maintaining the viability of PDAC. PDAC cells use cysteine to synthesize glutathione and coenzyme A, which combine to inhibit ferroptosis. In mice with a deletion of the cellular cystine transport system (Slc7a11) tumor-selective ferroptosis occurred and inhibited PDAC growth. This was also accomplished with the administration of the enzyme cyst(e)inase, which depleted cysteine and cystine, demonstrating a strategy that could be tested in clinical trials (Badgley et al. 2020). Cystine deprivation also inhibited tumor growth and has been shown to improve survival in three tumor-bearing mouse models: EGFR-mutant NSCLC xenografts (Poursaitidis et al. 2017). Cyst(e)inase suppressed the growth of prostate carcinoma allografts, reduced tumor growth in both prostate and breast cancer xenografts and doubled the median survival time of TCL1-Tg:p53-/- mice, which develop cancer resembling human chronic lymphocytic leukemia. It was observed that enzyme-mediated depletion of the serum L-cysteine and L-cystine pool suppressed the growth of multiple tumors, yet was very well tolerated (Cramer et al. 2017). These studies suggest that cyst(e)inase represents a safe and effective therapeutic modality for inactivating antioxidant cellular responses in a wide range of malignancies. Although these studies used pharmacological depletion of cystine by enzymatic degradation in animals, a similar result might be partially achieved through dietary restriction in terms of systemic depletion of cystine.

Cancer cell reprogramming of metabolism in poorly vascularized microenvironments leads to a role for glutamine and its immediate downstream metabolite glutamate in energy production for cancer cell proliferation through several metabolic pathways. Glutamine contributes to nucleotide biosynthesis and is essential for glutathione synthesis and maintenance of the redox balance in cells (Cluntun et al. 2017). Under hypoxic conditions, glutamine and glutamate also contribute to lipid synthesis (Metallo et al. 2011). Renal cell lines deficient in the von Hippel-Lindau tumor suppressor preferentially use reductive glutamine metabolism for lipid biosynthesis even at normal oxygen levels. The first step of glutamine catabolism is conversion to glutamate, which is catalyzed by cytosolic glutamine amidotransferases or by mitochondrial glutaminases. A number of approaches are conceivable, including depletion of glutamine in blood serum, blockade of cellular glutamine uptake, and inhibition of enzymes involved in glutamine synthesis or catabolism (Strekalova et al. 2015). Many transformed cells and embryonic stem cells are dependent on the biosynthesis of the universal methyl-donor S-adenosylmethionine (SAM) from methionine by the enzyme MAT2A to maintain their epigenome. Cancer stem cells (CSCs) rely on SAM biosynthesis and the combination of methionine depletion and MAT2A inhibition was tested in human triple (ER/PR/HER2)-negative breast carcinoma (TNBC) cell lines cultured as CSC-enriched mammospheres in control or methionine-free media. MAT2A was inhibited with siRNAs or cycloleucine. Methionine restriction inhibited mammosphere formation and reduced the CD44hi/C24low CSC population, and the combination of methionine restriction and cycloleucine was more effective than either alone at suppressing primary and lung metastatic tumor burden in a murine TNBC model (Strekalova et al. 2019).

L-asparaginases are routinely used to treat patients with acute lymphocytic leukemia (ALL); the incorporation of L-asparaginase as routine therapy for this disorder has significantly increased the overall survival rates to approximately 90%. This enzyme catalyzes the deamidation of both asparagine and glutamine, leading to depletion of both of these amino acids in serum. Since most ALL cells are auxotrophic for asparagine, L-asparaginase effectively starves them of this nutrient resulting in cell cycle arrest and apoptosis in ALL cells without affecting normal tissues. (Lopes et al. 2017, Sun et al. 2019). The therapeutic progress of aspariganase in ALL had encouraged its studies in solid tumors. Clinical trials reported intolerable toxicity in patients and resistance to asparaginase action in depleting asparagine and glutamine. Aspariganase treatment of PC3 prostate cancer cells triggered asparagine shortage accompanied by increased asparagine production through upregulation of asparagine synthesis as indicated by ribosomal and transcriptional profiling (Loayza-Puch and Agami 2016). This feedback loop under asparagine depleted conditions did not explain the resistance to asparagine action, since the PC3 cells remained proliferative despite asparagine depletion. A functional genetic screen in PC3 cells identified SLC1A3, an aspartate/glutamate transporter, as a novel contributor to asparaginase resistance, as well as tumor initiation and progression in a mouse model for breast cancer metastasis (Sun et al. 2019).

One-carbon unit metabolic pathways are used for nucleotide synthesis, methylation, and reductive metabolism which support cancer cell proliferation. Antifolates such as methotrexate that target one-carbon metabolism have a history of use dating back to the beginnings of chemotherapy. In 1948, Sidney Farber observed that dietary folate deficiency in children with acute leukemia induced temporary remissions (Farber and Diamond 1948). Amino acids such as serine are a major one-carbon source, and cancer cells are particularly susceptible to deprivation of one-carbon units by serine restriction or inhibition of de novo serine synthesis. Serine deprivation has also been shown to enhance cancer therapy by inhibiting the mitochondrial complex I which is needed for oxidative phosphorylation and production of energy to maintain cell viability. Normally, cells respond to the metformin or phenformin reduction of oxidative phosphorylation by increasing glucose consumption and glycolysis. However, serine-deprived cells cannot induce this compensatory increase in glucose metabolism and cannot produce the necessary energy for survival. When tested in vivo, either phenformin treatment or serine deprivation alone did not inhibit the growth of colon adenocarcinoma xenografts in mice, but their combination resulted in significant inhibition (Gravel et al. 2014). Unfortunately, phenformin coupled with serine deprivation is toxic, and the effect achieved by phenformin was not observed with low-dose metformin for the treatment of intestinal tumors in mice (Maddocks et al. 2017). Dietary deprivation of serine for inhibition of tumor progression is promising and should be tested in combination with cancer therapies and in various genetic backgrounds.

Serine synthesis from glycine, which is induced by low levels of cellular serine, reverses the action of the one-carbon metabolism enzyme serine hydroxymethyltransferase (SHMT). The conversion of glycine to serine by SHMT prevents efficient nucleotide synthesis and compromises the proliferation rate of serine-deprived cells (Pacold et al. 2016). Serine deprivation is a promising candidate as an anticancer strategy with the potential to slow tumor progression owing to the induction of serine synthesis, which is harmful for rapidly proliferating cancer cells.

Although dietary deprivation of amino acids has shown a clear preclinical benefit, and some restrictions of amino acids have shown promise in limited studies in humans, there are still no clear guidelines or proven regimens for dietary modification for patients with cancer. More clinical work and preclinical research focusing on understanding how amino acid modifications inhibit cancer in vivo must be completed before these types of dietary interventions become a common approach to cancer therapy.

CONCLUSION

Underpinning precision oncology is the concept of somatic mutations as the foundation of cancer development. Mutations in oncogenes rendering them constitutively active are considered driver mutations and are central control points for progression of malignancies. Conversely, tumor suppressor genes, involved naturally in controlling tumor pathogenesis, can cause cancer progression when inactivated through mutation or allele loss. Multiple processes result in dysregulation of the genetic machinery in DNA, RNA, or protein, leading to altered expression of the protein coded for by the gene. To capture the entire spectrum of potential alterations, multiple technologies are needed. The vast number of choices of technologies, commercial entities offering testing, and sometimes conflicting results have overwhelmed clinicians looking to obtain molecular information that will result in clinical utility for their patients. Even in academic centers, oncologists report varying confidence in their ability to use the genomic findings appropriately. So the challenge remains to optimize the information on safety and efficacy of these integrated approaches. It may be possible that the nutrition of the cancer patient via effects on cancer cell metabolism or the microbiome may offer a new integrated approach that links precision oncology and precision nutrition.

REFERENCES

Badgley, M. A., D. M. Kremer, H. C. Maurer, K. E. DelGiorno, H. J. Lee, V. Purohit, I. R. Sagalovskiy, A. Ma, J. Kapilian, C. E. M. Firl, A. R. Decker, S. A. Sastra, C. F. Palermo, L. R. Andrade, P. Sajjakulnukit, L. Zhang, Z. P. Tolstyka, T. Hirschhorn, C. Lamb, T. Liu, W. Gu, E. S. Seeley, E. Stone, G. Georgiou, U. Manor, A. Iuga, G. M. Wahl, B. R. Stockwell, C. A. Lyssiotis, and K. P. Olive. 2020. "Cysteine depletion induces pancreatic tumor ferroptosis in mice." *Science* 368 (6486):85–89. doi: 10.1126/science.aaw9872.

Barok, M., H. Joensuu, and J. Isola. 2014. "Trastuzumab emtansine: mechanisms of action and drug resistance." *Breast Cancer Res* 16 (2):209. doi: 10.1186/bcr3621.

Bernstein, I. D., M. R. Tam, and R. C. Nowinski. 1980. "Mouse leukemia: therapy with monoclonal antibodies against a thymus differentiation antigen." *Science* 207 (4426):68–71. doi: 10.1126/science.6965328.

Cheng, L., A. Lopez-Beltran, F. Massari, G. T. MacLennan, and R. Montironi. 2018. "Molecular testing for BRAF mutations to inform melanoma treatment decisions: a move toward precision medicine." *Mod Pathol* 31 (1):24–38. doi: 10.1038/modpathol.2017.104.

Choe, J. H., J. Z. Williams, and W. A. Lim. 2020. "Engineering T cells to treat cancer: the convergence of immuno-oncology and synthetic biology." *Annu Rev Cancer Biol* 4 (4):121–139. doi: 10.1146/annurev-cancerbio-030419-033657.

Choo, J. R., and S. C. Lee. 2018. "CDK4-6 inhibitors in breast cancer: current status and future development." *Expert Opin Drug Metab Toxicol* 14 (11):1123–1138. doi: 10.1080/17425255.2018.1541347.

Chung, A., M. Choi, B. C. Han, S. Bose, X. Zhang, L. Medina-Kauwe, J. Sims, R. Murali, M. Taguiam, M. Varda, R. Schiff, A. Giuliano, and X. Cui. 2015. "Basal protein expression is associated with worse outcome and trastuzamab resistance in HER2+ invasive breast cancer." *Clin Breast Cancer* 15 (6):448–457. e2. doi: 10.1016/j.clbc.2015.06.001.

Cluntun, A. A., M. J. Lukey, R. A. Cerione, and J. W. Locasale. 2017. "Glutamine metabolism in cancer: understanding the heterogeneity." *Trends Cancer* 3 (3):169–180. doi: 10.1016/j.trecan.2017.01.005.

Coffin, J. M., and H. Fan. 2016. "The discovery of reverse transcriptase." *Annu Rev Virol* 3 (1):29–51. doi: 10.1146/annurev-virology-110615-035556.

Cohen, C. W., K. R. Fontaine, R. C. Arend, T. Soleymani, and B. A. Gower. 2018. "Favorable effects of a ketogenic diet on physical function, perceived energy, and food cravings in women with ovarian or endometrial cancer: a randomized, controlled trial." *Nutrients* 10 (9):1187. doi: 10.3390/nu10091187.

Coiffier, B., E. Lepage, J. Briere, R. Herbrecht, H. Tilly, R. Bouabdallah, P. Morel, E. Van Den Neste, G. Salles, P. Gaulard, F. Reyes, P. Lederlin, and C. Gisselbrecht. 2002. "CHOP chemotherapy plus rituximab compared with CHOP alone in elderly patients with diffuse large-B-cell lymphoma." *N Engl J Med* 346 (4):235–242. doi: 10.1056/NEJMoa011795.

Cramer, S. L., A. Saha, J. Liu, S. Tadi, S. Tiziani, W. Yan, K. Triplett, C. Lamb, S. E. Alters, S. Rowlinson, Y. J. Zhang, M. J. Keating, P. Huang, J. DiGiovanni, G. Georgiou, and E. Stone. 2017. "Systemic depletion of L-cyst(e)ine with cyst(e)inase increases reactive oxygen species and suppresses tumor growth." *Nat Med* 23 (1):120–127. doi: 10.1038/nm.4232.

Farber, S., and L. K. Diamond. 1948. "Temporary remissions in acute leukemia in children produced by folic acid antagonist, 4-aminopteroyl-glutamic acid." *N Engl J Med* 238 (23):787–793. doi: 10.1056/NEJM194806032382301.

Ferrara, N., and W. J. Henzel. 1989. "Pituitary follicular cells secrete a novel heparin-binding growth factor specific for vascular endothelial cells." *Biochem Biophys Res Commun* 161 (2):851–858. doi: 10.1016/0006-291x(89)92678-8.

Gao, X., S. M. Sanderson, Z. Dai, M. A. Reid, D. E. Cooper, M. Lu, J. P. Richie, Jr., A. Ciccarella, A. Calcagnotto, P. G. Mikhael, S. J. Mentch, J. Liu, G. Ables, D. G. Kirsch, D. S. Hsu, S. N. Nichenametla, and J. W. Locasale. 2019. "Dietary methionine influences therapy in mouse cancer models and alters human metabolism." *Nature* 572 (7769):397–401. doi: 10.1038/s41586-019-1437-3.

Giovannucci, E. 2018. "Nutritional epidemiology and cancer: a tale of two cities." *Cancer Causes Control* 29 (11):1007–1014. doi: 10.1007/s10552-018-1088-y.

Gopalakrishnan, V., C. N. Spencer, L. Nezi, A. Reuben, M. C. Andrews, T. V. Karpinets, P. A. Prieto, D. Vicente, K. Hoffman, S. C. Wei, A. P. Cogdill, L. Zhao, C. W. Hudgens, D. S. Hutchinson, T. Manzo, M. Petaccia de Macedo, T. Cotechini, T. Kumar, W. S. Chen, S. M. Reddy, R. Szczepaniak Sloane,

J. Galloway-Pena, H. Jiang, P. L. Chen, E. J. Shpall, K. Rezvani, A. M. Alousi, R. F. Chemaly, S. Shelburne, L. M. Vence, P. C. Okhuysen, V. B. Jensen, A. G. Swennes, F. McAllister, E. Marcelo Riquelme Sanchez, Y. Zhang, E. Le Chatelier, L. Zitvogel, N. Pons, J. L. Austin-Breneman, L. E. Haydu, E. M. Burton, J. M. Gardner, E. Sirmans, J. Hu, A. J. Lazar, T. Tsujikawa, A. Diab, H. Tawbi, I. C. Glitza, W. J. Hwu, S. P. Patel, S. E. Woodman, R. N. Amaria, M. A. Davies, J. E. Gershenwald, P. Hwu, J. E. Lee, J. Zhang, L. M. Coussens, Z. A. Cooper, P. A. Futreal, C. R. Daniel, N. J. Ajami, J. F. Petrosino, M. T. Tetzlaff, P. Sharma, J. P. Allison, R. R. Jenq, and J. A. Wargo. 2018. "Gut microbiome modulates response to anti-PD-1 immunotherapy in melanoma patients." *Science* 359 (6371):97–103. doi: 10.1126/science.aan4236.

Gordon, M. S., K. Margolin, M. Talpaz, G. W. Sledge, Jr., E. Holmgren, R. Benjamin, S. Stalter, S. Shak, and D. Adelman. 2001. "Phase I safety and pharmacokinetic study of recombinant human anti-vascular endothelial growth factor in patients with advanced cancer." *J Clin Oncol* 19 (3):843–850. doi: 10.1200/JCO.2001.19.3.843.

Gravel, S. P., L. Hulea, N. Toban, E. Birman, M. J. Blouin, M. Zakikhani, Y. Zhao, I. Topisirovic, J. St-Pierre, and M. Pollak. 2014. "Serine deprivation enhances antineoplastic activity of biguanides." *Cancer Res* 74 (24):7521–7533. doi: 10.1158/0008-5472.CAN-14-2643-T.

Hanahan, D., and J. Folkman. 1996. "Patterns and emerging mechanisms of the angiogenic switch during tumorigenesis." *Cell* 86 (3):353–364. doi: 10.1016/s0092-8674(00)80108-7.

Hasskarl, J. 2018. "Everolimus." *Recent Results Cancer Res* 211:101–123. doi: 10.1007/978-3-319-91442-8_8.

Herrmann, E., S. Bierer, J. Gerss, T. Kopke, L. Hertle, and C. Wulfing. 2008. "Prospective comparison of sorafenib and sunitinib for second-line treatment of cytokine-refractory kidney cancer patients." *Oncology* 74 (3–4):216–222. doi: 10.1159/000151369.

Hochhaus, A., R. A. Larson, F. Guilhot, J. P. Radich, S. Branford, T. P. Hughes, M. Baccarani, M. W. Deininger, F. Cervantes, S. Fujihara, C. E. Ortmann, H. D. Menssen, H. Kantarjian, S. G. O'Brien, B. J. Druker, and Iris Investigators. 2017. "Long-term outcomes of imatinib treatment for chronic myeloid leukemia." *N Engl J Med* 376 (10):917–927. doi: 10.1056/NEJMoa1609324.

Hurvitz, S. A., M. Martin, W. F. Symmans, K. H. Jung, C. S. Huang, A. M. Thompson, N. Harbeck, V. Valero, D. Stroyakovskiy, H. Wildiers, M. Campone, J. F. Boileau, M. W. Beckmann, K. Afenjar, R. Fresco, H. J. Helms, J. Xu, Y. G. Lin, J. Sparano, and D. Slamon. 2018. "Neoadjuvant trastuzumab, pertuzumab, and chemotherapy versus trastuzumab emtansine plus pertuzumab in patients with HER2-positive breast cancer (KRISTINE): a randomised, open-label, multicentre, phase 3 trial." *Lancet Oncol* 19 (1):115–126. doi: 10.1016/S1470-2045(17)30716-7.

Iida, N., A. Dzutsev, C. A. Stewart, L. Smith, N. Bouladoux, R. A. Weingarten, D. A. Molina, R. Salcedo, T. Back, S. Cramer, R. M. Dai, H. Kiu, M. Cardone, S. Naik, A. K. Patri, E. Wang, F. M. Marincola, K. M. Frank, Y. Belkaid, G. Trinchieri, and R. S. Goldszmid. 2013. "Commensal bacteria control cancer response to therapy by modulating the tumor microenvironment." *Science* 342 (6161):967–970. doi: 10.1126/science.1240527.

Imbulgoda, A., D. Y. Heng, and C. Kollmannsberger. 2014. "Sunitinib in the treatment of advanced solid tumors." *Recent Results Cancer Res* 201:165–184. doi: 10.1007/978-3-642-54490-3_9.

Ivanov, I. I., and K. Honda. 2012. "Intestinal commensal microbes as immune modulators." *Cell Host Microbe* 12 (4):496–508. doi: 10.1016/j.chom.2012.09.009.

Ji, R. R., S. D. Chasalow, L. S. Wang, O. Hamid, H. Schmidt, J. Cogswell, S. Alaparthy, D. Berman, M. Jure-Kunkel, N. O. Siemers, J. R. Jackson, and V. Shahabi. 2012. "An immune-active tumor microenvironment favors clinical response to ipilimumab." *Cancer Immunol Immunother* 61 (7):1019–1031. doi: 10.1007/s00262-011-1172-6.

Klein, M. E., M. Kovatcheva, L. E. Davis, W. D. Tap, and A. Koff. 2018. "CDK4/6 inhibitors: the mechanism of action may not be as simple as once thought." *Cancer Cell* 34 (1):9–20. doi: 10.1016/j.ccell.2018.03.023.

Kochenderfer, J. N., and S. A. Rosenberg. 2013. "Treating B-cell cancer with T cells expressing anti-CD19 chimeric antigen receptors." *Nat Rev Clin Oncol* 10 (5):267–276. doi: 10.1038/nrclinonc.2013.46.

Kulakowski, A. 2011. "The contribution of Marie Sklodowska-Curie to the development of modern oncology." *Anal Bioanal Chem* 400 (6):1583–1586. doi: 10.1007/s00216-011-4712-1.

Kuwana, Y., Y. Asakura, N. Utsunomiya, M. Nakanishi, Y. Arata, S. Itoh, F. Nagase, and Y. Kurosawa. 1987. "Expression of chimeric receptor composed of immunoglobulin-derived V regions and T-cell receptor-derived C regions." *Biochem Biophys Res Commun* 149 (3):960–968. doi: 10.1016/0006-291x(87)90502-x.

Lambert, G. K., A. K. Duhme-Klair, T. Morgan, and M. K. Ramjee. 2013. "The background, discovery and clinical development of BCR-ABL inhibitors." *Drug Discov Today* 18 (19–20):992–1000. doi: 10.1016/j.drudis.2013.06.001.

Lee, L., T. Ito, and R. T. Jensen. 2018. "Everolimus in the treatment of neuroendocrine tumors: efficacy, side-effects, resistance, and factors affecting its place in the treatment sequence." *Expert Opin Pharmacother* 19 (8):909–928. doi: 10.1080/14656566.2018.1476492.

Lievre, M. 2006. "Evaluation of adverse treatment effects in controlled trials." *Joint Bone Spine* 73 (6):624–626. doi: 10.1016/j.jbspin.2006.09.006.

Lin, J., C. M. Gan, X. Zhang, S. Jones, T. Sjoblom, L. D. Wood, D. W. Parsons, N. Papadopoulos, K. W. Kinzler, B. Vogelstein, G. Parmigiani, and V. E. Velculescu. 2007. "A multidimensional analysis of genes mutated in breast and colorectal cancers." *Genome Res* 17 (9):1304–1318. doi: 10.1101/gr.6431107.

Loayza-Puch, F., and R. Agami. 2016. "Monitoring amino acid deficiencies in cancer." *Cell Cycle* 15 (17):2229–2230. doi: 10.1080/15384101.2016.1191256.

Lopes, A. M., L. Oliveira-Nascimento, A. Ribeiro, C. A. Tairum, Jr., C. A. Breyer, M. A. Oliveira, G. Monteiro, C. M. Souza-Motta, P. O. Magalhaes, J. G. Avendano, A. M. Cavaco-Paulo, P. G. Mazzola, C. O. Rangel-Yagui, L. D. Sette, A. Converti, and A. Pessoa. 2017. "Therapeutic l-asparaginase: upstream, downstream and beyond." *Crit Rev Biotechnol* 37 (1):82–99. doi: 10.3109/07388551.2015.1120705.

LoRusso, P. M., D. Weiss, E. Guardino, S. Girish, and M. X. Sliwkowski. 2011. "Trastuzumab emtansine: a unique antibody-drug conjugate in development for human epidermal growth factor receptor 2-positive cancer." *Clin Cancer Res* 17 (20):6437–6447. doi: 10.1158/1078-0432.CCR-11-0762.

Maddocks, O. D. K., D. Athineos, E. C. Cheung, P. Lee, T. Zhang, N. J. F. van den Broek, G. M. Mackay, C. F. Labuschagne, D. Gay, F. Kruiswijk, J. Blagih, D. F. Vincent, K. J. Campbell, F. Ceteci, O. J. Sansom, K. Blyth, and K. H. Vousden. 2017. "Modulating the therapeutic response of tumours to dietary serine and glycine starvation." *Nature* 544 (7650):372–376. doi: 10.1038/nature22056.

Makita, S., and K. Tobinai. 2017. "Mogamulizumab for the treatment of T-cell lymphoma." *Expert Opin Biol Ther* 17 (9):1145–1153. doi: 10.1080/14712598.2017.1347634.

Maloney, D. G., T. M. Liles, D. K. Czerwinski, C. Waldichuk, J. Rosenberg, A. Grillo-Lopez, and R. Levy. 1994. "Phase I clinical trial using escalating single-dose infusion of chimeric anti-CD20 monoclonal antibody (IDEC-C2B8) in patients with recurrent B-cell lymphoma." *Blood* 84 (8):2457–2466.

Metallo, C. M., P. A. Gameiro, E. L. Bell, K. R. Mattaini, J. Yang, K. Hiller, C. M. Jewell, Z. R. Johnson, D. J. Irvine, L. Guarente, J. K. Kelleher, M. G. Vander Heiden, O. Iliopoulos, and G. Stephanopoulos. 2011. "Reductive glutamine metabolism by IDH1 mediates lipogenesis under hypoxia." *Nature* 481 (7381):380–384. doi: 10.1038/nature10602.

Modest, D. P., S. Pant, and A. Sartore-Bianchi. 2019. "Treatment sequencing in metastatic colorectal cancer." *Eur J Cancer* 109:70–83. doi: 10.1016/j.ejca.2018.12.019.

Nadler, L. M., P. Stashenko, R. Hardy, W. D. Kaplan, L. N. Button, D. W. Kufe, K. H. Antman, and S. F. Schlossman. 1980. "Serotherapy of a patient with a monoclonal antibody directed against a human lymphoma-associated antigen." *Cancer Res* 40 (9):3147–3154.

Nicholson, R. I., J. M. Gee, and M. E. Harper. 2001. "EGFR and cancer prognosis." *Eur J Cancer* 37 (Suppl 4):S9–S15. doi: 10.1016/s0959-8049(01)00231-3.

Pacold, M. E., K. R. Brimacombe, S. H. Chan, J. M. Rohde, C. A. Lewis, L. J. Swier, R. Possemato, W. W. Chen, L. B. Sullivan, B. P. Fiske, S. Cho, E. Freinkman, K. Birsoy, M. Abu-Remaileh, Y. D. Shaul, C. M. Liu, M. Zhou, M. J. Koh, H. Chung, S. M. Davidson, A. Luengo, A. Q. Wang, X. Xu, A. Yasgar, L. Liu, G. Rai, K. D. Westover, M. G. Vander Heiden, M. Shen, N. S. Gray, M. B. Boxer, and D. M. Sabatini. 2016. "A PHGDH inhibitor reveals coordination of serine synthesis and one-carbon unit fate." *Nat Chem Biol* 12 (6):452–458. doi: 10.1038/nchembio.2070.

Poulin-Costello, M., L. Azoulay, E. Van Cutsem, M. Peeters, S. Siena, and M. Wolf. 2013. "An analysis of the treatment effect of panitumumab on overall survival from a phase 3, randomized, controlled, multicenter trial (20020408) in patients with chemotherapy refractory metastatic colorectal cancer." *Target Oncol* 8 (2):127–136. doi: 10.1007/s11523-013-0271-z.

Poursaitidis, I., X. Wang, T. Crighton, C. Labuschagne, D. Mason, S. L. Cramer, K. Triplett, R. Roy, O. E. Pardo, M. J. Seckl, S. W. Rowlinson, E. Stone, and R. F. Lamb. 2017. "Oncogene-selective sensitivity to synchronous cell death following modulation of the amino acid nutrient cystine." *Cell Rep* 18 (11):2547–2556. doi: 10.1016/j.celrep.2017.02.054.

Reff, M. E., K. Carner, K. S. Chambers, P. C. Chinn, J. E. Leonard, R. Raab, R. A. Newman, N. Hanna, and D. R. Anderson. 1994. "Depletion of B cells in vivo by a chimeric mouse human monoclonal antibody to CD20." *Blood* 83 (2):435–445.

Schwartzberg, L., E. S. Kim, D. Liu, and D. Schrag. 2017. "Precision oncology: who, how, what, when, and when not?" *Am Soc Clin Oncol Educ Book* 37:160–169. doi: 10.14694/EDBK_174176; doi: 10.1200/EDBK_174176.

Sgambato, A., F. Casaluce, P. Maione, and C. Gridelli. 2018. "Targeted therapies in non-small cell lung cancer: a focus on ALK/ROS1 tyrosine kinase inhibitors." *Expert Rev Anticancer Ther* 18 (1):71–80. doi: 10.1080/14737140.2018.1412260.

Sivan, A., L. Corrales, N. Hubert, J. B. Williams, K. Aquino-Michaels, Z. M. Earley, F. W. Benyamin, Y. M. Lei, B. Jabri, M. L. Alegre, E. B. Chang, and T. F. Gajewski. 2015. "Commensal Bifidobacterium promotes antitumor immunity and facilitates anti-PD-L1 efficacy." *Science* 350 (6264):1084–1089. doi: 10.1126/science.aac4255.

Strekalova, E., D. Malin, D. M. Good, and V. L. Cryns. 2015. "Methionine deprivation induces a targetable vulnerability in triple-negative breast cancer cells by enhancing TRAIL receptor-2 expression." *Clin Cancer Res* 21 (12):2780–2791. doi: 10.1158/1078-0432.CCR-14-2792.

Strekalova, E., D. Malin, E. M. M. Weisenhorn, J. D. Russell, D. Hoelper, A. Jain, J. J. Coon, P. W. Lewis, and V. L. Cryns. 2019. "S-adenosylmethionine biosynthesis is a targetable metabolic vulnerability of cancer stem cells." *Breast Cancer Res Treat* 175 (1):39–50. doi: 10.1007/s10549-019-05146-7.

Strosberg, J., G. El-Haddad, E. Wolin, A. Hendifar, J. Yao, B. Chasen, E. Mittra, P. L. Kunz, M. H. Kulke, H. Jacene, D. Bushnell, T. M. O'Dorisio, R. P. Baum, H. R. Kulkarni, M. Caplin, R. Lebtahi, T. Hobday, E. Delpassand, E. Van Cutsem, A. Benson, R. Srirajaskanthan, M. Pavel, J. Mora, J. Berlin, E. Grande, N. Reed, E. Seregni, K. Oberg, M. Lopera Sierra, P. Santoro, T. Thevenet, J. L. Erion, P. Ruszniewski, D. Kwekkeboom, E. Krenning, and Netter-Trial Investigators. 2017. "Phase 3 trial of (177)Lu-Dotatate for midgut neuroendocrine tumors." *N Engl J Med* 376 (2):125–135. doi: 10.1056/NEJMoa1607427.

Sun, J., R. Nagel, E. A. Zaal, A. P. Ugalde, R. Han, N. Proost, J. Y. Song, A. Pataskar, A. Burylo, H. Fu, G. J. Poelarends, M. van de Ven, O. van Tellingen, C. R. Berkers, and R. Agami. 2019. "SLC1A3 contributes to L-asparaginase resistance in solid tumors." *EMBO J* 38 (21):e102147. doi: 10.15252/embj.2019102147.

Tumeh, P. C., C. L. Harview, J. H. Yearley, I. P. Shintaku, E. J. M. Taylor, L. Robert, B. Chmielowski, M. Spasic, G. Henry, V. Ciobanu, A. N. West, M. Carmona, C. Kivork, E. Seja, G. Cherry, A. J. Gutierrez, T. R. Grogan, C. Mateus, G. Tomasic, J. A. Glaspy, R. O. Emerson, H. Robins, R. H. Pierce, D. A. Elashoff, C. Robert, and A. Ribas. 2014. "PD-1 blockade induces responses by inhibiting adaptive immune resistance." *Nature* 515 (7528):568–571. doi: 10.1038/nature13954.

Varmus, H. 2019. "Of oncogenes and open science: an interview with Harold Varmus." *Dis Model Mech* 12 (3):dmm038919. doi: 10.1242/dmm.038919.

Venter, J. C., M. D. Adams, E. W. Myers, P. W. Li, R. J. Mural, G. G. Sutton, H. O. Smith, M. Yandell, C. A. Evans, R. A. Holt, J. D. Gocayne, P. Amanatides, R. M. Ballew, D. H. Huson, J. R. Wortman, Q. Zhang, C. D. Kodira, X. H. Zheng, L. Chen, M. Skupski, G. Subramanian, P. D. Thomas, J. Zhang, G. L. Gabor Miklos, C. Nelson, S. Broder, A. G. Clark, J. Nadeau, V. A. McKusick, N. Zinder, A. J. Levine, R. J. Roberts, M. Simon, C. Slayman, M. Hunkapiller, R. Bolanos, A. Delcher, I. Dew, D. Fasulo, M. Flanigan, L. Florea, A. Halpern, S. Hannenhalli, S. Kravitz, S. Levy, C. Mobarry, K. Reinert, K. Remington, J. Abu-Threideh, E. Beasley, K. Biddick, V. Bonazzi, R. Brandon, M. Cargill, I. Chandramouliswaran, R. Charlab, K. Chaturvedi, Z. Deng, V. Di Francesco, P. Dunn, K. Eilbeck, C. Evangelista, A. E. Gabrielian, W. Gan, W. Ge, F. Gong, Z. Gu, P. Guan, T. J. Heiman, M. E. Higgins, R. R. Ji, Z. Ke, K. A. Ketchum, Z. Lai, Y. Lei, Z. Li, J. Li, Y. Liang, X. Lin, F. Lu, G. V. Merkulov, N. Milshina, H. M. Moore, A. K. Naik, V. A. Narayan, B. Neelam, D. Nusskern, D. B. Rusch, S. Salzberg, W. Shao, B. Shue, J. Sun, Z. Wang, A. Wang, X. Wang, J. Wang, M. Wei, R. Wides, C. Xiao, C. Yan, A. Yao, J. Ye, M. Zhan, W. Zhang, H. Zhang, Q. Zhao, L. Zheng, F. Zhong, W. Zhong, S. Zhu, S. Zhao, D. Gilbert, S. Baumhueter, G. Spier, C. Carter, A. Cravchik, T. Woodage, F. Ali, H. An, A. Awe, D. Baldwin, H. Baden, M. Barnstead, I. Barrow, K. Beeson, D. Busam, A. Carver, A. Center, M. L. Cheng, L. Curry, S. Danaher, L. Davenport, R. Desilets, S. Dietz, K. Dodson, L. Doup, S. Ferriera, N. Garg, A. Glucksmann, B. Hart, J. Haynes, C. Haynes, C. Heiner, S. Hladun, D. Hostin, J. Houck, T. Howland, C. Ibegwam, J. Johnson, F. Kalush, L. Kline, S. Koduru, A. Love, F. Mann, D. May, S. McCawley, T. McIntosh, I. McMullen, M. Moy, L. Moy, B. Murphy, K. Nelson, C. Pfannkoch, E. Pratts, V. Puri, H. Qureshi, M. Reardon, R. Rodriguez, Y. H. Rogers, D. Romblad, B. Ruhfel, R. Scott, C. Sitter, M. Smallwood, E. Stewart, R. Strong, E. Suh, R. Thomas, N. N. Tint, S. Tse, C. Vech, G. Wang, J. Wetter, S. Williams, M. Williams, S. Windsor, E. Winn-Deen, K. Wolfe, J. Zaveri, K. Zaveri, J. F. Abril, R. Guigo, M. J. Campbell, K. V. Sjolander, B. Karlak, A. Kejariwal, H. Mi, B. Lazareva, T. Hatton, A. Narechania, K. Diemer, A. Muruganujan, N. Guo, S. Sato, V. Bafna, S. Istrail, R. Lippert, R. Schwartz, B. Walenz, S. Yooseph, D. Allen, A. Basu, J. Baxendale, L. Blick, M. Caminha, J. Carnes-Stine, P. Caulk, Y. H. Chiang, M. Coyne, C. Dahlke, A. Mays, M. Dombroski, M. Donnelly, D. Ely, S. Esparham, C. Fosler, H. Gire, S. Glanowski, K. Glasser, A. Glodek, M. Gorokhov, K. Graham, B. Gropman, M. Harris, J. Heil, S. Henderson, J. Hoover, D. Jennings, C. Jordan, J. Jordan, J. Kasha, L. Kagan, C. Kraft, A. Levitsky, M. Lewis, X. Liu, J. Lopez, D. Ma, W. Majoros, J. McDaniel, S. Murphy, M. Newman, T. Nguyen, N.

Nguyen, M. Nodell, S. Pan, J. Peck, M. Peterson, W. Rowe, R. Sanders, J. Scott, M. Simpson, T. Smith, A. Sprague, T. Stockwell, R. Turner, E. Venter, M. Wang, M. Wen, D. Wu, M. Wu, A. Xia, A. Zandieh, and X. Zhu. 2001. "The sequence of the human genome." *Science* 291 (5507):1304–1351. doi: 10.1126/science.1058040.

Vetizou, M., J. M. Pitt, R. Daillere, P. Lepage, N. Waldschmitt, C. Flament, S. Rusakiewicz, B. Routy, M. P. Roberti, C. P. Duong, V. Poirier-Colame, A. Roux, S. Becharef, S. Formenti, E. Golden, S. Cording, G. Eberl, A. Schlitzer, F. Ginhoux, S. Mani, T. Yamazaki, N. Jacquelot, D. P. Enot, M. Berard, J. Nigou, P. Opolon, A. Eggermont, P. L. Woerther, E. Chachaty, N. Chaput, C. Robert, C. Mateus, G. Kroemer, D. Raoult, I. G. Boneca, F. Carbonnel, M. Chamaillard, and L. Zitvogel. 2015. "Anticancer immunotherapy by CTLA-4 blockade relies on the gut microbiota." *Science* 350 (6264):1079–1084. doi: 10.1126/science.aad1329.

Viaud, S., F. Saccheri, G. Mignot, T. Yamazaki, R. Daillere, D. Hannani, D. P. Enot, C. Pfirschke, C. Engblom, M. J. Pittet, A. Schlitzer, F. Ginhoux, L. Apetoh, E. Chachaty, P. L. Woerther, G. Eberl, M. Berard, C. Ecobichon, D. Clermont, C. Bizet, V. Gaboriau-Routhiau, N. Cerf-Bensussan, P. Opolon, N. Yessaad, E. Vivier, B. Ryffel, C. O. Elson, J. Dore, G. Kroemer, P. Lepage, I. G. Boneca, F. Ghiringhelli, and L. Zitvogel. 2013. "The intestinal microbiota modulates the anticancer immune effects of cyclophosphamide." *Science* 342 (6161):971–976. doi: 10.1126/science.1240537.

Vieira, A. T., M. M. Teixeira, and F. S. Martins. 2013. "The role of probiotics and prebiotics in inducing gut immunity." *Front Immunol* 4:445. doi: 10.3389/fimmu.2013.00445.

Vincenzi, B., A. Zoccoli, F. Pantano, O. Venditti, and S. Galluzzo. 2010. "Cetuximab: from bench to bedside." *Curr Cancer Drug Targets* 10 (1):80–95. doi: 10.2174/156800910790980241.

von Minckwitz, G., C. S. Huang, M. S. Mano, S. Loibl, E. P. Mamounas, M. Untch, N. Wolmark, P. Rastogi, A. Schneeweiss, A. Redondo, H. H. Fischer, W. Jacot, A. K. Conlin, I. L. Wapnir, C. Jackisch, M. P. DiGiovanna, P. A. Fasching, J. P. Crown, P. Wulfing, Z. Shao, E. Rota Caremoli, H. Wu, L. H. Lam, D. Tesarowski, M. Smitt, H. Douthwaite, S. M. Singel, C. E. Geyer, Jr., and Katherine Investigators. 2019. "Trastuzumab emtansine for residual invasive HER2-positive breast cancer." *N Engl J Med* 380 (7):617–628. doi: 10.1056/NEJMoa1814017.

Wakai, T., P. Prasoon, Y. Hirose, Y. Shimada, H. Ichikawa, and M. Nagahashi. 2019. "Next-generation sequencing-based clinical sequencing: toward precision medicine in solid tumors." *Int J Clin Oncol* 24 (2):115–122. doi: 10.1007/s10147-018-1375-3.

Weber, D. D., S. Aminzadeh-Gohari, J. Tulipan, L. Catalano, R. G. Feichtinger, and B. Kofler. 2020. "Ketogenic diet in the treatment of cancer - where do we stand?" *Mol Metab* 33:102–121. doi: 10.1016/j.molmet.2019.06.026.

Werner, R. J., A. D. Kelly, and J. J. Issa. 2017. "Epigenetics and precision oncology." *Cancer J* 23 (5):262–269. doi: 10.1097/PPO.0000000000000281.

4 Phytonutrients and Cancer

David Heber
UCLA Center for Human Nutrition

Navindra Seeram
University of Rhode Island

CONTENTS

INTRODUCTION

Since ancient times, fruits, vegetables, herbs, and spices have been thought to have specific health benefits (Buyel 2018). Modern nutrition science has developed a great deal of evidence on the role of phytonutrients from foods and supplements in fighting cancer, but much remains to be done. Evidence has been developed from population studies, basic studies in cells and animals, and a limited number of human intervention trials.

Epidemiological observations have shown an inverse relationship between the consumption of plant foods, rich in phytonutrients and the incidence of cancer. Basic and clinical studies on the effects of phytonutrients on cellular function and carcinogenesis have reinforced public health advice from the National Cancer Institute, the World Cancer Research Fund, and many other government and nongovernment agencies around the world to consume more colorful fruits and vegetables without specifying classes of phytonutrients. One step in this direction of public health information has been the classification of families of phytonutrients by color linked to lists of commonly consumed fruits and vegetables (Heber and Bowerman 2001).

Many phytochemicals are colorful, providing an easy way to communicate increased diversity of fruits and vegetables to the public. Red foods contain lycopene, the pigment in tomatoes, which is localized in the prostate gland and fat. Yellow-green vegetables, such as corn and leafy greens, contain lutein and zeaxanthin, which are localized in the retina and the brain. Red-purple foods contain anthocyanins and ellagitannins, which are powerful antioxidants found in pomegranate, grapes, berries, and red wine. Orange foods, including carrots, mangos, apricots, pumpkin, and winter squash, contain beta-carotene. Orange-yellow foods, including oranges, tangerines, and lemons, contain citrus flavonoids. Green foods, including broccoli, Brussels sprouts, and kale, contain glucosinolates. White-green foods in the onion family contain allyl sulfides. Consumers are advised to ingest one serving of each of the above groups daily, putting this recommendation within the National Cancer Institute and American Institute for Cancer Research guidelines of five to nine servings per day. The color code provides simplification, but it is also important as a way to help consumers find common fruits and vegetables easily while traveling, eating in restaurants or working. A diet with 400–600 g/day of fruits and vegetables is associated with reduced incidence of many common forms of cancer (Clinton, Giovannucci, and Hursting 2020).

Beyond specific phytonutrients acting as antioxidants and bioactives, increased amounts of fruits and vegetables in the diet provide fiber, water, vitamins, and minerals. This change in the dietary proportions of macronutrients in the diet displaces foods with hidden fat, sugar, and refined carbohydrates. Herbs and spices provide significant amounts of phytonutrients when only a few grams are consumed. Dietary botanical supplements made from standardized extracts further concentrate specific phytonutrients enabling meaningful clinical research studies by eliminating the natural and inherent variation in plants due to variable growing conditions.

The advice to consume more colorful fruits, vegetables, and spices as part of a healthy cancer preventive diet is universally endorsed. Unfortunately, phytonutrients in concentrated supplement form as capsules, tablets, juices, and tonics are often critically reviewed in the popular press and some scientific and medical journals by emphasizing misuse and adverse events over the potential benefits (Ronis, Pedersen, and Watt 2018).

PHYTONUTRIENTS

Phytonutrients are defined as bioactive nonnutrient compounds in fruits, vegetables, grains, and other plants (Durazzo et al. 2018). Bioactive compounds are compounds that occur in nature within the food chain and have the ability to interact with one or more compounds of living tissue while also demonstrating an effect on human health (Biesalski et al. 2009). To date, about 10,000 phytonutrients have been identified, but it is likely that a larger number of phytonutrients remain unknown (see Figure 4.1).

Research determining the impact of bioactive nutrients in foods and supplements on tumor angiogenesis, tumor progression, metastasis, and responses to chemotherapy may lead to phytonutrients playing an adjunctive role in cancer treatment and a primary role in cancer prevention and survivorship (Reglero and Reglero 2019, Marian 2017, Vernieri et al. 2018). Some phytonutrients, such as resveratrol, sulforaphane, curcumin, quercetin, and genistein, may enhance the action of chemotherapeutic agents used to treat cancer (Burnett et al. 2017, Hour et al. 2002, Li et al. 2018, Satoh et al. 2003, Zhou et al. 2019).

Phytonutrients are divided into chemical classes including phenolic acids, alkaloids, nitrogen-containing compounds, organosulfur compounds (OSCs), phytosterols, and carotenoids. Among the polyphenols there are phenolic acids, stilbenes, lignans, coumarins, tannins, and flavonoids. Tannins of note include hydrolysable tannins such as ellagitannins found in pomegranate and walnuts and condensed tannins found in cocoa. OSCs include isothiocyanates (ITC), indoles, allyl sulfides, and sulforaphane. Phytosterols inhibit cholesterol absorption and include sitosterol, campesterol, and stigmasterol. Stilbenes include resveratrol and pterostilbene. Carotenoids include alpha- and beta-carotene, beta-cryptoxanthin, lutein, zeaxanthin, astaxanthin, and lycopene (Liu 2013).

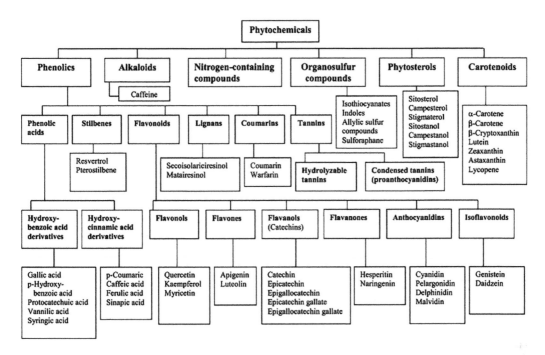

FIGURE 4.1 Phytochemicals classified by type. Also called phytonutrients, it is believed that there are more than 10,000 different compounds (Liu 2013).

Polyphenols and carotenoids are the major sources of antioxidants in commonly consumed foods and will be discussed first. The anticancer effects of phytonutrients have been attributed in part to their antioxidant activity (Chang, Sheen, and Lei 2015) since overproduction of oxidants (reactive oxygen species and reactive nitrogen species) in the human body with aging is integral to the pathogenesis of cancer (Zhang et al. 2015).

POLYPHENOLS

Polyphenol phytonutrients are the most abundant antioxidants in the human diet (Fu et al. 2011). Polyphenols are secondary metabolites that plants produce to protect themselves from other organisms. Dietary polyphenols have been shown to play important roles in human health. High intakes of fruits, vegetables, and whole grains, which are rich in polyphenols, have been linked to lowered risks of many chronic diseases including cancer. Polyphenol phytonutrients can scavenge reactive oxygen and nitrogen species secondary to the hydroxyl groups in the aromatic rings of their phenolics. The concentration of polyphenols available in foods depends on plant variety, growing season and region, processing and storage.

Inflammation plays a key role in cancer cell growth and metastasis. In addition to reactive oxygen and nitrogen species mentioned above, inflammation is modulated by polyphenols through interaction with several immune mediators including Nuclear factor kappa B (NF-κB), a proinflammatory transcription factor that modulates the expression of proteins including cytokines interleukin (IL)-1, IL-2, and interferon-γ. These proteins are involved in multiple cell signaling pathways associated with cancer progression and inflammation. Phosphorylated NF-κB binds to DNA and initiates the transcription of oncogenes which block apoptosis and promote cellular proliferation and angiogenesis. Polyphenols such as pomegranate ellagitannins and curcumin suppress NF-κB activity by inhibiting the phosphorylation by I kappa B kinase and impeding nuclear translocation of the NF-κB p65 subunit. The transcriptional factor AP-1 (Activator Protein-1) mediates the antiapoptotic, mitogenic, and proangiogenic genes but is downregulated by some polyphenols in cancer cells. One protein transcription factor in the Signal Transducer and Activator of Transcription (STAT) protein transcription factor in member of the STAT family, STAT3, contributes to the growth and survival of cancer cells by increasing the expression of antiapoptotic proteins such as Bcl-2 and Bcl-xL and blocking apoptosis. STAT 3 is activated by IL-6, the epidermal growth factor receptor (EGFR), platelet derived growth factor (PDGF), leukemia inhibitory factor (LIF), oncostatin M, and the ciliary neurotrophic factor (CNTF) family of cytokines. STAT3 is reported to be a molecular target of polyphenols in several tumors, both directly and indirectly by inhibition of IL-6. In addition, tumor necrosis factor alpha (TNF-α) activates NF-κB and the inflammatory genes (5-LOX, COX-2), inflammatory cytokines, molecules that adhere to cells, and inducible nitric oxide synthase (iNOS). Polyphenols can also impact the level of cyclin D, a regulator of cell cycle progression by inhibition of NF-κB. Importantly, the immunomodulatory effects of polyphenols affect cellular components in the tumor microenvironment including macrophages, dendritic cells, and both T and B lymphocytes (Giordano and Tommonaro 2019).

Dietary polyphenols are classified into chemically related groups such as flavonoids, phenolic acids, stilbenes, tannins, and coumarins. These classification groups do not capture all the polyphenols which have been studied for their role in human health and those are discussed as additional polyphenols below including curcumin (Zhou, Zheng, et al. 2016).

FLAVONOIDS

Flavonoids are the largest class of polyphenols comprising the anthocyanins/anthocyanidins, flavonols, flavones, flavanols (catechins), flavanones, and isoflavonoids. In turn, the flavanols include catechins, epicatechins, and proanthocyanidins which in turn include procyanidins and prodelphinidins (Chang, Sheen, and Lei 2015) (see Figure 4.2). Anthocyanins and ellagitannins are the major antioxidant polyphenols found in red-purple berries of all kinds including raspberries, pomegranate, and strawberries (Overall et al. 2017, Wu and Tian 2017). The antioxidant activity of different fruits is directly and closely related to total phenolic content. Therefore, fruits with higher total phenolic contents possess stronger antioxidant activity (Derakhshan et al. 2018). Each of these classes and other polyphenol research related to cancer is discussed below.

ANTHOCYANINS

Anthocyanins are the most abundant flavonoids in nature and provide the visible colors of red-purple and blue fruits and flowers. For example, strawberries, grapes, apples, and pomegranates can be different shades of red, blue, or purple and comprise one of seven color groups based on phytonutrient families (Heber and Bowerman 2001). There are over 500 different anthocyanins identified in 27 families and 72 genera of plants (Fang 2015). Anthocyanins are glycosylated with glucose, galactose, or rhamnose (Liu et al. 2015), while the anthocyanidins are the unglycosylated constituents of the B-ring structure (see Figure 4.3), and can be divided into at least six common types, such as pelargonidin, cyanidin, delphinidin, peonidin, petunidin, and malvidin, according to the different substituent groups on the flavylium B-ring.

Anthocyanins are highly unstable and very susceptible to degradation. Oxygen, temperature, light, enzymes, and pH are among the many factors that may affect the chemistry of anthocyanins and, consequently, their stability and color. The color of anthocyanins may vary according to different substituent groups present on the B ring, and color saturation increases with increasing number of hydroxyl groups and decreases with the addition of methoxyl groups (Kamiloglu et al. 2015).

The potential anticancer effects are mediated through antioxidant; anti-inflammation; antimutagenesis; differentiation; and inhibition of proliferation by modulating signal transduction pathways, inducing cell cycle arrest and stimulating apoptosis or autophagy of cancer cells; anti-invasion; antimetastasis; reversing drug resistance of cancer cells and increasing their sensitivity to chemotherapy. Anthocyanins/anthocyanidins (A/A) also inhibit the proinflammatory NF-κB pathway,

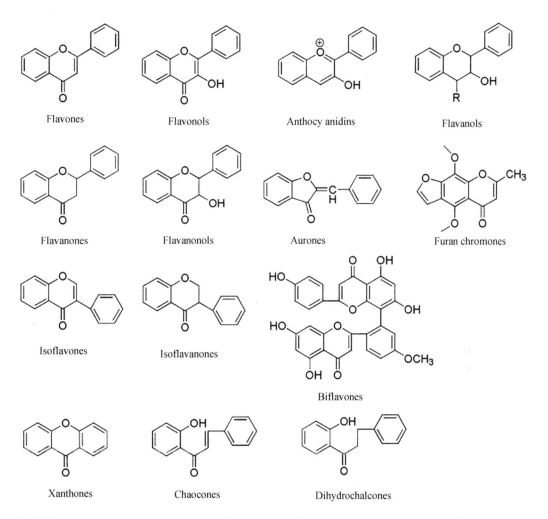

Flavones

Flavonols

Anthocy anidins

Flavanols

Flavanones

Flavanonols

Aurones

Furan chromones

Isoflavones

Isoflavanones

Biflavones

Xanthones

Chaocones

Dihydrochalcones

FIGURE 4.2 Chemical structures of the different types of flavonoids, the largest class of polyphenols with over 5,000 identified to date (Wang, Li, and Bi 2018).

attenuate Wnt signaling, and suppress abnormal epithelial cell proliferation. In addition, A/A induce mitochondrial-mediated apoptosis and downregulate Akt/mTOR (mammalian target of rapamycin) pathway. Furthermore, activation of AMP-activated protein kinase (AMPK) and sirtuin 1 (SIRT1) also contributes to the anticarcinogenic effects of A/A. Finally, downregulation of matrix metalloproteinases by A/A inhibits tumor invasion and metastasis. Therefore, A/A induce their antitumor effects against tumor cells via multiple steps in the process of carcinogenesis making A/A, an interesting candidate for future research in nutrition and cancer (Li et al. 2017).

Overexpression of the human epidermal growth factor receptor 2 (HER2) tyrosine kinase receptor gene has been identified as a negative prognostic factor for node-positive early breast cancer (Slamon et al. 1987). Trastuzumab (Herceptin®) is a recombinant humanized monoclonal antibody that is targeted against the HER2 tyrosine kinase receptor. Cyanidin-3-glucoside and peonidin-3-glucoside chosen for study from a large library based on cellular assays were able to inhibit phosphorylation of HER2, induce apoptosis, suppress migration and invasion, and inhibit tumor cell growth in trastuzumab-resistant breast cancer cells in vitro and in vivo. Patients who initially respond often demonstrate disease progression after 1 year, raising the possibility that a nontoxic anthocyanin might be used in conjunction with precision oncologic treatment of breast cancer (Li et al. 2016).

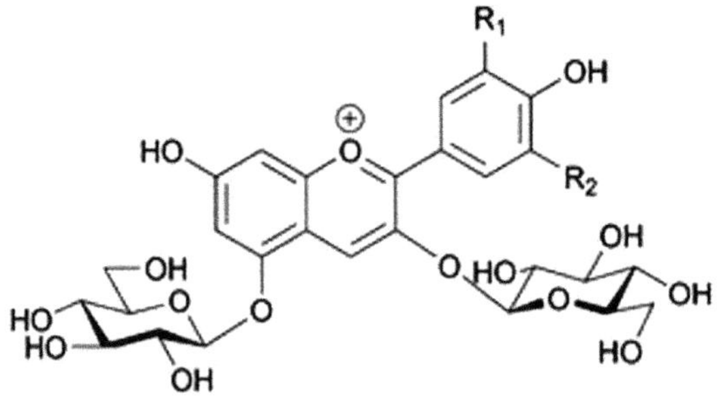

R$_1$	R$_2$	Anthocyanin	Aglycon
H	H	Pelargonin	Pelargonidin
OH	H	Cyanin	Cyanidin
OCH$_3$	H	Peonin	Peonidin
OH	OH	Delphin	Delphinidin
OCH$_3$	OH	Petunin	Petunidin
OCH$_3$	OCH$_3$	Malvin	Malvidin

FIGURE 4.3 Anthocyanins are glycosylated as shown in this figure, while anthocyanidins are the unglycosylated or aglycon structures above. This distinction is sometimes missed in the medical literature with all of the related structures referred to as anthocyanins. Cyanin means "blue", and most blue and purple plant colors are due to anthocyanins. Nearly 1,000 such pigments have been reported (Yoshida, Mori, and Kondo 2009).

FLAVANOLS (CATECHINS)

Flavanols include tea catechins which have been extensively studied with regard to their effects in cancer (Yang and Wang 2016). Tea is the second most commonly consumed beverage in the world after water. All different varieties of tea including white, green, oolong, and black teas (BT) are manufactured from the leaves of *Camellia sinensis*. For the production of green tea (GT), the leaves are heat-treated to retain the typical monomeric polyphenols, also known as flavan-3-ols, including (-)-epigallocatechin, (-)-epigallocatechin-3-gallate (EGCG), (-)-epicatechin, and (-)-epicatechin-3-gallate . For the production of BT; the leaves undergo fermentation in moist and warm conditions where endogenous oxidizing enzymes enhance the formation of polymers such as theaflavins and thearubigens. Oolong tea is fermented for a shorter time and so is intermediate between GT and BT. There are many other varieties of tea including white tea which is GT made from small new leaves.

Therefore, while GT is rich in monomeric catechins, BT contains a relatively small amount of these monomeric polyphenols along with a number of larger BT polymers such as theaflavins and thearubigins which are poorly absorbed. These polymers are metabolized by the intestinal microflora into phenolic acids. After consumption of GT higher concentrations of polyphenols are found in the circulation while after BT consumption the phenolic acid levels in the circulation are higher.

The majority of in vitro cell culture, in vivo animal, and human intervention studies have examined the effects of extracts of either GT or purified EGCG on carcinogenesis. The effects of GT polyphenols (GTPs) have been examined against a variety of cancers including lung, liver, prostate, colon, pancreatic, breast, and kidney cancers (Henning, Wang, and Heber 2011, Yang and Wang 2016). The demonstration of these anticarcinogenic effects has been largely carried out in cell culture and in animal models, since it is only possible to achieve relatively low concentrations of GTPs in humans through consumption of tea or tea supplements (Henning et al. 2004). In addition to their low bioavailability, GTPs are extensively methylated in the liver and excreted. GTPs undergo methylation, glucuronidation, and sulfation in in vitro systems and in animals and humans (Feng 2006).

Bioactive compounds from GT such as EGCG have been shown to alter DNA methyltransferase activity in studies of esophageal, oral, skin, lung, breast, and prostate cancer (PCa) cells, which may contribute to the chemopreventive effect of GT. Mouse model studies have confirmed the inhibitory effect of EGCG on DNA methylation. A human study also demonstrated that decreased methylation of CDX2 and BMP-2 in gastric carcinoma was associated with higher GT consumption (Henning et al. 2013).

GT and BT also support weight management which indirectly affects cancer risk through the hormonal effects of obesity. While caffeine in teas affects energy expenditure, decaffeinated GTP and BTP were shown to inhibit weight gain in mice fed with an obesogenic diet. Both BTP and GTP induced weight loss in mice eating an obesogenic high-fat/high-sugar diet in association with alterations of the microbiota (increased *Bifidobacteria* species and reduced *Firmicutes* species) and increased hepatic AMPK phosphorylation (Henning et al. 2018).

ISOFLAVONOIDS

Isoflavonoid polyphenols are found in legumes including the soybean bound to sugars as glycosides, e.g., genistein and daidzein. Their aglycones are genistin and daidzin, respectively.

These isoflavones have both estrogenic and antiestrogenic activities depending on the concentration of other estrogens in the microenvironment and the type of estrogenic receptor in the cells being studied. Whether an estrogenic effect is significant in terms of alleged tumor promotion or the phytoestrogen is acting as a weak estrogen agonist antagonizing endogenous estrogens is entirely dependent on which estrogen receptor (ER) is being referenced and the concentration of the isoflavone being studied as discussed below. To simply classify all isoflavones as "phytoestrogens" implying a cancer promoting estrogenic effect is misleading. However, some carefully designed experiments under nonphysiological conditions in ovariectomized mice (Allred et al. 2001) have given this misimpression to many oncologists and the public.

The physiological functions of plant-derived estrogenic compounds are modulated largely by the ER subtypes alpha (ERα) and beta (ERβ). These proteins have actions in the cell nucleus, regulating transcription of specific target genes by binding to associated DNA regulatory sequences. In humans, both receptor subtypes are expressed in many cells and tissues. ERα is present mainly in mammary gland, uterus, ovary, bone, testes, epididymis, prostate stroma, liver, and adipose tissue. By contrast, ERβ is found mainly in the prostate epithelium, bladder, ovarian granulosa cells, colon, adipose tissue, and immune cells. The beta subtype seems to have a more profound effect on the central nervous and immune systems, and it generally counteracts the ERα-promoted cell hyperproliferation in tissues such as the breast and the uterus (Paterni et al. 2014).

Epidemiological and migratory evidence suggests that dietary soy consumption can lower the risk for the breast cancer and PCa (Sahin et al. 2019). Soy isoflavones have been suggested to have cancer preventive effects. Epidemiological studies have shown a significant difference in cancer incidence among different ethnic groups, which could be attributed in part to dietary habits. For example, the incidence of breast cancer and PCa is much higher in the United States and Europe where dietary soy intake is low as compared with countries such as China and Japan, where dietary consumption of soy products is much higher. Genistein, a predominant isoflavone in soy, has been shown to inhibit cancer development, growth, and metastasis in animal models. It may act by modulating the genes related to cell cycle control and apoptosis (Zhang et al. 2013).

Lifetime soy consumption at a moderate level may prevent breast cancer recurrence through mechanisms that change the biology of tumors. For example, women who consumed soy during childhood develop breast cancers that express significantly reduced HER2 levels. More research is needed to understand why soy intake during early life may both reduce breast cancer risk and the risk of recurrence (Hilakivi-Clarke, Andrade, and Helferich 2010).

Human and animal data provide evidence for several anticancer properties of soy and/or its isoflavones. Soy isoflavones do not function as an estrogen, but rather exhibit antiestrogenic properties.

However, their metabolism differs between humans and animals, and therefore, the outcomes of animal studies may not be applicable to humans. Ovariectomized mice but not humans have undetectable levels of circulating estrogens making the weak estrogen-like effect of soy phytoestrogens detectable as they are at low concentrations in cell culture. In both male and female humans, circulating estrogens are not low due to the aromatization of adrenal androgens by adipose tissue, and soy isoflavones act as antiestrogens on alpha receptor but proestrogens on the beneficial beta-receptor. The majority of breast cancer cases are estrogen-alpha receptor-positive; therefore, soy isoflavones should be considered a potential anticancer therapeutic agent and warrant further investigation (Douglas, Johnson, and Arjmandi 2013).

Equol, a gut microbial metabolite produced from daidzein, is the isoflavone-derived metabolite with the greatest estrogenic and antioxidant activity associated with soy isoflavone consumption (Danciu et al. 2018). The conversion of daidzein into equol takes place in the intestine via the action of reductase enzymes belonging to ten species of gut bacteria. Both individuals who produce equol following soy consumption and nonproducers have been recognized for many years in clinical and population studies. Only 20%–30% of people in Western countries are classified as producers based on measures of equol excretion into urine, but 40%–60% of people in Asian countries where more soy and particularly daidzein are consumed are producers. The excretion of equol in the urine has been associated in epidemiological studies with decreased risks of breast, prostate, and colon cancers (Tseng et al. 2013).

The prevalence of bacterial species in the gut microbiota that convert daidzein to equol between the equol producers and nonproducers was studied in 1,044 Japanese individuals including 458 equol producers (Iino et al. 2019). It was found that the bacteria that convert daidzein to equol were present in both equol producers and nonproducers. However, the relative abundance and the prevalence of two species *Asaccharobacter celatus* and *Slackia isoflavoniconvertens* were significantly higher in equol producers than in nonproducers. It was concluded that the increased equol production observed with increased daidzein intake was associated with equol production status through an increase of *A. celatus* and *S. isoflavoniconvertens* in the gut microbiota.

FLAVONOLS

Flavonols are the predominant polyphenols in onions. At least 25 different flavonols have been characterized, and quercetin derivatives are the most predominant in all onion cultivars. Quercetin is widely distributed in plant foods and is one of the most abundant dietary flavonoids with an average daily consumption of 25–50 mg. Quercetin is the aglycone form of a number of other flavonoid glycosides, such as rutin and quercitrin, found in citrus fruit, buckwheat, and onions. Quercetin-4′-glucoside and quercetin-3,4′-diglucoside are the major flavonols described (Slimestad, Fossen, and Vagen 2007). Analogous derivatives of kaempferol and isorhamnetin have been identified as minor polyphenols. Recent reports indicate that the outer dry layers of onion bulbs contain oligomeric structures of quercetin in addition to condensation products of quercetin and protocatechuic acid.

Quercetin has demonstrated chemopreventive effects in colon cancer cells in vitro and in vivo through effects on cell cycle arrest, increases in apoptosis, antioxidant actions, modulation of ERs, regulation of signaling pathways, inhibition of metastasis and angiogenesis (Darband et al. 2018). Quercetin elicits biphasic, dose-dependent effects. It acts as an antioxidant and thus elicits chemopreventive effects at low concentrations, but functions as a pro-oxidant and may therefore elicit chemotherapeutic effects at high concentrations.

Quercetin has multiple intracellular molecular targets. Studies suggest that quercetin binds to several receptors that play important roles in carcinogenesis, regulates expression of various genes, induces epigenetic changes, and interferes with enzymes that metabolize chemical carcinogens. In addition, it also elicits anti-inflammatory and antiviral effects. The ability of quercetin to induce apoptosis of cancer cells without affecting noncancer cells has been documented using various cell lines. Quercetin also has antiangiogenic and antimetastatic properties.

When used in combination with chemotherapy and radiotherapy, quercetin can act as a sensitizer and protect noncancer cells from the side effects of currently used cancer therapies. The bioavailability of quercetin in humans is low and highly variable (0%–50%), and it is rapidly cleared with an elimination half-life of 1–2 hours after ingesting quercetin in foods or supplements.

The safety and potential usefulness of quercetin for the prevention and treatment of cancer have been documented in both animal experiments and a phase I clinical trial. Current studies are focused on nanoformulations to overcome the low bioavailability of natural quercetin, which limits its clinical use as an antitumor agent (Jana et al., 2018)

FLAVANONES

Citrus fruit and juices contain phytonutrients with health-promoting properties including supporting immune function. Citrus can be classified into multiple types, including mandarins, tangerines, oranges, pomelos, hybrids, lemons, and limes. All varieties of citrus originate from crosses of mandarin orange, citron, and pomelo.

Among the phytonutrients in citrus fruits and juices, flavanones (such as hesperetin, naringenin, eriodictyol, isosakuranetin, and their respective glycosides) are present in amounts ranging from 180 to 740 mg/L depending on the Citrus species and cultivar. The flavanones support and enhance the body's defenses against oxidative stress with potential for the prevention of cancer (Wang et al. 2017). Citrus flavanones from citrus fruits and juices modulate signal cascades relevant to carcinogenesis both in vitro and in vivo (Barreca et al. 2017, Zhao, Liu, and Xu 2018, Cirmi et al. 2018, Wang et al. 2017).

Isoprenoids such as limonene and geraniol are found in the lipid fraction of citrus peels and are used as flavoring agents. They inhibit the rate-limiting step in de novo cholesterogenesis at a posttranslational level and have been studied in cell culture and in limited numbers of breast cancer patients (Mo et al. 2018, Haag, Lindstrom, and Gould 1992).

PHENOLIC ACIDS

Phenolic acids are secondary plant metabolites that may have protective effects against oxidative stress, inflammation, and cancer in experimental studies. Phenolic acids are divided into two major classes: hydroxybenzoic and hydroxycinnamic acids. Each class may contain up to hundreds of individual compounds that have been demonstrated, to a various extent, to regulate several cellular molecular pathways leading to antioxidative, antiproliferative, and anti-inflammatory effects (Russo et al. 2017, Crozier, Del Rio, and Clifford 2010). Polyphenol-rich foods, such as coffee and tea, have demonstrated substantial association with decreased risk of cancer mortality (Grosso et al. 2016). In particular, growing evidence suggested that coffee may play an important role in cancer prevention (Grosso et al. 2017). Hydroxycinnamic acid largely comes from both caffeinated and decaffeinated coffee while hydroxybenzoic acid largely comes from nuts. Most basic and clinical research on polyphenols and cancer has been conducted on flavonoids, while epidemiological data on phenolic acids and cancer are limited.

The intake of phenolic acids and their food sources and associated lifestyle factors were studied in the European Prospective Investigation into Cancer and Nutrition (EPIC) study (Zamora-Ros et al. 2013). Phenolic acid intakes were estimated for 36,037 subjects aged 35–74 years and recruited between 1992 and 2000 in ten European countries using standardized 24 hours recall software (EPIC-Soft). The food sources of phenolics were also identified. Coffee was the main food source of phenolic acids and accounted for 55%–80% of the total phenolic acid intake, followed by fruits, vegetables, and nuts. The hydroxycinnamic acid subclass was the main contributor to the total phenolic acid intake, accounting for about 85%–95% of intake depending on the region. Hydroxybenzoic acids accounted for about 5%–14%; hydroxyphenylacetic acids up to 8% and hydroxyphenylpropanoic acids were less than 0.1% for all regions.

A case–control study in Sicily and Southern Italy found that the increased consumption of caffeic acid and ferulic acid was associated with a reduced risk of PCa. Furthermore, they focused their results on the intakes of caffeic acid and ferulic acid in this regard. However, further clinical studies designed to modify serum concentrations of these compounds in subjects at risk of PCa should be performed.

Colonic bacteria convert flavonoids into smaller phenolic acids, which can be absorbed into the circulation and may contribute to the chemopreventive activity of the parent compounds. Flavonoids from GT and BT, citrus fruit with rutin and soy supplements were exposed to the same conditions as in the colon in a dynamic in vitro model (TIM-2, TNO, Triskelion Zeist, The Netherlands). In this artificial colon the parent phytonutrients formed the same phenolic acid products of microbial metabolism as observed in human samples. Among the various phenolic acids formed, only 3,4-dihydroxyphenylacetic acid (3,4-DHPAA) exhibited antiproliferative activity in prostate and colon cancer cells. 3,4-DHPAA was also significantly ($P < 0.005$) more inhibitory in colon cancer cells (HCT116) compared with an immortalized normal intestinal epithelial cell line (IEC6) (Gao et al. 2006).

ELLAGITANNINS

Ellagitannins are found in walnuts and pomegranate, and in some berries such as strawberries and red and black raspberries. Extensive research was done between 2002 and the present on the effects of pomegranate ellagitannins on PCa. The wonderful variety of pomegranate is the major commercial variety sold in the United States and has been extensively studied as a potential antioxidant and anti-inflammatory phytonutrient. This variety originated in Iran and the fruit consists of deep red-purple seeds embedded in a white spongy astringent membrane surrounded by a thick skin, or pericarp. The pericarp constitutes almost 50% of the fruit weight and is a rich source of bioactive constituents including phenolics, flavonoids, ellagitannins, and anthocyanins which can be made into a popular refrigerated juice by pressing whole pomegranates. The remaining 50% by weight of the fruit consists of seeds and arils comprising 10% and 40% of the fruit weight, respectively.

Pomegranate juice (PJ) made from the whole fruit has a unique profile of anthocyanins including delphinidin-3-glucoside, cyanidin-3-glucoside, delphinidin-3,5-diglucoside, cyanidin-3,5-diglucoside, pelargonidin-3,5-diglucoside, and pelargonidin-3-glucoside as well as the ellagitannins, punicalagin, pedunculagin, punicalin, gallagic acid, ellagic acid (EA), and their related esters of glucose. Various organic acids such as ascorbic acid, citric acid, and malic acid are also present in the juice as well as minerals including potassium, nitrogen, calcium, phosphorus, magnesium, and sodium. PJ made from whole fruit has a different composition than supplements made from extracts of the squeezed pomegranate fruit (POMx) which is an important distinction in examining research results. Ellagitannins are also found in oak-aged beverages such as brandy and oak-aged red wine, and in some medicinal plants, but these have not had extensive study.

Upon hydrolysis in the small intestine, ellagitannins release EA partly absorbed into the circulation. Ellagitannin bioavailability is low, and gut microbiota metabolize them into simpler metabolites called urolithins. Urolithin metabolism was first noted to vary among individuals when healthy volunteers were given 180 mL of PJ concentrate and then had blood and urine samples collected and analyzed for 24–56 hours to study the pharmacokinetics of absorption and metabolism of ellagitannins to urolithins (Seeram et al. 2006). Urolithins formed by intestinal bacteria were shown to persist in plasma and tissues. Urolithins were judged to account for some of the health benefits noted after chronic PJ consumption. As gut microbiota vary among individuals, such interindividual variability should be considered as a moderating factor in clinical trials. Individuals who make different urolithins are called metabotypes (Tomas-Barberan, Selma, and Espin 2016, Selma et al. 2018, Romo-Vaquero et al. 2019).

PJ and extract show neuroprotective effects against Alzheimer's disease (AD) in several reported animal studies and a placebo-controlled clinical imaging study in humans (Braidy et al. 2016,

Essa et al. 2015, Hartman et al. 2006, Kwak et al. 2005, Siddarth et al. 2020, Subash et al. 2014, 2015). From a pomegranate extract, previously reported to show anti-AD effects in vivo in mice, 21 constituents, which were primarily ellagitannins, were isolated and identified (by HPLC, NMR, and HRESIMS). In silico computational studies, used to predict blood–brain barrier permeability, revealed that none of the PE constituents, but the urolithins, fulfilled criteria required for penetration (Yuan et al. 2016), prevented β-amyloid fibrillation in vitro and methyl-urolithin B (3-methoxy-6H-dibenzo[b,d]pyran-6-one), but not PE or its predominant ellagitannins, had a protective effect in *Caenorhabditis elegans* postinduction of amyloid β(1–42) induced neurotoxicity and paralysis. Therefore, urolithins are likely the brain absorbable compounds which contribute to pomegranate's anti-AD effects warranting further in vivo studies on these compounds.

A gastrointestinal simulation system (TWIN-SHIME) (Garcia-Villalba et al. 2017) was used to compare the metabolism of pomegranate polyphenols by the gut microbiota from two individuals with different urolithin metabotypes. Gut microbiota, ellagitannin metabolism, short-chain fatty acids (SCFA), transport of metabolites, and phase II metabolism using Caco-2 cells were explored. The simulation reproduced the in vivo metabolic profiles for each metabotype. The study demonstrated that microbial composition, metabolism of ellagitannins, and SCFA differ between metabotypes and along the large intestine. The assay also showed that pomegranate phenolics preserved intestinal cell integrity. Pomegranate polyphenols enhanced urolithin and propionate production, as well as *Akkermansia* and *Gordonibacter* prevalence with the highest effect in the descending colon. The results obtained by the system are consistent with previous human and animal studies and show that although urolithin metabolites are present along the gastrointestinal tract due to enterohepatic circulation, they are predominantly produced in the distal colon region (Selma et al. 2014).

PCa is the second major cause of cancer-related deaths in men in the United States. Studies both in vitro and in vivo over the last 15 years suggest that the potential protective effect of PJ against PCa is largely attributed to ellagitannins, representing the most abundant polyphenols present in PJ. Pantuck et al. (2006) performed the first clinical trial of PJ in PCa patients following surgery and radiation. The study reported that oral consumption of PJ had no adverse effects and significantly increased Prostate Specific Antigen (PSA) doubling times (PSADT) in men with PCa. A randomized, multicenter, double-blind phase II study was performed to determine the biological activity of two doses of POMx in PCa patients by monitoring PSADT following initial therapy for localized PCa. Treatment of PCa patients with POMx increased the PSADT by almost six months in both the treatment arms (Paller et al. 2013).

Following these positive clinical study results, studies of mechanism of action were carried out in mice with human PCa xenografts. Ellagitannin-rich extracts inhibited NF-κB and cell viability of PCa cell lines in a dose-dependent fashion in vitro. Maximal extract-induced apoptosis was dependent on extract-mediated NF-κB blockade. In the Los Angeles Prostate Cancer 4 (LAPC4) xenograft model, PE delayed the emergence of LAPC4 androgen-independent xenografts in castrated mice through an inhibition of proliferation and induction of apoptosis. Moreover, the observed increase in NF-κB activity during the transition from androgen dependence to androgen independence in the LAPC4 xenograft model was abrogated by extract treatment (Rettig et al. 2008, Seeram et al. 2007).

Several trials using PJ and POMx were conducted with patients on active surveillance, neoadjuvant treatment, patients with biochemical recurrence (BCR) following local therapy for PCa, and patients with metastatic castration-resistant prostate cancer (mCRPC). PJ and extract were shown to be safe but did not significantly improve outcomes in BCR patients in a large placebo-controlled trial (Pantuck et al. 2015). However, a subset of BCR patients with the Manganese Superoxide Dismutase AA genotype appeared to respond positively to the antioxidant effects of pomegranate treatment. Phase II trials of 100% pomegranate products in neoadjuvant patients and patients with mCRPC also did not demonstrate a benefit. A multicomponent food supplement containing pomegranate, broccoli, and turmeric extract showed promising results in a phase II study in active surveillance and BCR patients (Paller, Pantuck, and Carducci 2017, Thomas et al. 2014).

A phase II, randomized double-blind trial of men with PCa undergoing radical prostatectomy showed that there was no significant reduction in the level of 8-hydroxy-2'-deoxyguanosine in POMx treated group compared to the placebo-treated group. In addition, there were no differences in expression of p56, NFKB, or Ki67 within PCa tissues between arms (Freedland et al. 2013).

A phase IIb, double blinded, randomized placebo-controlled trial in patients with histologically confirmed PCa. Only patients with a PSA value ≥ 5 ng/mL were included. The subjects consumed 500 mL of PJ or 500 mL of placebo beverage every day for a 4-week period. Thereafter, all patients received 250 mL of the PJ daily for another 4 weeks. PSA values were taken at baseline, day 14, 28, and on day 56. The primary endpoint was the detection of a significant difference in PSA serum levels between the groups after one month of treatment. Pain scores and adherence to intervention were recorded using patient diaries. 102 patients were enrolled. The majority of patients had castration-resistant PCa (68%). 98 received either PJ or placebo between October 2008 and May 2011. Adherence to protocol was good, with 94 patients (96%) completing the first period and 87 patients (89%) completing both periods. No grade 3 or higher toxicities occurred within the study. No differences were detected between the two groups with regard to PSA kinetics and pain scores. Consumption of PJ as an adjunct intervention in men with advanced PCa does not result in significant PSA declines compared to placebo (Stenner-Liewen et al. 2013).

STILBENES

Resveratrol (3,4',5-trihydroxy stilbene) was originally identified as a phytoalexin made by plants as a defense against infection. This natural stilbene has been found in at least 185 plant species and is present in foods and beverages derived from them such as, for example, mulberries, peanuts, grapes, and red wine. There are more than 2,000 studies on resveratrol and cancer including both in vitro and in vivo carcinogenesis assays suggesting potential for the prevention of leukemia, breast, lung, colon, skin, prostate, ovarian, liver, oral, and thyroid cancers. Pterostilbene (trans 3,5-dimethoxy-4-hydroxystilbene) is a natural analog of resveratrol, but with higher bioavailability. Pterostilbene has been shown to inhibit growth, adhesion, and metastatic growth and to be an active apoptotic agent in different types of cancer cells including breast, lung, stomach, prostate, pancreas, and colon cancer (Sirerol et al. 2016).

LIGNANS

There is a growing interest in the presence of lignans in foods such as nuts, sesame, and flax, since they have antiestrogenic, antioxidant, and anticancer activities. Among edible plant foods, the most concentrated lignan sources are sesame and flax seeds. Flax seeds contain about 290 mg/100 g lignans; sesaminol is the major lignan in sesame seeds at about 540 mg/100 g. Only a handful of studies exist regarding lignan bioavailability in humans, including limited human pharmacokinetic studies. Plant lignans are metabolized by intestinal bacteria, undergoing transformation to the mammalian lignans, enterolactones, and enterodiols, prior to absorption. There is some data suggesting lignans decrease the risk of colon, prostate, and breast cancer (Rodriguez-Garcia et al. 2019).

ORGANOSULFURS

The organosulfur phytonutrients include ITC and indoles from cruciferous vegetables such as broccoli, broccoli sprouts, brussel sprouts, cabbage, and bok choy, and allyl sulfides from garlic, onions, chives, and asparagus.

A diet rich in cruciferous vegetables is associated with a lower risk of developing breast, lung, prostate, and colorectal cancer (Feskanich et al. 2000, Benabdelkrim, Djeffal, and Berredjem 2018). The chemoprotective effect of cruciferous vegetables is due to their high glucosinolate content and the capacity of glucosinolate metabolites, such as ITC and indoles, to modulate biotransformation enzyme systems (e.g., cytochromes P450 and conjugating enzymes). Data from molecular epide-miologic studies suggest that genetic and associated functional variations in biotransformation enzymes, particularly glutathione S-transferase (GST)M1 and GSTT1, which metabolize ITC, alter cancer risk in response to cruciferous vegetable exposure (Lampe and Peterson 2002).

The glucosinolates in cruciferous vegetables include glucoraphanin, glucobrassinin, and glu-conasturtun which release ITC, indole-3-carbinol, and phenylethylisothiocyanate, respectively. Among these several groups of metabolites, ITCs are the most common. Abundant evidence has suggested that ITCs are inhibitors of drug metabolizing phase I enzymes and potent inducers of phase II enzymes.

When cruciferous are consumed, myrosinase enzyme present in the plant hydrolyzes the gluco-sinolates in the proximal part of the gastrointestinal tract to various metabolites, such as ITC, nitriles, oxazolidine-2-thiones, and indole-3-carbinols (Bradlow 2008). Myrosinase is a β-thioglucosidase that is activated when the plant tissue containing glucosinolates is damaged, as is the case in food preparation (cutting, chopping, mixing) or chewing the vegetable. The enzyme is normally stored separately from glucosinolates in different cells, or in different intracellular compartments, depend-ing on the plant species. When cruciferous vegetables are cooked before consumption, myrosinase is inactivated as the enzyme protein is denatured and glucosinolates travel to the colon where they are hydrolyzed by the intestinal microbiota.

The metabolism of ITCs has been extensively studied. Absorbed ITCs are conjugated to gluta-thione in the liver and excreted in the urine as mercapturic acid. In humans, the formation of mer-capturic acids is the predominant metabolic pathway and the amount of mercapturic acid excreted is a good reflection of the amount of ITCs consumed and can be used as biomarkers of cruciferous vegetable intake. Because of these properties of ITCs, extensive research has examined the role of ITCs in the chemoprevention of various types of cancer (Abbaoui et al. 2018, Arumugam and Abdull Razis 2018, Zhang et al. 2018, Vanduchova, Anzenbacher, and Anzenbacherova 2019).

Sulforaphane is an ITC which has been the subject of extensive basic and clinical research. It is present in stored form in plant cells as stable glucoraphanin in cruciferous vegetables such as cabbage, cauliflower, kale, and broccoli, especially in broccoli sprouts. Sulforaphane is conju-gated with glutathione and undergoes further biotransformation, yielding metabolites. It has been shown that sulforaphane may protect against various types of cancer through both epidemiologi-cal, basic, and clinical research studies. Sulforaphane exerts antioxidative and anti-inflammatory effects by activating the nuclear factor E2-related factor (Nrf2), which subsequently induces phase II enzymes.

Broccoli-derived sulforaphane activates Nrf2 to induce the expression of a battery of cytoprotec-tive genes such as those playing key roles in cellular defense mechanisms including redox status and detoxification. Both its high bioavailability and significant Nrf2 inducer capacity contribute to the therapeutic potential of sulforaphane-yielding foods and supplements that contain both myrosinase and sulforaphane (Houghton 2019, Houghton, Fassett, and Coombes 2016).

Indoles are formed from the enzymatic breakdown of glucobrassicin by myrosinase during plant storage, preparation, or chewing. Indole-3-carbinol is unstable and polymerizes in the stomach at acid pH to oligomers that include diindoylmethane (DIM), which is the major indole bioactive compound, accounting for about 60% of the indole-3-carbinol end-products (Thomson, Ho, and Strom 2016).

Wattenberg and Loub first described the presence of DIM in crucifers, the cancer-preventive activity of freeze-dried broccoli, and the bioactivity of supplemental DIM in the prevention of carcinogen-induced breast cancer in animals (Wattenberg and Loub 1978). DIM selectively induced cell cycle arrest and apoptosis in both ER-positive and ER-negative breast cancer cells, without producing evidence of antiproliferative activity in normal breast epithelial cells. A wide array of mechanisms of cancer-related bioactivity of DIM have been described, including modulating car-cinogenesis at all stages of breast tumor development, including initiation, promotion, and progres-sion (Banerjee et al. 2011).

Studying the physiological responses to the intake of DIM is difficult, due in part to the variations in DIM content of different food sources. On average, 100 g of cruciferous vegetables contain up to 30 mg of glucobrassicin, which is estimated to convert to approximately 2 mg of DIM. However, the variation in DIM content between different cruciferous vegetables is considerable, with differences ranging from 5- to 8-fold (McNaughton and Marks 2003).

Much of the chemoprevention research on DIM has been carried out with dietary supplements containing microencapsulated DIM (Anderton et al. 2004). Despite these difficulties DIM can be measured in urine samples as a biomarker for epidemiological and clinical studies where urinary DIM discriminates between volunteers fed high and low doses of Brassica vegetables (Fujioka et al. 2016).

Another group of OSCs with a role in cancer prevention are the allyl sulfides from Allium vegetables such as garlic. Garlic consumption has been associated with reduced risks of various cancer types including gastric, colorectal, endometrial, lung, and prostate cancer (Puccinelli and Stan 2017).

Fresh garlic contains a mixture of water, fiber, carbohydrates, protein, and fat as well as more than 20 vitamins and minerals and at least 33 OSCs in two different groups. One group is lipid-soluble, including diallyl sulfide, diallyl disulfide, and diallyl trisulfide. The other group is water-soluble and includes S-allylcysteine (SAC) and S-allylmercaptocysteine (SAMC).

While standardized garlic supplements are needed for intervention studies in cancer prevention, there has been heterogeneity in the literature on garlic supplementation. Dried and pulverized whole garlic clove supplements have been used in a large number of controlled clinical trials since the mid-1980s, focusing primarily on serum cholesterol and blood pressure. The effects on serum lipids have been inconsistent, even for persons with high baseline cholesterol levels. Of 23 trials on serum cholesterol with a garlic powder product, 43% found no effect. These trials have been the subject of several meta-analyses (nine on serum lipids) concluding that the heterogeneity of dose, variable product types, identification of active compounds, standardization concerns, and unknown bioavailability impeding firm conclusions on the benefits of garlic supplements (Lawson and Hunsaker 2018).

The allyl thiosulfinates have been shown to be responsible for most of the pharmacological activity of crushed raw garlic cloves. Allicin is responsible for the antibacterial activity of garlic. Selective removal of allicin also removed all activities. Considerable evidence suggests that the allyl thiosulfinates, or their spontaneous transformation compounds (allyl polysulfides), or their common metabolite (allyl methyl sulfide, AMS) are responsible for most of the lipid-lowering, antioxidant, and anticancer effects of whole garlic, as observed in animals and humans. It is recommended that the minimum daily dose of a garlic powder supplement for possible health benefits should represent the equivalent of two grams of typical raw garlic by having an allicin potential of about 7–8 mg or an allicin content of 18–21 mg, and that the preferred dose for clinical trials should be two times this amount (Lawson and Wang 2005).

Aged garlic extract (AGE) is produced by immersion and extraction of sliced raw garlic in aqueous ethanol for over ten months at room temperature. During this process of aging, the odoriferous lipid-soluble compounds are converted into more stable and bioavailable water-soluble compounds. The contents of SAC and SAMC are high in AGE with low levels of lipid-soluble compounds. SAC is active against different human cancers including PCa, breast cancer, oral cancer, neuroblastoma, and nonsmall-cell lung carcinoma. Moreover, when SAC was administered to nude mice there was no toxicity noted. The molecular mechanisms underlying the anticancer properties of SAC, the predominant organosulfur component of AGE, include induction of carcinogen detoxification, inhibition of cell proliferation and growth, mediation of cell cycle arrest, induction of cell death, inhibition of epithelial-mesenchymal transition and cell invasion, suppression of metastasis, and induction of immunomodulation in cancer cells. The actions and mechanisms are not comprehensive, and important aspects of the anticancer activities of SAC still need to be explored. More specific studies, including clinical and epidemiological studies, are needed to advance the use of SAC for the prevention and treatment of cancer (Agbana et al. 2020).

CAROTENOIDS

Carotenoids absorb light in the visible spectrum resulting in yellow, orange, and red colors of fruits and vegetables. Lycopene, α-carotene, β-carotene, lutein, and cryptoxanthin are the main carotenoids in the diet (Xavier and Perez-Galvez 2016). In plants, the conjugate double-bond structure found in carotenoids absorbs light at ultraviolet and visible wavelengths during the energy production of photosynthesis protecting the plant cells containing carotenoids from the harmful effects of ultraviolet radiation. The presence of carotenoids also determines the characteristic color and absorption of light energy during photosynthesis to protect plants of origin from oxidant stress (Kirilovsky 2015). For example, red tomatoes are rich in lycopene, while orange carrots are rich in β-carotene, and their colors are determined by the absorption spectra of these two different carotenoids. More than 700 natural carotenoids have been identified. Carotenoids are found in red-, yellow-, and orange-colored fruits and vegetables as well as in all green leafy vegetables (Langi et al. 2018).

According to structures of carotenoids, two classes are distinguished as hydrocarbon carotenoids and xanthophylls. The carotenes include α-carotene, β-carotene, γ-carotene, lycopene, phytoene, and phytofluene. Xanthophylls contain oxygen and include lutein, zeaxanthin, β-cryptoxanthin, astaxanthin, and fucoxanthin (Rodriguez-Amaya 2016).

Overproduction of reactive oxygen and nitrogen species has been implicated in the development of breast, cervical, ovarian, and colorectal cancers. The antioxidant effects of carotenoids are the result of oxygen radical quenching by its double carbon–carbon bonds interacting with each other via conjugation and causing electrons in the molecule to move freely across each molecule. Increased consumption of fruits and vegetables rich in carotenoids has been associated with a reduced risk of breast, lung, head and neck, cervical, ovarian, colorectal, and prostate cancers (Eliassen et al. 2015, Van Hoang et al. 2018, Zhou, Wang, et al. 2016, Rowles et al. 2017).

Some of the carotenoids are also precursors of vitamin A and are converted into vitamin A in the body. From α-carotene and γ-carotene, one molecule of vitamin A while from β-carotene two molecules of vitamin A are synthesized (Shete and Quadro 2013). The chemical structure of vitamin A is one half of the structure of α-carotene. The second most common form of carotene, α-carotene, is found mostly in carrots, sweet potatoes, squash, tomatoes, red peppers, and dark green vegetables. β-Carotene is a fat-soluble provitamin as it is split to form vitamin A (Valko et al. 2007).

Lycopene has the highest antioxidant activity among the carotenoids. Lycopene is found in red tomatoes, watermelons, pink grapefruit, and rosehip. Since lycopene is fat soluble like the other carotenoids, its absorption is enhanced with the consumption of some olive oil or avocado at the same time (Unlu et al. 2005).

Lutein is concentrated in the macula and transported to the brain where it is the predominant carotenoid. Zeaxanthin and meso-zeaxanthin are also concentrated in the macula. The chemical structure of lutein and zeaxanthin is the same except for the position of a double bond in the end ring. Zeaxanthin is one of the most common carotenoid alcohols found in nature. It is a pigment that gives its color to maize, saffron, and many other plants. When zeaxanthin breaks down it forms picrocrocin, which is the carotenoid responsible for the taste and aroma of saffron.

Cryptoxanthin is closely related to β-carotene and has a characteristic color found in canteloupe. β-Cryptoxanthin is found in fruits and vegetables, such as mandarin, red pepper, and zucchini, and has important functions for human health. Its chemical structure is similar to β-carotene. While β-carotene is present in large quantities in a large number of fruits and vegetables, β-cryptoxanthin is present in a small number of food sources but at high concentrations.

Astaxanthin is a keto-carotenoid and is another zeaxanthin metabolite, containing both hydroxyl and ketone functional groups. Astaxanthin is found in microalgae, yeast, salmon, trout, shrimp, shellfish, and some birds' feathers such as those of the pink flamingo.

Fucoxantin is the carotenoid found in the chloroplasts of algae and mosses accounting for their brown or olive green color.

The activity of carotenoids as antioxidants is related to their interaction in the antioxidant network originated by Dr. Lester Packer at the University of California with other antioxidants, such as vitamins E and C. In addition, some carotenoids and their metabolites activate the nuclear factor-erythroid 2-related factor-2 (Nrf2) transcription factor, which triggers antioxidant gene expression in certain cells and tissues (Sahin et al. 2014). Carotenoids in forms of cancer characterized by oxidative stress, inflammation, and impaired mitochondrial function can reduce Nrf2 expression in some animal models. Prevention of low-density lipoproteins (LDL) oxidation by carotenoids has been suggested to be the basis of carotenoids' protective activity in some forms of cancer (Esterbauer et al. 1992).

The signaling pathways and molecules influenced by carotenoids to prevent various cancers include growth factor signaling, cell cycle-associated proteins, differentiation-related proteins, retinoid-like receptors, the antioxidant response element, nuclear receptors, AP-1 transcriptional complex, the Wnt/β-catenin pathway, angiogenic proteins, and inflammatory cytokines. The dose and the exposure time of β-carotene, lycopene, lutein, and zeaxanthin are important factors in determining cellular responses critical to cancer prevention.

AMIDES

Some polyphenols may have N-containing functional substituents. Two such groups of polyphenolic amides are of significance for being the major components of common foods: capsaicinoids in chili peppers (Chapa-Oliver and Mejia-Teniente 2016) and avenanthramides in oats (Sang and Chu 2017). Capsaicinoids such as capsaicin are responsible for the hotness of the chili peppers but have also been found to have strong antioxidant and anti-inflammatory properties, and they modulate the oxidative defense system in cells. Antioxidant activities including inhibition of LDL oxidation by avenanthramides have also been reported.

PHYTOSTEROLS

Phytosterols, which include plant sterols and stanols, are phytosteroids, similar in structure to cholesterol. Stanols are saturated sterols, having no double bonds in the sterol ring structure. More than 200 sterols and related compounds have been identified. Phytosterol-enriched foods and dietary supplements have been marketed for their ability to lower cholesterol.

Phytosterols lower serum cholesterol levels by reducing intestinal cholesterol absorption as a result of competing with cholesterol due to their structural similarities. Several in vivo studies have tested the efficacy of dietary phytosterol in the breast cancer development. Female immuno-deficient mice supplemented with 2% phytosterols and injected with MDA-MB-231 cells exhibited a reduction in serum cholesterol, accompanied with a reduction in tumor size and metastasis to lymph nodes and lungs. In ovariectomized athymic mice injected with MCF-7 cells, supplementation with β-sitosterol, the most common phytosterol, was also able to reduce tumor size. Another potential mechanism of action of phytosterols is the prevention of lipoprotein oxidation (Llaverias et al. 2013).

Numerous experimental in vitro studies demonstrated that phytosterols acted as anticancer compounds by modulating host systems to affect tumor surveillance or on tumors to affect tumor cell biology. Mechanisms affecting the tumors include slowing of cell cycle progression, induction of apoptosis, inhibition of tumor metastasis, altered signal transduction, and activation of angiogenesis. Host influences comprise enhancing immune recognition of cancer, influencing hormonal-dependent growth of endocrine tumors, and altering cholesterol metabolism.

Although the mechanism of action by which phytosterols may prevent cancer development is still under investigation, data from multiple experimental studies support the hypothesis that they may modulate proliferation and apoptosis of tumor cells. Phytosterols including sitosterol, campesterol, stigmasterol, and sitosterol are generally considered safe for human consumption and may also be added to a broad spectrum of foods. Few interventional studies have evaluated the relationship between the efficacy of different types and forms of phytosterols in cancer prevention (Blanco-Vaca, Cedo, and Julve 2019).

CURCUMIN

There are a number of nonflavonoid polyphenols found in foods that are considered important to human health. Curcumin is a natural yellow-color compound extracted from rhizome of the turmeric plant *Curcuma longa*, which belongs to the Zingiberaceae family and is widely grown in Southeast Asia. Studies on curcumin and cancer in vitro and in animals have been extensively reported in thousands of publications with curcumin demonstrated to modulate growth factors, enzymes, transcription factors, kinase, inflammatory cytokines, and proapoptotic (by upregulation) and antiapoptotic (by downregulation) proteins in cancer cells (Giordano and Tommonaro 2019).

Curcumin exhibits anticancer activity by targeting different cell signaling pathways including growth factors, cytokines, transcription factors, and genes modulating cellular proliferation and apoptosis. Curcumin has poor bioavailability due to low absorption, rapid metabolism, and systemic elimination that limit its potential efficacy. Further studies and clinical trials in humans are needed to validate curcumin as an effective anticancer agent.

Ursolic acid is a naturally synthesized pentacyclic triterpenoid, widely distributed in different fruits and vegetables. Ursolic acid and its derivatives have demonstrated in vitro anticancer activity, anti-inflammatory effects, and induction of apoptosis in several human cancer cell lines. In particular, ursolic acid inhibited breast cancer proliferation by inducing cell G1/G2 arrest and regulating the expression of key proteins in signal transduction pathways. In addition, ursolic acid induced apoptosis in human breast cancer cells through intrinsic and extrinsic apoptotic pathways (Yin et al. 2018). Ursolic acid exerted a dose- and time-dependent inhibitory effect on the migration and invasion of highly metastatic breast MDAMB231 cells at noncytotoxic concentrations. This effect was associated with reduced activities of matrix metalloproteinase-2 (MMP-2) which correlated with enhanced expression of tissue inhibitor of MMP-2 and plasminogen activator inhibitor-1, respectively. Ursolic acid suppressed the phosphorylation of Jun N-terminal kinase, Akt, and mTOR. The anti-invasive effects of ursolic acid on MDAMB231 cells might be through the inhibition of Jun N-terminal kinase, Akt, and mTOR phosphorylation and a reduction of the level of NF-κB protein in the nucleus, ultimately leading to downregulation of MMP-2. These results suggest that ursolic acid has the potential as a chemopreventive agent for metastatic breast cancer, but further research including clinical studies will be needed to confirm its efficacy (Jaman and Sayeed 2018, Yin et al. 2018).

CONCLUSION

With a rapidly expanding elderly population and relatively underdeveloped cancer research, treatment, and care programs, less developed nations are likely to be the hardest hit by the increase in cancer predicted in the next few decades. Therefore, prevention of cancer, specifically by means of food or other dietary agents, is likely the most cost-effective and sustainable method of dealing with this epidemic. The identification and characterization of dietary agents with chemopreventive potential are pivotal steps in this process. Traditional medicine systems such as Ayurveda and Traditional Chinese Medicine have deep roots in many of these underdeveloped communities and present a great opportunity for battling the global burden of cancer from the standpoint of primary prevention.

Discovery research on vitamins and minerals was largely considered settled by the 1950s, with the widespread marketing of multivitamin/multimineral tablets. While the public believed that the problem of nutritional deficiencies was solved with the disappearance of classical nutritional deficiency diseases such as scurvy, beriberi, and pellagra, we are now faced with unexpected nutrition problems primarily in the industrial West, which follow from an unappreciated deficiency of phyto-nutrients from colorful fruits and vegetables, an excess of dietary fats, and refining of grains.

The recognition that food-derived phytonutrient molecules can modulate intracellular molecular mechanisms has seen the emergence of the fields of nutrigenomics and nutrigenetics, disciplines derived from the interweaving of the sciences of nutrition, biochemistry, molecular biology, and genomics. It has been estimated that there are more than 10,000 phytonutrients present in foods, but our current knowledge is limited to the functions and potential preventive properties of the categories of phytonutrients reviewed above. There are few published clinical trials using phytonutrients for cancer prevention and only a small number of these withstand scientific scrutiny.

A careful review of the formulations of some available phytonutrient supplements reveals numerous problems with current regulation and accepted formulation and standardization practices. Even when the benefit for a compound has been demonstrated, it is common for commercial products to include the ingredient at doses much lower than that shown to be efficacious in either clinical trials or in traditional use by various cultures in the past. Consumers and uninformed clinicians may be easily fooled with citations for in vitro and animal studies, giving the false impression that the supplement is effective in humans.

The financial incentives and patent protection afforded to botanical dietary and phytonutrient supplements are far less than what is accorded to pharmaceuticals. Therefore, the commercial support of such research is lacking in quantity and quality. A government initiative to explore the benefits of phytonutrients in cancer prevention, treatment, and survival is needed for mankind to benefit from nature's pharmacy in the global fight against cancer.

REFERENCES

Abbaoui, B., C. R. Lucas, K. M. Riedl, S. K. Clinton, and A. Mortazavi. 2018. "Cruciferous vegetables, isothiocyanates, and bladder cancer prevention." *Mol Nutr Food Res* 62 (18):e1800079. doi: 10.1002/mnfr.201800079.

Agbana, Y. L., Y. Ni, M. Zhou, Q. Zhang, K. Kassegne, S. D. Karou, Y. Kuang, and Y. Zhu. 2020. "Garlic-derived bioactive compound S-allylcysteine inhibits cancer progression through diverse molecular mechanisms." *Nutr Res* 73:1–14 doi: 10.1016/j.nutres.2019.11.002.

Allred, C. D., K. F. Allred, Y. H. Ju, S. M. Virant, and W. G. Helferich. 2001. "Soy diets containing varying amounts of genistein stimulate growth of estrogen-dependent (MCF-7) tumors in a dose-dependent manner." *Cancer Res* 61 (13):5045–5050.

Anderton, M. J., M. M. Manson, R. Verschoyle, A. Gescher, W. P. Steward, M. L. Williams, and D. E. Mager. 2004. "Physiological modeling of formulated and crystalline 3,3'-diindolylmethane pharmacokinetics following oral administration in mice." *Drug Metab Dispos* 32 (6):632–638. doi: 10.1124/dmd.32.6.632.

Arumugam, A., and A. F. Abdull Razis. 2018. "Apoptosis as a mechanism of the cancer chemopreventive activity of glucosinolates: a review." *Asian Pac J Cancer Prev* 19 (6):1439–1448. doi: 10.22034/APJCP.2018.19.6.1439.

Banerjee, S., D. Kong, Z. Wang, B. Bao, G. G. Hillman, and F. H. Sarkar. 2011. "Attenuation of multi-targeted proliferation-linked signaling by 3,3'-diindolylmethane (DIM): from bench to clinic." *Mutat Res* 728 (1–2):47–66. doi: 10.1016/j.mrrev.2011.06.001.

Barreca, D., G. Gattuso, E. Bellocco, A. Calderaro, D. Trombetta, A. Smeriglio, G. Lagana, M. Daglia, S. Meneghini, and S. M. Nabavi. 2017. "Flavanones: citrus phytochemical with health-promoting properties." *Biofactors* 43 (4):495–506. doi: 10.1002/biof.1363.

Benabdelkrim, M., O. Djeffal, and H. Berredjem. 2018. "GSTM1 and GSTT1 Polymorphisms and susceptibility to prostate cancer: a case-control study of the Algerian population." *Asian Pac J Cancer Prev* 19 (10):2853–2858. doi: 10.22034/APJCP.2018.19.10.2853.

Biesalski, H. K., L. O. Dragsted, I. Elmadfa, R. Grossklaus, M. Muller, D. Schrenk, P. Walter, and P. Weber. 2009. "Bioactive compounds: definition and assessment of activity." *Nutrition* 25 (11–12):1202–1205. doi: 10.1016/j.nut.2009.04.023.

Blanco-Vaca, F., L. Cedo, and J. Julve. 2019. "Phytosterols in cancer: from molecular mechanisms to preventive and therapeutic potentials." *Curr Med Chem* 26 (37):6735–6749. doi: 10.2174/0929867325666180607093111.

Bradlow, H. L. 2008. "Review. Indole-3-carbinol as a chemoprotective agent in breast and prostate cancer." *In Vivo* 22 (4):441–445.

Braidy, N., M. M. Essa, A. Poljak, S. Selvaraju, S. Al-Adawi, T. Manivasagm, A. J. Thenmozhi, L. Ooi, P. Sachdev, and G. J. Guillemin. 2016. "Consumption of pomegranates improves synaptic function in a transgenic mice model of Alzheimer's disease." *Oncotarget* 7 (40):64589–64604. doi: 10.18632/oncotarget.10905.

Burnett, J. P., G. Lim, Y. Li, R. B. Shah, R. Lim, H. J. Paholak, S. P. McDermott, L. Sun, Y. Tsume, S. Bai, M. S. Wicha, D. Sun, and T. Zhang. 2017. "Sulforaphane enhances the anticancer activity of taxanes against triple negative breast cancer by killing cancer stem cells." *Cancer Lett* 394:52–64 doi: 10.1016/j.canlet.2017.02.023.

Buyel, J. F. 2018. "Plants as sources of natural and recombinant anti-cancer agents." *Biotechnol Adv* 36 (2):506–520. doi: 10.1016/j.biotechadv.2018.02.002.

Chang, H. P., L. Y. Sheen, and Y. P. Lei. 2015. "The protective role of carotenoids and polyphenols in patients with head and neck cancer." *J Chin Med Assoc* 78 (2):89–95. doi: 10.1016/j.jcma.2014.08.010.

Chapa-Oliver, A. M., and L. Mejia-Teniente. 2016. "Capsaicin: from plants to a cancer-suppressing agent." *Molecules* 21 (8), 931. doi: 10.3390/molecules21080931.

Cirmi, S., M. Navarra, J. V. Woodside, and M. M. Cantwell. 2018. "Citrus fruits intake and oral cancer risk: a systematic review and meta-analysis." *Pharmacol Res* 133:187–194. doi: 10.1016/j.phrs.2018.05.008.

Clinton, S. K., E. L. Giovannucci, and S. D. Hursting. 2020. "The World Cancer Research Fund/American Institute for Cancer Research third expert report on diet, nutrition, physical activity, and cancer: impact and future directions." *J Nutr* 150 (4):663–671. doi: 10.1093/jn/nxz268.

Crozier, A., D. Del Rio, and M. N. Clifford. 2010. "Bioavailability of dietary flavonoids and phenolic compounds." *Mol Aspects Med* 31 (6):446–467. doi: 10.1016/j.mam.2010.09.007.

Danciu, C., S. Avram, I. Z. Pavel, R. Ghiulai, C. A. Dehelean, A. Ersilia, D. Minda, C. Petrescu, E. A. Moaca, and C. Soica. 2018. "Main isoflavones found in dietary sources as natural anti-inflammatory agents." *Curr Drug Targets* 19 (7):841–853. doi: 10.2174/1389450118666171109150731.

Darband, S. G., M. Kaviani, B. Yousefi, S. Sadighparvar, F. G. Pakdel, J. A. Attari, I. Mohebbi, S. Naderi, and M. Majidinia. 2018. "Quercetin: a functional dietary flavonoid with potential chemo-preventive properties in colorectal cancer." *J Cell Physiol* 233 (9):6544–6560. doi: 10.1002/jcp.26595.

Derakhshan, Z., M. Ferrante, M. Tadi, F. Ansari, A. Heydari, M. S. Hosseini, G. O. Conti, and E. K. Sadrabad. 2018. "Antioxidant activity and total phenolic content of ethanolic extract of pomegranate peels, juice and seeds." *Food Chem Toxicol* 114:108–111. doi: 10.1016/j.fct.2018.02.023.

Douglas, C. C., S. A. Johnson, and B. H. Arjmandi. 2013. "Soy and its isoflavones: the truth behind the science in breast cancer." *Anticancer Agents Med Chem* 13 (8):1178–1187. doi: 10.2174/18715206113139990320.

Durazzo, A., L. D'Addezio, E. Camilli, R. Piccinelli, A. Turrini, L. Marletta, S. Marconi, M. Lucarini, S. Lisciani, P. Gabrielli, L. Gambelli, A. Aguzzi, and S. Sette. 2018. "From plant compounds to botanicals and back: a current snapshot." *Molecules* 23 (8):1844. doi: 10.3390/molecules23081844.

Eliassen, A. H., X. Liao, B. Rosner, R. M. Tamimi, S. S. Tworoger, and S. E. Hankinson. 2015. "Plasma carotenoids and risk of breast cancer over 20 y of follow-up." *Am J Clin Nutr* 101 (6):1197–1205. doi: 10.3945/ajcn.114.105080.

Essa, M. M., S. Subash, M. Akbar, S. Al-Adawi, and G. J. Guillemin. 2015. "Long-term dietary supplementation of pomegranates, figs and dates alleviate neuroinflammation in a transgenic mouse model of Alzheimer's disease." *PLoS One* 10 (3):e0120964. doi: 10.1371/journal.pone.0120964.

Esterbauer, H., G. Waeg, H. Puhl, M. Dieber-Rotheneder, and F. Tatzber. 1992. "Inhibition of LDL oxidation by antioxidants." *EXS* 62:145–157. doi: 10.1007/978-3-0348-7460-1_15.

Fang, J. 2015. "Classification of fruits based on anthocyanin types and relevance to their health effects." *Nutrition* 31 (11–12):1301–1306. doi: 10.1016/j.nut.2015.04.015.

Feng, W. Y. 2006. "Metabolism of green tea catechins: an overview." *Curr Drug Metab* 7 (7):755–809. doi: 10.2174/138920006778520552.

Feskanich, D., R. G. Ziegler, D. S. Michaud, E. L. Giovannucci, F. E. Speizer, W. C. Willett, and G. A. Colditz. 2000. "Prospective study of fruit and vegetable consumption and risk of lung cancer among men and women." *J Natl Cancer Inst* 92 (22):1812–1823. doi: 10.1093/jnci/92.22.1812.

Freedland, S. J., M. Carducci, N. Kroeger, A. Partin, J. Y. Rao, Y. Jin, S. Kerkoutian, H. Wu, Y. Li, P. Creel, K. Mundy, R. Gurganus, H. Fedor, S. A. King, Y. Zhang, D. Heber, and A. J. Pantuck. 2013. "A double-blind, randomized, neoadjuvant study of the tissue effects of POMx pills in men with prostate cancer before radical prostatectomy." *Cancer Prev Res (Phila)* 6 (10):1120–1127. doi: 10.1158/1940-6207.CAPR-12-0423.

Fu, L., B. T. Xu, X. R. Xu, R. Y. Gan, Y. Zhang, E. Q. Xia, and H. B. Li. 2011. "Antioxidant capacities and total phenolic contents of 62 fruits." *Food Chem* 129 (2):345–350. doi: 10.1016/j.foodchem.2011.04.079.

Fujioka, N., B. W. Ransom, S. G. Carmella, P. Upadhyaya, B. R. Lindgren, A. Roper-Batker, D. K. Hatsukami, V. A. Fritz, C. Rohwer, and S. S. Hecht. 2016. "Harnessing the power of cruciferous vegetables: developing a biomarker for brassica vegetable consumption using urinary 3,3'-diindolylmethane." *Cancer Prev Res (Phila)* 9 (10):788–793. doi: 10.1158/1940-6207.CAPR-16-0136.

Gao, K., A. Xu, C. Krul, K. Venema, Y. Liu, Y. Niu, J. Lu, L. Bensoussan, N. P. Seeram, D. Heber, and S. M. Henning. 2006. "Of the major phenolic acids formed during human microbial fermentation of tea, citrus, and soy flavonoid supplements, only 3,4-dihydroxyphenylacetic acid has antiproliferative activity." *J Nutr* 136 (1):52–57. doi: 10.1093/jn/136.1.52.

Garcia-Villalba, R., H. Vissenaekens, J. Pitart, M. Romo-Vaquero, J. C. Espin, C. Grootaert, M. V. Selma, K. Raes, G. Smagghe, S. Possemiers, J. Van Camp, and F. A. Tomas-Barberan. 2017. "Gastrointestinal simulation model TWIN-SHIME shows differences between human urolithin-metabotypes in gut microbiota composition, pomegranate polyphenol metabolism, and transport along the intestinal tract." *J Agric Food Chem* 65 (27):5480–5493. doi: 10.1021/acs.jafc.7b02049.

Giordano, A., and G. Tommonaro. 2019. "Curcumin and cancer." *Nutrients* 11 (10):2376. doi: 10.3390/nu11102376.

Grosso, G., J. Godos, F. Galvano, and E. L. Giovannucci. 2017. "Coffee, caffeine, and health outcomes: an umbrella review." *Annu Rev Nutr* 37:131–156. doi: 10.1146/annurev-nutr-071816-064941.

Grosso, G., A. Micek, J. Godos, S. Sciacca, A. Pajak, M. A. Martinez-Gonzalez, E. L. Giovannucci, and F. Galvano. 2016. "Coffee consumption and risk of all-cause, cardiovascular, and cancer mortality in smokers and non-smokers: a dose-response meta-analysis." *Eur J Epidemiol* 31 (12):1191–1205. doi: 10.1007/s10654-016-0202-2.

Haag, J. D., M. J. Lindstrom, and M. N. Gould. 1992. "Limonene-induced regression of mammary carcinomas." *Cancer Res* 52 (14):4021–4026.

Hartman, R. E., A. Shah, A. M. Fagan, K. E. Schwetye, M. Parsadanian, R. N. Schulman, M. B. Finn, and D. M. Holtzman. 2006. "Pomegranate juice decreases amyloid load and improves behavior in a mouse model of Alzheimer's disease." *Neurobiol Dis* 24 (3):506–515. doi: 10.1016/j.nbd.2006.08.006.

Heber, D., and S. Bowerman. 2001. "Applying science to changing dietary patterns." *J Nutr* 131 (11 Suppl):3078S–3081S. doi: 10.1093/jn/131.11.3078S.

Henning, S. M., Y. Niu, N. H. Lee, G. D. Thames, R. R. Minutti, H. Wang, V. L. Go, and D. Heber. 2004. "Bioavailability and antioxidant activity of tea flavanols after consumption of green tea, black tea, or a green tea extract supplement." *Am J Clin Nutr* 80 (6):1558–1564. doi: 10.1093/ajcn/80.6.1558.

Henning, S. M., P. Wang, C. L. Carpenter, and D. Heber. 2013. "Epigenetic effects of green tea polyphenols in cancer." *Epigenomics* 5 (6):729–741. doi: 10.2217/epi.13.57.

Henning, S. M., P. Wang, and D. Heber. 2011. "Chemopreventive effects of tea in prostate cancer: green tea versus black tea." *Mol Nutr Food Res* 55 (6):905–920. doi: 10.1002/mnfr.201000648.

Henning, S. M., J. Yang, M. Hsu, R. P. Lee, E. M. Grojean, A. Ly, C. H. Tseng, D. Heber, and Z. Li. 2018. "Decaffeinated green and black tea polyphenols decrease weight gain and alter microbiome populations and function in diet-induced obese mice." *Eur J Nutr* 57 (8):2759–2769. doi: 10.1007/s00394-017-1542-8.

Hilakivi-Clarke, L., J. E. Andrade, and W. Helferich. 2010. "Is soy consumption good or bad for the breast?" *J Nutr* 140 (12):2326S–2334S. doi: 10.3945/jn.110.124230.

Houghton, C. A. 2019. "Sulforaphane: its "Coming of Age" as a clinically relevant nutraceutical in the prevention and treatment of chronic disease." *Oxid Med Cell Longev* 2019:2716870. doi: 10.1155/2019/2716870.

Houghton, C. A., R. G. Fassett, and J. S. Coombes. 2016. "Sulforaphane and other nutrigenomic Nrf2 activators: can the clinician's expectation be matched by the reality?" *Oxid Med Cell Longev* 2016:7857186. doi: 10.1155/2016/7857186.

Hour, T. C., J. Chen, C. Y. Huang, J. Y. Guan, S. H. Lu, and Y. S. Pu. 2002. "Curcumin enhances cytotoxicity of chemotherapeutic agents in prostate cancer cells by inducing p21(WAF1/CIP1) and C/EBPbeta expressions and suppressing NF-kappaB activation." *Prostate* 51 (3):211–218. doi: 10.1002/pros.10089.

Iino, C., T. Shimoyama, K. Iino, Y. Yokoyama, D. Chinda, H. Sakuraba, S. Fukuda, and S. Nakaji. 2019. "Daidzein intake is associated with equol producing status through an increase in the intestinal bacteria responsible for equol production." *Nutrients* 11 (2):433. doi: 10.3390/nu11020433.

Jaman, M. S., and M. A. Sayeed. 2018. "Ellagic acid, sulforaphane, and ursolic acid in the prevention and therapy of breast cancer: current evidence and future perspectives." *Breast Cancer* 25 (5):517–528. doi: 10.1007/s12282-018-0866-4.

Jana, N., G. Bretislav, S. Pavel, and U. Pavla. 2018. "Potential of the flavonoid quercetin to prevent and treat cancer - current status of research." *Klin Onkol* 31 (3):184–190. doi: 10.14735/amko2018184.

Kamiloglu, S., E. Capanoglu, C. Grootaert, and J. Van Camp. 2015. "Anthocyanin absorption and metabolism by human intestinal caco-2 cells--a review." *Int J Mol Sci* 16 (9):21555–21574. doi: 10.3390/ijms160921555.

Kirilovsky, D. 2015. "Photosynthesis: dissipating energy by carotenoids." *Nat Chem Biol* 11 (4):242–243. doi: 10.1038/nchembio.1771.

Kwak, H. M., S. Y. Jeon, B. H. Sohng, J. G. Kim, J. M. Lee, K. B. Lee, H. H. Jeong, J. M. Hur, Y. H. Kang, and K. S. Song. 2005. "Beta-Secretase (BACE1) inhibitors from pomegranate (Punica granatum) husk." *Arch Pharm Res* 28 (12):1328–1332. doi: 10.1007/BF02977896.

Lampe, J. W., and S. Peterson. 2002. "Brassica, biotransformation and cancer risk: genetic polymorphisms alter the preventive effects of cruciferous vegetables." *J Nutr* 132 (10):2991–2994. doi: 10.1093/jn/131.10.2991.

Langi, P., S. Kiokias, T. Varzakas, and C. Proestos. 2018. "Carotenoids: from plants to food and feed industries." *Methods Mol Biol* 1852:57–71. doi: 10.1007/978-1-4939-8742-9_3.

Lawson, L. D., and S. M. Hunsaker. 2018. "Allicin bioavailability and bioequivalence from garlic supplements and garlic foods." *Nutrients* 10 (7):812. doi: 10.3390/nu10070812.

Lawson, L. D., and Z. J. Wang. 2005. "Allicin and allicin-derived garlic compounds increase breath acetone through allyl methyl sulfide: use in measuring allicin bioavailability." *J Agric Food Chem* 53 (6):1974–1983. doi: 10.1021/jf048323s.

Li, D., P. Wang, Y. Luo, M. Zhao, and F. Chen. 2017. "Health benefits of anthocyanins and molecular mechanisms: update from recent decade." *Crit Rev Food Sci Nutr* 57 (8):1729–1741. doi: 10.1080/10408398.2015.1030064.

Li, X., J. Xu, X. Tang, Y. Liu, X. Yu, Z. Wang, and W. Liu. 2016. "Anthocyanins inhibit trastuzumab-resistant breast cancer in vitro and in vivo." *Mol Med Rep* 13 (5):4007–4013. doi: 10.3892/mmr.2016.4990.

Li, S., S. Yuan, Q. Zhao, B. Wang, X. Wang, and K. Li. 2018. "Quercetin enhances chemotherapeutic effect of doxorubicin against human breast cancer cells while reducing toxic side effects of it." *Biomed Pharmacother* 100:441–447. doi: 10.1016/j.biopha.2018.02.055.

Liu, R. H. 2013. "Health-promoting components of fruits and vegetables in the diet." *Adv Nutr* 4 (3):384S–392S. doi: 10.3945/an.112.003517.

Liu, Y. E., D. H. Tan, C. C. Tong, Y. B. Zhang, Y. Xu, X. W. Liu, Y. Gao, and M. X. Hou. 2015. "Blueberry anthocyanins ameliorate radiation-induced lung injury through the protein kinase RNA-activated pathway." *Chemico-Biological Interactions* 242:363–371. doi: 10.1016/j.cbi.2015.11.001.

Llaverias, G., J. C. Escola-Gil, E. Lerma, J. Julve, C. Pons, A. Cabre, M. Cofan, E. Ros, J. L. Sanchez-Quesada, and F. Blanco-Vaca. 2013. "Phytosterols inhibit the tumor growth and lipoprotein oxidizability induced by a high-fat diet in mice with inherited breast cancer." *J Nutr Biochem* 24 (1):39–48. doi: 10.1016/j.jnutbio.2012.01.007.

Marian, M. J. 2017. "Dietary supplements commonly used by cancer survivors: are there any benefits?" *Nutr Clin Pract* 32 (5):607–627. doi: 10.1177/0884533617721687.

McNaughton, S. A., and G. C. Marks. 2003. "Development of a food composition database for the estimation of dietary intakes of glucosinolates, the biologically active constituents of cruciferous vegetables." *Br J Nutr* 90 (3):687–697. doi: 10.1079/bjn2003917.

Mo, H., R. Jeter, A. Bachmann, S. T. Yount, C. L. Shen, and H. Yeganehjoo. 2018. "The potential of isoprenoids in adjuvant cancer therapy to reduce adverse effects of statins." *Front Pharmacol* 9:1515. doi: 10.3389/fphar.2018.01515.

Overall, J., S. A. Bonney, M. Wilson, A. Beermann, M. H. Grace, D. Esposito, M. A. Lila, and S. Komarnytsky. 2017. "Metabolic effects of berries with structurally diverse anthocyanins." *Int J Mol Sci* 18 (2). doi: 10.3390/ijms18020422.

Paller, C. J., A. Pantuck, and M. A. Carducci. 2017. "A review of pomegranate in prostate cancer." *Prostate Cancer Prostatic Dis* 20 (3):265–270. doi: 10.1038/pcan.2017.19.

Paller, C. J., X. Ye, P. J. Wozniak, B. K. Gillespie, P. R. Sieber, R. H. Greengold, B. R. Stockton, B. L. Hertzman, M. D. Efros, R. P. Roper, H. R. Liker, and M. A. Carducci. 2013. "A randomized phase II study of pomegranate extract for men with rising PSA following initial therapy for localized prostate cancer." *Prostate Cancer Prostatic Dis* 16 (1):50–55. doi: 10.1038/pcan.2012.20.

Pantuck, A. J., J. T. Leppert, N. Zomorodian, W. Aronson, J. Hong, R. J. Barnard, N. Seeram, H. Liker, H. Wang, R. Elashoff, D. Heber, M. Aviram, L. Ignarro, and A. Belldegrun. 2006. "Phase II study of pomegranate juice for men with rising prostate-specific antigen following surgery or radiation for prostate cancer." *Clin Cancer Res* 12 (13):4018–4026. doi: 10.1158/1078-0432.CCR-05-2290.

Pantuck, A. J., C. A. Pettaway, R. Dreicer, J. Corman, A. Katz, A. Ho, W. Aronson, W. Clark, G. Simmons, and D. Heber. 2015. "A randomized, double-blind, placebo-controlled study of the effects of pomegranate extract on rising PSA levels in men following primary therapy for prostate cancer." *Prostate Cancer Prostatic Dis* 18 (3):242–248. doi: 10.1038/pcan.2015.32.

Paterni, I., C. Granchi, J. A. Katzenellenbogen, and F. Minutolo. 2014. "Estrogen receptors alpha (ERalpha) and beta (ERbeta): subtype-selective ligands and clinical potential." *Steroids* 90:13–29. doi: 10.1016/j.steroids.2014.06.012.

Puccinelli, M. T., and S. D. Stan. 2017. "Dietary bioactive diallyl trisulfide in cancer prevention and treatment." *Int J Mol Sci* 18 (8):1645. doi: 10.3390/ijms18081645.

Reglero, C., and G. Reglero. 2019. "Precision nutrition and cancer relapse prevention: a systematic literature review." *Nutrients* 11 (11):2799. doi: 10.3390/nu11112799.

Rettig, M. B., D. Heber, J. An, N. P. Seeram, J. Y. Rao, H. Liu, T. Klatte, A. Belldegrun, A. Moro, S. M. Henning, D. Mo, W. J. Aronson, and A. Pantuck. 2008. "Pomegranate extract inhibits androgen-independent prostate cancer growth through a nuclear factor-kappaB-dependent mechanism." *Mol Cancer Ther* 7 (9):2662–71. doi: 10.1158/1535–7163.MCT–08–0136.

Rodriguez-Amaya, D. B. 2016. "Structures and analysis of carotenoid molecules." *Subcell Biochem* 79:71–108. doi: 10.1007/978-3-319-39126-7_3.

Rodriguez-Garcia, C., C. Sanchez-Quesada, E. Toledo, M. Delgado-Rodriguez, and J. J. Gaforio. 2019. "Naturally lignan-rich foods: a dietary tool for health promotion?" *Molecules* 24 (5):917. doi: 10.3390/molecules24050917.

Romo-Vaquero, M., A. Cortes-Martin, V. Loria-Kohen, A. Ramirez-de-Molina, I. Garcia-Mantrana, M. C. Collado, J. C. Espin, and M. V. Selma. 2019. "Deciphering the human gut microbiome of urolithin metabotypes: association with enterotypes and potential cardiometabolic health implications." *Mol Nutr Food Res* 63 (4):e1800958. doi: 10.1002/mnfr.201800958.

Ronis, M. J. J., K. B. Pedersen, and J. Watt. 2018. "Adverse effects of nutraceuticals and dietary supplements." *Annu Rev Pharmacol Toxicol* 58:583–601. doi: 10.1146/annurev-pharmtox-010617-052844.

Rowles, J. L., 3rd, K. M. Ranard, J. W. Smith, R. An, and J. W. Erdman, Jr. 2017. "Increased dietary and circulating lycopene are associated with reduced prostate cancer risk: a systematic review and meta-analysis." *Prostate Cancer Prostatic Dis* 20 (4):361–377. doi: 10.1038/pcan.2017.25.

Russo, G. I., D. Campisi, M. Di Mauro, F. Regis, G. Reale, M. Marranzano, R. Ragusa, T. Solinas, M. Madonia, S. Cimino, and G. Morgia. 2017. "Dietary consumption of phenolic acids and prostate cancer: a case-control study in Sicily, Southern Italy." *Molecules* 22 (12). doi: 10.3390/molecules22122159.

Sahin, I., B. Bilir, S. Ali, K. Sahin, and O. Kucuk. 2019. "Soy isoflavones in integrative oncology: increased efficacy and decreased toxicity of cancer therapy." *Integr Cancer Ther* 18. doi: 10.1177/1534735419835310.

Sahin, K., C. Orhan, M. Tuzcu, N. Sahin, S. Ali, I. H. Bahcecioglu, O. Guler, I. Ozercan, N. Ilhan, and O. Kucuk. 2014. "Orally administered lycopene attenuates diethylnitrosamine-induced hepatocarcinogenesis in rats by modulating Nrf-2/HO-1 and Akt/mTOR pathways." *Nutr Cancer* 66 (4):590–598. doi: 10.1080/01635581.2014.894092.

Sang, S., and Y. Chu. 2017. "Whole grain oats, more than just a fiber: role of unique phytochemicals." *Mol Nutr Food Res* 61 (7). doi: 10.1002/mnfr.201600715.

Satoh, H., K. Nishikawa, K. Suzuki, R. Asano, N. Virgona, T. Ichikawa, K. Hagiwara, and T. Yano. 2003. "Genistein, a soy isoflavone, enhances necrotic-like cell death in a breast cancer cell treated with a chemotherapeutic agent." *Res Commun Mol Pathol Pharmacol* 113–114:149–158.

Seeram, N. P., W. J. Aronson, Y. Zhang, S. M. Henning, A. Moro, R. P. Lee, M. Sartippour, D. M. Harris, M. Rettig, M. A. Suchard, A. J. Pantuck, A. Belldegrun, and D. Heber. 2007. "Pomegranate ellagitannin-derived metabolites inhibit prostate cancer growth and localize to the mouse prostate gland." *J Agric Food Chem* 55 (19):7732–7737. doi: 10.1021/jf071303g.

Seeram, N. P., S. M. Henning, Y. Zhang, M. Suchard, Z. Li, and D. Heber. 2006. "Pomegranate juice ellagitannin metabolites are present in human plasma and some persist in urine for up to 48 hours." *J Nutr* 136 (10):2481–2485. doi: 10.1093/jn/136.10.2481.

Selma, M. V., D. Beltran, R. Garcia-Villalba, J. C. Espin, and F. A. Tomas-Barberan. 2014. "Description of urolithin production capacity from ellagic acid of two human intestinal Gordonibacter species." *Food Funct* 5 (8):1779–1784. doi: 10.1039/c4fo00092g.

Selma, M. V., A. Gonzalez-Sarrias, J. Salas-Salvado, C. Andres-Lacueva, C. Alasalvar, A. Orem, F. A. Tomas-Barberan, and J. C. Espin. 2018. "The gut microbiota metabolism of pomegranate or walnut ellagitannins yields two urolithin-metabotypes that correlate with cardiometabolic risk biomarkers: Comparison between normoweight, overweight-obesity and metabolic syndrome." *Clin Nutr* 37 (3):897–905. doi: 10.1016/j.clnu.2017.03.012.

Shete, V., and L. Quadro. 2013. "Mammalian metabolism of beta-carotene: gaps in knowledge." *Nutrients* 5 (12):4849–68. doi: 10.3390/nu5124849.

Siddarth, P., Z. Li, K. J. Miller, L. M. Ercoli, D. A. Merril, S. M. Henning, D. Heber, and G. W. Small. 2020. "Randomized placebo-controlled study of the memory effects of pomegranate juice in middle-aged and older adults." *Am J Clin Nutr* 111 (1):170–177. doi: 10.1093/ajcn/nqz241.

Sirerol, J. A., M. L. Rodriguez, S. Mena, M. A. Asensi, J. M. Estrela, and A. L. Ortega. 2016. "Role of Natural Stilbenes in the Prevention of Cancer." *Oxid Med Cell Longev* 2016:3128951. doi: 10.1155/2016/3128951.

Slamon, D. J., G. M. Clark, S. G. Wong, W. J. Levin, A. Ullrich, and W. L. McGuire. 1987. "Human breast cancer: correlation of relapse and survival with amplification of the HER-2/neu oncogene." *Science* 235 (4785):177–182. doi: 10.1126/science.3798106.

Slimestad, R., T. Fossen, and I. M. Vagen. 2007. "Onions: a source of unique dietary flavonoids." *J Agric Food Chem* 55 (25):10067–10080. doi: 10.1021/jf0712503.

Stenner-Liewen, F., H. Liewen, R. Cathomas, C. Renner, U. Petrausch, T. Sulser, K. Spanaus, H. H. Seifert, R. T. Strebel, A. Knuth, P. Samaras, and M. Muntener. 2013. "Daily pomegranate intake has no impact on PSA levels in patients with advanced prostate cancer - results of a phase IIb randomized controlled trial." *J Cancer* 4 (7):597–605. doi: 10.7150/jca.7123.

Subash, S., N. Braidy, M. M. Essa, A. B. Zayana, V. Ragini, S. Al-Adawi, A. Al-Asmi, and G. J. Guillemin. 2015. "Long-term (15 mo) dietary supplementation with pomegranates from Oman attenuates cognitive and behavioral deficits in a transgenic mice model of Alzheimer's disease." *Nutrition* 31 (1):223–229. doi: 10.1016/j.nut.2014.06.004.

Subash, S., M. M. Essa, A. Al-Asmi, S. Al-Adawi, R. Vaishnav, N. Braidy, T. Manivasagam, and G. J. Guillemin. 2014. "Pomegranate from Oman alleviates the brain oxidative damage in transgenic mouse model of Alzheimer's disease." *J Tradit Complement Med* 4 (4):232–238. doi: 10.4103/2225-4110.139107.

Thomas, R., M. Williams, H. Sharma, A. Chaudry, and P. Bellamy. 2014. "A double-blind, placebo-controlled randomised trial evaluating the effect of a polyphenol-rich whole food supplement on PSA progression in men with prostate cancer--the U.K. NCRN Pomi-T study." *Prostate Cancer Prostatic Dis* 17 (2):180–6. doi: 10.1038/pcan.2014.6.

Thomson, C. A., E. Ho, and M. B. Strom. 2016. "Chemopreventive properties of 3,3'-diindolylmethane in breast cancer: evidence from experimental and human studies." *Nutr Rev* 74 (7):432–443. doi: 10.1093/nutrit/nuw010.

Tomas-Barberan, F. A., M. V. Selma, and J. C. Espin. 2016. "Interactions of gut microbiota with dietary polyphenols and consequences to human health." *Curr Opin Clin Nutr Metab Care* 19 (6):471–476. doi: 10.1097/MCO.0000000000000314.

Tseng, M., C. Byrne, M. S. Kurzer, and C. Y. Fang. 2013. "Equol-producing status, isoflavone intake, and breast density in a sample of U.S. Chinese women." *Cancer Epidemiol Biomarkers Prev* 22 (11):1975–1983. doi: 10.1158/1055-9965.EPI-13-0593.

Unlu, N. Z., T. Bohn, S. K. Clinton, and S. J. Schwartz. 2005. "Carotenoid absorption from salad and salsa by humans is enhanced by the addition of avocado or avocado oil." *J Nutr* 135 (3):431–436. doi: 10.1093/jn/135.3.431.

Valko, M., D. Leibfritz, J. Moncol, M. T. Cronin, M. Mazur, and J. Telser. 2007. "Free radicals and antioxidants in normal physiological functions and human disease." *Int J Biochem Cell Biol* 39 (1):44–84. doi: 10.1016/j.biocel.2006.07.001.

Van Hoang, D., N. M. Pham, A. H. Lee, D. N. Tran, and C. W. Binns. 2018. "Dietary carotenoid intakes and prostate cancer risk: a case-control study from Vietnam." *Nutrients* 10 (1). doi: 10.3390/nu10010070.

Vanduchova, A., P. Anzenbacher, and E. Anzenbacherova. 2019. "Isothiocyanate from broccoli, sulforaphane, and its properties." *J Med Food* 22 (2):121–126. doi: 10.1089/jmf.2018.0024.

Vernieri, C., F. Nichetti, A. Raimondi, S. Pusceddu, M. Platania, F. Berrino, and F. de Braud. 2018. "Diet and supplements in cancer prevention and treatment: clinical evidences and future perspectives." *Crit Rev Oncol Hematol* 123:57–73. doi: 10.1016/j.critrevonc.2018.01.002.

Wang, T. Y., Q. Li, and K. S. Bi. 2018. "Bioactive flavonoids in medicinal plants: Structure, activity and biological fate." *Asian J Pharm Sci* 13 (1):12–23. doi: 10.1016/j.ajps.2017.08.004.

Wang, Y., J. Qian, J. Cao, D. Wang, C. Liu, R. Yang, X. Li, and C. Sun. 2017. "Antioxidant capacity, anticancer ability and flavonoids composition of 35 citrus (Citrus reticulata Blanco) varieties." *Molecules* 22 (7):1114. doi: 10.3390/molecules22071114.

Wattenberg, L. W., and W. D. Loub. 1978. "Inhibition of polycyclic aromatic hydrocarbon-induced neoplasia by naturally occurring indoles." *Cancer Res* 38 (5):1410–1413.

Wu, S., and L. Tian. 2017. "Diverse phytochemicals and bioactivities in the ancient fruit and modern functional food pomegranate (Punica granatum)." *Molecules* 22 (10):1606. doi: 10.3390/molecules22101606.

Xavier, A. A., and A. Perez-Galvez. 2016. "Carotenoids as a source of antioxidants in the diet." *Subcell Biochem* 79:359–375. doi: 10.1007/978-3-319-39126-7_14.

Yang, C. S., and H. Wang. 2016. "Cancer preventive activities of tea catechins." *Molecules* 21 (12):1679. doi: 10.3390/molecules21121679.

Yin, R., T. Li, J. X. Tian, P. Xi, and R. H. Liu. 2018. "Ursolic acid, a potential anticancer compound for breast cancer therapy." *Crit Rev Food Sci Nutr* 58 (4):568–574. doi: 10.1080/10408398.2016.1203755.

Yoshida, K., M. Mori, and T. Kondo. 2009. "Blue flower color development by anthocyanins: from chemical structure to cell physiology." *Nat Prod Rep* 26 (7):884–915. doi: 10.1039/b800165k.

Yuan, T., H. Ma, W. Liu, D. B. Niesen, N. Shah, R. Crews, K. N. Rose, D. A. Vattem, and N. P. Seeram. 2016. "Pomegranate's neuroprotective effects against Alzheimer's disease are mediated by urolithins, its ellagitannin-gut microbial derived metabolites." *ACS Chem Neurosci* 7 (1):26–33. doi: 10.1021/acschemneuro.5b00260.

Zamora-Ros, R., J. A. Rothwell, A. Scalbert, V. Knaze, I. Romieu, N. Slimani, G. Fagherazzi, F. Perquier, M. Touillaud, E. Molina-Montes, J. M. Huerta, A. Barricarte, P. Amiano, V. Menendez, R. Tumino, M. S. de Magistris, D. Palli, F. Ricceri, S. Sieri, F. L. Crowe, K. T. Khaw, N. J. Wareham, V. Grote, K. Li, H. Boeing, J. Forster, A. Trichopoulou, V. Benetou, K. Tsiotas, H. B. Bueno-de-Mesquita, M. Ros, P. H. Peeters, A. Tjonneland, J. Halkjaer, K. Overvad, U. Ericson, P. Wallstrom, I. Johansson, R. Landberg, E. Weiderpass, D. Engeset, G. Skeie, P. Wark, E. Riboli, and C. A. Gonzalez. 2013. "Dietary intakes and food sources of phenolic acids in the European Prospective Investigation into Cancer and Nutrition (EPIC) study." *Br J Nutr* 110 (8):1500–1511. doi: 10.1017/S0007114513000688.

Zhang, Y. J., R. Y. Gan, S. Li, Y. Zhou, A. N. Li, D. P. Xu, and H. B. Li. 2015. "Antioxidant phytochemicals for the prevention and treatment of chronic diseases." *Molecules* 20 (12):21138–21156. doi: 10.3390/molecules201219753.

Zhang, N. Q., S. C. Ho, X. F. Mo, F. Y. Lin, W. Q. Huang, H. Luo, J. Huang, and C. X. Zhang. 2018. "Glucosinolate and isothiocyanate intakes are inversely associated with breast cancer risk: a case-control study in China." *Br J Nutr* 119 (8):957–964. doi: 10.1017/S0007114518000600.

Zhang, Z., C. Z. Wang, G. J. Du, L. W. Qi, T. Calway, T. C. He, W. Du, and C. S. Yuan. 2013. "Genistein induces G2/M cell cycle arrest and apoptosis via ATM/p53-dependent pathway in human colon cancer cells." *Int J Oncol* 43 (1):289–296. doi: 10.3892/ijo.2013.1946.

Zhao, W., L. Liu, and S. Xu. 2018. "Intakes of citrus fruit and risk of esophageal cancer: a meta-analysis." *Medicine (Baltimore)* 97 (13):e0018. doi: 10.1097/MD.0000000000010018.

Zhou, C., W. Qian, J. Ma, L. Cheng, Z. Jiang, B. Yan, J. Li, W. Duan, L. Sun, J. Cao, F. Wang, E. Wu, Z. Wu, Q. Ma, and X. Li. 2019. "Resveratrol enhances the chemotherapeutic response and reverses the stemness induced by gemcitabine in pancreatic cancer cells via targeting SREBP1." *Cell Prolif* 52 (1):e12514. doi: 10.1111/cpr.12514.

Zhou, Y., T. Wang, Q. Meng, and S. Zhai. 2016. "Association of carotenoids with risk of gastric cancer: a meta-analysis." *Clin Nutr* 35 (1):109–116. doi: 10.1016/j.clnu.2015.02.003.

Zhou, Y., J. Zheng, Y. Li, D. P. Xu, S. Li, Y. M. Chen, and H. B. Li. 2016. "Natural polyphenols for prevention and treatment of cancer." *Nutrients* 8 (8):515. doi: 10.3390/nu8080515.

5 Nutrition and Immune Function

Emily Truong and Berkeley N. Limketkai
David Geffen School of Medicine at UCLA

CONTENTS

INTRODUCTION

The integral role that nutrition plays in immunity has given rise to nutritional immunology, a field that has focused on understanding the interactions between nutrition and the immune system. The importance of this relationship is highlighted by the clinical impact of nutrition on immune function, immune-mediated disease, and associated complications. Malnutrition and severe deficiencies of even single micronutrients (e.g., vitamin A and vitamin C) have been shown to cause profound illness and death. On the other hand, excess consumption of certain nutrients, such as saturated fats or refined carbohydrates, has been associated with increased risk of immune-mediated conditions, such as diabetes, allergy, psoriasis, and inflammatory bowel disease (IBD). Besides avoiding purportedly detrimental nutrients to help treat disease, select nutrients also have intrinsic therapeutic benefits through their immune-boosting, anti-inflammatory, or antioxidant properties.

The interaction between nutrients and immunity relies on broad and complex mechanisms. For one, a deficiency of nutrient substrates critical for maintenance of the innate or adaptive arms of the immune system can lead to a breakdown of immune function and a subsequent increased susceptibility to infections. Nutrient-derived metabolites can directly bind and regulate immune cells; alternatively, they could act as substrates or cofactors along pro- or anti-inflammatory pathways.

Food constituents can also indirectly influence inflammation through their beneficial or detrimental effects on intestinal microbial composition and mucosal health. Intestinal dysbiosis may favor enrichment of more pathogenic strains of bacteria and/or synthesis of proinflammatory metabolites. Moreover, compromise of mucosal integrity (increased intestinal permeability) would facilitate bacterial antigen translocation with local activation of mucosal immune cells and/or distal immune activation by systemically circulating antigens.

The diet strongly influences the gut microbiota, a mediator in the nutrition-immune function axis. The symbiotic relationship between host and gut microbiota involves a delicate trade-off between maintaining self-tolerance and eliminating harmful pathogens. Categorization of gut microbiota depends on secreted immunoglobulin A (IgA). In the small intestine, dendritic cells sample commensal antigens from gut microbiota and cause differentiation of regulatory T cells and IgA-producing B cells, which travel to Peyer's patches to stimulate further class switching and production of IgA specific for commensal antigens (Macpherson and Uhr 2004). The host benefits from developing self-tolerance to gut microbiota, which regulate both innate and adaptive immune homeostasis. Commensal bacteria promote induction of both regulatory T cells and Th17 cells while limiting inflammation (Round et al. 2011). For instance, upon encountering microbial ligands in the tissue, inflammatory monocytes can generate prostaglandin E_2 (PGE_2) to limit tissue damage from neutrophil activation (Grainger et al. 2013). Alongside regulating immune homeostasis, gut microbiota beneficially curb pathogenic microbes by competing for scarce nutrients, creating antimicrobial peptides, or inducing T and C cell responses against pathogens (Belkaid and Hand 2014). Alteration in the diverse, continually evolving gut microbiota communities often leads to weakened immunity, immune dysregulation, and the development of autoimmune disorders, whether intestinal or systemic. Certain microbial profiles have been associated with intestinal inflammation, such as the general increase in Bacteroidetes, Proteobacteria, and *Escherichia coli* and the reduction in Firmicutes, although cause or effect has not yet been established (Walker et al. 2011, Ott et al. 2004). Studies have also shown that malnutrition or deficiency of nutrients such as vitamin A adversely influences the microbiota population in a manner that leads to downregulation of Th17 cells and T cell migration to the gastrointestinal tract in response to antigens (Ott et al. 2004, Hall et al. 2011, Cha et al. 2010). As the intestine remains the primary site of nutrient absorption, the gut microbiome, immune system, and nutritional status share an exquisitely sensitive, multidirectional relationship.

This chapter will discuss several nutrients or food constituents with demonstrated effects on immune function, the theoretical basis for their effect, and their role in the pathogenesis of immune-mediated disease. This chapter then concludes with a discussion on our current understanding of immunonutrition in cancer prevention and treatment. Familiarity with this diversity of nutritional effects on the immune system underlies the strategic approach to recommending diets for immune health and treatment of disease, while identifying promising avenues for further investigation.

NUTRIENT–IMMUNE SYSTEM INTERACTIONS

VITAMIN A

The family of vitamin A comprises dietary retinol, its esterified form, and carotenoid precursors (Limketkai, Matarese, and Mullin 2020). The critical role of vitamin A for immunity is evident through the detrimental effects of vitamin A deficiency on immune function and infections. Supporting the innate immune system, vitamin A appears to regulate the mucosal epithelium and production of the mucus layer; a deficiency in vitamin A leads to a compromise of the mucosal barrier and increased risk and severity of infections in the respiratory and gastrointestinal tracts (Amit-Romach et al. 2009, McDaniel et al. 2015, Xing et al. 2020). Vitamin A additionally promotes development of natural killer cells and neutrophils, whereby low vitamin A concentrations have been associated with reduced titers and lytic activity of natural killer cells, impaired phagocytosis, and decreased bactericidal activity (Stephensen 2001). For the adaptive immune system, vitamin A regulates development of T helper (Th) lymphocytes and B lymphocytes. Vitamin A deficiency can lead to dysfunction in the cell-mediated and humoral immune responses, respectively. Besides vitamin A, β-carotene, a provitamin A molecule, has also been shown to regulate cell-mediated and humoral immunity. Moreover, provitamin A and nonprovitamin A carotenoids possess broader antioxidant properties that modulate cellular injury from reactive oxygen species (ROS), particularly in the setting of stress or an active infection (Chew and Park 2004). As such, dietary deprivation of vitamin A can lead to an increase in infection-related deaths in rodents, while vitamin A supplementation in children from impoverished countries has been shown to reduce the incidence of diarrhea, measles, and death (Green and Mellanby 1928, Mayo-Wilson et al. 2011).

Vitamin C

Vitamin C (ascorbic acid) is an essential micronutrient in humans due to our lack of L-gulono-1,4-γ-lactone oxidase that converts glucose to ascorbic acid (Limketkai, Matarese, and Mullin 2020). The major manifestation of vitamin C deficiency is scurvy, characterized by hemorrhage, bleeding gums, abnormal wound healing, impaired immunity, and death. Early recognition of its importance occurred in 1593 when Sir Richard Hawkins observed oranges and lemons to be most effective at staving off the scourge of scurvy among his sailors (Tickner and Medvei 1958). In 1601, Captain James Lancaster of the East India Company inadvertently stocked only one of his four vessels with lemon juice on a voyage to the East Indies. The health and survival of the crew on his flagship vessel, compared with the other accompanying vessels, was later attributed to the lemon juice. In 1757, James Lind, physician of the Royal Navy, published the first recorded prospective controlled clinical trial, where he found oranges and lemon to be more effective than other elixirs to treat scurvy.

Vitamin C possesses important effects on the synthesis of collagen and other connective tissues, thus conferring it an important role in the maintenance of the epithelial barriers of the innate immune system (Limketkai, Matarese, and Mullin 2020). Vitamin C additionally enhances neutrophil activity, lymphocyte development, and antibody/complement production (Prinz et al. 1977, Anderson et al. 1980, Manning et al. 2013). Experiments on the effects of vitamin C deficiency found that among guinea pigs exposed to *Mycobacterium tuberculosis* in their feed, those that received a diet partially deficient in vitamin C were more prone to developing intestinal tuberculosis than those with adequate vitamin C (McConkey and Smith 1933). Inversely, vitamin C supplementation has been found to improve infections. In a randomized controlled trial (RCT) of 57 geriatric patients admitted for acute respiratory infections, those who were administered 200 mg/day of vitamin C improved better than those who received placebo (Hunt et al. 1994). A systematic review and meta-analysis performed by the Cochrane Collaboration found that 200 mg/day of vitamin C might reduce the duration and severity of the common cold (Hemilä and Chalker 2013). Vitamin C was also found to reduce the common cold among those who experience severe physical stress, but not in the general population. These findings suggest that routine vitamin C supplementation might not be helpful, particularly among those without a vitamin C deficiency, although there are certain scenarios where supplementation may provide a low-risk, low-cost benefit.

Vitamin D

Vitamin D is a fat-soluble secosteroid that includes ergocalciferol (vitamin D_2) and cholecalciferol (vitamin D_3) (Limketkai et al. 2017). In humans, ergocalciferol can only be derived from exogenous dietary sources, while cholecalciferol can either be derived from diet, supplementation, or endogenous production through ultraviolet light exposure. Vitamin D is hydroxylated in the liver to 25-hydroxyvitamin D and, in the kidneys, to its active metabolite: 1,25-dihydroxyvitamin D. The function of vitamin D had historically been attributed to the maintenance of bone health, although more recent studies revealed immune-related functions as well (Abe et al. 1981, Provvedini et al. 1983). As an innate immune response, when the epithelial barrier is compromised, vitamin D promotes expression of Toll-like receptors and downstream production of antimicrobial peptides (Schauber et al. 2007). Vitamin also directly induces expression of human cathelicidin antimicrobial peptide and defensin β_2 (Wang et al. 2004, Gombart, Borregaard, and Koeffler 2005). The vitamin D receptor has been shown to regulate the development of B lymphocytes, T lymphocytes, macrophages, and natural killer cells (Kreutz et al. 1993, Chen et al. 2007, Yu and Cantorna 2008, Cantorna et al. 2015). Despite these demonstrated effects of vitamin D, the evidence demonstrating an association between vitamin D and infections is still tenuous. Ecological studies have relied on the north-south gradient (where residents of more northern regions receive less sunlight) or seasonal variations of vitamin D deficiency and the incidence of influenza to suggest an association between the two (Cannell et al. 2006). A large number of observational studies also found an inverse relationship between vitamin D concentrations and self-reported upper respiratory infections (Ginde, Mansbach, and Camargo 2009). However, randomized controlled trials that compared vitamin D supplementation with placebo inconsistently showed benefit for reducing the incidence of influenza (Urashima et al. 2010, Arihiro et al. 2019, Loeb et al. 2019). Given its immunomodulatory properties, vitamin D has nonetheless been implicated in multiple immune-mediated conditions, such as multiple sclerosis (MS), rheumatoid arthritis, IBD, and asthma (Limketkai, Matarese, and Mullin 2020).

ZINC

Zinc is among the most abundant trace elements in the body and serves as an enzymatic cofactor for a broad host of cellular processes (Limketkai, Matarese, and Mullin 2020). For innate immunity, zinc appears to play a critical role for wound healing and maintenance of the epithelial barrier, neutrophil chemotaxis, and neutrophil bactericidal activity (through ROS and neutrophil extracellular traps) (Vruwink et al. 1991, Hasegawa et al. 2000, Hasan, Rink, and Haase 2013). Interestingly, the immune system manipulates zinc availability as a host defense mechanism. Chelation of zinc by neutrophil-derived calprotectin has been shown to inhibit bacterial growth; in response, *Neisseria meningitidis* secretes protein receptors for calprotectin to not only elude zinc deprivation but to even capitalize on this rich source of protein-bound zinc (Corbin et al. 2008, Stork et al. 2013). Macrophages also rely on zinc transporters to deplete zinc from phagosomes where microorganisms are trapped (Subramanian Vignesh et al. 2013). Inversely, high zinc concentrations have been hypothesized to possess bactericidal properties. For the adaptive immune system, zinc influences development and proliferation of B lymphocytes and T lymphocytes, lymphocyte function, and antibody production (Fraker, Haas, and Luecke 1977, Dowd, Kelleher, and Guillou 1986, Moulder and Steward 1989, Cook-Mills and Fraker 1993, Maywald et al. 2017). Zinc deficiency can also lead to vitamin A deficiency that then interferes with vitamin A-associated immune functions (Limketkai, Matarese, and Mullin 2020). The immune benefits of zinc have been suggested in studies of zinc supplementation. Data from several studies suggest that zinc supplementation might reduce the duration of the common cold, although these findings have not been consistent (Godfrey, Godfrey, and Novick 1996, Mossad et al. 1996, Eby and Halcomb 2006).

COPPER

Copper is an essential trace mineral that serves as an enzymatic cofactor for numerous cellular and physiologic processes (Limketkai, Matarese, and Mullin 2020). Copper possesses important roles in connective tissue synthesis that is integral to maintaining the epithelial barrier for the innate immune system. Although uncommon in humans, copper deficiency leads to an arrest in the maturation of granulocytes, resulting in neutropenia (Dunlap, James, and Hume 1974, Zidar et al. 1977). Lack of adequate copper stores also adversely impacts neutrophil and macrophage function by decreasing phagocytic activity, superoxide dismutase activity, and overall killing capacity, whereas copper treatment strengthens intracellular killing of bacteria such as *Escherichia coli* (Babu and Failla 1990, Xin et al. 1991, White et al. 2009). In the adaptive immune system, copper deficiency is characterized by decreased antibody production by spleen cells (Koller et al. 1987, Lukasewycz and Prohaska 1990). This altered proliferation response is secondary to reduced concentrations of interleukin (IL)-2, leading to impaired mitogen-induced synthesis of DNA, which remains apparent even in states of marginal copper deficiency (Bala and Failla 1992). However, it remains unclear why IL-2 concentrations are decreased in patients with copper deficiency.

Iron

Essential for almost all living organisms, iron functions as an important cofactor in numerous oxidation-reduction reactions in its versatile states: ferrous (Fe^{2+}) or ferric (Fe^{3+}). Ferric iron is absorbed in the proximal duodenum, reduced to ferrous iron, and transported into the enterocyte through the divalent metal transporter 1 (DMT1). Ferrous iron can then be used for intracellular processes, stored, or exit the cell through the FPN1 transporter. Though iron functions as a limiting growth factor in its insoluble oxide form, which is not taken up readily, iron remains cytotoxic at high concentrations due to the formation of oxidative radicals through the Fenton reaction. As iron is critical for cell proliferation and activation in both host and pathogen cells, iron sequestration has long been recognized an important immune defense. During infection or inflammation, immune cells upregulate expression of mediators such as IL-1, IL-6, interferon-gamma, and tumor necrosis factor-alpha (TNF-α) and stimulate liver release of hepcidin (Nemeth et al. 2004, Lee et al. 2005, Weiss 2005, Nairz et al. 2010). Modulation of iron metabolism through both hepcidin-independent and hepcidin-dependent mechanisms inhibits FPN1 transport and iron efflux, thereby fortifying iron sequestration defenses and resulting in the commonly encountered anemia of chronic disease. Deprived of the iron necessary for growth and proliferation, pathogens evolved to counteract this innate immune defense by developing heme uptake systems, producing siderophores to chelate iron from host proteins, or utilizing transferrin or lactoferrin receptors (Schryvers and Morris 1988, Miyamoto et al. 2009, Cassat and Skaar 2012). Both deficiency and excess of iron can adversely impact immune functions. Iron deficiency impairs T lymphocyte proliferation, delayed hypersensitivity, and respiratory burst (Kuvibidila, Baliga, and Suskind 1981, Ahluwalia et al. 2004). On the other hand, iron excess is associated with increased susceptibility to infection due to increased hepcidin and ferritin levels, as well as decreased production of nitric oxide and IL-12 (Mencacci et al. 1997, Magnus et al. 1999, Gangaidzo et al. 2001, Singh and Sun 2008). Furthermore, iron-related proteins such as lactoferrin and transferrin have been shown to affect Th1/Th2 cell activities and early T-cell differentiation, respectively (Macedo et al. 2004, Fischer et al. 2006). Numerous mechanisms involved in iron homeostasis and transport are integral to immunity and continue to be investigated.

Tryptophan

As an essential amino acid found in many protein-rich foods, tryptophan serves as a broad host of metabolic purposes including nitrogen homeostasis and production of niacin and serotonin, the precursor for melatonin. Tryptophan is predominantly degraded through the kynurenine pathway, which utilizes indoleamine 2,3-dioxygenase 1(IDO1) and tryptophan-2,3-dioxygenase as rate-limiting enzymes. Recently, these enzymes and their roles in tryptophan catabolism have emerged as vital mechanisms for immune tolerance, such as the prevention of fetal rejection during pregnancy and protection against inflammatory arthritis (Munn et al. 1998, Grohmann et al. 2003, Ogbechi et al. 2020). The proposed mechanisms involve (1) tryptophan depletion and (2) the accumulation of tryptophan catabolites. The prevailing view holds that tryptophan depletion inhibits both T-cell replication (by causing arrest during the G1 phase of the cell cycle) and T-cell proliferation (by inactivating the mTOR pathway) (Munn et al. 1998, Mellor and Munn 2004, Metz et al. 2012). Downstream production of tryptophan's metabolic byproducts, known as kynurenines, have been implicated in inducing apoptosis of Th1, but not Th2, cells (Fallarino et al. 2002, Terness et al. 2002). Tryptophan catabolites additionally induce differentiation of regulatory T lymphocytes, which crucially regulate self-reactive T lymphocytes in the periphery (Fallarino et al. 2006). Interestingly, dietary supplements such as probiotics, omega-3 polyunsaturated fatty acids (ω-3 PUFAs), and antioxidants decrease IDO activity and thus inhibit activation of Th1-type immune cascades (Weyh, Krüger, and Strasser 2020). However, attempts to supplement tryptophan through dietary protein enrichment in hospitalized older patients with hip fractures failed to improve elevated Th1-type immune responses, illustrating that further research is necessary to investigate the role of tryptophan and its catabolites in the diet (Strasser et al. 2020).

FIBER

Fiber's numerous health benefits have long been recognized. Higher intake of dietary fiber contributes to enhanced laxation, lower body weight, improved satiation, increased uptake of minerals, and decreased risk of cardiovascular disease, colon cancer, and diabetes (Klosterbuer, Roughead, and Slavin 2011). Prebiotics, an important fiber subset predominantly consisting of oligosaccharides, resist digestion in the small intestine and undergo fermentation in the colon, thereby altering gastrointestinal microflora (Gibson et al. 2004). In turn, the gut microflora contributes to innate immunity by maintaining the integrity of the mucosal barrier that inhibits gastrointestinal tract invasion of pathogenic bacteria. Prebiotics further reduce potentially pathogenic bacterial populations. For instance, wheat dextrin increases proliferation of lactobacilli and inhibits *Clostridium perfringens* (Lefranc-Millot et al. 2012). Fermentable fibers increase mucin production and thereby prevent bacterial translocation across the gut barrier (Satchithanandam et al. 1990). Both prebiotics and fermentable fibers that do not fall under the prebiotic category produce short-chain fatty acids (SCFAs), which decrease colonic pH, enhance growth of beneficial bacteria (such as bifidobacteria and lactobacilli), and prevent proliferation of potentially pathogenic bacteria. Numerous animal studies have demonstrated that adding SCFAs to parenteral feeding not only increases macrophages, antibodies, neutrophils, and Th cells but also strengthens natural killer cells' cytotoxic activity (Schley and Field 2002). Moreover, SCFA-producing bacteria may change pathogen-associated molecular patterns, causing secretion of proinflammatory cytokines and nuclear factor-kappa B (NF-κB) activation (Akira, Takeda, and Kaisho 2001, Abreu 2003). Increased fiber intake strengthens resistance to infection (including infectious diarrhea, antibiotic-associated diarrhea, and febrile illness associated with diarrhea or respiratory infection) and alleviates the severity and symptoms of inflammatory conditions, such as irritable bowel syndrome and IBD (Cummings, Christie, and Cole 2001, Saavedra and Tschernia 2002, Parisi et al. 2002, Lewis, Burmeister, and Brazier 2005, Konikoff and Denson 2006).

FATTY ACIDS

Consumption of ω-3 PUFAs, such as α-linolenic acid, eicosapentaenoic acid, and docosahexaenoic acid, has been shown to reduce fasting serum levels of C-reactive protein (CRP), IL-6, and TNF-α among patients with chronic nonautoimmune disease and healthy individuals (Li et al. 2014). On the other hand, ω-6 PUFAs, such as linoleic acid (LA), have proinflammatory effects and consumption of a diet rich in saturated fats increases plasma concentrations of proinflammatory cytokines, such as IL-1β and IL-6. Metabolism of LA leads to the synthesis of arachidonic acid (AA), a substrate strongly implicated in inflammation. AA is converted by cyclooxygenase and lipoxygenase to several proinflammatory eicosanoid mediators, such as prostaglandin E_2, thromboxane A_2, and leukotriene B_4 (Innes and Calder 2018). By contrast, ω-3 PUFAs confer anti-inflammatory benefits by competing with AA and shifting to production of eicosanoids associated with milder inflammation or inhibition of inflammation (Calder 2017). The interactions of PUFAs are nonetheless more complex and an ideal ratio of ω-6 to ω-3 PUFAs has been estimated to be 4:1 (Simopoulos 2002). This contrasts from the standard Western diet where the ratio is closer to 10:1.

NUTRITION AND IMMUNE-MEDIATED DISEASES

ASTHMA

Asthma is a chronic respiratory disorder associated with airway inflammation, involving a complex interplay between genetic and environmental factors, including nutrition. Intake of vitamins D and E during pregnancy has been shown to reduce the risk of childhood wheeze, yet do not affect childhood asthma (Beckhaus et al. 2015). Fish oil supplementation during pregnancy reduces both childhood wheeze and asthma (Bisgaard et al. 2016). Breastfeeding transfers allergens, immunosuppressive cytokines, and immune complexes to the baby, thus decreasing susceptibility to asthma development (Dogaru et al. 2014). In addition to influencing asthma risk, nutrition has profound effects on asthma control and outcomes. The Western diet, characterized by high fat or processed foods, increases systemic and airway inflammation and adversely impacts gut microbiota (Guilleminault et al. 2017). As such, the Western diet is associated with increased asthma risk and negative asthma outcomes (Varraso et al. 2009, Tromp et al. 2012, Patel et al. 2014). On the other hand, the Mediterranean diet and higher intake of fruits and vegetables improve asthma by decreasing proinflammatory cytokines, reducing airway neutrophils in patients with asthma, and beneficially altering gut microbiota. These microbial changes lead to the production of SCFAs that activate G protein-coupled receptors, enhance regulatory T cell titers and function, and subsequently suppress airway inflammation (Wood et al. 2008, Romieu et al. 2009, Thorburn et al. 2015, Zhang et al. 2016, McAleer and Kolls 2018). Both childhood and adult intake of fruits and vegetable protect against development of asthma, improve asthma symptom control, and improve lung function (Wood et al. 2008, Uddenfeldt et al. 2010, Wood et al. 2012, Iikura et al. 2013, Sexton et al. 2013, Patel et al. 2014, Papadopoulou et al. 2015). RCTs of vitamin D supplementation in school-aged children found a reduction in the number of asthma exacerbations, steroid requirements, and emergency visits when compared with placebo, although there was no clear benefit on lung function (Riverin, Maguire, and Li 2015).

FOOD ALLERGY

Food allergies are increasingly common with peanuts, tree nuts, seeds, soy, wheat, shellfish, fish, egg, and milk-bearing responsibility for most of the more serious health consequences (Eigenmann et al. 2020). Because initial priming exposure to an allergen early in development was previously thought to cause allergic reaction upon subsequent exposure, allergen avoidance was advocated as the main strategy for preventing food allergy for many years. Recent studies overturned this principle and demonstrated that early introduction of allergenic foods does not lead to sensitization, but rather is protective against food allergy and promotes development of immune tolerance through increased expression of regulatory T cells (Roduit et al. 2014). The European Academy of Allergy and Clinical Immunology (EAACI) and the American Academy of Pediatrics recommend that the introduction of allergenic foods should not be delayed or avoided during pregnancy, lactation, or complementary feeding (Greer et al. 2008 and hydrolyzed formulas, Muraro et al. 2014). The EAACI nonetheless recommends that high-risk children, defined as those with a parent or sibling with a history of allergy, use hypoallergenic formula with a documented preventive effect in the first 4 months of life (Muraro et al. 2014). Furthermore, utilizing a validated food allergy outcome measure, the Australian HealthNuts study demonstrated that infantile vitamin D deficiency may be a risk factor for food allergy, specifically peanut and egg due to vitamin D's role in general immune tolerance and maintenance of the gastrointestinal epithelial barrier (Vassallo and Camargo 2010, Allen et al. 2013, Allen and Koplin 2016). The diet as a whole is also associated with food allergy (Roduit et al. 2014, Grimshaw et al. 2014). Specifically, high intake of vegetables, fruits, and foods prepared at home is associated with lower rates of food allergy by 2 years of age, possibly attributable to higher levels of prebiotics and altered gut microbiota (Gibson et al. 2004, Grimshaw et al. 2014). However, neonatal prebiotic supplementation fails to affect food allergy development, but instead beneficially impacts other allergic conditions, such as eczema (Osborn and Sinn 2013). Finally, supplementation with ω-3 PUFAs during pregnancy, lactation, and infancy exerts a protective influence against food sensitization and food allergies (Kull et al. 2006, Clausen et al. 2018).

ATOPIC DERMATITIS

Atopic dermatitis is a chronic inflammatory skin condition influenced by immune dysregulation, hereditary predispositions, and environmental factors. Nutrition plays an essential role in proper immunologic functioning and health. Several studies have demonstrated that vitamin D, which extensively contributes to skin barrier integrity and immune tolerance, positively influences both the prevalence and symptom severity of atopic dermatitis (Wang et al. 2004, Sidbury et al. 2008, Borzutzky and Camargo 2013, El Taieb et al. 2013, Wang et al. 2014, Su et al. 2017, Sánchez-Armendáriz et al. 2018). Additional studies have investigated correlations between maternal serum vitamin D level, maternal vitamin D intake, or vitamin D levels in umbilical cord blood and the incidence of atopic dermatitis, yet these findings remain conflicting (Erkkola et al. 2009, Weisse et al. 2013, Miyake et al. 2014, Baïz et al. 2014, Chiu et al. 2015). Vitamin E levels are negatively correlated with risk for atopic dermatitis; vitamin E supplementation decreases serum IgE and may effectively serve as adjunctive therapy for atopic dermatitis (Tsoureli-Nikita et al. 2002, Oh et al. 2010, Jaffary et al. 2015). There are contradictory findings concerning the effect of vitamin C levels in breast milk, vitamin C intake, and vitamin C levels in infants on risk of atopic dermatitis development in children (Martindale et al. 2005, Laitinen et al. 2005, Hoppu et al. 2005, Oh et al. 2010). As an anti-inflammatory suppressor of cytokine production, zinc is inversely correlated with the risk of atopic dermatitis, given lower zinc levels in the serum, erythrocytes, and hair of those with atopic dermatitis (David et al. 1984, Di Toro et al. 1987, Kim et al. 2014, Karabacak et al. 2016). Selenium deficiency in either the infant or mother worsens risk for atopic dermatitis (Yamada et al. 2013). Associations between copper, iron, or strontium and atopic dermatitis remain inconclusive (David et al. 1984, el-Kholy et al. 1990, Yamada et al. 2013). Overall, diets high in processed foods, meat, and instant noodles are associated with increased prevalence of atopic dermatitis in an adult population (Park, Choi, and Bae 2016). On the other hand, a maternal Mediterranean diet appears to protect against atopic dermatitis (Chatzi et al. 2008, Netting, Middleton, and Makrides 2014). Moreover, although nearly 40% of those with moderate to severe atopic dermatitis have a concurrent IgE-mediated food allergy, only a small subset experience atopic dermatitis symptom exacerbation from those foods (Eigenmann et al. 2020). To manage symptoms, many patients with atopic dermatitis turn to dietary modification, most commonly excluding junk foods, dairy, and gluten or adding fruits, vegetables, and fish oil (Nosrati et al. 2017). However, because food avoidance is correlated with increased risk of developing immediate reactions to that food, further studies are necessary to investigate dietary elimination as a treatment strategy (Chang et al. 2016).

INFLAMMATORY BOWEL DISEASE

The pathogenesis of Crohn's disease (CD) and ulcerative colitis (UC) is complex and yet unclear, although the diet has been implicated. Several epidemiologic studies have found that increased consumption of refined carbohydrates and saturated fats to be associated with an increased risk of IBD. By contrast, consumption of fiber and ω-3 PUFAs has been associated with a lower risk of

IBD. Among patients with established and active IBD, dietary interventions may influence intestinal inflammation. Exclusive enteral nutrition is effective for the induction of remission in CD and has been recommended by the European Crohn's and Colitis Organisation and European Society for Clinical Nutrition and Metabolism as a first-line treatment for pediatric CD (Lochs et al. 2006, Narula et al. 2018, Ruemmele et al. 2014). However, beyond enteral nutrition, there is currently insufficient evidence supporting the use of dietary interventions, at least as monotherapy, for the induction or maintenance of remission in IBD (Limketkai et al. 2019). The effect of dietary supplements on intestinal inflammation has also been explored. Vitamin D possesses immunomodulatory properties and has gained significant interest as a therapeutic agent, although the largest RCT thus far to evaluate the effect of vitamin D supplementation on CD found similar relapse rates between intervention arms (Jorgensen et al. 2010). For ω-3 PUFAs, in the two largest RCTs of fish oil supplementation for CD, relapse rates were also similar between intervention arms (Feagan et al. 2008). A meta-analysis by the Cochrane Collaboration on the use of fish oil for UC found no difference in relapse rates (Turner et al. 2007). There is emerging evidence on a potential benefit of curcumin, the active constituent in turmeric, and probiotics for UC, although more research is needed before these become routinely recommended therapies (Hanai et al. 2006, Shen, Zuo, and Mao 2014).

MULTIPLE SCLEROSIS

MS is a chronic autoimmune disease that involves the central nervous system, resulting in a variety of neurological symptoms that vary in type and severity. Although its cause is unknown, MS is influenced by a combination of immune abnormalities, genetic susceptibility, and environmental factors. MS has long had a connection to vitamin D. Low vitamin D concentrations, whether through lack of dietary intake or sunlight exposure, are associated with increased risk of disease development, exacerbations, relapse, and disability (Expanded Disability Status Scale [EDSS] score >3), whereas higher vitamin D concentrations tend to slow MS progression (Munger et al. 2006, Lucas et al. 2015, Mazdeh et al. 2013, Soilu-Hänninen et al. 2005). Through both immune modulation and anti-inflammatory metabolism, vitamin D inhibits regulatory $CD4^+$ T cells (Sánchez-Armendariz et al. 2018). High maternal milk intake during pregnancy may be associated with reduced risk of MS development in the offspring, yet intake of whole milk during adolescence is associated with an increased risk (Munger et al. 2011, Mirzaei et al. 2011). Although vitamin B12 plays important roles in the central nervous system ranging from immunomodulation and myelin sheath formation to conversion of homocysteine to methionine, study findings concerning vitamin B12's association with MS remain inconsistent (Najafi et al. 2012, Moghaddasi et al. 2013). Overall dietary patterns low in whole grain and dominated by sugar and fat are associated with postprandial inflammation and results in both higher MS prevalence and worsening of the inflammatory disease process (Margioris 2009, Jahromi et al. 2012, Bagur et al. 2017). Low-fat diet appears to protect against disease development, alleviate symptoms (using measures such as fatigue and the EDSS score), and reduce rates of relapse (Mauriz et al. 2013, Pantzaris et al. 2013, Jelinek et al. 2013, Hadgkiss et al. 2015). Animal studies illustrate that the fasting mimicking diet effectively enhances oligodendrocyte regeneration in several MS models and inhibits autoimmunity through reduction of proinflammatory cytokines and induction of lymphocyte apoptosis (Choi et al. 2016).

IMMUNONUTRITION IN CANCER PREVENTION AND TREATMENT

The immune system has etiologic and abortive influences on carcinogenesis. On one hand, chronic inflammation stemming from dysregulated immune function is associated with oxidative stress and carcinogenesis, such as in the case of UC and colorectal cancer (Kay et al. 2019, Axelrad, Lichtiger, and Yajnik 2016). On the other hand, immunosurveillance represents a forefront of the innate and adaptive immune system's anti-tumor effects (Zitvogel, Tesniere, and Kroemer 2006). In the early stages of oncogenesis, premalignant or malignant cell antigens are processed by antigen presenting cells and activate T-cell mediated immunity. Cytotoxic CD8$^+$ T lymphocytes detect and lyse tumor cells. Such features of the anti-tumor immune response form the basis for the use of cancer immunotherapy (Couzin-Frankel 2013). However, when tumor cells are able to evade immunosurveillance, they are able to proliferate, invade the tissues, and eventually metastasize.

Given the relationship between immune function and tumor cell survival, nutritional interventions have been considered as adjunctive strategies for cancer prevention and treatment. Antiinflammatory nutrients as described previously would hypothetically reduce inflammation and subsequent carcinogenesis. A retrospective analysis of 225,090 individuals with CD and 188,420 individuals with UC found that the use of antitumor necrosis factor therapy was associated with a lower incidence of colorectal cancer, reflecting the benefit of immunomodulation on cancer risk (PMID 33051651). Immune-boosting and modulating formulae have also been considered in cancer therapeutics. In addition to the components of standard enteral nutrition, immunonutrition formulae include components believed to influence the immune system: arginine (substrate for lymphocytes), omega-3 fatty acids (anti-inflammatory properties), glutamine (whose deficiency can adversely affect immune function), and nucleotides (involved in lymphocyte proliferation and activation).

There is still a great dearth of data on the use of immunonutrition for cancer treatment, although some preliminary data exist. In an early observational study of 31 patients with head and neck squamous cell carcinoma, immunonutrition provided prior to each chemotherapy cycle was associated with a reduction in CRP and α-1 acid glycoprotein, although there was no difference in inflammatory markers during chemoradiation therapy (Machon et al. 2012). The investigators nonetheless found a benefit in reducing the incidence of severe acute mucositis. A subsequent randomized controlled trial on 71 individuals with esophageal cancer undergoing chemoradiation therapy found that those in the immunonutrition group had lower inflammatory markers than those in the control group (Sunpaweravong et al. 2014). In another randomized controlled trial of 28 patients with head, neck, and esophageal cancer, investigators concluded that immunonutrition helped patients undergoing chemoradiation therapy adapt better to the oxidative stress and systemic inflammation (Talvas et al. 2015). Immunonutrition has theoretical benefits for immunosurveillance and immunotherapy by potentiating the antitumor immune response. However, much more research is needed to clarify the role of immunonutrition in this capacity.

CONCLUSION

Nutrients are indispensable components in the development, maintenance, and function of human biological processes, including the immune system. Some mechanisms that underlie nutrients' effects on these processes include serving as substrates or metabolic cofactors, preserving the epithelial barrier in innate immunity, regulating cellular proliferation and differentiation, and interacting with cellular receptors. The diet also exerts a strong effect on the intestinal microbiome, which itself can influence the inflammatory state. The impact of nutrients on biologic functions can be observed through diseases that could arise from deficiencies and toxicities, although these relationships between nutrition and disease pathogenesis are highly complex and still not yet clearly elucidated. Nonetheless, the optimization of nutritional status is critical for improving and maintaining health of the immune system. As the immune system exerts an influence on carcinogenesis and tumor progression, modulating inflammation and optimizing immune function have become important considerations in cancer prevention and treatment. Our knowledge on this interaction between nutrition, the immune system, and cancer just scratches the surface, thus motivating the need for much more research at the intersection of nutritional immunology and immuno-oncology.

REFERENCES

Abe, E., C. Miyaura, H. Sakagami, M. Takeda, K. Konno, T. Yamazaki, S. Yoshiki, and T. Suda. 1981. "Differentiation of mouse myeloid leukemia cells induced by 1 alpha,25-dihydroxyvitamin D3." *Proceedings of the National Academy of Sciences of the United States of America* 78 (8):4990–4994. doi: 10.1073/pnas.78.8.4990.

Abreu, M. T. 2003. "Immunologic regulation of toll-like receptors in gut epithelium." *Current Opinion in Gastroenterology* 19 (6):559–564. doi: 10.1097/00001574-200311000-00008.

Ahluwalia, N., J. Sun, D. Krause, A. Mastro, and G. Handte. 2004. "Immune function is impaired in iron-deficient, homebound, older women." *The American Journal of Clinical Nutrition* 79 (3):516–521. doi: 10.1093/ajcn/79.3.516.

Akira, S., K. Takeda, and T. Kaisho. 2001. "Toll-like receptors: critical proteins linking innate and acquired immunity." *Nature Immunology* 2 (8):675–680. doi: 10.1038/90609.

Allen, K. J., and J. J. Koplin. 2016. "Prospects for prevention of food allergy." *The Journal of Allergy and Clinical Immunology: In Practice* 4 (2):215–220. doi: 10.1016/j.jaip.2015.10.010.

Allen, K. J., J. J. Koplin, A.-L. Ponsonby, L. C. Gurrin, M. Wake, P. Vuillermin, P. Martin, M. Matheson, A. Lowe, M. Robinson, D. Tey, N. J. Osborne, T. Dang, H.-T. T. Tan, L. Thiele, D. Anderson, H. Czech, J. Sanjeevan, G. Zurzolo, T. Dwyer, M. L. K. Tang, D. Hill, and S. C. Dharmage. 2013. "Vitamin D insufficiency is associated with challenge-proven food allergy in infants." *The Journal of Allergy and Clinical Immunology* 131 (4):1109–1116e1–6. doi: 10.1016/j.jaci.2013.01.017.

Amit-Romach, E., Z. Uni, S. Cheled, Z. Berkovich, and R. Reifen. 2009. "Bacterial population and innate immunity-related genes in rat gastrointestinal tract are altered by vitamin A-deficient diet." *The Journal of Nutritional Biochemistry* 20 (1):70–77. doi: 10.1016/j.jnutbio.2008.01.002.

Anderson, R., R. Oosthuizen, R. Maritz, A. Theron, and A. J. Van Rensburg. 1980. "The effects of increasing weekly doses of ascorbate on certain cellular and humoral immune functions in normal volunteers." *The American Journal of Clinical Nutrition* 33 (1):71–76. doi: 10.1093/ajcn/33.1.71.

Arihiro, S., A. Nakashima, M. Matsuoka, S. Suto, K. Uchiyama, T. Kato, J. Mitobe, N. Komoike, M. Itagaki, Y. Miyakawa, S. Koido, A. Hokari, M. Saruta, H. Tajiri, T. Matsuura, and M. Urashima. 2019. "Randomized trial of vitamin D supplementation to prevent seasonal influenza and upper respiratory infection in patients with inflammatory bowel disease." *Inflammatory Bowel Disease* 25 (6):1088–1095. doi: 10.1093/ibd/izy346.

Axelrad, J. E., S. Lichtiger, and V. Yajnik. 2016. "Inflammatory bowel disease and cancer: the role of inflammation, immunosuppression, and cancer treatment." *World Journal of Gastroenterology* 22 (20):4794–4801. doi: 10.3748/wjg.v22.i20.4794.

Babu, U., and M. L. Failla. 1990. "Respiratory burst and candidacidal activity of peritoneal macrophages are impaired in copper-deficient rats." *The Journal of Nutrition* 120 (12):1692–1699. doi: 10.1093/jn/120.12.1692.

Bagur, M. José, M. Antonia Murcia, A. M. Jiménez-Monreal, J. A. Tur, M. Mar Bibiloni, G. L. Alonso, and M. Martínez-Tomé. 2017. "Influence of diet in multiple sclerosis: a systematic review." *Advances in Nutrition (Bethesda, MD)* 8 (3):463–472. doi: 10.3945/an.116.014191.

Baïz, N., P. Dargent-Molina, J. D. Wark, J.-C. Souberbielle, I. Annesi-Maesano, and Eden Mother-Child Cohort Study Group. 2014. "Cord serum 25-hydroxyvitamin D and risk of early childhood transient wheezing and atopic dermatitis." *The Journal of Allergy and Clinical Immunology* 133 (1):147–153. doi: 10.1016/j.jaci.2013.05.017.

Bala, S., and M. L. Failla. 1992. "Copper deficiency reversibly impairs DNA synthesis in activated T lymphocytes by limiting interleukin 2 activity." *Proceedings of the National Academy of Sciences of the United States of America* 89 (15):6794–6797. doi: 10.1073/pnas.89.15.6794.

Beckhaus, A. A., L. Garcia-Marcos, E. Forno, R. M. Pacheco-Gonzalez, J. C. Celedón, and J. A. Castro-Rodriguez. 2015. "Maternal nutrition during pregnancy and risk of asthma, wheeze, and atopic diseases during childhood: a systematic review and meta-analysis." *Allergy* 70 (12):1588–1604. doi: 10.1111/all.12729.

Belkaid, Y., and T. W. Hand. 2014. "Role of the microbiota in immunity and inflammation." *Cell* 157 (1):121–41. doi: 10.1016/j.cell.2014.03.011.

Bisgaard, H., Jakob Stokholm, B. L. Chawes, N. H. Vissing, E. Bjarnadóttir, A.-M. M. Schoos, H. M. Wolsk, T. M. Pedersen, R. K. Vinding, S. Thorsteinsdóttir, N. V. Følsgaard, N. R. Fink, J. Thorsen, A. G. Pedersen, J. Waage, M. A. Rasmussen, K. D. Stark, S. F. Olsen, and K. Bønnelykke. 2016. "Fish oil-derived fatty acids in pregnancy and wheeze and asthma in offspring." *The New England Journal of Medicine* 375 (26):2530–2539. doi: 10.1056/NEJMoa1503734.

Borzutzky, A., and C. A. Camargo. 2013. "Role of vitamin D in the pathogenesis and treatment of atopic dermatitis." *Expert Review of Clinical Immunology* 9 (8):751–760. doi: 10.1586/1744666X.2013.816493.

Calder, P. C. 2017. "Omega-3 fatty acids and inflammatory processes: from molecules to man." *Biochemical Society Transactions* 45 (5):1105–1115. doi: 10.1042/BST20160474.

Cannell, J. J., R. Vieth, J. C. Umhau, M. F. Holick, W. B. Grant, S. Madronich, C. F. Garland, and E. Giovannucci. 2006. "Epidemic influenza and vitamin D." *Epidemiology and Infection* 134 (6):1129–1140. doi: 10.1017/S0950268806007175.

Cantorna, M. T., L. Snyder, Y.-D. Lin, and L. Yang. 2015. "Vitamin D and 1,25(OH)2D regulation of T cells." *Nutrients* 7 (4):3011–3021. doi: 10.3390/nu7043011.

Cassat, J. E., and E. P. Skaar. 2012. "Metal ion acquisition in Staphylococcus aureus: overcoming nutritional immunity." *Seminars in Immunopathology* 34 (2):215–235. doi: 10.1007/s00281-011-0294-4.

Cha, H. R., S. Y. Chang, J. H. Chang, J. O. Kim, J. Y. Yang, C. H. Kim, and M. N. Kweon. 2010. "Downregulation of Th17 cells in the small intestine by disruption of gut flora in the absence of retinoic acid." *J Immunol* 184 (12):6799–806. doi: 10.4049/jimmunol.0902944.

Chang, A., R. Robison, M. Cai, and A. M. Singh. 2016. "Natural history of food-triggered atopic dermatitis and development of immediate reactions in children." *The Journal of Allergy and Clinical Immunology: In Practice* 4 (2):229–236.e1. doi: 10.1016/j.jaip.2015.08.006.

Chatzi, L., M. Torrent, I. Romieu, R. Garcia-Esteban, C. Ferrer, J. Vioque, M. Kogevinas, and J. Sunyer. 2008. "Mediterranean diet in pregnancy is protective for wheeze and atopy in childhood." *Thorax* 63 (6):507–513. doi: 10.1136/thx.2007.081745.

Chen, S., G. P. Sims, X. X. Chen, Y. Y. Gu, S. Chen, and P. E. Lipsky. 2007. "Modulatory effects of 1,25-dihydroxyvitamin D3 on human B cell differentiation." *Journal of Immunology (Baltimore, Md.: 1950)* 179 (3):1634–1647. doi: 10.4049/jimmunol.179.3.1634.

Chew, B. P., and J. S. Park. 2004. "Carotenoid action on the immune response." *The Journal of Nutrition* 134 (1):257S–261S. doi: 10.1093/jn/134.1.257S.

Chiu, C.-Y., S.-Y. Huang, Y.-C. Peng, M.-H. Tsai, M.-C. Hua, T.-C. Yao, K.-W. Yeh, and J.-L. Huang. 2015. "Maternal vitamin D levels are inversely related to allergic sensitization and atopic diseases in early childhood." *Pediatric Allergy and Immunology* 26 (4):337–343. doi: 10.1111/pai.12384.

Choi, I. Y., L. Piccio, P. Childress, B. Bollman, A. Ghosh, S. Brandhorst, J. Suarez, A. Michalsen, A. H. Cross, T. E. Morgan, M. Wei, F. Paul, M. Bock, and V. D. Longo. 2016. "A diet mimicking fasting promotes regeneration and reduces autoimmunity and multiple sclerosis symptoms." *Cell Reports* 15 (10):2136–2146. doi: 10.1016/j.celrep.2016.05.009.

Clausen, M., K. Jonasson, T. Keil, K. Beyer, and S. T. Sigurdardottir. 2018. "Fish oil in infancy protects against food allergy in Iceland-Results from a birth cohort study." *Allergy* 73 (6):1305–1312. doi: 10.1111/all.13385.

Cook-Mills, J. M., and P. J. Fraker. 1993. "Functional capacity of the residual lymphocytes from zinc-deficient adult mice." *The British Journal of Nutrition* 69 (3):835–848. doi: 10.1079/bjn19930084.

Corbin, B. D., E. H. Seeley, A. Raab, J. Feldmann, M. R. Miller, V. J. Torres, K. L. Anderson, B. M. Dattilo, P. M. Dunman, R. Gerads, R. M. Caprioli, W. Nacken, W. J. Chazin, and E. P. Skaar. 2008. "Metal chelation and inhibition of bacterial growth in tissue abscesses." *Science (New York, N.Y.)* 319 (5865):962–965. doi: 10.1126/science.1152449.

Couzin-Frankel, J. 2013. "Breakthrough of the year 2013. Cancer immunotherapy." *Science* 342 (6165):1432–1433. doi: 10.1126/science.342.6165.1432.

Cummings, J. H., S. Christie, and T. J. Cole. 2001. "A study of fructo oligosaccharides in the prevention of travellers' diarrhoea." *Alimentary Pharmacology & Therapeutics* 15 (8):1139–1145. doi: 10.1046/j.1365-2036.2001.01043.x.

David, T. J., F. E. Wells, T. C. Sharpe, and A. C. Gibbs. 1984. "Low serum zinc in children with atopic eczema." *The British Journal of Dermatology* 111 (5):597–601. doi: 10.1111/j.1365-2133.1984.tb06630.x.

Di Toro, R., G. Galdo Capotorti, G. Gialanella, M. M. del Giudice, R. Moro, and L. Perrone. 1987. "Zinc and copper status of allergic children." *Acta Paediatrica Scandinavica* 76 (4):612–617. doi: 10.1111/j.1651-2227.1987.tb10530.x.

Dogaru, C. M., D. Nyffenegger, A. M. Pescatore, B. D. Spycher, and C. E. Kuehni. 2014. "Breastfeeding and childhood asthma: systematic review and meta-analysis." *American Journal of Epidemiology* 179 (10):1153–1167. doi: 10.1093/aje/kwu072.

Dowd, P. S., J. Kelleher, and P. J. Guillou. 1986. "T-lymphocyte subsets and interleukin-2 production in zinc-deficient rats." *The British Journal of Nutrition* 55 (1):59–69. doi: 10.1079/bjn19860010.

Dunlap, W. M., G. W. James, and D. M. Hume. 1974. "Anemia and neutropenia caused by copper deficiency." *Annals of Internal Medicine* 80 (4):470–476. doi: 10.7326/0003-4819-80-4-470.

Eby, G. A., and W. W. Halcomb. 2006. "Ineffectiveness of zinc gluconate nasal spray and zinc orotate lozenges in common-cold treatment: a double-blind, placebo-controlled clinical trial." *Alternative Therapies in Health and Medicine* 12 (1):34–38.

Eigenmann, P. A., K. Beyer, G. Lack, A. Muraro, P. Y. Ong, S. H. Sicherer, and H. A. Sampson. 2020. "Are avoidance diets still warranted in children with atopic dermatitis?" *Pediatric Allergy and Immunology* 31 (1):19–26. doi: 10.1111/pai.13104.

el-Kholy, M. S., M. A. Gas Allah, S. el-Shimi, F. el-Baz, H. el-Tayeb, and M. S. Abdel-Hamid. 1990. "Zinc and copper status in children with bronchial asthma and atopic dermatitis." *The Journal of the Egyptian Public Health Association* 65 (5–6):657–668.

El Taieb, M. A., H. M. Fayed, S. S. Aly, and A. K. Ibrahim. 2013. "Assessment of serum 25-hydroxyvitamin d levels in children with atopic dermatitis: correlation with SCORAD index." *Dermatitis: Contact, Atopic, Occupational, Drug* 24 (6):296–301. doi: 10.1097/DER.0000000000000010.

Erkkola, M., M. Kaila, B. I. Nwaru, C. Kronberg-Kippilä, S. Ahonen, J. Nevalainen, R. Veijola, J. Pekkanen, J. Ilonen, O. Simell, M. Knip, and S. M. Virtanen. 2009. "Maternal vitamin D intake during pregnancy is inversely associated with asthma and allergic rhinitis in 5-year-old children." *Clinical and Experimental Allergy* 39 (6):875–882. doi: 10.1111/j.1365-2222.2009.03234.x.

Fallarino, F., U. Grohmann, C. Vacca, R. Bianchi, C. Orabona, A. Spreca, M. C. Fioretti, and P. Puccetti. 2002. "T cell apoptosis by tryptophan catabolism." *Cell Death and Differentiation* 9 (10):1069–1077. doi: 10.1038/sj.cdd.4401073.

Fallarino, F., U. Grohmann, S. You, B. C. McGrath, D. R. Cavener, C. Vacca, C. Orabona, R. Bianchi, M. L. Belladonna, C. Volpi, P. Santamaria, M. C. Fioretti, and P. Puccetti. 2006. "The combined effects of tryptophan starvation and tryptophan catabolites down-regulate T cell receptor zeta-chain and induce a regulatory phenotype in naive T cells." *Journal of Immunology (Baltimore, Md.: 1950)* 176 (11):6752–6761. doi: 10.4049/jimmunol.176.11.6752.

Feagan, B. G., W. J. Sandborn, U. Mittmann, S. Bar-Meir, G. D'Haens, M. Bradette, A. Cohen, C. Dallaire, T. P. Ponich, J. W. McDonald, X. Hebuterne, P. Pare, P. Klvana, Y. Niv, S. Ardizzone, O. Alexeeva, A. Rostom, G. Kiudelis, J. Spleiss, D. Gilgen, M. K. Vandervoort, C. J. Wong, G. Y. Zou, A. Donner, and P. Rutgeerts. 2008. "Omega-3 free fatty acids for the maintenance of remission in Crohn disease: the EPIC randomized controlled trials." *JAMA* 299 (14):1690–1697. doi: 10.1001/jama.299.14.1690.

Fischer, R., H. Debbabi, M. Dubarry, P. Boyaka, and D. Tomé. 2006. "Regulation of physiological and pathological Th1 and Th2 responses by lactoferrin." *Biochemistry and Cell Biology* 84 (3):303–311. doi: 10.1139/o06-058.

Fraker, P. J., S. M. Haas, and R. W. Luecke. 1977. "Effect of zinc deficiency on the immune response of the young adult A/J mouse." *The Journal of Nutrition* 107 (10):1889–1895. doi: 10.1093/jn/107.10.1889.

Francis C. Okeke, Danielle Flug Capalino, Laura E. Matarese, Gerard E. Mullin Vitamins and Minerals (Pages: 556-586) in Yamada's Textbook of Gastroenterology 7th edition (Editors: Daniel K. Podolsky MD, Michael Camilleri MD, J. Gregory Fitz MD FAASLD, Anthony N. Kalloo MD, Fergus Shanahan MD, Timothy C. Wang MD) 2016, John Wiley & Sons, Ltd.

Gangaidzo, I. T., V. M. Moyo, E. Mvundura, G. Aggrey, N. L. Murphree, H. Khumalo, T. Saungweme, I. Kasvosve, Z. A. Gomo, T. Rouault, J. R. Boelaert, and V. R. Gordeuk. 2001. "Association of pulmonary tuberculosis with increased dietary iron." *The Journal of Infectious Diseases* 184 (7):936–939. doi: 10.1086/323203.

Gibson, G. R., H. M. Probert, J. Van Loo, R. A. Rastall, and M. B. Roberfroid. 2004. "Dietary modulation of the human colonic microbiota: updating the concept of prebiotics." *Nutrition Research Reviews* 17 (2):259–275. doi: 10.1079/NRR200479.

Ginde, A. A., J. M. Mansbach, and C. A. Camargo. 2009. "Association between serum 25-hydroxyvitamin D level and upper respiratory tract infection in the Third National Health and Nutrition Examination Survey." *Archives of Internal Medicine* 169 (4):384–390. doi: 10.1001/archinternmed.2008.560.

Godfrey, J. C., N. J. Godfrey, and S. G. Novick. 1996. "Zinc for treating the common cold: review of all clinical trials since 1984." *Alternative Therapies in Health and Medicine* 2 (6):63–72.

Gombart, A. F., N. Borregaard, and H. P. Koeffler. 2005. "Human cathelicidin antimicrobial peptide (CAMP) gene is a direct target of the vitamin D receptor and is strongly up-regulated in myeloid cells by 1,25-dihydroxyvitamin D3." *FASEB Journal* 19 (9):1067–1077. doi: 10.1096/fj.04-3284com.

Grainger, J. R., E. A. Wohlfert, I. J. Fuss, N. Bouladoux, M. H. Askenase, F. Legrand, L. Y. Koo, J. M. Brenchley, I. D. Fraser, and Y. Belkaid. 2013. "Inflammatory monocytes regulate pathologic responses to commensals during acute gastrointestinal infection." *Nat Med* 19 (6):713–721. doi: 10.1038/nm.3189.

Green, H. N., and E. Mellanby. 1928. "Vitamin A as an anti-infective agent." *British Medical Journal* 2 (3537):691–696. doi: 10.1136/bmj.2.3537.691.

Greer, F. R., S. H. Sicherer, A. Wesley Burks, Nutrition American Academy of Pediatrics Committee on, Allergy American Academy of Pediatrics Section on, and Immunology. 2008. "Effects of early nutritional interventions on the development of atopic disease in infants and children: the role of maternal dietary restriction, breastfeeding, timing of introduction of complementary foods, and hydrolyzed formulas." *Pediatrics* 121 (1):183–191. doi: 10.1542/peds.2007-3022.

Grimshaw, K. E. C., J. Maskell, E. M. Oliver, R. C. G. Morris, K. D. Foote, E. N. Clare Mills, B. M. Margetts, and G. Roberts. 2014. "Diet and food allergy development during infancy: birth cohort study findings using prospective food diary data." *The Journal of Allergy and Clinical Immunology* 133 (2):511–519. doi: 10.1016/j.jaci.2013.05.035.

Grohmann, U., F. Fallarino, R. Bianchi, C. Orabona, C. Vacca, M. C. Fioretti, and P. Puccetti. 2003. "A defect in tryptophan catabolism impairs tolerance in nonobese diabetic mice." *The Journal of Experimental Medicine* 198 (1):153–160. doi: 10.1084/jem.20030633.

Guilleminault, L., E. J. Williams, H. A. Scott, B. S. Berthon, M. Jensen, and L. G. Wood. 2017. "Diet and asthma: is it time to adapt our message?" *Nutrients* 9 (11):1227. doi: 10.3390/nu9111227.

Hadgkiss, E. J., G. A. Jelinek, T. J. Weiland, N. G. Pereira, C. H. Marck, and D. M. van der Meer. 2015. "The association of diet with quality of life, disability, and relapse rate in an international sample of people with multiple sclerosis." *Nutritional Neuroscience* 18 (3):125–136. doi: 10.1179/1476830514Y.0000000117.

Hall, J. A., J. R. Grainger, S. P. Spencer, and Y. Belkaid. 2011. "The role of retinoic acid in tolerance and immunity." *Immunity* 35 (1):13–22. doi: 10.1016/j.immuni.2011.07.002.

Hanai, H., T. Iida, K. Takeuchi, F. Watanabe, Y. Maruyama, A. Andoh, T. Tsujikawa, Y. Fujiyama, K. Mitsuyama, M. Sata, M. Yamada, Y. Iwaoka, K. Kanke, H. Hiraishi, K. Hirayama, H. Arai, S. Yoshii, M. Uchijima, T. Nagata, and Y. Koide. 2006. "Curcumin maintenance therapy for ulcerative colitis: randomized, multicenter, double-blind, placebo-controlled trial." *Clin Gastroenterol Hepatol* 4 (12):1502–1506. doi: 10.1016/j.cgh.2006.08.008.

Hasan, R., L. Rink, and H. Haase. 2013. "Zinc signals in neutrophil granulocytes are required for the formation of neutrophil extracellular traps." *Innate Immunity* 19 (3):253–264. doi: 10.1177/1753425912458815.

Hasegawa, H., K. Suzuki, K. Suzuki, S. Nakaji, and K. Sugawara. 2000. "Effects of zinc on the reactive oxygen species generating capacity of human neutrophils and on the serum opsonic activity in vitro." *Luminescence* 15 (5):321–327. doi: 10.1002/1522-7243(200009/10)15:5<321::AID-BIO605>3.0.CO;2-O.

Hemilä, H., and E. Chalker. 2013. "Vitamin C for preventing and treating the common cold." *The Cochrane Database of Systematic Reviews* (1):CD000980. doi: 10.1002/14651858.CD000980.pub4.

Hoppu, U., M. Rinne, P. Salo-Väänänen, A. M. Lampi, V. Piironen, and E. Isolauri. 2005. "Vitamin C in breast milk may reduce the risk of atopy in the infant." *European Journal of Clinical Nutrition* 59 (1):123–128. doi: 10.1038/sj.ejcn.1602048.

Hunt, C., N. K. Chakravorty, G. Annan, N. Habibzadeh, and C. J. Schorah. 1994. "The clinical effects of vitamin C supplementation in elderly hospitalised patients with acute respiratory infections." *International Journal for Vitamin and Nutrition Research. Internationale Zeitschrift Fur Vitamin- Und Ernahrungsforschung. Journal International De Vitaminologie et de Nutrition* 64 (3):212–219.

Iikura, M., S. Yi, Y. Ichimura, A. Hori, S. Izumi, H. Sugiyama, K. Kudo, T. Mizoue, and N. Kobayashi. 2013. "Effect of lifestyle on asthma control in Japanese patients: importance of periodical exercise and raw vegetable diet." *PLoS One* 8 (7):e68290. doi: 10.1371/journal.pone.0068290.

Innes, J. K., and P. C. Calder. 2018. "Omega-6 fatty acids and inflammation." *Prostaglandins, Leukotrienes, and Essential Fatty Acids* 132:41–48. doi: 10.1016/j.plefa.2018.03.004.

Jaffary, F., G. Faghihi, A. Mokhtarian, and S. M. Hosseini. 2015. "Effects of oral vitamin E on treatment of atopic dermatitis: a randomized controlled trial." *Journal of Research in Medical Sciences* 20 (11):1053–1057. doi: 10.4103/1735-1995.172815.

Jahromi, S. R., M. Toghae, M. J. Razeghi Jahromi, and M. Aloosh. 2012. "Dietary pattern and risk of multiple sclerosis." *Iranian Journal of Neurology* 11 (2):47–53.

Jelinek, G. A., E. J. Hadgkiss, T. J. Weiland, N. G. Pereira, C. H. Marck, and D. M. van der Meer. 2013. "Association of fish consumption and Ω 3 supplementation with quality of life, disability and disease activity in an international cohort of people with multiple sclerosis." *The International Journal of Neuroscience* 123 (11):792–800. doi: 10.3109/00207454.2013.803104.

Jorgensen, S. P., J. Agnholt, H. Glerup, S. Lyhne, G. E. Villadsen, C. L. Hvas, L. E. Bartels, J. Kelsen, L. A. Christensen, and J. F. Dahlerup. 2010. "Clinical trial: vitamin D3 treatment in Crohn's disease - a randomized double-blind placebo-controlled study." *Alimentary Pharmacology & Therapeutics* 32 (3):377–383. doi: 10.1111/j.1365-2036.2010.04355.x.

Karabacak, E., E. Aydin, A. Kutlu, O. Ozcan, T. Muftuoglu, A. Gunes, B. Dogan, and S. Ozturk. 2016. "Erythrocyte zinc level in patients with atopic dermatitis and its relation to SCORAD index." *Postepy Dermatologii I Alergologii* 33 (5):349–352. doi: 10.5114/ada.2016.62841.

Kay, J., E. Thadhani, L. Samson, and B. Engelward. 2019. "Inflammation-induced DNA damage, mutations and cancer." *DNA Repair (Amst)* 83:102673. doi: 10.1016/j.dnarep.2019.102673.

Kim, J. E., S. R. Yoo, M. G. Jeong, J. Y. Ko, and Y. S. Ro. 2014. "Hair zinc levels and the efficacy of oral zinc supplementation in patients with atopic dermatitis." *Acta Dermato-Venereologica* 94 (5):558–562. doi: 10.2340/00015555-1772.

Klosterbuer, A., Z. F. Roughead, and J. Slavin. 2011. "Benefits of dietary fiber in clinical nutrition." *Nutrition in Clinical Practice* 26 (5):625–635. doi: 10.1177/0884533611416126.

Koller, L. D., S. A. Mulhern, N. C. Frankel, M. G. Steven, and J. R. Williams. 1987. "Immune dysfunction in rats fed a diet deficient in copper." *The American Journal of Clinical Nutrition* 45 (5):997–1006. doi: 10.1093/ajcn/45.5.997.

Konikoff, M. R., and L. A. Denson. 2006. "Role of fecal calprotectin as a biomarker of intestinal inflammation in inflammatory bowel disease." *Inflammatory Bowel Disease* 12 (6):524–534. doi: 10.1097/00054725-200606000-00013.

Kreutz, M., R. Andreesen, S. W. Krause, A. Szabo, E. Ritz, and H. Reichel. 1993. "1,25-dihydroxyvitamin D3 production and vitamin D3 receptor expression are developmentally regulated during differentiation of human monocytes into macrophages." *Blood* 82 (4):1300–1307.

Kull, I., A. Bergström, G. Lilja, G. Pershagen, and M. Wickman. 2006. "Fish consumption during the first year of life and development of allergic diseases during childhood." *Allergy* 61 (8):1009–1015. doi: 10.1111/j.1398-9995.2006.01115.x.

Kuvibidila, S. R., B. S. Baliga, and R. M. Suskind. 1981. "Effects of iron deficiency anemia on delayed cutaneous hypersensitivity in mice." *The American Journal of Clinical Nutrition* 34 (12):2635–2640. doi: 10.1093/ajcn/34.12.2635.

Laitinen, K., M. Kalliomäki, T. Poussa, H. Lagström, and E. Isolauri. 2005. "Evaluation of diet and growth in children with and without atopic eczema: follow-up study from birth to 4 years." *The British Journal of Nutrition* 94 (4):565–574. doi: 10.1079/bjn20051503.

Lee, P., H. Peng, T. Gelbart, L. Wang, and E. Beutler. 2005. "Regulation of hepcidin transcription by interleukin-1 and interleukin-6." *Proceedings of the National Academy of Sciences of the United States of America* 102 (6):1906–1910. doi: 10.1073/pnas.0409808102.

Lefranc-Millot, C., L. Guérin-Deremaux, D. Wils, C. Neut, L. E. Miller, and M. H. Saniez-Degrave. 2012. "Impact of a resistant dextrin on intestinal ecology: how altering the digestive ecosystem with NUTRIOSE®, a soluble fibre with prebiotic properties, may be beneficial for health." *The Journal of International Medical Research* 40 (1):211–224. doi: 10.1177/147323001204000122.

Lewis, S., S. Burmeister, and J. Brazier. 2005. "Effect of the prebiotic oligofructose on relapse of Clostridium difficile-associated diarrhea: a randomized, controlled study." *Clinical Gastroenterology and Hepatology* 3 (5):442–448. doi: 10.1016/s1542-3565(04)00677-9.

Li, K., T. Huang, J. Zheng, K. Wu, and D. Li. 2014. "Effect of marine-derived n-3 polyunsaturated fatty acids on C-reactive protein, interleukin 6 and tumor necrosis factor α: a meta-analysis." *PLoS One* 9 (2):e88103. doi: 10.1371/journal.pone.0088103.

Limketkai, B. N., Z. Iheozor-Ejiofor, T. Gjuladin-Hellon, A. Parian, L. E. Matarese, K. Bracewell, J. K. MacDonald, M. Gordon, and G. E. Mullin. 2019. "Dietary interventions for induction and maintenance of remission in inflammatory bowel disease." *Cochrane Database Syst Rev* (2):CD012839. doi: 10.1002/14651858.CD012839.pub2.

Limketkai, B. N., G. E. Mullin, D. Limsui, and A. M. Parian. 2017. "Role of vitamin D in inflammatory bowel disease." *Nutrition in Clinical Practice* 32 (3):337–345. doi: 10.1177/0884533616674492.

Lochs, H., C. Dejong, F. Hammarqvist, X. Hebuterne, M. Leon-Sanz, T. Schutz, W. van Gemert, A. van Gossum, L. Valentini, D. H. Lubke, S. Bischoff, N. Engelmann, P. Thul, and Espen. 2006. "ESPEN guidelines on enteral nutrition: gastroenterology." *Clinical Nutrition* 25 (2):260–274. doi: 10.1016/j.clnu.2006.01.007.

Loeb, M., A. D. Dang, V. D. Thiem, V. Thanabalan, B. Wang, N. B. Nguyen, H. T. M. Tran, T. M. Luong, P. Singh, M. Smieja, J. Maguire, and E. Pullenayegum. 2019. "Effect of vitamin D supplementation to reduce respiratory infections in children and adolescents in Vietnam: a randomized controlled trial." *Influenza Other Respir Viruses* 13 (2):176–183. doi: 10.1111/irv.12615.

Lucas, R. M., S. N. Byrne, J. Correale, S. Ilschner, and P. H. Hart. 2015. "Ultraviolet radiation, vitamin D and multiple sclerosis." *Neurodegenerative Disease Management* 5 (5):413–424. doi: 10.2217/nmt.15.33.

Lukasewycz, O. A., and J. R. Prohaska. 1990. "The immune response in copper deficiency." *Annals of the New York Academy of Sciences* 587:147–159. doi: 10.1111/j.1749-6632.1990.tb00142.x.

Macedo, M. Fatima, M. de Sousa, R. M. Ned, C. Mascarenhas, N. C. Andrews, and M. Correia-Neves. 2004. "Transferrin is required for early T-cell differentiation." *Immunology* 112 (4):543–549. doi: 10.1111/j.1365-2567.2004.01915.x.

Machon, C., S. Thezenas, A. M. Dupuy, E. Assenat, F. Michel, E. Mas, P. Senesse, and J. P. Cristol. 2012. "Immunonutrition before and during radiochemotherapy: improvement of inflammatory parameters in head and neck cancer patients." *Support Care Cancer* 20 (12):3129–3135. doi: 10.1007/s00520-012-1444-5.

Macpherson, A. J., and T. Uhr. 2004. "Induction of protective IgA by intestinal dendritic cells carrying commensal bacteria." *Science* 303 (5664):1662–1665. doi: 10.1126/science.1091334.

Magnus, S. A., I. R. Hambleton, F. Moosdeen, and G. R. Serjeant. 1999. "Recurrent infections in homozygous sickle cell disease." *Archives of Disease in Childhood* 80 (6):537–541. doi: 10.1136/adc.80.6.537.

Manning, J., B. Mitchell, D. A. Appadurai, A. Shakya, L. J. Pierce, H. Wang, V. Nganga, P. C. Swanson, J. M. May, D. Tantin, and G. J. Spangrude. 2013. "Vitamin C promotes maturation of T-cells." *Antioxidants & Redox Signaling* 19 (17):2054–2067. doi: 10.1089/ars.2012.4988.

Margioris, A. N. 2009. "Fatty acids and postprandial inflammation." *Current Opinion in Clinical Nutrition and Metabolic Care* 12 (2):129–137. doi: 10.1097/MCO.0b013e3283232a11.

Martindale, S., G. McNeill, G. Devereux, D. Campbell, G. Russell, and A. Seaton. 2005. "Antioxidant intake in pregnancy in relation to wheeze and eczema in the first two years of life." *American Journal of Respiratory and Critical Care Medicine* 171 (2):121–128. doi: 10.1164/rccm.200402-220OC.

Mauriz, E., A. Laliena, D. Vallejo, M. J. Tuñón, J. M. Rodríguez-López, R. Rodríguez-Pérez, and M. C. García-Fernández. 2013. "Effects of a low-fat diet with antioxidant supplementation on biochemical markers of multiple sclerosis long-term care residents." *Nutricion Hospitalaria* 28 (6):2229–2235. doi: 10.3305/nutr hosp.v28in06.6983.

Mayo-Wilson, E., A. Imdad, K. Herzer, M. Y. Yakoob, and Z. A. Bhutta. 2011. "Vitamin A supplements for preventing mortality, illness, and blindness in children aged under 5: systematic review and meta-analysis." *BMJ (Clinical Research Ed.)* 343:d5094. doi: 10.1136/bmj.d5094.

Maywald, M., S. K. Meurer, R. Weiskirchen, and L. Rink. 2017. "Zinc supplementation augments TGF-β1-dependent regulatory T cell induction." *Molecular Nutrition & Food Research* 61 (3). doi: 10.1002/mnfr.201600493.

Mazdeh, M., S. Seifirad, N. Kazemi, M. A. Seifrabie, A. Dehghan, and H. Abbasi. 2013. "Comparison of vitamin D3 serum levels in new diagnosed patients with multiple sclerosis versus their healthy relatives." *Acta Medica Iranica* 51 (5):289–292.

McAleer, J. P., and J. K. Kolls. 2018. "Contributions of the intestinal microbiome in lung immunity." *European Journal of Immunology* 48 (1):39–49. doi: 10.1002/eji.201646721.

McConkey, M., and D. T. Smith. 1933. "The relation of vitamin c deficiency to intestinal tuberculosis in the guinea pig." *The Journal of Experimental Medicine* 58 (4):503–512. doi: 10.1084/jem.58.4.503.

McDaniel, K. L., K. H. Restori, J. W. Dodds, M. J. Kennett, A. C. Ross, and M. T. Cantorna. 2015. "Vitamin A-deficient hosts become nonsymptomatic reservoirs of Escherichia coli-like enteric infections." *Infection and Immunity* 83 (7):2984–2991. doi: 10.1128/IAI.00201-15.

Mellor, A. L., and D. H. Munn. 2004. "IDO expression by dendritic cells: tolerance and tryptophan catabolism." *Nature Reviews. Immunology* 4 (10):762–774. doi: 10.1038/nri1457.

Mencacci, A., E. Cenci, J. R. Boelaert, P. Bucci, P. Mosci, C. Fè d'Ostiani, F. Bistoni, and L. Romani. 1997. "Iron overload alters innate and T helper cell responses to Candida albicans in mice." *The Journal of Infectious Diseases* 175 (6):1467–1476. doi: 10.1086/516481.

Metz, R., S. Rust, J. B. Duhadaway, M. R. Mautino, D. H. Munn, N. N. Vahanian, C. J. Link, and G. C. Prendergast. 2012. "IDO inhibits a tryptophan sufficiency signal that stimulates mTOR: a novel IDO effector pathway targeted by D-1-methyl-tryptophan." *Oncoimmunology* 1 (9):1460–1468. doi: 10.4161/onci.21716.

Mirzaei, F., K. B. Michels, K. Munger, E. O'Reilly, T. Chitnis, M. R. Forman, E. Giovannucci, B. Rosner, and A. Ascherio. 2011. "Gestational vitamin D and the risk of multiple sclerosis in offspring." *Annals of Neurology* 70 (1):30–40. doi: 10.1002/ana.22456.

Miyake, Y., K. Tanaka, H. Okubo, S. Sasaki, and M. Arakawa. 2014. "Maternal consumption of dairy products, calcium, and vitamin D during pregnancy and infantile allergic disorders." *Annals of Allergy, Asthma & Immunology* 113 (1):82–87. doi: 10.1016/j.anai.2014.04.023.

Miyamoto, K., K. Kosakai, S. Ikebayashi, T. Tsuchiya, S. Yamamoto, and H. Tsujibo. 2009. "Proteomic analysis of Vibrio vulnificus M2799 grown under iron-repleted and iron-depleted conditions." *Microbial Pathogenesis* 46 (3):171–177. doi: 10.1016/j.micpath.2008.12.004.

Moghaddasi, M., M. Mamarabadi, N. Mohebi, H. Razjouyan, and M. Aghaei. 2013. "Homocysteine, vitamin B12 and folate levels in Iranian patients with multiple sclerosis: a case control study." *Clinical Neurology and Neurosurgery* 115 (9):1802–1805. doi: 10.1016/j.clineuro.2013.05.007.

Mossad, S. B., M. L. Macknin, S. V. Medendorp, and P. Mason. 1996. "Zinc gluconate lozenges for treating the common cold. A randomized, double-blind, placebo-controlled study." *Annals of Internal Medicine* 125 (2):81–88. doi: 10.7326/0003-4819-125-2-199607150-00001.

Moulder, K., and M. W. Steward. 1989. "Experimental zinc deficiency: effects on cellular responses and the affinity of humoral antibody." *Clinical and Experimental Immunology* 77 (2):269–274.

Munger, K. L., L. I. Levin, B. W. Hollis, N. S. Howard, and A. Ascherio. 2006. "Serum 25-hydroxyvitamin D levels and risk of multiple sclerosis." *JAMA* 296 (23):2832–2838. doi: 10.1001/jama.296.23.2832.

Munger, K. L., T. Chitnis, A. L. Frazier, E. Giovannucci, D. Spiegelman, and A. Ascherio. 2011. "Dietary intake of vitamin D during adolescence and risk of multiple sclerosis." *Journal of Neurology* 258 (3):479–485. doi: 10.1007/s00415-010-5783-1.

Munn, D. H., M. Zhou, J. T. Attwood, I. Bondarev, S. J. Conway, B. Marshall, C. Brown, and A. L. Mellor. 1998. "Prevention of allogeneic fetal rejection by tryptophan catabolism." *Science (New York, N.Y.)* 281 (5380):1191–1193. doi: 10.1126/science.281.5380.1191.

Muraro, A., S. Halken, S. H. Arshad, K. Beyer, A. E. J. Dubois, G. Du Toit, P. A. Eigenmann, K. E. C. Grimshaw, A. Hoest, G. Lack, L. O'Mahony, N. G. Papadopoulos, S. Panesar, S. Prescott, G. Roberts, D. de Silva, C. Venter, V. Verhasselt, A. C. Akdis, A. Sheikh, EAACI Food Allergy, and Group Anaphylaxis Guidelines. 2014. "EAACI food allergy and anaphylaxis guidelines. Primary prevention of food allergy." *Allergy* 69 (5):590–601. doi: 10.1111/all.12398.

Nairz, M., A. Schroll, T. Sonnweber, and G. Weiss. 2010. "The struggle for iron - a metal at the host-pathogen interface." *Cellular Microbiology* 12 (12):1691–1702. doi: 10.1111/j.1462-5822.2010.01529.x.

Najafi, M. R., V. Shaygannajad, M. Mirpourian, and A. Gholamrezaei. 2012. "Vitamin B(12) deficiency and multiple sclerosis; is there any association?" *International Journal of Preventive Medicine* 3 (4):286–289.

Narula, N., A. Dhillon, D. Zhang, M. E. Sherlock, M. Tondeur, and M. Zachos. 2018. "Enteral nutritional therapy for induction of remission in Crohn's disease." *Cochrane Database Syst Rev* (4):CD000542. doi: 10.1002/14651858.CD000542.pub3.

Nemeth, E., S. Rivera, V. Gabayan, C. Keller, S. Taudorf, B. K. Pedersen, and T. Ganz. 2004. "IL-6 mediates hypoferremia of inflammation by inducing the synthesis of the iron regulatory hormone hepcidin." *The Journal of Clinical Investigation* 113 (9):1271–1276. doi: 10.1172/JCI20945.

Netting, M. J., P. F. Middleton, and M. Makrides. 2014. "Does maternal diet during pregnancy and lactation affect outcomes in offspring? A systematic review of food-based approaches." *Nutrition (Burbank, Los Angeles County, Calif.)* 30 (11–12):1225–1241. doi: 10.1016/j.nut.2014.02.015.

Nosrati, A., L. Afifi, M. J. Danesh, K. Lee, D. Yan, K. Beroukhim, R. Ahn, and W. Liao. 2017. "Dietary modifications in atopic dermatitis: patient-reported outcomes." *The Journal of Dermatological Treatment* 28 (6):523–538. doi: 10.1080/09546634.2016.1278071.

Ogbechi, J., F. I. Clanchy, Y.-S. Huang, L. M. Topping, T. W. Stone, and R. O. Williams. 2020. "IDO activation, inflammation and musculoskeletal disease." *Experimental Gerontology* 131:110820. doi: 10.1016/j.exger.2019.110820.

Oh, S. Y., J. Chung, M. K. Kim, S. O. Kwon, and B. H. Cho. 2010. "Antioxidant nutrient intakes and corresponding biomarkers associated with the risk of atopic dermatitis in young children." *European Journal of Clinical Nutrition* 64 (3):245–252. doi: 10.1038/ejcn.2009.148.

Osborn, D. A., and J. K. H. Sinn. 2013. "Prebiotics in infants for prevention of allergy." *The Cochrane Database of Systematic Reviews* (3):CD006474. doi: 10.1002/14651858.CD006474.pub3.

Ott, S. J., M. Musfeldt, D. F. Wenderoth, J. Hampe, O. Brant, U. R. Folsch, K. N. Timmis, and S. Schreiber. 2004. "Reduction in diversity of the colonic mucosa associated bacterial microflora in patients with active inflammatory bowel disease." *Gut* 53 (5):685–693. doi: 10.1136/gut.2003.025403.

Pantzaris, M. C., G. N. Loukaides, E. E. Ntzani, and I. S. Patrikios. 2013. "A novel oral nutraceutical formula of omega-3 and omega-6 fatty acids with vitamins (PLP10) in relapsing remitting multiple sclerosis: a randomised, double-blind, placebo-controlled proof-of-concept clinical trial." *BMJ Open* 3 (4):e002170. doi: 10.1136/bmjopen-2012-002170.

Papadopoulou, A., D. B. Panagiotakos, G. Hatziagorou, G. Antonogeorgos, V. N. Matziou, J. N. Tsanakas, C. Gratziou, S. Tsabouri, and K. N. Priftis. 2015. "Antioxidant foods consumption and childhood asthma and other allergic diseases: The Greek cohorts of the ISAAC II survey." *Allergologia Et Immunopathologia* 43 (4):353–360. doi: 10.1016/j.aller.2014.03.002.

Parisi, G. C., M. Zilli, M. P. Miani, M. Carrara, E. Bottona, G. Verdianelli, G. Battaglia, S. Desideri, A. Faedo, C. Marzolino, A. Tonon, M. Ermani, and G. Leandro. 2002. "High-fiber diet supplementation in patients with irritable bowel syndrome (IBS): a multicenter, randomized, open trial comparison between wheat bran diet and partially hydrolyzed guar gum (PHGG)." *Digestive Diseases and Sciences* 47 (8):1697–1704. doi: 10.1023/a:1016419906546.

Park, S., H.-S. Choi, and J.-H. Bae. 2016. "Instant noodles, processed food intake, and dietary pattern are associated with atopic dermatitis in an adult population (KNHANES 2009-2011)." *Asia Pacific Journal of Clinical Nutrition* 25 (3):602–613. doi: 10.6133/apjcn.092015.23.

Patel, S., A. Custovic, J. A. Smith, A. Simpson, G. Kerry, and C. S. Murray. 2014. "Cross-sectional association of dietary patterns with asthma and atopic sensitization in childhood - in a cohort study." *Pediatric Allergy and Immunology* 25 (6):565–571. doi: 10.1111/pai.12276.

Prinz, W., R. Bortz, B. Bregin, and M. Hersch. 1977. "The effect of ascorbic acid supplementation on some parameters of the human immunological defence system." *International Journal for Vitamin and Nutrition Research. Internationale Zeitschrift Fur Vitamin- Und Ernahrungsforschung. Journal International De Vitaminologie Et De Nutrition* 47 (3):248–257.

Provvedini, D. M., C. D. Tsoukas, L. J. Deftos, and S. C. Manolagas. 1983. "1,25-dihydroxyvitamin D3 receptors in human leukocytes." *Science (New York, N.Y.)* 221 (4616):1181–1183. doi: 10.1126/science.6310748.

Riverin, B. D., J. L. Maguire, and P. Li. 2015. "Vitamin D supplementation for childhood asthma: a systematic review and meta-analysis." *PloS One* 10 (8):e0136841. doi: 10.1371/journal.pone.0136841.

Roduit, C., R. Frei, M. Depner, B. Schaub, G. Loss, J. Genuneit, P. Pfefferle, A. Hyvärinen, A. M. Karvonen, J. Riedler, J.-C. Dalphin, J. Pekkanen, E. von Mutius, C. Braun-Fahrländer, R. Lauener, and Pasture Study Group. 2014. "Increased food diversity in the first year of life is inversely associated with allergic diseases." *The Journal of Allergy and Clinical Immunology* 133 (4):1056–1064. doi: 10.1016/j.jaci.2013.12.1044.

Romieu, I., A. Barraza-Villarreal, C. Escamilla-Núñez, J. L. Texcalac-Sangrador, L. Hernandez-Cadena, D. Díaz-Sánchez, J. De Batlle, and B. E. Del Rio-Navarro. 2009. "Dietary intake, lung function and airway inflammation in Mexico City school children exposed to air pollutants." *Respiratory Research* 10:122. doi: 10.1186/1465-9921-10-122.

Round, J. L., S. M. Lee, J. Li, G. Tran, B. Jabri, T. A. Chatila, and S. K. Mazmanian. 2011. "The Toll-like receptor 2 pathway establishes colonization by a commensal of the human microbiota." *Science* 332 (6032):974–977. doi: 10.1126/science.1206095.

Ruemmele, F. M., G. Veres, K. L. Kolho, A. Griffiths, A. Levine, J. C. Escher, J. Amil Dias, A. Barabino, C. P. Braegger, J. Bronsky, S. Buderus, J. Martin-de-Carpi, L. De Ridder, U. L. Fagerberg, J. P. Hugot, J. Kierkus, S. Kolacek, S. Koletzko, P. Lionetti, E. Miele, V. M. Navas Lopez, A. Paerregaard, R. K. Russell, D. E. Serban, R. Shaoul, P. Van Rheenen, G. Veereman, B. Weiss, D. Wilson, A. Dignass, A. Eliakim, H. Winter, D. Turner, Crohn's European, Organisation Colitis, Hepatology European Society of Pediatric Gastroenterology, and Nutrition. 2014. "Consensus guidelines of ECCO/ESPGHAN on the medical management of pediatric Crohn's disease." *Journal of Crohn's & Colitis* 8 (10):1179–207. doi: 10.1016/j.crohns.2014.04.005.

Saavedra, J. M., and A. Tschernia. 2002. "Human studies with probiotics and prebiotics: clinical implications." *British Journal of Nutrition* 87 Suppl 2:S241–S246. doi: 10.1079/BJNBJN/2002543.

Sánchez-Armendáriz, K., A. García-Gil, C. A. Romero, J. Contreras-Ruiz, M. Karam-Orante, D. Balcazar-Antonio, and J. Domínguez-Cherit. 2018. "Oral vitamin D3 5000 IU/day as an adjuvant in the treatment of atopic dermatitis: a randomized control trial." *International Journal of Dermatology* 57 (12):1516–1520. doi: 10.1111/ijd.14220.

Satchithanandam, S., M. Vargofcak-Apker, R. J. Calvert, A. R. Leeds, and M. M. Cassidy. 1990. "Alteration of gastrointestinal mucin by fiber feeding in rats." *The Journal of Nutrition* 120 (10):1179–1184. doi: 10.1093/jn/120.10.1179.

Schauber, J., R. A. Dorschner, A. B. Coda, A. S. Büchau, P. T. Liu, D. Kiken, Y. R. Helfrich, S. Kang, H. Z. Elalieh, A. Steinmeyer, U. Zügel, D. D. Bikle, R. L. Modlin, and R. L. Gallo. 2007. "Injury enhances TLR2 function and antimicrobial peptide expression through a vitamin D-dependent mechanism." *The Journal of Clinical Investigation* 117 (3):803–811. doi: 10.1172/JCI30142.

Schley, P. D., and C. J. Field. 2002. "The immune-enhancing effects of dietary fibres and prebiotics." *The British Journal of Nutrition* 87 Suppl 2:S221–230. doi: 10.1079/BJNBJN/2002541.

Schryvers, A. B., and L. J. Morris. 1988. "Identification and characterization of the transferrin receptor from Neisseria meningitidis." *Molecular Microbiology* 2 (2):281–288. doi: 10.1111/j.1365-2958.1988.tb00029.x.

Sexton, P., P. Black, P. Metcalf, C. R. Wall, S. Ley, L. Wu, F. Sommerville, S. Brodie, and J. Kolbe. 2013. "Influence of mediterranean diet on asthma symptoms, lung function, and systemic inflammation: a randomized controlled trial." *The Journal of Asthma* 50 (1):75–81. doi: 10.3109/02770903.2012. 740120.

Shen, J., Z. X. Zuo, and A. P. Mao. 2014. "Effect of probiotics on inducing remission and maintaining therapy in ulcerative colitis, Crohn's disease, and pouchitis: meta-analysis of randomized controlled trials." *Inflammatory Bowel Disease* 20 (1):21–35. doi: 10.1097/01.MIB.0000437495.30052.be.

Sidbury, R., A. F. Sullivan, R. I. Thadhani, and C. A. Camargo. 2008. "Randomized controlled trial of vitamin D supplementation for winter-related atopic dermatitis in Boston: a pilot study." *The British Journal of Dermatology* 159 (1):245–247. doi: 10.1111/j.1365-2133.2008.08601.x.

Simopoulos, A. P. 2002. "The importance of the ratio of omega-6/omega-3 essential fatty acids." *Biomedicine & Pharmacotherapy = Biomedecine & Pharmacotherapie* 56 (8):365–379. doi: 10.1016/s0753-3322(02)00253-6.

Singh, N., and H.-Y. Sun. 2008. "Iron overload and unique susceptibility of liver transplant recipients to disseminated disease due to opportunistic pathogens." *Liver Transplantation* 14 (9):1249–1255. doi: 10.1002/lt.21587.

Soilu-Hänninen, M., L. Airas, I. Mononen, A. Heikkilä, M. Viljanen, and A. Hänninen. 2005. "25-Hydroxyvitamin D levels in serum at the onset of multiple sclerosis." *Multiple Sclerosis (Houndmills, Basingstoke, England)* 11 (3):266–271. doi: 10.1191/1352458505ms1157oa.

Stephensen, C. B. 2001. "Vitamin A, infection, and immune function." *Annual Review of Nutrition* 21:167–192. doi: 10.1146/annurev.nutr.21.1.167.

Stork, M., J. Grijpstra, M. P. Bos, C. M. Torres, N. Devos, J. T. Poolman, W. J. Chazin, and J. Tommassen. 2013. "Zinc piracy as a mechanism of Neisseria meningitidis for evasion of nutritional immunity." *PLoS Pathogens* 9 (10):e1003733. doi: 10.1371/journal.ppat.1003733.

Strasser, B., G. Kohlboeck, M. Hermanky, and M. Leitzmann. 2020. "Role of dietary protein and exercise on biomarkers of immune activation in older patients during hospitalization." *Aging Clinical and Experimental Research* 32:2419–2423. doi: 10.1007/s40520-019-01461-7.

Su, O., A. G. Bahalı, A. D. Demir, D. B. Ozkaya, S. Uzuner, D. Dizman, and N. Onsun. 2017. "The relationship between severity of disease and vitamin D levels in children with atopic dermatitis." *Postepy Dermatologii I Alergologii* 34 (3):224–227. doi: 10.5114/pdia.2017.66054.

Subramanian Vignesh, K., J. A. L. Figueroa, A. Porollo, J. A. Caruso, and G. S. Deepe. 2013. "Granulocyte macrophage-colony stimulating factor induced Zn sequestration enhances macrophage superoxide and limits intracellular pathogen survival." *Immunity* 39 (4):697–710. doi: 10.1016/j.immuni.2013.09.006.

Sunpaweravong, S., P. Puttawibul, S. Ruangsin, S. Laohawiriyakamol, P. Sunpaweravong, D. Sangthawan, J. Pradutkanchana, P. Raungkhajorn, and A. Geater. 2014. "Randomized study of antiinflammatory and immune-modulatory effects of enteral immunonutrition during concurrent chemoradiotherapy for esophageal cancer." *Nutrition and Cancer* 66 (1):1–5. doi: 10.1080/01635581.2014.847473.

Talvas, J., G. Garrait, N. Goncalves-Mendes, J. Rouanet, J. Vergnaud-Gauduchon, F. Kwiatkowski, P. Bachmann, C. Bouteloup, J. Bienvenu, and M. P. Vasson. 2015. "Immunonutrition stimulates immune functions and antioxidant defense capacities of leukocytes in radiochemotherapy-treated head & neck and esophageal cancer patients: a double-blind randomized clinical trial." *Clinical Nutrition* 34 (5):810–817. doi: 10.1016/j.clnu.2014.12.002.

Terness, P., T. M. Bauer, L. Röse, C. Dufter, A. Watzlik, H. Simon, and G. Opelz. 2002. "Inhibition of allogeneic T cell proliferation by indoleamine 2,3-dioxygenase-expressing dendritic cells: mediation of suppression by tryptophan metabolites." *The Journal of Experimental Medicine* 196 (4):447–457. doi: 10.1084/jem.20020052.

Thorburn, A. N., C. I. McKenzie, S. Shen, D. Stanley, L. Macia, L. J. Mason, L. K. Roberts, C. H. Y. Wong, R. Shim, R. Robert, N. Chevalier, J. K. Tan, E. Mariño, R. J. Moore, L. Wong, M. J. McConville, D. L. Tull, L. G. Wood, V. E. Murphy, P. Mattes, P. G. Gibson, and C. R. Mackay. 2015. "Evidence that asthma is a developmental origin disease influenced by maternal diet and bacterial metabolites." *Nature Communications* 6:7320. doi: 10.1038/ncomms8320.

Tickner, F. J., and V. C. Medvei. 1958. "Scurvy and the health of European crews in the Indian Ocean in the seventeenth century." *Medical History* 2 (1):36–46. doi: 10.1017/s0025727300023255.

Tromp, I. I. M., J. C. Kiefte-de Jong, J. H. de Vries, V. W. V. Jaddoe, H. Raat, A. Hofman, J. C. de Jongste, and H. A. Moll. 2012. "Dietary patterns and respiratory symptoms in pre-school children: the Generation R study." *The European Respiratory Journal* 40 (3):681–689. doi: 10.1183/09031936.00119111.

Tsoureli-Nikita, E., J. Hercogova, T. Lotti, and G. Menchini. 2002. "Evaluation of dietary intake of vita-min E in the treatment of atopic dermatitis: a study of the clinical course and evaluation of the immunoglobulin E serum levels." *International Journal of Dermatology* 41 (3):146–150. doi: 10.1046/j.1365-4362.2002.01423.x.

Turner, D., S. H. Zlotkin, P. S. Shah, and A. M. Griffiths. 2007. "Omega 3 fatty acids (fish oil) for maintenance of remission in Crohn's disease." *Cochrane Database Syst Rev* (2):CD006320. doi: 10.1002/14651858. CD006320.pub2.

Uddenfeldt, M., C. Janson, E. Lampa, M. Leander, D. Norbäck, L. Larsson, and A. Rask-Andersen. 2010. "High BMI is related to higher incidence of asthma, while a fish and fruit diet is related to a lower-Results from a long-term follow-up study of three age groups in Sweden." *Respiratory Medicine* 104 (7):972–980. doi: 10.1016/j.rmed.2009.12.013.

Urashima, M., T. Segawa, M. Okazaki, M. Kurihara, Y. Wada, and H. Ida. 2010. "Randomized trial of vitamin D supplementation to prevent seasonal influenza A in schoolchildren." *Am J Clin Nutr* 91 (5):1255–1260. doi: 10.3945/ajcn.2009.29094.

Varraso, R., F. Kauffmann, B. Leynaert, N. Le Moual, M. C. Boutron-Ruault, F. Clavel-Chapelon, and I. Romieu. 2009. "Dietary patterns and asthma in the E3N study." *The European Respiratory Journal* 33 (1):33–41. doi: 10.1183/09031936.00130807.

Vassallo, M. F., and C. A. Camargo. 2010. "Potential mechanisms for the hypothesized link between sun-shine, vitamin D, and food allergy in children." *The Journal of Allergy and Clinical Immunology* 126 (2):217–222. doi: 10.1016/j.jaci.2010.06.011.

Vruwink, K. G., M. P. Fletcher, C. L. Keen, M. S. Golub, A. G. Hendrickx, and M. E. Gershwin. 1991. "Moderate zinc deficiency in rhesus monkeys. An intrinsic defect of neutrophil chemotaxis corrected by zinc repletion." *Journal of Immunology (Baltimore, Md.: 1950)* 146 (1):244–249.

Walker, A. W., J. D. Sanderson, C. Churcher, G. C. Parkes, B. N. Hudspith, N. Rayment, J. Brostoff, J. Parkhill, G. Dougan, and L. Petrovska. 2011. "High-throughput clone library analysis of the mucosa-associated microbiota reveals dysbiosis and differences between inflamed and non-inflamed regions of the intes-tine in inflammatory bowel disease." *BMC Microbiol* 11:7. doi: 10.1186/1471-2180-11-7.

Wang, S. S., K. L. Hon, A. P.-S. Kong, H.N.-H. Pong, G. W.-K. Wong, and T. F. Leung. 2014. "Vitamin D deficiency is associated with diagnosis and severity of childhood atopic dermatitis." *Pediatric Allergy and Immunology* 25 (1):30–35. doi: 10.1111/pai.12167.

Wang, T.-T., F. P. Nestel, V. Bourdeau, Y. Nagai, Q. Wang, J. Liao, L. Tavera-Mendoza, R. Lin, J. W. Hanrahan, S. Mader, J. H. White, and J. H. Hanrahan. 2004. "Cutting edge: 1,25-dihydroxyvitamin D3 is a direct inducer of antimicrobial peptide gene expression." *Journal of Immunology (Baltimore, Md.: 1950)* 173 (5):2909–2912. doi: 10.4049/jimmunol.173.5.2909.

Weiss, G. 2005. "Modification of iron regulation by the inflammatory response." *Best Practice & Research. Clinical Haematology* 18 (2):183–201. doi: 10.1016/j.beha.2004.09.001.

Weisse, K., S. Winkler, F. Hirche, G. Herberth, D. Hinz, M. Bauer, S. Röder, U. Rolle-Kampczyk, M. von Bergen, S. Olek, U. Sack, T. Richter, U. Diez, M. Borte, G. I. Stangl, and I. Lehmann. 2013. "Maternal and newborn vitamin D status and its impact on food allergy development in the German LINA cohort study." *Allergy* 68 (2):220–228. doi: 10.1111/all.12081.

Weyh, C., K. Krüger, and B. Strasser. 2020. "Physical activity and diet shape the immune system during aging." *Nutrients* 12 (3). doi: 10.3390/nu12030622.

White, C., J. Lee, T. Kambe, K. Fritsche, and M. J. Petris. 2009. "A role for the ATP7A copper-transporting ATPase in macrophage bactericidal activity." *The Journal of Biological Chemistry* 284 (49):33949–33956. doi: 10.1074/jbc.M109.070201.

Wood, L. G., M. L. Garg, H. Powell, and P. G. Gibson. 2008. "Lycopene-rich treatments modify noneosino-philic airway inflammation in asthma: proof of concept." *Free Radical Research* 42 (1):94–102. doi: 10.1080/10715760701767307.

Wood, L. G., M. L. Garg, J. M. Smart, H. A. Scott, D. Barker, and P. G. Gibson. 2012. "Manipulating antioxi-dant intake in asthma: a randomized controlled trial." *The American Journal of Clinical Nutrition* 96 (3):534–543. doi: 10.3945/ajcn.111.032623.

Xin, Z., D. F. Waterman, R. W. Hemken, and R. J. Harmon. 1991. "Effects of copper status on neutrophil func-tion, superoxide dismutase, and copper distribution in steers." *Journal of Dairy Science* 74 (9):3078–3085. doi: 10.3168/jds.S0022-0302(91)78493-2.

Xing, Y., K. Sheng, X. Xiao, J. Li, H. Wei, L. Liu, W. Zhou, and X. Tong. 2020. "Vitamin A deficiency is asso-ciated with severe Mycoplasma pneumoniae pneumonia in children." *Annals of Translational Medicine* 8 (4):120. doi: 10.21037/atm.2020.02.33.

Yamada, T., T. Saunders, S. Kuroda, K. Sera, T. Nakamura, T. Takatsuji, Obstetricians Fukuoka College of, Pediatric Association of Fukuoka District Gynecologists, T. Hara, and Y. Nose. 2013. "Cohort study for prevention of atopic dermatitis using hair mineral contents." *Journal of Trace Elements in Medicine and Biology* 27 (2):126–131. doi: 10.1016/j.jtemb.2012.08.003.

Yu, S., and M. T. Cantorna. 2008. "The vitamin D receptor is required for iNKT cell development." *Proceedings of the National Academy of Sciences of the United States of America* 105 (13):5207–5212. doi: 10.1073/pnas.0711558105.

Zhang, Z., L. Shi, W. Pang, W. Liu, J. Li, H. Wang, and G. Shi. 2016. "Dietary fiber intake regulates intestinal microflora and inhibits ovalbumin-induced allergic airway inflammation in a mouse model." *PLoS One* 11 (2):e0147778. doi: 10.1371/journal.pone.0147778.

Zidar, B. L., R. K. Shadduck, Z. Zeigler, and A. Winkelstein. 1977. "Observations on the anemia and neutropenia of human copper deficiency." *American Journal of Hematology* 3:177–185. doi: 10.1002/ajh.2830030209.

Zitvogel, L., A. Tesniere, and G. Kroemer. 2006. "Cancer despite immunosurveillance: immunoselection and immunosubversion." *Nature Reviews Immunology* 6 (10):715–727. doi: 10.1038/nri1936.

6 Personalized Nutrition and Cancer

Zhaoping Li and David Heber
UCLA Center for Human Nutrition

CONTENTS

INTRODUCTION

Personalized nutrition is defined as an approach that uses information on individual characteristics to develop targeted nutritional advice, products, or services to assist individuals in achieving a lasting dietary behavior change that is beneficial for health (Ordovas et al. 2018). Personalized nutrition is often associated or confused with precision nutrition, nutrigenomics, nutrigenetics, and nutritional genomics. It is important to define the difference between personalized nutrition and these closely related terms in order to implement personalized nutrition in the setting of cancer. Nutrigenetics is that part of personalized nutrition that studies the association of different phenotypic responses such as body weight, blood pressure, plasma cholesterol, or glucose levels to a specific diet or nutrient challenge depending on individual genotypic differences. Nutrigenomics is a broader term which includes the impact of nutrition and individual nutrients on all gene products and their metabolic consequences. Nutrigenomic epigenetic changes including methylation, histone modification, and microRNAs can modify the expression and function of an individual without affecting genotype. These changes can occur in utero as well as later in life and can be inherited affecting predisposition to obesity and cancer as the result of nutrient or hormone exposure. Metabolomics is the study and analysis of the numerous small metabolites and metabolic pathways related to genomic and epigenetic differences. The discovery of the gut microbiome and the metabolic products of bacterial communities in the gut has added an additional layer of complexity to nutrigenetics and nutrigenomics. Just to add one final "ome" to this discussion, the impact of environmental factors, such as stress, physical activity and diet, to which an individual is exposed and which may affect health have been called the exposome.

More and more dimensions or characteristics are being uncovered as necessary to achieve the goal of utilizing precision nutrition. The complexity of relationships between individual diet and phenotype has required the use of a wide range of approaches including machine learning and artificial intelligence. An instructive example of the ability to integrate complex characteristics into personalized nutrition is the ability to predict individual postprandial glucose elevations in response to different foods. Elevated postprandial blood glucose levels constitute a global epidemic and a major risk factor for prediabetes and type 2 diabetes mellitus. To develop specific dietary recommendations to control blood sugar after meals, researchers continuously monitored week-long glucose levels in an 800-person cohort and measured responses to 46,898 meals (Zeevi et al. 2015). They found high variability in the responses to identical meals in different individuals but reproducible responses in the same individuals, suggesting that universal dietary recommendations may sometimes have limited benefits for individuals (see Figure 6.1). A machine-learning algorithm was

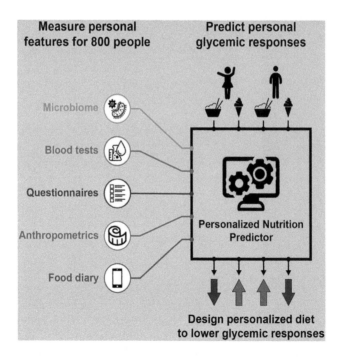

FIGURE 6.1 People eating identical meals present high variability in postmeal blood glucose response. Personalized diets created with the help of an accurate predictor of blood glucose response that integrates parameters such as dietary habits, physical activity, and gut microbiota successfully lowered postmeal blood glucose and its long-term metabolic consequences. (From Zeevi et al. 2015.)

used that integrated blood parameters, dietary habits, anthropometrics, physical activity, and gut microbiota measured in this cohort and it was able to accurately predict personalized postprandial glycemic response to real-life meals. They validated these predictions in an independent 100-person cohort, and conducted a blinded randomized controlled dietary intervention based on this algorithm which resulted in significantly lower postprandial glucose responses and consistent alterations to gut microbiota configuration in the intervention group compared to controls who received generalized advice. These results suggest that personalized diets may successfully modify elevated postprandial blood glucose and its metabolic consequences including increased cancer risk.

High glycemic index (GI) diets, which chronically raise postprandial blood glucose, may increase cancer risk making the individualized responses to foods relevant to cancer risk. Cancer risk and dietary GI were studied in the EPIC-Italy cohort. After a median 14.9 years, 5,112 incident cancers and 2,460 deaths were identified among 45,148 recruited adults. High GI was associated with increased risk of colon and bladder cancer. High intake of carbohydrate from high GI foods was significantly associated with increased risk of colon and diabetes-related cancers, but decreased risk of stomach cancer; whereas high intake of carbohydrates from low GI foods was associated with reduced colon cancer risk. In a Mediterranean population with high and varied carbohydrate intake, carbohydrates that strongly raise postprandial blood glucose were associated with increased colon and bladder cancer risk, while the quantity of carbohydrate consumed was associated with diabetes-related cancers (Sieri et al. 2017). This example relevant to nutrition and cancer risk illustrates the potential of precision nutrition for rises in blood glucose after meals.

The personalized responses to dietary composition (PREDICT 1) clinical trial recruited 1,002 twins and unrelated healthy adults in the United Kingdom to the PREDICT 1 study and assessed postprandial metabolic responses in a clinical setting and at home (Berry et al. 2020). The study was designed to quantify and predict individual variations in postprandial triglyceride, glucose, and insulin responses to standardized meals. PREDICT 1 examined the influence of genetic, metabolic, microbiome, meal composition, and meal context data in order to distinguish predictors of individual responses to meals. These predictions were validated in an independent cohort of adults from the United States. Large interindividual variability was observed as measured by the population coefficient of variation (standard deviation/mean, %) in postprandial responses of blood triglyceride (103%), glucose (68%), and insulin (59%) following identical meals. Person-specific factors, such as gut microbiome, had a greater influence (7.1% of variance) than did meal macronutrients (3.6%) for postprandial lipemia, but not for postprandial glycemia (6.0% and 15.4%, respectively). Genetic variants had a modest impact on predictions (9.5% for glucose, 0.8% for triglyceride, 0.2% for C-peptide). Findings were independently validated in a US cohort (n = 100 people). Using the huge amounts of data from the trial, a machine-learning model was developed that predicted both triglyceride (r = 0.47) and glycemic (r = 0.77) responses to food intake. These findings may be informative for developing personalized diet strategies in the future. However, the generalization of these findings will require validation in people of non-European ancestry, older adults, and people with diseases that affect metabolism, and will ultimately require appropriately powered longitudinal studies.

Precision nutrition is not yet available for all the complex relationships between an individual, their food consumption, their genotype, and their phenotype. The degree of scientific certainty required for precision nutrition is much greater than that required for personalized nutrition using established phenotypic and genomic data which will be described in this chapter.

There are well-established phenotypic differences between individuals in physical dimensions such as height and weight and differences in lean body mass and fat mass which can be determined by bioelectrical impedance and other anthropometric methods that have come into widespread use over the last 20 years. Both lean mass and fat mass can affect the risk of cancer and survival from malnutrition associated with advanced cancer. Lean mass can be used to prescribe personalized protein prescriptions leading to personalized meal plans. In cancer survivors, many of the same obesity-associated diseases that occur in the general population can affect cancer survivors making personalized weight management relevant to cancer survivors. Ethnicity and gender in turn affect fat distribution and the metabolic activity of fat especially in terms of inflammation mediated by intra-abdominal or visceral fat which may lead to insights into cancer risk reduction with personalized nutrition approaches. These basic insights which simply refer to phenotypic differences can be utilized for a more personalized approach in cancer and nutrition research and treatment. The future prospect that the development of precision nutrition will enhance precision oncology will require much more research and advances in analytical methods including artificial intelligence.

In this chapter, personalized nutrition advice will stay within the generalized broad guidelines, but will customize advice in an attempt to help individuals with cancer achieve a better diet and lifestyle that meets their individual goals for health and quality of life. There has been a positive evolution of the dietary guidelines over the last few decades, and this chapter is not a criticism of the dedicated professionals who developed the recommendations. The process developing dietary guidelines and information on dietary patterns will continue, but will always follow and not lead nutritional science. Since nutrition advice can be helpful when integrated with individual clinical information and personal preferences oncologists, primary care physicians, dietitians, and other healthcare providers can move now to include the personalized guidelines reviewed in this chapter.

NUTRIGENOMICS AND NUTRIGENOMICS

Nutrigenomics and Nutrigenomics include both nutrigenetics, which is the association of genetic variants with observed nutritional differences, and nutrigenomics which denotes the different outcomes of nutritional interventions in patients with different genetics due to the effects of nutrition on gene expression. Personalized nutrition based on inherited metabolic disorders has been implemented for decades based on well-established and defined genetic variants including those for lactose intolerance, phenylketonuria, and celiac disease leading to recommendations to avoid lactose, phenylalanine, and gluten in the diet. In nutrigenetic association studies, single-nucleotide variants also called single-nucleotide polymorphisms (SNPs) have been associated with common chronic diseases including obesity and cancer through interactions with the intakes of macro and micronutrients, or with the consumption of particular foods and dietary patterns. The challenge for personalized nutrition in cancer is to extend that principle to the complex multifactorial genetics of obesity, lipid disorders, glucose metabolism, and inflammation to the process of carcinogenesis and to create nutritional recommendations based on that knowledge.

For example, common variants in genes regulating homocysteine metabolism, such as methylenetetrahydrofolate reductase (MTHFR), and methionine synthase (MTR), have been linked to increased risk for breast cancer in individuals with low intakes of folate, vitamin B6, and vitamin B1 2 (Jiang-Hua et al. 2014). In this study, MTHFR genotype was linked with breast cancer in a Chinese population case–control study of 535 patients with newly diagnosed breast cancer and 673 controls. The MTHFR 667TT genotype and T allele were correlated with a significant increased risk of breast cancer when compared with the CC genotype. Individuals carrying the MTR 2756GG genotype and G allele had a higher risk of breast cancer when compared with subjects with the AA genotype. The MTHFR 667 T allele and MTR 2756 G allele were associated with a higher risk of breast cancer in individuals with low folate intake, vitamin B6, and vitamin B12, but the association disappeared among subjects with moderate and high intake of folate, vitamin B6, and vitamin B12. While this case–control study found that the MTHFR C677T and MTR A2756G polymorphisms are associated with risk of breast cancer, that risk could be reduced with increased intakes of folate, vitamin B6, and vitamin B12 even at moderate levels suggesting the potential impact of nutritional supplementation on a genetic predisposition to breast cancer.

The primary form of circulating vitamin D, 25-hydroxy-vitamin D (25(OH)D) is a modifiable quantitative trait associated with multiple medical outcomes, including osteoporosis, multiple sclerosis, selected malignancies, and especially colorectal cancer, with rickets being the most common expression of severe clinical vitamin D deficiency in children (DeLuca 2016). The concentration of 25(OH)D in blood, which reflects endogenous generation through ultraviolet B (UVB) exposure as well as exogenous dietary and supplemental vitamin D intake, is considered the best indicator of vitamin D status. Following metabolic activation to 1,25-dihydroxy-vitamin D [1,25(OH)2D] through multiple hydroxylation steps, vitamin D has pleiotropic effects in addition to its traditional role in calcium homeostasis; for example, vitamin D receptor response elements directly or indirectly influence cell cycling and proliferation, differentiation, and apoptosis (Christakos et al. 2016). Vitamin D status can be influenced by several polymorphisms in vitamin D pathway genes which modulate its effects on cell differentiation. Common genetic variants that influence circulating 25(OH)D levels could be important for identifying persons at risk for vitamin D deficiency and enhancing our understanding of the observed associations between vitamin D status and cancer discussed further below. In a very large randomized clinical trial of vitamin D supplementation in which genetic variations were not considered, supplementation with vitamin D did not result in a lower incidence of invasive cancer compared to placebo (Manson, Cook et al. 2019). This placebo-controlled intervention study illustrated that even large studies might fail to demonstrate benefits for cancer in general when genetic variation in blood levels, metabolism, and actions of 25OHD are not considered. Given the known variations in vitamin D metabolism and the common occurrence of vitamin D deficiencies in a subclinical range, the genetics of vitamin D and cancer deserve further study.

SNPs in genes encoding lipid proteins such as apolipoprotein C3 and apolipoprotein AI conferred a higher risk of metabolic syndrome (MS) in subjects with a Western dietary pattern (Hosseini-Esfahani et al. 2015). In nutrigenomic studies, gene-based personalized nutrition targeting the apolipoprotein E (APOE) gene was more effective in reducing saturated fat intake compared with standard dietary advice (Celis-Morales et al. 2017). Adherence to Mediterranean diet was greater among participants who received gene-based personalized nutrition targeting specific variants in five nutrient-responsive genes compared with those who received dietary advice on the basis of current diet plus phenotype (Livingstone et al. 2016). Genetic information regarding angiotensin I converting enzyme genotype revealed to subjects for personalized nutrition intervention resulted in greater changes in sodium intake compared to general population-based dietary advice (Nielsen et al. 2017). Gene expression can also be affected by diet relevant to cancer risk. For example, high meat consumption was associated with gene networks linked to cancer in colon tissue (Bouchard-Mercier et al. 2013). These nutrigenomic studies demonstrate some association with SNPs but in many cases while the provision of genetic information results in statistically significant differences in results of intervention, the differences are not large enough to be clinically significant based on current evidence.

Nutrigenomics documents the alteration of gene expression in part through epigenetic changes. Epigenetic changes are programmed throughout life and may explain in part the increased risks of cancer with aging. The epigenetics of cancer and aging may differ in the types of histone methylation observed based on studies of 98,857 CpG sites differentially methylated in aging and 286,746 in cancer as part of the NIH Roadmap Epigenomics and ENCODE projects (Perez, Tejedor et al. 2018). It is possible that the process of aging through small defects in transmitting epigenetic information through successive cell divisions, or maintaining it in differentiated cells, accumulates in a process that could be considered "epigenetic drift" intrinsic to aging. Epigenetic changes occur more frequently and at a faster rate than that corresponding genetic mutations, since the consequences for survival of the organism and species are less drastic and so fewer repair and defense mechanisms have evolved to protect the epigenome. Some of these changes may also be inherited and passed on to subsequent generations (Grossniklaus, Kelly et al. 2013). Epigenetics could explain the increased susceptibility of some populations to changes in diet and lifestyle following migration.

Illustrating the importance of personalized nutrition and environment on epigenetics and cancer risk, the patterns of epigenetic modifications in identical or monozygotic twins with identical genomes diverge as they become older. Differences in epigenetic changes such as DNA methylation in genetically identical individuals could be due to external and internal factors including smoking habits, physical activity, and nutritional habits (Schulz 2014). About one-third of monozygotic twins in one study exhibited differences in epigenetic markers which were more distinct in identical twins who were older, had different lifestyles, and had spent less of their lives together emphasizing the significant role of environmental and dietary factors in translating a common genotype into a different phenotype (Martin 2005).

An animal experiment which clearly illustrates the impact of nutrition on gene expression via methylation and epigenetics was carried out in the Agouti mouse. In a homozygous state, the Agouti gene is lethal but in the heterozygous state an inbred strain of Agouti mice generates a protein in utero that predisposes the animal to obesity, a change in coat color from brown to yellow and a predisposition to age-related chronic diseases including cancer (Waterland and Jirtle 2003). The change in coat color is related to the effect of melanocyte stimulating hormone on skin and also on food intake via effects on the hypothalamic centers controlling food intake (Wolff, Roberts et al. 1999). If you treat an obese yellow pregnant agouti mother mouse with methyl donor nutrients including folate, choline, betaine, and vitamin B12, she will give birth to normal brown babies without the Agouti protein due to inhibition of gene expression in utero (Wolff, Kodell et al. 1998). These animals are normal and have no increased risk of cancer. These epigenetic changes may be heritable for some genes such as the agouti gene even though many epigenetic changes are cleared at the time of implantation.

Nutrients can influence the epigenome during adult life as well within cancer cells. The interaction between the epigenetic makeup of an individual and his/her environmental exposure record or exposome is accepted as increasing the risk for a significant proportion of human malignancies. Recent studies have highlighted the key role of epigenetic mechanisms in mediating gene–environment interactions and translating exposures into tumorigenesis (Herceg et al. 2018). The epigenome is modified through several mechanisms including DNA methylation, histone modification, and micro RNA-mediated gene silencing. Changes observed in epigenetic markers have been observed in associated with either increased or decreased risks for cancer development suggesting that there is much more we need to learn about DNA methylation and cancer. There is convincing evidence indicating that several foods have protective roles in cancer prevention, through epigenetic changes that affect the tumor directly or the tumor microenvironment by creating conditions that favor tumor initiation and the multistep process of carcinogenesis.

DNA methylation is the most widely studied epigenetic modification relevant to cancer. DNA is methylated throughout the genome at intergenic regions and more densely at CpG islands (CGIs), DNA repair genes, or oncogenes (Supic, Jagodic et al. 2013). The aberrant methylation of promoter regions near tumor suppressor genes could influence gene expression, and abnormal levels of global methylation are associated with numerous cancers.

Chronological age is both the strongest demographic risk factor for cancer and the most important factor in the development of DNA methylation signatures in population-based studies. Age-associated epigenetic changes have been identified and provide the basis for an "epigenetic clock" (Horvath and Raj 2018). Aging also leads to molecular changes that trigger malignant transformation. The DNA methylation clock may be affected by different external and endogenous factors. Those exposures may contribute to methylation drift and "accelerated" aging, but caloric restriction in animal models leads to a reduction in this epigenetic drift (Maegawa et al. 2017). Diet and lifestyle were implicated in observed variations in the rate of aging among 1,000 healthy individuals followed prospectively between the ages of 26 and 38 (Belsky et al. 2015). Some individuals aged at half the normal rate while others aged at twice the normal rate based on 14 physiological and biochemical biomarkers (see Figure 6.2).

As DNA methylation landscape is altered as a function of age independently of exposures, there may be synergistic epigenetic effects between age and environmental exposures relevant to cancer. For instance, DNA methylation profiling in a large prospective cohort revealed an association between the epigenetic age acceleration and breast cancer risk and accelerated methylation in adjacent normal tissue in breast cancer patients (Hofstatter et al. 2018, Ambatipudi et al. 2017).

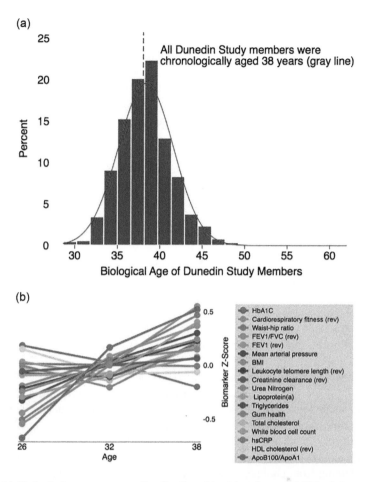

FIGURE 6.2 (a) Biological age was normally distributed in this cohort of 1,000 adults aged 38 years. (b) Biomarker values were standardized to have mean=0 and SD=1 across the 12 years of follow-up (Z scores). Z scores were coded so that higher values corresponded to older levels of the biomarkers; i.e., Z scores for cardiorespiratory fitness, lung function (FEV1 and FEV1/FVC), leukocyte telomere length, creatinine clearance, and HDL cholesterol, which decline with age, were reverse coded so that higher Z scores correspond to lower levels (From Belsky et al. 2015.)

Aberrant DNA methylation in cancer can be generated either prior to or following cell transformation through mutations. Increasing evidence suggests, however, that most methylation changes are generated in a programmed manner and occur in a subpopulation of tissue cells during normal aging, probably predisposing them for tumorigenesis (Klutstein, Nejman et al. 2016). It is likely that this methylation contributes to the tumor state by inhibiting the plasticity of cell differentiation processes. Despite some observations suggesting that this occurs mainly at promoter regions of tumor suppressor genes and is a result of growth selection, it now appears that this is a widespread programmed process that may be based on a relatively universal mechanism. Vertebrate CGIs are short interspersed DNA sequences that deviate significantly from the average genomic pattern by being GC-rich, CpG-rich, and predominantly nonmethylated. Most, perhaps all, CGIs are sites of transcription initiation, including thousands that are remote from currently annotated promoters. Although there are over 13,000 constitutively unmethylated CGIs in the human genome, approximately 2,000 of these are marked with polycomb, a protein complex that operates as a repressor by bringing about local heterochromatinization. In tumors, this complex appears to be responsible for recruiting the enzymes, DNA methyltransferases 3A and 3B (Moritz and Trievel 2018).

The DNA of each cell is wrapped around histone octamers. These histone proteins have tails that project from the nucleosome and many residues in these tails can be post-translationally modified, influencing all DNA-based processes, including chromatin compaction, nucleosome dynamics, and transcription. Histone tails together with other epigenetic changes determine whether the chromatin is active or inactive and this in turn affects the expression status of the genes within that chromatin region (Lawrence, Daujat, and Schneider 2016). Small noncoding RNA can also undergo DNA methylation or histone modification, thereby influencing the expression status of various genes promoting cancer development (Romano et al. 2017).

The excitement around the sequencing of the human genome in a small number of individuals in the late twentieth century created the impression that genomics was determinant in cancer and many other diseases. We now know that nutrition and lifestyle in a broad sense can influence gene expression, the rate of aging, and the multistep process of carcinogenesis.

CHOLINE

Choline can be acquired from the diet and via de novo biosynthesis through the methylation of phosphatidylethanolamine to phosphatidylcholine accounting for its not having been listed traditionally as a B vitamin. However, de novo synthesis of choline alone is not sufficient to meet human requirements. The US Recommended Dietary Intakes vary by age and gender, but is 550 mg/day in adult men, 425 mg/day in adult women, 450 mg/day in pregnant women, and 550 mg/day in lactating women (Yates, Schlicker, and Suitor 1998). Choline dietary intakes do not achieve adequate levels in many people (Zeisel and da Costa 2009).

Choline can modulate methylation and affect epigenetic regulation of gene expression because, via betaine homocysteine methyltransferase (BHMT), this nutrient together with its metabolite, betaine, and other methyl-group donors regulate the concentrations of 5-adenosylhomocysteine and 5-adenosylmethionine. As already discussed, the epigenetic mechanisms that modify gene expression without modifying the genetic code depend in part on the methylation of DNA or of histones. DNA and histone methylases are directly influenced by the availability of methyl-groups derived from the diet including from choline, betaine, methyl-folate, and methionine. These nutrients are the precursors that are converted to the universal methyl-donor 5-adenosylmethionine (Zeisel 2017).

Functional polymorphisms in genes encoding choline-related one-carbon metabolism enzymes, including phosphatidylethanolamine N-methyltransferase (PEMT), choline dehydrogenase (CHDH), and BHMT, have important roles in choline metabolism (Ganz et al. 2017) and may thus interact with dietary choline and betaine intake to modify cancer risk under conditions of dietary choline restriction. The interactive effect of polymorphisms in PEMT, BHMT, and CHDH genes with choline/betaine intake on breast cancer risk Chinese women was examined in a hospital-based case–control study of 570 cases with histologically confirmed breast cancer and 576 age-matched controls (Xu et al. 2008). Choline and betaine intakes were assessed by a validated FFQ, and genotyping was conducted for PEMT rs7946, CHDH rs9001, and BHMT rs3733890. Compared with the highest quartile of choline intake, the lowest intake quartile showed a significant increased risk of breast cancer. The SNP PEMT rs7946, CHDH rs9001, and BHMT rs3733890 had no overall association with breast cancer, but a significant risk reduction was observed among postmenopausal women with AA genotype of BHMT rs3733890 (OR 0.49; 95% CI 0.25, 0.98). Significant interactions were observed between choline intake and SNP PEMT rs7946 (P interaction=0·029) and BHMT rs3733890 (P interaction=0·006) in relation to breast cancer risk.

A population-based study of 1,508 cases of breast cancer and 1,556 controls examined the associations of the dietary intake of choline and two related micronutrients, methionine and betaine, and the risk of breast cancer. The highest quintile of choline consumption was associated with a lower risk of breast cancer (OR: 0.76; 95% confidence interval (CI): 0.58–1.00) compared with the lowest quintile. Two putatively functional SNPs of choline-metabolizing genes, PEMT-774G>C (rs12325817) and CHDH +432G>T (rs12676), were also found be related to breast cancer risk.

Compared with the PEMT GG genotype, the variant CC genotype was associated with an increased risk of breast cancer (OR: 1.30; 95% CI: 1.01–1.67). The CHDH minor T allele was also associated with an increased risk (OR: 1.19; 95% CI: 1.00–1.41) compared with the major G allele. The BHMT rs3733890 polymorphism was also examined but was found not to be associated with breast cancer risk. A significant interaction was found between dietary betaine intake and the PEMT rs7926 polymorphism (P(interaction)=0.04). These observations suggest that choline metabolism may play an important role in breast cancer etiology.

Animal experiments also support a role for choline and other methyl-donors in carcinogenesis, and provide some understanding of the underlying mechanisms involved. Rodents fed low choline, low methyl donor diets were observed 25 years ago to develop liver cancers (Zeisel et al. 1995). Choline-methyl-deficient diets resulted in decreased DNA methylation at many sites including at the oncogene c-myc (Shimizu et al. 2007). Down-regulation of microRNAs (miR-122 and miR-29) and up-regulation of miR-34a, miR-155, and miR-221 occurred in methyl-deficient liver (Pogribny, James, and Beland 2012, de Conti et al. 2017). These microRNAs act to modify the expression and translation of specific gene products involved in hepatocarcinogenesis.

Hepatocellular carcinoma (HCC) is a common cancer worldwide and represents one potential outcome of the natural history of chronic liver disease. The growing rates of HCC may be partially attributable to increased numbers of people with nonalcoholic fatty liver disease (NAFLD) and nonalcoholic steatohepatitis (NASH) (Ikawa-Yoshida et al. 2017) secondary to the global obesity epidemic. Liver cancer is the fifth most common cancer worldwide and the second most common cause of cancer mortality.

HCC is a major histological subtype and accounts for 70%–85% of primary liver cancers. The majority of HCC cases are due to chronic viral hepatitis B and C infections. Rigorous efforts to control viral hepatitis are succeeding with the spread of vaccination and innovative drugs (Chen et al. 2017). In developed countries, HCC traditionally associated with chronic hepatitis viral infection is expected to decline in the future (Anstee et al. 2019). However, obesity and MS are increasing globally due to dietary and lifestyle changes and NAFLD and NASH have emerged as relevant risk factors for HCC It has been estimated that between 4% and 22% of HCC cases can be ascribed to NAFLD (Michelotti, Machado, and Diehl 2013).

A meta-analysis of 11 studies in people calculated that diets low in choline increased the overall relative risk for developing cancer with the largest reported effects found for lung (30% increase); nasopharyngeal (58% increase); and breast cancer (60% increase). An increment in dietary intake of 100 mg/day of choline and betaine (a metabolite derived from choline) was estimated to be able to reduce cancer incidence by 11% (Sun et al. 2016, Ying et al. 2013, Du et al. 2016).

OBESITY

There are now ten common forms of cancer associated with obesity including postmenopausal breast, endometrial, ovarian, advanced prostate, colorectal, renal, pancreatic, liver, gallbladder cancers, and esophageal adenocarcinoma. The most widely held view of the mechanism underlying this association is that excess adiposity, estimated by the practical approximate variable of body mass index (BMI) or weight divided by height squared, is associated with reduced cancer survival. A number of studies have emerged challenging this by demonstrating that overweight and early obese states judged by BMI are associated with improved survival. This finding is termed the "obesity paradox" and is well recognized in the cardiovascular literature (Horwich, Fonarow, and Clark 2018).

BMI is a relatively crude measure of body adiposity and body composition and does not differentiate between lean mass and fat mass. In turn, body composition varies with age, sex, and ethnicity (Arnold et al. 2015), such that there are currently no specific age-gender-ethnicity indices to define obesity in a standardized manner. Thus, for example, in a cancer population, overweight individuals as defined by BMI, might have higher muscle mass compared with normal weight patients, explaining their better outcome compared with normal weight patients. While the obesity paradox was present in 175 patients with various cancers (breast, gynecological, head and neck, lung, and gastrointestinal) when obesity was assessed using BMI, the obesity paradox disappeared when obesity was defined using fat mass index and fat-free mass index, measures that consider differences in muscle and lean body mass (Gonzalez et al. 2014).

While genetics has revolutionized Precision Oncology, the ability of genetics to lead to personalized approaches to weight management have not yet advanced to practical application. A Genetic Risk Score (GRS) has been developed for obesity studies since no single gene explains obesity risk or approaches to obesity treatment. The GRS is a summary measure of a set of 16 genetic variants previously associated with obesity in population studies on BMI (rs9939609, FTO; rs17782313, MC4R; rs1801282, PPARG; rs1801133, MTHFR and rs894160, PLIN1) and lipid metabolism disturbances (rs1260326, GCKR; rs662799, APOA5; rs4939833, LIPG; rs18005881, UPC, rs328, LPL; rs12740374, CELSR2; rs429358 and rs7412, APOE; rs1799983, NOS3; rs1800777, CETP and rs1800206, PPARA). The GRS was validated by demonstrating that a high risk group of subjects with more than 7 risk alleles demonstrated increased BMI (0.93 kg/m^2 greater BMI), body fat mass (1.69% greater BFM), waist circumference (1.94 cm larger WC), and waist-to-hip ratio (0.01 greater waist-to-hip ratio) compared to the controls without those variants. Moreover, the associations of GRS and obesity are affected by differences in macronutrient intake underlining the importance of gene-nutrient interaction in obesity and obesity-associated cancer. For example, higher intakes of animal proteins were significantly associated with higher BFM in individuals within the high-risk GRS group (P interaction=0.032), whereas higher vegetable protein consumption had a protective effect among subjects in the low-risk group (P interaction=0.003), as these individuals were characterized by a lower percentage of BFM (Ramos-Lopez et al. 2017). Similar trends were reported by Rukh et al. (2013), where total protein intake was found to modulate GRS association with obesity in women (P interaction=0.039). Other studies on gene-macronutrients interactions, in which a GRS developed on the basis of BMI-associated SNPs was used, have revealed that high intake of sugar-sweetened beverages (Olsen et al. 2016, Rukh et al. 2013, Qi et al. 2012), fried foods (Qi et al. 2014), or saturated fatty-acids (Casas-Agustench et al. 2014) are also able to modulate the risk to develop obesity.

At present, personalized nutrition approaches to overweight and obese cancer patients are unlikely to be practically aided in the foreseeable future by genetic analysis. Nonetheless, consideration of variations in lean body mass that can affect risk and survival also affects calorie expenditure, nutritional requirements, and the ability of individuals to adhere to dietary advice. An individual with 150 pounds of lean body mass and a resting metabolism of 2,100 calories/day will have a much easier time adhering to a calorically restricted diet at 1,200 or 1,500 calories/day than an individual with 70 pounds of lean body mass and a resting metabolism of 1,000 calories/day. Therefore, in addition to any genetic predisposition, personalized approaches to weight management in cancer patients or survivors must take into account resting metabolic rate and lean body mass.

INSULIN RESISTANCE

Insulin resistance can be defined as the inability of insulin to stimulate glucose disposal and is often accompanied by hyperinsulinemia defined as fasting insulin levels of ≥10 µU/mL (Robbins et al. 1996). Insulin-mediated glucose disposal varies continuously throughout a population of apparently healthy individuals, with at least a six-fold variation between the most insulin sensitive and most insulin resistant of these individuals.

The concept of insulin resistance provides a conceptual framework with which to place a substantial number of apparently unrelated biological events into a single concept of the MS in which adipose tissue (AT) dysfunction plays a key role in the development of IR. While there are strong lifestyle determinants for the development of both insulin resistance and the MS, it is increasingly clear that an individual's risk of developing insulin resistance and aspects of the MS are also determined by genetic factors. Apparently, symptom-free individuals can have immune-metabolic phenotypes related to impaired angiogenesis and hypoxia, inflammation, inappropriate extracellular matrix remodeling and macrophage polarization as part of a molecular construct coined as AT dysfunction which triggers the early events leading to the development of insulin resistance. Clearly, these pathophysiological changes could influence the multistep process of carcinogenesis.

In an effort to identify new variants associated with insulin resistance, large-scale meta-analyses of GWAS have been performed using multiple cohorts which have measures of insulin sensitivity, processing and secretion. The Meta-Analyses of Glucose and Insulin-related traits Consortium performed meta-analyses on GWAS from 21 cohorts of nondiabetic individuals including 46,186 individuals with measures of fasting glucose and 38,238 with measures of fasting insulin and HOMA-IR as an index of insulin resistance. Twenty-five SNPs were followed up in a further 76,558 individuals with this approach identifying 16 loci associated with fasting glucose and two with fasting insulin. This study confirmed loci near GCKR and a newly identified loci near insulin-like growth factor-1 (IGF-1) as being associated with insulin resistance (Chen et al. 2017) with these findings being replicated in a further 14 cohorts comprising 29,084 nondiabetic individuals with detailed measures of fasting proinsulin, insulin secretion and sensitivity (Ingelsson et al. 2010).

Among 6,718 nonobese participants (2,057 with hyperinsulinemia [30.6%]) and 3,060 obese participants (2,303 with hyperinsulinemia [75.3%]) included in a prospective cohort study using data from the National Health and Nutrition Examination Survey 1999–2010 and followed up the participants until December 31, 2011 (Tsujimoto, Kajio, and Sugiyama 2017). Among all study participants, cancer mortality was significantly higher in those with hyperinsulinemia than in those without hyperinsulinemia (adjusted HR 2.04, 95% CI 1.24–3.34, p=0.005). Similarly, among nonobese participants, multivariate analysis showed that cancer mortality was significantly higher in those with hyperinsulinemia than in those without (adjusted HR 1.89, 95% CI 1.07–3.35, p=0.02). Considering that nonobese people with hyperinsulinemia were at higher risk of cancer mortality than those without hyperinsulinemia, improvement of hyperinsulinemia may be an important approach for preventing cancer regardless of the presence or absence of obesity.

A number of factors have been proposed to contribute to the increased risk of cancer development and mortality in the setting of obesity and pre-diabetes where insulin resistance is evident. These include hyperglycemia, insulin resistance, hyperinsulinemia, increased IGF-1 levels, dyslipidemia, inflammatory cytokines, increased leptin, and decreased adiponectin (Onitilo, Stankowski et al. 2014).

Phytonutrients A diet rich in cruciferous vegetables is associated with a lower risk of developing breast, lung, prostate, and colorectal cancer (Feskanich et al. 2000, Benabdelkrim, Djeffal, and Berredjem 2018). The chemoprotective effect of cruciferous vegetables is due to their high glucosinolate content and the capacity of glucosinolate metabolites, such as isothiocyanates (ITCs) and indoles, to modulate biotransformation enzyme systems (e.g., cytochromes P450 and conjugating enzymes). Data from molecular epidemiologic studies suggest that very common genetic and associated functional variations in biotransformation enzymes, particularly glutathione S-transferase (GST)M1 and GSTT1, which metabolize ITC, alter cancer risk in response to cruciferous vegetable exposure (Lampe and Peterson 2002). The organosulfur phytonutrients include ITCs and indoles from cruciferous vegetables such as broccoli, broccoli sprouts, brussel sprouts, cabbage,and bok choy, and allyl sulfides from garlic, onions, chives, and asparagus. The glucosinolates in cruciferous vegetables include glucoraphanin, glucobrassinin, and gluconasturtun which release ITC, indole-3 carbinol, and phenylethylisothiocyanate, respectively. Among these several groups of metabolites, ITCs are the most common. Abundant evidence has suggested that ITCs are inhibitors of drug metabolizing phase I enzymes and potent inducers of phase II enzymes.

GSTs are a multigene family of enzymes that inactivate toxins in glutathione-coupling reactions. They are responsible for cellular detoxification of environmental pollutants, carcinogens, chemotherapeutics, reactive oxygen species, and a wide spectrum of xenobiotics. Enzyme activity loss or reduction inhibits toxin neutralization. Null mutations are extremely common in the general population with up to 50% of individuals having a null mutation in GST M1 which slightly increases the risk of cancer in the absence of intake of cruciferous vegetables but markedly reduces risk by up to 50% when cruciferous vegetables which hyperinduce other members of the GST enzyme family in individuals with the null mutation compared to the general population (Brauer et al. 2011, Zhang et al. 2020). Many tumor studies including studies of colorectal, prostate, head and neck, leukemia, and oral cancers and precancers focus on three of the eight transferase classes, namely, theta (θ), mu (μ), and pi (π), encoded by genes GSTT1, GSTM1, and GSTP1, respectively (Klusek et al. 2018, Li et al. 2019, Benabdelkrim, Djeffal, and Berredjem 2018, Wang, Wu, and Sun 2019, Li et al. 2018, Bathi, Rao, and Mutalik 2009).

IMPLEMENTATION

Personalized nutrition is implemented using information based on generally accepted macronutrient ranges according to the Institute of Medicine guidelines and on clinical trials which show a lack of adverse events when these nutrients have been provided from foods or supplements. As will be repeatedly emphasized in this text, the cancer patient is a vulnerable individual and easily subject to nutritional claims for curing cancer from unqualified and sometimes dangerous practitioners. Patient's families also read about the promise of nutrition for cancer in the popular press and must be educated as to its realistic and potential benefits, as well as limitations and potential harms, for each patient's situation.

Government guidelines are based on established but incomplete nutrition science. They fail to account for the many aspects of the emerging science of nutrition including the benefits of phyto-nutrients, antioxidants, the microbiome, and the wealth of information emerging on the role of the microbiome in intermediary metabolism (Millen et al. 2016).

Dietary guidelines are meant to be broad in nature and not too far out in front of the science. Others are politically motivated compromises that do not even reflect the science that is known. There is also a natural bias towards foods and against dietary supplements among many authorities in nutrition which does not reflect the knowledge, attitudes, and behaviors of the public or the extensive body of data on micronutrient supplementation (Ronis, Pedersen, and Watt 2018, Dwyer, Coates, and Smith 2018).

While malnutrition in its later stages is visible, there is also what is known as "hidden hunger", a term popularized by Dr. Hans Biesalski of the University of Hohenheim in Germany to indicate the intracellular and sometimes localized deficiency of vitamins and minerals that is not easily diagnosed using typical forms of clinical inspection (Biesalski 2013).

Dietary supplements are meant to be an addition to the diet and they do not substitute for a poor dietary pattern. It is also true that obtaining all the micronutrients that have been implicated in healthy lifestyle by simply eating a healthy dietary pattern (formerly the four or five basic food groups) is no longer possible given the explosion of nutrition knowledge. Supplements can be a use-ful way to ensure that aspects of the dietary guidelines are being met such as those for minerals and micronutrients. Fears of toxicity are overblown and safe levels of supplements will be discussed further in this chapter (Andres et al. 2018, Asher, Corbett, and Hawke 2017).

Government advice on diet and physical activity is well-meaning, but it is too general to be very useful in advising individuals (Piercy et al. 2018). Personalized physical activity prescriptions are part of personalized nutrition as well based on individual physiology and preferences. In imple-menting all aspects of personalized nutrition, the recommendations in this text will stay within all of the general guidelines but will also personalize them to help individuals achieve a better diet and lifestyle that meets their individual goals for health and quality of life.

Dietary Guidelines The 2015–2020 Dietary Guidelines issued by the United States Department of Agriculture provided five overarching Guidelines that encourage healthy eating patterns. The Guidelines also embody the idea that a healthy eating pattern is not a rigid prescription, but rather, an adaptable framework in which individuals can enjoy foods that meet their personal, cultural, and traditional preferences and fit within their budget. Several examples of healthy eating patterns that translate and integrate the recommendations in overall healthy ways to eat are provided.

The overarching guidelines can easily be met while personalizing your patient's nutrition prescription. The guidelines are as follows:

1. Follow a healthy eating pattern across the lifespan. All food and beverage choices matter. Choose a healthy eating pattern at an appropriate calorie level to help achieve and maintain a healthy body weight, support nutrient adequacy, and reduce the risk of chronic disease.
2. Focus on variety, nutrient density (high content of nutrients per calorie), and amount. To meet nutrient needs within calorie limits, choose a variety of nutrient-dense foods across and within all food groups in recommended amounts.
3. Limit calories from added sugars and saturated fats and reduce sodium intake. Consume an eating pattern low in added sugars, saturated fats, and sodium. Cut back on foods and beverages higher in these components to amounts that fit within healthy eating patterns.
4. Shift to healthier food and beverage choices. Choose nutrient-dense foods and beverages across and within all food groups in place of less healthy choices. Consider cultural and personal preferences to make these shifts easier to accomplish and maintain.
5. Support healthy eating patterns for all. Everyone has a role in helping to create and support healthy eating patterns in multiple settings nationwide, from home to school to work to communities.

Key recommendations on a healthy eating patterns include: (1) a variety of vegetables from all of the subgroups including dark green, red and orange, legumes (beans and peas); (2) fruits, especially whole fruits; (3) grains, at least half of which are whole grains; (4) fat-free or low-fat dairy, including milk, yogurt, cheese, and/or fortified soy beverages; (5) a variety of protein foods, including seafood, lean meats and poultry, eggs, legumes (beans and peas), and nuts, seeds, and soy products; and healthy oils. It also limits saturated fats and trans fats, added sugars, and sodium.

Key recommendations that are quantitative are provided for several components of the diet that should be limited. These components are of particular public health concern in the United States, and the specified limits can help individuals achieve healthy eating patterns within calorie limits as follows: (1) consume less than 10% of calories/day from added sugars; (2) consume less than 10% of calories/day from saturated fats; (3) consume less than 2,300 mg/day of sodium; (4) if alcohol is consumed, it should be consumed in moderation—up to one drink per day for women and up to two drinks per day for men—and only by adults of legal drinking age.

To get away from individual nutrients such as fats, carbohydrates, and proteins, the Dietary Guidelines shifted to recommending dietary patterns. There are many different healthy eating patterns. The Healthy Mediterranean-Style Eating Pattern and Healthy Vegetarian Eating Pattern, which were developed by modifying the Healthy U.S.-Style Eating Pattern, are two examples of healthy eating patterns individuals that are provided in the guidelines. Similar to the Healthy U.S.-Style Eating Pattern, these patterns were designed to consider the types and proportions of foods Americans typically consume, but in nutrient-dense forms and appropriate amounts, which result in eating patterns that are attainable and relevant in the U.S. population. Other cultural preferences will apply in other countries. Additionally, healthy eating patterns can be flexible with respect to the intake of carbohydrate, protein, and fat within the context of the broad criteria for macronutrient intakes of protein, carbohydrate, and fat-enabling personalization based on body composition and food preferences.

PROTEIN

Protein is the macronutrient often called "the First Nutrient" is the most satiating of the macronutrients and in combination with exercise can maintain or build muscle mass. It is the only one of the macronutrients with a relevant dietary requirement daily and at every meal (Traylor, Gorissen, and Phillips 2018). Body composition analysis has uncovered the common occurrence of excess body fat and reduces lean mass. Dr. Jimmy Bell and colleagues at Hammersmith Hospital and Imperial College in London found that 40% of apparently healthy individuals with a normal BMI and normal WC had excess intraabdominal fat based on magnetic resonance imaging studies (Thomas, Parkinson et al. 2012).

Increasing or maintaining muscle mass has significant positive effects on metabolism and joint health. Aging and sedentary lifestyle lead to a loss of muscle which can be partially restored with adequate protein intake and purposeful exercises (Nowson and O'Connell 2015). Muscle cells take up glucose independent of insulin reducing stress on the pancreas even while glucose levels are normal in individuals with prediabetes or MS (Ebeling, Koistinen, and Koivisto 1998, Borghouts and Keizer 2000, Magnone et al. 2020).

Accurate skeletal muscle mass measurement in human subjects appeared at about the same time as the introduction of the sarcopenia concept in the late 1980s. Since then computed tomography and magnetic resonance imaging (MRI), have been used to gain insights into older methods such as anthropometry and urinary markers and more recently developed and refined methods including ultrasound. Bioimpedance analysis and dual-energy X-ray absorptiometry have been used to quantify regional and total body lean mass (Heymsfield, Gonzalez et al. 2015). Deuterated-creatine (D3-Cr) dilution provides a direct and accurate measurement of creatine pool size and skeletal muscle mass with no radiation. In a recent study in older men participating in the MrOS cohort study, D3-Cr muscle mass was associated with functional capacity and risk of injurious falls and disability, while assessments of lean body mass (LBM) or appendicular lean mass by dual energy x-ray absorptiomertry (DXA) were only weakly or not associated with these outcomes. Inaccurate measurements of muscle mass by DXA and other methods have led to inconsistent results and potentially erroneous conclusions about the importance of skeletal muscle mass in health and disease (Evans, Hellerstein et al. 2019). While there are many research methods available, bioimpedance with the weakness that it measures body water as lean or fat-free mass is still the most practical available method to estimate lean body mass. This estimate of lean body mass is central to developing diets to maintain optimal body composition and can be practically utilized both in outpatient and inpatient settings.

Bioelectrical impedance analysis (BIA) depends on the fact that muscle is about 70% water and conducts electricity while fat is an insulator. The most commonly used machines are modified scales with four contact points. By placing two contact points on the hands and two on the feet and separating these by a wide distance, it is possible to pass an alternating microcurrent at 50 cycles per second (50 Hz) through the body and assess impedance. The computer in the machine using proprietary algorithms then estimates both lean body mass and fat mass. The lean body mass measurement is accurate with 5%–10% while the body fat measurement is an estimate and does not specify the location of the fat as was done with MRI. BIA is a practical and cost-effective way to assess lean body mass which includes both muscle mass, organs, and bone mass (Kyle, Bosaeus et al. 2004). The amount of lean body mass is related directly to estimated resting energy expenditure as each pound of lean body mass burns about 14 calories/pound/day (or 30 calories/kg/day) while each pound of fat burns only about 3 calories/pound/day (or 6 calories/kg/day) (Cunningham 1980).

While the Dietary Guidelines suggest that Americans get adequate protein in their diet, the evidence suggests that the pattern of intake at each meal leads to insufficient amounts to maintain muscle protein synthesis throughout the day (Mamerow et al. 2014). Many Americans eat too little protein at breakfast, a little more for lunch and a large amount at dinner much of which is not utilized by the muscles for protein synthesis. A balanced distribution of protein throughout the day provides support of muscle protein synthesis (Layman et al. 2015).

The amount of lean body mass can be used to prescribe an adequate intake of lean protein to both control hunger and maintain lean body mass. In the University of California, Los Angeles (UCLA) Risk Factor Obesity Program, we utilize a nutrition prescription of 1 g/pound of lean body mass determined by BIA. The variations in body composition can be significant and affect resting energy expenditure and this is does not correlate with BMI. It has been established that lean body mass (also called Fat Free Mass (FFM)) is the strongest correlate of resting energy expenditure (Wang et al. 2000).

While Resting Energy Expenditure is not the same as total energy expenditure, it does accurately describe the greatest personal differences in the ability to lose or gain weight among individuals. A loss of 10 pounds of fat-free mass due to sedentary lifestyle and inadequate protein intake leads to a reduction in resting energy expenditure of 140 calories/day. This can be significant for a small woman who burns 1,500 calories/day at age 25 but loses 20 pounds of lean body mass by age 40 and then burns only 1,250 calories at rest. This results in the common clinical paradigm of a middle-aged women stating that she is gaining weight while still eating the same number of calories.

The Recommended Dietary Allowance (RDA) for protein was determined using a method called nitrogen balance. In this method the average protein is considered to have 1 g of nitrogen per 6.25 g of protein in the diet (Dickerson 2016). This is an obvious approximation since there are 21 different amino acids some having two nitrogen atoms while most have only one. Urinary urea excretion is the primary method of nitrogen exit from the body. While some exists as ammonia or creatinine, and some nitrogen is excreted through loss of intestinal cells in stool, urinary urea nitrogen is an acceptable clinical method to test for adequacy of protein intake.

Dr. Vernon Young at the Massacusetts Institute of Technology studied young healthy men eating egg whites and found that they achieved positive nitrogen balance at an intake of 0.8 g/kg body weight per day (Wayler et al. 1983, Young et al. 1973). Young healthy men eating 0.8 g/kg body weight went into positive nitrogen balance. This was assumed to hold for all men leading to a recommendation of 56 g/day for men and 46 g/day for women as the established RDA and this value has been used by governments around the world.

However, studies in 1989 found that in endurance athletes over 1.2 g/kg/day was needed to achieve positive nitrogen balance (Meredith et al. 1989). In weightlifters who clearly have a larger lean body mass than endurance athletes, a higher amount of over 2 g/kg body weight was needed (Lemon et al. 1992).

Taken together, these observations led to the conclusion that the RDA of 0.8 g/kg of body weight per day was too low and too general. The protein in the diet must be increased when lean body mass is increased. While the body tends to conserve lean body mass during starvation, optimal lean body mass can only be achieved with resistance exercise and surplus protein intake as evidenced by elimination of excess urinary urea nitrogen.

It turns out that a reasonable recommendation to implement is 1 g/pound of lean body mass per day. Lean body mass can be estimated with BIA which is widely available. The calculation of percent energy from protein indicates that this level of protein intake represents 29% of resting energy expenditure. Therefore, as a percent of total energy expenditure, this amounts to somewhere around 25% of the total including exercise, dietary thermogenesis, and fidgeting. This recommended amount of protein intake per day is well within the acceptable macronutrient range of 10%–35% established by the Institute of Medicine of the National Academy of Sciences and the Acceptable range of protein intake within the DRI for protein (Fulgoni 2008).

AMINO ACIDS

There are 21 common amino acids and while some amino acids can be made from other amino acids in the liver through a chemical exchange called transamination; 9 amino acids are essential and must be obtained from the diet similar to essential vitamins and minerals (Carter 1979). Some amino acids are called conditionally essential, because they must be consumed in the diet during growth to provide adequate growth rates, but become nonessential in adults who are not growing (Stifel and Herman 1972). One such amino acid is histidine, which is essential for growing rats but not adult rats.

Much of the data on essentiality of amino acids are obtained from rats, where single amino acid elimination is a way of determining whether a given amino acid is essential. For example, lysine and threonine cannot be made from other amino acids by transamination and must be included in the diet. The essential amino acids include phenylalanine, leucine, isoleucine, valine, lysine, threonine, tryptophan, methionine, and histidine (conditionally essential).

Proteins containing all of the essential amino acids and nonessential amino acids in proper amounts are called complete, while proteins missing some essential amino acids are called incomplete. Two incomplete proteins such as those found in corn and beans or rice and beans can be combined to produce a mixed protein with higher protein quality.

The original biological value tables found in many nutrition textbooks were assessed in animals and did not evaluate digestibility leading to the impression that soy protein, the highest quality protein in the plant world had a biological value of 73 compared to egg white which has a value of 100. The protein digestibility-corrected amino acid score (PDCAAS) has been adopted by Food and Agriculture Organization of the United Nations/World Health Organization as the preferred method for the measurement of protein quality in human nutrition (Schaafsma 2005). The method is based on a comparison of the concentration of the first limiting essential amino acid in the test protein with the concentration of that amino acid in a reference scoring pattern. This scoring pattern is derived from the essential amino acid requirements of the preschool-age child. The chemical score obtained in this way is corrected for true digestibility of the test protein. PDCAAS values higher than 100% are not accepted as such but are truncated to 100%. Using this method soy protein, whey protein, and egg white all have a biological value of 100% (Schaafsma 2005).

CARBOHYDRATES

A carbohydrate contains carbon, hydrogen and oxygen but no nitrogen, and can be broken down into sugars such as glucose and fructose or excreted from the body in undigested form. The term carbohydrate while useful for classifying macronutrients includes both the carbohydrates that have been industrially processed to a refined form as well as the indigestible carbohydrates found in fruits, vegetables, and whole grains. Refined carbohydrates in ultraprocessed foods (see below for definition) are often free of vitamins, minerals, and phytonutrients unless they are fortified. Moreover, fruits and vegetables as noted in the above diet plan have much lower calorie density such that a 100 g serving of a vegetable provides only 50 calories, fruit provides 70 calories, while a 100 g serving of a refined carbohydrate such as white rice provides 250 calories.

Simple sugars include glucose, fructose, lactose, and sucrose. These are listed as sugars on food labels, while the so-called complex carbohydrates are not included in this list despite the similarity discussed above. Lactose and sucrose are disaccharides made up of galactose/glucose and glucose/fructose, respectively. The tastes of corn sugar, sucrose or table sugar, and fructose are different. Fructose is the sweetest tasting sugar and is the one found in fruits such as oranges. Corn sugar tastes like pancake syrup and is the primary sweetener in colas in the US. In some countries such as Mexico, sucrose is used to sweeten colas and they taste distinctly different from their U.S. counterparts.

The term "complex carbohydrate" usually means a long-chain carbohydrate made up of many glucose or carbohydrate molecules linked together. According to the FDA, maltodextrin, or corn sugar, made up of 15 glucose molecules linked together, is a complex carbohydrate. In fact, as soon as corn sugar is dissolved in stomach acid it breaks up, giving exactly the same glucose release into the blood as table sugars.

From the standpoint of dental health, corn sugar can promote tooth decay (Jenkins et al. 1981). The original patent on maltodextrin claimed that it would enable infants to get more calories with less diarrhea since each maltodextrin molecule had 15 times the calories of an equivalent caloric load of glucose with much less osmolality (the physical chemical property of dissolved chemicals which draws fluid into the colon). In fact, this does help, but many infants still have colicky diarrhea as the infant expression of stress and food intolerance. Declaration of the different types of carbohydrates, especially of maltodextrin/corn syrup is insufficient in some products and consequently the consumer is not alerted to their cariogenic potential when used in older children. Complex carbohydrates by the FDA definition help neither dental health nor the development of diabetes.

In 1981, Dr. David Jenkins of the University of Toronto developed the GI (Jenkins et al. 1981). To determine GI, you compare how much the blood sugar rises over a several hour period by comparison to a fixed dose of pure corn sugar (or dextrose). In practice, a plot is made of the values of blood sugar over a 2-hour period, and the dots are connected creating a curve. The area under the curve of blood sugars after the administration of a fixed portion of carbohydrate (usually 50 g) of the test food is calculated and compared to the area under the curve following the administration of the same number of grams of carbohydrate from glucose which is given an arbitrary score of 100. The higher the number, the greater the blood sugar response and the resulting emotional impact on sugar craving. So a low GI food will cause a small rise, while a high GI food will trigger a dramatic spike in blood sugar. Here is a list of common foods with their GI (see Table 6.1).

TABLE 6.1
The GI, GL, and Total Calories of Foods

	GI	GL	Serving Size	Calories
Low GI (<55) and Low GL (<16) Foods (lowest calorie (110 calories per serving or less))				
Most vegetables	<20	<5	1 cup, cooked	40
Apple	40	6	1 average	75
Banana	52	12	1 average	90
Cherries	22	3	15 cherries	85
Grapefruit	25	5	1 average fruit	75
Kiwi	53	6	1 average fruit	45
Mango	51	14	1 small fruit	110
Orange	48	5	1 average fruit	65
Peach	42	7	1 average fruit	70
Plums	39	5	2 medium	70
Strawberries	40	1	1 cup	50
Tomato juice	38	4	1 cup	40
High GI (>55) but Low GL (<16) Foods (all low calorie (110 or less per serving))				
Apricots	57	6	4 medium	70
Orange juice	57	15	1 cup	110
Papaya	60	9	1 cup cubes	55
Pineapple	59	7	1 cup cubes	75
Pumpkin	75	3	1 cup, mashed	85
Shredded Wheat	75	15	1 cup mini squares	110
Toasted oats	74	15	1 cup	110
Watermelon	72	7	1 cup cubes	50
Moderate Calorie Low GI, Low GL (110–135 calories per serving or less)				
Apple juice	40	12	1 cup	135
Grapefruit juice	48	9	1 cup	115
Pear	33	10	1 medium	125
Peas	48	3	1 cup	135
Pineapple juice	46	15	1 cup	130
Whole-grain bread	51	14	1 slice	80–120
Higher Calorie, Low GI, Low GL (160–300 calories per serving)				
Barley	25	11	1 cup, cooked	190
Black beans	20	8	1 cup, cooked	235
Brown rice	50	16	1 cup	215
Garbanzo beans	28	13	1 cup, cooked	285

(Continued)

TABLE 6.1 (*Continued*)
The GI, GL, and Total Calories of Foods Are Listed Here

	GI	GL	Serving Size	Calories
Grapes	46	13	40 grapes	160
Kidney beans	23	10	1 cup, cooked	210
Lentils	29	7	1 cup, cooked	230
Soybeans	18	1	1 cup, cooked	300
Yam	37	13	1 cup, cooked	160
Low GI and Low GL, but High Fat and High Calorie				
Cashews	22	4	½ cup	395
Premium ice cream	38	10	1 cup	360
Low fat ice cream	37–50	13	1 cup	220
Peanuts	14	1	½ cup	330
Potato chips	54	15	2 ounces	345
Whole milk	27	3	1 cup	150
Vanilla pudding	44	16	1 cup	250
Fruit yogurt	31	9	1 cup	200+
Soy yogurt	50	13	1 cup	200+
High GI>55 High GL>16 (many higher calorie)				
Baked potato	85	34	1 small	220
Cola	63	33	16 ounce bottle	200
Corn	60	20	1 ear, 1 cup kernels	130
Corn chips	63	21	2 ounces	350
Corn flakes	92	24	1 cup	100
Cream of wheat	74	22	1 cup, cooked	130
Croissant	67	17	1 average	275
French fries	75	25	1 large order	515
Macaroni & cheese	64	46	1 cup	285
Oatmeal	75	17	1 cup, cooked	140
Pizza	60	20	1 large slice	300
Pretzels	83	33	1 ounce	115
Raisin bran	61	29	1 cup	185
Raisins	66	42	½ cup	250
Soda crackers	74	18	12 crackers	155
Waffles	76	18	1 average	150
White bread	73	20	2 small slices	160
White rice	64	23	1 cup, cooked	210

Source: Adapted from Foster-Powell, Holt et al. (2002).

The GI of foods is based on the GI—where glucose is set to equal 100. The other is the GL, which is the GI divided by 100 multiplied by its available carbohydrate content (i.e., carbohydrates minus fiber) in grams per serving.

Reliable tables of GIGI compiled from the scientific literature are instrumental in improving the quality of research examining the relation between GI, GL, and health. The GI has proven to be a more useful nutritional concept than is the chemical classification of carbohydrate (as simple or complex, as sugars or starches, or as available or unavailable), permitting new insights into the relation between the physiologic effects of carbohydrate-rich foods and health. Several prospective observational studies have shown that the chronic consumption of a diet with a high GL (GI×dietary carbohydrate content) is independently associated with an increased risk of developing type 2 diabetes, cardiovascular disease, and certain cancers. This revised table contains almost three times the number of foods listed in the original table (first published in this Journal in 1995) and contains nearly 1,300 data entries derived from published and unpublished verified sources, representing >750 different types of foods tested with the use of standard methods. The revised table also lists the GL associated with the consumption of specified serving sizes of different foods.

One problem with the GI is that it only detects carbohydrate quality, not quantity (Augustin et al. 2015). A GI value tells you only how rapidly a particular carbohydrate turns into sugar. It does not tell you how much of that carbohydrate is in a usual serving of a particular food. You need to know both things to understand a food's effect on blood sugar. The best example of this is the carrot. The form of sugar in the carrot has a high GI, but the total carbohydrate content of the carrot in a usual serving is low, so it does not add have much effect on blood sugar.

Glycemic Load (GL) takes into consideration a food's GI as well as the amount of carbohydrates per serving (see Table 6.1). A carrot has only 4 g of carbohydrate. To get 50 g, you would have to eat about a pound and a half of them. GL takes the GI value and multiplies it by the actual number of carbohydrates in a typical serving. While this number is useful for research studies, especially epidemiological studies, for the purpose of educating patients in primary care practice, it is enough to encourage the intake of healthy carbohydrates from low GI foods such as fruits, vegetables, whole grains while advising reductions in foods with refined carbohydrates such as cookies, candy bars, cakes, and pastries. These foods typically have hidden fats as well. Reducing the intake of sugar-sweetened drinks such as colas which have high GI is also vital as about one-third of all sugar in the diets of Americans come from this one source. Substituting water and unsweetened teas when not exercising is an important piece of advice. During prolonged exercise that is vigorous, sports drinks with added sugar are needed to maintain muscle glycogen, but for most minimal exercise simply drinking water to maintain hydration is adequate.

The studies of the effects and potential benefits of eating foods with a low GI require taking into account glucose load (GL). A food with a low GL is defined by consensus as one with a value of less than 16. GL has been found to be an important variable in epidemiological studies of diet and the risk of chronic disease. Population eating a diet which has a high GL, such as the U.S. diet of processed grains and few fruits and vegetables, have a higher risk of diabetes and heart disease than those in some Asian countries where they eat lots of fruits and vegetables with few processed foods. This has been documented both in population studies such as those conducted by the Harvard School of Public Health (Bhupathiraju et al. 2014). Diets high in GIGI and GL have been related to an increased risk of selected cancers reviewed in a meta-analysis of 21 studies (Turati et al. 2019).

The above findings support the hypothesis that diets with a high GL and a low cereal fiber content increase the risk of non-insulin dependent diabetes mellitus (NIDDM) in men as recently reviewed by an international group of nutrition experts (Augustin et al. 2015). Further, they concluded that grains should be consumed in a minimally refined form to reduce the incidence of NIDDM. Those foods with more dietary fiber, such as natural fruits and vegetables, are less likely to lead to obesity and diabetes than modern refined and processed carbohydrates with the fiber removed.

To design and implement effective measures to reduce added sugars, Monteiro, Mozaffarian, and colleagues examined data from the United States Department of Agriculture National Health and Nutrition Examination Survey (NHANES) survey to assess the contribution of ultraprocessed foods to sugar intake in the American diet (Martinez Steele et al. 2016). Ultraprocessed foods were defined as industrial formulations which, besides salt, sugar, oils, and fats, include substances not used in culinary preparations, in particular additives used to imitate sensorial qualities of minimally processed foods and their culinary preparations. Added sugars represented 1 of every 5 calories in the average ultraprocessed food (21.1%), far higher than the content of added sugars in processed foods (2.4%) and in unprocessed or minimally processed foods, and processed culinary ingredients grouped together (3.7%). A strong linear relationship was found between the dietary contribution of ultraprocessed foods and the dietary content of added sugars.

FIBER

Those carbohydrates excreted in undigested form or those partially or completely digested by colonic bacteria are referred to as dietary fibers. Since they are not digested, dietary fibers do not contribute directly to the nutritive value of foods in terms of calories, but they have many effects on human physiology.

Dietary fiber is classified as either soluble or insoluble dietary fiber. Insoluble dietary fibers such as cellulose (a structural carbohydrate making up plant cell walls) are not digested in the intestine and pass out in the stool where they can be found intact. Soluble carbohydrates such as pectin, guar, and starches are digested by bacteria in the colon. Stool mass is determined by the mass of fibers and the mass of bacteria in stool. A significant portion of stool mass is bacteria. Soluble fibers contribute to stool mass by promoting the growth of the bacteria that digest the soluble fiber and use it as fuel. Ancient humans ate a great deal of fiber and this fiber resulted in numerous large bulky stools that filled the colon and caused it to contract against a large volume load. Many people in developed countries eat only a small amount of fiber, approximately 10–15 g/day, compared to 35 g/day in a healthy plant-based diet and well over 50 g/day in ancient diets. In addition to the benefits on intestinal muscle function resulting from the bulk of fiber, soluble fiber found in fruits, vegetables, and some whole grains acts as a prebiotic nourishing healthy bacteria in the gut (Holscher 2017).

One consequence of eating a low fiber diet is that the colonic muscles contract against a smaller volume of stool and so exert higher pressures. It is generally believed that these higher pressures account for the common occurrence of diverticulosis (outpouching of mucosa between strands of muscle) in the colons of elderly individuals. Constipation is also very common in modern society, since a low fiber diet does not stimulate intestinal motility as well as a higher fiber diet does (Yang et al. 2012).

This slowing of transit time—the time it takes foods to get through the gastrointestinal tract—also permits greater reabsorption of substances normally excreted through the intestines. Constipation through several mechanisms may increase the risk of cancer (Sundboll et al. 2019). For example, estrogen is excreted in the bile from the liver into the intestine. In the intestine it is bound to fibers and excreted in the stool. Women with low fiber diets and constipation reabsorb this estrogen in the distal small intestine, called the ileum, rather than excreting the estrogen. This is not a minor effect and results in 20% higher blood estrogen levels in women on a low fiber diet compared to those consuming a high fiber diet (Rose et al. 1991).

FATS AND OILS

Fats and oils provide the most concentrated source of calories of any food stuff at 9 calories/g. Fats provide essential fatty acids which are called essential, because they are not made in the body and must be consumed similar to vitamins. However, they required in such small amounts that fatty acid deficiency does not occur in humans with an intact intestine eating a variety of foods (Spector and Kim 2015).

The essential fatty acids are linoleic, an omega-6 fatty acid, and linolenic acid, an omega-3 fatty which are precursors for longer chain fatty acids that enter a metabolic pathway in which the two types of fatty acids (omega-3 and omega-6 compete to form eicosanoids including prostaglandins, thromboxanes, and leukotrienes which are either anti-inflammatory or pro-inflammatory. It is the balance of omega-6 and omega-3 in the body fat and cell membranes which determines the types and balance of eicosanoids. In turn, the diet determines the balance of omega-3 and omega-6 fatty acids in the tissues (Strandjord, Lands, and Hibbeln 2018).

Ninety-five percent or more of the fats you eat and store are triglycerides. These fats have a three-carbon backbone and three fatty acids esterified at each of the three positions. When all the fatty acids on a triglyceride are the same they are called simple, otherwise they are called mixed triglycerides, which are more common (See Table 6.2). Fats are called saturated, polyunsaturated, or monounsaturated based on the characteristics of two of three fatty acids. The distinction between fats and fatty acids, while important, is often overlooked in discussions of dietary fats and foods.

The principal dietary sources of fat are meats, dairy products, poultry, fish, nuts, and vegetable oils and fats used in processed foods. Vegetables and fruits contain only small amounts of fat, so that vegetable oils are only sources of fat due to processing of vegetables. The most commonly used oils and fats for salad oil, cooking oils, shortenings, and margarines in the U.S. include soybean,

TABLE 6.2
Fatty Acid Composition in Commonly Eaten Fats

	Sat Fat	(18:2 n-6)	(18:3 n-3)	Mono
Olive oil	14%	9%	1%	74%
Avocado oil	12%	13%	1%	71%
Corn oil	13%	58%	1%	24%
Soybean oil	14%	51%	7%	23%
Peanut oil	17%	32%	0%	46%
Safflower oil	6%	75%	0%	14%
Sunflower oil	10%	66%	0%	20%
Palm oil	49%	9%	0%	37%
Lard				
Beef tallow	50%	3%	1%	42%
Butterfat	62%	2%	1%	29%
Coconut oil	87%	2%	0%	6%

Source: U.S. Department of Agriculture, Agricultural Research Service. 2003. USDA Nutrient Database for Standard
     Reference, Release 16. Nutrient Data Laboratory Home Page, http://www.nal.usda.gov/fnic/foodcomp.
*If a fat contains among the three fatty acids predominantly saturated, monounsaturated, or saturated fats shown above,
     then we use the shorthand of calling these saturated, monounsaturated, or saturated fats. Commonly eaten fats all
     have varying mixtures of the fatty acids above in their triglyceride lipids, the primary dietary source of fatty acids.*
Sat Fat, *saturated fatty acids;* 18:2 n-6, linoleic acid; 18:3 n-3, linolenic acid; Mono, monounsaturated omega-9 fatty acids.

corn, cottonseed, palm, peanut, olive, canola (low erucic acid rapeseed oil), safflower, sunflower, coconut, palm kernel, tallow, and lard. These fats and oils contain varying compositions of fatty acids which have particular physiological properties.

The cellular balance between the 20 and 22-carbon omega-6 (also called n-6) and omega-3 (also called n-3) polyunsaturated fatty acids can affect immune function. Humans are very inefficient in converting the 18 carbon fatty acids to 20 and 22-carbon length n-3 fatty acids so these must be consumed from the diet as ocean-caught fish or from fish oil supplements.

Excess calories, regardless of source, are stored as triglycerides. In the body, triglycerides are digested and the fatty acids incorporated into body fat where over a period of time, the chemical composition of the fat correlates with dietary fat structures to a certain extent.

Bioactive lipids also promote processes associated with malignant progression. For example, up-regulation of sphingosine kinase 1 in gastric cancer patients is associated with poor survival and increased progression (Li et al. 2009). The eicosanoid PGE2 promotes colorectal cancer progression (Wang and Dubois 2010). Similarly, lipids are also known to promote chronic inflammation, a process that drives carcinogenesis (Murata 2018).

Fats also require prolonged digestion and contribute to satiety, carry fat-soluble vitamins, and concentrate the tastes of foods to make them more palatable. The key problem for most people eating a Western diet is an excess of fat from processed foods which are rich in proinflammatory omega-6 fatty acids.

The simple solution for modern times is to select low fat fish, white meat of poultry, and occasional very lean meat, preferably grass-fed. The omega-6 to omega-3 ratio for fish is not comparable to those in the table above. Wild salmon has a ratio of 0.08 and farmed salmon has a ratio of 0.29. Addition of just 3 ounces of ocean caught fish (e.g., herring or sardines) or 3 g of fish oil capsules to a low fat diet will reduce the proportion of predicted omega-6 fatty acids in tissues from 80% to 40% (Lands 2014). This amazing impact of fish oils is a potent argument for including fish and fish oil supplements in a healthy diet.

PERSONALIZATION

Personalization of the macronutrient recommendation on the basis of lean body mass can used to very simply determine protein and calorie requirements. Once that has been determined, it is possible to build a personalized diet incorporating a variety of fruits, vegetables, whole grains, and healthy fats. Colorful fruits and vegetables and spices provide antioxidant phytonutrients with little impact on overall calorie intake. Many of the phytonutrients identified have established cellular actions, but for others there is much more to learn.

For those who wish to begin with the end in mind, the box immediately below describes how to build a diet based on these principles while the following sections provide the rationale based on nutrition science that is known at this time.

The first step in personalization is prescribing protein intake per day based on lean body mass. The concept is that the minimum protein is about 15% of total calories which is approximately 0.8 g/kg body weight per day. Optimum protein for weight management or building muscle with exercise is about 30% of total calories or approximately 2.0 g/kg body weight per day. LBM can be estimated from the BMI or measured using bioelectrical impedance where the lean body mass is also described as FFM. A simple prescription using lean body mass for 30% of total calories is about 1 g/pound or 2 g/kg of LBM or FFM.

Protein content is listed on food labels and can be found in many data bases, but is listed here to provide some simple examples of how to reach a personalized protein goal (see Table 6.3).

TABLE 6.3
Protein and Calorie Contents of Common Foods

Food Item	One Unit	Calories	Protein (g)
	Breakfast		
Egg whites	7 whites	115	25
Greek yogurt (0% fat)	1 cup	130	23
Without fruit added			
Nonfat cottage cheese	1 cup	140	28
	Vegetarian		
Soy Canadian bacon	4 slices	80	21 (varies)
Soy protein powder	1 ounce	110	20–25
Soy cereal	½ cup	140	25 (varies)
	Lunch and Dinner		
Poultry breast	3 ounces, cooked weight	115–140	25
Ocean-caught fish	4 ounces, cooked weight	130–170	25–31
Shrimp, crab, lobster	4 ounces, cooked weight	120	22–24
Tuna	4 ounces, water pack	145	27
Scallops	4 ounces, cooked weight	135	25
Egg whites	7 whites	115	25
Nonfat cottage cheese	1 cup	140	28
	Vegetarian		
Soy protein powder	1 ounce	110	20–25
Soy hot dog	2 links	110	22 (varies)
Soy ground round	¾ cup	120	24
Morningstar farms Better'n Burgers	2 patties	160	26
Tofu, firm	½ cup	180	20 (varies)
Vegetarian burgers	2 patties	180–220	26–28

Carbohydrates and fiber can largely come from seven servings per day of colorful fruits and vegetables with a typical 100 g serving of vegetable providing about 50 calories and a 100 g serving of fruit providing about 70 calories. The approximate calorie and fiber content for commonly eaten fruits and vegetables can be organized according to the color grouping to achieve greater dietary diversity (see Table 6.4).

Whole grain and refined grain foods provide about 250 calories/100 g so breads, cakes, pastries, and cookies should be minimized in the diet when reducing excess body fat through calorie restriction. Two slices of whole grain sprouted bread will have 140–200 calories while providing 4–8 g of protein. Instead of breads and cereals as the base of the diet with six to eight servings per day, reduce starch intakes by recommending more fruits and vegetables and fewer refined grains. This will both increase fiber intake and provide more vitamins, minerals, and phytonutrients to the diet

TABLE 6.4
Calorie and Fiber Content of Fruits and Vegetables Organized According to the Color Grouping

Food Item	Portion	Calories	Fiber
Red			
Tomato juice	1 cup	40	1
Tomato sauce/puree	1 cup	100	5
Tomato soup, made with water	1 cup	85	0
Tomato vegetable juice	1 cup	45	2
Tomatoes, cooked	1 cup	70	3
Tomatoes, raw	1 large	40	2
Watermelon	1 cup balls	50	1
Red/Purple			
Beets, cooked	1 cup	75	3
Blackberries	1 cup	75	8
Blueberries	1 cup	110	5
Cranberries	1 cup raw	60	5
Cranberry Sauce	1/4 cup	100	1
Eggplant, cooked	2 cups	60	5
Peppers, red	1 large	45	3
Plums	3 small	100	3
Red apple	1 medium	100	4
Red cabbage, cooked	2 cups	60	6
Red pear	1 medium	100	4
Red wine	4 oz. glass	80	0
Strawberries	1 1/2 cups, sliced	75	6
Orange			
Acorn squash, baked	1 cup	85	6
Apricot	5 whole	85	4
Cantaloupe	½ medium	80	2
Carrots, cooked	1 cup	70	5
Carrots, raw	3 medium	75	6
Mango	½ large	80	3
Pumpkin, cooked	1 cup	50	3
Winter squash, baked	1 cup	70	7

(Continued)

TABLE 6.4 (*Continued*)
Calorie and Fiber Content of Fruits and Vegetables Organized According to the Color Grouping

Food Item	Portion	Calories	Fiber
	Orange/Yellow		
Nectarine	1 large	70	2
Orange	1 large	85	4
Papaya	½ large	75	3
Peach	1 large	70	3
Peach nectar	⅔ cup	90	1
Pineapple	1 cup, diced	75	2
Tangerine	2 medium	85	5
Yellow grapefruit	1 fruit	75	2
	Yellow/Green		
Avocado	¼ average fruit	80	2
Banana	1 average	90	2
Collard greens, ckd	2 cups	100	10
Corn	½ cup kernels or 1 ear	75	2
Cucumber	1 average	40	2
Green beans, ckd	2 cups	85	8
Green peas	½ cup	70	4
Green peppers	1 large	45	3
Honeydew	¼ large melon	100	2
Kiwi	1 large	55	3
Mustard greens, ckd	2 cups	40	6
Romaine lettuce	4 cups	30	4
Spinach, cooked	2 cups	80	8
Spinach, raw	4 cups	30	4
Turnip greens, ckd	2 cups	60	10
Yellow peppers	1 large	50	2
Zucchini with skin, ckd	2 cups	60	5
	Green		
Broccoli, cooked	2 cups	85	9
Brussels sprouts	1 cup	60	4
Cabbage, cooked	2 cups	70	8
Cabbage, raw	2 cups	40	4
Cauliflower, ckd	2 cups	55	6
Chinese cabbage, ckd	2 cups	40	5
Kale, cooked	2 cups	70	5
Swiss chard	2 cups	70	7
	White/Green		
Artichoke	1 medium	60	6
Asparagus	18 spears	60	4
Celery	3 large stalks	30	3
Chives	2 tablespoons	2	0
Endive, raw	½ head	45	8
Garlic	1 clove	5	0
Leeks, cooked	1 medium	40	1
Mushrooms, cooked	1 cup	40	3
Onion	1 large	60	3

TABLE 6.5

Whole Grain and Refined Grain Calories, Fiber, and Protein Content per Serving

Grain /Starch	Serving Size	Calories	Fiber (g)	Protein (g)
Cooked beans	1 cup, cooked	230–280	10–14	14
Brown rice	1 cup, cooked	220	4	6
Lentils	1 cup, cooked	230	16	18
Potato, baked	1 medium	220	8	4
Sweet potato	1 small	100	2	2
Whole grain pasta	1 cup cooked		2	6
Plain instant oatmeal	1 packet	100	3	4
Shredded wheat, bite size	¾ cup	85	3	4
Fiber one cereal	¾ cup	90	21	4
All bran with extra fiber cereal	¾ cup	75	18	5
Kashi Go Lean Cereal	¾ cup	120	10	8
Kashi Good Friends Cereal	¾ cup	90	8	3
Kellogg's All Bran Cereal	¾ cup	120	15	6
Bran Chex Cereal	¾ cup	120	5	4
Kellogg Bran Buds Cereal	1/3 cup	85	12	2
Bread, Vogel	1 slice	100	3	5
Bread, Ezekiel sprouted wheat	1 slice	80	3	4

for healthy individuals and those with overweight and obesity who are trying to optimize their body composition (see Table 6.5).

There is no recommended dietary intake for carbohydrates but most people eating a Western Dietary pattern over-eat refined carbohydrates and do not meet the recommended intakes of fruits and vegetables. From a physiological point of view, the body can balance fat and carbohydrate with the minimum amounts of fat in the diet of 5%–10% of calories easily attained as long as the gastro-intestinal tract functions to absorb fat from foods. The key to personalizing fat in the diet is to balance omega-6 and omega-3 fatty acids in foods. This can be simply accomplished by reducing total fat to about 25% of total calories which includes hidden trans-fats and omega-6 fats in most processed foods while consuming about 2 g of fish oils from fish oil supplements or ocean-caught fish.

If a higher fat diet is desired with reduced carbohydrates, then omega-9 or monounsaturated fats should be used from olive oil or avocados, since these are neutral fats that do not upset the balance of omega-3 and omega-6. All fats have about 135 calories/15 mL (one tablespoon) and calories should be considered when adding fat to recipes.

This method of personalizing the diet is simple enough to enable personal choices of foods to obtain a diet that will help maintain healthy body composition when combined with physical activity, It begins from the assumption that most Americans and those consuming a Western Dietary pattern around the world are struggling to keep from storing excess body fat due to a sedentary lifestyle and omnipresent high fat, high sugar foods. Providing choices for a wide variety of foods while keeping some basic principles of nutrition and physiology in mind will allow for personalization that includes personal preferences within a healthy dietary pattern.

SUPPLEMENTS

Dietary supplement products are commonly used by adults in the United States (Kim et al. 2014). Less than 25% of all supplement products used are taken at the recommendation of a healthcare provider (Bailey et al. 2013). The use of supplements is motivated, in part, by evidence suggesting that increased intake of some dietary constituents not eaten as foods may be associated with reduced risk of cancer and other age-related diseases (Giovannucci et al. 2002). The Physicians' Health Study II RCT demonstrated that daily multivitamin/multimineral (MVMM) use modestly reduced total cancer incidence in men (Gaziano et al. 2012).

On the other hand, increasing skepticism of antioxidant supplements followed widely some very widely publicized observational studies claiming no benefits or even adverse effects of dietary supplements (Lippman et al. 2009, Omenn et al. 1996, Gaziano et al. 2009, Hennekens et al. 1996).

A study of supplement use by 38,024 adults was carried out using in-home interviews to determine use of supplements in the prior 30 days within the United States National Health and Nutrition Examination Surveys (NHANES) between 1999 and 2012 (Kantor et al. 2016). Supplement use was evaluated across seven NHANES cycles for use of any supplements, use of MVMM supplements, as defined by a product containing ≥10 vitamins and/or minerals, as well as use of individual vitamins, minerals, and nonvitamin, nonmineral supplements.

Overall, use of supplements remained stable between 1999 and 2012, with 52% of US adults reporting use of any supplements in 2011–2012. The use of MVMM decreased over time, with 37% reporting use of MVMM in 1999–2000 and 31% reporting use in 2011–2012 (difference: −5.7, p-trend < 0.001). Vitamin D supplementation from sources other than MVMM increased from 5.1% to 19% (difference: 14%, p-trend < 0.001) and use of fish oil supplements increased from 1.3% to 12% (difference: 11%, p-trend < 0.001) over the study period.

Use of lycopene-containing supplements also increased. A significant increase in lycopene use was observed in 2005–2006, at which time lycopene was used by 25% of men. This increase in the early 2000s followed well-publicized research suggesting that consumption of lycopene-rich tomato products was associated with reduced risk of prostate cancer (Giovannucci et al. 2002).This trend was almost entirely driven by MVMM due to the increased inclusion of lycopene in MVMM formulations, not increased use of individual lycopene supplements.

A marked increase in vitamin D supplement use was observed in this study independent of the vitamin D contained in MVMM. This increase coincided with a growing number of publications evaluating the potential benefits of vitamin D on outcomes including cancer (Keum and Giovannucci 2014). This research increased public awareness of the potential benefits of vitamin D and testing for vitamin D insufficiency by physicians (Shahangian et al. 2014) contributed to the increased consumption of vitamin D (Qato et al. 2016).

Preventing or treating obesity, as well as adhering to healthy dietary patterns, should be recommended to both the general population and cancer survivors because they are convincingly associated with reduced risk of primary or second cancers and, in some cases, with reduced cancer recurrences (Vernieri et al. 2018).

Nutritional supplements are widely used among patients with cancer who perceive them to be anticancer agents or as supportive of health during cancer treatment. Nutritional supplementation tailored to an individual's background diet, genetics, tumor histology, and treatments may yield benefits in subsets of patients is part of personalized nutrition which will increase in coming years and the application of genomics to nutrition leads to precision nutrition in practice settings.

Clinicians should have an open dialogue with patients about the nutritional supplements they are using. Supplement advice needs to be individualized and come from a credible source (Harvie 2014). Oncologists need to know the basics of vitamins, minerals, and supplements to be able to have such discussions in a credible fashion. The information below is provided with this purpose in mind.

VITAMINS

Vitamin deficiency diseases in the United States were relatively common prior to World War II. Today, with the fortification of the food supply, classical vitamin deficiency diseases such as scurvy and rickets are rare outside the setting of specific disease states, drug-nutrient interactions, or extreme malnutrition due to poverty.

The 2007–2010 National Health and Nutrition Examination Survey (NHANES) study found that the large majority of Americans despite having a high prevalence of obesity failed to get adequate levels of micronutrients through their diet. Vitamin D and Vitamin E intakes were below the Estimated Average Requirement (EAR) in 94% and 88% of the population respectively. In addition, 33%–50% of Americans had inadequate intakes of magnesium, calcium, and vitamins A and C. This was noted in the 2015 Dietary Guidelines Scientific Advisory Committee report which also stated that Vitamins A, D, E, C as well as folate, calcium, magnesium, fiber, and potassium were nutrients of concern. While all of these data are based on self-report, it is remarkable that 90% of adults consumed an inadequate amount of vitamin D.

Significant portions of the population with common chronic diseases also have inadequate intakes of micronutrients. Obesity is associated with inadequate absorption of vitamins A, C, D, and E as wells as calcium and magnesium and vitamin D deficiency (Thomas-Valdes et al. 2017, Hussain Gilani et al. 2019).

Despite the uncommon occurrence of classical vitamin deficiencies sufficient to cause acute disease in healthy individuals, a familiarity with the roles of the various common vitamins and minerals, and some knowledge of their assessment in the clinical laboratory, will aid in the assessment of the hospitalized or ambulatory cancer patient with suspected nutritional deficiency.

VITAMIN A

Night blindness was well-recognized in ancient Egypt where it was treated with juice from cooked liver or by including liver in the diet. The active agent, vitamin A, was discovered as a fat-soluble growth factor necessary for the rat in 1914 and structurally analyzed in 1930 (Blakermore et al. 1957).

The parent compound of the vitamin A family is all-trans retinol. Its aldehyde and acid forms are retinal and retinoic acid (RA). The active form of vitamin A for vision is 11-cis retinal which is converted to trans-retinal following the absorption of the energy of a light photon. Called photoisomerization, this light-mediated change in conformation from the cis- to the trans-form results in the dissociation of the protein rhodopsin which results in nerve impulses through the optic nerve to regions in the visual cortex when sight is formed from the integration of these impulses.

A second active function for vitamin A is cellular differentiation. RA is a morphogen derived from retinol (vitamin A) that plays important roles in cell growth, differentiation, organogenesis, and carcinogenesis. The production of RA from retinol requires two consecutive enzymatic reactions catalyzed by different sets of dehydrogenases. The retinol is first oxidized into retinal, which is then oxidized into RA. The RA interacts with retinoic acid receptor (RAR) and retinoic acid X receptor which then regulate the target gene expression within the nucleus of cells where they promote differentiation.

The recent discovery of four retinoic acid receptors (termed RAR-alpha through RAR-gamma) in the nucleus of cells has begun to elucidate the molecular mechanisms by which vitamin A induces differentiation of many types of cells (Conserva et al. 2019). A number of retinoids or synthetic vitamin A analogs (the best known is 13-cis RA or accutane) are used to treat acne and have been studied for their differentiating activities in the prevention and treatment of premalignant lesions of the skin, and cervix (Ianhez et al. 2019, Helm et al. 2013).

The term "vitamin A" applies to all compounds with biological activity similar to that of vitamin A. The interconversion and pharmacology of these various vitamin As is controversial and still under study (Baggerly et al. 2015, Pludowski et al. 2018). The international units (IU) apply only to animal experiments under standardized conditions. In the IU system, 0.3 μg of retinol or 0.34 μg of retinyl acetate or 0.6 μg of beta-carotene correspond to 1 IU. Diet can provide numerous vitamin A-like substances. Requirements and intakes are listed as retinal activity equivalents (RAE): 1 mg RAE = 1 mg retinal, 1.15 mg retinal acetate, 6 mg beta-carotene, 3,000 IU vitamin A.

Low plasma concentrations of retinol (<0.35 μmol/L) are associated with clinical symptoms of vitamin A deficiency (Biesalski, 1989). The Recommended Dietary Allowance for vitamin A is 5,000 IU (800–1,000 μg retinol equivalents, or RE) per day, and toxicity has been reported at intakes of 25,000 IU/day. This makes vitamin A one of the most toxic vitamins known.

VITAMIN D

There are two forms of vitamin D, vitamin D3 and vitamin D2. Vitamin D3 (cholecalciferol) occurs in some foods but is primarily produced in the skin on exposure to sunlight (Baggerly et al. 2015, Holick 2017). Vitamin D2 (ergocalciferol) does not occur naturally but is manufactured by the ultraviolet irradiation of ergosterol, which occurs in molds, yeasts, and plants. Vitamin D3 differs from vitamin D2 in that D2 has a double bond between carbon 22 and carbon 23 and a methyl group on carbon 24.

Only a few foods (cod liver oil, fatty fish, and egg yolks) contain substantial amounts of naturally occurring vitamin D3. The amount of vitamin D typically obtained from food sources other than fortified foods and skin synthesis often is insufficient. For this reason food is supplemented with vitamin D in most developed countries. In North America, food is supplemented with both vitamin D2 and vitamin D3, with milk being the principal fortified dietary component. Since dairy products have been fortified with vitamins A and D, dietary rickets has become rare in the US. Vitamin D acts to enhance calcium absorption from the intestine and has been shown to have differentiating effects on a number of different cell types including white blood cells and prostate cancer cells. The active form of vitamin D is 1,25 dihydroxyvitamin D3 formed from 25-hydroxyvitamin D in the kidneys. 25-hydroxyvitamin D is a large inactive pool formed and stored in the liver. The kidney also has an inactivation enzyme (24 hydroxylase) which converts 25 (OH) D to inactive 24,25 dihydroxyvitamin D. When 1,25 dihydroxyvitamin D acts at the nucleus it turns on the genes necessary to produce the 24 hydroxylase enzyme. Whenever there is such a branch point in the body, there is additional protection from toxicity and it indicates a substance with important metabolic roles in analogy to the conversion of thyroid hormone to active triiodothyronine (T3) or reverse T3 in response to nutritional status (Holick 2017).

As people age, the skin becomes less effective in forming vitamin D and people are advised to use sunscreens and avoid sun exposure to prevent skin cancer (Kockott et al. 2016). Vitamin D3 as a supplement is preferable to D2. D2 is less bioavailable than D3, but is used by vegans who insist on plant sources of vitamins. D2 is synthesized in plants including mushrooms exposed to ultraviolet light (Cardwell et al. 2018). Taking a dose of 2,000 IU/day is not toxic since it translates into an increase in 25OHD levels of only 24 ng/mL (see Table 6.6 below for desirable blood levels of vitamin D).

However, toxicity is only noted at doses greater than 20,000 U/day and many consumers take 1,000–5,000 U daily to take advantage of emerging science on the actions of vitamin D beyond its role in calcium absorption.

It is now estimated that approximately 1 billion people worldwide have blood concentrations of vitamin D that are considered suboptimal. Low vitamin D serum concentrations are linked to several types of cancers, cardiovascular disease, diabetes, upper respiratory tract infections, and all-cause mortality.

TABLE 6.6
Vitamin D Assessment Using Blood Levels of 25-Hydroxyvitamin D

25-Hydroxyvitamin D	Concentrations (ng/mL) (nmol/L)
Deficiency	<20 (<50)
Insufficiency	20–32 (50–80)
Sufficiency	32–100 (80–250)
Excess	>100 (>250)
Intoxication	>150 (>325)

Source: Adapted from Dr. Michael Holick, personal communication.

Immune effects of vitamin D have been recognized for over a century and is are now appreciated as having had a role in the use of sunlight in the therapy of tuberculosis in the preantibiotic era. Topical application of vitamin D cutaneous tuberculosis resulted in disappearance of lesions. In the last few years the significance of these observations to normal human physiology has become apparent (Hewison 2012).

There are increasing data linking vitamin insufficiency with prevalent immune disorders. Improved awareness of low circulating levels of precursor 25-hydroxyvitamin D in populations across the globe has prompted investigations of health problems associated with vitamin D insufficiency. Prominent among these are autoimmune diseases such as multiple sclerosis, type 1 diabetes, and Crohn's disease, but more recent studies indicate that infections such as tuberculosis may also be linked to low 25-hydroxyvitamin D levels.

Moreover, it is now clear that cells from the immune system contain all the machinery needed to convert 25-hydroxyvitamin D to active 1,25-dihydroxyvitamin D, and for subsequent responses to 1,25-dihydroxyvitamin D. Mechanisms such as this are important for promoting antimicrobial responses to pathogens in macrophages, and for regulating the maturation of antigen-presenting dendritic cells. The latter may be a key pathway by which vitamin D controls T-lymphocyte (T-cell) function. However, T-cells also exhibit direct responses to 1,25-dihydroxyvitamin D, notably the development of suppressor regulatory T-cells. Collectively these observations suggest that vitamin D is a key factor linking innate and adaptive immunity, and both of these functions may be compromised under conditions of vitamin D insufficiency.

Vitamin D is not just a vitamin but a hormone that like the retinoids travels to the nucleus to program the transcription of specific proteins. Research over the last three decades has brought to light many additional functions of vitamin D and redefined what is considered optimal vitamin D nutrition.

Several observational studies and a few prospectively randomized controlled trials have demonstrated that adequate levels of vitamin D can decrease the risk and improve survival rates for several types of cancers including breast, rectum, ovary, prostate, stomach, bladder, esophagus, kidney, lung, pancreas, uterus, non-Hodgkin lymphoma, and multiple myeloma (Jeon and Shin 2018). Individuals with serum vitamin D concentrations less than 20 ng/mL are considered most at risk, whereas those who achieve levels of 32–100 ng/mL are considered to have sufficient serum vitamin D concentrations (see Table 6.6) (Holick et al. 2011, Holick 2009).

Vitamin D can be obtained from exposure to the sun, through dietary intake, and via supplementation. Obtaining a total of approximately 4,000 IU/day of vitamin D3 from all sources has been shown to achieve serum concentrations considered to be in the sufficient range. Most individuals will require a dietary supplement of 2,000 IU/day of vitamin D3 to achieve sufficient levels as up to 20,000 IU/day is considered safe. Vitamin D3 is available as an over-the-counter product at most pharmacies and is relatively inexpensive, especially when compared with potential and demonstrated benefits. Since vitamin D fat soluble, it disperses into AT and overfat individuals are known to have decreased levels compared to lean individuals and to require higher doses to normalize blood levels of vitamin D.

VITAMIN E

A group of fat-soluble substances, the tocopherols are referred to as vitamin E. However, the vitamin E in the form of α-tocopherol was discovered about 100 years ago when it was found to be essential in preventing fetal resorption in pregnant, vitamin E-deficient rats fed lard-containing diets that were easily oxidized. The human diet contains eight different vitamin E-related molecules synthesized by plants; despite the fact that all of these molecules are peroxyl radical scavengers, the human body prefers α-tocopherol. The biological activity of vitamin E is highly dependent upon regulatory mechanisms that serve to retain α-tocopherol and excrete the non-α-tocopherol forms. This preference is dependent upon the combination of the function of α-tocopherol transfer protein (α-TTP) to enrich the plasma with α-tocopherol and the metabolism of non-α-tocopherols (Niki and Traber 2012).

α-TTP is critical for human health because mutations in this protein lead to severe vitamin E deficiency characterized by neurologic abnormalities, especially ataxia and eventually death if vitamin E is not provided in large quantities to overcome the lack of α-TTP. α-Tocopherol serves as a peroxyl radical scavenger that protects polyunsaturated fatty acids in membranes and lipoproteins. Although specific pathways and specific molecular targets have been sought in a variety of studies, the most likely explanation as to why humans require vitamin E is that it is a fat-soluble antioxidant. Alpha-D-tocopherol deficiency in rodents causes infertility.

Tocopherols have antioxidant properties protecting tissues and substances from the effects of oxygen. For example, these compounds can prevent in vitro oxidation of cholesterol, polyunsaturated fats, and other membrane lipids and proteins. In clinical studies, the antioxidant effects of vitamin E have been demonstrated only at doses that cannot be derived from usual diets but can only be achieved using supplement capsules (Aune et al. 2018).

In humans, severe vitamin E deficiency occurs as a result of genetic defects in the α-TTP, causing ataxia (Ulatowski and Manor 2015). The lack of functional α-TTP results in the rapid depletion of plasma a-tocopherol (Gohil et al. 2003), thereby demonstrating that α-TTP is needed to maintain plasma a-tocopherol concentrations. Fat malabsorption also leads to vitamin E deficiency including patients with cholestatic liver disease or cystic fibrosis (Traber and Manor 2012). Human vitamin E deficiency in addition to spinocerebellar ataxia which gets worse over time, there is also muscle deterioration including cardiomyopathy, ultimately resulting in death.

The use of vitamin E supplements has been associated with lower cardiovascular disease risk in males and has also been used effectively to retard the oxygen-induced damage to the eye in infants given 100% oxygen known as retrolental fibroplasias. There is increased interest in using vitamin E as an antioxidant for prevention of cardiovascular disease and common forms of cancer. The Recommended Dietary Allowance for vitamin E is between 8 and 12 μg equivalents/day to prevent rarely seen vitamin E deficiency, but many individuals take 400–800 IU supplements without ill effects.

A recent analysis of multiple studies found that above 330 IU/day was associated with a 5% increase in overall mortality from cardiovascular disease (Miller et al. 2005). These results have been discounted by many nutrition scientists and remain controversial (Biesalski et al. 2010). Studies have shown evidence of benefits of tocotrienols as well as tocopherols, but most supplements and multivitamins provide only synthetic alpha-D-tocopherol.

VITAMIN K

Vitamin K is a fat-soluble vitamin. The "K" is derived from the Danish word "koagulation". Coagulation refers to blood clotting, because vitamin K is essential for the functioning of several proteins involved in blood clotting. Vitamin K acts on target proteins in the clotting cascade by adding a gamma-carboxyl group to activate clotting proteins. Half of vitamin K comes from the diet, and the other half is synthesized from precursors by intestinal bacteria. Spinach, green leafy vegetables, cabbage, potatoes, cereals, and liver are good sources (Shearer, Fu, and Booth 2012).

Since vitamin K is found in so many foods and is also formed by intestinal bacteria, deficiency is rare. Individuals receiving prolonged antibiotic therapy destroying intestinal bacteria, and individuals with fat malabsorption are at risk for vitamin K deficiency. The Recommended Dietary Allowance for adults ranges between 45 and 80 μg/day.

Because warfarin antagonizes the action of vitamin K, rich dietary sources of vitamin K are restricted in patients on warfarin also known as coumadin (Violi et al. 2016). For patients whose blood tests called the INR vary greatly, it is an art to adjust the warfarin dose as dose adjustments often require 36 hours to be manifest.

There are two naturally occurring forms of vitamin K. Plants synthesize phylloquinone, also known as vitamin K1. Bacteria synthesize a range of vitamin K forms, using repeating 5-carbon units in the side chain of the molecule. These forms of vitamin K are designated menaquinone-n (MK-n), where n stands for the number of 5-carbon units. MK-n are collectively referred to as vitamin K2. The synthetic compound known as menadione (vitamin K3) is a provitamin that needs to be converted to menaquinone-4 (MK-4) to be active. MK-4 is not produced in significant amounts by bacteria, but appears to be synthesized by animals (including humans) from phylloquinone, which is found in plants (Nakagawa 2013). MK-4 is found in a number of organs other than the liver at higher concentrations than phylloquinone. This fact, along with the existence of a unique pathway for its synthesis, suggests there is some unique function of MK-4 that is yet to be discovered.

Vitamin K2 acts in bone as a cofactor for γ-carboxylase which converts the glutamic acid in in osteocalcin molecules to gamma-carboxyglutamic acid (Myneni and Mezey 2017). It is also a transcriptional regulator of bone-specific genes that act through steroid and xenobiotic receptors to favor the expression of osteoblastic markers. Vitamin K deficiency has been shown to be a risk factor for hip fracture in the elderly and vitamin K2 supplementation increases serum levels of osteocalcin and has a modest effect on bone mineral density.

VITAMIN B1

Vitamin B1 or thiamin deficiency disease, still seen today in alcoholics, is known as beriberi (Lonsdale 2018). This disease, which damages the nervous and cardiovascular systems, is found in two forms, wet beriberi with edema and congestive heart failure, and dry beriberi characterized by muscle atrophy due to nerve damage. In alcoholics, Wernicke-Korsakoff syndrome, characterized by mental confusion, memory disturbances, ataxia, opthalmoplegia, and nystagmus, can be fatal if not treated with intravenous thiamin (Polegato et al. 2019).

The dietary vitamin is phosphorylated by transfer of a high energy phosphate from adenosine triphosphate to form thiamin pyrophosphate in the intestine. Its primary function is to act as a coenzyme for the oxidative decarboxylation of alpha-keto-acids to carboxylic acids (e.g., pyruvate to acetyl coenzyme A (CoA)) and the transketolase reaction of the pentose phosphate shunt. The latter pathway is important for nucleic acid synthesis and the formation of NADPH for fatty acid synthesis and other reactions. Decreased transketolase activity in red cells can be detected early in the course of thiamin deficiency. The Recommended Dietary Allowance of thiamin is 0.5 mg/1,000 kcal and this is four times the intake at which deficiency signs are observed.

VITAMIN B2

Riboflavin known as vitamin B2 is a yellow fluorescent compound found throughout the animal and plant kingdoms. Humans and other mammals cannot synthesize these compounds which function in numerous enzyme complexes (including flavin mononucleotide and flavin adenine dinucleotide) involved in electron transport oxidation-reduction reactions. It is the central component of the cofactors flavin adenine dinucleotide (FAD) and flavin mononucleotide (FMN) (see below) and as such required for a variety of flavoproteoin enzyme reactions including activation of other vitamins (Pinto and Zempleni 2016).

Flavins are transported in the blood by albumin and by immunoglobulins. Uncomplicated riboflavin deficiency is uncommon, but dietary lack of the vitamin can lead to a deficit, not only in flavin coenzyme functions but also in the conversion of vitamin B-6 to pyridoxal 5′-phosphate. The recommended dietary allowance for riboflavin ranges between 1.2 and 1.8 mg/day for adults.

VITAMIN B6

The active form of pyridoxine (PN) or vitamin B6 is PLP, and this coenzyme is involved in over 60 different enzymatic reactions in the body including such common reactions as decarboxylation and aminotransferase reactions.

Isolated deficiencies of vitamin B-6 are rare, and it is most common to see deficiencies of multiple B vitamins. The best measure of vitamin B-6 status is plasma PLP which can be measured by HPLC. An intake of 2 mg/day is recommended in the RDA, and doses greater than 1 mg must be given to change PLP levels. At intakes of greater than 25 mg, PLP levels do not change further with the excess vitamin B-6 excreted in the urine as pyridoxal and pyridoxic acid. Very large doses (e.g., 500 mg/day) can cause peripheral neuropathy by inducing a conditioned deficiency of other B-vitamins catabolized in a manner similar to the excess vitamin B-6 ingested.

Vitamin B6 exists as six vitamers, including PN, pyridoxamine (PM), pyridoxine 5′-phosphate (PNP), pyridoxamine 5′-phosphate (PMP), PLP, and pyridoxal (PL)8. Dietary PN and PM serve as the main source of PNP and PMP. Oxidation of PNP and PMP produces PLP which can be further metabolized to PL through enzymatic hydrolysis (Zhang et al. 2017).

PLP, an active form of vitamin B6, is an essential cofactor required by many enzymes for metabolic processes including metabolism of carbohydrates, fats, and proteins 11–13. PNP oxidase (PNPO), also known as PMP oxidase, is a key enzyme in vitamin B6 metabolism and converts PNP and PMP into PLP.

The PNPO gene is located on chromosome 17q21.3215 and the level of PNPO mRNA expression is relatively high in human liver, skeletal muscle, and kidney, but low in lung and ovary16. PNPO has known to play a role in human epilepsy. PNPO has been implicated in breast, ovarian, and colorectal cancers (Zhang et al. 2017).

Niacin Vitamin B3, also known as niacin/nicotinic acid, can be synthesized by the body from tryptophan. The nickname niacin came from linking several letters in the words nicotinic, acid, and vitamin. When the properties of nicotinic acid, made by oxidation of nicotine, were first discovered it was decided that vitamin B3 or nicotinic acid should be named in such a way as to dissociate it from nicotine and not to create the impression that either smoking provided this vitamin or that wholesome food contained a poison (Jacobson and Jacobson 2018).

Once again, niacin refers to both nicotinic acid and nicotinamide, although sometimes used just to indicate niacin. Nicotinamide is converted to the Nicotinamide Adenine Dinucleotide cofactors (NAD and NADH) essential for a number of enzymatic reactions and is essential to electron transport. Niacin causes flushing and can reduce triglyceride levels in individuals with dyslipidemia at high doses of 500 mg three times a day, usually taken with aspirin to reduce the flushing reaction or in a long-acting form (Adiels et al. 2018). Nicotinamide does not have these lipid-lowering effects.

The deficiency disease, pellagra, was observed to occur in populations consuming a maize-based diet deficient in the amino acid tryptophan, which is the precursor for endogenous niacin formation (Rivadeneira, Moyer, and Salciccioli 2019). Large doses of nicotinic acid (1.5–3 g/day) but not nicotinamide will lower cholesterol and triglyceride levels and raise HDL levels in subgroups of hypercholesterolemic individuals. However, long-acting forms of niacin in large doses have been associated with liver damage, facial flushing, and worsening of hyperglycemia in diabetics. The recommended dietary allowance for niacin ranges between 13 and 20 mg/day for adults.

FOLIC ACID

Folate is a micronutrient, once called vitamin M, which frequently is deficient in American diets since it is derived from dark green, leafy vegetables. The root of the name folic comes from the Latin word for leaf. Folic acid acts in cell maturation and differentiates epithelial tissues. In the lung and the cervical epithelium prodifferentiation effects have been demonstrated. Folic acid has also been associated with the prevention of neural tube defects such as spina bifida through its effects in epigenetic methylation in utero (Viswanathan et al. 2017). It is included in all prenatal vitamins at an enhanced level.

Folate supplementation is restricted to 400 µg per tablet in over the counter vitamins given that fear that excessive folate in someone with B12 deficiency (see below) will develop subacute combined spinal degeneration and paralysis (Pavlov et al. 2019). Patients with pernicious anemia are among those susceptible to subacute combined spinal degeneration from excess folate intake as are those who have had a gastric bypass operation or gastrectomy.

Folate and folic acid are NOT interchangeable terms (Scaglione and Panzavolta 2014). Folic acid is the oxidized form found in fortified foods and supplements while folate is the reduced form found naturally in foods as polyglutamates which must be cleaved and converted in a series of steps to 5-methyl-tetrahydrofolate which plays a key role in methyl donor reactions.

Food sources of folate include mushrooms and green vegetables. Raw foods have higher amounts than cooked foods. Enrichment of white flour began in 1998 and is now the major source of folate in the American diet. The bioavailability of dietary folate is about 50%.

One Dietary Folate Equivalent (DFE) is equal to: 1 μg of food folate; 0.6 μg of folic acid from a supplement or fortified food consumed with a meal; or 0.5 μg of folic acid from a supplement taken without food (empty stomach). Stated alternately, DFE=μg food folate+(1.7×μg folic acid).

The MTHFR (Methyl Tetrahydrofolate Reductase) C677T polymorphism in folate metabolism leads to the amino acid alanine being replaced by valine (p.Ala222Val) and the production of a thermolabile variant of MTHFR with 30% less enzyme activity (Liew and Gupta 2015). The MTHFR C677T polymorphism has been suspected to induce hypomethylation and then activate proto-oncogenes, which could explain the association between this polymorphism and some types of cancer including oral cancer (Sailasree et al. 2011).

VITAMIN B12

Vitamin B12 also called cyanocobalamin is needed to make red blood cells and is necessary for the synthesis of nerve sheaths, fatty acids, and DNA. Since this vitamin is stored in the liver, nutritional deficiency usually takes years to develop. It is much more common to see metabolic deficiencies. Most commonly an anemia due to B12 deficiency results from an autoimmune disease called pernicious anemia in which the parietal cells in the stomach that make a binding protein (intrinsic factor) necessary for B12 absorption are destroyed (Bunn 2014). The healthy individuals most at risk of a dietary vitamin B12 deficiency are vegetarians, since there is no B12 in any plant product. There is also a decreased capability for absorption of vitamin B12 in the elderly due to decreased gastric acid secretion (Stabler 2013).

Vitamin B12 levels need to be measured in individuals at risk, since folate administered to an individual with B12 deficiency will result in subacute combined degeneration of the spine and paralysis. The Recommended Dietary Allowance for adults is only 2–2.6 μg/day.

Vitamin B12 consists of a class of chemically related compounds, all of which have vitamin activity. It contains the biochemically rare element cobalt sitting in the center of a planar tetrapyrrole ring called a corrin ring. More recently, hydroxocobalamin, methylcobalamin, and adenosylcobalamin can be found in more expensive pharmacological products and food supplements. The extra utility of these compounds is currently controversial.

CHOLINE

Choline as already discussed above is not formally considered a B vitamin since a portion of the choline requirement can be met via endogenous de novo synthesis of phosphatidylcholine catalyzed by PEMT in the liver. A recommended dietary intake for choline of 550 mg/day in humans was set in 1998, and though many foods contain choline, 90% of Americans do not get enough in their diets (Zeisel, Klatt, and Caudill 2018).

When deprived of dietary choline, most adult men and postmenopausal women developed signs of organ dysfunction such as fatty liver, liver or muscle cell damage, and reduced capacity to handle a methionine load, resulting in elevated homocysteine levels in the blood.

Only some premenopausal women with a genetic polymorphism develop problems, because estrogen induces expression of the PEMT gene and allows premenopausal women to make more of their needed choline endogenously. The dietary requirement for choline can vary based on common polymorphisms in genes of choline and folate metabolism including the MTHFR gene. The CC polymorphism is the most common and protects individuals from choline deficiency. The less common TT polymorphism in about 10% of individuals does not protect individuals from choline deficiency.

Along with folate and B12 deficiency, inadequate consumption of choline can lead to high homocysteine and all the risks associated with that including cardiovascular disease, and neuropsychiatric illness (Alzheimer's disease, schizophrenia). Inadequate choline intake can also lead to fatty liver or NAFLD in combination with overweight and obesity. As reviewed earlier, inadequate choline intake from the diet is associated with an increased risk of common forms of cancer. The issues around choline illustrate the impact of nutrigenetics, the differences among individuals impacting risk of age-related chronic diseases.

VITAMIN B5

Pantothenic acid is also called pantothenate or vitamin B5. Pantothenic acid is required to synthesize CoA which is intrinsic to the synthesis of proteins, carbohydrates, and fats (Snyder et al. 2015). The structure of pantothenic acid is made up of an amide linkage between pantoic acid and alanine. Its name derives from a Greek root meaning "from everywhere", since small quantities of pantothenic acid are found in nearly every food, with high amounts in avocado, whole grains, legumes, eggs, and meats. It commonly occurs in its alcohol form, pantothenol, and as calcium pantothenate. Pantothenic acid is used as an ingredient in some hair and skin care products, since it is reputed with no proof to prevent graying of the hair. It was discovered by Dr. Roger Williams in 1933 (Lanska 2012).

Within cells, pyruvate produced from the breakdown of glucose via the glycolytic pathway is transported into mitochondria for the production of ATP via oxidative phosphorylation as discussed earlier in the course. When oxygen is available, pyruvate is converted into a two-carbon acetyl group (acetyl CoA) which is then picked up by CoA. Acetyl CoA can be used in a variety of ways by the cell, but its major function is to deliver the acetyl group derived from pyruvate to the Krebs cycle of glucose catabolism to produce ATP energy for the cell.

In all living organisms, CoA is synthesized in a five-step process that requires four molecules of ATP, from pantothenate and cysteine. The structure of CoA was identified in the early 1950s at the Lister Institute in London together with workers at the Massachusetts General Hospital and Harvard Medical School (Theodoulou et al. 2014).

Since CoA contains a sulfhydryl group it can react with carboxylic acid group to form a thioester which can be used to help transfer fatty acids with over ten carbons from the cytoplasm to the mitochondria. A molecule of CoA carrying an acetyl group is also referred to as acetyl-CoA. Examples of uses of CoA include fatty acyl-CoAs (proprionyl-CoA, butyryl-CoA, myristoyl-CoA, crotonyl-CoA, acetoacetyl-CoA, benzoyl-CoA, phenylacetyl-CoA), malonyl-Co-A, succinyl-CoA, hydroxymethylglutaryl CoA. The last compound is involved in the rate-limiting step in cholesterol biosynthesis which is HMG-CoA-reductase.

BIOTIN

Biotin, also known as vitamin B7, vitamin H, and or coenzyme R, is a coenzyme for carboxylase enzymes, involved in the synthesis of fatty acids, isoleucine, and valine, and in gluconeogenesis (Mock 2017). Biotin exists in food as protein-bound form or biocytin. Proteolysis by protease is required prior to absorption. This process assists free biotin release from biocytin and protein-bound biotin. The biotin present in corn is readily available; however, most grains have about a 20%–40% bioavailability of biotin. Biotin is found in a wide variety of foods with high biotin content include peanuts, Swiss chard, liver, Saskatoon berries, and leafy green vegetables.

Symptoms of biotin deficiency include hair loss, dermatitis, and conjunctivitis. The reason is called vitamin H which is from the German for Hair and Skin ("Haut"), since these are characteristic of biotin deficiency. Neurological and psychological symptoms can occur with only mild deficiencies. Dermatitis, conjunctivitis, and hair loss will generally occur only when deficiency becomes more severe. Pregnant women tend to have a high risk of biotin deficiency. Nearly half of pregnant women have abnormal increases of 3-hydroxyisovaleric acid, which reflects reduced status of biotin. Biotin deficiency can also be caused by inborn metabolic errors affecting biotin-related enzymes. In animals fed raw egg white, biotin deficiency occurs due to a protein called avidin which binds biotin. Avidin is denatured with cooking so cooked egg white does not affect biotin availability. Patients with gastric bypass or gastrectomy can develop biotin deficiency in the absence of supplementation since proteolysis is required in the stomach to release protein-bound biotin found in foods (Saleem and Soos 2020).

CONCLUSION

Advances in genomics, metabolomics, and proteomics are improving our understanding regarding cancer metabolic diversity, resulting in detailed classifications of tumors and raising the effectiveness of precision medicine. Likewise, the growing knowledge of interactions between nutrients and the expression of certain genes could ultimately lead to altered cancer therapies based on precision nutrition strategies. Numerous epidemiological studies have provided evidence linking diet and lifestyle with cancer prevention, carcinogenesis, tumor growth, and relapse. Precision nutrition is an emerging science that relies on well-established factors such as genetic and epigenetic variation and the microbiome reviewed in this chapter.

However, we must recognize that the field of personalized nutrition will require much more scientific evidence to find its proper place in precision oncology. In the meantime, all healthcare providers can use existing tools and patient preferences to optimize nutritional consultation for cancer patients. It can never be emphasized enough that the cancer patient population is a vulnerable population and should be treated with empathy and humility in promoting personalized nutrition in cancer.

REFERENCES

Adiels, M., M. J. Chapman, P. Robillard, M. Krempf, M. Laville, J. Boren, and Group Niacin Study. 2018. "Niacin action in the atherogenic mixed dyslipidemia of metabolic syndrome: insights from metabolic biomarker profiling and network analysis." *J Clin Lipidol* 12 (3):810–821.el. doi: 10.1016/j. jacl.2018.03.083.

Ambatipudi, S., S. Horvath, F. Perrier, C. Cuenin, H. Hernandez-Vargas, F. Le Calvez-Kelm, G. Durand, G. Byrnes, P. Ferrari, L. Bouaoun, A. Sklias, V. Chajes, K. Overvad, G. Severi, L. Baglietto, F. Clavel-Chapelon, R. Kaaks, M. Barrdahl, H. Boeing, A. Trichopoulou, P. Lagiou, A. Naska, G. Masala, C. Agnoli, S. Polidoro, R. Tumino, S. Panico, M. Dolle, P. H. M. Peeters, N. C. Onland-Moret, T. M. Sandanger, T. H. Nost, E. Weiderpass, J. R. Quiros, A. Agudo, M. Rodriguez-Barranco, J. M. Huerta Castano, A. Barricarte, A. M. Fernandez, R. C. Travis, P. Vineis, D. C. Muller, E. Riboli, M. Gunter, I. Romieu, and Z. Herceg. 2017. "DNA methylome analysis identifies accelerated epigenetic ageing associated with postmenopausal breast cancer susceptibility." *Eur J Cancer* 75:299–307 doi: 10.1016/j. ejca.2017.01.014.

Andres, S., S. Pevny, R. Ziegenhagen, N. Bakhiya, B. Schafer, K. I. Hirsch-Ernst, and A. Lampen. 2018. "Safety aspects of the use of quercetin as a dietary supplement." *Mol Nutr Food Res* 62 (1). doi: 10.1002/ mnfr.201700447.

Anstee, Q. M., H. L. Reeves, E. Kotsiliti, O. Govaere, and M. Heikenwalder. 2019. "From NASH to HCC: current concepts and future challenges." *Nat Rev Gastroenterol Hepatol* 16 (7):411–428. doi: 10.1038/ s41575-019-0145-7.

Arnold, M., N. Pandeya, G. Byrnes, P. A. G. Renehan, G. A. Stevens, P. M. Ezzati, J. Ferlay, J. J. Miranda, I. Romieu, R. Dikshit, D. Forman, and I. Soerjomataram. 2015. "Global burden of cancer attributable to high body-mass index in 2012: a population-based study." *Lancet Oncol* 16 (1):36–46. doi: 10.1016/ S1470-2045(14)71123-4.

Asher, G. N., A. H. Corbett, and R. L. Hawke. 2017. "Common herbal dietary supplement-drug interactions." *Am Fam Physician* 96 (2):101–107.

Augustin, L. S., C. W. Kendall, D. J. Jenkins, W. C. Willett, A. Astrup, A. W. Barclay, I. Bjorck, J. C. Brand-Miller, F. Brighenti, A. E. Buyken, A. Ceriello, C. La Vecchia, G. Livesey, S. Liu, G. Riccardi, S. W. Rizkalla, J. L. Sievenpiper, A. Trichopoulou, T. M. Wolever, S. Baer-Sinnott, and A. Poli. 2015. "Glycemic index, glycemic load and glycemic response: An International Scientific Consensus Summit from the International Carbohydrate Quality Consortium (ICQC)." *Nutr Metab Cardiovasc Dis* 25 (9):795–815. doi: 10.1016/j.numecd.2015.05.005.

Aune, D., N. Keum, E. Giovannucci, L. T. Fadnes, P. Boffetta, D. C. Greenwood, S. Tonstad, L. J. Vatten, E. Riboli, and T. Norat. 2018. "Dietary intake and blood concentrations of antioxidants and the risk of cardiovascular disease, total cancer, and all-cause mortality: a systematic review and dose-response meta-analysis of prospective studies." *Am J Clin Nutr* 108 (5):1069–1091. doi: 10.1093/ajcn/nqy097.

Baggerly, C. A., R. E. Cuomo, C. B. French, C. F. Garland, E. D. Gorham, W. B. Grant, R. P. Heaney, M. F. Holick, B. W. Hollis, S. L. McDonnell, M. Pittaway, P. Seaton, C. L. Wagner, and A. Wunsch. 2015. "Sunlight and vitamin D: necessary for public health." *J Am Coll Nutr* 34 (4):359–365. doi: 10.1080/07315724.2015.1039866.

Bailey, R. L., J. J. Gahche, P. E. Miller, P. R. Thomas, and J. T. Dwyer. 2013. "Why US adults use dietary supplements." *JAMA Intern Med* 173 (5):355–361. doi: 10.1001/jamainternmed.2013.2299.

Bathi, R. J., R. Rao, and S. Mutalik. 2009. "GST null genotype and antioxidants: risk indicators for oral pre-cancer and cancer." *Indian J Dent Res* 20 (3):298–303. doi: 10.4103/0970-9290.57365.

Belsky, D. W., A. Caspi, R. Houts, H. J. Cohen, D. L. Corcoran, A. Danese, H. Harrington, S. Israel, M. E. Levine, J. D. Schaefer, K. Sugden, B. Williams, A. I. Yashin, R. Poulton, and T. E. Moffitt. 2015. "Quantification of biological aging in young adults." *Proc Natl Acad Sci U S A* 112 (30):E4104–10. doi: 10.1073/pnas.1506264112.

Benabdelkrim, M., O. Djeffal, and H. Berredjem. 2018. "GSTM1 and GSTT1 polymorphisms and suscepti-bility to prostate cancer: a case-control study of the Algerian population." *Asian Pac J Cancer Prev* 19 (10):2853–2858. doi: 10.22034/APJCP.2018.19.10.2853.

Berry, S. E., A. M. Valdes, D. A. Drew, F. Asnicar, M. Mazidi, J. Wolf, J. Capdevila, G. Hadjigeorgiou, R. Davies, H. Al Khatib, C. Bonnett, S. Ganesh, E. Bakker, D. Hart, M. Mangino, J. Merino, I. Linenberg, P. Wyatt, J. M. Ordovas, C. D. Gardner, L. M. Delahanty, A. T. Chan, N. Segata, P. W. Franks, and T. D. Spector. 2020. "Human postprandial responses to food and potential for precision nutrition." *Nat Med* 26 (6):964–973. doi: 10.1038/s41591-020-0934-0.

Bhupathiraju, S. N., D. K. Tobias, V. S. Malik, A. Pan, A. Hruby, J. E. Manson, W. C. Willett, and F. B. Hu. 2014. "Glycemic index, glycemic load, and risk of type 2 diabetes: results from 3 large US cohorts and an updated meta-analysis." *Am J Clin Nutr* 100 (1):218–232. doi: 10.3945/ajcn.113.079533.

Biesalski, H. K. 1989. "Comparative assessment of the toxicology of vitamin A and retinoids in man." *Toxicology* 57(2):117–161. doi: 10.1016/0300-483x(89)90161-3. PMID: 2665185.

Biesalski, H. K. 2013. "International congress 'Hidden Hunger', March 5–9, 2013, Stuttgart-Hohenheim, Germany." *Ann Nutr Metab* 62 (4):298–302. doi: 10.1159/000351078.

Biesalski, H. K., T. Grune, J. Tinz, I. Zollner, and J. B. Blumberg. 2010. "Reexamination of a meta-analysis of the effect of antioxidant supplementation on mortality and health in randomized trials." *Nutrients* 2 (9):929–949. doi: 10.3390/nu2090929.

Blakermore, F., C. W. Ottaway, K. C. Sellers, E. Eden, and T. Moore. 1957. "The effects of a diet deficient in vitamin A on the development of the skull, optic nerves and brain of cattle." *J Comp Pathol* 67 (3):277–288. doi: 10.1016/s0368-1742(57)80027-7.

Borghouts, L. B., and H. A. Keizer. 2000. "Exercise and insulin sensitivity: a review." *Int J Sports Med* 21 (1):1–12. doi: 10.1055/s-2000-8847.

Bouchard-Mercier, A., A. M. Paradis, I. Rudkowska, S. Lemieux, P. Couture, and M. C. Vohl. 2013. "Associations between dietary patterns and gene expression profiles of healthy men and women: a cross-sectional study." *Nutr J* 12:24. doi: 10.1186/1475-2891-12-24.

Brauer, H. A., T. E. Libby, B. L. Mitchell, L. Li, C. Chen, T. W. Randolph, Y. Y. Yasui, J. W. Lampe, and P. D. Lampe. 2011. "Cruciferous vegetable supplementation in a controlled diet study alters the serum pepti-dome in a GSTM1-genotype dependent manner." *Nutr J* 10:11. doi: 10.1186/1475-2891-10-11.

Bunn, H. F. 2014. "Vitamin B12 and pernicious anemia--the dawn of molecular medicine." *N Engl J Med* 370 (8):773–776. doi: 10.1056/NEJMcibr1315544.

Cardwell, G., J. F. Bornman, A. P. James, and L. J. Black. 2018. "A review of mushrooms as a potential source of dietary Vitamin D." *Nutrients* 10 (10):1498. doi: 10.3390/nu10101498.

Carter, H. E. 1979. "Essential amino acids." *Ann N Y Acad Sci* 325:236–251. doi: 10.1111/j.1749-6632.1979. tb14138.x.

Casas-Agustench, P., D. K. Arnett, C. E. Smith, C. Q. Lai, L. D. Parnell, I. B. Borecki, A. C. Frazier-Wood, M. Allison, Y. D. Chen, K. D. Taylor, S. S. Rich, J. I. Rotter, Y. C. Lee, and J. M. Ordovas. 2014. "Saturated fat intake modulates the association between an obesity genetic risk score and body mass index in two US populations." *J Acad Nutr Diet* 114 (12):1954–1966. doi: 10.1016/j.jand.2014.03.014.

Celis-Morales, C., K. M. Livingstone, C. F. Marsaux, A. L. Macready, R. Fallaize, C. B. O'Donovan, C. Woolhead, H. Forster, M. C. Walsh, S. Navas-Carretero, R. San-Cristobal, L. Tsirigoti, C. P. Lambrinou, C. Mavrogianni, G. Moschonis, S. Kolossa, J. Hallmann, M. Godlewska, A. Surwillo, I. Traczyk, C. A. Drevon, J. Bouwman, B. van Ommen, K. Grimaldi, L. D. Parnell, J. N. Matthews, Y. Manios, H. Daniel, J. A. Martinez, J. A. Lovegrove, E. R. Gibney, L. Brennan, W. H. Saris, M. Gibney, J. C. Mathers, and Study Food4Me. 2017. "Effect of personalized nutrition on health-related behaviour change: evidence from the Food4Me European randomized controlled trial." *Int J Epidemiol* 46 (2):578–588. doi: 10.1093/ije/dyw186.

Chen, D. F., W. J. Sun, K. J. Liu, and L. Z. Wen. 2017. "[Current epidemiology and pathogenesis of non-alcoholic fatty liver disease-associated liver cancer]." *Zhonghua Gan Zang Bing Za Zhi* 25 (2):111–114. doi: 10.3760/cma.j.issn.1007-3418.2017.02.006.

Christakos, S., P. Dhawan, A. Verstuyf, L. Verlinden, and G. Carmeliet. 2016. "Vitamin D: metabolism, molecular mechanism of action, and pleiotropic effects." *Physiol Rev* 96 (1):365–408. doi: 10.1152/physrev.00014.2015.

Conserva, M. R., L. Anelli, A. Zagaria, G. Specchia, and F. Albano. 2019. "The pleiotropic role of retinoic acid/retinoic acid receptors signaling: from vitamin A metabolism to gene rearrangements in acute promyelocytic leukemia." *Int J Mol Sci* 20 (12):2921. doi: 10.3390/ijms20122921.

Cunningham, J. J. 1980. "A reanalysis of the factors influencing basal metabolic rate in normal adults." *Am J Clin Nutr* 33 (11):2372–2374. doi: 10.1093/ajcn/33.11.2372.

de Conti, A., J. F. Ortega, V. Tryndyak, K. Dreval, F. S. Moreno, I. Rusyn, F. A. Beland, and I. P. Pogribny. 2017. "MicroRNA deregulation in nonalcoholic steatohepatitis-associated liver carcinogenesis." *Oncotarget* 8 (51):88517–88528. doi: 10.18632/oncotarget.19774.

DeLuca, H. F. 2016. "Vitamin D: historical overview." *Vitam Horm* 100:1–20. doi: 10.1016/bs.vh.2015.11.001.

Dickerson, R. N. 2016. "Nitrogen balance and protein requirements for critically ill older patients." *Nutrients* 8 (4):226. doi: 10.3390/nu8040226.

Du, Y. F., W. P. Luo, F. Y. Lin, Z. Q. Lian, X. F. Mo, B. Yan, M. Xu, W. Q. Huang, J. Huang, and C. X. Zhang. 2016. "Dietary choline and betaine intake, choline-metabolising genetic polymorphisms and breast cancer risk: a case-control study in China." *Br J Nutr* 116 (6):961–968. doi: 10.1017/S0007114516002956.

Dwyer, J. T., P. M. Coates, and M. J. Smith. 2018. "Dietary supplements: regulatory challenges and research resources." *Nutrients* 10 (1):41. doi: 10.3390/nu10010041.

Ebeling, P., H. A. Koistinen, and V. A. Koivisto. 1998. "Insulin-independent glucose transport regulates insulin sensitivity." *FEBS Lett* 436 (3):301–303. doi: 10.1016/s0014-5793(98)01149-1.

Evans, W. J., M. Hellerstein, E. Orwoll, S. Cummings, and P. M. Cawthon. 2019. "D3 -Creatine dilution and the importance of accuracy in the assessment of skeletal muscle mass." *J Cachexia Sarcopenia Muscle* 10(1):14–21. doi: 10.1002/jcsm.12390. Epub 2019 Mar 21. PMID: 30900400; PMCID: PMC6438329.

Feskanich, D., R. G. Ziegler, D. S. Michaud, E. L. Giovannucci, F. E. Speizer, W. C. Willett, and G. A. Colditz. 2000. "Prospective study of fruit and vegetable consumption and risk of lung cancer among men and women." *J Natl Cancer Inst* 92 (22):1812–1823. doi: 10.1093/jnci/92.22.1812. PMID: 11078758.

Foster-Powell, K., Holt, S. H. A., Brand-Miller, J. C. 2002. "International table of GI and GL values: 2002." Am J Clin Nutr 76 (1): 5–56.

Fulgoni, V. L., 3rd. 2008. "Current protein intake in America: analysis of the National Health and Nutrition Examination Survey, 2003–2004." *Am J Clin Nutr* 87 (5):1554S–1557S. doi: 10.1093/ajcn/87.5.1554S.

Ganz, A. B., V. V. Cohen, C. C. Swersky, J. Stover, G. A. Vitiello, J. Lovesky, J. C. Chuang, K. Shields, V. G. Fomin, Y. S. Lopez, S. Mohan, A. Ganti, B. Carrier, O. V. Malysheva, and M. A. Caudill. 2017. "Genetic variation in choline-metabolizing enzymes alters choline metabolism in young women consuming choline intakes meeting current recommendations." *Int J Mol Sci* 18 (2):252. doi: 10.3390/ijms18020252.

Gaziano, J. M., R. J. Glynn, W. G. Christen, T. Kurth, C. Belanger, J. MacFadyen, V. Bubes, J. E. Manson, H. D. Sesso, and J. E. Buring. 2009. "Vitamins E and C in the prevention of prostate and total cancer in men: the Physicians' Health Study II randomized controlled trial." *JAMA* 301 (1):52–62. doi: 10.1001/jama.2008.862.

Gaziano, J. M., H. D. Sesso, W. G. Christen, V. Bubes, J. P. Smith, J. MacFadyen, M. Schvartz, J. E. Manson, R. J. Glynn, and J. E. Buring. 2012. "Multivitamins in the prevention of cancer in men: the Physicians' Health Study II randomized controlled trial." *JAMA* 308 (18):1871–1880. doi: 10.1001/jama.2012.14641.

Giovannucci, E., E. B. Rimm, Y. Liu, M. J. Stampfer, and W. C. Willett. 2002. "A prospective study of tomato products, lycopene, and prostate cancer risk." *J Natl Cancer Inst* 94 (5):391–398. doi: 10.1093/jnci/94.5.391.

Gohil, K., B. C. Schock, A. A. Chakraborty, Y. Terasawa, J. Raber, R. V. Farese, Jr., L. Packer, C. E. Cross, and M. G. Traber. 2003. "Gene expression profile of oxidant stress and neurodegeneration in transgenic mice deficient in alpha-tocopherol transfer protein." *Free Radic Biol Med* 35 (11):1343–1354. doi: 10.1016/s0891-5849(03)00509-4.

Gonzalez, M. C., C. A. Pastore, S. P. Orlandi, and S. B. Heymsfield. 2014. "Obesity paradox in cancer: new insights provided by body composition." *Am J Clin Nutr* 99 (5):999–1005. doi: 10.3945/ajcn.113.071399.

Harvie, M. 2014. "Nutritional supplements and cancer: potential benefits and proven harms." *Am Soc Clin Oncol Educ Book*:e478–e486. doi: 10.14694/EdBook_AM.2014.34.e478.

Helm, C. W., D. J. Lorenz, N. J. Meyer, W. W. Rising, and J. L. Wulff. 2013. "Retinoids for preventing the progression of cervical intra-epithelial neoplasia." *Cochrane Database Syst Rev* (6):CD003296. doi: 10.1002/14651858.CD003296.pub3.

Hennekens, C. H., J. E. Buring, J. E. Manson, M. Stampfer, B. Rosner, N. R. Cook, C. Belanger, F. LaMotte, J. M. Gaziano, P. M. Ridker, W. Willett, and R. Peto. 1996. "Lack of effect of long-term supplementation with beta carotene on the incidence of malignant neoplasms and cardiovascular disease." *N Engl J Med* 334 (18):1145–1149. doi: 10.1056/NEJM199605023341801.

Herceg, Z., A. Ghantous, C. P. Wild, A. Sklias, L. Casati, S. J. Duthie, R. Fry, J. P. Issa, R. Kellermayer, I. Koturbash, Y. Kondo, J. Lepeule, S. C. S. Lima, C. J. Marsit, V. Rakyan, R. Saffery, J. A. Taylor, A. E. Teschendorff, T. Ushijima, P. Vineis, C. L. Walker, R. A. Waterland, J. Wiemels, S. Ambatipudi, D. Degli Esposti, and H. Hernandez-Vargas. 2018. "Roadmap for investigating epigenome deregulation and environmental origins of cancer." *Int J Cancer* 142 (5):874–882. doi: 10.1002/ijc.31014.

Hewison, M. 2012. "Vitamin D and immune function: an overview." *Proc Nutr Soc* 71 (1):50–61. doi: 10.1017/S0029665111001650.

Heymsfield, S. B., M. C. Gonzalez, J. Lu, G. Jia, and J. Zheng. 2015. "Skeletal muscle mass and quality: evolution of modern measurement concepts in the context of sarcopenia." *Proc Nutr Soc* 74(4):355–366. doi: 10.1017/S0029665115000129. Epub 2015 Apr 8. PMID: 25851205.

Hofstatter, E. W., S. Horvath, D. Dalela, P. Gupta, A. B. Chagpar, V. B. Wali, V. Bossuyt, A. M. Storniolo, C. Hatzis, G. Patwardhan, M. K. Von Wahlde, M. Butler, L. Epstein, K. Stavris, T. Sturrock, A. Au, S. Kwei, and L. Pusztai. 2018. "Increased epigenetic age in normal breast tissue from luminal breast cancer patients." *Clin Epigenetics* 10 (1):112. doi: 10.1186/s13148-018-0534-8.

Holick, M. F. 2009. "Vitamin D status: measurement, interpretation, and clinical application." *Ann Epidemiol* 19 (2):73–78. doi: 10.1016/j.annepidem.2007.12.001.

Holick, M. F. 2017. "The vitamin D deficiency pandemic: approaches for diagnosis, treatment and prevention." *Rev Endocr Metab Disord* 18 (2):153–165. doi: 10.1007/s11154-017-9424-1.

Holick, M. F., N. C. Binkley, H. A. Bischoff-Ferrari, C. M. Gordon, D. A. Hanley, R. P. Heaney, M. H. Murad, C. M. Weaver, and Society Endocrine. 2011. "Evaluation, treatment, and prevention of vitamin D deficiency: an Endocrine Society clinical practice guideline." *J Clin Endocrinol Metab* 96 (7):1911–1930. doi: 10.1210/jc.2011-0385.

Holscher, H. D. 2017. "Dietary fiber and prebiotics and the gastrointestinal microbiota." *Gut Microbes* 8 (2):172–184. doi: 10.1080/19490976.2017.1290756.

Horvath, S., and K. Raj. 2018. "DNA methylation-based biomarkers and the epigenetic clock theory of ageing." *Nat Rev Genet* 19 (6):371–384. doi: 10.1038/s41576-018-0004-3.

Horwich, T. B., G. C. Fonarow, and A. L. Clark. 2018. "Obesity and the obesity paradox in heart failure." *Prog Cardiovasc Dis* 61 (2):151–156. doi: 10.1016/j.pcad.2018.05.005.

Hosseini-Esfahani, F., P. Mirmiran, M. S. Daneshpour, Y. Mehrabi, M. Hedayati, M. Soheilian-Khorzoghi, and F. Azizi. 2015. "Dietary patterns interact with APOA1/APOC3 polymorphisms to alter the risk of the metabolic syndrome: the Tehran Lipid and Glucose Study." *Br J Nutr* 113 (4):644–653. doi: 10.1017/S0007114514003687.

Grossniklaus, U., W. G. Kelly, B. Kelly, A. C. Ferguson-Smith, and M. Pembrey, and S. Lindquist. 2013. "Transgenerational epigenetic inheritance: how important is it?" *Nat Rev Genet.* 14(3):228–235. doi: 10.1038/nrg3435. Erratum in: *Nat Rev Genet.* 2013 Nov; 14(11):820. Erratum in: *Nat Rev Genet.* 2013 Sep; 14(9). doi:10.1038/nrg3595. Kelly, Bill [corrected to Kelly, William G]. PMID: 23416892; PMCID: PMC4066847.

Hussain Gilani, S. Y., S. Bibi, A. Siddiqui, S. R. Ali Shah, F. Akram, and M. U. Rehman. 2019. "Obesity and diabetes as determinants of vitamin D deficiency." *J Ayub Med Coll Abbottabad* 31 (3):432–435.

Ianhez, M., S. A. Pinto, H. A. Miot, and E. Bagatin. 2019. "A randomized, open, controlled trial of tretinoin 0.05% cream vs. low-dose oral isotretinoin for the treatment of field cancerization." *Int J Dermatol* 58 (3):365–373. doi: 10.1111/ijd.14363.

Ikawa-Yoshida, A., S. Matsuo, A. Kato, Y. Ohmori, A. Higashida, E. Kaneko, and M. Matsumoto. 2017. "Hepatocellular carcinoma in a mouse model fed a choline-deficient, L-amino acid-defined, high-fat diet." *Int J Exp Pathol* 98 (4):221–233. doi: 10.1111/iep.12240.

Ingelsson, E., C. Langenberg, M. F. Hivert, I. Prokopenko, V. Lyssenko, J. Dupuis, R. Magi, S. Sharp, A. U. Jackson, T. L. Assimes, P. Shrader, J. W. Knowles, B. Zethelius, F. A. Abbasi, R. N. Bergman, A. Bergmann, C. Berne, M. Boehnke, L. L. Bonnycastle, S. R. Bornstein, T. A. Buchanan, S. J. Bumpstead, Y. Bottcher, P. Chines, F. S. Collins, C. C. Cooper, E. M. Dennison, M. R. Erdos, E. Ferrannini, C. S. Fox, J. Graessler, K. Hao, B. Isomaa, K. A. Jameson, P. Kovacs, J. Kuusisto, M. Laakso, C. Ladenvall, K. L. Mohlke, M. A. Morken, N. Narisu, D. M. Nathan, L. Pascoe, F. Payne, J. R. Petrie, A. A. Sayer, P. E. Schwarz, L. J. Scott, H. M. Stringham, M. Stumvoll, A. J. Swift, A. C. Syvanen, T. Tuomi, J. Tuomilehto, A. Tonjes, T. T. Valle, G. H. Williams, L. Lind, I. Barroso, T. Quertermous, M. Walker, N. J. Wareham, J. B. Meigs, M. I. McCarthy, L. Groop, R. M. Watanabe, J. C. Florez, and Magic investigators. 2010. "Detailed physiologic characterization reveals diverse mechanisms for novel genetic Loci regulating glucose and insulin metabolism in humans." *Diabetes* 59 (5):1266–1275. doi: 10.2337/db09-1568.

Jacobson, M. K., and E. L. Jacobson. 2018. "Vitamin B3 in health and disease: toward the second century of discovery." *Methods Mol Biol* 1813:3–8. doi: 10.1007/978-1-4939-8588-3_1.

Jenkins, D. J., T. M. Wolever, R. H. Taylor, H. Barker, H. Fielden, J. M. Baldwin, A. C. Bowling, H. C. Newman, A. L. Jenkins, and D. V. Goff. 1981. "Glycemic index of foods: a physiological basis for carbohydrate exchange." *Am J Clin Nutr* 34 (3):362–366. doi: 10.1093/ajcn/34.3.362.

Jeon, S. M., and E. A. Shin. 2018. "Exploring vitamin D metabolism and function in cancer." *Exp Mol Med* 50 (4):20. doi: 10.1038/s12276-018-0038-9.

Jiang-Hua, Q., J. De-Chuang, L. Zhen-Duo, C. Shu-de, and L. Zhenzhen. 2014. "Association of methylenetetrahydrofolate reductase and methionine synthase polymorphisms with breast cancer risk and interaction with folate, vitamin B6, and vitamin B 12 intakes." *Tumour Biol* 35 (12):11895–11901. doi: 10.1007/s13277-014-2456-1.

Kantor, E. D., C. D. Rehm, M. Du, E. White, and E. L. Giovannucci. 2016. "Trends in dietary supplement use among US adults from 1999–2012." *JAMA* 316 (14):1464–1474. doi: 10.1001/jama.2016.14403.

Keum, N., and E. Giovannucci. 2014. "Vitamin D supplements and cancer incidence and mortality: a meta-analysis." *Br J Cancer* 111 (5):976–980. doi: 10.1038/bjc.2014.294.

Kim, H. J., E. Giovannucci, B. Rosner, W. C. Willett, and E. Cho. 2014. "Longitudinal and secular trends in dietary supplement use: nurses' health study and health professionals follow-up study, 1986–2006." *J Acad Nutr Diet* 114 (3):436–443. doi: 10.1016/j.jand.2013.07.039.

Klusek, J., A. Nasierowska-Guttmejer, A. Kowalik, I. Wawrzycka, P. Lewitowicz, M. Chrapek, and S. Gluszek. 2018. "GSTM1, GSTT1, and GSTP1 polymorphisms and colorectal cancer risk in Polish nonsmokers." *Oncotarget* 9 (30):21224–21230. doi: 10.18632/oncotarget.25031.

Klutstein, M., D. Nejman, R. Greenfield, and H. Cedar. 2016. "DNA Methylation in Cancer and Aging." *Cancer Res* 76(12):3446–3450. doi: 10.1158/0008-5472.CAN-15-3278. Epub 2016 Jun 2. PMID: 27256564.

Kockott, D., B. Herzog, J. Reichrath, K. Keane, and M. F. Holick. 2016. "New approach to develop optimized sunscreens that enable cutaneous vitamin D formation with minimal erythema risk." *PLoS One* 11 (1):e0145509. doi: 10.1371/journal.pone.0145509.

Kyle, U. G., I. Bosaeus, A. D. De Lorenzo, P. Deurenberg, M. Elia, G. J. Manuel, H. B. Lilienthal, L. Kent-Smith, J. C. Melchior, M. Pirlich, H. Scharfetter, A. M. W. J. Schols, and C. Pichard C; ESPEN. 2004. "Bioelectrical impedance analysis-part II: utilization in clinical practice." *Clin Nutr* 23(6):1430–1453. doi: 10.1016/j.clnu.2004.09.012. PMID: 15556267.

Lampe, J.W. and S. Peterson. 2002. Brassica, biotransformation and cancer risk: genetic polymorphisms alter the preventive effects of cruciferous vegetables. *J Nutr* 132(10):2991–2994. doi: 10.1093/jn/131.10.2991. PMID: 12368383.

Lands, B. 2014. "Dietary omega-3 and omega-6 fatty acids compete in producing tissue compositions and tissue responses." *Mil Med* 179 (11 Suppl):76–81. doi: 10.7205/MILMED-D-14-00149.

Lanska, D. J. 2012. "The discovery of niacin, biotin, and pantothenic acid." *Ann Nutr Metab* 61 (3):246–253. doi: 10.1159/000343115.

Lawrence, M., S. Daujat, and R. Schneider. 2016. "Lateral thinking: how histone modifications regulate gene expression." *Trends Genet* 32 (1):42–56. doi: 10.1016/j.tig.2015.10.007.

Layman, D. K., T. G. Anthony, B. B. Rasmussen, S. H. Adams, C. J. Lynch, G. D. Brinkworth, and T. A. Davis. 2015. "Defining meal requirements for protein to optimize metabolic roles of amino acids." *Am J Clin Nutr* 101 (6):1330S–1338S. doi: 10.3945/ajcn.114.084053.

Lemon, P. W., M. A. Tarnopolsky, J. D. MacDougall, and S. A. Atkinson. 1992. "Protein requirements and muscle mass/strength changes during intensive training in novice bodybuilders." *J Appl Physiol (1985)* 73 (2):767–775. doi: 10.1152/jappl.1992.73.2.767.

Li, J. Y., L. N. Huang, H. L. Xue, Q. Q. Zhu, and C. H. Li. 2018. "Glutathione S-transferase mu-1, glutathione S-transferase theta-1 null genotypes, and oral cancer risk: a meta-analysis in the Chinese population." *J Cancer Res Ther* 14 (Suppl):S1052–S1056. doi: 10.4103/0973-1482.199786.

Li, S., F. Xue, Y. Zheng, P. Yang, S. Lin, Y. Deng, P. Xu, L. Zhou, Q. Hao, Z. Zhai, Y. Wu, Z. Dai, and S. Chen. 2019. "GSTM1 and GSTT1 null genotype increase the risk of hepatocellular carcinoma: evidence based on 46 studies." *Cancer Cell Int* 19:76. doi: 10.1186/s12935-019-0792-3.

Li, W., C. P. Yu, J. T. Xia, L. Zhang, G. X. Weng, H. Q. Zheng, Q. L. Kong, L. J. Hu, M. S. Zeng, Y. X. Zeng, M. Li, J. Li, and L. B. Song. 2009. "Sphingosine kinase 1 is associated with gastric cancer progression and poor survival of patients." *Clin Cancer Res* 15 (4):1393–1399. doi: 10.1158/1078-0432.CCR-08-1158.

Liew, S. C., and E. D. Gupta. 2015. "Methylenetetrahydrofolate reductase (MTHFR) C677T polymorphism: epidemiology, metabolism and the associated diseases." *Eur J Med Genet* 58 (1):1–10. doi: 10.1016/j.ejmg.2014.10.004.

Lippman, S. M., E. A. Klein, P. J. Goodman, M. S. Lucia, I. M. Thompson, L. G. Ford, H. L. Parnes, L. M. Minasian, J. M. Gaziano, J. A. Hartline, J. K. Parsons, J. D. Bearden, 3rd, E. D. Crawford, G. E. Goodman, J. Claudio, E. Winquist, E. D. Cook, D. D. Karp, P. Walther, M. M. Lieber, A. R. Kristal, A. K. Darke, K. B. Arnold, P. A. Ganz, R. M. Santella, D. Albanes, P. R. Taylor, J. L. Probstfield, T. J. Jagpal, J. J. Crowley, F. L. Meyskens, Jr., L. H. Baker, and C. A. Coltman, Jr. 2009. "Effect of selenium and vitamin E on risk of prostate cancer and other cancers: the Selenium and Vitamin E Cancer Prevention Trial (SELECT)." *JAMA* 301 (1):39–51. doi: 10.1001/jama.2008.864.

Livingstone, K. M., C. Celis-Morales, S. Navas-Carretero, R. San-Cristobal, A. L. Macready, R. Fallaize, H. Forster, C. Woolhead, C. B. O'Donovan, C. F. Marsaux, S. Kolossa, L. Tsirigoti, C. P. Lambrinou, G. Moschonis, M. Godlewska, A. Surwillo, C. A. Drevon, Y. Manios, I. Traczyk, E. R. Gibney, L. Brennan, M. C. Walsh, J. A. Lovegrove, W. H. Saris, H. Daniel, M. Gibney, J. A. Martinez, J. C. Mathers, and Study Food4Me. 2016. "Effect of an Internet-based, personalized nutrition randomized trial on dietary changes associated with the Mediterranean diet: the Food4Me study." *Am J Clin Nutr* 104 (2):288–297. doi: 10.3945/ajcn.115.129049.

Lonsdale, D. 2018. "Thiamin." *Adv Food Nutr Res* 83:1–56 doi: 10.1016/bs.afnr.2017.11.001.

Maegawa, S., Y. Lu, T. Tahara, J. T. Lee, J. Madzo, S. Liang, J. Jelinek, R. J. Colman, and J. J. Issa. 2017. "Caloric restriction delays age-related methylation drift." *Nat Commun* 8 (1):539. doi: 10.1038/s41467-017-00607-3.

Magnone, M., L. Emionite, L. Guida, T. Vigliarolo, L. Sturla, S. Spinelli, A. Buschiazzo, C. Marini, G. Sambuceti, A. De Flora, A. M. Orengo, V. Cossu, S. Ferrando, O. Barbieri, and E. Zocchi. 2020. "Insulin-independent stimulation of skeletal muscle glucose uptake by low-dose abscisic acid via AMPK activation." *Sci Rep* 10 (1):1454. doi: 10.1038/s41598-020-58206-0.

Mamerow, M. M., J. A. Mettler, K. L. English, S. L. Casperson, E. Arentson-Lantz, M. Sheffield-Moore, D. K. Layman, and D. Paddon-Jones. 2014. "Dietary protein distribution positively influences 24-h muscle protein synthesis in healthy adults." *J Nutr* 144 (6):876–880. doi: 10.3945/jn.113.185280.

Manson, J. E., N. R. Cook, I. M.Lee, W. Christen, S. S. Bassuk, S. Mora, H. Gibson, D. Gordon, T. Copeland, D. D'Agostino, G. Friedenberg, C. Ridge, V. Bubes, E. L. Giovannucci, W. C. Willett, and J. E. Buring; VITAL Research Group. 2019. "Vitamin D Supplements and Prevention of Cancer and Cardiovascular Disease." *N Engl J Med* 380(1):33–44. doi: 10.1056/NEJMoa1809944. Epub 2018 Nov 10. PMID: 30415629; PMCID: PMC6425757.

Martin, D. I., R. Ward, and C. M. Suter. 2005. "Germline epimutation: A basis for epigenetic disease in humans." *Ann N Y Acad Sci* 1054:68–77. doi: 10.1196/annals.1345.009. PMID: 16339653.

Martinez Steele, E., L. G. Baraldi, M. L. Louzada, J. C. Moubarac, D. Mozaffarian, and C. A. Monteiro. 2016. "Ultra-processed foods and added sugars in the US diet: evidence from a nationally representative cross-sectional study." *BMJ Open* 6 (3):e009892. doi: 10.1136/bmjopen-2015-009892.

Meredith, C. N., M. J. Zackin, W. R. Frontera, and W. J. Evans. 1989. "Dietary protein requirements and body protein metabolism in endurance-trained men." *J Appl Physiol (1985)* 66 (6):2850–2856. doi: 10.1152/jappl.1989.66.6.2850.

Michelotti, G. A., M. V. Machado, and A. M. Diehl. 2013. "NAFLD, NASH and liver cancer." *Nat Rev Gastroenterol Hepatol* 10 (11):656–665. doi: 10.1038/nrgastro.2013.183.

Millen, B. E., S. Abrams, L. Adams-Campbell, C. A. Anderson, J. T. Brenna, W. W. Campbell, S. Clinton, F. Hu, M. Nelson, M. L. Neuhouser, R. Perez-Escamilla, A. M. Siega-Riz, M. Story, and A. H. Lichtenstein. 2016. "The 2015 dietary guidelines advisory committee scientific report: development and major conclusions." *Adv Nutr* 7 (3):438–444. doi: 10.3945/an.116.012120.

Miller, E. R., 3rd, R. Pastor-Barriuso, D. Dalal, R. A. Riemersma, L. J. Appel, and E. Guallar. 2005. "Meta-analysis: high-dosage vitamin E supplementation may increase all-cause mortality." *Ann Intern Med* 142 (1):37–46. doi: 10.7326/0003-4819-142-1-200501040-00110.

Mock, D. M. 2017. "Biotin: from nutrition to therapeutics." *J Nutr* 147 (8):1487–1492. doi: 10.3945/jn.116.238956.

Moritz, L. E., and R. C. Trievel. 2018. "Structure, mechanism, and regulation of polycomb-repressive complex 2." *J Biol Chem* 293 (36):13805–13814. doi: 10.1074/jbc.R117.800367.

Murata, M. 2018. "Inflammation and cancer." *Environ Health Prev Med* 23 (1):50. doi: 10.1186/s12199-018-0740-1.

Myneni, V. D. and E. Mezey. 2017. "Regulation of bone remodeling by vitamin K2." *Oral Dis* 23(8):1021–1028. doi: 10.1111/odi.12624. Epub 2017 Apr 5. PMID: 27976475; PMCID: PMC5471136.

Nakagawa, K. 2013. "[Biological significance and metabolic activation of vitamin K]." *Yakugaku Zasshi* 133 (12):1337–1341. doi: 10.1248/yakushi.13-00228-1.

Nielsen, D. E., D. A. Carere, C. Wang, J. S. Roberts, R. C. Green, and P. Gen Study Group. 2017. "Diet and exercise changes following direct-to-consumer personal genomic testing." *BMC Med Genomics* 10 (1):24. doi: 10.1186/s12920-017-0258-1.

Niki, E., and M. G. Traber. 2012. "A history of vitamin E." *Ann Nutr Metab* 61 (3):207–212. doi: 10.1159/000343106.

Nowson, C., and S. O'Connell. 2015. "Protein requirements and recommendations for older people: a review." *Nutrients* 7 (8):6874–6899. doi: 10.3390/nu7085311.

Olsen, N. J., L. Angquist, S. C. Larsen, A. Linneberg, T. Skaaby, L. L. Husemoen, U. Toft, A. Tjonneland, J. Halkjaer, T. Hansen, O. Pedersen, K. Overvad, T. S. Ahluwalia, T. I. Sorensen, and B. L. Heitmann. 2016. "Interactions between genetic variants associated with adiposity traits and soft drinks in relation to longitudinal changes in body weight and waist circumference." *Am J Clin Nutr* 104 (3):816–826. doi: 10.3945/ajcn.115.122820.

Omenn, G. S., G. E. Goodman, M. D. Thornquist, J. Balmes, M. R. Cullen, A. Glass, J. P. Keogh, F. L. Meyskens, Jr., B. Valanis, J. H. Williams, Jr., S. Barnhart, M. G. Cherniack, C. A. Brodkin, and S. Hammar. 1996. "Risk factors for lung cancer and for intervention effects in CARET, the beta-carotene and retinol efficacy trial." *J Natl Cancer Inst* 88 (21):1550–1559. doi: 10.1093/jnci/88.21.1550.

Onitilo, A. A., R. V. Stankowski, R. L. Berg, J. M Engel, I. Glurich, G. M. Williams, and S. A. Doi. 2014. "Type 2 diabetes mellitus, glycemic control, and cancer risk." *Eur J Cancer Prev* 23(2):134–140. doi: 10.1097/CEJ.0b013e3283656394. PMID: 23962874.

Ordovas, J. M., L. R. Ferguson, E. S. Tai, and J. C. Mathers. 2018. "Personalised nutrition and health." *BMJ* 361:bmj.k2173. doi: 10.1136/bmj.k2173.

Pavlov, C. S., I. V. Damulin, Y. O. Shulpekova, and E. A. Andreev. 2019. "Neurological disorders in vitamin B12 deficiency." *Ter Arkh* 91 (4):122–129. doi: 10.26442/00403660.2019.04.000116.

Pérez, R. F., J. R. Tejedor, G. F.Bayón, A. F. Fernández, and M. F. Fraga. 2018. "Distinct chromatin signatures of DNA hypomethylation in aging and cancer." *Aging Cell* 17 (3):e12744. doi: 10.1111/acel.12744. Epub 2018 Mar 5. PMID: 29504244; PMCID: PMC5946083.

Piercy, K. L., R. P. Troiano, R. M. Ballard, S. A. Carlson, J. E. Fulton, D. A. Galuska, S. M. George, and R. D. Olson. 2018. "The physical activity guidelines for Americans." *JAMA* 320 (19):2020–2028. doi: 10.1001/jama.2018.14854.

Pinto, J. T., and J. Zempleni. 2016. "Riboflavin." *Adv Nutr* 7 (5):973–975. doi: 10.3945/an.116.012716.

Pludowski, P., M. F. Holick, W. B. Grant, J. Konstantynowicz, M. R. Mascarenhas, A. Haq, V. Povoroznyuk, N. Balatska, A. P. Barbosa, T. Karonova, E. Rudenka, W. Misiorowski, I. Zakharova, A. Rudenka, J. Lukaszkiewicz, E. Marcinowska-Suchowierska, N. Laszcz, P. Abramowicz, H. P. Bhattoa, and S. J. Wimalawansa. 2018. "Vitamin D supplementation guidelines." *J Steroid Biochem Mol Biol* 175:125–135 doi: 10.1016/j.jsbmb.2017.01.021.

Pogribny, I. P., S. J. James, and F. A. Beland. 2012. "Molecular alterations in hepatocarcinogenesis induced by dietary methyl deficiency." *Mol Nutr Food Res* 56 (1):116–125. doi: 10.1002/mnfr.201100524.

Polegato, B. F., A. G. Pereira, P. S. Azevedo, N. A. Costa, L. A. M. Zornoff, S. A. R. Paiva, and M. F. Minicucci. 2019. "Role of thiamin in health and disease." *Nutr Clin Pract* 34 (4):558–564. doi: 10.1002/ncp.10234.

Qato, D. M., J. Wilder, L. P. Schumm, V. Gillet, and G. C. Alexander. 2016. "Changes in prescription and over-the-counter medication and dietary supplement use among older adults in the United States, 2005 vs 2011." *JAMA Intern Med* 176 (4):473–482. doi: 10.1001/jamainternmed.2015.8581.

Qi, Q., A. Y. Chu, J. H. Kang, J. Huang, L. M. Rose, M. K. Jensen, L. Liang, G. C. Curhan, L. R. Pasquale, J. L. Wiggs, I. De Vivo, A. T. Chan, H. K. Choi, R. M. Tamimi, P. M. Ridker, D. J. Hunter, W. C. Willett, E. B. Rimm, D. I. Chasman, F. B. Hu, and L. Qi. 2014. "Fried food consumption, genetic risk, and body mass index: gene-diet interaction analysis in three US cohort studies." *BMJ* 348:g1610. doi: 10.1136/bmj.g1610.

Qi, Q., A. Y. Chu, J. H. Kang, M. K. Jensen, G. C. Curhan, L. R. Pasquale, P. M. Ridker, D. J. Hunter, W. C. Willett, E. B. Rimm, D. I. Chasman, F. B. Hu, and L. Qi. 2012. "Sugar-sweetened beverages and genetic risk of obesity." *N Engl J Med* 367 (15):1387–1396. doi: 10.1056/NEJMoa1203039.

Ramos-Lopez, O., F. I. Milagro, H. Allayee, A. Chmurzynska, M. S. Choi, R. Curi, R. De Caterina, L. R. Ferguson, L. Goni, J. X. Kang, M. Kohlmeier, A. Marti, L. A. Moreno, C. Perusse, C. Prasad, L. Qi, R. Reifen, J. I. Riezu-Boj, R. San-Cristobal, J. L. Santos, and J. A. Martinez. 2017. "Guide for current nutrigenetic, nutrigenomic, and nutriepigenetic approaches for precision nutrition involving the prevention and management of chronic diseases associated with obesity." *J Nutrigenet Nutrigenomics* 10 (1–2):43–62. doi: 10.1159/000477729.

Rivadeneira, A., P. Moyer, and J. D. Salciccioli. 2019. "Pellagra in the USA: unusual manifestations of a rare entity." *BMJ Case Rep* 12 (9):e230972. doi: 10.1136/bcr-2019-230972.

Robbins, D. C., L. Andersen, R. Bowsher, R. Chance, B. Dinesen, B. Frank, R. Gingerich, D. Goldstein, H. M. Widemeyer, S. Haffner, C. N. Hales, L. Jarett, K. Polonsky, D. Porte, J. Skyler, G. Webb, and K. Gallagher. 1996. "Report of the American Diabetes Association's Task Force on standardization of the insulin assay." *Diabetes* 45 (2):242–256. doi: 10.2337/diab.45.2.242.

Romano, G., D. Veneziano, M. Acunzo, and C. M. Croce. 2017. "Small non-coding RNA and cancer." *Carcinogenesis* 38 (5):485–491. doi: 10.1093/carcin/bgx026.

Ronis, M. J. J., K. B. Pedersen, and J. Watt. 2018. "Adverse effects of nutraceuticals and dietary supplements." *Annu Rev Pharmacol Toxicol* 58:583–601 doi: 10.1146/annurev-pharmtox-010617-052844.

Rose, D. P., M. Goldman, J. M. Connolly, and L. E. Strong. 1991. "High-fiber diet reduces serum estrogen concentrations in premenopausal women." *Am J Clin Nutr* 54 (3):520–525. doi: 10.1093/ajcn/54.3.520.

Rukh, G., E. Sonestedt, O. Melander, B. Hedblad, E. Wirfalt, U. Ericson, and M. Orho-Melander. 2013. "Genetic susceptibility to obesity and diet intakes: association and interaction analyses in the Malmo Diet and Cancer Study." *Genes Nutr* 8 (6):535–547. doi: 10.1007/s12263-013-0352-8.

Sailasree, R., K. R. Nalinakumari, P. Sebastian, and S. Kannan. 2011. "Influence of methylenetetrahydrofolate reductase polymorphisms in oral cancer patients." *J Oral Pathol Med* 40 (1):61–66. doi: 10.1111/j.1600-0714.2010.00943.x.

Saleem, F. and M. P. Soos. 2021. Biotin Deficiency. 2020 Apr 20. In: StatPearls [Internet]. Treasure Island (FL): StatPearls Publishing. PMID: 31613531.

Scaglione, F., and G. Panzavolta. 2014. "Folate, folic acid and 5-methyltetrahydrofolate are not the same thing." *Xenobiotica* 44 (5):480–488. doi: 10.3109/00498254.2013.845705.

Schulz, W. A. 2014. "Integrating epigenetics." *Biol Chem* 395 (11):1263–1264. doi: 10.1515/hsz-2014-0248. PMID: 25229415.

Schaafsma, G. 2005. "The protein digestibility-corrected amino acid score (PDCAAS)--a concept for describing protein quality in foods and food ingredients: a critical review." *J AOAC Int* 88 (3):988–994.

Shahangian, S., T. D. Alspach, J. R. Astles, A. Yesupriya, and W. K. Dettwyler. 2014. "Trends in laboratory test volumes for Medicare Part B reimbursements, 2000–2010." *Arch Pathol Lab Med* 138 (2):189–203. doi: 10.5858/arpa.2013-0149-OA.

Shearer, M. J., X. Fu, and S. L. Booth. 2012. "Vitamin K nutrition, metabolism, and requirements: current concepts and future research." *Adv Nutr* 3 (2):182–195. doi: 10.3945/an.111.001800.

Shimizu, K., M. Onishi, E. Sugata, Y. Sokuza, C. Mori, T. Nishikawa, K. Honoki, and T. Tsujiuchi. 2007. "Disturbance of DNA methylation patterns in the early phase of hepatocarcinogenesis induced by a choline-deficient L-amino acid-defined diet in rats." *Cancer Sci* 98 (9):1318–1322. doi: 10.1111/j.1349-7006.2007.00564.x.

Sieri, S., C. Agnoli, V. Pala, S. Grioni, F. Brighenti, N. Pellegrini, G. Masala, D. Palli, A. Mattiello, S. Panico, F. Ricceri, F. Fasanelli, G. Frasca, R. Tumino, and V. Krogh. 2017. "Dietary glycemic index, glycemic load, and cancer risk: results from the EPIC-Italy study." *Sci Rep* 7 (1):9757. doi: 10.1038/s41598-017-09498-2.

Snyder, N. W., G. Tombline, A. J. Worth, R. C. Parry, J. A. Silvers, K. P. Gillespie, S. S. Basu, J. Millen, D. S. Goldfarb, and I. A. Blair. 2015. "Production of stable isotope-labeled acyl-coenzyme A thioesters by yeast stable isotope labeling by essential nutrients in cell culture." *Anal Biochem* 474:59–65 doi: 10.1016/j.ab.2014.12.014.

Spector, A. A., and H. Y. Kim. 2015. "Discovery of essential fatty acids." *J Lipid Res* 56 (1):11–21. doi: 10.1194/jlr.R055095.

Stabler, S. P. 2013. "Clinical practice. Vitamin B12 deficiency." *N Engl J Med* 368 (2):149–160. doi: 10.1056/NEJMcp1113996.

Stifel, F. B., and R. H. Herman. 1972. "Is histidine an essential amino acid in man?" *Am J Clin Nutr* 25 (2):182–185. doi: 10.1093/ajcn/25.2.182.

Strandjord, S. E., B. Lands, and J. R. Hibbeln. 2018. "Validation of an equation predicting highly unsaturated fatty acid (HUFA) compositions of human blood fractions from dietary intakes of both HUFAs and their precursors." *Prostaglandins Leukot Essent Fatty Acids* 136:171–176 doi: 10.1016/j.plefa.2017.03.005.

Sun, S., X. Li, A. Ren, M. Du, H. Du, Y. Shu, L. Zhu, and W. Wang. 2016. "Choline and betaine consumption lowers cancer risk: a meta-analysis of epidemiologic studies." *Sci Rep* 6:35547. doi: 10.1038/srep35547.

Sundboll, J., S. K. Thygesen, K. Veres, D. Liao, J. Zhao, H. Gregersen, and H. T. Sorensen. 2019. "Risk of cancer in patients with constipation." *Clin Epidemiol* 11:299–310 doi: 10.2147/CLEP.S205957.

Supic, G., M. Jagodic, Z. Magic. 2013. "Epigenetics: a new link between nutrition and cancer." *Nutr Cancer* 65(6):781–792. doi: 10.1080/01635581.2013.805794. PMID: 23909721.

Theodoulou, F. L., O. C. Sibon, S. Jackowski, and I. Gout. 2014. "Coenzyme A and its derivatives: renaissance of a textbook classic." *Biochem Soc Trans* 42 (4):1025–1032. doi: 10.1042/BST20140176.

Thomas, E. L., J. R. Parkinson, G. S., Frost, A. P. Goldstone, C. J. Doré, J. P. McCarthy, A. L. Collins, J. A. Fitzpatrick, G. Durighel, S. D. Taylor-Robinson, and J. D. Bell. 2012. "The missing risk: MRI and MRS phenotyping of abdominal adiposity and ectopic fat." *Obesity (Silver Spring)* 20 (1):76–87. doi: 10.1038/oby.2011.142. Epub 2011 Jun 9. PMID: 21660078.

Thomas-Valdes, S., Mdgv Tostes, P. C. Anunciacao, B. P. da Silva, and H. M. P. Sant'Ana. 2017. "Association between vitamin deficiency and metabolic disorders related to obesity." *Crit Rev Food Sci Nutr* 57 (15):3332–3343. doi: 10.1080/10408398.2015.1117413.

Traylor, D. A., S. H. M. Gorissen, and S. M. Phillips. 2018. "Perspective: protein requirements and optimal intakes in aging: are we ready to recommend more than the recommended daily allowance?" *Adv Nutr* 9 (3):171–182. doi: 10.1093/advances/nmy003.

Tsujimoto, T., H. Kajio, and T. Sugiyama. 2017. "Association between hyperinsulinemia and increased risk of cancer death in nonobese and obese people: a population-based observational study." *Int J Cancer* 141 (1):102–111. doi: 10.1002/ijc.30729.

Turati, F., C. Galeone, L. S. A. Augustin, and C. La Vecchia. 2019. "Glycemic index, glycemic load and cancer risk: an updated meta-analysis." *Nutrients* 11 (10):2342. doi: 10.3390/nu11102342.

Ulatowski, L. M., and D. Manor. 2015. "Vitamin E and neurodegeneration." *Neurobiol Dis* 84:78–83. doi: 10.1016/j.nbd.2015.04.002.

Vernieri, C., F. Nichetti, A. Raimondi, S. Pusceddu, M. Platania, F. Berrino, and F. de Braud. 2018. "Diet and supplements in cancer prevention and treatment: Clinical evidences and future perspectives." *Crit Rev Oncol Hematol* 123:57–73. doi: 10.1016/j.critrevonc.2018.01.002.

Violi, F., G. Y. Lip, P. Pignatelli, and D. Pastori. 2016. "Interaction between dietary vitamin K intake and anticoagulation by vitamin K antagonists: is it really true?: a systematic review." *Medicine (Baltimore)* 95 (10):e2895. doi: 10.1097/MD.0000000000002895.

Viswanathan, M., K. A. Treiman, J. Kish-Doto, J. C. Middleton, E. J. Coker-Schwimmer, and W. K. Nicholson. 2017. "Folic acid supplementation for the prevention of neural tube defects: an updated evidence report and systematic review for the US Preventive Services Task Force." *JAMA* 317 (2):190–203. doi: 10.1001/jama.2016.19193.

Wang, D., and R. N. Dubois. 2010. "Eicosanoids and cancer." *Nat Rev Cancer* 10 (3):181–193. doi: 10.1038/nrc2809.

Wang, Z., S. Heshka, D. Gallagher, C. N. Boozer, D. P. Kotler, and S. B. Heymsfield. 2000. "Resting energy expenditure-fat-free mass relationship: new insights provided by body composition modeling." *Am J Physiol Endocrinol Metab* 279 (3):E539–E545. doi: 10.1152/ajpendo.2000.279.3.E539.

Wang, J., D. Wu, and A. Sun. 2019. "Effects of GST null genotypes on individual susceptibility to leukemia: a meta-analysis." *Exp Mol Pathol* 108:137–142. doi: 10.1016/j.yexmp.2019.01.004.

Waterland, R. A., and R. L. Jirtle. 2003. "Transposable elements: targets for early nutritional effects on epigenetic gene regulation." *Mol Cell Biol* 23 (15):5293–5300. doi: 10.1128/mcb.23.15.5293-5300.2003.

Wayler, A., E. Queiroz, N. S. Scrimshaw, F. H. Steinke, W. M. Rand, and V. R. Young. 1983. "Nitrogen balance studies in young men to assess the protein quality of an isolated soy protein in relation to meat proteins." *J Nutr* 113 (12):2485–2491. doi: 10.1093/jn/113.12.2485.

Wolff, G. L., R. L. Kodell, J. A. Kaput, and W. J. Visek. 1999. "Caloric restriction abolishes enhanced metabolic efficiency induced by ectopic agouti protein in yellow mice." *Proc Soc Exp Biol Med* 221(2):99–104. doi: 10.1046/j.1525-1373.1999.d01-61.x. PMID: 10352119.

Wolff, G. L., R. L. Kodell, S. R. Moore, and C. A. Cooney. 1998. "Maternal epigenetics and methyl supplements affect agouti gene expression in Avy/a mice." *FASEB J* 12(11):949–957. PMID: 9707167.

Xu, X., M. D. Gammon, S. H. Zeisel, Y. L. Lee, J. G. Wetmur, S. L. Teitelbaum, P. T. Bradshaw, A. I. Neugut, R. M. Santella, and J. Chen. 2008. "Choline metabolism and risk of breast cancer in a population-based study." *FASEB J* 22 (6):2045–2052. doi: 10.1096/fj.07-101279.

Yang, J., H. P. Wang, L. Zhou, and C. F. Xu. 2012. "Effect of dietary fiber on constipation: a meta analysis." *World J Gastroenterol* 18 (48):7378–7383. doi: 10.3748/wjg.v18.i48.7378.

Yates, A. A., S. A. Schlicker, and C. W. Suitor. 1998. "Dietary reference intakes: the new basis for recommendations for calcium and related nutrients, B vitamins, and choline." *J Am Diet Assoc* 98 (6):699–706. doi: 10.1016/S0002-8223(98)00160-6.

Ying, J., M. H. Rahbar, D. M. Hallman, L. M. Hernandez, M. R. Spitz, M. R. Forman, and O. Y. Gorlova. 2013. "Associations between dietary intake of choline and betaine and lung cancer risk." *PLoS One* 8 (2):e54561. doi: 10.1371/journal.pone.0054561.

Young, V. R., Y. S. Taylor, W. M. Rand, and N. S. Scrimshaw. 1973. "Protein requirements of man: efficiency of egg protein utilization at maintenance and submaintenance levels in young men." *J Nutr* 103 (8):1164–1174. doi: 10.1093/jn/103.8.1164.

Zeevi, D., T. Korem, N. Zmora, D. Israeli, D. Rothschild, A. Weinberger, O. Ben-Yacov, D. Lador, T. Avnit-Sagi, M. Lotan-Pompan, J. Suez, J. A. Mahdi, E. Matot, G. Malka, N. Kosower, M. Rein, G. Zilberman-Schapira, L. Dohnalova, M. Pevsner-Fischer, R. Bikovsky, Z. Halpern, E. Elinav, and E. Segal. 2015. "Personalized nutrition by prediction of glycemic responses." *Cell* 163 (5):1079–1094. doi: 10.1016/j.cell.2015.11.001.

Zeisel, S. 2017. "Choline, other methyl-donors and epigenetics." *Nutrients* 9 (5):445. doi: 10.3390/nu9050445.

Zeisel, S. H., and K. A. da Costa. 2009. "Choline: an essential nutrient for public health." *Nutr Rev* 67 (11):615–623. doi: 10.1111/j.1753-4887.2009.00246.x.

Zeisel, S. H., K. A. da Costa, C. D. Albright, and O. H. Shin. 1995. "Choline and hepatocarcinogenesis in the rat." *Adv Exp Med Biol* 375:65–74. doi: 10.1007/978-1-4899-0949-7_6.

Zeisel, S. H., K. C. Klatt, and M. A. Caudill. 2018. "Choline." *Adv Nutr* 9 (1):58–60. doi: 10.1093/advances/nmx004.

Zhang, N. Q., X. F. Mo, F. Y. Lin, X. X. Zhan, X. L. Feng, X. Zhang, H. Luo, and C. X. Zhang. 2020. "Intake of total cruciferous vegetable and its contents of glucosinolates and isothiocyanates, GST polymorphisms, and breast cancer risk: a case-control study in China." *Br J Nutr* 124:548–557. doi: 10.1017/S0007114520001348.

Zhang, L., D. Zhou, W. Guan, W. Ren, W. Sun, J. Shi, Q. Lin, J. Zhang, T. Qiao, Y. Ye, Y. Wu, Y. Zhang, X. Zuo, K. L. Connor, and G. Xu. 2017. "Pyridoxine 5'-phosphate oxidase is a novel therapeutic target and regulated by the TGF-beta signalling pathway in epithelial ovarian cancer." *Cell Death Dis* 8 (12):3214. doi: 10.1038/s41419-017-0050-3.

7 Epidemiology of Nutrition, Diet, and Cancer Risk

David Heber and Qing-Yi Lu
UCLA Center for Human Nutrition

Zuo-Feng Zhang
UCLA Fielding School of Public Health

CONTENTS

INTRODUCTION

The theory that nutrition might be involved in the causes and prevention of cancer goes back over 100 years when laboratory studies first demonstrated that changes in diet could affect tumor growth in animals. Epidemiology is the science that examines associations between factors including diet, nutrition, behaviors, and environmental factors that may be causal. Epidemiological plus experimental evidence can be employed to establish cause-and-effect relationship. Epidemiological observations integrated with knowledge from many disciplines including chemistry, animal studies, and clinical observations can provide new insights into nutrition and cancer risk. During the mid-twentieth century, the major focus of cancer epidemiology was on the role of tobacco and alcohol in cancer. It was not until the early 1960s, when studies were first conducted to examine the relationship between diet and cancer, especially gastric cancer. Following a widely recognized study from Doll and Peto published in 1981 on the causes of cancer deaths they identified using epidemiological associations (Peto et al. 1981), major research programs on nutrition and cancer were initiated and pursued by academic institutions. Research studies on tobacco and lung cancer went beyond epidemiology by combining a series of studies using human genetics, biology and biochemistry, and animal studies to enhance our understanding of the epidemiological associations which clearly indicated an association. Resistance from the tobacco industry to these findings took decades to overcome in the United States through government action and yet smoking remains a major cause of cancer globally.

In the last few decades, findings from extensive epidemiologic and experimental investigation have linked obesity and to varying extents the consumption of several foods and nutrients to the risk of common forms of cancer including colorectal, post-menopausal breast, ovarian, and pancreatic cancers. There is substantial evidence for the potential preventive effects of a diet rich in fruits and vegetables and this became a major area of research for many laboratories supported by the National Cancer Institute in the US. Attempts to study individual antioxidants such as beta-carotene and lycopene in blood samples associated with yellow, orange, and red fruit and vegetable intakes have yielded associations with skin cancer, prostate cancer, and breast cancer. Vitamin D, folate, calcium, and fiber have been studied in relation to colorectal cancer (CRC). Nutrients and foods may also interact, as a dietary pattern, to influence cancer risk. Diet likely influences carcinogenesis through several interacting mechanisms. These include the direct effects on immune responsiveness and inflammation, and the indirect effects of excess body fat in overweight and obese individuals on hormones that drive cancer development and progression. Evidence suggested that the gut microbiota may play an important role in the relationship between diet and cancer. Studies of cancer risk and prognosis, diet, and nutrients may provide guidance for the development of dietary modifications with the promise of reducing overall cancer burden and better prognosis. The evolution of the evidence that nutrition can impact carcinogenesis is a theme throughout this book, but this chapter will detail the contributions of epidemiology to the development of scientific insight into the impacts of diet and nutrition on cancer risk and prevention.

THE TOBACCO MODEL

The epidemiology of tobacco and lung cancer set the stage for the development of study designs and methods to study nutrition and cancer risk in populations around the world. In the early 1950s, a series of epidemiologic studies revealed a strong statistical association between lung cancer and smoking, particularly cigarettes (Doll and Hill 1950, Wynder and Graham 1985). Weaker associations were observed by additional studies between cigarette smoking and cancers of the oral cavity, larynx, and esophagus, which comprises the logical pathway for of cigarette smoke inhalation and the deposition of particulates. However, many other potential human carcinogens had been shown to generate tumors in a variety of laboratory animals (Wogan et al. 2004). In human cancers there is a 20- to 30-year lag time between the exposure to a carcinogen and the clinical diagnosis of a malignant tumor. This lag time cannot possibly be studied in animals effectively. A smoking machine was employed by Wynder and colleagues in order to mimic inhalation of tobacco smoke by humans and to collect the resultant tobacco tars, which were then placed onto the skins of mice at weekly intervals and observed skin papillomas after 8 months. In addition, 44% of the mice had histologically documented skin cancers. This study provided a working tool for the identification of carcinogenic agents in cigarette smoke (Bock, Moore, and Clark 1965). Among more than 8,000 chemical compounds inhaled during smoking, there were 81 carcinogens identified by International Agency for Research on Cancer (IARC) in tobacco smoke. There were various levels of certainty assigned to different carcinogens by this group depending on the level of evidence (Hecht 2003). This historical evolution of epidemiological data in combination with laboratory and animal studies paved the way for the studies of nutrients and chemicals in the multistep process of carcinogenesis (Smith et al. 2016).

Tobacco carcinogenic materials may directly interact with DNA and may be metabolized from procarcinogen to carcinogen by cellular enzymes that form covalent adducts with nucleotides in DNA (Conney 1982), causing DNA damage. Tobacco-specific nitrosamines can act directly on DNA nucleotides without further metabolism of carcinogens. These modified nucleotides are miscode or stall DNA replication, resulting in point mutations and chromosomal rearrangements or deletions, respectively, leading to mutations throughout the genome, including genes that encode proteins that maintain genetic stability (Wood, Mitchell, and Lindahl 2005, Wood and Doublie 2016). DNA damages if unrepaired can have impact on the efficiency of DNA repair or the fidelity of DNA synthesis. DNA damage as a consequence secondary to smoking cigarettes can lead to a "mutator phenotype" accounting for tens of thousands of mutations found in human lung cancer (Fox and Loeb 2010, Loeb 2011, Jiang and Xu 2019). Nicotine is the primary addictive substance in tobacco but it has not been shown to be carcinogenic. Nicotine can promote cell proliferation and cell division while also inhibiting apoptosis processes which could interact with the carcinogens in cigarette smoke to enhance mutagenesis (Murphy et al. 2011).

Polymorphisms in the genes of enzymes responsible for the metabolic activation (phase 1 enzymes) or detoxification (phase 2 enzymes) of chemical carcinogens may be responsible for some of the variations in the susceptibility of different human populations to cigarette-induced lung cancers (Park et al. 2005, Wang et al. 2010, Boldry et al. 2017). The development of new technology and the advancement of biochemical sciences enhanced the ability to quantify human exposure to cigarette smoke. A panel of tobacco carcinogens and related metabolites as well as toxicant metabolites such as hair and urinary cotinine level can be measured by ultrasensitive mass spectrometry (Chadwick and Keevil 2007, Yuan et al. 2017). Major factors in driving biological mechanistic studies on DNA repair and mutagenesis include identification of tobacco-related chemical carcinogens, their association with cancer risk, potential interactions with cellular metabolic processes, and the adducts formed in DNA. Most altered nucleotides in DNA are excised and the DNA sequence is restored prior to cell division by DNA repair system of human body. The Nobel Prize in Chemistry was awarded in 2015 to Drs. Lindahl, Sancar, and Modrich for their pioneering contributions, respectively, to the delineation of pathways for base excision repair, nucleotide excision repair, and mismatch repair. These DNA repair processes result in most tobacco-induced alterations in DNA nucleotides prior to cellular replication. DNA damage is measured by digestion of cellular DNA and detection of modified nucleotides by high-pressure liquid chromatography, mass spectrometry, and postlabeling (Loft et al. 2012, Villalta, Hochalter, and Hecht 2017). Changes in DNA repair enzymes have been proposed as a biomarker for smoking (Sevilya et al. 2014, Ma, Chen, and Petersen 2017). These methods can help epidemiologists determining the likelihood of developing lung cancer in smokers as well as the potential tobacco–gene interactions on the risk of lung cancer which is related to effectiveness of different approaches to genetic-based individualized chemoprevention including nutrition and dietary supplements.

This topic is current on a global basis where smoking remains the predominant cause of lung and 13 other smoking-related cancers. The prevalence of tobacco smoking has been decreasing in the United States and the developed world, however, increasing in the developing countries. It is estimated that there are 1.3 billion smokers worldwide (WHO, 2020) and more than 1 million people die of tobacco-induced lung cancer each year. This is a major worldwide epidemic that is entirely caused by human behavior. An equal number of smokers succumb to other smoking-related cancers, emphysema, cardiovascular diseases, and other tobacco-associated diseases each year. Recent data suggest that susceptibility to coronavirus infections including SARS COVID-19 is increased in smokers (Vardavas and Nikitara 2020). The success in reducing tobacco-associated diseases in the United States could be duplicated in many other countries that lack adequate resources to combat the powerful advertising launched by tobacco industries to addict new smokers.

BRADFORD HILL CRITERIA

The Bradford Hill criteria proposed in 1965 are the most widely cited framework for causal inference (Fedak et al. 2015) and include the following nine criteria to help determine if observed epidemiologic associations are causal: (1) strength of the Association—the larger an association between exposure and disease, the higher likelihood that the association is causal. The example given is that scrotal cancer in chimney sweeps was 200 times more frequent than in other occupations; (2) consistency—multiple epidemiologic studies using a variety of locations, populations, and methods should show a consistent association between exposure and disease with respect to the null hypothesis. A critical aspect is the replicate observed associations in independent studies, because causal relationship cannot be depended on a single study because of potential issues of internal validity;

(3) specificity—Hill also suggested that associations are more likely to be causal when they are specific, meaning the exposure causes only one disease. This is less directly relevant today when many forms of cancer are associated with multiple exposures and have commonalities even at the molecular level regardless of organ of origin. However, there are good examples that meet this criterion such as asbestos and mesothelioma as well as specific infectious agents associated with specific diseases; (4) temporality is a universally accepted criteria and states that for an exposure–disease relationship to be causal, exposure must precede the onset of disease. For exposures that affect epigenetics including DNA methylation and histone modification the same principle applies, since the effects of the exposures occur after prior exposure in specific periods of development in utero or even in previous generations, the effects occur in offspring; (5) biological gradient—if a dose–response is seen, it is more likely that the association is causal. This can be complex when there are threshold doses for an observed effect or other nonlinear dose–response relationships; (6) biological plausibility—the general concept of plausibility supports causal inference when there is a logical sequence that meets current understanding of biological mechanisms. In particular, molecular epidemiological advancements have enabled researchers to illuminate more intermediate steps in the cause–effect chain of events contributing to an improved understanding of biological plausibility for suggested causal relationships; (7) coherence—a coherent story among several avenues of study design support a causal connection and molecular epidemiology can been used to demonstrate a comprehensible story regarding various aspects of the cause-and-effect hypothesized; (8) experiment—epidemiologic studies in disease risk decline following an intervention or cessation of exposure may lead, if successful, to the strongest support for causal inference; (9) analogy—this criterion has been interpreted to mean that when one causal agent is known, the standards of evidence are lowered for a second causal agent with a similar structure or function. The Bradford Hill Criteria remain one of the most cited concepts in health research but do not represent a checklist to be completed (Phillips and Goodman 2004). However, they are still upheld as valid tools for aiding causal inference and remain an important way for researchers to compare and discuss epidemiological data. The way each criterion can be applied and interpreted in the setting of multidisciplinary data must be carefully measured against the varied and often novel types of data available in each unique situation to determine the strength of the causal inferences that can be made.

While the Bradford Hill criteria were developed in an earlier era of epidemiology when much of our current knowledge of cancer was not available, they still serve as a guidepost to remind us that association is not always causation. The incorporation of recent developments in nutritional "omics" technologies in studies of nutrition and cancer will largely be beneficial to nutritional epidemiology. "Omics" technologies include a collection of high-throughput methods for assessing a large number of genomic, epigenomic, transcriptomic, proteomic, metabolomic, and microbiomic traits from biological specimens including tissues and body fluids. The integration of these technologies into traditional nutritional epidemiology through a "systems epidemiology" approach (see Figure 7.1) can improve study designs and provide additional insights on biological mechanistic pathways, which will enhance the traditional nutritional epidemiologic approach. All of these areas require an interdisciplinary approach integrating emerging scientific knowledge on cancer risk and progression assessment and prediction.

Dietary intake in epidemiological studies and food item intakes are derived from self-report. With self-reporting questionnaires, the study participants may intentionally or unintentionally over-report or under-report a particular food item. Direct recording of all food intakes over several days often results in reactive effects such as participants simplifying their diets to reduce the burden of record-keeping. A commonly used tool in nutritional epidemiology is the food frequency questionnaire where participants are asked to complete the food questionnaires indicating how often they ate a particular food on a daily, weekly, or monthly basis, which may represent usual patterns of their dietary intake. In case–control studies, the exposure to dietary factors must occur prior to the diagnosis. Typically, the reference period used is a year prior to diagnosis. It is possible in case–control studies that 1 year may be insufficient and that dietary habits for the distant past prior to diagnosis might have affected initiation and progression of the disease but were difficult to be collected.

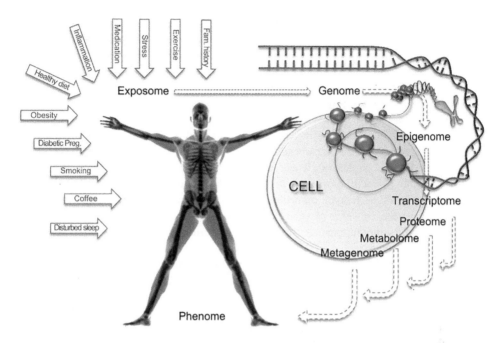

FIGURE 7.1 A future direction in nutritional epidemiologic research: a systems epidemiology approach to the discovery of interactions between the exposome (all nongenetic elements to which we are exposed) and the quantifiable elements of the human physiome [Reproduced with permission from Franks et al., 2013].

In case–control studies there can also be a difference in participation rates between cases and controls, which might be due to the fact that cases are more eager to participate in a study related to their diseases than participating population controls. Controls that agree to participate might have a healthier diet and lifestyle and therefore are more eager to participate in a case–control study asking about their lifestyle choices and dietary habits. It is notable that participation bias where healthier individuals participate in diet studies which can affect the associations under study. Another potential bias in nutritional epidemiology of cancer is misclassification bias; however, it is most likely that nondifferential misclassification leads to underestimate of the observed associations.

Large prospective cohort studies are valuable sources of information because dietary exposures occur prior to disease endpoint. However, these studies are limited by the difficulties in collecting and measuring dietary intake in free-living individuals and populations. Individual diets are made up of complex foods with many ingredients. Often foods also contain poorly characterized components that are consumed in varying amounts and combinations by different individuals. Diets, individual dietary habits, and food composition change over time make dietary assessment difficult. Most dietary assessment methods include errors due to day-to-day, diurnal, and seasonal variations over time. The omission of foods eaten either in the food frequency questionnaire (FFQ) or during dietary data collecting process is a common source of error.

Several widely accepted techniques are utilized to characterize dietary intake of nutrients, foods, and even dietary patterns despite their known limitations in large studies. Inherent shortcomings of a method are corrected with factors that are derived after comparing results from two different methods, such as food-frequency questionnaires and food records. However, errors in both methods used for measuring diet may be correlated, so that results from the reference method are not independent of those that are derived from the test method leading to an underestimate of the error in measurement. Nutritional biomarkers have been developed in order that more accurate factors for correction of dietary records can be realized, but these are limited in number and are not always useful. If an appropriate biomarker for a study can be identified such as blood lycopene levels, then the estimated nutrients such as lycopene level from dietary questionnaire or records will be compared with blood level of the biomarker so that some validation of results can be carried out.

Biomarker levels of a particular nutrient do not depend solely on dietary consumption since they can be affected by lifestyle, physiology, metabolism, and common genetic polymorphisms. In addition, plasma levels of micronutrients may not be ideal for cancer epidemiological studies, because they only represent current exposure levels and may not reflect past dietary pattern, if considering the long duration of latency for cancer development.

The cost of keeping diet records in large-scale epidemiologic studies may not be feasible. However, because dietary records can ascertain detailed dietary information accurately, they are useful in validation studies of other diet assessment instruments, and in monitoring compliance in clinical trials. In addition, diet record process may change an individual's diet, resulting in the data atypical of usual intake. However, estimated intakes of dietary items and nutrients from diet records have been found to correlate reasonably well with those from multiple 24-hours recalls (Hebert et al. 2014). Repeated 24-hours recalls involve a participant reporting all foods consumed in the previous 24 hours or calendar day to a trained interviewer in person or over the phone. Although reliance on the participant's memory leaves room for measurement error, a skilled interviewer can produce highly detailed and useful nutritional data comparable to a diet record (Julian-Almarcegui et al. 2016). This method has been widely used in nutritional intervention studies or clinical trials. It is also employed in national surveys to monitor trends in dietary and nutritional intake. In nutritional epidemiologic studies of cancer, FFQ is the most frequently used method in the measurement of dietary history, which is relatively simple in large-scale data collection and can acquire past dietary history and patterns.

In prognostic studies of nutritional oncology, we can use already collected dietary history from cancer patients of either cohort or case–control studies. Dietary collection instruments include food frequency questionnaire, food records, or 24-hour food recall if dietary data are not available from nutritional epidemiological studies. However, if existing dietary data are available, most likely they are collected by FFQ. The study design of prognostic studies is prospective, the study population are cancer patients, and the potential disease endpoints include recurrence, prognosis, metastasis, and deaths. The limitations of case–control studies discussed above such as selection bias and recall bias would be minimized in cancer prognostic studies because the study will not include controls and the dietary data are collected before the clinical endpoint. Additional advantage is that if adopting nutritional data from case–control or cohort studies, a variety of risk factors or potential confounding factors have already been collected and can be utilized in prognostic studies.

DIET AND CANCER

Although substantial studies in nutritional epidemiology have been conducted in recent years, the role of dietary factors in promoting or inhibiting cancers is largely unknown. Sufficient evidence has been discovered that the increased risk of liver cancer is associated with exposure to aflatoxin, a contaminant of foods produced by some fungi that grow on moldy nuts and grains. In many developing countries without widespread refrigeration this contaminant combines with hepatitis virus infection to promote liver cancer. The IARC has classified that naturally occurring aflatoxins are carcinogenic to humans (IARC 1993). Aflatoxin is the first group 1 carcinogen identified from foods classified by IARC. Increased ingestion of processed meat was found to be a convincing evidence for an increased risk of CRC, and high intake of red meat to probably increase the risk. IARC classified processed meat intake as group 1 and red meat intake as group 2A carcinogen (IARC 2015). World Cancer Research Fund (WCRF) and American Institute of Cancer Research (AICR) reported that increased intake of dietary fiber and whole grains probably decrease the risk of CRC (WCRF/AICR 2018).

CAROTENOIDS

A strong theme in the epidemiological study of nutrition and cancer risk concerns the effects of phytonutrients including beta-carotene and lycopene. In 1981, an epidemiological study reported that individuals who consumed a greater amount of green leafy and yellow vegetables exhibited a lower risk for cancer (Peto et al. 1981). Beta-carotene was suggested to be responsible for the anticancer effect observed. Later, that same year, a report of a 19-year longitudinal cohort study with 33 lung cancer patients concluded that smokers had a much greater incidence of lung cancer than nonsmokers and that the greatest incidence occurred in the quartile that reflected the lowest carotene intake but did not separate the effects of alpha- and beta-carotene (Shekelle et al. 1981). A large number of prospective and retrospective epidemiological studies of either the intake of foods rich in beta-carotene or high blood levels of beta-carotene reported a strong association with reduced risks of various kinds of cancers including lung, skin, colon, breast, and prostate (Shekelle et al. 1981, Vainio and Rautalahti 1998). For example, almost all of nine major case–control studies of lung cancer associated a lower risk for persons with a higher intake of carotenoids (Vainio and Rautalahti 1998). Furthermore, significant inverse associations of lung cancer with blood (plasma or serum) beta-carotene concentrations were found in seven prospective nested case–control studies (Vainio and Rautalahti 1998).

Based on consistent observed associations by epidemiological studies, consensus had been reached among scientists and National Institutes of Health (NIH) to conduct interventional studies using beta-carotene to prevent lung cancer. A randomized intervention trial using 2 by 2 factorial design was conducted to test whether alpha-tocopherol (50 mg/day), beta-carotene (20 mg/day) (ATBC) can be used as supplements for Lung Cancer Prevention. The study was a double-blind and placebo-controlled; total and disease-specific mortality and incidence of various diseases and symptoms were monitored for safety (Julian-Almarcegui et al. 2016). A total of 29,133 male smokers aged between 50 and 69 years old were recruited from 1985 to 1993 and randomized into four arms: with placebo capsules, with beta-carotene only, with alpha-tocopherol only, and with both beta-carotene and alpha-tocopherol. All participants were followed-up for maximum 8 years with a median of 6.1 years and 169,751 person-years. A total of 876 lung cancer patients were newly diagnosed during the study. Individuals receiving alpha-tocopherol were not associated with reduced risk of lung cancer. It was unexpected that a higher incidence of lung cancer was observed among men who were in beta-carotene group compared with these in placebo group. No clear interaction was observed between alpha-tocopherol and beta-carotene on risk of lung cancer. Men who received alpha-tocopherol had fewer prostate cancer diagnoses than among those who did not. Beta-carotene appeared to have no effect on the incidence of other cancer sites. Alpha-tocopherol had no clear effect on total mortality, although more deaths from hemorrhagic stroke. Beta-carotene was associated with 8% increase total mortality, primarily because more deaths from lung cancer and ischemic heart disease were in beta-carotene group. This trial highlighted the difficulty in taking even a supported scientific hypothesis into a clinical trial. In this case, the single-dose level of beta-carotene used was supraphysiological. Smoking was known to alter beta-carotene plasma levels and subsequent studies in a model using smoking ferrets where it was demonstrated that lung cell metaplasia occurred with a dose of beta-carotene similar to what was used in the ATBC trial adjusted for body weight (Liu et al. 2000). Interestingly, when a lower dose that would be obtained from a recommended intake of fruits and vegetables at 6 mg was administered alone or with smoking. There was no increase of lung metaplasia observed. Extensive epidemiological data formed the basis for the enthusiasm that beta-carotene would act as an anti-cancer agent in lung cancer. However, the study of the molecular mechanisms affecting beta-carotene has demonstrated pro-oxidant activities in microenvironments affected by smoking (Black et al. 2020). Whereas a diet rich in carotenoid-containing fruits and vegetables may be beneficial in the fight against some diseases, there are potential risks when supraphysiological doses of beta-carotene are supplemented. According to 2018 WCRF/AICR report, high-dose beta-carotene supplements are associated with lung cancer risk with convincing evidence (WCRF/AICR, 2018). It has been suggested that tobacco smokers should avoid beta-carotene supplement.

Lycopene, a carotenoid with multiple bioactivities, is found abundantly in tomato, tomato-based products, pink grapefruit, and watermelon. An early study of aggressive prostate cancer found that lycopene-rich foods such as tomato and tomato-based products evidenced by dietary intake analysis and increased blood levels of lycopene reduced prostate cancer risk (Giovannucci et al. 2002). In a meta-analysis of studies published up to 2003 (Etminan, Takkouche, and Caamano-Isorna 2004), high intakes of tomato or tomato-based products were associated with a 10% to 20% reduction in prostate cancer risk, and high serum or plasma concentrations of lycopene were associated with a 25% reduced risk. Among more recent studies of lycopene and prostate cancer, some support an inverse association, whereas others present null findings. The heterogeneity of less aggressive and more aggressive prostate cancers diagnosed in the Prostate Specific Antigen (PSA) era may contribute to this inconsistency (Giovannucci 2007).

As more studies were done, it became apparent that the inverse association between lycopene intake and prostate cancer risk was weak for endpoints enriched with indolent cancers such as those identified through PSA screening rather than palpation, and was stronger for lethal prostate cancer than for total prostate cancer. This overall pattern suggests that lycopene may be primarily influencing progression of prostate cancers.

Studies conducted in the United States before the widespread use of PSA screening (Ilic, Forbes, and Hassed 2011) or in other areas where the PSA screening is not prevalent (Key et al. 2007, Huang et al. 2003) generally support a positive role of lycopene in prostate cancer prevention. In settings where incident cases were primarily diagnosed through PSA screening, the studies generally yielded null findings (Mills et al. 1989, Key et al. 1997). Further, in the observational study component of the Prostate Cancer Prevention Trial (Kirsh et al. 2006, Pourmand et al. 2007), a reanalysis showed no association between lycopene level and cancers that had shown no evidence of progression but were detected by an end-of-study biopsy. Interestingly, lycopene was associated with cancers that showed signs of progression during the study through symptoms, growth, or rise in PSA (Giovannucci 2011). In 2018, the WCRF/AICR did not perform an expert review on lycopene given the weak nature of the evidence of a direct association with cancer in recent studies (WCRF/AICR 2018).

OBESITY

Obesity is clearly associated globally with common forms of cancer. For example, it has been estimated that 11.9% of cancers in men and 13.1% of cancers in women could be due to obesity. Many studies have associated excess body fat with an increased risk for cancer. More than 13 anatomic sites of cancer are associated with obesity, including endometrial, esophageal, renal, and pancreatic adenocarcinomas; hepatocellular carcinoma (HCC); gastric cancer; meningioma; multiple myeloma; colorectal, postmenopausal breast, ovarian, gallbladder, and thyroid cancers (Avgerinos et al. 2019). Obesity was found to be a risk factor for several malignancies in epidemiologic investigations carried out in the 1990s as the obesity epidemic in the United States was recognized.

Obesity has taken its place alongside other well-established cancer risk factors such as genetic predisposition, ionizing radiation, tobacco use, infections, unhealthy diet, alcohol consumption, sedentary lifestyle, and environmental toxin exposures. As obesity and metabolic syndrome increase with aging population around the world, common forms of cancer are also expected to increase. Tobacco cessation and weight management may represent the two most important lifestyle changes impacting the burden of postmenopausal breast cancer and CRC, which represent two of the most frequent malignancies at a global level. Obesity could soon surpass smoking and infections as a significant preventable cause of cancer (Ligibel et al. 2014).

Visceral fat is associated with insulin resistance (IR) in overweight and obese individuals. IR contributes to the development of Metabolic Syndrome, a collection of risk factors (high blood sugar, high blood pressure, and dyslipidemia) that has been associated with an increased risk of cancer (Uzunlulu, Telci Caklili, and Oguz 2016). IR associated with visceral fat also stresses the pancreas over time and in many individuals leads to the development of type 2 diabetes mellitus (T2DM) which itself is associated with an increased risk of cancer (Tsilidis et al. 2015). The visceral adipose tissue is an endocrine organ that produces free fatty acids, interleukin-6, monocyte chemoattractant protein, plasminogen activator inhibitor 1 (PAI-1), adiponectin, leptin, and tumor necrosis factor α. These molecules increase cancer cell proliferation and decrease antitumor immunity (Barchetta et al. 2019).

The epidemiological literature suggests that IR, hyperinsulinemia, and increased levels of insulin-like growth factors place patients with T2DM at greater risk of cancer. The American Diabetes Association and American Cancer Society reported an approximately two-fold increased risk of cancers of the liver, pancreas, and endometrium and a 1.2- to 1.5-fold increased risk of cancers of the colon and rectum, breast, and bladder in patients with T2DM (Giovannucci et al. 2010). Several observational studies found that newly diagnosed cancer patients have a higher prevalence of diabetes (Ballotari et al. 2017, Liu et al. 2015, Huang et al. 2020), and a bidirectional association between these diseases has been suggested (Satija et al. 2015).

The WCRF/AICR third expert report in 2018 suggested strong evidence that body fatness and weight gain increased the risk of cancer. Convincing evidence based on epidemiological studies was observed between adult fatness and increased risk of cancers of the esophagus (adenocarcinoma), pancreas, liver, colorectum, breast (postmenopause), endometrium, and kidney as well as between adult weight gain and postmenopausal breast cancer (WCRF/AICR 2018).

VITAMIN D

The first observations relating vitamin D to cancer by Apperly in 1941 demonstrated an inverse correlation between sunlight exposure and overall cancer incidence and mortality in North America (Kricker and Armstrong 2006). By the 1980s, the first epidemiological studies linking low sunlight exposure and high risk of colon and prostate cancers were reported suggesting vitamin D as the hormonal factor reducing colon cancer risk (Garland and Garland 1980). Similar observations followed for prostate cancer (Hanchette and Schwartz 1992). Since then, many epidemiological studies have supported and extended the ultraviolet-B–vitamin D–cancer hypothesis in 18 different types of cancers (Grant and Mohr 2009). The evidence has been further supported by studies showing the direct association between vitamin D intake and cancer risk. Several lines of population-based studies revealed an inverse correlation between serum 25-hydroxyvitamin D (25(OH)D) levels and high risk of colon (Garland et al. 2009), breast (Abbas et al. 2013), prostate (Tretli et al. 2009, Mondul et al. 2017), gastric, and other cancers.

25(OH)D which is measured to estimate vitamin D status is actually a prehormone which is converted to 1,25 dihydroxyvitamin D or calcitriol in the kidney. Calcitriol has cellular actions throughout the body using the same mechanism to induce gene expression in the nucleus as steroid hormones binding first to a cytoplasmic vitamin D receptor protein which has a nuclear binding site that activates gene transcription. Calcitriol influences numerous cellular pathways that could have a role in determining cancer risk and prognosis. Epidemiological and early clinical trials are inconsistent. While most studies are based on blood levels of 25(OH) D, further metabolism of 25(OH)D in target tissues is mediated by two key enzymes: 1α-hydroxylase (CYP27B1), which catalyzes the synthesis of calcitriol from 25(OH)D or 24-hydroxylase (CYP24) which leads to inactive 24,25 dihydroxyvitamin D. Therefore, the conversion of calcitriol into less active compounds can complicate associations of blood levels of 25(OH)D and cancer (Swami, Krishnan, and Feldman 2011). A number of preclinical and clinical studies strongly suggested that vitamin D deficiency would increase the risk of developing cancer and that avoiding deficiency and adding vitamin D supplements might be a safe way to reduce cancer incidence and improve cancer prognosis and outcome. Unfortunately, the single large randomized trial of vitamin D supplementation in which vitamin D3 (cholecalciferol) at a dose of 2,000 IU/day and marine n-3 (also called omega-3) fatty acids at a dose of 1 g/day were administered to 25,871 participants for the prevention of cancer and cardiovascular disease among men 50 years of age or older and women 55 years of age or older in the United States failed to demonstrate a reduced incidence of invasive cancer over a median follow-up of 5.3 years (Manson et al. 2019). Nonetheless, there was no toxicity noted in this large trial and some experts still suggest that suboptimal levels of 25(OH)D are extremely common and deserve assessment and supplementation with a view to reducing cancer risk (Holick 2017).

Based on epidemiologic studies of dietary intake, supplements, and plasma or serum levels of vitamin D, the 2018 WCRF/AICR expert review stated that vitamin D is associated with suggested decreased risk of CRC with limited evidence (WCRF/AICR 2018).

CALCIUM

A nutritional calcium deficit combined with a compromised vitamin D status (reviewed above) is a risk factor for multiple chronic diseases, including various types of malignancy. While these two factors often coexist, there is evidence that poor calcium nutrition is a significant risk factor for total cancer incidence. The associations between intake of dairy food and calcium intakes and total cancer as well as cancer at individual sites were examined in the NIH-AARP (American Association of Retired Persons) Diet and Health Study (Park et al. 2009). Intakes of dairy food and calcium from foods and supplements were assessed with a FFQ. Over 7 years of follow-up, 36,965 incident cancer cases in men and 16,605 in women were identified through state cancer registries. Calcium intake was not associated with total cancer in men but was nonlinearly associated with total cancer in women. The risk decreased up to 1,300 mg/day dairy food and calcium intakes were found to be inversely associated with cancers of the digestive system in both men and women (multivariate relative risk for the highest quintile of total calcium vs the lowest, 0.84; 95% CI, 0.77–0.92 in men, and 0.77; 95% CI, 0.69–0.91 in women). Decreased risk was particularly pronounced for CRC. Intake of calcium supplemental was also inversely associated with CRC risk.

Increases in dietary calcium have been shown to inhibit large-bowel carcinogenesis in animal models (Pence et al. 1995), and several epidemiologic studies have shown lower risks of CRC and adenomas in association with higher calcium intake (Song, Garrett, and Chan 2015). Trials of calcium supplementation for adenoma prevention have shown reduced risks (Gao et al. 2018). Moreover, calcium and vitamin D may have synergistic chemopreventive effects against colorectal neoplasia (Barbachano et al. 2017). Low calcium intake has been associated with varying degrees with the development of gastric, pancreatic, ovarian, endometrial, lung, and prostate cancer, as well as multiple myeloma (Rahmati et al. 2018).

A large randomized, multicenter, double-blind, placebo-controlled trial at 11 academic medical centers and associated medical practices in the United States conducted between July 2004 through July 2008 enrolled patients 45–75 years of age who were in good general health, did not have familial CRC syndromes or serious intestinal disease, had at least one colorectal adenoma removed within 4 months before enrollment, had no remaining polyps after a complete colonoscopy, and were expected to have a 3- or 5-year colonoscopic follow-up examination. There was a mean net increase in serum 25-hydroxyvitamin D levels of 7.83 ng/mL, relative to control group with placebo. During follow-up, 43% of participants had one or more adenomas diagnosed. The adjusted risk ratios for recurrent adenomas were 0.99 (95% confidence interval [CI], 0.89–1.09) when vitamin D group compared with no vitamin D group; 0.95 (95% CI, 0.85–1.06) with calcium versus no calcium, and 0.93 (95% CI, 0.80–1.08) with both agents versus neither agent. Similar findings were observed for advanced adenomas. There were few serious adverse events. This large intervention trial failed to show a reduction in the risk of recurrent colorectal adenomas over a period of 3–5 years with calcium and vitamin D supplementation (Baron, Barry et al. 2015).

Once again, a simple randomized controlled trial in large numbers of subjects did not show a positive result. This is not surprising given what we know of the molecular heterogeneity of colon polyps and the influence of diet on the microbiota which can influence carcinogenesis locally in the colon (O'Keefe 2016, Garrett 2019, Flemer et al. 2017). The risk of CRC is increased by processed and red meat consumption but suppressed by fiber. Food composition affects colonic health and cancer risk through the change in microbial metabolism in the colon. The gut microbiota ferment complex dietary carbohydrates that are resistant to digestion by intestinal enzymes. While providing energy to support the microbiota, this process also results in the release of short-chain fatty acids including butyrate, which can be utilized for the metabolic needs of the colon and the body.

Butyrate has antineoplastic properties and is a preferred energy source for colonocytes. Butyrate promotes colonic health by maintaining mucosal integrity and suppressing inflammation and carcinogenesis through effects on immunity, gene expression, and epigenetic modulation. Protein residues and fat-stimulated bile acids are also metabolized by the microbiota to inflammatory and/or carcinogenic metabolites, which increase the risk of cancer. Tumor genetics has also been increasingly used in choosing targeted therapies and in the prediction of drug response, but there are still few validated biomarkers of CRC. The discovery of noninvasive, sensitive, and specific biomarkers is an urgent need, and translational proteomics play a key role in this process, as these markers may enable better comprehension of colorectal carcinogenesis, identification of potential markers, and subsequent validation of observations in nutritional intervention trials (Alves Martins et al. 2019). Strong evidence was suggested that calcium supplement is a probable protective factor for CRC risk (WCRF/AICR 2018).

FIBER

Plant foods containing fiber have long been thought to protect against cancer. Most prominent among the hypotheses is hat fruit and vegetables or their components may protect against cancer. Fiber, which is found in high amounts in fruit, vegetables, and whole grains, is also hypothesized to protect against some cancers. On the basis of case–control studies, the 1997 report from the WCRF/AICR concluded that there was convincing evidence that fruit and vegetables decreased the risk of cancers of the mouth and pharynx, esophagus, stomach, and lung (Glade 1999).

In the second report published in 2007, the judgment for fruit and vegetables was downgraded: there were no cancer sites for which the evidence of a protective effect of fruit and vegetables was deemed to be convincing (Demeyer, Honikel, and De Smet 2008). The downgrade was mainly due to the inclusion of results from cohort studies that became available after the first report. For fiber, in the 1997 report there were no cancer sites for which the evidence of a protective effect of fiber was judged to be convincing or probable; in the 2007 report foods containing dietary fiber were judged to probably decrease the risk of CRC (Demeyer, Honikel, and De Smet 2008). A 20% decrease in cancer-specific mortality in participants with the highest adherence to the 2007 WCRF/AICR cancer prevention recommendations compared with those with the lowest adherence was demonstrated in the European Prospective Investigation into Nutrition and Cancer (EPIC) cohort (Jankovic et al. 2017) (Shams-White et al. 2019).

The EPIC study, designed to investigate the relations between diet, lifestyle, and environmental factors and the incidence of different cancers, is one such cohort that has investigated fruit, vegetable, and fiber consumption in relation to cancer risk. The study recruited half a million participants, and over 60,000 incident cases of cancer have been identified. One of the major strengths of EPIC is the inclusion of study centers in ten European countries, giving substantial variation in dietary intakes within the cohort (Ferrari et al. 2004). Many articles from EPIC in this research area have been published since the 2007 WCRF/AICR report.

The associations between fruit, vegetable, or fiber consumption and the risk of cancer at 14 different sites have been reported (Bradbury, Appleby, and Key 2014). The risks of cancers of the upper gastrointestinal tract were inversely associated with fruit intake but not associated with vegetable intake. The risk of CRC was inversely associated with intakes of total fruit and vegetables and total fiber, and the risk of liver cancer was also inversely associated with the intake of total fiber. The risk of cancer of the lung was inversely associated with fruit intake but was not associated with vegetable intake; this association with fruit intake was restricted to smokers and might be influenced by residual confounding due to smoking. There was a borderline inverse association of fiber intake with breast cancer risk. For the other nine cancer sites studied (stomach, biliary tract, pancreas, cervix, endometrium, prostate, kidney, bladder, and lymphoma) there were no reported significant associations of risk with intakes of total fruit, vegetables, or fiber. Since the composition of plant foods in the marketplace varies widely in terms of fiber and phytonutrient content, work on biomarkers of fruit and vegetable intake such as carotenoids and polyphenol metabolites already discussed in this chapter may help to further inform these associations.

It is also difficult to separate the impact of fruit and vegetables as part of a plant-based dietary pattern along with the impacts of physical activity on energy expenditure and obesity which are known to impact cancer risk. In a separate study of participants in the EPIC study from ten countries found that baseline fruit and vegetable intakes were not associated with weight change overall. However, baseline fruit and vegetable intakes were inversely associated with weight change in men and women who quit smoking during follow-up. Also weak positive associations between vegetable intake and weight change were found in women who were overweight, were former smokers, or had high prudent dietary pattern scores and weak inverse associations between fruit intake and weight change were noted in women who were >50 years of age, were of normal weight, were never smokers, or had low prudent dietary pattern scores (Vergnaud et al. 2012).

The International Head and Neck Cancer Epidemiology consortium was established in 2004 to elucidate the etiology of Head and Neck Cancers (HNCs) through pooled analyses of individual-level data on HNCs on a large scale. To date, it includes 35 case–control studies, for a total of 25,478 cases and 37,111 controls. An inverse association with HNC risk was found for higher intakes of fruit and vegetables, while no association was observed for some cereal and grain products. In addition, higher intakes of selected micronutrients and food components from natural sources, such as vitamin E, vitamin C, folate, and carotenoids, have been previously found to reduce HNCs risk. Fiber intake was also inversely associated with oral and pharyngeal cancer risks combined and with laryngeal cancer. Inverse associations were consistently observed for the subsites of oral and pharyngeal cancers. These findings from a multicenter large-scale pooled analysis suggest that a greater intake of fiber may lower HNC risk (Kawakita et al. 2017).

In a systematic review of 20 studies examining whole grains and cancer, 6 studies reported a statistically significant 6%–47% reduction in risk, but 14 studies showed no association. In a review of 29 studies examining cereal fiber intake in relation to cancer, 8 showed a statistically significant 6%–49% reduction in risk, whereas 21 studies reported no association (Makarem et al. 2016). Therefore, while whole grains and cereal fiber may protect against gastrointestinal cancers, the studies to date require further confirmation.

The 2017 WCRF/AICR report concluded that there is strong evidence that wholegrain and foods containing dietary fiber probably decrease the risk of CRC. In a dose–response meta-analysis with six studies published in 2017 (page 40), a statistic significant of 17% decrease in the risk CRC with 90 g increase in wholegrains intake per day (RR 0.83 (95% CI = 0.78–0.89), n = 8,320 cases) was observed.

A cohort study of 125,455 participants in the United States, which included 141 patients with HCC and had an average follow-up of 24.2 years, reported that increased intake of whole grains was associated with a reduced risk of HCC. A nonsignificant inverse HCC association was observed for total bran but not for germ; increased intake of cereal fiber but not fruit or vegetable fiber was associated with a nonsignificant lower risk of HCC (Yang et al. 2019).

Endometrial cancer is the most common gynecologic cancer especially in economically developed countries (Torre et al. 2016). Long-lasting unopposed estrogen exposure increases the chance of development of endometrial cancer, and since dietary fiber is involved in absorption and reabsorption of sterols, this was chosen as a potentially fruitful area of investigation. Fiber is known to influence the metabolism of estrogens (Bagga et al. 1995). Therefore, it is biologically plausible to hypothesize an inverse association of dietary fiber intake with the risk of endometrial cancer (Chen et al. 2018). Dietary fiber has been proposed to decrease the risk of multiple cancers, such as CRC, breast cancer, and pancreatic cancer. Several biological mechanisms have been proposed to support the effects of dietary fiber in reducing cancer risk, including decreasing cholesterol levels in plasma, decreasing postprandial blood sugar, and enhancing bacterial fermentation of fiber to short-chain fatty acids. Higher dietary fiber intake also reduces body fatness as reflected either by body mass index, weight, or waist circumference, hip circumference, and waist-to-hip ratio (Aune et al. 2015).

In 2018, the WCRF/AICR issued revised recommendations for cancer prevention. The relation between adherence to these recommendations and the risk of total cancer were examined in two large population-based Swedish prospective cohorts (Kaluza et al. 2020). During some 15 years of follow-up, 12,693 incident cancers occurred among some 50,000 subjects in the cohort. The Standardized-WCRF/AICR 2018 Score for dietary habits was used to assess the association of these habits and cancer. Both the overall score and the increases noted in the score as a result of adherence to these dietary recommendations were associated with a decreased risk of cancer. It was noted that 90% of the participants did not meet the WCRF/AICR guidelines regarding consumption of plant foods, limited consumption of red/processed meat, and fast foods or similar processed foods. Not surprisingly given the global epidemic of obesity, less than half of participants met acceptable weight and physical activity recommendations. Therefore, the factors promoting obesity and overweight in the study subjects may have compromised the ability to separately analyze recommendations on plant foods and fiber which interact.

CRUCIFEROUS VEGGIES

A number of studies investigating the association of vegetable consumption with the risk of breast cancer found that cruciferous vegetables consumption was associated with a reduced risk of breast cancer. Further research attributed this association to the phytonutrients sulforaphane and indole-3-carbinol. Sulforaphane is an isothiocyanate precursor found in cruciferous vegetables with multiple molecular targets relevant to cancer. These include various anti-inflammatory, antioxidant, and anti-cancer cellular targets. Several studies have demonstrated that sulforaphane acts on modulating and/or regulating the cell cycle

through induction of cell cycle arrest, activation of programmed cell death, and disruption of signaling within the tumor microenvironment (Atwell et al. 2015).

A meta-analysis of 13 epidemiologic studies concluded based on evidence from 11 case–control and 2 cohort studies that increased consumption of cruciferous vegetables was significantly associated with reduction in breast cancer risk (Liu and Lv 2013). In a study conducted on Chinese women involving 1,485 cases and 1,506 controls, intake of cruciferous vegetables reduced the breast cancer risk by almost 50%.

In another case–control study in 1,491 patients with breast cancer and 1,482 controls, increased cruciferous vegetable intake was associated with a 32% reduction in breast cancer risk. A meta-analysis, comprises studies conducted over 18 years in Europe including a total of 3,034 breast cancer patients and 11,492 controls, demonstrated a reduced risk of breast cancer as a result of consumption of cruciferous vegetables (Bosetti et al. 2012). In a case–control study involving 740 Caucasian women with breast cancer and 810 controls, inverse associations were found between consumption of cruciferous vegetables and breast cancer risk, predominantly among premenopausal women (Ambrosone et al. 2004).

The association between cruciferous vegetable consumption and CRC development was demonstrated among Japanese adults aged between 45 and 74 years in the Japan Public Health Center-based Prospective Study (Mori et al. 2019). Over 1,325,853 person-years of follow-up, 2,612 cases were identified. No significant associations were observed in this study between the highest cruciferous vegetable intake quartile (compared with the lowest) CRC risk in men and women. There was a trend in women that had a P value of 0.08 between cruciferous vegetable intake and the risk of colon cancer after excluding participants who developed colon cancer in the first 3 years of follow-up, but a positive association was found with proximal colon cancer in men.

Twenty-four case–control and 11 prospective studies were included in an analysis of the association of cruciferous vegetable intake and CRC (Wu et al. 2013). When all the studies were combined in the association study, a statistically significant inverse association between cruciferous vegetable intake and CRC risk was noted. Specific subanalysis for consumption of cabbage and broccoli yielded similar results. When separately analyzed, case–control studies of cruciferous vegetable intake yielded similar results. The results from prospective studies that were analyzed showed borderline statistical significance. Moreover, significant inverse associations were noted for colon cancer and distal CRC both among prospective and case–control studies. The distal location could be consistent with greater exposure to carcinogens and a greater defense reaction against them.

The chemoprevention benefit of cruciferous diet is largely attributed to sulforaphane and indole-3-carbinol, and both dietary supplements and sulforaphane-enriched broccoli have been developed (Zhang et al. 2018). Cruciferous vegetables contain high concentrations of glucosinolates that must be hydrolyzed by the intestinal microflora to release the active isothiocyanates (Zhang et al. 2018). Since enzymatic activation by myrosinase of sulforaphane is required, simple dehydration of broccoli and encapsulation as well as heating of broccoli in processing can eliminate any benefit unless myrosinase is included and activated in the supplement after digestion. Eating broccoli and other cruciferous vegetables activates myrosinase during chewing and digestion and isothiocyanate can be detected in urine samples.

FOLATE

The association of folate and cancer risk has been studied extensively due to its role in methylation and nucleotide synthesis. Folate is a key source of the one carbon group in the process of DNA methylation, which belongs to epigenetic modification pathways critical to normal genomic regulation and development. Normal mammalian development is dependent on DNA methylation, supporting the importance of changes in folate intake both as a biomarker for folate status and as a mechanistic link to cancer risk. Lower folate intake or folate deficiency is associated with elevated risk of cancers of many sites. Folic acid supplementation as well as higher serum levels of folic acid were related to an increased prostate cancer risk. Polymorphisms of genes in the one-carbon pathway may have some impact on risk of cancers in certain ethnic groups (Pieroth et al. 2018).

Following the action of the U.S. Centers for Disease Control and legislation mandating folic acid fortification of enriched cereal-grain products in 1998 in the US, safety concerns were raised that excess consumption of folic acid and high blood folate biomarkers assayed in participants may be related to an increased risk of certain types of cancer. In the National Health and Nutrition Examination Survey conducted between 1999 and 2002, baseline data were collected from about 1,400 participants aged 57 or older (Hu, Juan, and Sahyoun 2016) with 8,114 person-years of follow-up. The study found that in 125 cancer cases after adjusting for confounders, the highest quartile versus the second quartile of RBC folate and dietary folate equivalents demonstrated a reduced risk of cancer. When using continuous variables, levels of serum and RBC folate were associated with reduced risk of cancer ($p < 0.01$). No significant associations were observed between the presence of unmetabolized folic acid, intake of naturally occurring food folate or folic acid separately, and cancer incidence. Therefore, in this large study, both high total folate intake and folate biomarkers in older adults appeared to be associated with reduced cancer risk in the years after folic acid fortification of processed grain products. There was no evidence of a negative impact at the current level of folic acid fortification on cancer risk. Several bacteria in the gastrointestinal tract can synthesize B-vitamins, including folate, in quantities that resemble dietary intake. The impact of bacterial folate biosynthesis concerning human health and disease remains unexplored and the study of the effects on the microbiome of folate fortification remains to be established (Kok et al. 2020).

SELENIUM

Selenium is found naturally in soil, foods, and water, and is a micronutrient essential to human health that has been associated with cancer prevention. Effects of selenium are thought to be mediated by selenium-containing proteins known as selenoproteins. Selenoproteins have antioxidant activity which can attenuate cancer development by minimizing oxidative insult and resultant DNA damage. Dr. Larry Clark and co-workers (Clark, Cantor, and Allaway 1991) suggested that individuals with high plasma and nail selenium would have a lower incidence of cancer. Studies in poorly nourished individuals in rural China, U.S. nonmelanoma skin cancer patients, and the Health Professional Follow-Up

Study in prostate cancer subjects (Vinceti et al. 2017) were all in agreement with the possibility that intake of high concentrations of selenium at levels above those needed to correct selenium deficiency could possibly inhibit carcinogenesis (Vinceti et al. 2014, Clark et al. 1996). An extensive review published in 2018 of 93 separate studies testing this hypothesis found little evidence of any effect of selenium supplementation on cancer risk. Two randomized controlled trials with 19,009 participants indicated that CRC was unaffected by selenium administration. Similarly, no beneficial effects were found in nonmelanoma skin cancer, lung cancer, breast cancer, bladder cancer, and prostate cancer (Vinceti et al. 2018). However, when 15 additional observational cohort studies were included, it was found that both lower cancer incidence (summary odds ratio and lower cancer mortality were associated with the highest selenium exposure compared with the lowest. While the observations in this study demonstrated a decrease in the risk of site-specific cancers for stomach, colorectal, lung, breast, bladder, and prostate cancers (Vinceti et al. 2018), the hypothesis that increasing selenium intake may reduce cancer risk was not supported strongly by the epidemiological evidence.

GREEN TEA

Studies of carcinogenesis in animal models have demonstrated that green tea, black tea, and their constituents could act on multiple targets in the multistage process of carcinogenesis including angiogenesis. An epidemiological study of 49,920 men in Japan between the ages of 40 and 69 recording their green tea consumption habits established that drinking five or more cups of tea per day compared with less than one cup per day was associated with a decreased risk of advanced prostate cancer (Kurahashi et al. 2008).

In a study of 455,981 participants between the ages of 30 and 79 in the China Kadoorie Biobank prospective cohort (Li et al. 2019), daily tea consumers were more likely to be current smokers and daily alcohol consumers in this population. A total of 22,652 incident cancers occurred during 10.1 years follow-up. When the subsequent analysis was limited to nonsmokers and nonexcessive alcohol consumers to minimize confounding, tea consumption was not associated with total cancers, lung cancer, CRC, or liver cancer. On the other hand, tea consumption tended to be associated with an increased risk of stomach cancer. In all the individuals studied, cancer risk increased with increases in the amount of tobacco smoked or alcohol consumed. These findings suggest that in the way that tea is consumed by over 500,000 Chinese individuals studied, there may be no beneficial effect of tea consumption on overall cancer incidence or most common forms of cancer.

In common with most Japanese green tea studies, the China Kadoorie study employed drinking green tea less than weekly as a reference group in their analysis, which mixed nongreen tea drinkers and less frequent green tea drinkers so that the results could be underestimating the beneficial effects of green tea on cancer risk.

Despite the lack of clear epidemiological evidence of an association of green tea drinking with reduced cancer risk, it is widely believed among the Chinese people that tea consumption is beneficial for cancer prevention. Some health channels in mass media specifically recommend drinking tea to reduce the harm of tobacco use. This commonly held idea together with other cultural and social factors has been associated in part with the habits of smoking, alcohol, and tea consumption among Chinese men. The most recent system review on the relationship between green tea drinking and cancer risk indicated that conflicting results were observed from experimental and nonexperimental epidemiological studies with limited evidence for the beneficial effect of green tea drinking on all cancer or on specific cancer risk (Filippini et al. 2020).

CONCLUSION

Nutritional epidemiology has led to an increased understanding of how diet and nutritional factors can reduce or increase cancer risk using methods that have been modified from traditional epidemiology in order to study diverse and interacting dietary factors which are more complex and different from discrete exposures such as chimney soot, tobacco, or alcohol. Measurement error is an inherent challenge in studies of nutritional epidemiology especially when it comes to dietary intake and its related biomarkers. Careful study design and well-developed dietary assessment tools coupled with specific biomarkers and innovative statistical analysis can aid future studies which may lead to new useful insights on diet and cancer risks in free-living populations. Prospective cohort studies are often considered the strongest observational study design, but these large studies conducted over many years cannot reflect demographic changes duet to immigration and behavior changes during the follow-up. As a result, these studies may not be representative of current ethnically diverse populations in terms of health status and socioeconomic factors that affect cancer risk. Healthier individuals from higher socioeconomic strata are also known to volunteer for these large prospective cohort studies, leading to potential selection bias. Major studies have led in many cases to the development of dietary advice communicated by international organizations and governments to help decrease the risks of common forms of cancer through changes in diet and lifestyle based on associations seen in these large cohorts.

Randomized controlled trials in nutrition have been touted as the highest form of evidence in nutritional science. However, randomized controlled trials have inherent challenges. There are a number of issues in defining a control or placebo group for nutrition. There are also challenges as well in designing the intervention group by randomization to balance confounding conditions between intervention and placebo groups. One solution that has been explored is to assign participants to consume different amounts of a nutrient with comparisons made of high and low intakes between intervention and control groups. For some nutrients, this solution is problematic as it may not be ethical to give a very low dose or create a nutritional deficiency of an essential substance in the control group. Often these challenges result in too narrow a contrast in nutrient intakes between the control and intervention groups so that the effects of the nutrient on cancer are underestimated. The randomized controlled drug trial is not easily adapted directly in nutritional intervention studies. While epidemiological studies "adjust" for confounding nutrients, a change in one macronutrient such as carbohydrate forces a change in another macronutrient such as fat when calories and protein are held constant. Compensatory changes among macronutrients and other substances such as fiber complicate attempts to study epidemiological insights within the construct of a randomized controlled clinical study.

Intervention studies of dietary or nutritional factors on cancer risk are also very challenging in view of the decades that it takes cancers to develop in humans. As a result, it is very difficult to observe true endpoints in a diet in a clinical study. This issue has been seen in several large intervention studies where analyses after 10 years demonstrated different results than the earlier analyses. Another major challenge for dietary intervention studies with free-living individuals is adherence to trial design and dropouts resulting in missing data that must be handled using specialized statistical methods.

Evidence from prospective cohort studies and clinical nutrition intervention trials monitoring intermediate endpoints can both be used together to develop some reasonable conclusions on the influence of diet and lifestyle on cancer. These conclusions can then be used to inform public policy to reduce cancer risks. Unlike smoking cessation, this Public Health Nutrition has implications beyond the individual including food manufacturing, availability of foods, and social equality which are beyond the scope of this chapter. Summarizing this evidence in systematic reviews and meta-analyses can be especially helpful in understanding a vast evidence base and informing policy. The late Dr. David Kritchevsky, a legend of modern nutrition with a great sense of humor, used to joke that "meta-analysis is to analysis as metaphysics is to physics". This notion applies whenever studies with different levels of evidence are combined as if they were comparable. It is vital that meta-analyses and systematic reviews should be conducted with caution and interpreted in light of the broader context of the field of nutritional science and cancer adapting the aspects of the Bradford Hill criteria that make sense in the modern context of all the disciplines considered in epidemiological studies or diet, nutrition, and cancer risk.

REFERENCES

Abbas, S., J. Linseisen, S. Rohrmann, J. Chang-Claude, P. H. Peeters, P. Engel, M. Brustad, E. Lund, G. Skeie, A. Olsen, A. Tjonneland, K. Overvad, M. C. Boutron-Ruault, F. Clavel-Chapelon, G. Fagherazzi, R. Kaaks, H. Boeing, B. Buijsse, G. Adarakis, V. Ouranos, A. Trichopoulou, G. Masala, V. Krogh, A. Mattiello, R. Tumino, C. Sacerdote, G. Buckland, M. V. Suarez, M. J. Sanchez, M. D. Chirlaque, A. Barricarte, P. Amiano, J. Manjer, E. Wirfalt, P. Lenner, M. Sund, H. B. Bueno-de-Mesquita, F. J. van Duijnhoven, K. T. Khaw, N. Wareham, T. J. Key, V. Fedirko, I. Romieu, V. Gallo, T. Norat, P. A. Wark, and E. Riboli. 2013. "Dietary intake of vitamin D and calcium and breast cancer risk in the European Prospective Investigation into Cancer and Nutrition." *Nutr Cancer* 65 (2):178–187. doi: 10.1080/01635581.2013.752018.

Alves Martins, B. A., G. F. de Bulhoes, I. N. Cavalcanti, M. M. Martins, P. G. de Oliveira, and A. M. A. Martins. 2019. "Biomarkers in colorectal cancer: the role of translational proteomics research." *Front Oncol* 9:1284. doi: 10.3389/fonc.2019.01284.

Ambrosone, C. B., S. E. McCann, J. L. Freudenheim, J. R. Marshall, Y. Zhang, and P. G. Shields. 2004. "Breast cancer risk in premenopausal women is inversely associated with consumption of broccoli, a source of isothiocyanates, but is not modified by GST genotype." *J Nutr* 134 (5):1134–1138. doi: 10.1093/jn/134.5.1134.

Atwell, L. L., L. M. Beaver, J. Shannon, D. E. Williams, R. H. Dashwood, and E. Ho. 2015. "Epigenetic regulation by sulforaphane: opportunities for breast and prostate cancer chemoprevention." *Curr Pharmacol Rep* 1 (2):102–111. doi: 10.1007/s40495-014-0002-x.

Aune, D., T. Norat, M. Leitzmann, S. Tonstad, and L. J. Vatten. 2015. "Physical activity and the risk of type 2 diabetes: a systematic review and dose-response meta-analysis." *Eur J Epidemiol* 30 (7):529–542. doi: 10.1007/s10654-015-0056-z.

Avgerinos, K. I., N. Spyrou, C. S. Mantzoros, and M. Dalamaga. 2019. "Obesity and cancer risk: emerging biological mechanisms and perspectives." *Metabolism* 92:121–135. doi: 10.1016/j.metabol.2018.11.001.

Bagga, D., J. M. Ashley, S. P. Geffrey, H. J. Wang, R. J. Barnard, S. Korenman, and D. Heber. 1995. "Effects of a very low fat, high fiber diet on serum hormones and menstrual function. Implications for breast cancer prevention." *Cancer* 76 (12):2491–2496. doi: 10.1002/1097-0142(19951215)76:12<2491::aid-cncr2820761213>3.0.co;2-r.

Ballotari, P., M. Vicentini, V. Manicardi, M. Gallo, S. Chiatamone Ranieri, M. Greci, and P. Giorgi Rossi. 2017. "Diabetes and risk of cancer incidence: results from a population-based cohort study in northern Italy." *BMC Cancer* 17 (1):703. doi: 10.1186/s12885-017-3696-4.

Barbachano, A., A. Fernandez-Barral, G. Ferrer-Mayorga, A. Costales-Carrera, M. J. Larriba, and A. Munoz. 2017. "The endocrine vitamin D system in the gut." *Mol Cell Endocrinol* 453:79–87 doi: 10.1016/j.mce.2016.11.028.

Barchetta, I., F. A. Cimini, G. Ciccarelli, M. G. Baroni, and M. G. Cavallo. 2019. "Sick fat: the good and the bad of old and new circulating markers of adipose tissue inflammation." *J Endocrinol Invest* 42 (11):1257–1272. doi: 10.1007/s40618-019-01052-3.

Baron J.A., E. L. Barry, L. A., Mott, J. R. Rees, R. S. Sandler, D.C. Snover, R.M. Bostick, A. Ivanova, B. F. Cole, D. J. Ahnen, G. J. Beck, R. S. Bresalier, C. A. Burke, T.R. Church, M. Cruz-Correa, J. C. Figueiredo, M. Goodman, A. S. Kim, D. J. Robertson, R. Rothstein, A. Shaukat, M. E. Seabrook, R. W. Summers. 2015. A Trial of Calcium and Vitamin D for the Prevention of Colorectal Adenomas. *The New England Journal of Medicine* 373(16):1519–1530. doi: 10.1056/NEJMoa1500409. PMID: 26465985; PMCID: PMC4643064.

Black, H. S., F. Boehm, R. Edge, and T. G. Truscott. 2020. "The benefits and risks of certain dietary carotenoids that exhibit both anti- and pro-oxidative mechanisms-a comprehensive review." *Antioxidants (Basel)* 9 (3):264. doi: 10.3390/antiox9030264.

Bock, F. G., G. E. Moore, and P. C. Clark. 1965. "Carcinogenic activity of cigarette smoke condensate. 3. Biological activity of refined tar from several types of cigarettes." *J Natl Cancer Inst* 34:481–493.

Boldry, E. J., Y. M. Patel, S. Kotapati, A. Esades, S. L. Park, M. Tiirikainen, D. O. Stram, L. Le Marchand, and N. Tretyakova. 2017. "Genetic determinants of 1,3-butadiene metabolism and detoxification in three populations of smokers with different risks of lung cancer." *Cancer Epidemiol Biomarkers Prev* 26 (7):1034–1042. doi: 10.1158/1055-9965.EPI-16-0838.

Bosetti, C., M. Filomeno, P. Riso, J. Polesel, F. Levi, R. Talamini, M. Montella, E. Negri, S. Franceschi, and C. La Vecchia. 2012. "Cruciferous vegetables and cancer risk in a network of case-control studies." *Ann Oncol* 23 (8):2198–2203. doi: 10.1093/annonc/mdr604.

Bradbury, K. E., P. N. Appleby, and T. J. Key. 2014. "Fruit, vegetable, and fiber intake in relation to cancer risk: findings from the European Prospective Investigation into Cancer and Nutrition (EPIC)." *Am J Clin Nutr* 100 (Suppl 1):394S–398S. doi: 10.3945/ajcn.113.071357.

Chadwick, C. A., and B. Keevil. 2007. "Measurement of cotinine in urine by liquid chromatography tandem mass spectrometry." *Ann Clin Biochem* 44 (Pt 5):455–462. doi: 10.1258/000456307781645996.

Chen, K., Q. Zhao, X. Li, J. Zhao, P. Li, S. Lin, H. Wang, J. Zang, Y. Xiao, W. Xu, F. Chen, and Y. Gao. 2018. "Dietary fiber intake and endometrial cancer risk: a systematic review and meta-analysis." *Nutrients* 10 (7). doi: 10.3390/nu10070945.

Clark, L. C., K. P. Cantor, and W. H. Allaway. 1991. "Selenium in forage crops and cancer mortality in U.S. counties." *Arch Environ Health* 46 (1):37–42. doi: 10.1080/00039896.1991.9937427.

Clark, L. C., G. F. Combs, Jr., B. W. Turnbull, E. H. Slate, D. K. Chalker, J. Chow, L. S. Davis, R. A. Glover, G. F. Graham, E. G. Gross, A. Krongrad, J. L. Lesher, Jr., H. K. Park, B. B. Sanders, Jr., C. L. Smith, and J. R. Taylor. 1996. "Effects of selenium supplementation for cancer prevention in patients with carcinoma of the skin. A randomized controlled trial. Nutritional Prevention of Cancer Study Group." *JAMA* 276 (24):1957–1963.

Conney, A. H. 1982. "Induction of microsomal enzymes by foreign chemicals and carcinogenesis by polycyclic aromatic hydrocarbons: G. H. A. Clowes Memorial Lecture." *Cancer Res* 42 (12):4875–4917.

Demeyer, D., K. Honikel, and S. De Smet. 2008. "The World Cancer Research Fund report 2007: a challenge for the meat processing industry." *Meat Sci* 80 (4):953–959. doi: 10.1016/j.meatsci.2008.06.003.

Doll, R., and A. B. Hill. 1950. "Smoking and carcinoma of the lung; preliminary report." *Br Med J* 2 (4682):739–748. doi: 10.1136/bmj.2.4682.739.

Etminan, M., B. Takkouche, and F. Caamano-Isorna. 2004. "The role of tomato products and lycopene in the prevention of prostate cancer: a meta-analysis of observational studies." *Cancer Epidemiol Biomarkers Prev* 13 (3):340–345.

Fedak, K. M., A. Bernal, Z. A. Capshaw, and S. Gross. 2015. "Applying the Bradford Hill criteria in the 21st century: how data integration has changed causal inference in molecular epidemiology." *Emerg Themes Epidemiol* 12:14. doi: 10.1186/s12982-015-0037-4.

Ferrari, P., R. Kaaks, M. T. Fahey, N. Slimani, N. E. Day, G. Pera, H. C. Boshuizen, A. Roddam, H. Boeing, G. Nagel, A. Thiebaut, P. Orfanos, V. Krogh, T. Braaten, E. Riboli, Cancer European Prospective Investigation into, and study Nutrition. 2004. "Within- and between-cohort variation in measured macronutrient intakes, taking account of measurement errors, in the European Prospective Investigation into Cancer and Nutrition study." *Am J Epidemiol* 160 (8):814–822. doi: 10.1093/aje/kwh280.

Filippini, T., M. Malavolti, F. Borrelli, A. A. Izzo, S. J. Fairweather-Tait, M. Horneber, and M. Vinceti. 2020. "Green tea (Camellia sinensis) for the prevention of cancer." *Cochrane Database of Systematic Reviews* (3):CD005004. doi: 10.1002/14651858.CD005004.pub3.

Flemer, B., D. B. Lynch, J. M. Brown, I. B. Jeffery, F. J. Ryan, M. J. Claesson, M. O'Riordain, F. Shanahan, and P. W. O'Toole. 2017. "Tumour-associated and non-tumour-associated microbiota in colorectal cancer." *Gut* 66 (4):633–643. doi: 10.1136/gutjnl-2015-309595.

Fox, E. J., and L. A. Loeb. 2010. "Lethal mutagenesis: targeting the mutator phenotype in cancer." *Semin Cancer Biol* 20 (5):353–359. doi: 10.1016/j.semcancer.2010.10.005.

Franks PW, Pearson E, Florez JC. Gene-environment and gene-treatment interactions in type 2 diabetes: progress, pitfalls, and prospects. *Diabetes Care* 2013;36:1413–21.

Gao, Y., C. Y. Um, V. Fedirko, R. E. Rutherford, M. E. Seabrook, E. L. Barry, J. A. Baron, and R. M. Bostick. 2018. "Effects of supplemental vitamin D and calcium on markers of proliferation, differentiation, and apoptosis in the normal colorectal mucosa of colorectal adenoma patients." *PLoS One* 13 (12):e0208762. doi: 10.1371/journal.pone.0208762.

Garland, C. F., and F. C. Garland. 1980. "Do sunlight and vitamin D reduce the likelihood of colon cancer?" *Int J Epidemiol* 9 (3):227–231. doi: 10.1093/ije/9.3.227.

Garland, C. F., E. D. Gorham, S. B. Mohr, and F. C. Garland. 2009. "Vitamin D for cancer prevention: global perspective." *Ann Epidemiol* 19 (7):468–483. doi: 10.1016/j.annepidem.2009.03.021.

Garrett, W. S. 2019. "The gut microbiota and colon cancer." *Science* 364 (6446):1133–1135. doi: 10.1126/science.aaw2367.

Giovannucci, E. 2007. "Does prostate-specific antigen screening influence the results of studies of tomatoes, lycopene, and prostate cancer risk?" *J Natl Cancer Inst* 99 (14):1060–1062. doi: 10.1093/jnci/djm048.

Giovannucci, E. 2011. "Commentary: Serum lycopene and prostate cancer progression: a re-consideration of findings from the prostate cancer prevention trial." *Cancer Causes Control* 22 (7):1055–1059. doi: 10.1007/s10552-011-9776-x.

Giovannucci, E., D. M. Harlan, M. C. Archer, R. M. Bergenstal, S. M. Gapstur, L. A. Habel, M. Pollak, J. G. Regensteiner, and D. Yee. 2010. "Diabetes and cancer: a consensus report." *Diabetes Care* 33 (7):1674–1685. doi: 10.2337/dc10-0666.

Giovannucci, E., E. B. Rimm, Y. Liu, M. J. Stampfer, and W. C. Willett. 2002. "A prospective study of tomato products, lycopene, and prostate cancer risk." *J Natl Cancer Inst* 94 (5):391–398. doi: 10.1093/jnci/94.5.391.

Glade, M. J. 1999. "Food, nutrition, and the prevention of cancer: a global perspective. American Institute for Cancer Research/World Cancer Research Fund, American Institute for Cancer Research, 1997." *Nutrition* 15 (6):523–526. doi: 10.1016/s0899-9007(99)00021-0.

Grant, W. B., and S. B. Mohr. 2009. "Ecological studies of ultraviolet B, vitamin D and cancer since 2000." *Ann Epidemiol* 19 (7):446–454. doi: 10.1016/j.annepidem.2008.12.014.

Hanchette, C. L., and G. G. Schwartz. 1992. "Geographic patterns of prostate cancer mortality. Evidence for a protective effect of ultraviolet radiation." *Cancer* 70 (12):2861–2869. doi: 10.1002/1097-0142(19921215)70:12<2861::aid-cncr2820701224>3.0.co;2-g.

Hebert, J. R., T. G. Hurley, S. E. Steck, D. R. Miller, F. K. Tabung, K. E. Peterson, L. H. Kushi, and E. A. Frongillo. 2014. "Considering the value of dietary assessment data in informing nutrition-related health policy." *Adv Nutr* 5 (4):447–455. doi: 10.3945/an.114.006189.

Hecht, S. S. 2003. "Tobacco carcinogens, their biomarkers and tobacco-induced cancer." *Nat Rev Cancer* 3 (10):733–744. doi: 10.1038/nrc1190.

Holick, M. F. 2017. "The vitamin D deficiency pandemic: approaches for diagnosis, treatment and prevention." *Rev Endocr Metab Disord* 18 (2):153–165. doi: 10.1007/s11154-017-9424-1.

Hu, J., W. Juan, and N. R. Sahyoun. 2016. "Intake and biomarkers of folate and risk of cancer morbidity in older adults, NHANES 1999–2002 with Medicare linkage." *PLoS One* 11 (2):e0148697. doi: 10.1371/journal.pone.0148697.

Huang, B. Z., S. J. Pandol, C. Y. Jeon, S. T. Chari, C. A. Sugar, C. R. Chao, Z. F. Zhang, B. U. Wu, and V. W. Setiawan. 2020. "New-onset diabetes, longitudinal trends in metabolic markers, and risk of pancreatic cancer in a heterogeneous population." *Clin Gastroenterol Hepatol* 18 (8):1812–1821.e7. doi: 10.1016/j.cgh.2019.11.043.

Huang, H. Y., A. J. Alberg, E. P. Norkus, S. C. Hoffman, G. W. Comstock, and K. J. Helzlsouer. 2003. "Prospective study of antioxidant micronutrients in the blood and the risk of developing prostate cancer." *Am J Epidemiol* 157 (4):335–344. doi: 10.1093/aje/kwf210.

IARC. 1993. *Some Naturally Occurring Substances: Food Items and Constituents, Heterocyclic Aromatic Amines and Mycotoxins. IARC Monographs on the Evaluation of Carcinogenic Risks to Humans.* Vol. 56.

IARC. 2015. *Red Meat and Processed Meat IARC Monographs on the Evaluation of Carcinogenic Risks to Humans.* Vol. 114.

Ilic, D., K. M. Forbes, and C. Hassed. 2011. "Lycopene for the prevention of prostate cancer." *Cochrane Database Syst Rev* (11):CD008007. doi: 10.1002/14651858.CD008007.pub2.

Jankovic, N., A. Geelen, R. M. Winkels, B. Mwungura, V. Fedirko, M. Jenab, A. K. Illner, H. Brenner, J. M. Ordonez-Mena, J. C. Kiefte de Jong, O. H. Franco, P. Orfanos, A. Trichopoulou, P. Boffetta, A. Agudo, P. H. Peeters, A. Tjonneland, G. Hallmans, H. B. Bueno-de-Mesquita, Y. Park, E. J. Feskens, L. C. de Groot, E. Kampman, Health Consortium on, Europe Ageing: Network of Cohorts in, and States the United. 2017. "Adherence to the WCRF/AICR dietary recommendations for Cancer Prevention and Risk of Cancer in Elderly from Europe and the United States: a meta-analysis within the CHANCES project." *Cancer Epidemiol Biomarkers Prev* 26 (1):136–144. doi: 10.1158/1055-9965.EPI-16-0428.

Jiang, N., and X. Xu. 2019. "Exploring the survival prognosis of lung adenocarcinoma based on the cancer genome atlas database using artificial neural network." *Medicine (Baltimore)* 98 (20):e15642. doi: 10.1097/MD.0000000000015642.

Julian-Almarcegui, C., S. Bel-Serrat, M. Kersting, G. Vicente-Rodriguez, G. Nicolas, K. Vyncke, C. Vereecken, W. De Keyzer, L. Beghin, S. Sette, L. Halstrom, E. Grammatikaki, M. Gonzalez-Gross, S. Crispim, N. Slimani, L. Moreno, S. De Henauw, and I. Huybrechts. 2016. "Comparison of different approaches to calculate nutrient intakes based upon 24-h recall data derived from a multicenter study in European adolescents." *Eur J Nutr* 55 (2):537–545. doi: 10.1007/s00394-015-0870-9.

Kaluza, J., H. R. Harris, N. Hakansson, and A. Wolk. 2020. "Adherence to the WCRF/AICR 2018 recommendations for cancer prevention and risk of cancer: prospective cohort studies of men and women." *Br J Cancer* 122 (10):1562–1570. doi: 10.1038/s41416-020-0806-x.

Kawakita, D., Y. A. Lee, F. Turati, M. Parpinel, A. Decarli, D. Serraino, K. Matsuo, A. F. Olshan, J. P. Zevallos, D. M. Winn, K. Moysich, Z. F. Zhang, H. Morgenstern, F. Levi, K. Kelsey, M. McClean, C. Bosetti, W. Garavello, S. Schantz, G. P. Yu, P. Boffetta, S. C. Chuang, M. Hashibe, M. Ferraroni, C. La Vecchia, and V. Edefonti. 2017. "Dietary fiber intake and head and neck cancer risk: a pooled analysis in the International Head and Neck Cancer Epidemiology consortium." *Int J Cancer* 141 (9):1811–1821. doi: 10.1002/ijc.30886.

Key, T. J., P. N. Appleby, N. E. Allen, R. C. Travis, A. W. Roddam, M. Jenab, L. Egevad, A. Tjonneland, N. F. Johnsen, K. Overvad, J. Linseisen, S. Rohrmann, H. Boeing, T. Pischon, T. Psaltopoulou, A. Trichopoulou, D. Trichopoulos, D. Palli, P. Vineis, R. Tumino, F. Berrino, L. Kiemeney, H. B. Bueno-de-Mesquita, J. R. Quiros, C. A. Gonzalez, C. Martinez, N. Larranaga, M. D. Chirlaque, E. Ardanaz, P. Stattin, G. Hallmans, K. T. Khaw, S. Bingham, N. Slimani, P. Ferrari, S. Rinaldi, and E. Riboli. 2007. "Plasma carotenoids, retinol, and tocopherols and the risk of prostate cancer in the European Prospective Investigation into Cancer and Nutrition study." *Am J Clin Nutr* 86 (3):672–681. doi: 10.1093/ajcn/86.3.672.

Key, T. J., P. B. Silcocks, G. K. Davey, P. N. Appleby, and D. T. Bishop. 1997. "A case-control study of diet and prostate cancer." *Br J Cancer* 76 (5):678–687. doi: 10.1038/bjc.1997.445.

Kirsh, V. A., S. T. Mayne, U. Peters, N. Chatterjee, M. F. Leitzmann, L. B. Dixon, D. A. Urban, E. D. Crawford, and R. B. Hayes. 2006. "A prospective study of lycopene and tomato product intake and risk of prostate cancer." *Cancer Epidemiol Biomarkers Prev* 15 (1):92–98. doi: 10.1158/1055-9965.EPI-05-0563.

Kok, D. E., W. T. Steegenga, E. J. Smid, E. G. Zoetendal, C. M. Ulrich, and E. Kampman. 2020. "Bacterial folate biosynthesis and colorectal cancer risk: more than just a gut feeling." *Crit Rev Food Sci Nutr* 60 (2):244–256. doi: 10.1080/10408398.2018.1522499.

Kricker, A., and B. Armstrong. 2006. "Does sunlight have a beneficial influence on certain cancers?" *Prog Biophys Mol Biol* 92 (1):132–139. doi: 10.1016/j.pbiomolbio.2006.02.015.

Kurahashi, N., S. Sasazuki, M. Iwasaki, M. Inoue, S. Tsugane, and JPHC Study Group. 2008. "Green tea consumption and prostate cancer risk in Japanese men: a prospective study." *Am J Epidemiol* 167 (1):71–77. doi: 10.1093/aje/kwm249.

Li, X., C. Yu, Y. Guo, Z. Bian, Z. Shen, L. Yang, Y. Chen, Y. Wei, H. Zhang, Z. Qiu, J. Chen, F. Chen, Z. Chen, J. Lv, L. Li, and Group China Kadoorie Biobank Collaborative. 2019. "Association between tea consumption and risk of cancer: a prospective cohort study of 0.5 million Chinese adults." *Eur J Epidemiol* 34 (8):753–763. doi: 10.1007/s10654-019-00530-5.

Ligibel, J. A., C. M. Alfano, K. S. Courneya, W. Demark-Wahnefried, R. A. Burger, R. T. Chlebowski, C. J. Fabian, A. Gucalp, D. L. Hershman, M. M. Hudson, L. W. Jones, M. Kakarala, K. K. Ness, J. K. Merrill, D. S. Wollins, and C. A. Hudis. 2014. "American Society of Clinical Oncology position statement on obesity and cancer." *J Clin Oncol* 32 (31):3568–3574. doi: 10.1200/JCO.2014.58.4680.

Liu, C., X. D. Wang, R. T. Bronson, D. E. Smith, N. I. Krinsky, and R. M. Russell. 2000. "Effects of physiological versus pharmacological beta-carotene supplementation on cell proliferation and histopathological changes in the lungs of cigarette smoke-exposed ferrets." *Carcinogenesis* 21 (12):2245–2253. doi: 10.1093/carcin/21.12.2245.

Liu, X., K. Hemminki, A. Forsti, K. Sundquist, J. Sundquist, and J. Ji. 2015. "Cancer risk in patients with type 2 diabetes mellitus and their relatives." *Int J Cancer* 137 (4):903–910. doi: 10.1002/ijc.29440.

Liu, X., and K. Lv. 2013. "Cruciferous vegetables intake is inversely associated with risk of breast cancer: a meta-analysis." *Breast* 22 (3):309–313. doi: 10.1016/j.breast.2012.07.013.

Loeb, L. A. 2011. "Human cancers express mutator phenotypes: origin, consequences and targeting." *Nat Rev Cancer* 11 (6):450–457. doi: 10.1038/nrc3063.

Loft, S., P. Svoboda, H. Kawai, H. Kasai, M. Sorensen, A. Tjonneland, U. Vogel, P. Moller, K. Overvad, and O. Raaschou-Nielsen. 2012. "Association between 8-oxo-7,8-dihydroguanine excretion and risk of lung cancer in a prospective study." *Free Radic Biol Med* 52 (1):167–172. doi: 10.1016/j.freeradbiomed.2011.10.439.

Ma, Y., Y. Chen, and I. Petersen. 2017. "Expression and promoter DNA methylation of MLH1 in colorectal cancer and lung cancer." *Pathol Res Pract* 213 (4):333–338. doi: 10.1016/j.prp.2017.01.014.

Makarem, N., J. M. Nicholson, E. V. Bandera, N. M. McKeown, and N. Parekh. 2016. "Consumption of whole grains and cereal fiber in relation to cancer risk: a systematic review of longitudinal studies." *Nutr Rev* 74 (6):353–373. doi: 10.1093/nutrit/nuw003.

Manson, J. E., N. R. Cook, I. M. Lee, W. Christen, S. S. Bassuk, S. Mora, H. Gibson, D. Gordon, T. Copeland, D. D'Agostino, G. Friedenberg, C. Ridge, V. Bubes, E. L. Giovannucci, W. C. Willett, J. E. Buring, and Vital Research Group. 2019. "Vitamin D supplements and prevention of cancer and cardiovascular disease." *N Engl J Med* 380 (1):33–44. doi: 10.1056/NEJMoa1809944.

Mills, P. K., W. L. Beeson, R. L. Phillips, and G. E. Fraser. 1989. "Cohort study of diet, lifestyle, and prostate cancer in Adventist men." *Cancer* 64 (3):598–604. doi: 10.1002/1097-0142(19890801)64:3<598::aid-cncr2820640306>3.0.co;2-6.

Mondul, A. M., S. J. Weinstein, T. M. Layne, and D. Albanes. 2017. "Vitamin D and cancer risk and mortality: state of the science, gaps, and challenges." *Epidemiol Rev* 39 (1):28–48. doi: 10.1093/epirev/mxx005.

Mori, N., N. Sawada, T. Shimazu, T. Yamaji, A. Goto, R. Takachi, J. Ishihara, M. Iwasaki, M. Inoue, S. Tsugane, and JPHC Study Group. 2019. "Cruciferous vegetable intake and colorectal cancer risk: Japan public health center-based prospective study." *Eur J Cancer Prev* 28 (5):420–427. doi: 10.1097/CEJ.0000000000000491.

Murphy, S. E., L. B. von Weymarn, M. M. Schutten, F. Kassie, and J. F. Modiano. 2011. "Chronic nicotine consumption does not influence 4-(methylnitrosamino)-1-(3-pyridyl)-1-butanone-induced lung tumorigenesis." *Cancer Prev Res (Phila)* 4 (11):1752–1760. doi: 10.1158/1940-6207.CAPR-11-0366.

O'Keefe, S. J. 2016. "Diet, microorganisms and their metabolites, and colon cancer." *Nat Rev Gastroenterol Hepatol* 13 (12):691–706. doi: 10.1038/nrgastro.2016.165.

Park, J. Y., L. Chen, A. Elahi, P. Lazarus, and M. S. Tockman. 2005. "Genetic analysis of microsomal epoxide hydrolase gene and its association with lung cancer risk." *Eur J Cancer Prev* 14 (3):223–230. doi: 10.1097/00008469-200506000-00005.

Park, Y., M. F. Leitzmann, A. F. Subar, A. Hollenbeck, and A. Schatzkin. 2009. "Dairy food, calcium, and risk of cancer in the NIH-AARP Diet and Health Study." *Arch Intern Med* 169 (4):391–401. doi: 10.1001/archinternmed.2008.578.

Pence, B. C., D. M. Dunn, C. Zhao, M. Landers, and M. J. Wargovich. 1995. "Chemopreventive effects of calcium but not aspirin supplementation in cholic acid-promoted colon carcinogenesis: correlation with intermediate endpoints." *Carcinogenesis* 16 (4):757–765. doi: 10.1093/carcin/16.4.757.

Peto, R., R. Doll, J. D. Buckley, and M. B. Sporn. 1981. "Can dietary beta-carotene materially reduce human cancer rates?" *Nature* 290 (5803):201–208. doi: 10.1038/290201a0.

Phillips, C. V., and K. J. Goodman. 2004. "The missed lessons of Sir Austin Bradford Hill." *Epidemiol Perspect Innov* 1 (1):3. doi: 10.1186/1742-5573-1-3.

Pieroth, R., S. Paver, S. Day, and C. Lammersfeld. 2018. "Folate and its impact on cancer risk." *Curr Nutr Rep* 7 (3):70–84. doi: 10.1007/s13668-018-0237-y.

Pourmand, G., S. Salem, A. Mehrsai, M. Lotfi, M. A. Amirzargar, H. Mazdak, A. Roshani, A. Kheirollahi, E. Kalantar, N. Baradaran, B. Saboury, F. Allameh, A. Karami, H. Ahmadi, and Y. Jahani. 2007. "The risk factors of prostate cancer: a multicentric case-control study in Iran." *Asian Pac J Cancer Prev* 8 (3):422–428.

Rahmati, S., M. Azami, A. Delpisheh, M. R. Hafezi Ahmadi, and K. Sayehmiri. 2018. "Total calcium (dietary and supplementary) intake and prostate cancer: a systematic review and meta-analysis." *Asian Pac J Cancer Prev* 19 (6):1449–1456. doi: 10.22034/APJCP.2018.19.6.1449.

Satija, A., D. Spiegelman, E. Giovannucci, and F. B. Hu. 2015. "Type 2 diabetes and risk of cancer." *BMJ* 350:g7707. doi: 10.1136/bmj.g7707.

Sevilya, Z., Y. Leitner-Dagan, M. Pinchev, R. Kremer, D. Elinger, H. S. Rennert, E. Schechtman, L. S. Freedman, G. Rennert, T. Paz-Elizur, and Z. Livneh. 2014. "Low integrated DNA repair score and lung cancer risk." *Cancer Prev Res (Phila)* 7 (4):398–406. doi: 10.1158/1940-6207.CAPR-13-0318.

Shams-White, M. M., N. T. Brockton, P. Mitrou, D. Romaguera, S. Brown, A. Bender, L. L. Kahle, and J. Reedy. 2019. "Operationalizing the 2018 World Cancer Research Fund/American Institute for Cancer Research (WCRF/AICR) Cancer Prevention Recommendations: a standardized scoring system." *Nutrients* 11 (7):1572. doi: 10.3390/nu11071572.

Shekelle, R. B., M. Lepper, S. Liu, C. Maliza, W. J. Raynor, Jr., A. H. Rossof, O. Paul, A. M. Shryock, and J. Stamler. 1981. "Dietary vitamin A and risk of cancer in the Western Electric study." *Lancet* 2 (8257):1185–1190. doi: 10.1016/s0140-6736(81)91435-5.

Smith, M. T., K. Z. Guyton, C. F. Gibbons, J. M. Fritz, C. J. Portier, I. Rusyn, D. M. DeMarini, J. C. Caldwell, R. J. Kavlock, P. F. Lambert, S. S. Hecht, J. R. Bucher, B. W. Stewart, R. A. Baan, V. J. Cogliano, and K. Straif. 2016. "Key characteristics of carcinogens as a basis for organizing data on mechanisms of carcinogenesis." *Environ Health Perspect* 124 (6):713–721. doi: 10.1289/ehp.1509912.

Song, M., W. S. Garrett, and A. T. Chan. 2015. "Nutrients, foods, and colorectal cancer prevention." *Gastroenterology* 148 (6):1244–1260.e16. doi: 10.1053/j.gastro.2014.12.035.

Swami, S., A. V. Krishnan, and D. Feldman. 2011. "Vitamin D metabolism and action in the prostate: implications for health and disease." *Mol Cell Endocrinol* 347 (1–2):61–69. doi: 10.1016/j.mce.2011.05.010.

Torre, L. A., R. L. Siegel, E. M. Ward, and A. Jemal. 2016. "Global cancer incidence and mortality rates and trends--an update." *Cancer Epidemiol Biomarkers Prev* 25 (1):16–27. doi: 10.1158/1055-9965. EPI-15-0578.

Tretli, S., E. Hernes, J. P. Berg, U. E. Hestvik, and T. E. Robsahm. 2009. "Association between serum 25(OH) D and death from prostate cancer." *Br J Cancer* 100 (3):450–454. doi: 10.1038/sj.bjc.6604865.

Tsilidis, K. K., J. C. Kasimis, D. S. Lopez, E. E. Ntzani, and J. P. Ioannidis. 2015. "Type 2 diabetes and cancer: umbrella review of meta-analyses of observational studies." *BMJ* 350:g7607. doi: 10.1136/bmj.g7607.

Uzunlulu, M., O. Telci Caklili, and A. Oguz. 2016. "Association between metabolic syndrome and cancer." *Ann Nutr Metab* 68 (3):173–179. doi: 10.1159/000443743.

Vainio, H., and M. Rautalahti. 1998. "An international evaluation of the cancer preventive potential of carotenoids." *Cancer Epidemiol Biomarkers Prev* 7 (8):725–728.

Vardavas, C. I., and K. Nikitara. 2020. "COVID-19 and smoking: a systematic review of the evidence." *Tob Induc Dis* 18:20. doi: 10.18332/tid/119324.

Vergnaud, A. C., T. Norat, D. Romaguera, T. Mouw, A. M. May, I. Romieu, H. Freisling, N. Slimani, M. C. Boutron-Ruault, F. Clavel-Chapelon, S. Morois, R. Kaaks, B. Teucher, H. Boeing, B. Buijsse, A. Tjonneland, J. Halkjaer, K. Overvad, M. U. Jakobsen, L. Rodriguez, A. Agudo, M. J. Sanchez, P. Amiano, J. M. Huerta, A. B. Gurrea, N. Wareham, K. T. Khaw, F. Crowe, P. Orfanos, A. Naska, A. Trichopoulou, G. Masala, V. Pala, R. Tumino, C. Sacerdote, A. Mattiello, H. B. Bueno-de-Mesquita, F. J. van Duijnhoven, I. Drake, E. Wirfalt, I. Johansson, G. Hallmans, D. Engeset, T. Braaten, C. L. Parr, A. Odysseos, E. Riboli, and P. H. Peeters. 2012. "Fruit and vegetable consumption and prospective weight change in participants of the European Prospective Investigation into Cancer and Nutrition-Physical Activity, Nutrition, Alcohol, Cessation of Smoking, Eating Out of Home, and Obesity study." *Am J Clin Nutr* 95 (1):184–193. doi: 10.3945/ajcn.111.019968.

Villalta, P. W., J. B. Hochalter, and S. S. Hecht. 2017. "Ultrasensitive high-resolution mass spectrometric analysis of a DNA adduct of the carcinogen benzo[a]pyrene in human lung." *Anal Chem* 89 (23):12735–12742. doi: 10.1021/acs.analchem.7b02856.

Vinceti, M., G. Dennert, C. M. Crespi, M. Zwahlen, M. Brinkman, M. P. Zeegers, M. Horneber, R. D'Amico, and C. Del Giovane. 2014. "Selenium for preventing cancer." *Cochrane Database Syst Rev* (3):CD005195. doi: 10.1002/14651858.CD005195.pub3.

Vinceti, M., T. Filippini, S. Cilloni, and C. M. Crespi. 2017. "The epidemiology of selenium and human cancer." *Adv Cancer Res* 136:1–48 doi: 10.1016/bs.acr.2017.07.001.

Vinceti, M., T. Filippini, C. Del Giovane, G. Dennert, M. Zwahlen, M. Brinkman, M. P. Zeegers, M. Horneber, R. D'Amico, and C. M. Crespi. 2018. "Selenium for preventing cancer." *Cochrane Database Syst Rev* (1):CD005195. doi: 10.1002/14651858.CD005195.pub4.

Wang, X., B. N. Chorley, G. S. Pittman, S. R. Kleeberger, J. Brothers, 2nd, G. Liu, A. Spira, and D. A. Bell. 2010. "Genetic variation and antioxidant response gene expression in the bronchial airway epithelium of smokers at risk for lung cancer." *PLoS One* 5 (8):e11934. doi: 10.1371/journal.pone.0011934.

WCRF/AICR. 2018. "Diet, Nutrition, Physical Activity and Cancer: a Global Perspective. Continuous Update Project Expert Report 2018." www.aicr.org and www.wcrf.org.

WHO. 2020. "Tobacco." https://www.who.int/news-room/fact-sheets/detail/tobacco.

Wogan, G. N., S. S. Hecht, J. S. Felton, A. H. Conney, and L. A. Loeb. 2004. "Environmental and chemical carcinogenesis." *Semin Cancer Biol* 14 (6):473–486. doi: 10.1016/j.semcancer.2004.06.010.

Wood, R. D., and S. Doublie. 2016. "DNA polymerase theta (POLQ), double-strand break repair, and cancer." *DNA Repair (Amst)* 44:22–32 doi: 10.1016/j.dnarep.2016.05.003.

Wood, R. D., M. Mitchell, and T. Lindahl. 2005. "Human DNA repair genes, 2005." *Mutat Res* 577 (1–2):275–283. doi: 10.1016/j.mrfmmm.2005.03.007.

Wu, Q. J., Y. Yang, E. Vogtmann, J. Wang, L. H. Han, H. L. Li, and Y. B. Xiang. 2013. "Cruciferous vegetables intake and the risk of colorectal cancer: a meta-analysis of observational studies." *Ann Oncol* 24 (4):1079–1087. doi: 10.1093/annonc/mds601.

Wynder, E. L., and E. A. Graham. 1985. "Landmark article May 27, 1950: tobacco smoking as a possible etiologic factor in bronchiogenic carcinoma. A study of six hundred and eighty-four proved cases. By Ernest L. Wynder and Evarts A. Graham." *JAMA* 253 (20):2986–2994. doi: 10.1001/jama.253.20.2986.

Yang, W., Y. Ma, Y. Liu, S. A. Smith-Warner, T. G. Simon, D. Q. Chong, Q. Qi, J. A. Meyerhardt, E. L. Giovannucci, A. T. Chan, and X. Zhang. 2019. "Association of intake of whole grains and dietary fiber with risk of hepatocellular carcinoma in US adults." *JAMA Oncol* 5 (6):879–886. doi: 10.1001/jamaoncol.2018.7159.

Yuan, J. M., H. H. Nelson, S. G. Carmella, R. Wang, J. Kuriger-Laber, A. Jin, J. Adams-Haduch, S. S. Hecht, W. P. Koh, and S. E. Murphy. 2017. "CYP2A6 genetic polymorphisms and biomarkers of tobacco smoke constituents in relation to risk of lung cancer in the Singapore Chinese Health Study." *Carcinogenesis* 38 (4):411–418. doi: 10.1093/carcin/bgx012.

Zhang, N. Q., S. C. Ho, X. F. Mo, F. Y. Lin, W. Q. Huang, H. Luo, J. Huang, and C. X. Zhang. 2018. "Glucosinolate and isothiocyanate intakes are inversely associated with breast cancer risk: a case-control study in China." *Br J Nutr* 119 (8):957–964. doi: 10.1017/S0007114518000600.

8 Oxidant Stress and Carcinogenesis

Susanne Henning
UCLA Center for Human Nutrition

CONTENTS

INTRODUCTION

Humans and many organisms evolved over millions of years by adaptation to an increasing concentration of oxygen in the atmosphere by developing a complex network of defense against oxidant stress. Oxygen comprises approximately 20% of the air we breathe and the air that bathes the plants that surround us. In nature, free oxygen is produced by the light-driven splitting of water during oxygenic photosynthesis. Green algae and cyanobacteria in marine environments provide about 70% of the free oxygen produced on earth and the rest is produced by terrestrial plants (1). Free oxygen is also dissolved in the world's oceans and lakes. The increased solubility of oxygen at lower temperatures has important implications for ocean life, as polar oceans support a much higher density of life due to their higher oxygen content.

Both the animal and the plant worlds use oxygen in many ways but have to defend against its potentially damaging effects, as demonstrated when an apple is cut open and exposed to the air. The browning of an apple in minutes of exposure to air demonstrates that activating oxidases such as the polyphenol oxidase in the apple's chloroplast can induce secondary chemically modified sugars and polyphenols that react with amino acids or proteins once the protective colorful peel no longer protects the flesh of the apple (2).

In vertebrates, oxygen is diffused through membranes in the lungs and into red blood cells. Hemoglobin binds oxygen, changing its color from bluish red to bright red. A liter of blood can dissolve $200 \, cm^3$ of oxygen. Within the cells of our bodies, oxidation reactions are used to produce energy within the mitochondria, in enzymatic reactions that detoxify drugs and phytochemicals and redox reactions in signaling pathways (3,4). The challenge of managing the potential threat of oxidative damage has led to the development of multiple defense mechanisms against this outcome within all living organisms. Unbalanced oxidation would lead to the destruction of all the critical cellular elements that permit life, including cellular lipids, proteins, and carbohydrates.

Oxidation is the gain of oxygen or loss of electrons, and reduction is loss of oxygen or gain of electrons. Oxidation and reduction reactions must occur in pairs. When one atom or molecule is oxidized, another is reduced to defend against the potentially damaging effects of free radicals. Reactive oxygen species (ROS) consist of molecules that have been oxidized and now have an unpaired electron which can oxidize other molecules. In turn, these molecules that were previously stable become unstable ROS expanding the oxidative changes to more molecules in a chain reaction.

A free radical is any chemical species with an unpaired electron that can be neutral, positively charged, or negatively charged. Although a few stable free radicals are known, most are very reactive. In free radical chain reactions, the radical product of one reaction becomes the starting material for another, propagating free radical damage (5).

SOURCE OF FREE RADICALS AND OXIDATIVE STRESS

The term "oxidative stress" refers to a significant imbalance between ROS production and antioxidant defenses. Helmut Sies defined it as "a disturbance in the pro-oxidant–antioxidant balance in favor of the former, leading to potential damage" (6).

ROS is an umbrella term for an array of derivatives of molecular oxygen that occur as a normal attribute of aerobic life. There are four major ROS in biological systems that are free radicals: superoxide anion $\left((O_2^-)\right)$, hydrogen peroxide (H_2O_2), hydroxyl radical (OH^-), and singlet oxygen ($^1O_2$). In addition, peroxynitrite ($ONOO^-$) and nitric oxide (NO) and other reactive nitrogen species (RNS) are called free radicals (7).

These free radicals can be generated via a number of mechanisms, including normal physiological processes and processes resulting from external factors. A ubiquitous source of free radicals is the mitochondrial electron transport chain (ETC). Complexes I, II, and IV all "pump" protons (i.e., H^+) into the mitochondrial space between the inner and outer mitochondrial membrane, establishing a proton gradient across the inner mitochondrial membrane (8). As the protons pass through Complex V, the osmotic energy of the gradient is converted into chemical energy, in the form of ATP. Complex I and in part complex II release O_2—H_2O_2 toward the mitochondrial matrix and complex III toward the cristae lumen (9). Superoxide anion $\left(O_2^{-*}\right)$ radical may reduce cytochrome C in the intermembrane space or may be converted to hydrogen peroxide (H_2O_2) and oxygen (10,11). Oxidation-reduction reactions involve the transfer of electrons between two materials and are mediated by cofactors (coenzymes).

Another important source of ROS are enzyme reactions. Overall, in human cells, more than 40 H_2O_2- and/or O_2^--generating enzymes have been identified, and this list is increased to well over 50 by inclusion of enzymes generating other ROS such as lipid hydroperoxides or nitric oxide (NO) and hypochlorous acid (9). The major endogenous enzymatic sources of O_2^- and H_2O_2 are transmembrane nicotinamide adenine dinucleotide phosphate (NADPH) oxidases (NOXs) (9). NOXs have also been associated with specialized redox-active endosomes (redoxosomes), which form in response to specific extracellular stimuli, such as nutrients, growth factors, and cytokines, and allow compartmentalization of H_2O_2 for local redox-mediated regulation (microdomains) or cell signaling from cell-surface receptors (9).

Metabolism is not the only source of free radicals. Environmental pollutants are sources for free radicals including nitrogen dioxide, ozone, cigarette smoke, radiation, halogenated hydrocarbons, heavy metals, and certain pesticides. Alcohol consumption can induce oxidative reactions in the liver. Certain chemotherapeutic agents including doxorubicin, cyclophosphamide, 5-fluorouracil, methotrexate, and vincristine can produce oxygen radicals at doses used in cancer patients. Increased physical activity can generate free radicals as the result of increased oxygen consumption during exercise.

ANTIOXIDANTS

The human body is equipped with a variety of antioxidant defense mechanisms that serve to counterbalance the effect of oxidants. In general, these can be divided into two categories: nonenzymatic and enzymatic. Nonenzymatic antioxidants include low-molecular weight compounds provided by foods (vitamin C and E, carotenoids, polyphenols, and other phytochemicals [see Chapter 4 in this book]) and components of metabolic processes (uric acid, cysteine, lipoic acid, glutathione, and coenzyme Q10) (12). The main enzymes contributing to the antioxidant defense are superoxide dismutase (SOD), catalase, and glutathione peroxidase (13). SOD converts superoxide to H_2O_2, and catalase or glutathione peroxidase eliminates H_2O_2. With glutathione (GSH) as the reducing substrate, GSH peroxidase also catalyzes the reduction of lipid peroxyl radicals to lipid hydroperoxides. The resulting oxidized form of GSH, glutathione disulfide (GSSG), is reverted to GSH by GSH reductase, with the electrons coming from NADPH (14). Cells exposed to ROS also activate the transcription factor and master regulator of antioxidant response, nuclear factor erythroid 2-related factor 2 (NRF2). ROS-mediated NRF2 response triggers gene expression of antioxidant enzyme systems (glutathione peroxidase, glutathione reductase, thioredoxin reductase, ferritin, NADPH: quinone oxidoreductase 1, peroxiredoxin-thioredoxin, etc.) (15).

Vitamin E and other lipid soluble antioxidants are located in the lipid bilayer of the cell membrane, and are effective inhibitors of lipid peroxidation that helps to maintain membrane integrity. With the reduction of a lipid peroxy radical to lipid hydroperoxide, α-tocopherol itself is converted to α-tocopheroxyl radical, which can be reduced by water-soluble antioxidants such as ascorbic acid to regenerate α-tocopherol. Through this mechanism, the two vitamins work together to protect against cellular oxidative damage. Ascorbic acid, in turn, can be regenerated from its oxidized forms by a number of enzymatic and nonenzymatic mechanisms (16).

This network of lipid- and water-soluble antioxidants is supported by a wide spectrum of naturally occurring water- and lipid-soluble antioxidants from our food. Thousands of dietary compounds such as carotenoids (lutein, lycopene), flavonoids (anthocyanins, phloretin), flavonols (keampferol, quercetin), flavanols (catechin, epicatechin), flavanones (eriodictyol, hesperetin), flavones (luteolin), isoflavonoids (daidzein,genistein), organosulfur compounds (allicin), phenolic acids (caffeic acid, chlorogenic acid), polyphenols (curcumin, resveratrol), stilbenes (tetrahydroxy-stilbene glucoside), and tannins (ellagitannins) affect oxidative metabolism and oxidative stress (17,18).

Another group of compounds has been referred to as "indirect antioxidants" such as isothiocyanates and triterpenoids, which can trigger nuclear-factor-erythroid-2-p45-re-lated-factor-2 (Nrf2)-regulated antioxidant and cytoprotective enzymes. Nrf2 is a transcription factor that responds to cellular stresses and is subject to regulation at different levels. Some antioxidants induce indirect antioxidant activity by stimulating antioxidant enzymes (14).

Due to the large network of interacting antioxidant systems, a holistic approach is needed to understand the nutritional impact upon oxidative stress when investigating the effect of nutrition on oxidative stress. Recent advances in omics and data analysis methods provide viable tools for systems nutrition approaches (18).

PRO-OXIDANTS

Antioxidants have the ability to scavenge radicals and protect biomolecules, such as lipids, proteins, and DNA against oxidative damage. On the contrary, their ability to accept and donate electrons also enables them to act as pro-oxidants under certain conditions and causing oxidative damage to biomolecules (19). High concentrations of certain antioxidants have been considered to have pro-oxidant properties. Whether these pro-oxidant properties are physiologically relevant, in vivo is unclear. In vitro, vitamin C, β-carotene, and green tea polyphenol have been documented to have pro-oxidant properties in different milieus and a high antioxidant dose and oxidizing environment (such as that of a smoker's lung) can promote their pro-oxidant behavior (14,20–24).

Originally, dietary antioxidants were considered as beneficial in cancer prevention. A seminal study, in 1981, reported that individuals that consumed a greater amount of green leafy and yellow vegetables exhibited a lower risk for cancer (25). Since these types of vegetables are rich in carotenoids, particularly β-carotene, which are able to quench singlet oxygen and have strong antioxidant capacity, the investigators suggested that β-carotene might be responsible for the anticancer effect observed. However, the protective function of certain carotenoids, particularly β-carotene and lycopene, and α-tocopherol has been challenged by results from the α-Tocopherol, β-Carotene Cancer Prevention Study (ATBC) and β-Carotene and Retinol Efficacy Trial (CARET) in lung cancer in heavy smokers (15,26,27). Results showed significantly increased incidence of lung cancer and have raised concern regarding the safety of β-carotene supplementation and the warning that it should not be used in cancer prevention in the general population (20). The chemical background of the anti- and pro-oxidant activity of carotenoids has been described in detail by Black et al. (20).

Recently, anticancer therapies that induce oxidative stress by increasing ROS and/or inhibiting antioxidant processes have received significant attention. The acceleration of accumulative ROS disrupts redox homeostasis and causes severe damage in cancer cells. In the review by Kim et al., ROS-inducing cancer therapy and the anticancer mechanism employed by pro-oxidative agents have been extensively described (28).

ROLE OF ROS IN REDOX SIGNALING

ROS are not only toxic molecules, but are fundamentally involved in intercellular and intracellular signaling during normal metabolism. The major mechanism by which ROS mediate their biological effects in redox regulation is through thiol-based modification of target proteins (8). Sies et al. provide an excellent summary of basic mechanisms of ROS signaling (7).

The critical initial step in redox signaling through proteins is the reaction of H_2O_2 with cysteine (Cys) thiolate (S^-) to form the sulfenate (SO^-). This reaction leads to a change in function of the protein, and it can lead to further reactions leading to intramolecular or intermolecular disulfide (SS) formation or glutathionylation (SSG) of the reactive cysteine. In addition, superoxide anion radicals $\left(O_2^-\right)$ can react with Fe–S clusters in proteins, such as in aconitase, which also can lead to a change in function. When O_2^- is generated concomitantly with nitric oxide (NO), peroxynitrite ($ONOO^-$) is formed efficiently, leading to nitration of tyrosine (Tyr) residues in proteins, again causing functional modifications (9).

Since reversibility is an essential feature in redox signaling, disulfides and glutathionylated, nitrosylated as well as persulfidated cysteines can be reduced back to the original thiol either through the thioredoxin system or through the glutathione (GSH) system. Sulfenate can be further oxidized to sulfinate and sulfonate.

Redox signaling affects protein function, leading to changes in signaling outputs, enzyme activity, gene transcription, and membrane and genome integrity, to just name a few examples. Regarding the total number of cellular cysteines, Sies et al. showed that about 10%–20% thiols of the full 214,000 thiols in the cellular cysteine proteome are readily oxidized under aerobic conditions.

Signal transduction through redox signaling occurs in multiple locations in the cell such as plasma membrane, mitochondria, peroxisomes, and endoplasmic reticulum (ER) (7). The plasma membrane is a key platform for cell signaling, integrating, and transmitting signals between the extracellular space and the intracellular space. The plasma membrane is a major site of oxidant generation (mediated by NOXs, xanthine oxidase, etc.) and transport (via aquaporins). It is also the site where signaling receptors (importantly including receptor tyrosine kinases) and ion channels are subject to redox regulation. In the context of membranes, oxidants also target lipids. The resulting lipid peroxidation generates lipid hydroperoxides and lipid-derived second messengers, which then can attack key regulatory proteins (e.g., the NRF2 system) or heat shock response pathways, generating lipid–protein adducts in a process known as lipoxidation.

Signals from the plasma membrane and other cellular sites control activation of gene transcription in the nucleus, many of which are aimed at homeostasis maintenance and are regulated by oxidants via master switches such as NRF2 and NF-κB. The overall redox environment in the nucleus is more reduced than in the cytosol, and gene expression is sensitive to oxidants, as is DNA replication.

As mentioned earlier, mitochondria are key cellular sources of O_2^- and H_2O_2. The physiological role of mitochondrial redox metabolism spans numerous fundamental aspects beyond energy capture, as diverse as participating in anabolic and catabolic pathways, apoptosis, and having a role in epigenetic cell regulation. Mitochondria themselves respond to oxidant exposure with functional consequences. Several mitochondrial proteins, importantly including ETC components, contain Fe–S clusters, which are highly reactive toward O_2^-, leads to a change in the function of the enzyme. Changes in oxidant availability will inevitably impact mitochondrial functions in metabolism, including respiration and subsequent oxidant generation.

The role of peroxisomes in the metabolism of lipids and H_2O_2 has led to interesting new perspectives in redox signaling. Peroxisomes contain a number of H_2O_2-generating oxidases, such as fatty acyl-CoA oxidase and D-amino acid oxidase, as well as H_2O_2-reducing enzymes, such as catalase and peroxiredoxin 5. While peroxisomal H_2O_2 metabolism obviously relates to regulation of peroxisomal functions, it also addresses extraperoxisomal redox targets such as FOXO3 or PTEN. In addition, peroxisomal catalases are able to modulate oxidative stress at the cellular level, and catalase can even be secreted, which has been associated with malignant transformation. The abundance and distribution of peroxisomes are highly variable among cell types, raising the possibility of an important role in cell-specific redox signaling.

In the context of protein metabolism, a major process is the formation of disulfide bridges, which for proteins that enter the secretory route occurs in the ER during oxidative protein folding. For every disulfide formed in a reaction catalyzed by protein disulfide isomerases, there is production of one oxidizing equivalent, H_2O_2, resulting from reoxidation of protein disulfide isomerases catalyzed by endoplasmic oxidoreductin 1 (ERO1). Hence, H_2O_2 is a by-product of protein folding. Different cell types have different secretory products dependent on these ER systems. For instance, plasma cells use H_2O_2 to support antibody production, and pancreatic islets use H_2O_2 to support insulin production.

The NRF2–KEAP1 system is the paradigm for a physiological thiol-based sensor–effector apparatus responding to oxidant challenge with a role in maintaining redox homeostasis in eukaryotes. It is a major sensor for oxidative and electrophilic stresses, whereby KEAP1, which functions as an NRF2 inhibitor, harbors several cysteine residues that can be subject to oxidation. The NRF2–KEAP1 system is regulated by thioredoxin reductase 1 and by the sirtuin family of deacetylases. Furthermore, redox-sensitive microRNAs modulate the NRF2 system.

Another well-characterized system is the NF-κB pathway. NF-κB serves as a master switch of inflammation, which is associated with extensive H_2O_2 production. Cytosolic H_2O_2 can activate the NF-κB pathway, and this occurs via H_2O_2-mediated oxidation and activation of the inhibitor of NF-κB (IκB) kinases, which negatively control the stability of I-κB.

The third example is hypoxia-inducible factor (HIF), which is a transcription factor that serves as the master regulator of transcriptional responses to decreased oxygen levels. Hypoxia (oxygen deficiency) has been associated with an increase in O_2^- (and subsequent H_2O_2) generation due to inhibition of the mitochondrial ETC (15).

ROS ARE PART OF METABOLIC PHENOTYPE OF CANCER CELLS

The metabolic phenotype of cancer cells is transformed to upregulate nucleotide synthesis and glycolysis, while changes in oxidative phosphorylation can be more variable (29). Otto Warburg was the first to characterize cancer as having a more glycolytic metabolism despite the availability of oxygen, which was labeled the "Warburg effect" or aerobic glycolysis. Aerobic glycolysis is a cardinal feature of many tumors (29). ROS are a key determinant of cancer's metabolic phenotype. Studies have shown that cancer cells have higher steady-state ROS levels (30).

Extensive investigations have addressed the question why cancer cells perform aerobic glycolysis even though less energy is produced per glucose molecule when compared to oxidative phosphorylation. Although glycolytic shunts are important for nucleotide synthesis during proliferation, this does not explain the massive amount of glucose that is shifted down the central glycolytic pathway and excreted as lactate. One explanation is that glycolysis allows rapid ATP production while reducing the growth-limiting ROS associated with oxidative phosphorylation. Furthermore, glucose can be diverted to the pentose phosphate pathway (PPP), which generates the cofactor NADPH, needed for the antioxidant activity of glutathione. A key mediator of glycolysis activation is the hypoxia-inducible factor 1 (HIF-1), which can be activated by both hypoxia and ROS itself. Nrf2 is another transcription factor heavily implicated in both metabolism and redox. It is activated by both ROS and oncogenes such as Kras, Braf, and Myc (31). It induces the production of the NADPH cofactor through the PPP, which simultaneously enhances proliferation through increased nucleotide synthesis (32).

Both glycolysis and antioxidant upregulation may provide the greatest survival advantage and allow cancers to thrive under extreme conditions. This is possible through the ROS-dependent induction of both HIF-1 and the transcription factor Nrf2, which itself increases HIF-1 activation (29).

Since each patient's cancer is unique, metabolic and redox profiling of biopsies could help guide individualized treatments. Assays previously used for the direct measurement of ROS include the oxidation of dihydroethidine to measure superoxide levels and CDCFH2 for hydrogen peroxides is not sensitive enough due to the unstable and reactive nature of ROS. A more stable downstream marker of ROS would be the level of advanced oxidation protein products. In addition, analysis of NADPH/NAD ratios as well as the expression of specific antioxidant enzymes might be superior for an understanding of a cancer's adaptive antioxidant response (29).

Furthermore, the role of glutamine as an alternative form of energy production has also been investigated extensively (29). Aggressive cancers in particular are found to have a dependence on glutamine availability. While glutaminolysis does play an important role in replenishing metabolic intermediates, its importance for redox is underappreciated. Glutamine can increase antioxidant capacity since it is a precursor for glutathione. In addition, glutamine can be used to generate NADPH through the malate pathway, providing a multitude of substrates for the glutathione system.

Glutamine (Gln) is converted by glutaminases (GLS and GLS2) into glutamate (Glu), which gives rise to α-ketoglutarate in the mitochondria matrix. The Gln pathway is reprogrammed in cancer to increase production of glutathione (GSH) and oxidized glutathione (GSSG), which ratio is regulated by glutathione reductase (GR) and glutathione peroxidase (GPx). Together with thioredoxin (Trx) redox system, they reduce mitochondrial oxidative stress.

L-glutamine, a nonessential amino acid, is the most abundant amino acid in human plasma (0.5–0.8 mM), consistent with its versatile usage as a biosynthetic substrate (33). Targeting glutaminolysis in combination with drugs that unbalance mitochondrial redox state are widely used for treating multiple types of cancers (34).

Activated Nrf2 increases metabolic flux from glutamine to GSH, enhancing its biosynthesis, utilization, and regeneration, as well as inducing the production of NADPH through the modulation of ME, in turn raising the malate oxidative decarboxylation to pyruvate to replenish the TCA cycle (35).

Many polyphenols and plant extracts have been shown to impair mitochondrial function and metabolism by modulating the redox state and leading to apoptosis and death in many types of cancer cells. In this context, curcumin, genistein, and gallic acid treatment affected mitochondrial functionality, by modulating mitochondrial membrane potential, activating caspase-3, -9, Bax, and p53, decreasing the cellular energy status Adenosine Triphosphate/Adenosine Diphosphate (ATP/ADP), arresting cell cycle, and promoting cytochrome c release in colorectal and acute myeloid leukemia cancer cells (35).

OXIDATIVE STRESS AND REDOX BALANCE IN CARCINOGENESIS

ROS have long been associated with cancer where different types of tumor cells have been shown to produce elevated levels of ROS compared to their normal counterparts (36,37). Elevated levels of ROS in cancer cells are formed by high metabolic activity, cellular signaling, peroxisomal activity, mitochondrial dysfunction, activation of oncogenes, and increased enzymatic activity of oxidases, cyclooxygenases, lipoxygenases, and thymidine phosphorylases (36). Elevated levels of ROS are thought to be oncogenic, causing increased receptor and oncogene activity, stimulation of growth factor-dependent pathways, or induce genetic instability (37). Moreover, excessive intracellular levels of ROS may damage lipids, proteins, and DNA (38).

As described above, ROS also act as signaling molecules in cancer, contributing to abnormal cell growth, metastasis, resistance to apoptosis, angiogenesis, and in some types of cancer a differentiation block. Increased levels of ROS are protumorigenic, resulting in the activation of prosurvival signaling pathways, loss of tumor suppressor gene-function, increased glucose metabolism, adaptations to hypoxia, and the generation of oncogenic mutations (38).

Dependent on ROS concentration, oxygen radicals influence cancer development in apparently contradictory ways, either initiating/stimulating tumorigenesis and supporting transformation/proliferation of cancer cells or in very high concentrations causing cell death. Tumor cells employ a variety of adaptation mechanisms in response to ROS and oxidative stress. To accommodate high ROS levels, tumor cells are able to upregulate their antioxidant defense utilizing reduced glutathione (GSH), thioredoxins (TXN1 and TXN2), NADPH generation, and the activity of antioxidant transcription factors (activator protein 1 [AP-1], HIF-1α, heat shock factor 1 [HSF1], nuclear factor kB [NF-kB], nuclear factor-erythroid 2 p45-related factor 2 [NRF2], and tumor protein p53). NRF2 provides a principal inducible defense against oxidative stress because it regulates a wide spectrum of antioxidant and detoxification genes (7,39). NRF2 activates a wide spectrum of antioxidant genes upon exposure to ROS or soft electrophiles. Hayes et al. provides an excellent review of the role of ROS in tumor development and cell death (39). During initiation, genetic changes enable cell survival under high ROS levels by activating antioxidant transcription factors or increasing NADPH via the PPP. During progression and metastasis, tumor cells adapt to oxidative stress by increasing NADPH in various ways, including activation of AMPK, the PPP, and reductive glutamine and folate metabolism (38–40).

For many years, numerous laboratories have investigated the possibility that antioxidant dietary compounds, when delivered in combination with certain cancer therapies, could function synergistically to eliminate cancer cells. However, despite promising findings suggesting synergy between chemotherapeutics and antioxidants against tumor cells, more recent findings depict numerous molecular mechanisms demonstrating that alterations in the intracellular antioxidant machinery in tumor cells facilitate cancer cell survival and promote resistance to chemotherapeutic agents. For instance, in a number of distinct cancer contexts, the stabilization of the Nrf2 transcription factor, a master regulator of the intracellular antioxidant program and redox homeostasis, can facilitate the development of chemoresistance (41).

In opposite, toxic levels of ROS production in cancers are antitumorigenic resulting in an increase of oxidative stress and induction of tumor cell death (38).

In reference to the nature of ROS behavior as a double-edged sword, even though several studies have documented the benefits of antioxidant drugs for cancer therapies, none has been supported by solid trials performed on a large scale (15).

An increasing number of therapeutic strategies are being developed to elevate ROS levels to overwhelm the redox adaptation of the same cells, inducing oxidative stress incompatible with cellular life (37).

Trials using therapeutic opportunities targeting ROS are under way either using antioxidants to reduce ROS or to induce ROS or inhibit antioxidant pathways to enhance ROS (15). Clinical trials using antioxidants or pro-oxidants are ongoing (15).

OBESITY, OXIDATIVE STRESS, AND CANCER

Obesity is an established risk factor for 13 different cancer sites (endometrial, postmenopausal breast, colorectal, esophageal, renal/kidneys, meningioma, pancreatic, gastric cardia, liver, multiple myeloma, ovarian, gallbladder, and thyroid) (42). The WCRF/AICR also highlighted that there is convincing and sufficient evidence that obesity is associated with an increased risk of endometrial, esophageal, colorectal, liver, pancreatic, postmenopausal breast, and renal/kidney cancers (43). Oxidative stress is one of the many biologic mechanisms whereby obesity, sedentary behavior, and physical activity are related to cancer incidence. Other mechanisms include endogenous sex steroids and metabolic hormones, insulin sensitivity, telomere length, DNA methylation, and gut microbiome (44).

Increased oxidative stress is a common pathophysiological characteristic of increased adiposity (45). Elevated mitochondrial substrate load consequently increases ETC activity and ROS production (46). Obese individuals exhibit higher levels of oxidative stress in white adipose tissue, including elevated ROS levels and decreased antioxidant activity coupled with alterations in adipokines (47).

ROS and RNS overload the homeostatic system resulting in proinflammatory adipokine secretion, immune-activation, and chronic inflammation. Excessive oxidative stress in the cell activates NRF2 which upregulates genes encoding major cytoprotective enzymes such as NAD(P)H:quinone oxidoreductase 1 (NQO1), heme oxygenase 1 (HO1), and glutathione S-transferases (GST) (45).

A recent study demonstrated that the total thiol levels, a marker of antioxidant defense capacity, showed statistically significant inverse linear associations with all weight measures including body mass index, waist-to-hip ratio, and waist circumference (48). Data were derived from 1,734 participants of a population-based cohort study of older adults (age range: 57–83 years) at two time points 3 years apart (48).

Obese patients undergoing bariatric surgery were recruited to compare markers of oxidative stress and damage before and after significant weight loss (49). Oxidative stress has been shown to play a key role in several obesity-related detrimental health consequences including DNA oxidation. The most common DNA oxidation lesion is 8-oxo-7,8-dihydroguanine (8-oxoG), which causes DNA-base mispairing leading to mutations (50). Some published studies already demonstrated elevated DNA damage in obesity (49,51,52). Overall, bariatric surgery induced significant reduction in excess body weight and improved the patients' health status, including reduced DNA strand breaks and slightly improved antioxidant status in some of the investigated endpoints, while cellular ROS formation and DNA oxidation damage stayed unaltered (49).

ANTIOXIDANT AND ANTI-INFLAMMATORY DIETS AND CANCER

Epidemiological studies have observed the association between dietary patterns and the risk of certain types of cancer (53). Extensive studies have been conducted on the cancer preventive activities of antioxidants from food and beverages. While laboratory research has shown impressive and promising results, such promising cancer preventive activities have not been demonstrated in many human intervention trials (54). The dietary antioxidants such as vitamin C, vitamin E, and carotenoids are among the most widely investigated antioxidants for their potential to decrease risk of cancer incidence.

Some epidemiological studies have indicated beneficial effects of vitamin C, vitamin E, carotenoids, and selenium in the prevention of cancer by inhibiting the formation of carcinogens, preventing DNA damage from oxidative stress and improving immune function (55–57). Many prospective studies found associations between dietary antioxidants including vitamin C, vitamin E, and carotenoids and total cancer (58,59), but other studies did not show an inverse association (60) or found no significant association (61). Some of the previous studies may have been too small and therefore underpowered to find a significant association (62).

A recent meta-analysis investigated the association of dietary intake and blood levels of antioxidants with coronary heart disease, stroke, cardiovascular disease, cancer, and/or all-cause mortality (63). The meta-analysis of 69 prospective studies found an inverse association with total cancer incidence between dietary intake and blood concentration of, vitamin C, blood concentrations of carotenoids (total, β-carotene, α-carotene, lycopene, β-cryptoxanthin), and blood concentrations of α-tocopherol, but not gamma tocopherol (63). An increase of 5 µg/mL in serum α-T level was linked to a 9% or 6% decrease in total cancer rate or total mortality rate, respectively (63).

Another recent meta-analysis, however, determined that in older adults evidence was inconclusive on the associations between dietary or supplemental intake of antioxidants and mortality in the older population (56).

VITAMIN E

Naturally occurring vitamin E exists in eight chemical forms (alpha-, beta-, gamma-, and delta-tocopherol and alpha-, beta-, gamma-, and delta-tocotrienol) that have varying levels of biological activity (64,65). Nuts, seeds, and vegetable oils are among the best sources of alpha-tocopherol, and significant amounts are available in green leafy vegetables and fortified cereals (66). Most vitamin E in American diets is in the form of gamma-tocopherol from soybean, canola, corn, and other vegetable oils and food products (67).

Several large-scale clinical intervention studies have been performed in the last 20 years using individual antioxidant compounds or combinations of antioxidants. An excellent overview of studies involving different forms of tocopherol has been provided by Yang et al. (68).

For example, the Women's Health Study (600 mg of α-T on alternate days) after 10 years of follow-up did not significantly affect the incidence of colon, lung, or total cancers (69). The Physicians' Health Study II (400 mg of α-T every other day) or vitamin C (500 mg synthetic ascorbic acid) to physicians for 8 years did not reduce the risk of prostate cancer or all other cancer (70). In addition the selenium and vitamin E cancer prevention trial (SELECT) failed to demonstrate a preventive effect against cancer (68,71).

More recently, however, a nested case–control study in the vitamin E intervention study (SELECT) determined that genetic variants involved in selenium or vitamin E metabolism or transport and anti-oxidant capacity may underlie the complex associations of selenium and vitamin E. Statistically significant ($P < 0.05$) interactions between selenium assignment and SNPs in several key antioxidant genes including CAT, SOD2, PRDX6, SOD3, and TXNRD2, and high-grade prostate cancer risk were found (72). Three SNP variations (SEC14L2, SOD1, and TTPA) were found to be associated with a lower risk of prostate cancer in subjects receiving vitamin E in the SELECT. The SNP variation for both SEC14L 2 and SOD1 was associated with significantly lowered prostate cancer risk. The SNP of TTPA, involved in the formation of the alpha-tocopherol transport protein, which results in lower levels of α-TTP and presumably lower α-T, was associated with increased risk of prostate cancer in the absence of vitamin E supplementation, and vitamin E supplementation seemed to offset this increased risk (68,72).

In addition other forms of vitamin E such as γ-tocopherol (γT), δ-tocopherol (δT), γ-tocotrienol (γTE), and δ-tocotrienol (δTE) can inhibit the growth and induce death of many types of cancer cells, and are capable of suppressing cancer development in preclinical cancer models (73).

Vitamin E is a fat-soluble vitamin and differences in its pharmacokinetic have been demonstrated depending on body fat (74). The data suggest that when obesity is accompanied by liver fat, meal-derived α-tocopherol as well as lipoprotein-derived α-tocopherol could be diverted to a liver fat depot, perhaps with diminished local availability. Especially after food ingestion, fat in hepatocytes might generate excess oxidants (75), precisely when there would be decreased availability of α-tocopherol for oxidant quenching, perhaps leading to chronic oxidant-induced liver damage (i.e., progression to inflammation, hepatocyte injury, and irreversible cirrhosis). Possibly, in obese individuals, low vitamin E levels might be found throughout the body contributing to insufficient response to oxidative stress (74).

CAROTENOIDS

Carotenoids are a diverse group of natural pigments and are present in many fruits and vegetables. Recent outstanding reviews have been published on the anticarcinogenic activity and its mechanism of carotenoids (76–78). A short overview and summary is presented here. Lycopene, β-carotene, α-carotene, lutein, zeaxanthin, and β-cryptoxanthin are the most common carotenoids in human serum (79). Due to their largely hydrocarbon structure, carotenoids tend to be nonpolar and need dietary fat to be absorbed into the intestinal lumen. Due to their excellent antioxidant properties, carotenoids can contribute to the promotion of human health. However, under unusual conditions of unbalanced intracellular redox status, high oxygen tension, and high carotenoid concentration, carotenoids can act as pro-oxidant molecules. At low oxygen pressures, carotenoids can act as potent chain-breaking antioxidants. At high pO_2, they are readily autoxidized, thus exhibiting pro-oxidant activities (20).

It has been well established that malignant cells innately maintain high intracellular ROS levels compared to normal cells. Under the higher levels of intracellular ROS in the cancer cells, the pro-oxidant activities of carotenoids predominate over their antioxidant activities, resulting in increased oxidative stress, which facilitates apoptosis of cancer cells. In contrast, under normal metabolic processes (in the normal cells), carotenoids can optimize the redox status, thus playing an essential role in maintaining the oxidative balance. Considering this dynamic antioxidant (in the normal cells) and pro-oxidant (in the cancer cells) actions, carotenoids are emerging as novel therapeutic agents for selective killing of cancer cells (80,81). In addition to their anti- and pro-oxidant activity carotenoids exhibit many other anticarcinogenic effects including induction of apoptosis, inhibition of cell cycle progression, metastasis, angiogenesis, alteration of gap junction intercellular communication, and multidrug resistance which has been extensively reviewed by Saini et al. (76).

Despite potential benefits that have been reported in the literature, epidemiological studies surrounding carotenoids and their role in protection from carcinogenesis and progression have yielded mixed results. Current results from the most updated meta-analyses indicate that higher lycopene consumption and circulating blood concentrations are associated with a decreased risk of prostate cancer (relative risk [RR] = 0.88, 95% confidence interval [CI] = 0.78–0.98 for both diet and blood) (82). There was also a linear dose–response for dietary lycopene such that the RR of prostate cancer decreased by 1% for each additional 1 mg of lycopene that was consumed (p = 0.026) (82).

A pooled analysis by Petimar et al. evaluated the associations between specific fruits, vegetables, and beans and prostate cancer risk in 15 prospective cohorts (83). These 15 cohorts utilized similar instruments (such as a food frequency questionnaire) to determine consumption patterns at baseline. No associations between tomato consumption and prostate cancer were observed in this study. Interestingly, Petimar et al. also indicated that the vast majority of studies did not assess tomato products with bio-available lycopene (83). These results are in line with the results from a recent meta-analysis from our laboratory (84). In this meta-analysis, it was found that raw tomatoes were not associated with a reduced risk of prostate cancer (RR = 0.95, 95%CI = 0.84–1.09); however, sources of bioavailable tomato were associated with a reduced risk of prostate cancer (RR = 0.84, 95%CI = 0.73–0.98). These data suggest that bioavailability of carotenoids affects the subsequent risk associations with cancer.

A recent expert of the World Cancer Research Fund (WCRF)/American Institute for Cancer Research (AICR) suggested that the foods containing carotenoids may protect against lung cancer and breast cancer (perimenopause and postmenopause) (43). As part of WCRF/AICR continuous update project (CUP), a systematic review of 17 prospective studies, including 458,434 participants (3,603 cases), revealed that the blood concentrations of retinol, α- and β-carotene, lycopene, and total carotenoids were inversely associated with lung cancer risk (90). In this systematic review, subjects with the highest concentrations of total carotenoids and retinol showed 19% and 34% lower RR of lung cancer, respectively, compared with the lowest blood concentrations. In the most recent CUP report, it was concluded that there is limited–suggestive evidence of a casual decrease in breast or lung cancers with foods containing carotenoids. For other cancer sites, evidence was reported as limited–no conclusion.

Another report from 18 prospective cohort analyses showed a weak inverse association between α-carotene, β-carotene, and lutein + zeaxanthin intake and risk of ER–, but not ER+, breast cancer (85). However, findings from a French E3N study involving 366 cases of invasive breast cancer (84 premenopausal women and 282 postmenopausal women) suggested that higher levels of lipophilic antioxidant micronutrients (carotenoids, tocopherols, and retinol) in serum did not protect against breast cancer, at least in postmenopausal women (86).

Although the epidemiological and preclinical data suggest that carotenoids are protective against cancer, the limited data from randomized controlled trials are conflicting. The two most relevant trials are the CARET and ATBC trials. As described in the section above on pro-oxidants, daily β-carotene was supplemented at 20 mg/day in the ATBC study and 30 mg/day in the CARET study (26) increase lung cancer risk in current smokers and individuals with occupational asbestos exposure (42–44). Importantly, however, the β-carotene that was supplemented in these trials was provided at a much higher dose than a normal person would consume. Daily β-carotene consumption ranges between 1 and 2 mg/day (NHANES2007–2014) (45,46). In contrast, β-carotene was supplemented at 20 mg/day in the ATBC study and 30 mg/day in the CARET study (42,43). These concentrations were approximately 10–20 times higher than an adult would naturally consume.

VITAMIN C

Vitamin C, also known as L-ascorbic acid, is a water-soluble vitamin that is naturally present in fruits and vegetable (66). Humans, unlike most animals, are unable to synthesize vitamin C endogenously, so it is an essential dietary component.

It may come as a surprise, that globally, vitamin C deficiency is prevalent in low-income countries and certain population subgroups in high-income countries (87).

In meta-analyses of prospective studies higher consumption of fruits and vegetables is associated with lower risk of total cancer, perhaps, in part, due to their high vitamin C content (63). Vitamin C can limit the formation of carcinogens, such as nitrosamines, in vivo; modulate immune response; and, through its antioxidant function, possibly attenuate oxidative damage that can lead to cancer (88,89).

During the 1970s, studies by Cameron, Campbell, and Pauling suggested that high-dose vitamin C has beneficial effects on quality of life and survival time in patients with terminal cancer (90,91). However, some subsequent studies—including a randomized, double-blind, placebo-controlled clinical trial by Moertel and colleagues at the Mayo Clinic (92)—did not support these findings. In the Moertel study, patients with advanced colorectal cancer who received 10 g/day vitamin C fared no better than those receiving a placebo.

Emerging research suggests that the route of vitamin C administration (intravenous (IV) vs. oral) could explain the conflicting findings (93). Most intervention trials, including the one conducted by Moertel and colleagues, used only oral administration, whereas Cameron and colleagues used a combination of oral and IV administration. Oral administration of vitamin C, even of very large doses, can raise plasma vitamin C concentrations to a maximum of only 220 μmol/L, whereas IV administration can produce plasma concentrations as high as 26,000 μmol/L (94). Concentrations of this magnitude are selectively cytotoxic to tumor cells in vitro.

There is a substantial body of literature that documents potential antitumor effects of ascorbate in in vitro and in vivo settings, with many reporting cytotoxicity toward cancer cells and a slowing of tumor growth in animal models (95). Human clinical studies, however, have been infrequent, with most recent phase I/II studies aiming to determine the tolerability of pharmacological doses of ascorbate for patients with advanced cancer (93,96).

Although data in animal models indicted a significant reduction in tumor growth, the administration of pharmacological vitamin C as a single agent was not curative. This emphasizes that a future trend may lie in a combination of vitamin C and chemotherapeutic agents. The review by Visser et al. summarizes results from clinical trials showing an additive effect with high concentrations of vitamin C in combination with the following chemotherapy agents: cisplatin, cyclophosphamide, doxorubicin, etoposide, fluorouracil, gemcitamine, irinotecan, paclitaxel, tamoxifen, vincristine, FOLFIRI14, and FOLFOX regimens.

FLAVONOIDS

Based on their chemical structure, flavonoids can be classified into six principal subclasses: flavonols (mainly including quercetin, kaempferol, myricetin, and isorhamnetin), flavones (apigenin and luteolin), flavanones (hesperetin and naringenin), flavan-3-ols (catechin, epicatechin, epigallocatechin, epicatechin-3-gallate, epigallocatechin-3-gallate), anthocyanins (cyanidin, delphinidin, malvidin, pelargonidin, petunidin, peonidin), and isoflavones (genistein and daidzein). Dietary flavonols mainly exist in tea, onions, broccoli, and various common fruits. Flavanones and flavones are in oranges and other citrus fruits or citrus juice. Flavones are also abundant in vegetables, such as celery, peppers, and lettuce. Flavan-3-ols are in green tea, apples, cocoa, red wine, grapes, and other fruits. Anthocyanidines are in colored berries, black currants, grapes, and some vegetables, such as eggplant and radishes. Unlike other flavonoids, isoflavones are mostly contained in soy products instead of fruits, vegetables, and tea (97). Many flavonoids have strong antioxidant activity (98,99).

Many epidemiological studies investigating the potential of flavonoids to decrease the risk of cancer have been performed. One recent epidemiological prospective cohort study including 56,048 participants of the Danish Diet, Cancer, and Health cohort cross-linked with Danish nationwide registries and followed for 23 years demonstrated that a moderate habitual intake of flavonoids is inversely associated with all-cause, cardiovascular-, and cancer-related mortality. This strong association plateaus at intakes of approximately 500 mg/day. Furthermore, the inverse associations between total flavonoid intake and mortality outcomes are stronger and more linear in smokers than in nonsmokers, as well as in heavy (>20 g/day) vs. low-moderate (<20 g/day) alcohol consumers (100). Krishnan et al. provides a review of clinical trials with flavonoid and other bioactive compounds including quercetin, curcumin, piperin, capsaicin, pigallocatechin gallate (EGCG), phenethyl isothiocyanate, and resveratrol in several types of cancer (101). This review also highlights the diverse mechanisms in addition to the antioxidant activity.

Green tea polyphenols are among the most commonly investigated flavonoids. A recent Cochrane review provided an excellent update on the use of green tea for cancer prevention. The review included 142 intervention and epidemiological studies. Overall, the evidence from the studies showed that the consumption of green tea consumption to reduce the risk of cancer was inconsistent (102). In particular, results from experimental studies suggested that green tea extract supplementation yielded a decreased risk for prostate cancer, but increased risk for gynecological cancer. Green tea supplementation seemed to slightly improve the quality of life compared with placebo, although it was associated with some adverse effects including gastrointestinal disorders, higher levels of liver enzymes, and, more rarely, insomnia, raised blood pressure and skin reactions. The evaluation of epidemiological studies comparing people consuming the highest amount of green tea to those in the lowest category of consumption, Filippini et al. found an indication of a lower occurrence of new cases of overall types of cancer, while no difference emerged for lethal cases (102).

Preclinical studies demonstrate that flavonoids, through their antioxidant activity, target many molecular signaling pathways by inducing Nerf2 activation, leading to apoptosis and cell cycle arrest or activation of tumor suppressor p53. In addition, flavonoids exhibit many anticarcinogenic effects independent of their antioxidant activity by inhibiting proliferation, deregulate hypoxia and glucose metabolism, and downregulation of inflammatory processes (103).

The dietary vitamin E (VE) intake in the above studies was mainly obtained from food frequency questionnaires. The food items rich in VE also contain vitamin C, selenium, and other constituents that may contribute to a reduction in cancer risk. Thus, the effects of "dietary VE" would also include the effects of other constituents from the food, and commercial VE supplements would not be as effective (68).

These antioxidants are mainly found in fruits and vegetable. For example, vitamin C is found abundantly in fruits, vegetables, especially berries, citrus fruits and juices, kiwi, broccoli, and peppers and some legumes. Carotenoids are mainly found in green and yellow fruits and vegetables. Fruits and vegetable in addition have a wide variety of other antioxidants and therefore evaluating the effect of fruit and vegetable consumption on risk of cancer might show a protective effect. Another meta-analysis by Aune et al. demonstrated a borderline protective effect of fruit and vegetable consumption with RR of 0.97 (95% CI: 0.95–0.99, I 2 = 49%, n = 12) for total cancer (63). Inverse associations were observed between the intake of green-yellow vegetables and cruciferous vegetables and total cancer risk (63).

As radical scavengers, dietary antioxidants suppress ROS generation. Antioxidants can be obtained externally and diets rich in fruits and vegetables play a crucial role in providing antioxidants such as vitamin C, vitamin E, carotenoids, including β-carotene, α-carotene, β-cryptoxanthin, lycopene, lutein, and zeaxanthin, and flavonoids. Considering that the usual diet consists of antioxidants in various chemical forms with different degrees of antioxidant capacities and that these combined antioxidants may exert cumulative or synergistic effects, dietary total antioxidant capacity (TAC) has received attention as a useful tool for assessing total antioxidant power in the diet (104). However, the utility of dietary TAC has been debated due to the fact that estimation of dietary TAC varies widely by measurement methodology and that dietary TAC might not directly reflect plasma TAC (105). Nevertheless, high-dietary TAC has been consistently reported to be associated with lower biomarkers indicative of oxidative stress and cancer (105–107).

An oxidative balance score (OBS) has been defined in multiple ways, ranging from inclusion of 3–28 components, and often including both dietary and nondietary lifestyle factors that have antioxidant or pro-oxidant effects. A mixture of predefined and population-dependent cut-points is used in the scoring algorithm. A comprehensive review published in 2019 reported a significantly reduced risk of colorectal cancer (two studies) and breast cancer (one study) in individuals with high "antioxidative" scores on the OBS (108). Data on the OBS and individual cancers are limited, and associations often reflect other lifestyle- related risk factors such as smoking, adiposity, and use of nonsteroidal anti-inflammatory drugs (53).

GLUTATHIONE AND GLUTATHIONE REACTIVE UNITS IN FOOD

The tripeptide GSH (L-γ-glutamyl-L-cysteinyl-glycine) is the most abundant low-molecular-mass thiol, essential in antioxidant defense (Matés et al. 2012b).

The ratio between the reduced and oxidized form (GSH/GSSG) is the primary redox couple that determines the antioxidant capacity of cells (109). GSH and GSH/GSSG regulate many cellular events such as cell proliferation and apoptosis. Cellular GSH homeostasis is provided through (1) de novo synthesis from precursor sulfur amino acids methionine and cysteine, (2) regeneration from its oxidized form GSSG utilizing NADPH as a reductant, and (3) uptake of extracellular GSH via a Na+-dependent transport systems (34). Glutathione serves several vital functions, including (1) scavenging peroxides, (2) modulating key processes as cell proliferation, apoptosis, microtubular related events, and immunological function, (3) maintaining the essential thiol status of proteins by preventing oxidation of –SH groups or by reducing disulfide bonds induced by oxidative stress, (4) detoxifying electrophiles, and (5) affording a reservoir for cysteine (110).

Optimizing glutathione levels has been proposed as a strategy for health promotion and disease prevention, although clear, causal relationships between glutathione status and disease risk or treatment remain to be clarified (111). Nonetheless, human clinical research suggests that nutritional interventions, including amino acids, vitamins, minerals, phytochemicals, and foods, can have important effects on circulating glutathione which may translate to clinical benefits. Importantly, genetic variations modify the glutathione status and influence the response to nutritional factors that impact glutathione levels (111).

A factor influencing glutathione status is the degree of variability in an individual's capacity to produce glutathione, mainly due to genetic variability in enzymes involved in its production and/ or regeneration. The enzymes that have received increased attention in the scientific literature and within clinical medicine include glutathione-S-transferase and gamma-glutamyl transferase (111). While there may be a need to increase low levels of glutathione, proper balance, rather than excess, is required.

Minich et al provides an extensive review of the role of nutrition in support of GSH concentration (111). Oral intake of GSH has not consistently proven useful since it may be degraded by intestinal peptidases (111). GSH content varies considerably among foods. For example, among fruits and vegetables, asparagus, avocado, green beans, and spinach are high in GSH (112).

Chemical analyses show that dairy products, cereals, and breads are generally low in GSH; fruits and vegetables have moderate to high amounts of GSH; and freshly prepared meats are relatively high in GSH. Frozen foods generally had GSH contents similar to fresh foods, whereas other forms of processing and preservation generally resulted in extensive loss of GSH (113).

Jones et al. not only determined the concentration of GSH in different foods, but also the concentration of reactive chemicals that react with GHS (GHS reactive units, GRU). GRUs represent the amount GSH lost when incubating food homogenates with a known amount of GSH (114). For instance, the study identified some foods (e.g., blueberries, cherries, and prunes) that have relatively high concentrations of reactive chemicals, and others (e.g., freshly prepared meats) that have abundant levels of GSH and no GSH-reactive chemicals. These results imply that a specific reactive chemical may be a health risk if consumed with a diet high in GRUs but present a lower risk if consumed with a diet high in GSH. An alternative possibility is that exposure to reactive chemicals in the diet may be beneficial. Many reactive chemicals trigger detoxification and antioxidant mechanisms; thus, the intake of foods containing GRUs could enhance protection.

Another option to increase plasma GSH is to provide cysteine, the amino acid, which is rate limiting in GSH formation. N-acetylcysteine (NAC) is frequently studied and suggested as a supplement for glutathione support. Although NAC is promising as a supplement to both boost glutathione levels and potentially mitigate some of the issues related to oxidative stress, studies supplementing NAC have not been conclusive (115,116).

CONCLUSION

ROS are very short lived and are ideal participants in the regulation of physiological functions leading to changes in signaling outputs, enzyme activity, gene transcription and membrane and genome integrity. One major goal is to achieve a balance between the generation of ROS in response to metabolic demand and the availability of antioxidants to protect from oxidative damage. In physiological processes, there are two aspects to free radicals. In high concentrations, ROS can induce damage to macromolecules (lipid, carbohydrate, protein, and DNA) and initiate and promote cancer development. In low concentrations, they provide important regulatory functions to sustain health. Similar aspects are observed with antioxidants that can also function as pro-oxidants under certain conditions. The antioxidant capacity depends on a large network of nonenzymatic dietary and endogenous antioxidants and enzymatic reactions regenerating free radicals. A wide variety of dietary lipid-soluble and water-soluble antioxidants from fruits, nuts, and vegetable are necessary to sustain this antioxidant network. In addition, dietary sources of sulfur containing amino acids are needed to support the formation of glutathione and provide cysteine, an important redox switch. The antioxidant bioactive compounds provided by these foods also contribute to other functions supporting health such as anti-inflammation, DNA repair, phase II xenobiotic detoxification, and more.

In cancer cells energy metabolism is transformed to aerobic glycolysis to supply nucleotides for proliferation, and also to reduce oxidative phosphorylation-limiting mitochondrial ROS. Cells also divert glucose to the PPP, which generates the cofactor NADPH, needed for the antioxidant activity of glutathione. Eating a large amount of foods providing a wide variety of antioxidants appears to be important for cancer prevention. A recent meta-analysis demonstrated that cancer risk was significantly decreased with increased consumption of antioxidant nutrients from fruits and vegetable. However, randomized clinical trials are needed to support this finding.

Based on the increased energy turnover, cancer cells have increased intercellular concentrations of ROS that renders them vulnerable to oxidative stress, but leaves nontransformed cells resistant to oxidative damage. This vulnerability can be targeted by chemotherapeutic drugs generating ROS and possibly in combination with pro-oxidant redox compounds/antioxidants. Using this pro-oxidant capacity of dietary compounds is a novel and promising approach to cancer treatment.

REFERENCES

1. Mazard S, Penesyan A, Ostrowski M, Paulsen IT, Egan S. Tiny microbes with a big impact: the role of Cyanobacteria and their metabolites in shaping our future. *Marine Drugs* 2016;14(5):97. doi: 10.3390/md14050097.

2. Serra S, Anthony B, Boscolo Sesillo F, Masia A, Musacchi S. Determination of Post-Harvest Biochemical Composition, Enzymatic Activities, and Oxidative Browning in 14 Apple Cultivars. *Foods.* 2021;10(1):186.

3. Dai DF, Chiao YA, Marcinek DJ, Szeto HH, Rabinovitch PS. Mitochondrial oxidative stress in aging and healthspan. *Longevity & Healthspan* 2014;3:6. doi: 10.1186/2046-2395-3-6.

4. Wang Y, Hekimi S. Mitochondrial dysfunction and longevity in animals: untangling the knot. *Science* 2015;350(6265):1204–1207. doi: 10.1126/science.aac4357.

5. Holmstrom KM, Finkel T. Cellular mechanisms and physiological consequences of redox-dependent signalling. *Nature Reviews Molecular Cell Biology* 2014;15(6):411–421. doi: 10.1038/nrm3801.

6. Halliwell B. Biochemistry of oxidative stress. *Biochemical Society Transactions* 2007;35(Pt 5):1147–1150. doi: 10.1042/BST0351147.

7. Sies H, Berndt C, Jones DP. Oxidative stress. *Annual Review of Biochemistry* 2017;86:715–748. doi: 10.1146/annurev-biochem-061516-045037.

8. Go YM, Fernandes J, Hu X, Uppal K, Jones DP. Mitochondrial network responses in oxidative physiology and disease. *Free Radical Biology & Medicine* 2018;116:31–40. doi: 10.1016/j.freeradbiomed.2018.01.005.

9. Sies H, Jones DP. Reactive oxygen species (ROS) as pleiotropic physiological signalling agents. *Nature Reviews Molecular Cell Biology* 2020;21(7):363–383. doi: 10.1038/s41580-020-0230-3.

10. Turrens JF. Mitochondrial formation of reactive oxygen species. *The Journal of Physiology* 2003;552(Pt 2):335–344. doi: 10.1113/jphysiol.2003.049478.

11. Raimondi V, Ciccarese F, Ciminale V. Oncogenic pathways and the electron transport chain: a dangeROS liaison. *British Journal of Cancer* 2020;122(2):168–181. doi: 10.1038/s41416-019-0651-y.

12. Vertuani S, Angusti A, Manfredini S. The antioxidants and pro-antioxidants network: an overview. *Current Pharmaceutical Design* 2004;10(14):1677–1694. doi: 10.2174/1381612043384655.

13. Ali SS, Ahsan H, Zia MK, Siddiqui T, Khan FH. Understanding oxidants and antioxidants: classical team with new players. *Journal of Food Biochemistry* 2020;44(3):e13145. doi: 10.1111/jfbc.13145.

14. Yang CS, Ho CT, Zhang J, Wan X, Zhang K, Lim J. Antioxidants: differing meanings in food science and health science. *Journal of Agricultural and Food Chemistry* 2018;66(12):3063–3068. doi: 10.1021/acs.jafc.7b05830.

15. Purohit V, Simeone DM, Lyssiotis CA. Metabolic regulation of redox balance in cancer. *Cancers* 2019;11(7):955. doi: 10.3390/cancers11070955.

16. Carr A, Frei B. Does vitamin C act as a pro-oxidant under physiological conditions? *FASEB Journal* 1999;13(9):1007–1024. doi: 10.1096/fasebj.13.9.1007.

17. Liskova A, Stefanicka P, Samec M, Smejkal K, Zubor P, Bielik T, Biskupska-Bodova K, Kwon TK, Danko J, Busselberg D, Adamek, A., Rodrigo, L., Kruzliak, P., Shleikin, A., Kubatka, P. Dietary phytochemicals as the potential protectors against carcinogenesis and their role in cancer chemoprevention. *Clinical and Experimental Medicine* 2020;20(2):173–190. doi: 10.1007/s10238-020-00611-w.

18. Dennis KK, Go YM, Jones DP. Redox systems biology of nutrition and oxidative stress. *The Journal of Nutrition* 2019;149(4):553–565. doi: 10.1093/jn/nxy306.

19. Bergstrom T, Ersson C, Bergman J, Moller L. Vitamins at physiological levels cause oxidation to the DNA nucleoside deoxyguanosine and to DNA--alone or in synergism with metals. *Mutagenesis* 2012;27(4):511–517. doi: 10.1093/mutage/ges013.

20. Black HS, Boehm F, Edge R, Truscott TG. The benefits and risks of certain dietary carotenoids that exhibit both anti- and pro-oxidative mechanisms-a comprehensive review. *Antioxidants* 2020;9(3):264. doi: 10.3390/antiox9030264.

21. Pawlowska E, Szczepanska J, Blasiak J. Pro- and antioxidant effects of vitamin C in cancer in correspondence to its dietary and pharmacological concentrations. *Oxidative Medicine and Cellular Longevity* 2019;2019:7286737. doi: 10.1155/2019/7286737.

22. Shin J, Song MH, Oh JW, Keum YS, Saini RK. Pro-oxidant actions of carotenoids in triggering apoptosis of cancer cells: a review of emerging evidence. *Antioxidants* 2020;9(6):532. doi: 10.3390/antiox9060532.

23. Eghbaliferiz S, Iranshahi M. Prooxidant activity of polyphenols, flavonoids, anthocyanins and carotenoids: updated review of mechanisms and catalyzing metals. *Phytotherapy Research* 2016;30(9):1379–1391. doi: 10.1002/ptr.5643.

24. Mao X, Xiao X, Chen D, Yu B, He J. Tea and its components prevent cancer: a review of the redox-related mechanism. *International Journal of Molecular Sciences* 2019;20(21):5249. doi: 10.3390/ijms20215249.

25. Peto R, Doll R, Buckley JD, Sporn MB. Can dietary beta-carotene materially reduce human cancer rates? *Nature* 1981;290(5803):201–208. doi: 10.1038/290201a0.

26. Omenn GS, Goodman GE, Thornquist MD, Balmes J, Cullen MR, Glass A, Keogh JP, Meyskens FL, Jr., Valanis B, Williams JH, Jr., Barnhart S, Cherniack MG, Brodkin CA, Hammar S. Risk factors for lung cancer and for intervention effects in CARET, the beta-carotene and retinol efficacy trial. *Journal of the National Cancer Institute* 1996;88(21):1550–1559. doi: 10.1093/jnci/88.21.1550.

27. Alpha-Tocopherol BCCPSG. The effect of vitamin E and beta carotene on the incidence of lung cancer and other cancers in male smokers. *The New England Journal of Medicine* 1994;330(15):1029–1035. doi: 10.1056/NEJM199404143301501.

28. Kim SJ, Kim HS, Seo YR. Understanding of ROS-inducing strategy in anticancer therapy. *Oxidative Medicine and Cellular Longevity* 2019;2019:5381692. doi: 10.1155/2019/5381692.

29. Rodic S, Vincent MD. Reactive oxygen species (ROS) are a key determinant of cancer's metabolic phenotype. *International Journal of Cancer* 2018;142(3):440–448. doi: 10.1002/ijc.31069.

30. Li P, Wu M, Wang J, Sui Y, Liu S, Shi D. NAC selectively inhibit cancer telomerase activity: a higher redox homeostasis threshold exists in cancer cells. *Redox Biology* 2016;8:91–97. doi: 10.1016/j.redox.2015.12.001.

31. DeNicola GM, Karreth FA, Humpton TJ, Gopinathan A, Wei C, Frese K, Mangal D, Yu KH, Yeo CJ, Calhoun ES, Scrimieri F, Winter JM, Hruban RH, Iacobuzio-Donahue C, Kern SE, Blair IA, Tuveson DA. Oncogene-induced Nrf2 transcription promotes ROS detoxification and tumorigenesis. *Nature* 2011;475(7354):106–109. doi: 10.1038/nature10189.

32. Mitsuishi Y, Taguchi K, Kawatani Y, Shibata T, Nukiwa T, Aburatani H, Yamamoto M, Motohashi H. Nrf2 redirects glucose and glutamine into anabolic pathways in metabolic reprogramming. *Cancer Cell* 2012;22(1):66–79. doi: 10.1016/j.ccr.2012.05.016.

33. Mates JM, Campos-Sandoval JA, de Los Santos-Jimenez J, Segura JA, Alonso FJ, Marquez J. Metabolic reprogramming of cancer by chemicals that target glutaminase isoenzymes. *Current Medicinal Chemistry* 2020;27:5317–5339. doi: 10.2174/0929867326666190416165004.

34. Mates JM, Campos-Sandoval JA, Santos-Jimenez JL, Marquez J. Dysregulation of glutaminase and glutamine synthetase in cancer. *Cancer Letters* 2019;467:29–39. doi: 10.1016/j.canlet.2019.09.011.

35. Quiles JL, Sanchez-Gonzalez C, Vera-Ramirez L, Giampieri F, Navarro-Hortal MD, Xiao J, Llopis J, Battino M, Varela-Lopez A. Reductive stress, bioactive compounds, redox-active metals, and dormant tumor cell biology to develop redox-based tools for the treatment of cancer. *Antioxidants & Redox Signaling* 2020;33:860–881. doi: 10.1089/ars.2020.8051.

36. Kumari S, Badana AK, G MM, G S, Malla R. Reactive oxygen species: a key constituent in cancer survival. *Biomarker Insights* 2018;13:1177271918755391. doi: 10.1177/1177271918755391.

37. Perillo B, Di Donato M, Pezone A, Di Zazzo E, Giovannelli P, Galasso G, Castoria G, Migliaccio A. ROS in cancer therapy: the bright side of the moon. *Experimental & Molecular Medicine* 2020;52(2):192–203. doi: 10.1038/s12276-020-0384-2.

38. Moloney JN, Cotter TG. ROS signalling in the biology of cancer. *Seminars in Cell & Developmental Biology* 2018;80:50–64. doi: 10.1016/j.semcdb.2017.05.023.

39. Hayes JD, Dinkova-Kostova AT, Tew KD. Oxidative stress in cancer. *Cancer Cell* 2020;38(2):167–197. doi: 10.1016/j.ccell.2020.06.001.

40. Cockfield JA, Schafer ZT. Antioxidant defenses: a context-specific vulnerability of cancer cells. *Cancers* 2019;11(8):1208. doi: 10.3390/cancers11081208.

41. Buti S, Bersanelli M, Sikokis A, Maines F, Facchinetti F, Bria E, Ardizzoni A, Tortora G, Massari F. Chemotherapy in metastatic renal cell carcinoma today? A systematic review. *Anti-Cancer Drugs* 2013;24(6):535–554. doi: 10.1097/CAD.0b013e3283609ec1.

42. Lauby-Secretan B, Scoccianti C, Loomis D, Grosse Y, Bianchini F, Straif K, International Agency for Research on Cancer Handbook Working G. Body Fatness and Cancer--Viewpoint of the IARC Working Group. *The New England Journal of Medicine* 2016;375(8):794–798. doi: 10.1056/NEJMsr1606602.

43. Clinton SK, Giovannucci EL, Hursting SD. The World Cancer Research Fund/American Institute for Cancer Research Third Expert Report on Diet, Nutrition, Physical Activity, and Cancer: impact and future directions. *The Journal of Nutrition* 2020;150(4):663–671. doi: 10.1093/jn/nxz268.

44. Friedenreich CM, Ryder-Burbidge C, McNeil J. Physical activity, obesity and sedentary behavior in cancer etiology: epidemiologic evidence and biologic mechanisms. *Molecular Oncology* 2020;15. doi: 10.1002/1878-0261.12772.

45. Vasileva LV, Savova MS, Amirova KM, Dinkova-Kostova AT, Georgiev MI. Obesity and NRF2-mediated cytoprotection: where is the missing link? *Pharmacological Research* 2020;156:104760. doi: 10.1016/j.phrs.2020.104760.

46. Masschelin PM, Cox AR, Chernis N, Hartig SM. The impact of oxidative stress on adipose tissue energy balance. *Frontiers in Physiology* 2019;10:1638. doi: 10.3389/fphys.2019.01638.

47. Furukawa S, Fujita T, Shimabukuro M, Iwaki M, Yamada Y, Nakajima Y, Nakayama O, Makishima M, Matsuda M, Shimomura I. Increased oxidative stress in obesity and its impact on metabolic syndrome. *The Journal of Clinical Investigation* 2004;114(12):1752–1761. doi: 10.1172/JCI21625.

48. Anusruti A, Jansen E, Gao X, Xuan Y, Brenner H, Schottker B. Longitudinal associations of body mass index, waist circumference, and waist-to-hip ratio with biomarkers of oxidative stress in older adults: results of a large cohort study. *Obesity Facts* 2020;13(1):66–76. doi: 10.1159/000504711.

49. Bankoglu EE, Gerber J, Kodandaraman G, Seyfried F, Stopper H. Influence of bariatric surgery induced weight loss on oxidative DNA damage. *Mutation Research* 2020;853:503194. doi: 10.1016/j.mrgentox.2020.503194.

50. Cooke MS, Evans MD, Dizdaroglu M, Lunec J. Oxidative DNA damage: mechanisms, mutation, and disease. *FASEB Journal* 2003;17(10):1195–1214. doi: 10.1096/fj.02-0752rev.

51. Luperini BC, Almeida DC, Porto MP, Marcondes JP, Prado RP, Rasera I, Oliveira MR, Salvadori DM. Gene polymorphisms and increased DNA damage in morbidly obese women. *Mutation Research* 2015;776:111–117. doi: 10.1016/j.mrfmmm.2015.01.004.

52. Donmez-Altuntas H, Sahin F, Bayram F, Bitgen N, Mert M, Guclu K, Hamurcu Z, Aribas S, Gundogan K, Diri H. Evaluation of chromosomal damage, cytostasis, cytotoxicity, oxidative DNA damage and their association with body-mass index in obese subjects. *Mutation Research Genetic Toxicology and Environmental Mutagenesis* 2014;771:30–36. doi: 10.1016/j.mrgentox.2014.06.006.

53. Steck SE, Murphy EA. Dietary patterns and cancer risk. *Nature Reviews Cancer* 2020;20(2):125–138. doi: 10.1038/s41568-019-0227-4.

54. Yang CS, Chen JX, Wang H, Lim J. Lessons learned from cancer prevention studies with nutrients and non-nutritive dietary constituents. *Molecular Nutrition & Food Research* 2016;60(6):1239–1250. doi: 10.1002/mnfr.201500766.

55. Key TJ. Fruit and vegetables and cancer risk. *British Journal of Cancer* 2011;104(1):6–11. doi: 10.1038/sj.bjc.6606032.

56. Das A, Hsu MSH, Rangan A, Hirani V. Dietary or supplemental intake of antioxidants and the risk of mortality in older people: a systematic review. *Nutrition & Dietetics* 2020;78:24–40. doi: 10.1111/1747-0080.12611.

57. Leenders M, Siersema PD, Overvad K, Tjonneland A, Olsen A, Boutron-Ruault MC, Bastide N, Fagherazzi G, Katzke V, Kuhn T, Boeing H, Aleksandrova K, Trichopoulou A, Lagiou P, Klinaki E, Masala G, Grioni S, Santucci De Magistris M, Tumino R, Ricceri F, Peeters PH, Lund E, Skeie G, Weiderpass E, Quirós JR, Agudo A, Sánchez MJ, Dorronsoro M, Navarro C, Ardanaz E, Ohlsson B, Jirström K, Van Guelpen B, Wennberg M, Khaw KT, Wareham N, Key TJ, Romieu I, Huybrechts I, Cross AJ, Murphy N, Riboli E, Bueno-de-Mesquita HB. Subtypes of fruit and vegetables, variety in consumption and risk of colon and rectal cancer in the European Prospective Investigation into Cancer and Nutrition. *International Journal of Cancer* 2015;137(11):2705–2714. doi: 10.1002/ijc.29640.

58. Bates CJ, Hamer M, Mishra GD. Redox-modulatory vitamins and minerals that prospectively predict mortality in older British people: the National Diet and Nutrition Survey of people aged 65 years and over. *The British Journal of Nutrition* 2011;105(1):123–132. doi: 10.1017/S0007114510003053.

59. Genkinger JM, Platz EA, Hoffman SC, Comstock GW, Helzlsouer KJ. Fruit, vegetable, and antioxidant intake and all-cause, cancer, and cardiovascular disease mortality in a community-dwelling population in Washington County, Maryland. *American Journal of Epidemiology* 2004;160(12):1223–1233. doi: 10.1093/aje/kwh339.

60. Shibata A, Paganini-Hill A, Ross RK, Henderson BE. Intake of vegetables, fruits, beta-carotene, vitamin C and vitamin supplements and cancer incidence among the elderly: a prospective study. *British Journal of Cancer* 1992;66(4):673–679. doi: 10.1038/bjc.1992.336.

61. Stepaniak U, Micek A, Grosso G, Stefler D, Topor-Madry R, Kubinova R, Malyutina S, Peasey A, Pikhart H, Nikitin Y, Bobak M, Pająk A. Antioxidant vitamin intake and mortality in three Central and Eastern European urban populations: the HAPIEE study. *European Journal of Nutrition* 2016;55(2):547–560. doi: 10.1007/s00394-015-0871-8.

62. Aune D, Keum N, Giovannucci E, Fadnes LT, Boffetta P, Greenwood DC, Tonstad S, Vatten LJ, Riboli E, Norat T. Dietary intake and blood concentrations of antioxidants and the risk of cardiovascular disease, total cancer, and all-cause mortality: a systematic review and dose-response meta-analysis of prospective studies. *The American Journal of Clinical Nutrition* 2018;108(5):1069–1091. doi: 10.1093/ajcn/nqy097.

63. Aune D, Giovannucci E, Boffetta P, Fadnes LT, Keum N, Norat T, Greenwood DC, Riboli E, Vatten LJ, Tonstad S. Fruit and vegetable intake and the risk of cardiovascular disease, total cancer and all-cause mortality-a systematic review and dose-response meta-analysis of prospective studies. *International Journal of Epidemiology* 2017;46(3):1029–1056. doi: 10.1093/ije/dyw319.

64. Traber MG, Atkinson J. Vitamin E, antioxidant and nothing more. *Free Radical Biology & Medicine* 2007;43(1):4–15. doi: 10.1016/j.freeradbiomed.2007.03.024.

65. Traber MG. Vitamin E regulatory mechanisms. *Annual Review of Nutrition* 2007;27:347–362. doi: 10.1146/annurev.nutr.27.061406.093819.

66. Bolling BW, McKay DL, Blumberg JB. The phytochemical composition and antioxidant actions of tree nuts. *Asia Pacific Journal of Clinical Nutrition* 2010;19(1):117–123.

67. Dietrich M, Traber MG, Jacques PF, Cross CE, Hu Y, Block G. Does gamma-tocopherol play a role in the primary prevention of heart disease and cancer? A review. *Journal of the American College of Nutrition* 2006;25(4):292–299. doi: 10.1080/07315724.2006.10719538.

68. Yang CS, Luo P, Zeng Z, Wang H, Malafa M, Suh N. Vitamin E and cancer prevention: studies with different forms of tocopherols and tocotrienols. *Molecular Carcinogenesis* 2020;59(4):365–389. doi: 10.1002/mc.23160.

69. Lee IM, Cook NR, Gaziano JM, Gordon D, Ridker PM, Manson JE, Hennekens CH, Buring JE. Vitamin E in the primary prevention of cardiovascular disease and cancer: the Women's Health Study: a randomized controlled trial. *JAMA* 2005;294(1):56–65. doi: 10.1001/jama.294.1.56.

70. Wang L, Sesso HD, Glynn RJ, Christen WG, Bubes V, Manson JE, Buring JE, Gaziano JM. Vitamin E and C supplementation and risk of cancer in men: posttrial follow-up in the Physicians' Health Study II randomized trial. *The American Journal of Clinical Nutrition* 2014;100(3):915–923. doi: 10.3945/ajcn.114.085480.

71. Lippman SM, Klein EA, Goodman PJ, Lucia MS, Thompson IM, Ford LG, Parnes HL, Minasian LM, Gaziano JM, Hartline JA, Parsons JK, Bearden JD 3rd, Crawford ED, Goodman GE, Claudio J, Winquist E, Cook ED, Karp DD, Walther P, Lieber MM, Kristal AR, Darke AK, Arnold KB, Ganz PA, Santella RM, Albanes D, Taylor PR, Probstfield JL, Jagpal TJ, Crowley JJ, Meyskens FL Jr, Baker LH, Coltman CA Jr. Effect of selenium and vitamin E on risk of prostate cancer and other cancers: the Selenium and Vitamin E Cancer Prevention Trial (SELECT). *JAMA* 2009;301(1):39–51. doi: 10.1001/jama.2008.864.

72. Chan JM, Darke AK, Penney KL, Tangen CM, Goodman PJ, Lee GM, Sun T, Peisch S, Tinianow AM, Rae JM, Klein, EA, Thompson Jr, IM, Kantoff, PM, Mucci, LA. Selenium- or vitamin E-related gene variants, interaction with supplementation, and risk of high-grade prostate cancer in SELECT. *Cancer Epidemiology, Biomarkers & Prevention* 2016;25(7):1050–1058. doi: 10.1158/1055-9965.EPI-16-0104.

73. Jiang Q. Natural forms of vitamin E and metabolites-regulation of cancer cell death and underlying mechanisms. *IUBMB Life* 2019;71(4):495–506. doi: 10.1002/iub.1978.

74. Violet PC, Ebenuwa IC, Wang Y, Niyyati M, Padayatty SJ, Head B, Wilkins K, Chung S, Thakur V, Ulatowski L, Atkinson J, Ghelfi M, Smith, S, Tu, H, Bobe, G, Liu, C-Y, Herion, DW, Shamburek,RD, Manor, D, Traber, MG, Levine, M. Vitamin E sequestration by liver fat in humans. *JCI Insight* 2020;5(1). doi: 10.1172/jci.insight.133309.

75. Suzuki A, Diehl AM. Nonalcoholic steatohepatitis. *Annual Review of Medicine* 2017;68:85–98. doi: 10.1146/annurev-med-051215-031109.

76. Saini RK, Keum YS, Daglia M, Rengasamy KR. Dietary carotenoids in cancer chemoprevention and chemotherapy: a review of emerging evidence. *Pharmacological Research* 2020;157:104830. doi: 10.1016/j.phrs.2020.104830.

77. Saini RK, Rengasamy KRR, Mahomoodally FM, Keum YS. Protective effects of lycopene in cancer, cardiovascular, and neurodegenerative diseases: an update on epidemiological and mechanistic perspectives. *Pharmacological Research* 2020;155:104730. doi: 10.1016/j.phrs.2020.104730.

78. Rowles JL, 3rd, Erdman JW, Jr. Carotenoids and their role in cancer prevention. *Biochimica et biophysica acta Molecular and Cell Biology of Lipids* 2020;1865(11):158613. doi: 10.1016/j.bbalip.2020.158613.

79. Shardell MD, Alley DE, Hicks GE, El-Kamary SS, Miller RR, Semba RD, Ferrucci L. Low-serum carotenoid concentrations and carotenoid interactions predict mortality in US adults: the Third National Health and Nutrition Examination Survey. *Nutrition Research* 2011;31(3):178–189. doi: 10.1016/j.nutres.2011.03.003.

80. Gansukh E, Nile A, Sivanesan I, Rengasamy KRR, Kim DH, Keum YS, Saini RK. Chemopreventive effect of beta-cryptoxanthin on human cervical carcinoma (HeLa) cells is modulated through oxidative stress-induced apoptosis. *Antioxidants* 2019;9(1):28. doi: 10.3390/antiox9010028.

81. Gansukh E, Mya KK, Jung M, Keum YS, Kim DH, Saini RK. Lutein derived from marigold (Tagetes erecta) petals triggers ROS generation and activates Bax and caspase-3 mediated apoptosis of human cervical carcinoma (HeLa) cells. *Food and Chemical Toxicology* 2019;127:11–18. doi: 10.1016/j.fct.2019.02.037.

82. Rowles JL, 3rd, Ranard KM, Smith JW, An R, Erdman JW, Jr. Increased dietary and circulating lycopene are associated with reduced prostate cancer risk: a systematic review and meta-analysis. *Prostate Cancer and Prostatic Diseases* 2017;20(4):361–377. doi: 10.1038/pcan.2017.25.

83. Petimar J, Wilson KM, Wu K, Wang M, Albanes D, van den Brandt PA, Cook MB, Giles GG, Giovannucci EL, Goodman GE, Håkansson,N, Helzlsouer, k, Key, TJ, Kolonel, LN, Liao, LM, Männistö, S, McCullough, ML, Milne, RL, Neuhouser, ML, Park, Y, Platz, EA, Riboli, E, Sawada, N, Schenk, JM, Tsugane, S, Verhage, B, Wang, Y, Wilkens, LR, Wolk, A, Ziegler, RG, Smith-Warner, SA. A pooled analysis of 15 prospective cohort studies on the association between fruit, vegetable, and mature bean consumption and risk of prostate cancer. *Cancer Epidemiology, Biomarkers & Prevention* 2017;26(8):1276–1287. doi: 10.1158/1055-9965.EPI-16-1006.

84. Rowles JL, 3rd, Ranard KM, Applegate CC, Jeon S, An R, Erdman JW, Jr. Processed and raw tomato consumption and risk of prostate cancer: a systematic review and dose-response meta-analysis. *Prostate Cancer and Prostatic Diseases* 2018;21(3):319–336. doi: 10.1038/s41391-017-0005-x.

85. Zhang X, Spiegelman D, Baglietto L, Bernstein L, Boggs DA, van den Brandt PA, Buring JE, Gapstur SM, Giles GG, Giovannucci E, Goodman G, Hankinson SE, Helzlsouer KJ, Horn-Ross PL, Inoue M, Jung S, Khudyakov P, Larsson SC, Lof M, McCullough ML, Miller AB, Neuhouser ML, Palmer JR, Park Y, Robien K, Rohan TE, Ross JA, Schouten LJ, Shikany JM, Tsugane S, Visvanathan K, Weiderpass E, Wolk A, Willett WC, Zhang SM, Ziegler RG, Smith-Warner SA. Carotenoid intakes and risk of breast cancer defined by estrogen receptor and progesterone receptor status: a pooled analysis of 18 prospective cohort studies. *The American Journal of Clinical Nutrition* 2012;95(3):713–725. doi: 10.3945/ajcn.111.014415.

86. Maillard V, Kuriki K, Lefebvre B, Boutron-Ruault MC, Lenoir GM, Joulin V, Clavel-Chapelon F, Chajes V. Serum carotenoid, tocopherol and retinol concentrations and breast cancer risk in the E3N-EPIC study. *International Journal of Cancer* 2010;127(5):1188–1196. doi: 10.1002/ijc.25138.

87. Rowe S, Carr AC. Global vitamin C status and prevalence of deficiency: a cause for concern? *Nutrients* 2020;12(7):2008. doi: 10.3390/nu12072008.

88. Frei B, England L, Ames BN. Ascorbate is an outstanding antioxidant in human blood plasma. *Proceedings of the National Academy of Sciences of the United States of America* 1989;86(16):6377–6381. doi: 10.1073/pnas.86.16.6377.

89. Hecht SS. Approaches to cancer prevention based on an understanding of N-nitrosamine carcinogenesis. *Proceedings of the Society for Experimental Biology and Medicine Society for Experimental Biology and Medicine* 1997;216(2):181–191. doi: 10.3181/00379727-216-44168.

90. Cameron E, Pauling L. The orthomolecular treatment of cancer. I. The role of ascorbic acid in host resistance. *Chemico-Biological Interactions* 1974;9(4):273–283. doi: 10.1016/0009-2797(74)90018-0.

91. Cameron E, Pauling L. Supplemental ascorbate in the supportive treatment of cancer: Prolongation of survival times in terminal human cancer. *Proceedings of the National Academy of Sciences of the United States of America* 1976;73(10):3685–3689. doi: 10.1073/pnas.73.10.3685.

92. Moertel CG, Fleming TR, Creagan ET, Rubin J, O'Connell MJ, Ames MM. High-dose vitamin C versus placebo in the treatment of patients with advanced cancer who have had no prior chemotherapy. A randomized double-blind comparison. *The New England Journal of Medicine* 1985;312(3):137–141. doi: 10.1056/NEJM198501173120301.

93. Abiri B, Vafa M. Vitamin C and cancer: the role of vitamin C in disease progression and quality of life in cancer patients. *Nutrition and Cancer* 2020:1–11. doi: 10.1080/01635581.2020.1795692.

94. Padayatty SJ, Riordan HD, Hewitt SM, Katz A, Hoffer LJ, Levine M. Intravenously administered vitamin C as cancer therapy: three cases. *CMAJ* 2006;174(7):937–942. doi: 10.1503/cmaj.050346.

95. Vissers MCM, Das AB. Potential mechanisms of action for vitamin C in cancer: reviewing the evidence. *Frontiers in Physiology* 2018;9:809. doi: 10.3389/fphys.2018.00809.

96. Hoffer LJ, Robitaille L, Zakarian R, Melnychuk D, Kavan P, Agulnik J, Cohen V, Small D, Miller WH, Jr. High-dose intravenous vitamin C combined with cytotoxic chemotherapy in patients with advanced cancer: a phase I-II clinical trial. *PLoS One* 2015;10(4):e0120228. doi: 10.1371/journal.pone.0120228.

97. Chang H, Lei L, Zhou Y, Ye F, Zhao G. Dietary flavonoids and the risk of colorectal cancer: an updated meta-analysis of epidemiological studies. *Nutrients* 2018;10(7):950. doi: 10.3390/nu10070950.

98. Pietta PG. Flavonoids as antioxidants. *Journal of Natural Products* 2000;63(7):1035–1042. doi: 10.1021/np9904509.

99. Griffiths K, Aggarwal BB, Singh RB, Buttar HS, Wilson D, De Meester F. Food antioxidants and their anti-inflammatory properties: a potential role in cardiovascular diseases and cancer prevention. *Diseases* 2016;4(3):28. doi: 10.3390/diseases4030028.

100. Bondonno NP, Dalgaard F, Kyro C, Murray K, Bondonno CP, Lewis JR, Croft KD, Gislason G, Scalbert A, Cassidy A, Piccini, JP, Overvad, K, Hodgson, JM, Dalgaard, F. Flavonoid intake is associated with lower mortality in the Danish Diet Cancer and Health Cohort. *Nature Communications* 2019;10(1):3651. doi: 10.1038/s41467-019-11622-x.

101. NavaneethaKrishnan S, Rosales JL, Lee KY. ROS-mediated cancer cell killing through dietary phytochemicals. *Oxidative Medicine and Cellular Longevity* 2019;2019:9051542. doi: 10.1155/2019/9051542.

102. Filippini T, Malavolti M, Borrelli F, Izzo AA, Fairweather-Tait SJ, Horneber M, Vinceti M. Green tea (Camellia sinensis) for the prevention of cancer. The Cochrane database of systematic reviews 2020;(3):CD005004. doi: 10.1002/14651858.CD005004.pub3.

103. Nosrati N, Bakovic M, Paliyath G. Molecular mechanisms and pathways as targets for cancer prevention and progression with dietary compounds. *International Journal of Molecular Sciences* 2017;18(10):2050. doi: 10.3390/ijms18102050.

104. Pellegrini N, Vitaglione P, Granato D, Fogliano V. Twenty-five years of total antioxidant capacity measurement of foods and biological fluids: merits and limitations. *Journal of the Science of Food and Agriculture* 2020;100:5064–5078. doi: 10.1002/jsfa.9550.

105. Ha K, Kim K, Sakaki JR, Chun OK. Relative validity of dietary total antioxidant capacity for predicting all-cause mortality in comparison to diet quality indexes in US adults. *Nutrients* 2020;12(5):1210. doi: 10.3390/nu12051210.

106. Lucas AL, Bosetti C, Boffetta P, Negri E, Tavani A, Serafini M, Polesel J, Serraino D, La Vecchia C, Rossi M. Dietary total antioxidant capacity and pancreatic cancer risk: an Italian case-control study. *British Journal of Cancer* 2016;115(1):102–107. doi: 10.1038/bjc.2016.114.

107. Vance TM, Wang Y, Su LJ, Fontham ET, Steck SE, Arab L, Bensen JT, Mohler JL, Chen MH, Chun OK. Dietary total antioxidant capacity is inversely associated with prostate cancer aggressiveness in a population-based study. *Nutrition and Cancer* 2016;68(2):214–224. doi: 10.1080/01635581.2016.1134596.

108. Hernandez-Ruiz A, Garcia-Villanova B, Guerra-Hernandez E, Amiano P, Ruiz-Canela M, Molina-Montes E. A review of a priori defined oxidative balance scores relative to their components and impact on health outcomes. *Nutrients* 2019;11(4):774. doi: 10.3390/nu11040774.

109. Lora J, Alonso FJ, Segura JA, Lobo C, Marquez J, Mates JM. Antisense glutaminase inhibition decreases glutathione antioxidant capacity and increases apoptosis in Ehrlich ascitic tumour cells. *European Journal of Biochemistry* 2004;271(21):4298–4306. doi: 10.1111/j.1432-1033.2004.04370.x.

110. Mates JM, Campos-Sandoval JA, de Los Santos-Jimenez J, Marquez J. Glutaminases regulate glutathione and oxidative stress in cancer. *Archives of Toxicology* 2020;94(8):2603–2623. doi: 10.1007/s00204-020-02838-8.

111. Minich DM, Brown BI. A review of dietary (phyto)nutrients for glutathione support. *Nutrients* 2019;11(9):2073. doi: 10.3390/nu11092073.

112. Demirkol O, Adams C, Ercal N. Biologically important thiols in various vegetables and fruits. *Journal of Agricultural and Food Chemistry* 2004;52(26):8151–8154. doi: 10.1021/jf040266f.

113. Jones DP, Coates RJ, Flagg EW, Eley JW, Block G, Greenberg RS, Gunter EW, Jackson B. Glutathione in foods listed in the National Cancer Institute's Health Habits and History Food Frequency Questionnaire. *Nutrition and Cancer* 1992;17(1):57–75. doi: 10.1080/01635589209514173.

114. He M, Openo K, McCullough M, Jones DP. Total equivalent of reactive chemicals in 142 human food items is highly variable within and between major food groups. *The Journal of Nutrition* 2004;134(5):1114–1119. doi: 10.1093/jn/134.5.1114.

115. Zhang Q, Ju Y, Ma Y, Wang T. N-acetylcysteine improves oxidative stress and inflammatory response in patients with community acquired pneumonia: A randomized controlled trial. *Medicine* 2018;97(45):e13087. doi: 10.1097/MD.0000000000013087.

116. Rushworth GF, Megson IL. Existing and potential therapeutic uses for N-acetylcysteine: the need for conversion to intracellular glutathione for antioxidant benefits. *Pharmacology & Therapeutics* 2014;141(2):150–159. doi: 10.1016/j.pharmthera.2013.09.006.

9 Nutrition, Angiogenesis, and Cancer

William W. Li and Elad Mashiach
The Angiogenesis Foundation

CONTENTS

INTRODUCTION

The origins of anti-cancer therapy based on the inhibition of angiogenesis or neovascularization were pioneered as an original concept in 1971 by Dr. Judah Folkman at the Harvard Medical School (Folkman 1971). The work of this visionary pioneer of angiogenesis research whose ideas were initially dismissed by the medical community established the fundamental laboratory tools to study blood vessel growth, starting with culturing vascular endothelial cells, developing in vivo models for angiogenesis, purifying the first angiogenic growth factors, and discovering the first angiogenesis inhibitors which could interfere with tumor growth. His research formed the foundation of antiangiogenic therapy (Li et al. 2018). There are now more than one dozen Food and Drug Administration (FDA)-approved antiangiogenic agents used routinely to treat thyroid, lung, brain, colorectal, renal, gastrointestinal stromal tumors, and other cancers.

The same methodologies used to develop antiangiogenic drugs have been used to validate the angiogenesis inhibitory effects of dietary factors. This chapter will review basic, clinical, and epidemiological studies relating nutrients and diets to the inhibition of angiogenesis. These insights now set the stage for a new approach to nutritional oncology through the application of antiangiogenic foods and nutrients.

NUTRIENTS AND ANGIOGENESIS

Vascular biologists led by Theodore Fotsis studied the urine of farmers in Japan and detected a chromatographic peak that could only have originated from dietary sources. The farmers, living in a village outside of Kyoto, were vegetarians who consumed a plant-based diet high in soy products. The peak was isolated and identified as the phytoestrogen genistein which is present in soy. Genistein was tested in cell cultures of vascular endothelial cells and found to potently inhibit angiogenesis (Fotsis et al. 1998). This study was the first to demonstrate that a factor present in foods could inhibit angiogenesis. Subsequently, bioactive molecules present in licorice, cinnamon, garlic, and many other plant-based and marine-sourced foods have also been described with antiangiogenic activity.

The Angiogenesis Foundation has evaluated more than 20 dietary factors studied in angiogenesis assays at the US National Cancer Institute and demonstrated their activity in suppressing vascular endothelial growth at levels comparable to some cancer drugs (Li et al. 2012). A further connection between natural sources and angiogenesis was recognized by Eric Dupont in Quebec who developed an antiangiogenic extract, AE941, from elasmobranchs, the family of cartilaginous fishes including sharks, rays, and skates—a bycatch of the Canadian fisheries industry. This compound showed significantly improved survival in patients with advanced lung, breast, and colorectal cancer (CRC) in Phase II clinical trials (Miller et al. 1998). Further commercial development of the compound was abandoned by the sponsor while it was in a Phase III study. A study of the labels found on 29 shark cartilage supplements on the market found that about half were in violation of labelling regulations for dietary supplements with the most common issue being unverified disease claims (Isaacs and Hellberg 2019). While compounds within the shark cartilage have been found to inhibit angiogenesis, its proper role in clinical cancer therapy has yet to be established.

ANGIOGENESIS AND CARCINOGENESIS

Angiogenesis is necessary for tumor growth and metastatic progression. The discovery of the first specific angiogenic cytokine, VEGF, in 1989 paved the way for the clinical approval of the first antiangiogenic tumor drug 15 years later. Understanding the various stages involved in the development of tumor blood vessels through angiogenesis, and the association with inflammation through the actions of endothelial cells sets the stage for exploring the effects of dietary factors on angiogenesis.

All cells in the body exist near capillaries at a distance of no more than 100–200 μm, and the diffusion limit of oxygen and reduced oxygenation in tumors leads to the development of blood vessels via angiogenesis (Vaupel and Mayer 2017). In addition to structural support for the circulatory delivery of oxygen and nutrients, the vascular endothelial cells lining blood vessels secrete paracrine and survival signals that maintain organ viability (Eelen et al. 2015). Cancer cells secrete high levels of proangiogenic factors which lead to the development of a vascular network made up of disorganized, immature, and permeable blood vessels, resulting in poor tumor perfusion (Zhang et al. 2019).

The hypoxic microenvironment created by impaired tumor perfusion can promote the selection of more invasive and aggressive tumor cells and can also impede the tumor-killing action of immune cells (Riera-Domingo et al. 2020, Barsoum et al. 2014). Reduced tumor perfusion as a result of disorganized vasculature also reduces the diffusion of chemotherapeutic drugs into the tumor as well as reducing the effectiveness of radiotherapy (Viallard and Larrivee 2017). Cancer cells have increased metabolic demands that require the induction of new blood vessels to facilitate malignant expansion (Intlekofer and Finley 2019, DeBerardinis and Chandel 2016). Targeting angiogenesis suppresses the growth of primary tumors and the occurrence of metastases (Zhao and Adjei 2015, Folkman 2002).

The association between inflammation and cancer is well-recognized, but what is less widely appreciated is that angiogenesis promotes both inflammation and carcinogenesis. In 1863, Rudolf Virchow reported that some cancers were infiltrated by white blood cells, leading to the hypothesis that inflammation is associated with cancer. Infections with a number of infectious agents including *Helicobacter pylori* and human papillomavirus (HPV) are causally linked to cancer. Chronic inflammation without infection can also be induced by asbestos, ultraviolet light, and silica crystals leading to tumor development (Aguilar-Cazares et al. 2019).

During chronic and sustained inflammation, pathological angiogenesis can be initiated (Carmeliet and Jain 2011) leading to immune cell interactions with endothelial cells which promote both angiogenesis and tumor development. Vascular endothelial growth factor (VEGF) modifies the endothelial barrier (Shibuya 2013, Melincovici et al. 2018). VEGF is secreted by neutrophils, platelets, macrophages, activated-T cells, dendritic cells, pericytes, and the endothelial cells themselves (Lapeyre-Prost et al. 2017). Five members of the VEGF family have been identified, namely, VEGF-A, VEGF-B, VEGF-C, VEGF-D, and placenta growth factor (PlGF) (Takahashi and Shibuya 2005, Melincovici et al. 2018). VEGF-A is the most potent stimulator of angiogenesis (Lapeyre-Prost et al. 2017). In addition to increased vascular permeability, vasodilatation, and the recruitment of inflammatory cells, VEGF triggers the inhibition of apoptosis and increases cellular proliferation (Lapeyre-Prost et al. 2017).

VEGF acts through high-affinity tyrosine kinase receptors VEGFR-1, VEGFR-2, and VEGFR-3. VEGFR-2 is expressed primarily in endothelial cells and its interaction with VEGF-A triggers increased vascular permeability. VEGFR-2 dimerization induces the autophosphorylation of tyrosine residues and the activation of specific signaling pathways, including the PI3K and p38 MAPK pathways (Takahashi and Shibuya 2005, Melincovici et al. 2018).

Three specific windows exist for targeting tumor angiogenesis with dietary strategies: (1) the prevascularized phase; (2) the angiogenic switch; and (3) the vascularized phase (see Figure 9.1).

During the prevascularized phase, incipient tumors with 60–80 cells obtain their nutrients and oxygen supply by diffusion. While this limits their growth potential, they can migrate toward existing host vessels through a process known as vessel co-option (Eelen et al. 2015, Folkman 2002). With this new supply of oxygen and nutrients, tumors remain largely microscopic containing 500,000–1,000,000 cells, expanding to at most 2 mm in diameter before metabolic demand outstrips their oxygen and nutrient supplies. This state corresponds to carcinoma *in situ*, where the rate of tumor cell proliferation is balanced by tumor cell apoptosis (Holmgren, O'Reilly, and Folkman 1995, Pezzuto and Carico 2018).

Cancer can exist in this dormant state for long periods. Immune surveillance as part of healthy immune function, and influenced by the gut microbiome, can eventually eliminate most of these dormant microscopic cancers without the development of clinically detectable tumors. Angiogenesis inhibitors can interrupt the multistep process of carcinogenesis at this stage and prevent further progression to clinically evident tumors (Lin, Zhang, and Luo 2016).

There are many examples of such preinvasive lesions, including breast ductal carcinoma *in situ*, cervical intraepithelial neoplasia, actinic keratosis in the skin, Barrett's esophagus, squamous metaplasia with dysplasia in bronchial mucosa, premalignant colon adenoma, and high-grade prostate intraepithelial neoplasia (HGPIN) (Solin 2019, Siegel, Korgavkar, and Weinstock 2017, Verlaat et al. 2018, Bujanda and Hachem 2018, Rigden et al. 2016, Thiruvengadam and Thiruvengadam 2018, Zhou 2018).

Microscopic cancers can also be found incidentally in patients undergoing surgery to resect a primary cancer. Up to 25% of colon cancer patients, for example, may eventually develop hepatic metastases after primary tumor resection (Qiu et al. 2015). Suppressing tumor neovascularization at subclinical stages can restrict cancer to a dormant, microscopic state to enable the immune system to eliminate malignant cells (Holmgren 1996, Naumov et al. 2008). Cancer chemoprevention utilizing drugs such as celecoxib (Celebrex), tamoxifen (Nolvadex), and raloxifene (Evista) that

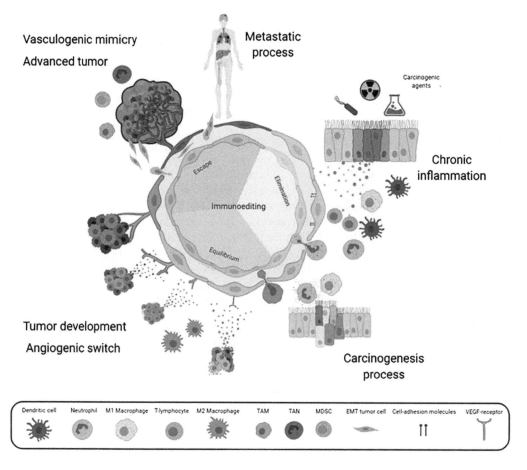

FIGURE 9.1 Angiogenesis, chronic inflammation, and cancer. Sustained inflammation leads to reactive oxygen species damage to cells and initiates carcinogenesis. The metabolic demands of tumor cells lead to hypoxia and stimulation of angiogenesis leading to the angiogenic switch; while, immune cell infiltration now promotes tumor growth (Escape phase). At advanced cancer stages, tumor mass viability is maintained by sustained angiogenesis. Leaky endothelium in the new blood vessels enables immune cell extravasation. The complex and dynamic tumor microenvironment promotes phenotypic changes into aggressive tumors generating metastatic foci. Three specific windows exist for targeting tumor angiogenesis with dietary strategies: the prevascularized phase; the angiogenic switch; and the vascularized phase. The intensity of the color represents the gradual activation of the endothelium in the figure above (Aguilar-Cazares et al. 2019).

are known to possess antiangiogenic activity (Garvin and Dabrosin 2003, Masferrer et al. 2000, Navarro, Mirkin, and Archer 2003) are already in clinical use. Foods with antiangiogenic properties could find application at this stage of cancer development as well.

Tumor progression from dormancy to clinical cancer is dependent on the recruitment of blood vessels through a process known as the angiogenic switch. Once new blood vessels are present with endothelial cells effects on the tumor microenvironment and its different components, progression to clinical cancer occurs. Therefore, the angiogenic switch is a potential target for inhibiting angiogenesis through drugs or dietary factors (Li et al. 2012, Baeriswyl and Christofori 2009).

Three classic studies have established the steps involved in this switch. The first study involved a mouse model (Rip1-Tag2 transgenic mice) of spontaneous β-islet cell tumor formation (Hanahan and Folkman 1996, Hanahan 1985). The transformed β-cells expressed an oncogene which resulted in up to 70% of these islets becoming hyperplastic. Angiogenesis was observed between the hyperplastic stage and the time at which subset islets became invasive cancers.

Notably, some of the islets remained nonangiogenic, and they did not grow beyond 0.6–0.8 mm^3 in size (Folkman et al. 1989). The second study involved a transgenic mouse model of dermal fibrosarcoma (Lacey, Alpert, and Hanahan 1986, Kandel et al. 1991). Distinct stages of cancer development were observed ranging from normal to hyperplasia with mild and aggressive fibromas to frank neoplasia with fibrosarcoma. The prevascular fibromas could only form as thin lesions, whereas the fibrosarcomas were invasive and rich with blood vessels. A third study in K14-HPV16 transgenic mice expressing the HPV type 16 oncogene targeted to basal cells of the epidermis, showed keratinocytes undergoing sequential changes ranging from normal with no vascularization to hyperplasia with mild vascularization from underlying dermis to dysplasia with abundant vessels, and ultimately to squamous cell carcinoma with intense angiogenesis (Bergers, Hanahan, and Coussens 1998). At all phases, angiogenesis was associated with mast cells containing angiogenic stimulatory factors including MCP-4, VEGF, bFGF, transforming growth factor-β (TGF-β), tumor necrosis factor-alpha (TNF-α), and IL-8 (Coussens et al. 1999, Norrby 2002, Cimpean et al. 2017). The angiogenic factor, VEGF, was increased in dysplasia and in carcinoma (Smith-McCune et al. 1997).

The angiogenic switch is a focal target for interference utilizing angiogenesis inhibitors. While it is pragmatically not feasible in the clinical setting to deliver an intervention just at the moment of angiogenic switching, the models described above lend themselves to laboratory and preclinical testing of drugs, nutrients, and whole food extracts with antiangiogenic activity.

At the next stage, during angiogenic tumor progression, pathological capillary growth toward cancer cells can be halted. The velocity of this capillary growth ranges from 0.223 to 0.8 mm/day, and their penetration of the tumor mass can support expansion (Folkman 1985, Wurschmidt, Beck-Bornholdt, and Vogler 1990, Yamaura, Yamada, and Matsuzawa 1976, Gimbrone et al. 1972). It is estimated that each endothelial cell can support the metabolic needs of up to 100 cancer cells, while these vessels occupy less than 2% of tumor volume (Folkman 1996, Modzelewski et al. 1994, Thompson et al. 1987). The same vascular network that feeds cancer cells also facilitates metastases through hematogenous spread (Fidler and Ellis 1994). Experimental studies have shown that a 1 cm tumor shed millions of cancer cells into the circulation every 24 hours (Butler and Gullino 1975). Most pharmacological inhibitors of angiogenesis have been studied and developed to interfere with tumor growth during in this vascularized phase of tumor growth (see Table 9.1).

TABLE 9.1
Pharmacological Inhibitors of Angiogenesis

	Indication (Country-If Abroad)	Mechanism of Action
Monoclonal Antibody Therapies		
Bevacizumab (Avastin®)	Metastatic colorectal cancer (mCRC), nonsmall-cell lung cancer (NSCLC), advanced breast cancer (Europe), glioblastoma, metastatic RCC, advanced ovarian cancer (Europe)	Humanized monoclonal antibody that binds VEGF and prevents its interaction with VEGF receptor (VEGFR-1 and VEGFR-2)
Ramucirumab (Cyramza®)	Advanced or metastatic gastric or gastroesophageal junction adenocarcinoma, metastatic NSCLC, and mCRC	Humanized monoclonal antibody that binds to VEGFR-2 and prevents VEGF from binding
Cetuximab (Erbitux®)	Metastatic Colorectal Cancer—second line, Locally Advanced or Metastatic Head and Neck Cancer	Cetuximab is a chimeric monoclonal antibody which binds to and inhibits epidermal growth factor receptor (EGFR)
Ziv-Aflibercept (ZALTRAP®)	In combination with other drugs for the treatment of patients with mCRC that is resistant to treatment with an oxaliplatin- containing regimen	Recombinant fusion protein that consists of VEGF-binding portions from the extracellular domains of human VEGF receptors 1 and 2 fused to the Fc portion of the human IgG1 immunoglobulin

(Continued)

TABLE 9.1 (*Continued*)
Pharmacological Inhibitors of Angiogenesis

	Indication (Country-If Abroad)	Mechanism of Action
Small Molecule Tyrosine Kinase Inhibitors (TKIs)		
Axitinib (Inlyta®)	Advanced RCC after failure of one prior systemic therapy	Oral multikinase inhibitor that targets VEGFR-1, -2, -3
Cabozantinib (Cometriq®)	Progressive, metastatic medullary thyroid cancer	Inhibitor of c-Met and VEGFR-2
Lenvatinib (Lenvima®)	Progressive, differentiated thyroid cancer whose disease progressed despite receiving radioactive iodine therapy	A multikinase inhibitor of FGF, VEGF, PDGFR-alpha, RET, and KIT
Pazopanib (Votrient®)	Advanced RCC	Small-molecule TK inhibitor of VEGF, PDGFR and c-kit
Regorafenib (Stivarga®)	Advanced mCRC that has progressed or has recurred after multiple treatments	Oral multikinase inhibitor that targets VEGFR-1, -2, -3, TIE2, PDGFR, and FGFR, KIT, RET, RAF, BRAF, and BRAFV600E
Sorafenib (Nexavar®)	Advanced RCC, advanced HCC, thyroid carcinoma	Small molecule TK inhibitor of VEGFR-1, VEGFR-2, VEGFR-3, PDGFR-β, and Raf-1
Sunitinib (Sutent®)	Advanced RCC, GIST, pancreatic neuroendocrine tumors	Small molecule TK inhibitor of VEGFR-1, VEGFR-2, VEGFR-3, PDGFR-β, and RET
Vandetanib (Caprelsa®)	Medullary Thyroid Cancer	Small molecule TK inhibitor of VEGFR and EGFR
Erlotinib (Tarceva®)	Locally advanced or metastatic NSCLC, pancreatic cancer	Inhibits EGFR via reversible binding to the ATP binding site of the receptor
Inhibitors of mTOR		
Temsirolimus (Torisel®)	Advanced RCC, Relapsed or refractory mantle cell lymphoma/NHL (European Union)	Inhibitor of mTOR (mammalian target of rapamycin), part of the PI3 kinase/AKT pathway involved in tumor cell proliferation and angiogenesis
Everolimus (Afinitor®)	Advanced RCC, pancreatic neuroendocrine tumors, subependymal giant cell astrocytoma	Inhibitor of mTOR , part of the PI3 kinase/AKT pathway involved in tumor cell proliferation and angiogenesis
Other Antiangiogenic Agents		
Interferon alfa (Intron® A and Roferon®)	Hairy cell leukemia, malignant melanoma, follicular lymphoma, AIDS-related Kaposi's sarcoma	Pharmacologic version of an endogenous cytokine with antiangiogenic activity
Lenalidomide (Revlimid®)	Myelodysplastic Syndrome associated with 5q deletion, Multiple myeloma	Possesses immunomodulatory, anti-inflammatory, and antiangiogenic properties, although the precise MOA is poorly understood
Thalidomide (Thalomid®)	Multiple myeloma	Possesses immunomodulatory, anti-inflammatory, and antiangiogenic properties, although the precise MOA is poorly understood
TAS-102 (Lonsurf®)	mCRC	A thymidine phosphorylase inhibitor
rhEndostatin (Endostar®)	NSCLC (China)	Endogenous angiogenesis inhibitor; recombinant protein; blocks VEGF-induced tyrosine phosphorylation of KDR-Flk-1 in endothelial cells, and down regulates MMP-2/9

DRUG TARGETS AND ANGIOGENIC FACTORS

Drugs designed to inhibit angiogenesis are directed against one or more of the following steps in blood vessel growth: (1) the production of angiogenic factors; (2) the binding of these factors to endothelial cell receptors; (3) endothelial signal transduction; (4) endothelial proliferation and migration; (5) vessel sprouting and three-dimensional tube formation; (6) vascular maturation by pericyte recruitment; and (7) mobilization of bone marrow-derived endothelial progenitor cells. These strategies provide directions for research evaluating the impact of nutrients and diets on the multistep process of tumor angiogenesis.

Targeting angiogenesis in tumors, regardless of strategy, has some unique advantages over the use of cytotoxic agents. The tumor vasculature is poorly constructed compared to normal healthy blood vessels, which are nonproliferating, so the side effects of cytotoxic agents, such as alopecia, myelosuppression, peripheral sensory neuropathy, renal toxicity, and severe gastrointestinal toxicity, are avoided (Eskens and Verweij 2006). Endothelial cells are available to drugs in the circulation avoiding the challenges of delivering drugs directly to tumor cells. Vascular endothelial cells have an extremely low mutation rate, so antiangiogenic interventions targeting various steps in blood vessel growth are less likely to induce drug resistance (Auerbach and Auerbach 1994, Engerman, Pfaffenbach, and Davis 1967, Hobson and Denekamp 1984, Tannock 1970, Ausprunk and Folkman 1977).

Cancer cells produce and release angiogenic growth factors that activate endothelial cells in nearby blood vessels. More than 20 such growth factors have been identified, sequenced, and had their genes cloned. Virtually all share the ability to stimulate endothelial proliferation, migration, or capillary tube formation. The major angiogenic factors include: (1) fibroblast growth factor-2 (originally called basic FGF) was the first angiogenic factor to be identified from a tumor by Folkman and colleagues (Shing et al. 1984); (2) VEGF is the best studied and one of the most potent hypoxia-mediated endothelial mitogen known. VEGF also increases vessel permeability and induces the vascular survival factor, Bcl-2 (Senger et al. 1983, Leung et al. 1989, Nor et al. 1999). All tumors have the ability to produce VEGF and its receptor, Flk-1/KDR, is selectively expressed on vascular endothelial cells, making this a turn-key regulator for tumor angiogenesis (Risau 1997); and (3) PlGF plays a specific role in neovascularization by recruiting bone marrow-derived vascular stem cells to disease sites (Adini et al. 2002, Hattori et al. 2002). Other factors include platelet-derived growth factor (PDGF), platelet-derived endothelial cell growth factor (PD-ECGF), interleukin-3 (IL-3), IL-8, TGF-β, and TNF-α, neuregulin, a ligand for the ErbB receptor, and keratinocyte growth factor (KGF or FGF-7) (Folkman and Klagsbrun 1987, Thommen et al. 1997, Russell et al. 1999, Gillis et al. 1999).

In normal, healthy subjects' most angiogenic factors are present at low or undetectable levels in the circulation. By contrast, markedly elevated levels of factors such as bFGF, VEGF, and PD-ECGF are present in the serum, urine, and cerebrospinal fluid of cancer patients (Nguyen 1997).

Maturation of blood vessels involves the recruitment of perivascular cells (smooth muscle cells, pericytes) to provide architectural support and cell–cell signals that maintain integrity of the vasculature. The Ang/Tie system plays a critical role in controlling this type of remodeling and maturation and is involved in the transition between quiescent and activated blood vessels. Angiopoietin-1 (Ang-1) binds to the Tie-2 receptor, leading to expression of PDGF and other cytokines that stimulate pericytes to the abluminal surface of blood vessels (Folkman and D'Amore 1996). Angiopoietin-2 (Ang-2) is a competitive ligand to Ang1 and also binds to the Tie-2 receptor. This factor is mostly secreted by endothelial cells at sites of active vascular remodeling in tumors and acts in an autocrine manner. Ang-2 promotes the dissociation of pericytes from pre-existing vessels and increases vascular permeability (Hammes et al. 2004). This facilitates the infiltration of proteases, cytokines, and myeloid cells, and facilitates new sprout formation in the presence of VEGF. Ang-2 levels are elevated in a number of diseases associated with vascular dysfunction, including ocular neovascularization, kidney, disease, and sepsis (Augustin et al. 2009).

Ang-2 is another therapeutic target and trepanned is a peptide-Fc fusion protein, which inhibits angiogenesis by blocking the binding of both Ang-1 and Ang-2 to the Tie-2 receptor. In a randomized, double-blind, placebo-controlled phase 3 trial for recurrent ovarian cancer, trepanned in combination with paclitaxel inhibited angiogenesis, leading to prolongation of progression-free survival (Monk et al. 2014).

VASCULAR ENDOTHELIAL CELLS AND NEOVASCULARIZATION

Vascular endothelial cells proliferate and migrate toward the tumor, using integrins ($\alpha v \beta 3$, $\alpha v \beta 5$, $\alpha 5 \beta 1$) to attach to the extracellular matrix and other vascular cells. Inhibition of these integrins has been explored as an antiangiogenic approach. Because integrins-matrix attachment promotes vascular survival, interfering with integrin signaling has been shown to promote apoptosis (Marth et al. 2017). Such apoptotic signaling is another approach to disrupt tumor angiogenesis (van der Schaft et al. 2002, Nelson et al. 2000, Huang et al. 2001).

Matrix metalloproteinases (MMPs) are enzymes secreted by the tip cells of sprouting vessels, and they dissolve extracellular matrix to facilitate vascular invasion (Nelson et al. 2000). A number of MMPs (MMP-2, MMP-9, MMP-12, and MMP-21) are associated with physiological and pathological angiogenesis (Sang 1998, Koolwijk et al. 2001). Inhibition of MMP can suppress both angiogenesis as well as tumor cell invasion of the extracellular matrix.

Neovascularization can be inhibited by increasing the homeostatic regulators that normally suppress angiogenesis (Hanahan and Folkman 1996). Blood vessel growth can be suppressed with endogenous angiogenesis inhibitors that are dominant in the microvascular environment (Plate et al. 1993, Rastinejad, Polverini, and Bouck 1989, Ohno-Matsui et al. 2001). Such endogenous inhibitors of angiogenesis are ubiquitous throughout the body. Thrombospondin-1 is one such inhibitor, and deletion of the thrombospondin-1 gene in mice leads to more rapid tumor growth (Lawler and Lawler 2012). Thus, thrombospondin-1 has been regarded as a potential candidate for targeting tumor angiogenesis (Teodoro, Evans, and Green 2007, Dameron et al. 1994).

Many cytokines also inhibit angiogenesis and may play a role in tumor suppression. They include interferon-alpha (IFN-α) (Dameron et al. 1994), IFN-γ (Voest et al. 1995), chemokine grow-beta (Cao et al. 1995), platelet factor-4 (Maione et al. 1990), IL-12 (Voest et al. 1995) and IL-18 (Cao et al. 1999).

These observations on the cross-talk between the immune system effectors and angiogenesis further strengthen the rationale for studying the combination of antiangiogenic therapy with immunotherapy. Preclinical studies in pancreatic, breast, and brain tumor mouse models provide evidence that anti-PD-L1 therapy can sensitize tumors to antiangiogenic therapy and prolong its efficacy, and that antiangiogenic therapy can improve anti-PD-L1 treatment-inducing enhanced cytotoxic T-cell infiltration, activity, and tumor cell destruction (Allen et al. 2017).

NUTRITIONAL INHIBITION OF ANGIOGENESIS

Plant-based diets are becoming increasingly popular. In part, this increased popularity is due to the data demonstrating that a plant-based diet is a healthier alternative to a diet dominated by meats. In addition to genetic factors associated with endothelial dysfunction, many dietary and other lifestyle factors, such as tobacco use, high meat and fat intake, obesity, and oxidative stress, have been implicated through a combination of basic and epidemiological observations. Polyphenols and other phytonutrients derived from a plant-based diet can inhibit angiogenesis. A plant-based diet is by definition low in fat, cholesterol, salt, animal products, and sugar. It is a conscious and mindful individual decision to maximize the nutrients and health benefits per calorie of foods eaten while minimizing potential harmful exposures to prevent cancer and other age-related chronic diseases. Taste, cost, and convenience dominate the food choices in the Western diet producing profits from foods that are low in nutrient and high in fat and sugar. However, populations around the world are becoming more health conscious forcing a change in the foods available in the marketplace today.

The fundamental concepts of antiangiogenic nutritional strategies for cancer prevention, treatment, and prevention of relapse are based on the following principles: (1) all tumors, solid and hematological, are dependent upon angiogenesis for growth beyond 2–$3\,mm^3$ because new blood vessels bring oxygen, nutrients, and paracrine factors to cancer cells; (2) when angiogenesis is blocked, tumor growth is slowed or prevented; (3) early intervention with antiangiogenic factors can prevent cancer, while treatment of established cancer using antiangiogenic agents can stabilize disease and improve survival; (4) dietary factors present in food have shown potent antiangiogenic activity in assays used for antiangiogenic drug development; (5) clinical and epidemiological evidence support consuming whole foods containing antiangiogenic dietary factors lower the risk for cancer development or progression. The following sections will present the background supporting research on the clinical application of antiangiogenic foods in cancer.

SOY AND ISOFLAVONES

Soy consumption is associated with lowered risk for a number of angiogenesis-dependent diseases, including breast, prostate, and CRC (Yan, Spitznagel, and Bosland 2010, Shu et al. 2009, Applegate et al. 2018). A widespread belief that soy is dangerous for women to consume because of its phytoestrogens is fallacious. Plant phytoestrogens do not provoke breast cancer growth. To the contrary, the soy phytoestrogens genistein is a potent antiangiogenic bioactive (Lecomte et al. 2017). The Shanghai Breast Cancer Survival study enrolled 5,042 breast cancer survivors and followed them for 4 years. They documented the amount of soy these women consumed and correlated this with the recurrence of and death from breast cancer. Women with the highest level of soy intake had a reduction in their risk of cancer recurrence by 32% (Shu et al. 2009). The risk of mortality was decreased by 29%. These associations with soy consumption were seen irrespective of the estrogen receptor status of the patients.

Soy contains genistein, daidzein, equol, and glyceolins which have potent antiangiogenic activity. Many different types of soy food that are commonly consumed in Asian countries are dietary sources of these bioactives. Fermented soy products tofu, soy sauce, miso, and natto have higher concentrations of genistein than fresh soybeans (Lee et al. 2013). Dietary supplements have also been developed to exploit antiangiogenic soy isoflavones. Genistein concentrated polysaccharide (GCP) is one such supplement created by fermenting soy with a mushroom-derived polysaccharide. In preclinical studies, GCP has direct cytotoxicity to prostate cancer and lymphoma cells (Bemis et al. 2004). GCP exerts its antiangiogenic capabilities by targeting MMPs, VEGF, EGF, and ERK1/2, PI3-K/Akt, NF-κB signaling pathways (Varinska et al. 2015). *In vitro*, genistein can suppress the cellular production of mRNA level of MMP-2, MMP-3, MMP-13, and MMP-15 (Latocha et al. 2014). *In vivo* studies have also shown a soy isoflavone extract, when added to docetaxel, reduced the expression of VEGF2 and NF-κBp65 (Hejazi et al. 2015).

TEAS AND CATECHINS

Numerous studies have shown tea drinking correlates with reduced cancer risk. An Italian study followed men with HGPIN, a precursor to prostate cancer, and identified a protective effect from consuming daily green tea catechins over the course of a single year (Bettuzzi et al. 2006). The double-blind, placebo-control study randomized 60 men with HGPIN into a treatment arm receiving 600 mg of purified green tea catechins (equivalent to two to three cups of tea/day) or a placebo arm. After 1 year of follow-up, prostate biopsy results revealed that 30% of the placebo group progressed on to develop prostate cancer, while the green tea catechin-treatment arm had only a progression rate of only 3%. Another prostate cancer study found that short-term daily supplementation of green tea extract significantly reduced PSA, and detectable levels of VEGF, HGF, IGF-I (McLarty et al. 2009). Additionally, the reduction of CRC risk has been associated with consuming two to three cups of green tea daily (Yang et al. 2007). The chemopreventive effects of green tea have been observed for the treatment of precancerous oral (to prevent oral cancer) and cervical lesions (to prevent cervical cancer) (Ahn et al. 2003, Li et al. 1999). Polyphenon E, an extract from green tea leaves is in clinical trials for prostate, bladder, esophageal, lung, head and neck cancers, and leukemia. In its topical form, polyphenon E 15% ointment was approved by the U.S. FDA in 2006 as a treatment for external genital warts, which is an angiogenic premalignant neoplasm and a precursor to cervical cancer (Li and Li 2008).

Different teas possess variable levels of the antiangiogenic catechin epigallocatechin-3-gallate (EGCG). Green tea contains six-fold more EGCG compared to black tea.

Green tea is processed by steaming and heating the tea leaves to inactivate the naturally occurring oxidase enzymes in tea leaves. They are then rolled and dried which preserves the EGCG content. Black teas are prepared from tea leaves that are not steamed. The natural oxidation and fermentation is allowed to progress prior to drying. Earl Grey tea is a flavored tea, made from a blend of tea with Bergamot oil. Bergamot is a type of orange that mainly grows in Italy and France, and is said to be a hybrid of lemon and bitter orange plants. Earl Grey has been found to be a more potent angiogenesis inhibitor than Chinese jasmine (green) tea, and the jasmine tea was found to be more potent than Japanese sencha tea in studies done at the Angiogenesis Foundation. When jasmine tea was blended with sencha, the resulting mix had a synergistic effect on inhibiting blood vessel growth. These studies point out the complexity of the effects that can occur from commonly consumed tea varieties

The antioxidant polyphenols of green teas and black teas have been linked with a decreased risk of colon, prostate, lung, esophageal, and other cancers in mechanistic studies in cancer cells and animal models (Yang and Wang 1993, Yang et al. 1997, Wang et al. 1995). Tea leaves contain more than 2,000 bioactive compounds including catechins, gallic acid, and theaflavins. Studies conducted by the Angiogenesis Foundation demonstrated that these bioactives potently inhibited angiogenesis and are potentially chemopreventive (Li et al. 2012, Wang et al. 1989, Wang et al. 1995, Wang et al. 1992, Cao and Cao 1999, Liao et al. 2004, Sazuka et al. 1995). EGCG inhibits growth factor-stimulated endothelial cell proliferation and induces avascular zones in the chick chorioallantoic membrane assay (Cao and Cao 1999). EGCG also inhibits VEGF by decreasing its expression as well as inhibiting its receptor binding (Shirakami et al. 2009). In mice, green tea solution 0.6% administered orally results in decreased VEGF expression and lower microvessel density in lung adenomas, as well as fewer tumors induced by an experimental carcinogen (Liao et al. 2004). Angiogenesis and markers of oxidant stress were inhibited in prostate cancer xenografts in mice consuming green tea polyphenols in doses comparable to human green tea consumption (Henning et al. 2012). Interestingly, EGCG also modulates AK strain Transforming also known as Protein kinase B (AKT), NF-κB, MAP kinases, and micro-RNAs that also regulate angiogenesis (Hu, Wang, et al. 2019, Liao et al. 2020). Human tumor xenografts examined by microarray and Western blot analysis showed that EGCG downregulated VEGF and HIF1α levels via the PI3K/AKT/mTOR signaling pathways (Wang, Man, et al. 2018).

TOMATOES AND CAROTENOIDS

Tomatoes contain a large number of bioactive substances, including rutin, beta-crytoxanthin, and lycopene, among others. Lycopene, which has antiangiogenic activity, has been the best studied. A systematic review of more than 30 studies confirms an inverse relationship between lycopene consumption and prostate cancer (Rowles et al. 2018). One of the largest studies is the Harvard Health Professionals Follow-Up which examined 46,719 men for lycopene intake and found that consuming two to three cups of tomato sauce per week is associated with up to a 30% decreased risk of prostate cancer (Graff et al. 2016). Moreover, in men that eventually developed prostate cancer, those that ate more tomatoes by serving developed less aggressive cancers, with lower microvessel density, suggesting an impact not only for prevention but for altering the growth kinetics of prostate carcinogenesis (Zu et al. 2014).

Tomatoes contain a number of beneficial phytonutrients including lycopene, rutin, and beta-cryptoxanthin. Lycopene is the best studied of these. Lycopene is also found in papayas and watermelon. Preclinical and clinical studies have shown that lycopene has potent antiangiogenic effects by inhibiting VEGF, Platelet Activation Factor, and MMP-2 (Chen et al. 2012, Chiang et al. 2007). Lycopene treatment of prostate cancer cell lines inhibits their ability to matric adhesion and tumor cell migration at physiologically achievable concentrations in humans (Elgass, Cooper, and Chopra 2014). In vivo studies have also demonstrated that lycopene suppresses the growth of mammary, liver, and prostate cancer, and metastases (Seren et al. 2008).

POMEGRANATE, STRAWBERRIES, WALNUTS, PECANS, AND ELLAGIC ACID

Pomegranate, strawberries, walnuts, and pecans are rich in ellagitannins and ellagic acid (EA). The ellagitannins are hydrolyzed to EA in the small intestine and then EA is converted to smaller urolithins by the microbiome. Pomegranate juice and EA have been demonstrated to have antiangiogenic activity and can be metabolized by the microbiome to smaller polyphenols with potent antiangiogenic activity (Kowshik et al. 2014, Sartippour et al. 2008). In vitro studies of glioma models discovered that long-term application of EA downregulated gene expression and immunoreactivity of VEGF (Cetin and Biltekin 2019). In addition to EA, a number of other phenolics have been identified in extracts of strawberries including cyanidin-3-glucoside, pelargonidin, pelargonidin-3-glucoside, pelargonidin-3-rutinoside, kaempferol, quercetin, kaempferol-3-(6′-coumaroyl)glucoside), 3,4,5-trihydroxyphenyl-acrylic acid, glucose ester of (E)-p-coumaric acid (Seeram 2010) extracts. A number of berry extracts including strawberry, wild blueberry, and cranberry have been shown to activate Akt in a dose-dependent manner via PI3 kinase and induced cell migration and angiogenesis in vitro in human umbilical vein endothelial cells (HUVECs) (Tulio et al. 2012).

Pomegranate juice contains anthocyanins, ellagitannins, EA, and related polyphenols (Seeram et al. 2005). In a study done in mice with human prostate tumor xenografts given a human equivalent of 1.7 cups (8 oz) of pomegranate juice per day, pomegranate juice reduced tumor size and tumor microvessel density, compared to controls, and demonstrated a reduction in tumor angiogenesis (Sartippour et al. 2008). A clinical study in men with recurrent prostate cancer showed that those who consumed 1 cup of pomegranate juice per day had a significantly decreased prostate-specific antigen doubling time, from 15 to 54 months (Pantuck et al. 2006). For ovarian cancer, animal studies showed that EA at concentrations of 10–15 µg/mL markedly reduced expression of MMP-2 and MMP-9, enzymes critical for angiogenesis, and tumor invasion (Liu et al. 2017). In breast cancer cell lines, EA was shown to exert its antiangiogenic effects via inhibiting VEGF receptor 2 (VEGFR-2) phosphorylation and impeding tumor growth (Wang et al. 2012).

BERRIES AND ANTHOCYANINS

Anthocyanins are natural pigments possessing antiangiogenic activity that are present in cranberries, blueberries, black raspberries (BRB), grapes, and red wine. The concentration of anthocyanins varies and berries contain a variety of anthocyanins including cyanidins, delphinidins, malvidins, pelargonidins, peonidins, and petunidins which have been reported to alter metabolic and inflammatory markers in cells, animals, and humans (Tsakiroglou P et al 2019). Cranberry proanthocyanidins have been shown to inhibit angiogenesis in ovarian cancer cells (Kim et al. 2012). Anthocyanins at a concentration of 60 µg/mL inhibit endothelial cell migration by affecting cytoskeletal arrangement and cell adhesion (Tsakiroglou et al. 2019).

In a study of esophageal papillomas in rats, animals fed BRB had fewer papillomas, and those that developed were of smaller volume, and exhibited reduced cell proliferation. Expression of VEGF and HIF-1alpha was lower in the BRB-fed mice compared to the non-BRB-fed mice (Wang et al. 2011, Lu et al. 2006). DNA microarray studies of rat esophageal carcinogenesis showed that dietary BRB alter expression of angiogenic genes, including the cyclooxygenase and lipoxygenase pathways, as well as MMP-10 expression. Staining for CD34, a classical marker for endothelial cells in microvessels, was significantly reduced in the BRB diet animals (Wang et al. 2011, Stoner et al. 2006). An extract from BRB has been studied in human subjects diagnosed clinically with oral intraepithelial neoplasia. A 10% BRB gel was applied to the oral mucosa of patients four times daily. After 6 weeks, there was a reduced histological grade of dysplastic lesions in 50% of treated subjects and reduced expression of COX-2 and iNOS was seen in the lesions (Shumway et al. 2008).

RED WINE AND RESVERATROL

Red wine, which contains antiangiogenic resveratrol, has been examined in population studies for anticancer effects. The European Prospective Investigation into Cancer (EPIC)-Norfolk study followed 24,244 participants for 11 years and identified that consumption of one glass of red wine per day was associated with a decreased risk of CRC by 39% compared to nondrinkers (Park et al. 2009). A separate cohort study of 2,044 people found comparable results with less than a full glass of red wine per day (Crockett et al. 2011). An inverse relationship between red wine consumption and lung cancer incidence was found by the California Men's Health study. The researchers analyzed 84,000 men and discovered a 61% risk reduction of lung cancer in men drinking at least one glass of red wine per day (Chao et al. 2008). Additionally, the Health Professionals Follow-up Study identified a protective effect of red wine for prostate cancer, reporting a 36% risk reduction in men drinking two-to-four glasses of red wine per week (Sutcliffe et al. 2007). Although red wine contains hundreds of bioactives, resveratrol has been identified as a key factor for its preclinical and clinical benefits against cancer. A Phase I clinical trial of resveratrol in patients with colorectal showed the supplement increased apoptosis and a decrease in proliferation (Howells et al. 2011, Patel et al. 2010).

Resveratrol is a defense against fungi produced in in plants, as a part of their defense mechanism. Resveratrol is the best-known bioactive compound in red wine with both anticancer and cardiovascular benefits. Resveratrol is found in several dietary sources such as grapes, apples, raspberries, blueberries, plums, peanuts, and products made from these plants. Resveratrol can be isolated and purified from these biological sources or synthesized in a few steps with high yield.

Red wine contains many other polyphenols, including gallic acid, rutin, catechins, quercetin, and caffeic acid. Fresh grape skin contains 50–100 µg resveratrol per gram. The amount in Italian red wine is 1.5–3 mg/L (Markoski et al. 2016, Jang et al. 1997). Resveratrol's antiangiogenic activities including its ability to bind to VEGF thereby suppressing endothelial cell proliferation, migration, invasion, and tube formation (Hu, Chan, et al. 2019). Another pathway by which resveratrol inhibits angiogenesis is via inhibition of HIF1-alpha (Li, Cao, et al. 2016). Resveratrol has been found to inhibit a variety of cancers, including breast, prostate, stomach, colon, lung, pancreas cancer, melanoma, and glioma (Bishayee 2009, Shukla and Singh 2011, Chen et al. 2015, Anso et al. 2010, Pal et al. 2014, Sundarraj, Raghunath, and Perumal 2018).

BEER HOPS AND XANTHOHUMOL

Beer has unexpected associations with reduced cancer risk. A U.S. National Cancer Institute study enrolled 107,998 participants and examined the association between beer consumption and renal cell carcinoma (RCC). The results showed that people who drank five beers per week were associated with a 33% reduced risk for RCC (Karami, Daugherty, and Purdue 2015). Another study called the North Carolina Colon Study enrolled 2,044 subjects and demonstrated that consumption of less than seven beers per week was associated with 24% reduction in risk of CRC (Crockett et al. 2011).

The hop flower is rich in resins which give beer a bitterness when used early in the brewing process, and aroma when added at the end. Hops also act as a preservative in beer. Some brewers have boosted the hopping levels of their India Pale Ales to add a variety of bitterness levels and flavors to beers. Beer hops contain xanthohumol, which has antiangiogenic properties (Gallo et al. 2016, Albini et al. 2006). Studies of pancreatic cancer showed that xanthohumol downregulates pathologic angiogenesis via blocking the activation of Nf-κB, and by suppressing expression of VEGF and IL-8 (Saito et al. 2018). Xanthohumol also directly increases cancer cell apoptosis and activates the antiangiogenic 5' adenosine monophosphate-activated protein kinase pathway while inhibiting the pro-angiogenic AKT pathway (Liu et al. 2016, Gallo et al. 2016). Notably, xanthohumol was showed to be a more a potent angiogenesis inhibitor than EGCG, found in green tea (Gallo et al. 2016). In another study, xanthohumol was shown to suppress proliferation of medullary thyroid, breast, and glioblastoma cancer cells (Cook et al. 2010, Festa et al. 2011).

CRUCIFEROUS VEGETABLES AND GLUCOSINOLATES

Cruciferous vegetables are a large family containing glucosinolates and include broccoli, cauliflower, bok choy, cabbage, mustard green, Brussel sprouts, and radishes. When these plants are crushed before cooking, an enzyme called myrosinase within plant cell vesicles is activated and glucosinolates are cleaved to release the bioactive molecules isothiocyanate (ITC) and indole-3-carbinol, both of which are antiangiogenic. This enzymatic activation is an ancient defense mechanism of plants found in multiple species. In animal models of colorectal carcinoma, ITC inhibits pathological angiogenesis through the inhibition of VEGF and bFGF (Kwak, Lee, and Ju 2016). In particular, ITCs inhibit the expression of growth factor and protease production while inducing endothelial cell apoptosis and reducing expression of endothelial adhesion molecules (Li et al. 2012, Kunimasa et al. 2008, Hudson et al. 2012). Consumption of cruciferous vegetables is associated with a reduced risk of melanoma by 28%, non-Hodgkin's lymphoma (NHL) by 40%, lung cancer by 28%, breast cancer by 17%, esophageal cancer by 31%, and prostate cancer by 59% (Ollberding et al. 2013, Freedman et al. 2007, Mignone et al. 2009, Steinmetz, Potter, and Folsom 1993, Richman, Carroll, and Chan 2012, Micha et al. 2014, Millen et al. 2004).

Epidemiological evidence also supports the cancer preventative benefits of cruciferous vegetable. The EPIC study examined the dietary habits and health of 521,468 subjects across ten European countries between 1991 and 2000 (Buchner et al. 2010). After an average follow-up of 8.7 years, 1,830 people were diagnosed with lung cancer. EPIC showed that regular consumption of cauliflower and cabbage was associated with a 23% reduction in the risk for squamous cells carcinoma of the lung, among smokers. The study also revealed an almost 50% reduced risk of cancer of the upper digestive tract (oral cavity, pharynx, larynx, and esophagus) among people who ate the most cauliflower and cabbage (34 g/day) compared with those who ate the least (3 g/day) of these foods (Boeing et al. 2006). The Shanghai Men's Health study followed 61,491 adult males for 5½ years. The consumption of green leafy vegetables was associated with the reduced risk of lung cancer by 28% (Takata et al. 2013). The protective effect has been studied in smokers. A meta-analysis study showed that active smokers who regularly consume vegetables have a 13% reduced risk of developing lung cancer (Wang et al. 2019).

Cruciferous vegetable consumption is also associated with the reduced risk of hematological malignancies. A large prospective study of more than 35,000 women living in Iowa followed for 20 years found a 18% reduced risk for NHL among women who had the highest consumption of cruciferous vegetables. Specifically, the consumption of at least four servings per month of broccoli was associated with a 28% risk reduction for lymphoma (Thompson et al. 2010). The Nurses Health Study found among 67,000 women that frequent dietary intake of broccoli (at least two servings per week) was associated with a 33% risk reduction for ovarian cancer (Gates et al. 2009).

OMEGA-3 AND OMEGA-6 FATTY ACID BALANCE
FROM FOODS AND SUPPLEMENTS

Triglycerides are the major form of fat in the diet and stored in fat cells. They have three fatty acids and are classified as saturated, monounsaturated, or polyunsaturated fats based on the number of double bonds in the predominant fatty acid chains, polyunsaturated fatty acids with carbon atoms between 18 and 22 are classified as Omega-3 or Omega-6 based on the position of the first of two double bonds in the carbon chain. These two types of fatty acids compete for the same active sites on a series of enzymes leading to the formation of proinflammatory or anti-inflammatory eicosanoids including prostaglandins, thromboxanes, and leukotrienes. Inflammation is a normal process important in wound healing and fighting infections but when inflammation is maintained chronically, it leads to formation of reactive oxygen species and promotion of tumorigenesis and angiogenesis.

Two fatty acids with 20 and 22 carbon, respectively, have been most widely studies (EPA (eicosapentaenoic acid) and DHA (docosahexaenoic acid). While an 18 carbon fatty acid (ALA (alpha linolenic acid)) is an omega-3 fatty acid found in plant foods. However, in the context of a typical dietary pattern in developed countries, humans are inefficient in converting ALA into EPA and DHA. EPA and DHA are found predominantly in seafood and fish oil or algae-derived dietary supplements, while ALA is found in plant-based foods, such as flax seeds. The balance of eicosanoid precursors in human tissues differs widely, reflecting voluntary dietary choices among different groups worldwide and influencing the risk for age-related chronic diseases (Okuyama et al. 2007, Innes and Calder 2018, Micha et al. 2014).

Omega-3 PUFAs inhibit angiogenesis by downregulating the expression of VEGF mRNA, and they attenuate the VEGF-induced phosphorylation of VEGFR2 (Zhang et al. 2013). Metabolites of omega-3 PUFAs, notably epoxy docosapentaenoic acids (EDPs), have also been shown to potently inhibit neovascularization. In a Matrigel plug assay in mice, EDP inhibited VEGF-induced angiogenesis. 19,20-EDP, which is a major EDP isomer in tissues, inhibited VEGF-induced angiogenesis with an EC50 value of 0.3 µg/animal (Zhang et al. 2013). 19,20-EDP also suppressed basic fibroblast growth factor-induced angiogenesis in mice (Zhang et al. 2013). By contrast, omega-6 PUFAs have been shown to stimulate angiogenesis via endothelial migration (Li et al. 2012). Therefore, the most important factor for PUFA consumption is not just the absolute amount but the ratio between omega-3 to omega-6 PUFAs. Diet with higher omega-3 to omega-6 ratio provides more protection against cancer and inflammation (Kaliannan et al. 2015, Simopoulos 2002).

A large body of epidemiological evidence also provides evidence that omega-3 fatty acids have anti-inflammatory and angiogenesis inhibitory properties, and reduce the risk of cancer. The Singapore Chinese Health Study examined the health of 35,298 women and identified that eating three or more ounces of fish per day, the source of omega-3 fatty acids, was linked with a 26% reduced risk of breast cancer (Gago-Dominguez et al. 2004). Another prospective cohort study evaluating 68,109 persons showed that men who consumed omega-3 fatty acid-containing foods at least 4 days a week for up to 3 years in the study had a 78% reduced risk of developing CRC (Kantor et al. 2014).

LEAFY GREEN VEGETABLES AND VITAMINS K1 AND K2

Vitamin K1 is primarily found in leafy green vegetables, while K2 is most abundant in fermented foods and some animal products. High concentrations of vitamin K2 are also found in cheese, particularly Dutch Gouda, Swiss Emmental, and Norwegian Jarlsberg. Vitamin K2 is also formed from vitamin K1 by the microbiome after ingestion of vitamin K1 from green leafy vegetables (Fenn et al. 2017).

Vitamin K2 has greater bioavailability than vitamin K1. Vitamin K2 has been studied for its antiangiogenic effects in vitro and its consumption is associated with reduced risk of many forms of cancers. This vitamin induces cancer cell apoptosis so it suppresses cancer by inhibiting angiogenesis and tumor cell growth (Yoshiji et al. 2006, Kayashima et al. 2009). In vivo studies of protein S, a vitamin K2-dependent glycoprotein, demonstrated its anti-angiogenic capabilities via inhibition of VEGFR2-dependent vascularization. Moreover, protein S inhibits the capacity of endothelial cells to form capillary-like networks as well as VEGF-induced endothelial cell migration and proliferation (Fraineau et al. 2012). In addition to these cellular pathways, vitamin K also interferes with the STAT3 signaling pathway. Activation of STAT3 stimulates both tumor cell and endothelial cell proliferation (Fraineau et al. 2012). To further study its mechanism of action, a vitamin K analog called plumbagin was isolated from the herb chitrak. Plumbagin was found to downregulate VEGF expression (Sandur et al. 2010). Vitamin K2 also directly interferes with the growth of colon cancer cells and prostate cancer cells (Kayashima et al. 2010, Samykutty et al. 2013).

One of the largest epidemiological studies ever conducted of diet and cancer, EPIC, closely examined the effect of vitamin K2 on various cancers. EPIC researchers followed the health records and dietary patterns of 24,300 participants for up to 14 years (1994–2008), during which 1,775 cancers were diagnosed, of which 458 were fatal. Participants who consumed higher quantities of cheese (41 g or more/day) had a significantly reduced risk of dying from lung and prostate cancers compared to those that ate lower quantities (14 g/day) (Nimptsch et al. 2010). While the effects of dairy and cancer have remained controversial and unresolved, vitamin K2 is well established as an antiangiogenic vitamin. The chemopreventive properties of vitamin K2 extend beyond lung and prostate cancers. A Japanese study evaluated 40 women diagnosed with virus-associated liver cirrhosis and randomly assigned individuals to a vitamin K2 (45 mg/day) supplement intervention or a control group. Over the 7 years of the study, the group that received daily vitamin K2 had a 20% decreased risk of developing hepatocellular carcinoma (HCC) compared to control. On an annual incidence basis, HCC developed in only 1.6% in the treatment group compared with 8.8% incidence of cancer in the control group (Habu et al. 2004).

ANGIOGENESIS PREVENTION

Cancer prevention by eating antiangiogenic foods has been termed "angioprevention". A life-long dietary pattern of these foods would naturally yield the greatest benefit. Diversity of foods and consistency of healthy eating patterns is important. An estimated 30%–40% of cancers could be avoided through diet and lifestyle interventions (Donaldson 2004). Parental habits influence the later dietary behaviors of children, so cancer prevention through antiangiogenic foods can start early in life and be propagated across generations. Such an approach could be particularly useful in populations that are at high risk for developing specific cancer. The high consumption of papaya and other foods rich in antiangiogenic carotenoids has been found to reduce the risk of cervical cancers in high risk individuals (Siegel et al. 2010). Another study found that risk of squamous cell carcinoma of the lung was reduced by 23% in habitual smokers eating cruciferous vegetables (Boeing et al. 2006). The consumption of tomatoes and tomato juice, which contains antiangiogenic lycopene, was linked to a reduced risk of mesothelioma in individuals with a history of asbestos exposure and smoking (Muscat and Huncharek 1996). A multiethnic, case–control trial conducted in Hawaii found that the risk of developing endometrial cancer was lower in women who regularly consumed high amounts of soy foods despite pre-existing cancer risks (Goodman et al. 1997).

ADJUNCTIVE TREATMENT WITH ANTIANGIOGENIC FOODS

Antiangiogenic foods may be useful in adjunctively augmenting cancer treatments, including surgery, chemotherapy, radiotherapy, targeted therapy, and immunotherapy. A balanced diet rich in bioactive compounds can help accelerate the recovery from cancer and improve the quality of life. An epidemiological study examining 9,514 women diagnosed with invasive breast cancer found that consumption of soy isoflavones among breast cancer patients improved the efficacy of the pharmacological treatment while reducing the recurrence of cancer (Nechuta et al. 2012). Cancer patients are often keenly aware of the potential that diet could aid their treatment and recovery, but a significant gap of knowledge concerning nutrition exists among oncologists (Spiro et al. 2006). Accordingly, many oncologists do not provide accurate and up-to-date information and dietary guidance to their patients. Consequently, patients are left to their own devices to find dietary advice from the Internet that may even have an adverse effect on their recovery (Rauh et al. 2018). It is thus imperative that oncologists become educated and well-versed in nutrition and stay current on scientific and clinical developments surrounding foods with antiangiogenic activity.

Since the nutritional and dietary requirement for each patient may vary depending on the age, type, stage of cancer as well as the treatment protocol, the diet should be tailored to individual patients. Incorporating antiangiogenic foods into a patient's diet takes a patient-centered approach. Nutritional oncology is not aimed to replace current oncological treatment modalities, but rather to be additive to mainstream therapies. Generally speaking, antiangiogenic foods exert little interference with pharmacological agents, however, food-drug interactions should always be considered.

PREVENTION OF RELAPSE

Following successful cancer treatment, a dietary strategy may be useful to help cancer survivors remain in remission. Tumor recurrence is dependent upon growth of microscopic cancers through the angiogenic switch, so an antiangiogenic diet may be useful for secondary prevention.

Notably, the nutritional quality of cancer survivors can be inferior to that of healthy people (Zhang et al. 2015, Rock et al. 2012). An evidence-based approach is critical to establish postcancer nutrition guidelines. Intake of fruits, vegetables, and legumes such as soy has been found to reduce the risk of recurrence and improve the survival in breast cancer (Qiu and Jiang 2019, Clinton, Giovannucci, and Hursting 2019). Another study reports that a high-quality, low-fat diet improves patient recovery from breast cancer, while a western-style diet high in fat, starch, and red meat hinders progress (Schwedhelm et al. 2016). A compromised immune system in cancer survivors can increase their risk of recurrence and put them at an elevated risk for other diseases such as COVID, as well. The bioactives found in some antiangiogenic foods are also known to exert positive effects on immunity (Clinton, Giovannucci, and Hursting 2019, Boeing et al. 2006). A sound dietary strategy for cancer survivors can improve their overall health, suppress tumor regrowth, and quality of life.

MICROBIOTA, DIET, AND ANGIOGENESIS

Although we tend to think of ourselves as a single organism made up of trillions of human cells, until the discovery of the microbiome, we ignored over 14 trillion other organisms living symbiotically in and on our bodies. Humans are not a single organism but rather a holobiont defined as an organism that functions as an assemblage of multiple species that work together in symbiosis. The human body is a complex ecosystem that includes trillions of bacteria carrying 99% of the genetic material related to our bodies and residing in many organs, with a collective weight of approximately 3 pounds. Importantly, the microbiome can influence angiogenesis and tip the scale towards developing or resisting cancer.

The first studies reporting a mechanistic link between the gut microbiome and angiogenesis compared germ-free mice with ex-germ-free mice for their ability to develop intestinal capillary networks (Stappenbeck, Hooper, and Gordon 2002). Later studies showed that the regulation of the vessel density in the small intestine is mediated by tissue factor, a membrane receptor that promotes angiogenesis through the thrombin-PAR1 signaling pathway (Stappenbeck, Hooper, and Gordon 2002). It has been suggested that quorum sensing peptides, secreted by pathogenic gram-negative bacteria such as *E. coli*, promote angiogenesis and breast cancer cell invasion (De Spiegeleer et al. 2015). Inflammatory bowel disease (IBD) is another condition linking microbiome to angiogenesis. Studies of intestinal mucosal expression of VEGF-A demonstrated inflammation-induced angiogenesis occurs in patients with IBD (De Spiegeleer et al. 2015, Scaldaferri et al. 2009, Danese et al. 2007). In addition to VEGF, HIF-1α was also shown to be activated in infections such as *S aureus* and *E. coli* (Werth et al. 2010). Although *E. coli* is often associated with pathogenic, inflammatory, and angiogenesis-promoting infection, some of its actions are antagonistic. For example, *E. coli* STa activity has an inhibitory role on both VEGF and VCAM-1 expression (Werth et al. 2010). The antiangiogenic inhibitory effect of *E. coli* STa was shown to be part of the PKG-ERK42/44 pathway (Saha et al. 2008). *Pseudomonas aeruginosa* is another species that inhibits angiogenesis via its azurin, a secreted 128 amino acid redox protein. Azurin can penetrate HUVECs and colocalize with VEGFR-2, thus inhibiting VEGF-activated angiogenesis (Mehta et al. 2011).

Many species of gut bacteria are associated with cancer (Peek and Blaser 2002, Caygill et al. 1994, Lecuit et al. 2004, Ferreri et al. 2008). Because of the rich diversity of microbes in the colon, however, it is challenging to tease apart the relative importance of each microbe, as well as microbe–microbe interactions, to the etiology of cancer. In CRC, a simplified model hypothesizes that gut bacteria disrupt mucosal immunity and this leads to detrimental effects on gene expression and epithelial cell function, leading to carcinogenesis (Van Raay and Allen-Vercoe 2017). This intestinal microbiota adaptation hypothesis posits that the gut microbial system constantly exists in a state of dynamic equilibrium (Lozupone et al. 2012, Heiman and Greenway 2016). Any stressor, such as inflammation, leads to a rise in bacterial species that preferentially benefits from the new environment. Microbiota adaptations are relevant to cancer because they help to explain how changes in the microenvironment can drive a disease in a positive feedback loop. Current research focuses on understanding how these changes in the microenvironment shift it in favor of cancer-inhibiting microbiota to prevent tumorigenesis. Another prime example of bacteria that drives cancer through angiogenesis is *Helicobacter pylori*. Infection with *H. pylori* is classified as a carcinogen that can lead to gastric ulcer formation, gastric atrophy, and finally gastric cancer (Fox and Wang 2007). Currently, five major groups of angiogenic biomarkers are upregulated and associated with gastric cancer: VEGF family, angiopoietin (ANG)/endostatin family, ANG-like family, IL family and HIF family (Macedo et al. 2017).

The microbiome also influences malignancies beyond the gastrointestinal tract. *Fusobacterium nucleatum*, an oral bacteria previously thought to be confined to the gut, was discovered to colonize breast cancers and accelerate tumor growth (Macedo et al. 2017). Notably, one mechanism by which *F. nucleatum* drives tumorigenesis is via overexpression of MMP-9, an angiogenesis-promoting protease.

Current interventions directed at eliminating pathobionts such as *F. nucleatum* and *H. pylori* utilize antibiotics as the primary treatment. Antibiotics are too blunt an instrument to carry out such selective work, and their use also eliminates other beneficial bacterial species. A more superior approach is to understand and address the root causes of the dysbiosis and aim at restoring homeostatic balance of the microbiome. Dietary strategies and interventions to treat dysbiosis associated with cancer risk would transform the conventional approach to cancer.

The impact of nutrition on angiogenesis extends to the microbiome. Among the many substances our microbiota produce, the best-known are known as short-chain fatty acids (SCFAs). The SCFAs are produced when gut bacteria digest plant fibers. SCFAs have been found to have an array of health benefits. They protect the gut through their anti-inflammatory properties, and they have the ability to improve our body's ability to metabolize glucose and lipids (Morrison and Preston 2016). Their cancer protective effects are attributed to their antiangiogenic capabilities, notably sodium butyrate. When sodium butyrate was added to the highly vascular colon cancer cell line HT29, it inhibited VEGF expression and modulated the levels of HIF-1α (Coradini et al. 2000). A great way to increase the intake of sodium butyrate and other SCFAs is to seek out foods that are rich in dietary fiber. These foods increase the function of healthy gut bacteria by providing them with the food they need to thrive (Makki et al. 2018). Examples of such foods are raspberries, pears, green peas, chia seeds, split peas, lentils, and black beans.

FERMENTED FOODS AND ANGIOGENESIS

Fermented foods such as yogurt, kimchi, sauerkraut, and kombutcha that contain live bacteria are probiotic foods that can influence the gut microbiome. A prospective study evaluated the benefits of ingesting yogurt every 3–4 days over the course of 6 weeks (Lisko, Johnston, and Johnston 2017). Each serving provided approximately 1 billion beneficial bacteria. Fecal material analysis from these subjects revealed an increase in *Lactobacillus casei*, *Lactobacillus reuteri*, and *Lactobacillus rhamnosus*, indicating that eating yogurt can beneficially influence the gut microbiome (Lisko, Johnston, and Johnston 2017). *L. rhamnosus* GG, a probiotic strain with antiangiogenic properties, is often added to yogurt. An in vivo study uncovered the mechanism by which *L. rhamnosus* GG exerts its antiangiogenic effects by downregulating the secretion of IL-17 cytokine by Th17 lymphocytes (Li, Sung, et al. 2016). Studies have already demonstrated that IL-17 is a potent promoter of angiogenesis (Numasaki et al. 2003). In the same study, a probiotic supplement containing *L. rhamnosus* GG was shown to reduce HCC tumor size and weight by 40%, compared to a control. A double blind, placebo-controlled human conducted by researchers from the Karolinska Institute in Sweden sought to examine the effect of *L. rhamnosus* GG on colon cancer. The researchers administered a probiotic mixture including *L. rhamnosus* GG for 12 weeks and showed it reduced the risk of CRC and decreased a number of cancer biomarkers (Rafter et al. 2007).

Kimchi, a korean staple dish, consists of salted and fermented vegetables such as radishes, scallions, jeotgal, napa cabbage, and chile peppers is a traditional probiotic food. The antiangiogenic characteristics of Kimchi are attributed to the preponderance of *Lactobacillus* in the product (Park et al. 2012). Another bacteria named *Lentibacillus kimchi* is present in kimchi (Oh et al. 2016). This species produces vitamin K2, which is antiangiogenic. Moreover, studies of kimchi extracts have shown direct anticancer properties against hepatocellular and colon cancer cells, as well as leukemia (Kwak et al. 2014).

Certain cheeses contain useful bacteria that can foster antiangiogenic effects. Parmigiano-Reggiano is a traditional hard cheese from Parma, Italy, that is aged before being sold and eaten. This temporal aging allows for a rise and fall in bacteria species. Initially, many species are present, later as then cheese matures and the acidity changes, many bacteria disappear (Gala et al. 2008). Among the surviving species is *L. rhamnosus* GG, the same cancer protective and antiangiogenic bacteria found in yogurt (Lazzi et al. 2014). Gouda cheese also has a diverse profile of probiotic bacteria including *Lactobacillus casei* and *Lactobacillus plantarum* (Tiptiri-Kourpeti et al. 2016). As with Parmigiano-Reggiano, the bacterial population of Gouda changes as the cheese ages.

BERRY POLYPHENOLS

Various types of berries contain phenolic compounds such as flavonols, phenolic acids, and anthocyanins. These antiangiogenic molecules can exert many beneficial effects to combat tumor growth. Our gut microbiome can help to hydrolyze the polyphenols to enable them to be efficiently absorbed (Duenas et al. 2015). Among the bacteria that catalyze polyphenols are *Bacteroides* and *Eubacterium*, which together with *Lactobacillus*, *Bifidobacterium*, *Akkermansia* confer health benefits to the host. The relationship between the microbiome and the polyphenols is bilateral. Once in the colon, the polyphenols themselves can modulate bacterial populations (Cardona et al. 2013). Grape polyphenols dramatically increased the growth of *Akkermansia muciniphila* and decreased the proportion of Firmicutes to Bacteroidetes, changes in microbial community structure that protected mice from diet-induced obesity and metabolic disease (Roopchand et al. 2015). Human studies also show that antiangiogenic polyphenols can modulate the microbiota by modifying the microbiome (Molan, Liu, and Plimmer 2014).

CITRUS FRUITS

Neohesperidin (NHP), a flavanone found in citrus fruits, is responsible for strong bitter flavor. NHP has already been demonstrated to display a wide range of pharmacological properties, including suppression of osteoclast differentiation, anti-inflammation, ROS-scavenging activity, cardiovascular protection, protection from ROS, and neuroprotective effects (Benavente-Garcia and Castillo 2008, Jia et al. 2015, Wang, Yuan, et al. 2018). *In vivo* studies demonstrate that NHP possesses antiangiogenic potency and can prevent experimental colorectal tumorigenesis (Gong et al. 2019). The effects of a 12-week NHP diet significantly reduced vessel density in mice. Moreover, NHP was shown to modulate gut microbiota and favorably decrease the ratio of Bacteroidetes/Firmicutes which is associated with many pathologies (Gong et al. 2019). Taken together, the data suggest that NHP is an antiangiogenic compound that exerts its antitumor effects by reducing oncomicrobes and increasing beneficial gut bacteria.

CONCLUSION AND FUTURE DIRECTIONS

Angiogenesis is a clinically validated target for controlling tumor growth. Antiangiogenic therapy through nutrition intervention can help address the rising burden of cancer (Rahib et al. 2014, Heron 2019). Diet and cancer are inextricably linked, and negative dietary influences are estimated to contribute to 20%–60% of cancers worldwide, and approximately one-third of deaths from cancer in Western countries (McCullough and Giovannucci 2004, Doll 1992).

The identification of antiangiogenic dietary factors has been aided through observational epidemiologic studies, which have associated specific foods with reduced cancer risk. Large-scale screening of food-based antiangiogenic activity using computational models, artificial intelligence, and neural network algorithms will further increase efficiency and aid to pinpoint potent naturally occurring antiangiogenic biomolecules.

In conjunction with high-throughput bioactive identification, the identification of growing conditions that optimize food bioactivity should be carried out. Increasing productivity and nutrients in food can thus not only combat micronutrient deficiency but also cancer. For example, utilization of mutualistic fungi can increase the nutrient content of crops during their growth while decreasing pesticide usage. Identifying specific high-potency varietals, and naturally breeding them together could be studied to determine if this increases the content of their antiangiogenic biomolecules. Through agricultural breeding and enhanced growing conditions of foods, it may be possible to create generations of foods based on potency, similar to how there exist ever more potent generations of pharmaceutical agents.

Special attention should be paid to the impact of storage, preparation, and cooking of various foods in terms of impact on antiangiogenic activity. It is known, for example, that increase in temperature during canning of foods can be detrimental to water-soluble nutrients such as vitamins C and B. Frozen foods may retain nutrients initially despite processing but can display a decrease in nutrient content during storage due to oxidation. Future studies should elucidate if changes in temperature, oxygen, and moisture influence antiangiogenic molecules. Likewise, cooking conditions may have various effects on the bioavailability of antiangiogenic molecules. Cooking tomatoes, for example, converts trans-lycopene to cis-lycopene which allows for greater bioavailability (Unlu et al. 2005). Steaming of vegetables was shown to preserve more phytochemicals than other cooking modalities (Palermo, Pellegrini, and Fogliano 2014). Future studies should examine the impact of cooking and the net effect of combining foods to elucidate how their health benefits can be optimized.

The health benefit of antiangiogenic foods extends far beyond individual gain to the entire human civilization. As technological advancements enable long-duration space travel, humans will become extraterrestrial. Space flight and human settlement on the Moon and Mars and beyond will expose the body to galactic radiation, microgravity, shifts in microbiome, circulatory changes, and other threats. Food will be more than critical for nutrient supplementation, but what humans eat in space will become countermeasures to cancer and other diseases that arise from these threats. The availability and production of fresh food will be a challenge, so every food used in space should serve multiple purposes. Antiangiogenic foods will be an important part of a strategy to prevent and fight cancer. Interestingly, conditions in space have been shown to be conducive to amplifying the angiogenesis inhibitory properties of certain foods. To date, astronauts on the International Space Station have grown a few plants including Romaine Lettuce and Tokyo Bekana Chinese cabbage (Khodadad et al. 2020). Interestingly, some plants grown in microgravity exhibit higher levels of antiangiogenic phenolic acids than their counterparts on Earth (Khodadad et al. 2020). The long-term health and well-being of humans off planet depend on the development of functional foods. Antiangiogenic dietary strategies represent a novel approach to cancer prevention, treatment, and prevention of relapse.

REFERENCES

Adini, A., T. Kornaga, F. Firoozbakht, and L. E. Benjamin. 2002. "Placental growth factor is a survival factor for tumor endothelial cells and macrophages." *Cancer Res* 62 (10):2749–52.

Aguilar-Cazares, D., R. Chavez-Dominguez, A. Carlos-Reyes, C. Lopez-Camarillo, O. N. Hernadez de la Cruz, and J. S. Lopez-Gonzalez. 2019. "Contribution of angiogenesis to inflammation and cancer." *Front Oncol* 9:1399. doi: 10.3389/fonc.2019.01399.

Ahn, W. S., J. Yoo, S. W. Huh, C. K. Kim, J. M. Lee, S. E. Namkoong, S. M. Bae, and I. P. Lee. 2003. "Protective effects of green tea extracts (polyphenon E and EGCG) on human cervical lesions." *Eur J Cancer Prev* 12 (5):383–390. doi: 10.1097/00008469-200310000-00007.

Albini, A., R. Dell'Eva, R. Vene, N. Ferrari, D. R. Buhler, D. M. Noonan, and G. Fassina. 2006. "Mechanisms of the antiangiogenic activity by the hop flavonoid xanthohumol: NF-kappaB and Akt as targets." *FASEB J* 20 (3):527–529. doi: 10.1096/fj.05-5128fje.

Allen, E., A. Jabouille, L. B. Rivera, I. Lodewijckx, R. Missiaen, V. Steri, K. Feyen, J. Tawney, D. Hanahan, I. P. Michael, and G. Bergers. 2017. "Combined antiangiogenic and anti-PD-L1 therapy stimulates tumor immunity through HEV formation." *Sci Transl Med* 9 (385). doi: 10.1126/scitranslmed.aak9679.

Anso, E., A. Zuazo, M. Irigoyen, M. C. Urdaci, A. Rouzaut, and J. J. Martinez-Irujo. 2010. "Flavonoids inhibit hypoxia-induced vascular endothelial growth factor expression by a HIF-1 independent mechanism." *Biochem Pharmacol* 79 (11):1600–1609. doi: 10.1016/j.bcp.2010.02.004.

Applegate, C. C., J. L. Rowles, K. M. Ranard, S. Jeon, and J. W. Erdman. 2018. "Soy consumption and the risk of prostate cancer: an updated systematic review and meta-analysis." *Nutrients* 10 (1). doi: 10.3390/nu10010040.

Auerbach, W., and R. Auerbach. 1994. "Angiogenesis inhibition: a review." *Pharmacol Ther* 63 (3):265–311. doi: 10.1016/0163-7258(94)90027-2.

Augustin, H. G., G. Y. Koh, G. Thurston, and K. Alitalo. 2009. "Control of vascular morphogenesis and homeostasis through the angiopoietin-Tie system." *Nat Rev Mol Cell Biol* 10 (3):165–177. doi: 10.1038/nrm2639.

Ausprunk, D. H., and J. Folkman. 1977. "Migration and proliferation of endothelial cells in preformed and newly formed blood vessels during tumor angiogenesis." *Microvasc Res* 14 (1):53–65. doi: 10.1016/0026-2862(77)90141-8.

Baeriswyl, V., and G. Christofori. 2009. "The angiogenic switch in carcinogenesis." *Semin Cancer Biol* 19 (5):329–337. doi: 10.1016/j.semcancer.2009.05.003.

Barsoum, I. B., C. A. Smallwood, D. R. Siemens, and C. H. Graham. 2014. "A mechanism of hypoxia-mediated escape from adaptive immunity in cancer cells." *Cancer Res* 74 (3):665–674. doi: 10.1158/0008-5472.CAN-13-0992.

Bemis, D. L., J. L. Capodice, M. Desai, R. Buttyan, and A. E. Katz. 2004. "A concentrated aglycone isoflavone preparation (GCP) that demonstrates potent anti-prostate cancer activity in vitro and in vivo." *Clin Cancer Res* 10 (15):5282–5292. doi: 10.1158/1078-0432.CCR-03-0828.

Benavente-Garcia, O., and J. Castillo. 2008. "Update on uses and properties of citrus flavonoids: new findings in anticancer, cardiovascular, and anti-inflammatory activity." *J Agric Food Chem* 56 (15):6185–6205. doi: 10.1021/jf8006568.

Bergers, G., D. Hanahan, and L. M. Coussens. 1998. "Angiogenesis and apoptosis are cellular parameters of neoplastic progression in transgenic mouse models of tumorigenesis." *Int J Dev Biol* 42 (7):995–1002.

Bettuzzi, S., M. Brausi, F. Rizzi, G. Castagnetti, G. Peracchia, and A. Corti. 2006. "Chemoprevention of human prostate cancer by oral administration of green tea catechins in volunteers with high-grade prostate intraepithelial neoplasia: a preliminary report from a one-year proof-of-principle study." *Cancer Res* 66 (2):1234–1240. doi: 10.1158/0008-5472.CAN-05-1145.

Bishayee, A. 2009. "Cancer prevention and treatment with resveratrol: from rodent studies to clinical trials." *Cancer Prev Res (Phila)* 2 (5):409–418. doi: 10.1158/1940-6207.CAPR-08-0160.

Boeing, H., T. Dietrich, K. Hoffmann, T. Pischon, P. Ferrari, P. H. Lahmann, M. C. Boutron-Ruault, F. Clavel-Chapelon, N. Allen, T. Key, G. Skeie, E. Lund, A. Olsen, A. Tjonneland, K. Overvad, M. K. Jensen, S. Rohrmann, J. Linseisen, A. Trichopoulou, C. Bamia, T. Psaltopoulou, L. Weinehall, I. Johansson, M. J. Sanchez, P. Jakszyn, E. Ardanaz, P. Amiano, M. D. Chirlaque, J. R. Quiros, E. Wirfalt, G. Berglund, P. H. Peeters, C. H. van Gils, H. B. Bueno-de-Mesquita, F. L. Buchner, F. Berrino, D. Palli, C. Sacerdote, R. Tumino, S. Panico, S. Bingham, K. T. Khaw, N. Slimani, T. Norat, M. Jenab, and E. Riboli. 2006. "Intake of fruits and vegetables and risk of cancer of the upper aero-digestive tract: the prospective EPIC-study." *Cancer Causes Control* 17 (7):957–969. doi: 10.1007/s10552-006-0036-4.

Buchner, F. L., H. B. Bueno-de-Mesquita, J. Linseisen, H. C. Boshuizen, L. A. Kiemeney, M. M. Ros, K. Overvad, L. Hansen, A. Tjonneland, O. Raaschou-Nielsen, F. Clavel-Chapelon, M. C. Boutron-Ruault, M. Touillaud, R. Kaaks, S. Rohrmann, H. Boeing, U. Nothlings, A. Trichopoulou, D. Zylis, V. Dilis, D. Palli, S. Sieri, P. Vineis, R. Tumino, S. Panico, P. H. Peeters, C. H. van Gils, E. Lund, I. T. Gram, T. Braaten, C. Martinez, A. Agudo, L. Arriola, E. Ardanaz, C. Navarro, L. Rodriguez, J. Manjer, E. Wirfalt, G. Hallmans, T. Rasmuson, T. J. Key, A. W. Roddam, S. Bingham, K. T. Khaw, N. Slimani, P. Bofetta, G. Byrnes, T. Norat, D. Michaud, and E. Riboli. 2010. "Fruits and vegetables consumption and the risk of histological subtypes of lung cancer in the European Prospective Investigation into Cancer and Nutrition (EPIC)." *Cancer Causes Control* 21 (3):357–371. doi: 10.1007/s10552-009-9468-y.

Bujanda, D. E., and C. Hachem. 2018. "Barrett's esophagus." *Mo Med* 115 (3):211–213.

Butler, T. P., and P. M. Gullino. 1975. "Quantitation of cell shedding into efferent blood of mammary adeno-carcinoma." *Cancer Res* 35 (3):512–516.

Cao, R., H. L. Wu, N. Veitonmaki, P. Linden, J. Farnebo, G. Y. Shi, and Y. Cao. 1999. "Suppression of angio-genesis and tumor growth by the inhibitor K1-5 generated by plasmin-mediated proteolysis." *Proc Natl Acad Sci U S A* 96 (10):5728–5733. doi: 10.1073/pnas.96.10.5728.

Cao, Y., and R. Cao. 1999. "Angiogenesis inhibited by drinking tea." *Nature* 398 (6726):381. doi: 10.1038/18793.

Cao, Y., C. Chen, J. A. Weatherbee, M. Tsang, and J. Folkman. 1995. "gro-beta, a-C-X-C- chemokine, is an angiogenesis inhibitor that suppresses the growth of Lewis lung carcinoma in mice." *J Exp Med* 182 (6):2069–2077. doi: 10.1084/jem.182.6.2069.

Cardona, F., C. Andres-Lacueva, S. Tulipani, F. J. Tinahones, and M. I. Queipo-Ortuno. 2013. "Benefits of polyphenols on gut microbiota and implications in human health." *J Nutr Biochem* 24 (8):1415–1422. doi: 10.1016/j.jnutbio.2013.05.001.

Carmeliet, P., and R. K. Jain. 2011. "Molecular mechanisms and clinical applications of angiogenesis." *Nature* 473 (7347):298–307. doi: 10.1038/nature10144.

Caygill, C. P., M. J. Hill, M. Braddick, and J. C. Sharp. 1994. "Cancer mortality in chronic typhoid and para-typhoid carriers." *Lancet* 343 (8889):83–84. doi: 10.1016/s0140-6736(94)90816-8.

Cetin, A., and B. Biltekin. 2019. "Combining ellagic acid with temozolomide mediates the cadherin switch and angiogenesis in a glioblastoma model." *World Neurosurg* 132:e178–e184. doi: 10.1016/j.wneu.2019.08.228.

Chao, C., J. M. Slezak, B. J. Caan, and V. P. Quinn. 2008. "Alcoholic beverage intake and risk of lung can-cer: the California Men's Health Study." *Cancer Epidemiol Biomarkers Prev* 17 (10):2692–2699. doi: 10.1158/1055-9965.EPI-08-0410.

Chen, C. M., Y. H. Hsieh, J. M. Hwang, H. J. Jan, S. C. Hsieh, S. H. Lin, and C. Y. Lai. 2015. "Fisetin sup-presses ADAM9 expression and inhibits invasion of glioma cancer cells through increased phosphoryla-tion of ERK1/2." *Tumour Biol* 36 (5):3407–3415. doi: 10.1007/s13277-014-2975-9.

Chen, M. L., Y. H. Lin, C. M. Yang, and M. L. Hu. 2012. "Lycopene inhibits angiogenesis both in vitro and in vivo by inhibiting MMP-2/uPA system through VEGFR2-mediated PI3K-Akt and ERK/p38 signaling pathways." *Mol Nutr Food Res* 56 (6):889–899. doi: 10.1002/mnfr.201100683.

Chiang, H. S., W. B. Wu, J. Y. Fang, D. F. Chen, B. H. Chen, C. C. Huang, Y. T. Chen, and C. F. Hung. 2007. "Lycopene inhibits PDGF-BB-induced signaling and migration in human dermal fibroblasts through interaction with PDGF-BB." *Life Sci* 81 (21–22):1509–1517. doi: 10.1016/j.lfs.2007.09.018.

Cimpean, A. M., R. Tamma, S. Ruggieri, B. Nico, A. Toma, and D. Ribatti. 2017. "Mast cells in breast cancer angiogenesis." *Crit Rev Oncol Hematol* 115:23–26. doi: 10.1016/j.critrevonc.2017.04.009.

Clinton, S. K., E. L. Giovannucci, and S. D. Hursting. 2019. "The World Cancer Research Fund/American Institute for Cancer Research Third Expert Report on Diet, Nutrition, Physical Activity, and Cancer: impact and future directions." *J Nutr.* doi: 10.1093/jn/nxz268.

Cook, M. R., J. Luo, M. Ndiaye, H. Chen, and M. Kunnimalaiyaan. 2010. "Xanthohumol inhibits the neu-roendocrine transcription factor achaete-scute complex-like 1, suppresses proliferation, and induces phosphorylated ERK1/2 in medullary thyroid cancer." *Am J Surg* 199 (3):315–318; discussion 318. doi: 10.1016/j.amjsurg.2009.08.034.

Coradini, D., C. Pellizzaro, D. Marimpietri, G. Abolafio, and M. G. Daidone. 2000. "Sodium butyrate modu-lates cell cycle-related proteins in HT29 human colonic adenocarcinoma cells." *Cell Prolif* 33 (3):139–146. doi: 10.1046/j.1365-2184.2000.00173.x.

Coussens, L. M., W. W. Raymond, G. Bergers, M. Laig-Webster, O. Behrendtsen, Z. Werb, G. H. Caughey, and D. Hanahan. 1999. "Inflammatory mast cells up-regulate angiogenesis during squamous epithelial carcinogenesis." *Genes Dev* 13 (11):1382–1397. doi: 10.1101/gad.13.11.1382.

Crockett, S. D., M. D. Long, E. S. Dellon, C. F. Martin, J. A. Galanko, and R. S. Sandler. 2011. "Inverse relationship between moderate alcohol intake and rectal cancer: analysis of the North Carolina Colon Cancer Study." *Dis Colon Rectum* 54 (7):887–894. doi: 10.1007/DCR.0b013e3182125577.

Dameron, K. M., O. V. Volpert, M. A. Tainsky, and N. Bouck. 1994. "Control of angiogenesis in fibroblasts by p53 regulation of thrombospondin-1." *Science* 265 (5178):1582–1584. doi: 10.1126/science.7521539.

Danese, S., M. Sans, D. M. Spencer, I. Beck, F. Donate, M. L. Plunkett, C. de la Motte, R. Redline, D. E. Shaw, A. D. Levine, A. P. Mazar, and C. Fiocchi. 2007. "Angiogenesis blockade as a new therapeutic approach to experimental colitis." *Gut* 56 (6):855–862. doi: 10.1136/gut.2006.114314.

De Spiegeleer, B., F. Verbeke, M. D'Hondt, A. Hendrix, C. Van De Wiele, C. Burvenich, K. Peremans, O. De Wever, M. Bracke, and E. Wynendaele. 2015. "The quorum sensing peptides PhrG, CSP and EDF pro-mote angiogenesis and invasion of breast cancer cells in vitro." *PLoS One* 10 (3):e0119471. doi: 10.1371/journal.pone.0119471.

DeBerardinis, R. J., and N. S. Chandel. 2016. "Fundamentals of cancer metabolism." *Sci Adv* 2 (5):e1600200. doi: 10.1126/sciadv.1600200.

Doll, R. 1992. "The lessons of life: keynote address to the nutrition and cancer conference." *Cancer Res* 52 (7 Suppl):2024s–2029s.

Donaldson, M. S. 2004. "Nutrition and cancer: a review of the evidence for an anti-cancer diet." *Nutr J* 3:19. doi: 10.1186/1475-2891-3-19.

Duenas, M., I. Munoz-Gonzalez, C. Cueva, A. Jimenez-Giron, F. Sanchez-Patan, C. Santos-Buelga, M. V. Moreno-Arribas, and B. Bartolome. 2015. "A survey of modulation of gut microbiota by dietary polyphenols." *Biomed Res Int* 2015:850902. doi: 10.1155/2015/850902.

Eelen, G., P. de Zeeuw, M. Simons, and P. Carmeliet. 2015. "Endothelial cell metabolism in normal and diseased vasculature." *Circ Res* 116 (7):1231–1244. doi: 10.1161/CIRCRESAHA.116.302855.

Elgass, S., A. Cooper, and M. Chopra. 2014. "Lycopene treatment of prostate cancer cell lines inhibits adhesion and migration properties of the cells." *Int J Med Sci* 11 (9):948–954. doi: 10.7150/ijms.9137.

Engerman, R. L., D. Pfaffenbach, and M. D. Davis. 1967. "Cell turnover of capillaries." *Lab Invest* 17 (6):738–743.

Eskens, F. A., and J. Verweij. 2006. "The clinical toxicity profile of vascular endothelial growth factor (VEGF) and vascular endothelial growth factor receptor (VEGFR) targeting angiogenesis inhibitors; a review." *Eur J Cancer* 42 (18):3127–3139. doi: 10.1016/j.ejca.2006.09.015.

Fenn, K., P. Strandwitz, E. J. Stewart, E. Dimise, S. Rubin, S. Gurubacharya, J. Clardy, and K. Lewis. 2017. "Quinones are growth factors for the human gut microbiota." *Microbiome* 5 (1):161. doi: 10.1186/s40168-017-0380-5.

Ferreri, A. J., R. Dolcetti, G. P. Dognini, L. Malabarba, N. Vicari, E. Pasini, M. Ponzoni, M. G. Cangi, L. Pecciarini, A. G. Resti, C. Doglioni, S. Rossini, and S. Magnino. 2008. "Chlamydophila psittaci is viable and infectious in the conjunctiva and peripheral blood of patients with ocular adnexal lymphoma: results of a single-center prospective case-control study." *Int J Cancer* 123 (5):1089–1093. doi: 10.1002/ijc.23596.

Festa, M., A. Capasso, C. W. D'Acunto, M. Masullo, A. G. Rossi, C. Pizza, and S. Piacente. 2011. "Xanthohumol induces apoptosis in human malignant glioblastoma cells by increasing reactive oxygen species and activating MAPK pathways." *J Nat Prod* 74 (12):2505–2513. doi: 10.1021/np200390x.

Fidler, I. J., and L. M. Ellis. 1994. "The implications of angiogenesis for the biology and therapy of cancer metastasis." *Cell* 79 (2):185–188. doi: 10.1016/0092-8674(94)90187-2.

Folkman, J. 1971. "Tumor angiogenesis: therapeutic implications." *N Engl J Med* 285 (21):1182–1186. doi: 10.1056/NEJM197111182852108.

Folkman, J. 1985. "Tumor angiogenesis." *Adv Cancer Res* 43:175–203. doi: 10.1016/s0065-230x(08)60946-x.

Folkman, J. 1996. "Tumor angiogenesis and tissue factor." *Nat Med* 2 (2):167–168. doi: 10.1038/nm0296-167.

Folkman, J. 2002. "Role of angiogenesis in tumor growth and metastasis." *Semin Oncol* 29 (6 Suppl 16):15–18. doi: 10.1053/sonc.2002.37263.

Folkman, J., and P. A. D'Amore. 1996. "Blood vessel formation: what is its molecular basis?" *Cell* 87 (7):1153–1155. doi: 10.1016/s0092-8674(00)81810-3.

Folkman, J., and M. Klagsbrun. 1987. "Angiogenic factors." *Science* 235 (4787):442–447. doi: 10.1126/science.2432664.

Folkman, J., K. Watson, D. Ingber, and D. Hanahan. 1989. "Induction of angiogenesis during the transition from hyperplasia to neoplasia." *Nature* 339 (6219):58–61. doi: 10.1038/339058a0.

Fotsis, T., M. S. Pepper, R. Montesano, E. Aktas, S. Breit, L. Schweigerer, S. Rasku, K. Wahala, and H. Adlercreutz. 1998. "Phytoestrogens and inhibition of angiogenesis." *Baillieres Clin Endocrinol Metab* 12 (4):649–666. doi: 10.1016/s0950-351x(98)80009-8.

Fox, J. G., and T. C. Wang. 2007. "Inflammation, atrophy, and gastric cancer." *J Clin Invest* 117 (1):60–69. doi: 10.1172/JCI30111.

Fraineau, S., A. Monvoisin, J. Clarhaut, J. Talbot, C. Simonneau, C. Kanthou, S. M. Kanse, M. Philippe, and O. Benzakour. 2012. "The vitamin K-dependent anticoagulant factor, protein S, inhibits multiple VEGF-A-induced angiogenesis events in a Mer- and SHP2-dependent manner." *Blood* 120 (25):5073–5083. doi: 10.1182/blood-2012-05-429183.

Freedman, N. D., Y. Park, A. F. Subar, A. R. Hollenbeck, M. F. Leitzmann, A. Schatzkin, and C. C. Abnet. 2007. "Fruit and vegetable intake and esophageal cancer in a large prospective cohort study." *Int J Cancer* 121 (12):2753–2760. doi: 10.1002/ijc.22993.

Gago-Dominguez, M., J. E. Castelao, C. L. Sun, D. Van Den Berg, W. P. Koh, H. P. Lee, and M. C. Yu. 2004. "Marine n-3 fatty acid intake, glutathione S-transferase polymorphisms and breast cancer risk in post-menopausal Chinese women in Singapore." *Carcinogenesis* 25 (11):2143–2147. doi: 10.1093/carcin/bgh230.

Gala, E., S. Landi, L. Solieri, M. Nocetti, A. Pulvirenti, and P. Giudici. 2008. "Diversity of lactic acid bacteria population in ripened Parmigiano Reggiano cheese." *Int J Food Microbiol* 125 (3):347–351. doi: 10.1016/j.ijfoodmicro.2008.04.008.

Gallo, C., K. Dallaglio, B. Bassani, T. Rossi, A. Rossello, D. M. Noonan, G. D'Uva, A. Bruno, and A. Albini. 2016. "Hop derived flavonoid xanthohumol inhibits endothelial cell functions via AMPK activation." *Oncotarget* 7 (37):59917–59931. doi: 10.18632/oncotarget.10990.

Garvin, S., and C. Dabrosin. 2003. "Tamoxifen inhibits secretion of vascular endothelial growth factor in breast cancer in vivo." *Cancer Res* 63 (24):8742–8748.

Gates, M. A., A. F. Vitonis, S. S. Tworoger, B. Rosner, L. Titus-Ernstoff, S. E. Hankinson, and D. W. Cramer. 2009. "Flavonoid intake and ovarian cancer risk in a population-based case-control study." *Int J Cancer* 124 (8):1918–1925. doi: 10.1002/ijc.24151.

Gillis, P., U. Savla, O. V. Volpert, B. Jimenez, C. M. Waters, R. J. Panos, and N. P. Bouck. 1999. "Keratinocyte growth factor induces angiogenesis and protects endothelial barrier function." *J Cell Sci* 112 (Pt 12):2049–2057.

Gimbrone, M. A., Jr., S. B. Leapman, R. S. Cotran, and J. Folkman. 1972. "Tumor dormancy in vivo by prevention of neovascularization." *J Exp Med* 136 (2):261–276. doi: 10.1084/jem.136.2.261.

Gong, Y., R. Dong, X. Gao, J. Li, L. Jiang, J. Zheng, S. Cui, M. Ying, B. Yang, J. Cao, and Q. He. 2019. "Neohesperidin prevents colorectal tumorigenesis by altering the gut microbiota." *Pharmacol Res* 148:104460. doi: 10.1016/j.phrs.2019.104460.

Goodman, M. T., L. R. Wilkens, J. H. Hankin, L. C. Lyu, A. H. Wu, and L. N. Kolonel. 1997. "Association of soy and fiber consumption with the risk of endometrial cancer." *Am J Epidemiol* 146 (4):294–306. doi: 10.1093/oxfordjournals.aje.a009270.

Graff, R. E., A. Pettersson, R. T. Lis, T. U. Ahearn, S. C. Markt, K. M. Wilson, J. R. Rider, M. Fiorentino, S. Finn, S. A. Kenfield, M. Loda, E. L. Giovannucci, B. Rosner, and L. A. Mucci. 2016. "Dietary lycopene intake and risk of prostate cancer defined by ERG protein expression." *Am J Clin Nutr* 103 (3):851–860. doi: 10.3945/ajcn.115.118703.

Habu, D., S. Shiomi, A. Tamori, T. Takeda, T. Tanaka, S. Kubo, and S. Nishiguchi. 2004. "Role of vitamin K2 in the development of hepatocellular carcinoma in women with viral cirrhosis of the liver." *JAMA* 292 (3):358–361. doi: 10.1001/jama.292.3.358.

Hammes, H. P., J. Lin, P. Wagner, Y. Feng, F. Vom Hagen, T. Krzizok, O. Renner, G. Breier, M. Brownlee, and U. Deutsch. 2004. "Angiopoietin-2 causes pericyte dropout in the normal retina: evidence for involvement in diabetic retinopathy." *Diabetes* 53 (4):1104–1110. doi: 10.2337/diabetes.53.4.1104.

Hanahan, D. 1985. "Heritable formation of pancreatic beta-cell tumours in transgenic mice expressing recombinant insulin/simian virus 40 oncogenes." *Nature* 315 (6015):115–122. doi: 10.1038/315115a0.

Hanahan, D., and J. Folkman. 1996. "Patterns and emerging mechanisms of the angiogenic switch during tumorigenesis." *Cell* 86 (3):353–364. doi: 10.1016/s0092-8674(00)80108-7.

Hattori, K., B. Heissig, Y. Wu, S. Dias, R. Tejada, B. Ferris, D. J. Hicklin, Z. Zhu, P. Bohlen, L. Witte, J. Hendrikx, N. R. Hackett, R. G. Crystal, M. A. Moore, Z. Werb, D. Lyden, and S. Rafii. 2002. "Placental growth factor reconstitutes hematopoiesis by recruiting VEGFR1(+) stem cells from bone-marrow microenvironment." *Nat Med* 8 (8):841–849. doi: 10.1038/nm740.

Heiman, M. L., and F. L. Greenway. 2016. "A healthy gastrointestinal microbiome is dependent on dietary diversity." *Mol Metab* 5 (5):317–320. doi: 10.1016/j.molmet.2016.02.005.

Hejazi, E., J. Nasrollahzadeh, R. Fatemi, L. Barzegar-Yar Mohamadi, K. Saliminejad, Z. Amiri, M. Kimiagar, M. Houshyari, M. Tavakoli, and F. Idali. 2015. "Effects of combined soy isoflavone extract and docetaxel treatment on murine 4T1 breast tumor model." *Avicenna J Med Biotechnol* 7 (1):16–21.

Heron, M. 2019. "Deaths: leading causes for 2017." *Natl Vital Stat Rep* 68 (6):1–77.

Henning SM, P. Wang, J. Said, C. Magyar, B. Castor, N. Doan, C. Tosity, A. Moro, K. Gao, L. Li, and D. Heber. 2012. Polyphenols in brewed green tea inhibit prostate tumor xenograft growth by localizing to the tumor and decreasing oxidative stress and angiogenesis. *Journal of Nutritional Biochemistry.* 23 (11):1537–1542. doi: 10.1016/j.jnutbio.2011.10.007. Epub 2012 Mar 8. PMID: 22405694; PMCID: PMC3374889.

Hobson, B., and J. Denekamp. 1984. "Endothelial proliferation in tumours and normal tissues: continuous labelling studies." *Br J Cancer* 49 (4):405–413. doi: 10.1038/bjc.1984.66.

Holmgren, L. 1996. "Antiangiogenis restricted tumor dormancy." *Cancer Metastasis Rev* 15 (2):241–245. doi: 10.1007/BF00437478.

Holmgren, L., M. S. O'Reilly, and J. Folkman. 1995. "Dormancy of micrometastases: balanced proliferation and apoptosis in the presence of angiogenesis suppression." *Nat Med* 1 (2):149–153. doi: 10.1038/nm0295-149.

Howells, L. M., D. P. Berry, P. J. Elliott, E. W. Jacobson, E. Hoffmann, B. Hegarty, K. Brown, W. P. Steward, and A. J. Gescher. 2011. "Phase I randomized, double-blind pilot study of micronized resveratrol (SRT501) in patients with hepatic metastases--safety, pharmacokinetics, and pharmacodynamics." *Cancer Prev Res (Phila)* 4 (9):1419–1425. doi: 10.1158/1940-6207.CAPR-11-0148.

Hu, D. L., G. Wang, J. Yu, L. H. Zhang, Y. F. Huang, D. Wang, and H. H. Zhou. 2019. "Epigallocatechin3gallate modulates long noncoding RNA and mRNA expression profiles in lung cancer cells." *Mol Med Rep* 19 (3):1509–1520. doi: 10.3892/mmr.2019.9816.

Hu, W. H., G. K. Chan, R. Duan, H. Y. Wang, X. P. Kong, T. T. Dong, and K. W. Tsim. 2019. "Synergy of ginkgetin and resveratrol in suppressing VEGF-induced angiogenesis: a therapy in treating colorectal cancer." *Cancers (Basel)* 11 (12):1828. doi: 10.3390/cancers11121828.

Huang, S., C. A. Pettaway, H. Uehara, C. D. Bucana, and I. J. Fidler. 2001. "Blockade of NF-kappaB activity in human prostate cancer cells is associated with suppression of angiogenesis, invasion, and metastasis." *Oncogene* 20 (31):4188–4197. doi: 10.1038/sj.onc.1204535.

Hudson, T. S., S. N. Perkins, S. D. Hursting, H. A. Young, Y. S. Kim, T. C. Wang, and T. T. Wang. 2012. "Inhibition of androgen-responsive LNCaP prostate cancer cell tumor xenograft growth by dietary phenethyl isothiocyanate correlates with decreased angiogenesis and inhibition of cell attachment." *Int J Oncol* 40 (4):1113–1121. doi: 10.3892/ijo.2012.1335.

Innes, J. K., and P. C. Calder. 2018. "Omega-6 fatty acids and inflammation." *Prostaglandins Leukot Essent Fatty Acids* 132:41–48. doi: 10.1016/j.plefa.2018.03.004.

Intlekofer, A. M., and L. W. S. Finley. 2019. "Metabolic signatures of cancer cells and stem cells." *Nat Metab* 1 (2):177–188. doi: 10.1038/s42255-019-0032-0.

Isaacs, R. B., and R. S. Hellberg. 2019. "Shark cartilage supplement labeling practices and compliance with U.S. regulations." *J Diet Suppl* 18:44–56. doi: 10.1080/19390211.2019.1698687.

Jang, M., L. Cai, G. O. Udeani, K. V. Slowing, C. F. Thomas, C. W. Beecher, H. H. Fong, N. R. Farnsworth, A. D. Kinghorn, R. G. Mehta, R. C. Moon, and J. M. Pezzuto. 1997. "Cancer chemopreventive activity of resveratrol, a natural product derived from grapes." *Science* 275 (5297):218–220. doi: 10.1126/science.275.5297.218.

Jia, S., Y. Hu, W. Zhang, X. Zhao, Y. Chen, C. Sun, X. Li, and K. Chen. 2015. "Hypoglycemic and hypolipidemic effects of neohesperidin derived from Citrus aurantium L. in diabetic KK-A(y) mice." *Food Funct* 6 (3):878–886. doi: 10.1039/c4fo00993b.

Kaliannan, K., B. Wang, X. Y. Li, K. J. Kim, and J. X. Kang. 2015. "A host-microbiome interaction mediates the opposing effects of omega-6 and omega-3 fatty acids on metabolic endotoxemia." *Sci Rep* 5:11276. doi: 10.1038/srep11276.

Kandel, J., E. Bossy-Wetzel, F. Radvanyi, M. Klagsbrun, J. Folkman, and D. Hanahan. 1991. "Neovascularization is associated with a switch to the export of bFGF in the multistep development of fibrosarcoma." *Cell* 66 (6):1095–1104. doi: 10.1016/0092-8674(91)90033-u.

Kantor, E. D., J. W. Lampe, U. Peters, T. L. Vaughan, and E. White. 2014. "Long-chain omega-3 polyunsaturated fatty acid intake and risk of colorectal cancer." *Nutr Cancer* 66 (4):716–727. doi: 10.1080/01635581.2013.804101.

Karami, S., S. E. Daugherty, and M. P. Purdue. 2015. "A prospective study of alcohol consumption and renal cell carcinoma risk." *Int J Cancer* 137 (1):238–242. doi: 10.1002/ijc.29359.

Kayashima, T., M. Mori, R. Mizutani, K. Nishio, K. Kuramochi, K. Tsubaki, H. Yoshida, Y. Mizushina, and K. Matsubara. 2010. "Synthesis and biological evaluation of vitamin K derivatives as angiogenesis inhibitor." *Bioorg Med Chem* 18 (17):6305–6309. doi: 10.1016/j.bmc.2010.07.022.

Kayashima, T., M. Mori, H. Yoshida, Y. Mizushina, and K. Matsubara. 2009. "1,4-Naphthoquinone is a potent inhibitor of human cancer cell growth and angiogenesis." *Cancer Lett* 278 (1):34–40. doi: 10.1016/j.canlet.2008.12.020.

Khodadad, C. L. M., M. E. Hummerick, L. E. Spencer, A. R. Dixit, J. T. Richards, M. W. Romeyn, T. M. Smith, R. M. Wheeler, and G. D. Massa. 2020. "Microbiological and nutritional analysis of lettuce crops grown on the International Space Station." *Front Plant Sci* 11:199. doi: 10.3389/fpls.2020.00199.

Kim, K. K., A. P. Singh, R. K. Singh, A. Demartino, L. Brard, N. Vorsa, T. S. Lange, and R. G. Moore. 2012. "Anti-angiogenic activity of cranberry proanthocyanidins and cytotoxic properties in ovarian cancer cells." *Int J Oncol* 40 (1):227–235. doi: 10.3892/ijo.2011.1198.

Koolwijk, P., N. Sidenius, E. Peters, C. F. Sier, R. Hanemaaijer, F. Blasi, and V. W. van Hinsbergh. 2001. "Proteolysis of the urokinase-type plasminogen activator receptor by metalloproteinase-12: implication for angiogenesis in fibrin matrices." *Blood* 97 (10):3123–3131. doi: 10.1182/blood.v97.10.3123.

Kowshik, J., H. Giri, T. K. Kishore, R. Kesavan, R. N. Vankudavath, G. B. Reddy, M. Dixit, and S. Nagini. 2014. "Ellagic acid inhibits VEGF/VEGFR2, PI3K/Akt and MAPK signaling cascades in the hamster cheek pouch carcinogenesis model." *Anticancer Agents Med Chem* 14 (9):1249–1260. doi: 10.2174/187 1520614666140723114217.

Kunimasa, K., T. Kobayashi, S. Sugiyama, K. Kaji, and T. Ohta. 2008. "Indole-3-carbinol suppresses tumor-induced angiogenesis by inhibiting tube formation and inducing apoptosis." *Biosci Biotechnol Biochem* 72 (8):2243–2246. doi: 10.1271/bbb.80292.

Kwak, S. H., Y. M. Cho, G. M. Noh, and A. S. Om. 2014. "Cancer preventive potential of kimchi lactic acid bacteria (Weissella cibaria, Lactobacillus plantarum)." *J Cancer Prev* 19 (4):253–258. doi: 10.15430/ JCP.2014.19.4.253.

Kwak, Y., J. Lee, and J. Ju. 2016. "Anti-cancer activities of Brassica juncea leaves in vitro." *EXCLI J* 15:699–710. doi: 10.17179/excli2016-586.

Lacey, M., S. Alpert, and D. Hanahan. 1986. "Bovine papillomavirus genome elicits skin tumours in transgenic mice." *Nature* 322 (6080):609–612. doi: 10.1038/322609a0.

Lapeyre-Prost, A., M. Terme, S. Pernot, A. L. Pointet, T. Voron, E. Tartour, and J. Taieb. 2017. "Immunomodulatory activity of VEGF in cancer." *Int Rev Cell Mol Biol* 330:295–342. doi: 10.1016/ bs.ircmb.2016.09.007.

Latocha, M., J. Plonka, D. Kusmierz, M. Jurzak, R. Polaniak, and A. Nowosad. 2014. "Transcripional activity of genes encoding MMPs and TIMPs in breast cancer cells treated by genistein and in normal cancer-associated fibroblasts--in vitro studies." *Acta Pol Pharm* 71 (6):1095–1102.

Lawler, P. R., and J. Lawler. 2012. "Molecular basis for the regulation of angiogenesis by thrombospondin-1 and -2." *Cold Spring Harb Perspect Med* 2 (5):a006627. doi: 10.1101/cshperspect.a006627.

Lazzi, C., S. Turroni, A. Mancini, E. Sgarbi, E. Neviani, P. Brigidi, and M. Gatti. 2014. "Transcriptomic clues to understand the growth of Lactobacillus rhamnosus in cheese." *BMC Microbiol* 14:28. doi: 10.1186/1471-2180-14-28.

Lecomte, S., F. Demay, F. Ferriere, and F. Pakdel. 2017. "Phytochemicals targeting estrogen receptors: beneficial rather than adverse effects?" *Int J Mol Sci* 18 (7):1381. doi: 10.3390/ijms18071381.

Lecuit, M., E. Abachin, A. Martin, C. Poyart, P. Pochart, F. Suarez, D. Bengoufa, J. Feuillard, A. Lavergne, J. I. Gordon, P. Berche, L. Guillevin, and O. Lortholary. 2004. "Immunoproliferative small intestinal disease associated with Campylobacter jejuni." *N Engl J Med* 350 (3):239–248. doi: 10.1056/NEJMoa031887.

Lee, S. H., J. Lee, M. H. Jung, and Y. M. Lee. 2013. "Glyceollins, a novel class of soy phytoalexins, inhibit angiogenesis by blocking the VEGF and bFGF signaling pathways." *Mol Nutr Food Res* 57 (2):225–234. doi: 10.1002/mnfr.201200489.

Leung, D. W., G. Cachianes, W. J. Kuang, D. V. Goeddel, and N. Ferrara. 1989. "Vascular endothelial growth factor is a secreted angiogenic mitogen." *Science* 246 (4935):1306–1309. doi: 10.1126/science.2479986.

Li, J., C. Y. Sung, N. Lee, Y. Ni, J. Pihlajamaki, G. Panagiotou, and H. El-Nezami. 2016. "Probiotics modulated gut microbiota suppresses hepatocellular carcinoma growth in mice." *Proc Natl Acad Sci U S A* 113 (9):E1306–E1315. doi: 10.1073/pnas.1518189113.

Li, N., Z. Sun, C. Han, and J. Chen. 1999. "The chemopreventive effects of tea on human oral precancerous mucosa lesions." *Proc Soc Exp Biol Med* 220 (4):218–224. doi: 10.1046/j.1525-1373.1999.d01-37.x.

Li, T., G. Kang, T. Wang, and H. Huang. 2018. "Tumor angiogenesis and anti-angiogenic gene therapy for cancer." *Oncol Lett* 16 (1):687–702. doi: 10.3892/ol.2018.8733.

Li, V. W., and W. W. Li. 2008. "Antiangiogenesis in the treatment of skin cancer." *J Drugs Dermatol* 7 (1 Suppl 1):S17–S24.

Li, W., L. Cao, X. Chen, J. Lei, and Q. Ma. 2016. "Resveratrol inhibits hypoxia-driven ROS-induced invasive and migratory ability of pancreatic cancer cells via suppression of the Hedgehog signaling pathway." *Oncol Rep* 35 (3):1718–1726. doi: 10.3892/or.2015.4504.

Li, W. W., V. W. Li, M. Hutnik, and A. S. Chiou. 2012. "Tumor angiogenesis as a target for dietary cancer prevention." *J Oncol* 2012:879623. doi: 10.1155/2012/879623.

Liao, J., G. Y. Yang, E. S. Park, X. Meng, Y. Sun, D. Jia, D. N. Seril, and C. S. Yang. 2004. "Inhibition of lung carcinogenesis and effects on angiogenesis and apoptosis in A/J mice by oral administration of green tea." *Nutr Cancer* 48 (1):44–53. doi: 10.1207/s15327914nc4801_7.

Liao, Z. H., H. Q. Zhu, Y. Y. Chen, R. L. Chen, L. X. Fu, L. Li, H. Zhou, J. L. Zhou, and G. Liang. 2020. "The epigallocatechin gallate derivative Y6 inhibits human hepatocellular carcinoma by inhibiting angiogenesis in MAPK/ERK1/2 and PI3K/AKT/ HIF-1alpha/VEGF dependent pathways." *J Ethnopharmacol* 259:112852. doi: 10.1016/j.jep.2020.112852.

Lin, Z., Q. Zhang, and W. Luo. 2016. "Angiogenesis inhibitors as therapeutic agents in cancer: challenges and future directions." *Eur J Pharmacol* 793:76–81. doi: 10.1016/j.ejphar.2016.10.039.

Lisko, D. J., G. P. Johnston, and C. G. Johnston. 2017. "Effects of dietary yogurt on the healthy human gastro-intestinal (GI) microbiome." *Microorganisms* 5 (1):6. doi: 10.3390/microorganisms5010006.

Liu, H., Z. Zeng, S. Wang, T. Li, E. Mastriani, Q. H. Li, H. X. Bao, Y. J. Zhou, X. Wang, Y. Liu, W. Liu, S. Hu, S. Gao, M. Yu, Y. Qi, Z. Shen, H. Wang, T. Gao, L. Dong, R. N. Johnston, and S. L. Liu. 2017. "Main components of pomegranate, ellagic acid and luteolin, inhibit metastasis of ovarian cancer by down-regulating MMP2 and MMP9." *Cancer Biol Ther* 18 (12):990–999. doi: 10.1080/15384047.2017.1394542.

Liu, M., H. Yin, X. Qian, J. Dong, Z. Qian, and J. Miao. 2016. "Xanthohumol, a prenylated chalcone from hops, inhibits the viability and stemness of doxorubicin-resistant MCF-7/ADR cells." *Molecules* 22 (1):36. doi: 10.3390/molecules22010036.

Lozupone, C. A., J. I. Stombaugh, J. I. Gordon, J. K. Jansson, and R. Knight. 2012. "Diversity, stability and resilience of the human gut microbiota." *Nature* 489 (7415):220–230. doi: 10.1038/nature11550.

Lu, H., J. Li, D. Zhang, G. D. Stoner, and C. Huang. 2006. "Molecular mechanisms involved in chemopre-vention of black raspberry extracts: from transcription factors to their target genes." *Nutr Cancer* 54 (1):69–78. doi: 10.1207/s15327914nc5401_8.

Macedo, F., K. Ladeira, A. Longatto-Filho, and S. F. Martins. 2017. "Gastric cancer and angiogenesis: is VEGF a useful biomarker to assess progression and remission?" *J Gastric Cancer* 17 (1):1–10. doi: 10.5230/jgc.2017.17.e1.

Maione, T. E., G. S. Gray, J. Petro, A. J. Hunt, A. L. Donner, S. I. Bauer, H. F. Carson, and R. J. Sharpe. 1990. "Inhibition of angiogenesis by recombinant human platelet factor-4 and related peptides." *Science* 247 (4938):77–79. doi: 10.1126/science.1688470.

Makki, K., E. C. Deehan, J. Walter, and F. Backhed. 2018. "The impact of dietary fiber on gut microbiota in host health and disease." *Cell Host Microbe* 23 (6):705–715. doi: 10.1016/j.chom.2018.05.012.

Markoski, M. M., J. Garavaglia, A. Oliveira, J. Olivaes, and A. Marcadenti. 2016. "Molecular properties of red wine compounds and cardiometabolic benefits." *Nutr Metab Insights* 9:51–57. doi: 10.4137/NMI.S32909.

Marth, C., I. Vergote, G. Scambia, W. Oberaigner, A. Clamp, R. Berger, C. Kurzeder, N. Colombo, P. Vuylsteke, D. Lorusso, M. Hall, V. Renard, S. Pignata, R. Kristeleit, S. Altintas, G. Rustin, R. M. Wenham, M. R. Mirza, P. C. Fong, A. Oza, B. J. Monk, H. Ma, F. D. Vogl, and B. A. Bach. 2017. "ENGOT-ov-6/TRINOVA-2: randomised, double-blind, phase 3 study of pegylated liposomal doxorubicin plus treba-nanib or placebo in women with recurrent partially platinum-sensitive or resistant ovarian cancer." *Eur J Cancer* 70:111–121. doi: 10.1016/j.ejca.2016.09.004.

Masferrer, J. L., K. M. Leahy, A. T. Koki, B. S. Zweifel, S. L. Settle, B. M. Woerner, D. A. Edwards, A. G. Flickinger, R. J. Moore, and K. Seibert. 2000. "Antiangiogenic and antitumor activities of cyclooxygen-ase-2 inhibitors." *Cancer Res* 60 (5):1306–1311.

McCullough, M. L., and E. L. Giovannucci. 2004. "Diet and cancer prevention." *Oncogene* 23 (38):6349–6364. doi: 10.1038/sj.onc.1207716.

McLarty, J., R. L. Bigelow, M. Smith, D. Elmajian, M. Ankem, and J. A. Cardelli. 2009. "Tea polyphenols decrease serum levels of prostate-specific antigen, hepatocyte growth factor, and vascular endothelial growth factor in prostate cancer patients and inhibit production of hepatocyte growth factor and vascu-lar endothelial growth factor in vitro." *Cancer Prev Res (Phila)* 2 (7):673–682. doi: 10.1158/1940-6207.CAPR-08-0167.

Mehta, R. R., T. Yamada, B. N. Taylor, K. Christov, M. L. King, D. Majumdar, F. Lekmine, C. Tiruppathi, A. Shilkaitis, L. Bratescu, A. Green, C. W. Beattie, and T. K. Das Gupta. 2011. "A cell penetrating peptide derived from azurin inhibits angiogenesis and tumor growth by inhibiting phosphorylation of VEGFR-2, FAK and Akt." *Angiogenesis* 14 (3):355–369. doi: 10.1007/s10456-011-9220-6.

Melincovici, C. S., A. B. Bosca, S. Susman, M. Marginean, C. Mihu, M. Istrate, I. M. Moldovan, A. L. Roman, and C. M. Mihu. 2018. "Vascular endothelial growth factor (VEGF) - key factor in normal and patho-logical angiogenesis." *Rom J Morphol Embryol* 59 (2):455–467.

Micha, R., S. Khatibzadeh, P. Shi, S. Fahimi, S. Lim, K. G. Andrews, R. E. Engell, J. Powles, M. Ezzati, D. Mozaffarian, Nutrition Global Burden of Diseases, and D. E. Chronic Diseases Expert Group NutriCo. 2014. "Global, regional, and national consumption levels of dietary fats and oils in 1990 and 2010: a system-atic analysis including 266 country-specific nutrition surveys." *BMJ* 348:g2272. doi: 10.1136/bmj.g2272.

Mignone, L. I., E. Giovannucci, P. A. Newcomb, L. Titus-Ernstoff, A. Trentham-Dietz, J. M. Hampton, W. C. Willett, and K. M. Egan. 2009. "Dietary carotenoids and the risk of invasive breast cancer." *Int J Cancer* 124 (12):2929–2937. doi: 10.1002/ijc.24334.

Millen, A. E., M. A. Tucker, P. Hartge, A. Halpern, D. E. Elder, D. Guerry, E. A. Holly, R. W. Sagebiel, and N. Potischman. 2004. "Diet and melanoma in a case-control study." *Cancer Epidemiol Biomarkers Prev* 13 (6):1042–1051.

Miller, D. R., G. T. Anderson, J. J. Stark, J. L. Granick, and D. Richardson. 1998. "Phase I/II trial of the safety and efficacy of shark cartilage in the treatment of advanced cancer." *J Clin Oncol* 16 (11):3649–3655. doi: 10.1200/JCO.1998.16.11.3649.

Modzelewski, R. A., P. Davies, S. C. Watkins, R. Auerbach, M. J. Chang, and C. S. Johnson. 1994. "Isolation and identification of fresh tumor-derived endothelial cells from a murine RIF-1 fibrosarcoma." *Cancer Res* 54 (2):336–339.

Molan, A. L., Z. Liu, and G. Plimmer. 2014. "Evaluation of the effect of blackcurrant products on gut microbiota and on markers of risk for colon cancer in humans." *Phytother Res* 28 (3):416–422. doi: 10.1002/ptr.5009.

Monk, B. J., A. Poveda, I. Vergote, F. Raspagliesi, K. Fujiwara, D. S. Bae, A. Oaknin, I. Ray-Coquard, D. M. Provencher, B. Y. Karlan, C. Lhomme, G. Richardson, D. G. Rincon, R. L. Coleman, T. J. Herzog, C. Marth, A. Brize, M. Fabbro, A. Redondo, A. Bamias, M. Tassoudji, L. Navale, D. J. Warner, and A. M. Oza. 2014. "Anti-angiopoietin therapy with trebananib for recurrent ovarian cancer (TRINOVA-1): a randomised, multicentre, double-blind, placebo-controlled phase 3 trial." *Lancet Oncol* 15 (8):799–808. doi: 10.1016/S1470-2045(14)70244-X.

Morrison, D. J., and T. Preston. 2016. "Formation of short chain fatty acids by the gut microbiota and their impact on human metabolism." *Gut Microbes* 7 (3):189–200. doi: 10.1080/19490976.2015.1134082.

Muscat, J. E., and M. Huncharek. 1996. "Dietary intake and the risk of malignant mesothelioma." *Br J Cancer* 73 (9):1122–1125. doi: 10.1038/bjc.1996.215.

Naumov, G. N., J. Folkman, O. Straume, and L. A. Akslen. 2008. "Tumor-vascular interactions and tumor dormancy." *APMIS* 116 (7–8):569–585. doi: 10.1111/j.1600-0463.2008.01213.x.

Navarro, F. J., S. Mirkin, and D. F. Archer. 2003. "Effect of raloxifene, 17beta-estradiol, and progesterone on mRNA for vascular endothelial growth factor isoforms 121 and 165 and thrombospondin-1 in Ishikawa cells." *Fertil Steril* 79 (6):1409–1415. doi: 10.1016/s0015-0282(03)00350-9.

Nechuta, S. J., B. J. Caan, W. Y. Chen, W. Lu, Z. Chen, M. L. Kwan, S. W. Flatt, Y. Zheng, W. Zheng, J. P. Pierce, and X. O. Shu. 2012. "Soy food intake after diagnosis of breast cancer and survival: an in-depth analysis of combined evidence from cohort studies of US and Chinese women." *Am J Clin Nutr* 96 (1):123–132. doi: 10.3945/ajcn.112.035972.

Nelson, A. R., B. Fingleton, M. L. Rothenberg, and L. M. Matrisian. 2000. "Matrix metalloproteinases: biologic activity and clinical implications." *J Clin Oncol* 18 (5):1135–1149. doi: 10.1200/JCO.2000.18.5.1135.

Nguyen, M. 1997. "Angiogenic factors as tumor markers." *Invest New Drugs* 15 (1):29–37. doi: 10.1023/a:1005766511385.

Nimptsch, K., S. Rohrmann, R. Kaaks, and J. Linseisen. 2010. "Dietary vitamin K intake in relation to cancer incidence and mortality: results from the Heidelberg cohort of the European Prospective Investigation into Cancer and Nutrition (EPIC-Heidelberg)." *Am J Clin Nutr* 91 (5):1348–1358. doi: 10.3945/ajcn.2009.28691.

Nor, J. E., J. Christensen, D. J. Mooney, and P. J. Polverini. 1999. "Vascular endothelial growth factor (VEGF)-mediated angiogenesis is associated with enhanced endothelial cell survival and induction of Bcl-2 expression." *Am J Pathol* 154 (2):375–384. doi: 10.1016/S0002-9440(10)65284-4.

Norrby, K. 2002. "Mast cells and angiogenesis." *APMIS* 110 (5):355–371. doi: 10.1034/j.1600-0463.2002.100501.x.

Numasaki, M., J. Fukushi, M. Ono, S. K. Narula, P. J. Zavodny, T. Kudo, P. D. Robbins, H. Tahara, and M. T. Lotze. 2003. "Interleukin-17 promotes angiogenesis and tumor growth." *Blood* 101 (7):2620–2627. doi: 10.1182/blood-2002-05-1461.

Oh, Y. J., H. W. Lee, S. K. Lim, M. S. Kwon, J. Lee, J. Y. Jang, J. H. Lee, H. W. Park, Y. D. Nam, M. J. Seo, S. W. Roh, and H. J. Choi. 2016. "Lentibacillus kimchii sp. nov., an extremely halophilic bacterium isolated from kimchi, a Korean fermented vegetable." *Antonie Van Leeuwenhoek* 109 (6):869–876. doi: 10.1007/s10482-016-0686-5.

Ohno-Matsui, K., I. Morita, J. Tombran-Tink, D. Mrazek, M. Onodera, T. Uetama, M. Hayano, S. I. Murota, and M. Mochizuki. 2001. "Novel mechanism for age-related macular degeneration: an equilibrium shift between the angiogenesis factors VEGF and PEDF." *J Cell Physiol* 189 (3):323–333. doi: 10.1002/jcp.10026.

Okuyama, H., Y. Ichikawa, Y. Sun, T. Hamazaki, and W. E. Lands. 2007. "Omega3 fatty acids effectively prevent coronary heart disease and other late-onset diseases--the excessive linoleic acid syndrome." *World Rev Nutr Diet* 96:83–103. doi: 10.1159/000097809.

Ollberding, N. J., B. Aschebrook-Kilfoy, D. B. Caces, S. M. Smith, D. D. Weisenburger, and B. C. Chiu. 2013. "Dietary intake of fruits and vegetables and overall survival in non-Hodgkin lymphoma." *Leuk Lymphoma* 54 (12):2613–2619. doi: 10.3109/10428194.2013.784968.

Pal, H. C., S. Sharma, L. R. Strickland, S. K. Katiyar, M. E. Ballestas, M. Athar, C. A. Elmets, and F. Afaq. 2014. "Fisetin inhibits human melanoma cell invasion through promotion of mesenchymal to epithelial transition and by targeting MAPK and NFkappaB signaling pathways." *PLoS One* 9 (1):e86338. doi: 10.1371/journal.pone.0086338.

Palermo, M., N. Pellegrini, and V. Fogliano. 2014. "The effect of cooking on the phytochemical content of vegetables." *J Sci Food Agric* 94 (6):1057–1070. doi: 10.1002/jsfa.6478.

Pantuck, A. J., J. T. Leppert, N. Zomorodian, W. Aronson, J. Hong, R. J. Barnard, N. Seeram, H. Liker, H. Wang, R. Elashoff, D. Heber, M. Aviram, L. Ignarro, and A. Belldegrun. 2006. "Phase II study of pomegranate juice for men with rising prostate-specific antigen following surgery or radiation for prostate cancer." *Clin Cancer Res* 12 (13):4018–4026. doi: 10.1158/1078-0432.CCR-05-2290.

Park, E. J., J. Chun, C. J. Cha, W. S. Park, C. O. Jeon, and J. W. Bae. 2012. "Bacterial community analysis during fermentation of ten representative kinds of kimchi with barcoded pyrosequencing." *Food Microbiol* 30 (1):197–204. doi: 10.1016/j.fm.2011.10.011.

Park, J. Y., P. N. Mitrou, C. C. Dahm, R. N. Luben, N. J. Wareham, K. T. Khaw, and S. A. Rodwell. 2009. "Baseline alcohol consumption, type of alcoholic beverage and risk of colorectal cancer in the European Prospective Investigation into Cancer and Nutrition-Norfolk study." *Cancer Epidemiol* 33 (5):347–354. doi: 10.1016/j.canep.2009.10.015.

Patel, K. R., V. A. Brown, D. J. Jones, R. G. Britton, D. Hemingway, A. S. Miller, K. P. West, T. D. Booth, M. Perloff, J. A. Crowell, D. E. Brenner, W. P. Steward, A. J. Gescher, and K. Brown. 2010. "Clinical pharmacology of resveratrol and its metabolites in colorectal cancer patients." *Cancer Res* 70 (19):7392–7399. doi: 10.1158/0008-5472.CAN-10-2027.

Peek, R. M., Jr., and M. J. Blaser. 2002. "Helicobacter pylori and gastrointestinal tract adenocarcinomas." *Nat Rev Cancer* 2 (1):28–37. doi: 10.1038/nrc703.

Pezzuto, A., and E. Carico. 2018. "Role of HIF-1 in cancer progression: novel insights. A review." *Curr Mol Med* 18 (6):343–351. doi: 10.2174/1566524018666181109121849.

Plate, K. H., G. Breier, B. Millauer, A. Ullrich, and W. Risau. 1993. "Up-regulation of vascular endothelial growth factor and its cognate receptors in a rat glioma model of tumor angiogenesis." *Cancer Res* 53 (23):5822–5827.

Qiu, M., J. Hu, D. Yang, D. P. Cosgrove, and R. Xu. 2015. "Pattern of distant metastases in colorectal cancer: a SEER based study." *Oncotarget* 6 (36):38658–38666. doi: 10.18632/oncotarget.6130.

Qiu, S., and C. Jiang. 2019. "Soy and isoflavones consumption and breast cancer survival and recurrence: a systematic review and meta-analysis." *Eur J Nutr* 58 (8):3079–3090. doi: 10.1007/s00394-018-1853-4.

Rafter, J., M. Bennett, G. Caderni, Y. Clune, R. Hughes, P. C. Karlsson, A. Klinder, M. O'Riordan, G. C. O'Sullivan, B. Pool-Zobel, G. Rechkemmer, M. Roller, I. Rowland, M. Salvadori, H. Thijs, J. Van Loo, B. Watzl, and J. K. Collins. 2007. "Dietary synbiotics reduce cancer risk factors in polypectomized and colon cancer patients." *Am J Clin Nutr* 85 (2):488–496. doi: 10.1093/ajcn/85.2.488.

Rahib, L., B. D. Smith, R. Aizenberg, A. B. Rosenzweig, J. M. Fleshman, and L. M. Matrisian. 2014. "Projecting cancer incidence and deaths to 2030: the unexpected burden of thyroid, liver, and pancreas cancers in the United States." *Cancer Res* 74 (11):2913–2921. doi: 10.1158/0008-5472.CAN-14-0155.

Rastinejad, F., P. J. Polverini, and N. P. Bouck. 1989. "Regulation of the activity of a new inhibitor of angiogenesis by a cancer suppressor gene." *Cell* 56 (3):345–355. doi: 10.1016/0092-8674(89)90238-9.

Rauh, S., A. Antonuzzo, P. Bossi, R. Eckert, M. Fallon, A. Frobe, S. Gonella, R. Giusti, G. Lakatos, D. Santini, and A. Villarini. 2018. "Nutrition in patients with cancer: a new area for medical oncologists? A practising oncologist's interdisciplinary position paper." *ESMO Open* 3 (4):e000345. doi: 10.1136/esmoopen-2018-000345.

Richman, E. L., P. R. Carroll, and J. M. Chan. 2012. "Vegetable and fruit intake after diagnosis and risk of prostate cancer progression." *Int J Cancer* 131 (1):201–210. doi: 10.1002/ijc.26348.

Riera-Domingo, C., A. Audige, S. Granja, W. C. Cheng, P. C. Ho, F. Baltazar, C. Stockmann, and M. Mazzone. 2020. "Immunity, hypoxia, and metabolism-the menage a trois of cancer: implications for immunotherapy." *Physiol Rev* 100 (1):1–102. doi: 10.1152/physrev.00018.2019.

Rigden, H. M., A. Alias, T. Havelock, R. O'Donnell, R. Djukanovic, D. E. Davies, and S. J. Wilson. 2016. "Squamous metaplasia is increased in the bronchial epithelium of smokers with chronic obstructive pulmonary disease." *PLoS One* 11 (5):e0156009. doi: 10.1371/journal.pone.0156009.

Risau, W. 1997. "Mechanisms of angiogenesis." *Nature* 386 (6626):671–674. doi: 10.1038/386671a0.

Rock, C. L., C. Doyle, W. Demark-Wahnefried, J. Meyerhardt, K. S. Courneya, A. L. Schwartz, E. V. Bandera, K. K. Hamilton, B. Grant, M. McCullough, T. Byers, and T. Gansler. 2012. "Nutrition and physical activity guidelines for cancer survivors." *CA Cancer J Clin* 62 (4):243–274. doi: 10.3322/caac.21142.

Roopchand, D. E., R. N. Carmody, P. Kuhn, K. Moskal, P. Rojas-Silva, P. J. Turnbaugh, and I. Raskin. 2015. "Dietary polyphenols promote growth of the gut bacterium Akkermansia muciniphila and attenuate high-fat diet-induced metabolic syndrome." *Diabetes* 64 (8):2847–2858. doi: 10.2337/db14-1916.

Rowles, J. L., 3rd, K. M. Ranard, C. C. Applegate, S. Jeon, R. An, and J. W. Erdman, Jr. 2018. "Processed and raw tomato consumption and risk of prostate cancer: a systematic review and dose-response meta-analysis." *Prostate Cancer Prostatic Dis* 21 (3):319–336. doi: 10.1038/s41391-017-0005-x.

Russell, K. S., D. F. Stern, P. J. Polverini, and J. R. Bender. 1999. "Neuregulin activation of ErbB receptors in vascular endothelium leads to angiogenesis." *Am J Physiol* 277 (6):H2205–H2211. doi: 10.1152/ajpheart.1999.277.6.H2205.

Saha, S., P. Chowdhury, A. Pal, and M. K. Chakrabarti. 2008. "Downregulation of human colon carcinoma cell (COLO-205) proliferation through PKG-MAP kinase mediated signaling cascade by E. coli heat stable enterotoxin (STa), a potent anti-angiogenic and anti-metastatic molecule." *J Appl Toxicol* 28 (4):475–483. doi: 10.1002/jat.1297.

Saito, K., Y. Matsuo, H. Imafuji, T. Okubo, Y. Maeda, T. Sato, T. Shamoto, K. Tsuboi, M. Morimoto, H. Takahashi, H. Ishiguro, and S. Takiguchi. 2018. "Xanthohumol inhibits angiogenesis by suppressing nuclear factor-kappaB activation in pancreatic cancer." *Cancer Sci* 109 (1):132–140. doi: 10.1111/cas.13441.

Samykutty, A., A. V. Shetty, G. Dakshinamoorthy, R. Kalyanasundaram, G. Zheng, A. Chen, M. C. Bosland, A. Kajdacsy-Balla, and M. Gnanasekar. 2013. "Vitamin k2, a naturally occurring menaquinone, exerts therapeutic effects on both hormone-dependent and hormone-independent prostate cancer cells." *Evid Based Complement Alternat Med* 2013:287358. doi: 10.1155/2013/287358.

Sandur, S. K., M. K. Pandey, B. Sung, and B. B. Aggarwal. 2010. "5-hydroxy-2-methyl-1,4-naphthoquinone, a vitamin K3 analogue, suppresses STAT3 activation pathway through induction of protein tyrosine phosphatase, SHP-1: potential role in chemosensitization." *Mol Cancer Res* 8 (1):107–118. doi: 10.1158/1541-7786.MCR-09-0257.

Sang, Q. X. 1998. "Complex role of matrix metalloproteinases in angiogenesis." *Cell Res* 8 (3):171–177. doi: 10.1038/cr.1998.17.

Sartippour, M. R., N. P. Seeram, J. Y. Rao, A. Moro, D. M. Harris, S. M. Henning, A. Firouzi, M. B. Rettig, W. J. Aronson, A. J. Pantuck, and D. Heber. 2008. "Ellagitannin-rich pomegranate extract inhibits angiogenesis in prostate cancer in vitro and in vivo." *Int J Oncol* 32 (2):475–480.

Sazuka, M., S. Murakami, M. Isemura, K. Satoh, and T. Nukiwa. 1995. "Inhibitory effects of green tea infusion on in vitro invasion and in vivo metastasis of mouse lung carcinoma cells." *Cancer Lett* 98 (1):27–31.

Scaldaferri, F., S. Vetrano, M. Sans, V. Arena, G. Straface, E. Stigliano, A. Repici, A. Sturm, A. Malesci, J. Panes, S. Yla-Herttuala, C. Fiocchi, and S. Danese. 2009. "VEGF-A links angiogenesis and inflammation in inflammatory bowel disease pathogenesis." *Gastroenterology* 136 (2):585–595.e5. doi: 10.1053/j.gastro.2008.09.064.

Schwedhelm, C., H. Boeing, G. Hoffmann, K. Aleksandrova, and L. Schwingshackl. 2016. "Effect of diet on mortality and cancer recurrence among cancer survivors: a systematic review and meta-analysis of cohort studies." *Nutr Rev* 74 (12):737–748. doi: 10.1093/nutrit/nuw045.

Seeram, N. P. 2010. "Recent trends and advances in berry health benefits research." *J Agric Food Chem* 58 (7):3869–3870. doi: 10.1021/jf902806j.

Seeram, N. P., L. S. Adams, S. M. Henning, Y. Niu, Y. Zhang, M. G. Nair, and D. Heber. 2005. "In vitro antiproliferative, apoptotic and antioxidant activities of punicalagin, ellagic acid and a total pomegranate tannin extract are enhanced in combination with other polyphenols as found in pomegranate juice." *J Nutr Biochem* 16 (6):360–367. doi: 10.1016/j.jnutbio.2005.01.006.

Senger, D. R., S. J. Galli, A. M. Dvorak, C. A. Perruzzi, V. S. Harvey, and H. F. Dvorak. 1983. "Tumor cells secrete a vascular permeability factor that promotes accumulation of ascites fluid." *Science* 219 (4587):983–985. doi: 10.1126/science.6823562.

Seren, S., R. Lieberman, U. D. Bayraktar, E. Heath, K. Sahin, F. Andic, and O. Kucuk. 2008. "Lycopene in cancer prevention and treatment." *Am J Ther* 15 (1):66–81. doi: 10.1097/MJT.0b013e31804c7120.

Shibuya, M. 2013. "Vascular endothelial growth factor and its receptor system: physiological functions in angiogenesis and pathological roles in various diseases." *J Biochem* 153 (1):13–19. doi: 10.1093/jb/mvs136.

Shing, Y., J. Folkman, R. Sullivan, C. Butterfield, J. Murray, and M. Klagsbrun. 1984. "Heparin affinity: purification of a tumor-derived capillary endothelial cell growth factor." *Science* 223 (4642):1296–1299. doi: 10.1126/science.6199844.

Shirakami, Y., M. Shimizu, S. Adachi, H. Sakai, T. Nakagawa, Y. Yasuda, H. Tsurumi, Y. Hara, and H. Moriwaki. 2009. "(-)-Epigallocatechin gallate suppresses the growth of human hepatocellular carcinoma cells by inhibiting activation of the vascular endothelial growth factor-vascular endothelial growth factor receptor axis." *Cancer Sci* 100 (10):1957–1962. doi: 10.1111/j.1349-7006.2009.01241.x.

Shu, X. O., Y. Zheng, H. Cai, K. Gu, Z. Chen, W. Zheng, and W. Lu. 2009. "Soy food intake and breast cancer survival." *JAMA* 302 (22):2437–2443. doi: 10.1001/jama.2009.1783.

Shukla, Y., and R. Singh. 2011. "Resveratrol and cellular mechanisms of cancer prevention." *Ann N Y Acad Sci* 1215:1–8. doi: 10.1111/j.1749-6632.2010.05870.x.

Shumway, B. S., L. A. Kresty, P. E. Larsen, J. C. Zwick, B. Lu, H. W. Fields, R. J. Mumper, G. D. Stoner, and S. R. Mallery. 2008. "Effects of a topically applied bioadhesive berry gel on loss of heterozygosity indices in premalignant oral lesions." *Clin Cancer Res* 14 (8):2421–2430. doi: 10.1158/1078-0432.CCR-07-4096.

Siegel, E. M., J. L. Salemi, L. L. Villa, A. Ferenczy, E. L. Franco, and A. R. Giuliano. 2010. "Dietary consumption of antioxidant nutrients and risk of incident cervical intraepithelial neoplasia." *Gynecol Oncol* 118 (3):289–294. doi: 10.1016/j.ygyno.2010.05.022.

Siegel, J. A., K. Korgavkar, and M. A. Weinstock. 2017. "Current perspective on actinic keratosis: a review." *Br J Dermatol* 177 (2):350–358. doi: 10.1111/bjd.14852.

Simopoulos, A. P. 2002. "The importance of the ratio of omega-6/omega-3 essential fatty acids." *Biomed Pharmacother* 56 (8):365–379. doi: 10.1016/s0753-3322(02)00253-6.

Smith-McCune, K., Y. H. Zhu, D. Hanahan, and J. Arbeit. 1997. "Cross-species comparison of angiogenesis during the premalignant stages of squamous carcinogenesis in the human cervix and K14-HPV16 transgenic mice." *Cancer Res* 57 (7):1294–300.

Solin, L. J. 2019. "Management of ductal carcinoma in situ (DCIS) of the breast: present approaches and future directions." *Curr Oncol Rep* 21 (4):33. doi: 10.1007/s11912-019-0777-3.

Spiro, A., C. Baldwin, A. Patterson, J. Thomas, and H. J. Andreyev. 2006. "The views and practice of oncologists towards nutritional support in patients receiving chemotherapy." *Br J Cancer* 95 (4):431–434. doi: 10.1038/sj.bjc.6603280.

Stappenbeck, T. S., L. V. Hooper, and J. I. Gordon. 2002. "Developmental regulation of intestinal angiogenesis by indigenous microbes via Paneth cells." *Proc Natl Acad Sci U S A* 99 (24):15451–15455. doi: 10.1073/pnas.202604299.

Steinmetz, K. A., J. D. Potter, and A. R. Folsom. 1993. "Vegetables, fruit, and lung cancer in the Iowa Women's Health Study." *Cancer Res* 53 (3):536–543.

Stoner, G. D., T. Chen, L. A. Kresty, R. M. Aziz, T. Reinemann, and R. Nines. 2006. "Protection against esophageal cancer in rodents with lyophilized berries: potential mechanisms." *Nutr Cancer* 54 (1):33–46. doi: 10.1207/s15327914nc5401_5.

Sundarraj, K., A. Raghunath, and E. Perumal. 2018. "A review on the chemotherapeutic potential of fisetin: In vitro evidences." *Biomed Pharmacother* 97:928–940. doi: 10.1016/j.biopha.2017.10.164.

Sutcliffe, S., E. Giovannucci, M. F. Leitzmann, E. B. Rimm, M. J. Stampfer, W. C. Willett, and E. A. Platz. 2007. "A prospective cohort study of red wine consumption and risk of prostate cancer." *Int J Cancer* 120 (7):1529–1535. doi: 10.1002/ijc.22498.

Takahashi, H., and M. Shibuya. 2005. "The vascular endothelial growth factor (VEGF)/VEGF receptor system and its role under physiological and pathological conditions." *Clin Sci (Lond)* 109 (3):227–241. doi: 10.1042/CS20040370.

Takata, Y., Y. B. Xiang, G. Yang, H. Li, J. Gao, H. Cai, Y. T. Gao, W. Zheng, and X. O. Shu. 2013. "Intakes of fruits, vegetables, and related vitamins and lung cancer risk: results from the Shanghai Men's Health Study (2002-2009)." *Nutr Cancer* 65 (1):51–61. doi: 10.1080/01635581.2013.741757.

Tannock, I. F. 1970. "Population kinetics of carcinoma cells, capillary endothelial cells, and fibroblasts in a transplanted mouse mammary tumor." *Cancer Res* 30 (10):2470–2476.

Teodoro, J. G., S. K. Evans, and M. R. Green. 2007. "Inhibition of tumor angiogenesis by p53: a new role for the guardian of the genome." *J Mol Med (Berl)* 85 (11):1175–1186. doi: 10.1007/s00109-007-0221-2.

Thiruvengadam, R., and S. S. Thiruvengadam. 2018. "Pre-cancerous colon polyps in the young - incidental adenoma detection in average-risk persons forty and younger." *Scand J Gastroenterol* 53 (10–11):1418–1420. doi: 10.1080/00365521.2018.1514067.

Thommen, R., R. Humar, G. Misevic, M. S. Pepper, A. W. Hahn, M. John, and E. J. Battegay. 1997. "PDGF-BB increases endothelial migration on cord movements during angiogenesis in vitro." *J Cell Biochem* 64 (3):403–413.

Thompson, C. A., T. M. Habermann, A. H. Wang, R. A. Vierkant, A. R. Folsom, J. A. Ross, and J. R. Cerhan. 2010. "Antioxidant intake from fruits, vegetables and other sources and risk of non-Hodgkin's lymphoma: the Iowa Women's Health Study." *Int J Cancer* 126 (4):992–1003. doi: 10.1002/ijc.24830.

Thompson, W. D., K. J. Shiach, R. A. Fraser, L. C. McIntosh, and J. G. Simpson. 1987. "Tumours acquire their vasculature by vessel incorporation, not vessel ingrowth." *J Pathol* 151 (4):323–332. doi: 10.1002/path.1711510413.

Tiptiri-Kourpeti, A., K. Spyridopoulou, V. Santarmaki, G. Aindelis, E. Tompoulidou, E. E. Lamprianidou, G. Saxami, P. Ypsilantis, E. S. Lampri, C. Simopoulos, I. Kotsianidis, A. Galanis, Y. Kourkoutas, D. Dimitrellou, and K. Chlichlia. 2016. "Lactobacillus casei exerts anti-proliferative effects accompanied by apoptotic cell death and up-regulation of TRAIL in colon carcinoma cells." *PLoS One* 11 (2):e0147960. doi: 10.1371/journal.pone.0147960.

Tsakiroglou, P., J. Weber, S. Ashworth, C. Del Bo, and D. Klimis-Zacas. 2019. "Phenolic and anthocyanin fractions from wild blueberries (V. angustifolium) differentially modulate endothelial cell migration partially through RHOA and RAC1." *J Cell Biochem.* doi: 10.1002/jcb.28383.

Tulio, A. Z., Jr., C. Chang, I. Edirisinghe, K. D. White, J. E. Jablonski, K. Banaszewski, A. Kangath, R. K. Tadapaneni, B. Burton-Freeman, and L. S. Jackson. 2012. "Berry fruits modulated endothelial cell migration and angiogenesis via phosphoinositide-3 kinase/protein kinase B pathway in vitro in endothelial cells." *J Agric Food Chem* 60 (23):5803–5812. doi: 10.1021/jf3001636.

Unlu, N. Z., T. Bohn, S. K. Clinton, and S. J. Schwartz. 2005. "Carotenoid absorption from salad and salsa by humans is enhanced by the addition of avocado or avocado oil." *J Nutr* 135 (3):431–436. doi: 10.1093/jn/135.3.431.

van der Schaft, D. W., R. P. Dings, Q. G. de Lussanet, L. I. van Eijk, A. W. Nap, R. G. Beets-Tan, J. C. Bouma-Ter Steege, J. Wagstaff, K. H. Mayo, and A. W. Griffioen. 2002. "The designer anti-angiogenic peptide anginex targets tumor endothelial cells and inhibits tumor growth in animal models." *FASEB J* 16 (14):1991–1993. doi: 10.1096/fj.02-0509fje.

Van Raay, T., and E. Allen-Vercoe. 2017. "Microbial interactions and interventions in colorectal cancer." *Microbiol Spectr* 5 (3). doi: 10.1128/microbiolspec.BAD-0004-2016.

Varinska, L., P. Gal, G. Mojzisova, L. Mirossay, and J. Mojzis. 2015. "Soy and breast cancer: focus on angiogenesis." *Int J Mol Sci* 16 (5):11728–11749. doi: 10.3390/ijms160511728.

Vaupel, P., and A. Mayer. 2017. "Tumor oxygenation status: facts and fallacies." *Adv Exp Med Biol* 977:91–99. doi: 10.1007/978-3-319-55231-6_13.

Verlaat, W., R. W. Van Leeuwen, P. W. Novianti, E. Schuuring, Cjlm Meijer, A. G. J. Van Der Zee, P. J. F. Snijders, D. A. M. Heideman, R. D. M. Steenbergen, and G. B. A. Wisman. 2018. "Host-cell DNA methylation patterns during high-risk HPV-induced carcinogenesis reveal a heterogeneous nature of cervical pre-cancer." *Epigenetics* 13 (7):769–778. doi: 10.1080/15592294.2018.1507197.

Viallard, C., and B. Larrivee. 2017. "Tumor angiogenesis and vascular normalization: alternative therapeutic targets." *Angiogenesis* 20 (4):409–426. doi: 10.1007/s10456-017-9562-9.

Voest, E. E., B. M. Kenyon, M. S. O'Reilly, G. Truitt, R. J. D'Amato, and J. Folkman. 1995. "Inhibition of angiogenesis in vivo by interleukin 12." *J Natl Cancer Inst* 87 (8):581–586. doi: 10.1093/jnci/87.8.581.

Wang, C., T. Yang, X. F. Guo, and D. Li. 2019. "The associations of fruit and vegetable intake with lung cancer risk in participants with different smoking status: a meta-analysis of prospective cohort studies." *Nutrients* 11 (8). doi: 10.3390/nu11081791.

Wang, J., G. C. W. Man, T. H. Chan, J. Kwong, and C. C. Wang. 2018. "A prodrug of green tea polyphenol (-)-epigallocatechin-3-gallate (Pro-EGCG) serves as a novel angiogenesis inhibitor in endometrial cancer." *Cancer Lett* 412:10–20. doi: 10.1016/j.canlet.2017.09.054.

Wang, J., Y. Yuan, P. Zhang, H. Zhang, X. Liu, and Y. Zhang. 2018. "Neohesperidin prevents Abeta25-35-induced apoptosis in primary cultured hippocampal neurons by blocking the S-nitrosylation of protein-disulphide isomerase." *Neurochem Res* 43 (9):1736–1744. doi: 10.1007/s11064-018-2589-5.

Wang, L. S., A. A. Dombkowski, C. Seguin, C. Rocha, D. Cukovic, A. Mukundan, C. Henry, and G. D. Stoner. 2011. "Mechanistic basis for the chemopreventive effects of black raspberries at a late stage of rat esophageal carcinogenesis." *Mol Carcinog* 50 (4):291–300. doi: 10.1002/mc.20634.

Wang, N., Z. Y. Wang, S. L. Mo, T. Y. Loo, D. M. Wang, H. B. Luo, D. P. Yang, Y. L. Chen, J. G. Shen, and J. P. Chen. 2012. "Ellagic acid, a phenolic compound, exerts anti-angiogenesis effects via VEGFR-2 signaling pathway in breast cancer." *Breast Cancer Res Treat* 134 (3):943–955. doi: 10.1007/s10549-012-1977-9.

Wang, Z. Y., R. Agarwal, W. A. Khan, and H. Mukhtar. 1992. "Protection against benzo[a]pyrene- and N-nitrosodiethylamine-induced lung and forestomach tumorigenesis in A/J mice by water extracts of green tea and licorice." *Carcinogenesis* 13 (8):1491–1494. doi: 10.1093/carcin/13.8.1491.

Wang, Z. Y., W. A. Khan, D. R. Bickers, and H. Mukhtar. 1989. "Protection against polycyclic aromatic hydrocarbon-induced skin tumor initiation in mice by green tea polyphenols." *Carcinogenesis* 10 (2):411–415. doi: 10.1093/carcin/10.2.411.

Wang, Z. Y., L. D. Wang, M. J. Lee, C. T. Ho, M. T. Huang, A. H. Conney, and C. S. Yang. 1995. "Inhibition of N-nitrosomethylbenzylamine-induced esophageal tumorigenesis in rats by green and black tea." *Carcinogenesis* 16 (9):2143–2148. doi: 10.1093/carcin/16.9.2143.

Werth, N., C. Beerlage, C. Rosenberger, A. S. Yazdi, M. Edelmann, A. Amr, W. Bernhardt, C. von Eiff, K. Becker, A. Schafer, A. Peschel, and V. A. Kempf. 2010. "Activation of hypoxia inducible factor 1 is a general phenomenon in infections with human pathogens." *PLoS One* 5 (7):e11576. doi: 10.1371/journal. pone.0011576.

Wurschmidt, F., H. P. Beck-Bornholdt, and H. Vogler. 1990. "Radiobiology of the rhabdomyosarcoma R1H of the rat: influence of the size of irradiation field on tumor response, tumor bed effect, and neovascularization kinetics." *Int J Radiat Oncol Biol Phys* 18 (4):879–882. doi: 10.1016/0360-3016(90)90411-c.

Yamaura, H., K. Yamada, and T. Matsuzawa. 1976. "Radiation effect on the proliferating capillaries in rat transparent chambers." *Int J Radiat Biol Relat Stud Phys Chem Med* 30 (2):179–187. doi: 10.1080/09553007614550931.

Yan, L., E. L. Spitznagel, and M. C. Bosland. 2010. "Soy consumption and colorectal cancer risk in humans: a meta-analysis." *Cancer Epidemiol Biomarkers Prev* 19 (1):148–158. doi: 10.1158/1055-9965. EPI-09-0856.

Yang, C. S., and Z. Y. Wang. 1993. "Tea and cancer." *J Natl Cancer Inst* 85 (13):1038–1049. doi: 10.1093/ jnci/85.13.1038.

Yang, G., X. O. Shu, H. Li, W. H. Chow, B. T. Ji, X. Zhang, Y. T. Gao, and W. Zheng. 2007. "Prospective cohort study of green tea consumption and colorectal cancer risk in women." *Cancer Epidemiol Biomarkers Prev* 16 (6):1219–1223. doi: 10.1158/1055-9965.EPI-07-0097.

Yang, G., Z. Y. Wang, S. Kim, J. Liao, D. N. Seril, X. Chen, T. J. Smith, and C. S. Yang. 1997. "Characterization of early pulmonary hyperproliferation and tumor progression and their inhibition by black tea in a 4-(methylnitrosamino)-1-(3-pyridyl)-1-butanone-induced lung tumorigenesis model with A/J mice." *Cancer Res* 57 (10):1889–1894.

Yoshiji, H., S. Kuriyama, R. Noguchi, J. Yoshii, Y. Ikenaka, K. Yanase, T. Namisaki, M. Kitade, M. Yamazaki, T. Akahane, K. Asada, T. Tsujimoto, M. Uemura, and H. Fukui. 2006. "Amelioration of carcinogenesis and tumor growth in the rat liver by combination of vitamin K2 and angiotensin-converting enzyme inhibitor via anti-angiogenic activities." *Oncol Rep* 15 (1):155–159.

Zhang, F. F., S. Liu, E. M. John, A. Must, and W. Demark-Wahnefried. 2015. "Diet quality of cancer survivors and noncancer individuals: results from a national survey." *Cancer* 121 (23):4212–4221. doi: 10.1002/ cncr.29488.

Zhang, G., D. Panigrahy, L. M. Mahakian, J. Yang, J. Y. Liu, K. S. Stephen Lee, H. I. Wettersten, A. Ulu, X. Hu, S. Tam, S. H. Hwang, E. S. Ingham, M. W. Kieran, R. H. Weiss, K. W. Ferrara, and B. D. Hammock. 2013. "Epoxy metabolites of docosahexaenoic acid (DHA) inhibit angiogenesis, tumor growth, and metastasis." *Proc Natl Acad Sci U S A* 110 (16):6530–6535. doi: 10.1073/pnas.1304321110.

Zhang, T., C. Suo, C. Zheng, and H. Zhang. 2019. "Hypoxia and metabolism in metastasis." *Adv Exp Med Biol* 1136:87–95. doi: 10.1007/978-3-030-12734-3_6.

Zhao, Y., and A. A. Adjei. 2015. "Targeting angiogenesis in cancer therapy: moving beyond vascular endothelial growth factor." *Oncologist* 20 (6):660–673. doi: 10.1634/theoncologist.2014-0465.

Zhou, M. 2018. "High-grade prostatic intraepithelial neoplasia, PIN-like carcinoma, ductal carcinoma, and intraductal carcinoma of the prostate." *Mod Pathol* 31 (S1):S71–S79. doi: 10.1038/modpathol.2017.138.

Zu, K., L. Mucci, B. A. Rosner, S. K. Clinton, M. Loda, M. J. Stampfer, and E. Giovannucci. 2014. "Dietary lycopene, angiogenesis, and prostate cancer: a prospective study in the prostate-specific antigen era." *J Natl Cancer Inst* 106 (2):djt430. doi: 10.1093/jnci/djt430.

10 Cholesterol and Prostate Cancer

Smrruthi V. Venugopal
Cedars-Sinai Medical Center

Michael R. Freeman
Cedars-Sinai Medical Center

Stephen F. Freedland
Cedars-Sinai Medical Center
Durham VA Medical Center

Shafiq A. Khan
Clark Atlanta University

CONTENTS

INTRODUCTION

Prostate cancer (PC) is the most commonly diagnosed non-cutaneous cancer and the second leading cause of cancer-related death for men in the United States (Culp et al. 2020). While early detection of PC has made it one of the most curable cancers, progression to treatment-resistant disease, termed "castration-resistance", is typically lethal. There is an urgent need to develop innovative strategies to reduce both PC incidence and disease progression (Yap et al. 2016).

According to the American Cancer Society, there will be over 191,000 men diagnosed with PC, and 33,000 deaths from PC, in the United States in 2020 (Siegel, Miller, and Jemal 2020). PC typically appears in men 65 years or older, and African-American men are at higher risk than men of

European or Asian ancestry. The most well-established risk factors for PC development and progression are advanced age, race, inherited susceptibility, and certain environmental factors (Gurel et al. 2008, Shafi, Yen, and Weigel 2013).

Studies of migrants have provided evidence that environmental influences, such as nutrition, may have an effect on the rate of emergence and aggressiveness of PC. According to a study conducted by Cook et al., a 30-fold differential in the rate of PC incidence is seen between nations with the lowest PC mortality rates (China and Japan) and those with the highest rates (United States, Western and Northern Europe and Australia) (Cook et al. 1999a). It was also observed that migrant populations from countries with a low incidence of clinical PC tend to acquire the incidence rate of the new country (Cook et al. 1999a). First-generation Asian-Americans demonstrate a three- to five-fold increased risk of PC compared to their native counterparts in Japan and China, even though they experience rates of disease approximately one-third to one-half those of European-Americans (Cook et al. 1999b). Studies have also shown that PC incidence rates have risen in Asian countries that have undergone Westernization, such as South Korea, China, and Thailand (Han et al. 2015, Pu et al. 2004, Alvarez et al. 2018, Liu et al. 2019). These data suggest that environmental factors such as a Western diet, which includes substantial amounts of red meat and an excess of fat and cholesterol, can exacerbate PC risk.

Cholesterol is a neutral, steroidal lipid acquired externally through diet or synthesized in mammalian cells via the mevalonate pathway. Most bodily cholesterol is synthesized in the liver. It makes up to one-third of the lipid content of the plasma membrane and is essential for maintenance and integrity of lipid membranes in mammalian cells. Cholesterol, in addition to its structural role, is an essential precursor in the synthesis of endocrine signaling mediators, such as steroid hormones (Payne and Hales 2004). Due to its various functions in the cell, intracellular cholesterol levels are tightly regulated via multiple regulatory mechanisms, including cholesterol uptake, biosynthesis, and efflux, to maintain highly controlled intracellular concentrations. Additional downstream processes include conversion to esters, oxysterols, and bile acid (Huang, Song, and Xu 2020). It has been recognized for many years that homeostatic control over cholesterol metabolism in PC is disrupted, resulting in increased accumulation of cholesterol (Krycer, Kristiana, and Brown 2010). Cholesterol accumulation in PC has been associated with increased cell proliferation, inflammation, steroidogenesis, and decreased apoptosis (Huang, Song, and Xu 2020).

Here we will describe the metabolic and regulatory mechanisms involved in cholesterol synthesis and its intracellular accumulation, and the role cholesterol dysregulation is likely to play in PC progression. In addition, we will briefly explore the role of cholesterol in the changing landscape of clinical care for PC patients in the current era.

CHOLESTEROL SYNTHESIS AND REGULATION IN NORMAL CELLS

HOW CELLS ACQUIRE CHOLESTEROL

Mammalian cells acquire cholesterol in two ways: from dietary sources or by *de novo* synthesis from the mevalonate pathway. In this section, we will discuss these along with the mechanisms involved in the regulation of cholesterol synthesis.

DIETARY ORIGIN OF CHOLESTEROL

Cholesterol can be derived from dietary sources. Cholesterol is absorbed from food by Niemann–Pick type C1 (NPC1)-like 1 (NPC1L1) protein on the surface of enterocytes within the intestine (Altmann et al. 2004). The gut then releases cholesterol as chylomicrons, from which cholesterol is taken up by the liver. The liver, the major site of endogenous cholesterol biosynthesis, delivers both newly synthesized and exogenously acquired cholesterol to the bloodstream as very-low-density lipoproteins (VLDLs). After processing within bloodstream, the VLDLs generate circulating low-density lipoproteins (LDLs), which can be used by peripheral cells via receptor-mediated endo-cytosis (Goldstein and Brown 2009). Within the cell, cholesterol is dynamically transported between various organelles by vesicular and non-vesicular mechanisms to fulfill its multifaceted functions (Maxfield and van Meer 2010). Lipid-free or lipid-poor apolipoprotein A-I (apoA-I) acquires the surplus cholesterol produced by the liver, intestine, and pancreas via passive or active mechanisms to produce high-density lipoproteins (HDLs) (Phillips 2014). Excess cholesterol is esterified by acyl-coenzyme A cholesterol acyltransferase (ACAT) (also known as Sterol O-acyltransferase (SOAT)) to cholesteryl esters (Chang et al. 2009). Cholesterol esters are subsequently stored as a cholesterol reservoir in cytosolic lipid droplets or released as components of plasma lipoproteins, including chylomicrons, VLDLs, LDLs, and HDLs. HDLs are transported from peripheral tissues back to the liver and intestine, where cholesterol is recycled or eliminated. Cholesterol is also transported to steroidogenic organs, where it serves as a precursor for the biosynthesis of steroid hormones.

DE NOVO CHOLESTEROL SYNTHESIS

Cholesterol is also synthesized *de novo* via the mevalonate pathway (see Figure 10.1a). The first step of the pathway involves the condensation of three molecules of acetyl-coenzyme A (acetyl-CoA) (the end product of glycolysis) to 3-hydroxy-3-methylglutaryl-CoA (HMG-CoA). Subsequently, HMG-CoA, in the presence of 3-hydroxy-3-methylglutaryl-CoA reductase (HMGCR), is converted to mevalonate (Jeong et al. 2018). Mevalonate production by HMGCR is one of the two rate-limiting steps of this pathway and is targeted using cholesterol lowering drugs known as "statins". Mevalonate undergoes phosphorylation by mevalonate kinase and is then metabolized to isopentenyl pyrophosphate (IPP) (Gruenbacher and Thurnher 2015, 2018, Mullen et al. 2016). By facilitating IPP generation, the mevalonate pathway is critical for the production of farnesyl pyrophosphate (FPP) and geranylgeranyl pyrophosphate (GGPP), mediated by a cas-cade of several synthases, including farnesyl diphosphate synthase (FDPS) and GGPP synthase (Gruenbacher and Thurnher 2018, Wang and Casey 2016). FPP serves as a precursor of squalene (a cholesterol precursor) and the second-rate limiting step in the mevalonate pathway. The syn-thesis of cholesterol from squalene is further mediated by enzymes, such as squalene epoxidase/monooxygenase (SQLE) and squalene synthase (Thurnher, Nussbaumer, and Gruenbacher 2012, Brown et al. 2016).

Cholesterol plays a crucial role in the synthesis and function of cellular membranes as well as a precursor of steroid hormones, vitamin D, and bile acid (Narwal et al. 2019, Cruz et al. 2013). In addition, cholesterol is also essential for the biogenesis of lipid rafts, and plasma membrane microdomains consisting of lipids and proteins. These dynamic assemblies are involved in mem-brane trafficking, signal transduction, and cell polarization (Simons and Ehehalt 2002). Further downstream products of FPP are dolichol and ubiquinone, which are important for glycosylation of proteins and mitochondrial electron transport (Jeong et al. 2018, Awad et al. 2018). In addition, the synthesis of FPP and GGPP is also critical for post-translational modifications referred to as protein prenylation. Prenylation of proteins is mediated by farnesyltransferase (FTase) I and gera-nylgeranyl transferase (GGTase) I and II (Thurnher, Gruenbacher, and Nussbaumer 2013, Jeong et al. 2018). The localization, membrane anchoring, and activity of hundreds of effector proteins, such as kinases, are dependent on post-translational prenylation. Because of these many and diverse vital functions, cholesterol synthesis via the mevalonate pathway is tightly regulated.

REGULATION OF DE NOVO CHOLESTEROL SYNTHESIS

Fine-tuned regulation of cholesterol biosynthesis is important to ensure continuous production of isoprenoids as well as to protect cells from accumulation of toxic, free cholesterol. Regulation of cholesterol biosynthesis is achieved by feedback regulation and transcriptional regulation of cho-lesterol synthesis.

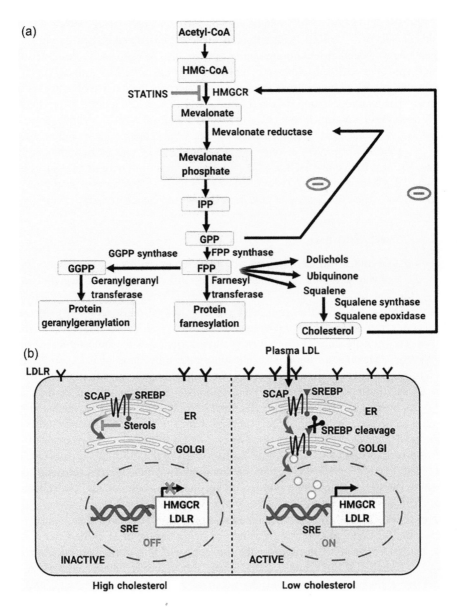

FIGURE 10.1 *De novo* cholesterol synthesis pathway and its transcriptional regulation: (a) *De novo* synthesis of cholesterol, dolichols, ubiquinone, FPP, and GGPP from the end product of glycolysis, acetyl-CoA. (b) Transcriptional regulation of the mevalonate pathway. HMGCR, 3-hydroxy-3-methylglutaryl-CoA reductase; ER, endoplasmic reticulum; LDL, low density lipoprotein; LDLR, low density lipoprotein receptor; SRE, sterol regulatory element; SREBP, sterol regulatory element binding protein; SCAP, SREBP cleavage activating proteins. (Adapted from Gobel et al. 2020.)

CHOLESTEROL FEEDBACK REGULATION

Early studies demonstrated that cholesterol is synthesized *de novo* by mice and dogs when fed a low cholesterol diet, and is produced at a reduced amount, and degraded, when cholesterol intake is high, a demonstration of a negative feedback loop in cholesterol metabolism (Gould et al. 1953).

The mevalonate pathway is regulated by several transcriptional and translational mechanisms (Sharpe and Brown 2013). The rate-limiting step of cholesterol production is mediated by HMGCR, which makes it the most controlled step of the pathway (Sharpe and Brown 2013). In cultured cells, HMGCR activity increases upon LDL starvation and is strongly suppressed when LDL is added back to the medium. The residual activity ensures critical mevalonate production for nonsterol end products, but is completely abolished with supplementation of LDL and mevalonate (Brown and Goldstein 1980). In addition, accumulation of mevalonate pathway products leads to accelerated HMGCR degradation, where the protein half-life is shortened to a few minutes (Leichner et al. 2009). In fibroblasts, compactin, a *Penicillium*-derived HMGCR-inhibitor, blocked enzymatic activity but concomitantly induced strong HMGCR protein expression (Brown et al. 1978). This effect is mediated by a synergy of enhanced HMGCR transcription and mRNA translation, as well as a prolonged protein half-life. In addition to HMGCR, negative feedback responses by GGPP, FPP, and IPP inhibit the activity of the mevalonate kinase gene (Hinson et al. 1997).

Transcriptional Master Regulators of Cholesterol Production

Identification and study of sterol regulatory element binding proteins (SREBPs) represented a breakthrough in understanding the regulation of mevalonate pathway genes (see Figure 10.1b). These transcription factors are synthesized as inactive precursors at the endoplasmic reticulum membrane, where they are attached to SREBP cleavage activating proteins (SCAP). SCAPs are sterol sensors, which escort SREBPs to the Golgi apparatus when intramembranous sterol levels are low. SREBPs are cleaved at the Golgi apparatus by two proteases (S1P and S2P), releasing the active fragment, which is then translocated to the nucleus and binds to sterol regulatory elements (SRE) in promotor regions of multiple target genes such as HMGCR and SQLE. These genes are involved in *de novo* cholesterol production and the synthesis of phospholipids, triglycerides, and fatty acids (Horton, Goldstein, and Brown 2002, Attie and Seidah 2005, Brown and Goldstein 2009, Brown and Goldstein 1997). When intracellular cholesterol storage is high, translocation of the SCAP-SREBP complex, and subsequent SREBP cleavage, is prevented. Loss of sterol sensing in cells carrying mutated SCAP proteins leads to failure of SREBP cleavage inhibition and overaccumulation of sterols (Hua et al. 1996). All these processes are fine-tuned by cholesterol derivatives, such as oxysterols or methylated sterols, as well as specific metabolic conditions, including hypoxia. Liver X receptor (LXR), whose activation decreases cellular cholesterol uptake, is a regulator of cholesterol synthesis (Baek and Nelson 2016). The complexity of these precisely controlled regulatory mechanisms ensures steady maintenance of cholesterol homeostasis within cells (Simons and Ikonen 2000).

Linking Cholesterol Accumulation to PC Progression

We have discussed how cholesterol metabolism is tightly regulated; however, increases in cholesterol content of prostate adenomas relative to normal tissue were reported by Swyer almost 80 years ago (Swyer 1942). Subsequent studies on human and animal prostate tissue also reported increases in cholesterol content in the prostate and prostatic secretions, correlating with disease, age, or presence of malignancy (Schaffner 1981). These older observations are in agreement with studies of the relative cholesterol content of human breast cancer as evaluated by Raman spectroscopy (Haka et al. 2009). Cholesterol accumulation may be a more general property of cancer and has been reported in a variety of cancer types (Krycer and Brown 2013). Cholesterol accumulation in cancer tissues is likely due to increased cholesterol absorption from the circulation, loss of feedback regulation of LDLRs, and overexpression and/or overactivation of SREBP2, HMGCR, and SQLE, key components of the *de novo* cholesterol synthesis pathway. In addition, androgen, which is essential for prostate development, also stimulates cholesterol and fatty acid synthesis in human PC cells directly by increasing transcription of HMGCR and fatty acid synthase (FASN) genes. Other components of the *de novo* cholesterol synthesis pathway, such as FDPS, are also regulated by androgen and play a role in the accumulation of cholesterol (Freeman and Solomon 2004). Excess accumulation of cholesterol arising from these mechanisms could potentially affect physiologic responses by

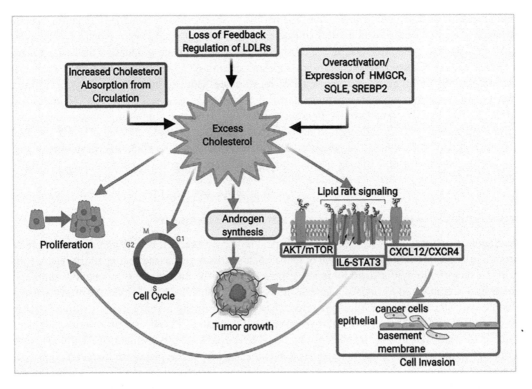

FIGURE 10.2 Cholesterol accumulation induces increased cell proliferation, cell cycle transit, growth, and invasion, all of which may promote PC progression. Red arrows indicate increase. LDLR, Low-density lipoprotein receptor; AKT, protein kinase B; mTOR, mammalian target of rapamycin; IL-6, interleukin-6; STAT3, signal inducer and activator of transcription factor 3; CXCL12, C-X-C motif chemokine; CXCR4, C-X-C chemokine receptor type 4 (Biorender 2020).

malignant prostate cells in numerous ways, including cell proliferation, steroidogenesis, and lipid raft signaling. In the next section, we discuss some of the possible consequences of cholesterol accumulation in PC (see Figure 10.2).

CELL PROLIFERATION

Cholesterol is essential for the proliferation of mammalian cells (Brown, Dana, and Goldstein 1974, Chen, Kandutsch, and Waymouth 1974, Chen, Heiniger, and Kandutsch 1975), and its synthesis is tightly synchronized to cell cycle progression (Chen, Heiniger, and Kandutsch 1975). Treatment of cells with statin drugs, which target HMGCR and inhibit the synthesis of cholesterol and its upstream intermediates, causes cells to arrest in G1 (Sivaprasad, Abbas, and Dutta 2006). However, these studies cannot be interpreted as demonstrating cholesterol dependence, as they did not determine whether cholesterol or an upstream intermediate (e.g., GGPP) is required. Further studies into the effects of statins on cell cycle progression have shown that lovastatin raises the level of p21 and p27 cyclin-dependent kinase inhibitors (Martínez-Botas et al. 2001). Consistent with these findings SREBP-1a has been shown to drive the expression of p21 (Inoue et al. 2005). Taken together, these studies demonstrate a mechanistic link between the cholesterol synthesis pathway and cell cycle regulation. Studies aimed at determining the specific effect of cholesterol in cell cycle progression have demonstrated that limiting concentrations of cholesterol cause cells to growth arrest at the G2 stage, possibly through specific effects on p34[cdc2] (Martínez-Botas et al. 1999). Whether lowering cholesterol levels in these cases cause growth arrest due to insufficient material for membrane synthesis, or a more specific regulatory role, is not known. However, certain observations suggest that a regulatory mechanism is likely involved. For example, in a number of different organisms (whether their main membrane sterol is cholesterol, ergosterol, or a phytosterol), absence of the primary sterol leads to growth arrest, regardless of the availability of a related, membrane-compatible sterol (e.g., replacing cholesterol with ergosterol). In these cases, a small amount of native sterol, insufficient for membrane synthesis, is required to repair cell cycle progression (Dahl, Biemann, and Dahl 1987, Whitaker and Nelson 1988). Moreover, blocking the cholesterol synthesis pathway downstream from HMGCR, thus allowing for a more specific effect on cholesterol synthesis to be examined, demonstrated that cells arrest at G2/M (Suárez et al. 2002, Fernández et al. 2005).

The concept that cholesterol accumulation is involved in cell cycle regulation in PC is supported by findings on nuclear localization and chromatin-associated cholesterol. Papadopoulos et al. have shown that the level of chromatin-associated cholesterol increases prior to the initiation of S-phase (Papadopoulos et al. 1997). The translocation of cholesterol into the nucleus is probably facilitated by the peripheral-type benzodiazepine receptor (PBR), which was previously reported to function as a regulator of cholesterol transport to the inner mitochondrial membrane, which is also a rate-determining step in steroid biosynthesis (Papadopoulos et al. 1997). Immunohistochemical analysis showed a preferentially increased PBR level around the nuclear periphery of cancerous cells when compared to the level found in prostate cells collected from unaffected sites. In the nucleus of PC cells, the ratio of nuclear cholesterol to cyclin E (a regulator of cell cycle progression, which remains expressed in cells allowing cells to move from G1 to S phase) was shown to be twice as high as in normal prostate cells (Singh et al. 2017). Therefore, increased cholesterol concentration within the cell nucleus could be a stimulus for cellular division.

Regardless of any role for cholesterol in cell cycle control, rapid growth of aggressive PC cells requires sustained metabolic flow of a substantial amount of cholesterol, which is dependent on the critical components and regulators (e.g., HMGCR, SREBP2) of the mevalonate pathway. Coculturing normal human prostate stromal cells with malignant PC cells was shown to induce HMGCR expression, thereby stimulating PC cell growth (Ashida, Kawada, and Inoue 2017). Studies from our laboratory demonstrated that inhibition of miR-185 and 342 (negative regulators of SREBP1/2 signaling) increases SREBP1, SEBP2 levels and expression of their downstream genes (e.g., FASN, HMGCR), thereby causing increased proliferation of LNCaP and C4-2B PC cells (Li et al. 2013). In addition to critical rate-limiting enzymes and transcription factors, metabolites of the mevalonate pathway also are instrumental in the proliferation of PC cells.

Collectively, these studies suggest that the cholesterol synthesis pathway plays an essential role in tumor cell proliferation.

STEROIDOGENESIS

PC cells respond to androgen through the action of the androgen receptor (AR), a nuclear receptor that controls PC development, and cancer cell survival and proliferation, at all stages of the disease. Indeed, the primary, long-standing clinical strategy to treat aggressive PC is androgen-deprivation therapy (ADT) (Feldman and Feldman 2001). Although clinical responses to ADT are typical, even with next-generation agents, more than 80% of these cancers will re-emerge (Rice, Malhotra, and Stoyanova 2019). The cancers that reappear are typically more clinically aggressive and respond progressively less well to AR signaling inhibitor therapy, resulting in a poor prognosis and progression to lethal disease (Feldman and Feldman 2001). This recurrent form of PC is termed castration-resistant PC (CRPC). Over the years, multiple lines of evidence have accumulated in support of the hypothesis that PC cells carry out intratumoral androgen synthesis (Locke et al. 2008, Dillard, Lin, and Khan 2008, Montgomery et al. 2008) sufficient to activate the AR, especially in CRPC. Studies have demonstrated that the enzymes necessary for *de novo* androgen synthesis are expressed in PC tumor xenografts and that androgen-starved PC cells have the capacity to synthesize dihydrotestosterone (DHT) from acetic acid, indicating that the entire mevalonate-steroidogenic pathway is functionally intact (Locke et al. 2008). Other reports have demonstrated that all enzymes necessary for testosterone and DHT synthesis are present in human primary and metastatic PC (Montgomery et al. 2008), implying that *de novo* steroidogenesis is not merely an experimental phenomenon, but instead a likely mechanism of disease progression in the hormone-repressed state.

An essential precursor in androgen synthesis is cholesterol. Consequently, it is possible that cholesterol promotes PC growth through effects on steroidogenesis. Dillard et al. reported that the expression of steroid metabolic machinery, including steroidogenic acute regulatory (StAR) protein, cytochrome P450 cholesterol side chain cleavage (P450scc), and cytochrome P450 family 17 subfamily A member 1 (CYP17A1) was found to be significantly higher in an androgen-independent LNCaP derivative (C81), compared to its androgen-dependent counterpart (C33). These studies were also able to demonstrate that C81 cells secreted 5-fold higher testosterone than C33 and that C81 was able to directly convert cholesterol to testosterone (Dillard, Lin, and Khan 2008). Our laboratory used an *in vivo* LNCaP PC xenograft model, and diet-induced hypocholesterolemia and hypercholesterolemia, to demonstrate that the xenograft tumors expressed the full spectrum of steroidogenic enzymes necessary for androgen biosynthesis, with the intratumoral cholesterol concentration directly correlating with expression of CYP17A, an enzyme essential for *de novo* androgen synthesis from cholesterol (Mostaghel et al. 2012). This suggests that cholesterol acts not only as a crucial precursor, but also as a pathway agonist, stimulating the upregulation of steroidogenic genes. These results are consistent with other studies demonstrating that proteins responsible for cholesterol regulation, LDLR, scavenger receptor (SR)B1, ATP-binding cassette (ABCA1, StAR, HMG-CoA), and the side-chain cleavage enzyme cytochrome P450 family 11 subfamily A member 1 (CYP11A1) are altered during PC progression to increase available cholesterol, coincident with an increase in androgens to physiologically relevant levels (Leon et al. 2010, Locke et al. 2009).

LIPID RAFT SIGNALING

Cholesterol-rich lipid rafts are defined as small, heterogeneous membrane domains formed by self-aggregation of cholesterol, sphingolipids, and glycolipids, transported from trans-Golgi network to the cell surface (Mollinedo and Gajate 2015). There are at least two morphologically distinguishable varieties of lipid rafts on the cell surface. The first variety identified as 50–100 nm invaginations in the plasma membrane is called caveolae. These rafts are characterized by the presence of structural proteins caveolins (caveolin-1, -2, and -3), which bind directly to cholesterol (Nassar and Parat 2020). The second variety are called flat or G rafts, which do not form a recognizable membrane structure, as they lack caveolins (Freeman and Solomon 2004). Both varieties of rafts are isolated biochemically using ice cold, nonionic detergents, such as Triton X-100 and Nonidet P-40, and have been shown to contain cohorts of (GPI)-anchored proteins, Src family kinases and other signaling proteins (Freeman and Solomon 2004). Association between lipid rafts and PC is supported by the identification of caveolin-1 (CAV1) as a marker for aggressive PC, a predictor of poor prognosis following surgery in lymph node-negative PC patients and a mediator of androgen insensitivity (Nassar and Parat 2020, Nasu et al. 1998).

The link to CAV1 shows that lipid rafts are potential sites for signal transduction relevant to PC progression (Hager, Solomon, and Freeman 2006). The possibility that the association between CAV1-localized lipid rafts and PC is functional, as opposed to correlative, was supported by the demonstration that anti-CAV1 antibodies suppressed PC metastasis in mice, suggesting that cholesterol may play a role in metastatic dissemination (Kuo et al. 2012). Further reports supporting the functional role of CAV1 in aggressive disease demonstrate that CAV1 reprograms transforming growth factor β (TGFβ) signaling from tumor suppressive to oncogenic in PC, by promoting the expression of oncogenic TGFβ targets snail family transcriptional repressor 2 (SLUG) and plasminogen activator inhibitor, type 1 (PAI-1), and suppressing the expression of tumor suppressive TGFβ targets E-cadherin (CDH1), desmoplakin, and cyclin-dependent kinase inhibitor type 1A (CDKN1A) (Pellinen et al. 2018). Furthermore, supporting its functional role, CAV1 knockdown using siRNA led to growth arrest and inhibition of invasion in PC cell lines DU145 and PC-3 (Pellinen et al. 2018). Lin et al. reported that CAV1 can promote PC growth via tumor-derived exosomes in a paracrine fashion (Lin et al. 2019). Furthermore, it has been reported that CAV1 may positively contribute to the upregulation of CRPC cell migration by inducing the expression of important cell motility genes, including vimentin, N-cadherin, matrix metalloproteinase 13 (MMP13), and Myc-related gene from lung cancer (MYCL) in PC-3 cells (Kamibeppu et al. 2018). A recent report also demonstrated that AR, along with transient receptor potential melastatin 8 (TRPM8), can accumulate in caveoli under low testosterone (T) concentration. Accumulation of AR and TRPM8 under low T causes decrease in TRPM8-mediated calcium influx and increases PC cell migration (Grolez et al. 2019). This report suggests that AR can function in a nongenomic mechanism when it localizes to lipid rafts. Collectively, these findings demonstrate that lipid rafts may regulate PC growth, migration, and invasion, as well as reprogram vital PC oncogenic programs by compartmentalizing signaling proteins essential for these functions within cholesterol-rich, plasma membrane domains.

Earlier studies showed that addition of LDL to PC3 PC cell cultures stimulated cell growth (Hughes-Fulford, Chen, and Tjandrawinata 2001). This result is intriguing when taking into consideration that some solid tumors accumulate excess cholesterol. Can these findings be interpreted in the context of lipid-raft signaling? Cholesterol has been shown to be an essential lipid raft component, as it promotes the functional integrity of caveolar and non-caveolar rafts. Studies have also shown that raft-dependent signaling can be inhibited by dispersing cholesterol or depleting cholesterol from the membrane using cholesterol depleting agents such as methyl-β-cyclodextrin (MβD) (Adam et al. 2007). In contrast, studies have also shown that liquid-ordered, sphyingomyelin-enriched lipid domains can exist in the absence of cholesterol. These cholesterol-deficient rafts can be disrupted by addition of cholesterol (Freeman and Solomon 2004). Lipid rafts are heterogenous in structure, function, and respond in numerous ways to changes in cholesterol levels, and excess cholesterol accumulation in PC leads to alteration of lipid-raft dependent signaling (Freeman and Solomon 2004). However, which signal transduction mechanisms are altered by cholesterol metabolism in PC, and how might cancer cells and tissues be affected by these changes?

Signals vital to PC cell survival, proliferation, and metastasis are transmitted through lipid rafts. Early reports associating lipid rafts with PC cell growth showed that the epidermal growth factor receptor (EGFR) is phosphorylated and active in membrane rafts (Zhuang et al. 2002). EGFR activation leads to activation of protein kinase B (AKT1), which in turn promotes survival of PC cells. Treatment of PC cells with statins disrupts lipid raft organization and interferes with EGFR signaling (Zhuang et al. 2005). When mice with LNCaP cell-derived xenografts were fed a high cholesterol diet, a lipid raft-dependent increase in AKT1 phosphorylation was observed, which promoted tumor growth and reduced apoptosis (Zhuang et al. 2005). Depletion of cholesterol from lipid raft domains not only inhibited EGFR/ AKT1 but also markedly altered the phosphorylation status of ERK and the mitochondrial apoptosis pathway (Oh et al. 2007).

In another study from our lab, we reported that membrane cholesterol directly regulated lipid raft resident AKT1, which influenced cell survival signals (Adam et al. 2007). In particular, myristoylated AKT1 (MyrAKT1, an oncogene), which predominantly localizes to rafts, was regulated by altering membrane cholesterol levels (Adam et al. 2007). Furthermore, lipid raft-resident MyrAKT1 exhibited markedly distinct substrate preference (toward histone H2B and MBP) compared to MyrAKT1 immunoprecipitated from cytosol and the non-raft fraction, suggesting a redirection of signaling when the protein is present in cholesterol-rich domains. Adam et al. also demonstrated that depletion of membrane cholesterol reduced the cytoprotective effect of MyrAKT1 in LNCaP cells exposed to a PI3K inhibitor (LY294002). Finally, the activation of downstream substrates of MyrAKT, such as ribosomal protein S6 kinase beta-1 (p70S6K), glycogen synthase kinase (GSK), and foxhead box protein O1A (FKHR) was attenuated upon depletion of membrane cholesterol. These studies identify rafts as an upstream site of discrete signals to the cell interior, and that rafts can sequester key signaling proteins, resulting in distinct patterns of signal transduction.

Additional studies of *in vivo* and *in vitro* models of PC showed LXRs as modulators of lipid raft signaling. Treatment of LNCaP cells and xenografts with synthetic LXR agonist T0901317 caused cholesterol export through ATP-building cassette subfamily G member 1 (ABCG1) upregulation (Pommier et al. 2010). This, in turn, downregulated phosphorylation of raft-associated AKT1 and caused apoptosis. Atomic force microscopy of the topography of the inner surface of the plasma membrane of LNCaP cells treated with the LXR agonist revealed a dispersion of membrane raft domains. Confocal microscopy also revealed changes in flotillin 2 staining compared to untreated cells. These results suggest that cholesterol export regulates lipid raft dynamics, which in turn affect AKT1 pathway signaling (Pommier et al. 2010).

One of the signaling pathways frequently activated in PC is the Hedgehog (Hh) pathway (Fan et al. 2004, Riobo 2012). The Hh receptor, which is a complex of patched (PTCH1) and smoothened (SMO) proteins, is localized within cholesterol-rich microdomains, where PTCH1 interacts with CAV1. The active form of sonic Hh (Shh) results from simultaneous autoproteolysis and covalent modification of the N-terminal part of the protein with a cholesterol molecule (Karpen et al. 2001). Several lines of evidence show that PTCH1 interaction with CAV1 recruits SMO to the receptor complex residing in raft domains. Cholesterol depletion experiments showed decreased amounts of both PTCH1 and CAV1 in caveolae, indicating that cholesterol is involved in recruiting both PTCH1 and CAV1 to sites of pathway activation (Karpen et al. 2001). These data indicate that CAV1 and cholesterol may be essential for downstream signaling from the Hh receptor complex (Karpen et al. 2001).

Another signaling pathway seen in PC that involves lipid rafts is the interleukin-6-janus kinase-signal inducer and activator of transcription proteins 3 (IL-6-JAK-STAT3) pathway. Kim et al. reported that disruption of lipid rafts by the cholesterol-binding compound, filipin, inhibited IL-6-mediated STAT3 activation in LNCaP cells (Kim et al. 2004). This study also showed that IL-6-induced phosphorylation of STAT3, its translocation to the nucleus, as well as promotor activity of the neuroendocrine marker, neuron enolase (NSE), and accumulation of NSE protein were partly dependent on intact lipid rafts (Kim et al. 2004). Phosphorylation of STAT3 is also predominantly localized to lipid rafts after stimulation of LNCaP cells with IL-6. Consequently, these findings represent another demonstration of a cholesterol-dependent signal transduction mechanism underlying a process relevant to PC progression. These data are consistent with two recently published studies by Alfaqih et al. and Dambal et al. in 2020. Alfaqih et al. reported that 27-hydroxcholesterol (27HC), a cholesterol metabolite, is a negative regulator of cellular cholesterol content and its dysregulation significantly contributes to PC progression (Alfaqih, Nelson, et al. 2017). Most recently, Dambal et al. demonstrated how 27HC affected anticancer activity in PC cells (Dambal et al. 2020). This report showed that 27HC treatment of DU145 PC cells led to a rapid and profound depletion of membrane cholesterol level and disruption of lipid raft size and architecture. This, in turn, impaired oncogenic signaling through the IL6-JAK-STAT3 pathway *in vitro* and *in vivo* and delayed *in vivo* tumor growth in a PC model with constitutively active STAT3 (Dambal et al. 2020). Furthermore, 27HC sensitized PC cells to STAT3 inhibitors and impaired migration and invasion. These data show that controlling intracellular cholesterol levels by 27HC can inhibit IL6-JAK-STAT3 signaling and may synergize with STAT3-targeted compounds in order to inhibit cell migration and invasion in PC cells (Dambal et al. 2020). Collectively, the above studies demonstrate that cholesterol in lipid rafts is essential for IL6-STAT3 signaling, suggesting that lipid raft signaling may operate in CRPC.

In most cases of advanced PC, metastases form in the bones and lymph nodes. One of the steps that triggers cancer cell spreading involves chemoattraction of circulating PC cells toward chemokines released by specific sites. Data show that the C-X-C motif chemokine 12/CXC chemokine receptor type 4 (CXCL12/CXCR4) interaction transactivates the human epidermal growth factor receptor 2 (HER2) in lipid rafts of PC cells by phosphorylating nonreceptor tyrosine kinase Src. Treatment of PC-3 cells with MβCD reduced the basal level and the CXCL12-mediated phosphorylation of HER2 in lipid rafts (Chinni et al. 2008). In addition, it was also observed that CXC4 levels were slightly decreased in lipid rafts, and elevated in cytosolic and membrane fractions, upon MβCD treatment (Chinni et al. 2008). Subsequent studies by Conley-LaComb et al. also reported that CXCL12/

CXCR4 transactivated both HER2 and EGFR and this transactivation occurred exclusively in the lipid raft microdomain (Conley-LaComb et al. 2016). These data demonstrate that intact lipid rafts are required for CXCL12/CXCR4-triggered activation of HER2 and induction of PC3 cell invasion.

Lipid rafts can selectively recruit signaling molecules associated with virus infection, apoptotic pathways, and death receptor activation signaling (Liu et al. 2015). Signal transduction can be affected by modifying the cholesterol content of the lipid rafts and enhance antitumor activity of drugs or efficacy of gene therapy for PC. Lui et al. reported that combining prostate-restricted replication competent adenovirus-mediated-TNF-related apoptosis-inducing ligand (PRRA-TRAIL) with lovastatin, a cholesterol-lowering drug, enhanced anti-tumor efficacy *in vivo* and *in vitro* through activation of apoptotic signaling (Liu et al. 2015). This study also reported that lovastatin enhanced infection efficiency of PRRA and virus-delivered TRAIL expression by increasing the expression level of Coxsackievirus and adenovirus receptor (CAR) and slightly increasing expression of integrins (Liu et al. 2015). Furthermore, lovastatin also enhanced TRAIL-induced apoptosis by increasing the expression of death receptor (DR) DR4. Interestingly, these effects of lovastatin on CAR, integrins, and DR4 expression levels were closely associated with lovastatin-mediated depletion of cholesterol in the lipid rafts of PC cells (Liu et al. 2015). These studies demonstrate that modulation of cholesterol can improve oncolytic adenovirus infection efficiency and antitumor efficacy of TRAIL. In another study by Hsu et al., para-toluenesulfonamide (PTS), a small molecule that inhibited cell proliferation of two CRPC cell lines (PC-3 and DU145), led to a decrease in lipid-raft associated total and phosphorylated forms of AKT1, mammalian target of rapamycin (mTOR), and p70S6K kinases (Hsu et al. 2018). In addition, supplementation with cholesterol rescued the PTS-induced inhibitory effect on these kinases. PTS is an antitumor agent with *in vitro* and *in vivo* efficacies through inhibition of both AKT-dependent and -independent mTOR/p70S6K signaling (Hsu et al. 2018). Disturbance of lipid rafts and cholesterol content may partly explain the PTS-mediated antitumor mechanism. Therefore, these studies reveal that modulating the cholesterol content of lipid rafts, in combination with drugs and gene therapy, can lead to activation of proapoptotic signaling pathways.

Collectively, these data suggest that accumulation of cholesterol in the plasma membrane, whether due to an increase in circulating cholesterol or dysregulation of cholesterol synthesis or sequestration, promotes formation of lipid raft domains, which in turn activate signaling pathways involved in PC growth, survival, and progression. In addition, they also suggest that cholesterol-lowering drugs are capable of modulating lipid raft architecture, thereby promoting sensitivity to proapoptotic signals.

CHOLESTEROL LOWERING DRUGS IN PC PREVENTION

Statins lower serum cholesterol by inhibiting HMGCR, the rate-limiting enzyme in the cholesterol synthesis, primarily in the liver. Statins are of two types: hydrophilic and lipophilic, depending on their solubility. Hydrophilic statins are more hepatoselective than lipophilic statins, as they are actively transported to the liver by organic anion transporting polypeptides (OATPs) (Alfaqih, Allott, et al. 2017). On the other hand, lipophilic statins are more readily taken up by non-hepatic tissues that do not express specific transporters, such as the prostate (Alfaqih, Allott, et al. 2017). Hence, lipophilic statins have been suggested to exert greater influence on the prostate than hydrophilic statins; however, this suggestion has not yet been supported by observational studies of statins and PC risk. Regardless of the type of statin used, during the past decade, preclinical, cell-based, and animal-based research has shown that statins, in general, can inhibit PC-associated inflammation, angiogenesis, cell proliferation, migration, and/or adhesion and invasion, and promote apoptosis via cholesterol- and non-cholesterol mediated pathways (Alfaqih, Allott, et al. 2017). Statins appear to induce apoptosis of PC cells independent of their effect on cholesterol levels (Boudreau, Yu, and Johnson 2010). Statins have been shown to inhibit cyclin-dependent kinase 2 and stimulate cell cycle arrest or activate specific proteases that can activate apoptosis-associated signals (Lee et al. 1998, Marcelli et al. 1998). Statins have also been shown to directly induce anti-inflammatory and antiangiogenic properties that might also inhibit PC growth and progression (Boudreau, Yu, and Johnson 2010). One study in a cohort of men undergoing radical prostatectomy observed that statin users were 69% less likely to express inflammation within their prostate tumors than nonusers, as shown by pathological evaluation of tumor sections (Bañez et al. 2010).

More than 30 observational studies have examined the link between statin use and PC. Most of the retrospective and prospective cohort studies showed an inverse relation between statin use and total PC risk (Alfaqih, Allott, et al. 2017). However, case-control studies, reported varying findings, from no association to elevated risk of total PC with statin use (Alfaqih, Allott, et al. 2017). In addition, meta-analyses of randomized controlled trials of statin use for the primary and secondary prevention of adverse cardiovascular outcome reported no association between statin use and PC risk (Fulcher et al. 2015). Factors that could explain these differences in association between statin use and PC risk reported by observational studies and randomized trials are: (1) participants in these trials and studies do not represent the general population; (2) both statin and non-statin users were under dietary intervention, such as foods low in fat, high in viscous fibers, plant sterols, vegetable protein foods, and nuts in all trails and studies; (3) the most common statin used in observational studies and randomized trials is pravastatin, which inhibits HMGCR more weakly than simvastatin (the most commonly prescribed statin in the United States), and (4) short follow-up periods for 27 statin trials to date (Fulcher et al. 2015, Alfaqih, Allott, et al. 2017).

All six large, prospective studies found that statin users exhibited reduced risk of advanced PC without any reduction or with an attenuated reduction, in total PC risk (Alfaqih, Allott, et al. 2017). A large observational study using the Health Professionals Follow-up cohort also found that statin users had 49% lower risk of advanced disease and up to 61% lower risk of fatal PC. Conversely, the study found no association with reduced risk of total PC (Platz et al. 2006). A prospective cohort study using data from the Cancer Preventive Study II Nutritional Survey observed that men who took statins for more than 5 years had 40% reduced rick of advanced PC. However, these findings were only slightly significant and did not reach significance in a follow up analysis of this data set (Jacobs et al. 2007). A large retrospective cohort study, which made use of men from the Veterans Affairs New England Healthcare System, also showed a 60% reduction in the risk of advanced PC among statin users (Farwell et al. 2011). Conversely, two other retrospective cohort and six case-control studies found no significant association between statin use and risk of advanced PC (Boudreau et al. 2008, Morote et al. 2014).

Isolating PC-specific mortality rate may be more informative, as most men with PC do not die from PC. A Danish registry-based population study found that PC patients who died of the disease, and who started taking a statin before PC diagnosis, had significantly lower PC-specific mortality than nonusers (Nielsen, Nordestgaard, and Bojesen 2013). A study that was designed to assess the association between beta-blockers and PC-specific mortality rate, and analyzed use of statins as a confounding factor, found that statin use inversely correlated with lethal PC (Grytli et al. 2014). Finally, an analysis of a population-based database in the UK found that use of statins was associated with lower risk of death from PC (Yu et al. 2014). In addition, the reduction in risk was higher in men taking statins before PC diagnosis. Overall, the existing literature at this writing suggests that statin use is inversely associated with PC specific mortality and may have a chem-preventative effect in some individuals.

In addition to their potential chemopreventive effects, statins are also being studied in the context of established PC therapy, such as brachytherapy and radiotherapy. A study of 938 men treated with brachytherapy compared treatment outcome of 191 men taking statins to those of nonusers (Moyad et al. 2006). This study found that statin users have smaller prostate volume, lower prostate specific antigen (prostate specific antigen (PSA) is directly regulated by AR and its level is used widely for PC screening), and lower tumor burden compared to nonusers (Moyad et al. 2006). Another study, composed of men with T1–3 PC treated with radiotherapy, included 382 men who were taking statins before PC diagnosis and found statin use was a predictor of improved 5-year PSA-failure free survival (Kollmeier et al. 2011). A retrospective study, examining the association between statin use and risk of biochemical recurrence in PC patients treated with brachytherapy, found that statin use significantly delayed the biochemical PC recurrence (Oh et al. 2015). Furthermore, meta-analyses of 13 studies that examined the association of statin use with biochemical recurrence, following treatment with radical prostatectomy or radiotherapy, found that statin use correlated with significant improvement in recurrence-free survival in radiotherapy patients, but not in patients who had undergone radical prostatectomy (Park et al. 2013). Taking all these studies into consideration, it appears that statin use can slow progression of PC in men treated with radiation. The likely mechanism is the sensitization of PC cells to the treatment. While existing data are encouraging, this conclusion needs further confirmation.

Although there is increasing evidence that statin use reduces risk of PC, especially advanced PC, this issue is still not resolved. Designing a large clinical trial remains a challenge because of the complex molecular mechanisms of action, uncertainty about the type of statin that should be tested, challenges with recruitment because of the widespread use of these drugs, and the long time to progression to lethal disease, which is a salient feature of PC. There is, however, substantial encouraging evidence that statins are beneficial in certain individuals, and as secondary or tertiary preventives in patients undergoing treatment with radiation.

ROLE OF CHOLESTEROL IN THE CHANGING LANDSCAPE OF PC PROGRESSION

PC at diagnosis is an androgen-driven disease, reliant on ligand-mediated signaling via the AR for tumor growth. Accordingly, ADT is standard-of-care therapy. The current clinical challenge is that virtually all PC patients treated with ADT eventually progress to CRPC (Stoykova and Schlaepfer 2019). A salient feature of CRPC is the reactivation of AR signaling. This is reflected by a progressive rise in serum PSA, which is transcriptionally regulated by AR. A number of studies have shown that many AR-regulated genes (androgen-response "hallmark" genes) are re-expressed in most CRPCs, and several mechanisms capable of maintaining AR activity (including genomic amplification of the AR locus, AR mutation, and AR splice variants, such as AR-V7) have been established (Davies, Beltran, and Zoubeidi 2018). Due to the essential role of AR signaling in advanced PC, drugs that suppress androgen or AR itself are still at the leading edge of drug development in this disease. Several drugs, including improved AR antagonists (enzalutamide) (Scher et al. 2012) and an inhibitor of androgen synthesis (abiraterone) (de Bono et al. 2011), modestly extend survival.

However, drug resistance ultimately ensues, which allows a subset of PC tumors to lose dependence on the AR pathway and co-opt alternative lineage programs to bypass therapeutic pressure and sustain tumor growth (Davies, Beltran, and Zoubeidi 2018). Clinically, this lineage reprogramming is associated with loss of epithelial identity and the transition from prostate adenocarcinoma to aggressive, neuroendocrine prostate cancer (NEPC) (Davies, Zoubeidi, and Selth 2020). A prominent example of NEPC features arising in the context of PC therapy was identified in a multi-institutional prospective study conducted by Aggarwal et al. A novel PC variant, referred to as treatment-emergent small cell neuroendocrine PC, was found to be associated with shortened survival, low AR activity, pure or mixed small cell histology and expression of neuroendocrine (NE) lineage markers, including chromogranin A (CHGA) and synaptophysin (SYP). This NE variant was found to be present in 17% of evaluable patients with metastatic CRPC (mCRPC), suggesting this is an important tumor type seen in treatment-resistant mCRPC (Aggarwal et al. 2018). Many of these specimens exhibited persistent nuclear localization of the AR, coexisting with lower AR transcriptional activity, indicating an "AR indifferent" phenotype. Collectively, these findings indicate that NE differentiation in PC can be a result of therapeutic pressure.

The vast majority of prostate adenocarcinomas are androgen-driven solid tumors, suggesting, from studies discussed above, that cholesterol may serve as an intratumoral reservoir of androgen precursor sufficient to activate the AR. However, with the recent rise in incidence of NEPC features in up to 15%–20% of advanced PC patients, the role of cholesterol in the context of AR indifference is unclear. A recent report by Gao et al. assessed potential differences in the lipid profile of prostate adenocarcinoma and NEPC using untargeted metabolomics, lipidomics, and transcriptomics using two PC cell line models: LNCaP, an androgen-dependent and hormonal therapy responsive model, and LASCPC-01, an NEPC model where N-Myc is the NE driver, with no expression of AR (Gao et al. 2019) (Figure 10.2). Citrate is exported from the mitochondria to the cytosol and subsequently cleaved by ATP citrate lyase (ACLY) to oxaloacetate and acetyl-CoA, which is the starting product of both cholesterol and fatty acid synthesis (Costello and Franklin 1991). Studies by Gao et al. demonstrated that citrate accumulated in LNCaP cells, which in turn caused higher expression of ACLY and FASN (essential for fatty acid accumulation in prostate adenocarcinoma). In addition, LNCaP cells also exhibited reduced levels of carnitine and short chain acylcarnitine (required for fatty acid oxidation), which may reduce fatty acid oxidation activity (Gao et al. 2019). In combination, these two mechanisms may cause the accumulation of cholesterol and fatty acids. In contrast, LASCPC-01 cells demonstrated reduced levels of FASN and elevated levels of carnitines, an indication that LASCPC-01 cells favor fatty acid oxidation vs fatty acid accumulation (Gao et al. 2019). The tendency toward fatty acid oxidation by the NEPC cell line LASCPC-01 may reflect the need for energy for tumor growth and the potential for enhancing cholesterol synthesis by increasing acetyl-CoA production (a byproduct of fatty acid oxidation). In aggregate, these studies demonstrated that lipid metabolism may be distinct between prostate adenocarcinoma and tumors with substantial NEPC differentiation.

Given the changing landscape of aggressive PC arising from new therapies, we believe there is an urgent need to reassess the role of cholesterol, and the complex web of cholesterol metabolism, in the context of emergent, low AR activity/AR-independent CRPC variants with NE features. It will be important to characterize in detail whether metabolic requirements and perturbations in these variants are distinct from those seen in adenocarcinoma and mCRPC. This can be done with existing technology, such as RNA-seq, metabolomic, and targeted lipidomic analyses, and other approaches. Uncovering such differences in cholesterol metabolic pathways may reveal new therapeutic options against certain types of CRPC arising in response to therapeutic challenge directed against the AR axis.

CONCLUDING REMARKS

Cholesterol metabolism is critical for the maintenance and integrity of cell membranes, signaling mediators, production of isoprenoids, and maintenance of cellular homeostasis. In addition, cholesterol is also vital in the growth and development of the prostate, as it acts as a precursor for the synthesis of androgens. Because of increased cholesterol absorption from the circulation, loss of feedback regulation, and overexpression and/or overactivation of SREBP2, HMGCR, and SQLE, cholesterol homeostasis is disrupted in PC. Evidence from many sources suggests that this dysregulation can lead to increased tumor cell proliferation, migration, alterations in membrane dynamics and upregulation of steroidogenesis, findings that collectively nominate cholesterol as a mediator of PC progression. New discoveries will be revealed when we learn more about the distinct metabolic characteristics and signaling mechanisms that drive treatment-resistant variants of CRPC.

REFERENCES

Adam, R. M., N. K. Mukhopadhyay, J. Kim, D. Di Vizio, B. Cinar, K. Boucher, K. R. Solomon, and M. R. Freeman. 2007. "Cholesterol sensitivity of endogenous and myristoylated Akt." *Cancer Res* 67 (13):6238–6246. doi: 10.1158/0008-5472.Can-07-0288.

Aggarwal, R., J. Huang, J. J. Alumkal, L. Zhang, F. Y. Feng, G. V. Thomas, A. S. Weinstein, V. Friedl, C. Zhang, O. N. Witte, P. Lloyd, M. Gleave, C. P. Evans, J. Youngren, T. M. Beer, M. Rettig, C. K. Wong, L. True, A. Foye, D. Playdle, C. J. Ryan, P. Lara, K. N. Chi, V. Uzunangelov, A. Sokolov, Y. Newton, H. Beltran, F. Demichelis, M. A. Rubin, J. M. Stuart, and E. J. Small. 2018. "Clinical and genomic characterization of treatment-emergent small-cell neuroendocrine prostate cancer: a multi-institutional prospective study." *J Clin Oncol* 36 (24):2492–2503. doi: 10.1200/jco.2017.77.6880.

Alfaqih, M. A., E. H. Allott, R. J. Hamilton, M. R. Freeman, and S. J. Freedland. 2017. "The current evidence on statin use and prostate cancer prevention: are we there yet?" *Nat Rev Urol* 14 (2):107–119. doi: 10.1038/nrurol.2016.199.

Alfaqih, M. A., E. R. Nelson, W. Liu, R. Safi, J. S. Jasper, E. Macias, J. Geradts, J. W. Thompson, L. G. Dubois, M. R. Freeman, C.-y. Chang, J.-T. Chi, D. P. McDonnell, and S. J. Freedland. 2017. "CYP27A1 loss dysregulates cholesterol homeostasis in prostate cancer." *Cancer Res* 77 (7):1662–1673. doi: 10.1158/0008-5472.Can-16-2738.

Altmann, S. W., H. R. Davis, L.-j. Zhu, X. Yao, L. M. Hoos, G. Tetzloff, S. P. N. Iyer, M. Maguire, A. Golovko, M. Zeng, L. Wang, N. Murgolo, and M. P. Graziano. 2004. "Niemann-Pick C1 like 1 protein is critical for intestinal cholesterol absorption." *Science* 303 (5661):1201–1204. doi: 10.1126/science.1093131.

Alvarez, C. S., S. Virani, R. Meza, L. S. Rozek, H. Sriplung, and A. M. Mondul. 2018. "Current and future burden of prostate cancer in Songkhla, Thailand: analysis of incidence and mortality trends from 1990 to 2030." *J Glob Oncol* 4:1–11 doi: 10.1200/jgo.17.00128.

Ashida, S., C. Kawada, and K. Inoue. 2017. "Stromal regulation of prostate cancer cell growth by mevalonate pathway enzymes HMGCS1 and HMGCR." *Oncol Lett* 14 (6):6533–6542. doi: 10.3892/ol.2017.7025.

Attie, A. D., and N. G. Seidah. 2005. "Dual regulation of the LDL receptor—some clarity and new questions." *Cell Metab* 1 (5):290–292. doi: 10.1016/j.cmet.2005.04.006.

Awad, A. M., M. C. Bradley, L. Fernández-del-Río, A. Nag, H. S. Tsui, and C. F. Clarke. 2018. "Coenzyme Q10 deficiencies: pathways in yeast and humans." *Essays Biochem* 62 (3):361–376. doi: 10.1042/EBC20170106.

Baek, A. E., and E. R. Nelson. 2016. "The contribution of cholesterol and its metabolites to the pathophysiology of breast cancer." *Horm Cancer* 7 (4):219–228. doi: 10.1007/s12672-016-0262-5.

Bañez, L. L., J. C. Klink, J. Jayachandran, A. L. Lark, L. Gerber, R. J. Hamilton, E. M. Masko, R. T. Vollmer, and S. J. Freedland. 2010. "Association between statins and prostate tumor inflammatory infiltrate in men undergoing radical prostatectomy." *Cancer Epidemiol Biomarkers Prev* 19 (3):722–728. doi: 10.1158/1055-9965.Epi-09-1074.

Biorender. 2020. Biorender.com.

Boudreau, D. M., O. Yu, D. S. M. Buist, and D. L. Miglioretti. 2008. "Statin use and prostate cancer risk in a large population-based setting." *Cancer Causes Control* 19 (7):767–774. doi: 10.1007/s10552-008-9139-4.

Boudreau, D. M., O. Yu, and J. Johnson. 2010. "Statin use and cancer risk: a comprehensive review." *Expert Opin Drug Saf* 9 (4):603–621. doi: 10.1517/14740331003662620.

Brown, D. N., I. Caffa, G. Cirmena, D. Piras, A. Garuti, M. Gallo, S. Alberti, A. Nencioni, A. Ballestrero, and G. Zoppoli. 2016. "Squalene epoxidase is a bona fide oncogene by amplification with clinical relevance in breast cancer." *Sci Rep* 6 (1):19435. doi: 10.1038/srep19435.

Brown, M. S., J. R. Faust, J. L. Goldstein, I. Kaneko, and A. Endo. 1978. "Induction of 3-hydroxy-3-methylglutaryl coenzyme A reductase activity in human fibroblasts incubated with compactin (ML-236B), a competitive inhibitor of the reductase." *J Biol Chem* 253 (4):1121–1128.

Brown, M. S., and J. L. Goldstein. 1980. "Multivalent feedback regulation of HMG CoA reductase, a control mechanism coordinating isoprenoid synthesis and cell growth." *J Lipid Res* 21 (5):505–517.

Brown, M. S., S. E. Dana, and J. L. Goldstein. 1974. "Regulation of 3-hydroxy-3-methylglutaryl coenzyme A reductase activity in cultured human fibroblasts. Comparison of cells from a normal subject and from a patient with homozygous familial hypercholesterolemia." *J Biol Chem* 249 (3):789–796.

Brown, M. S., and J. L. Goldstein. 1997. "The SREBP pathway: regulation of cholesterol metabolism by proteolysis of a membrane-bound transcription factor." *Cell* 89 (3):331–340. doi: 10.1016/s0092-8674(00)80213-5.

Brown, M. S., and J. L. Goldstein. 2009. "Cholesterol feedback: from Schoenheimer's bottle to Scap's MELADL." *J Lipid Res* 50 (Supplement):S15–S27. doi: 10.1194/jlr.R800054-JLR200.

Chang, T.-Y., B.-L. Li, C. C. Y. Chang, and Y. Urano. 2009. "Acyl-coenzyme A:cholesterol acyltransferases." *Am J Physiol Endocrinol Metab* 297 (1):E1–E9. doi: 10.1152/ajpendo.90926.2008.

Chen, H. W., H. J. Heiniger, and A. A. Kandutsch. 1975. "Relationship between sterol synthesis and DNA synthesis in phytohemagglutinin-stimulated mouse lymphocytes." *Proc Natl Acad Sci U S A* 72 (5):1950–1954. doi: 10.1073/pnas.72.5.1950.

Chen, H. W., A. A. Kandutsch, and C. Waymouth. 1974. "Inhibition of cell growth by oxygenated derivatives of cholesterol." *Nature* 251 (5474):419–421. doi: 10.1038/251419a0.

Chinni, S. R., H. Yamamoto, Z. Dong, A. Sabbota, R. D. Bonfil, and M. L. Cher. 2008. "CXCL12/CXCR4 transactivates HER2 in lipid rafts of prostate cancer cells and promotes growth of metastatic deposits in bone." *Mol Cancer Res* 6 (3):446–457. doi: 10.1158/1541-7786.Mcr-07-0117.

Conley-LaComb, M. K., L. Semaan, R. Singareddy, Y. Li, E. I. Heath, S. Kim, M. L. Cher, and S. R. Chinni. 2016. "Pharmacological targeting of CXCL12/CXCR4 signaling in prostate cancer bone metastasis." *Mol Cancer* 15 (1):68. doi: 10.1186/s12943-016-0552-0.

Cook, L. S., M. Goldoft, S. M. Schwartz, and N. S. Weiss. 1999b. "Incidence of adenocarcinoma of the prostate in Asian immigrants to the united states and their descendants." *J Urol* 161 (1):152–155. doi: 10.1016/S0022-5347(01)62086-X.

Costello, L. C., and R. B. Franklin. 1991. "Concepts of citrate production and secretion by prostate 1. Metabolic relationships." *Prostate* 18 (1):25–46. doi: 10.1002/pros.2990180104.

Cruz, P., H. Mo, W. McConathy, N. Sabnis, and A. Lacko. 2013. "The role of cholesterol metabolism and cholesterol transport in carcinogenesis: a review of scientific findings, relevant to future cancer therapeutics." *Front Pharmacol* 4: 119.

Culp, M. B., I. Soerjomataram, J. A. Efstathiou, F. Bray, and A. Jemal. 2020. "Recent global patterns in prostate cancer incidence and mortality rates." *Eur Urol* 77 (1):38–52. doi: 10.1016/j.eururo.2019.08.005.

Dahl, C., H. P. Biemann, and J. Dahl. 1987. "A protein kinase antigenically related to pp60v-src possibly involved in yeast cell cycle control: positive in vivo regulation by sterol." *Proc Natl Acad Sci U S A* 84 (12):4012–4016. doi: 10.1073/pnas.84.12.4012.

Dambal, S., M. Alfaqih, S. Sanders, E. Maravilla, A. Ramirez-Torres, G. C. Galvan, M. Reis-Sobreiro, M. Rotinen, L. M. Driver, M. S. Behrove, T. J. Talisman, J. Yoon, S. You, J. Turkson, J.-T. Chi, M. R. Freeman, E. Macias, and S. J. Freedland. 2020. "27-hydroxycholesterol impairs plasma membrane lipid raft signaling as evidenced by inhibition of IL6–JAK–STAT3 signaling in prostate cancer cells." *Mol Cancer Res* 18 (5):671–684. doi: 10.1158/1541-7786.Mcr-19-0974.

Davies, A., A. Zoubeidi, and L. A. Selth. 2020. "The epigenetic and transcriptional landscape of neuroendocrine prostate cancer." *Endocr Relat Cancer* 27 (2):R35–R50. doi: 10.1530/erc-19-0420.

Davies, A. H., H. Beltran, and A. Zoubeidi. 2018. "Cellular plasticity and the neuroendocrine phenotype in prostate cancer." *Nat Rev Urol* 15 (5):271–286. doi: 10.1038/nrurol.2018.22.

de Bono, J. S., C. J. Logothetis, A. Molina, K. Fizazi, S. North, L. Chu, K. N. Chi, R. J. Jones, O. B. Goodman, Jr., F. Saad, J. N. Staffurth, P. Mainwaring, S. Harland, T. W. Flaig, T. E. Hutson, T. Cheng, H. Patterson, J. D. Hainsworth, C. J. Ryan, C. N. Sternberg, S. L. Ellard, A. Fléchon, M. Saleh, M. Scholz, E. Efstathiou, A. Zivi, D. Bianchini, Y. Loriot, N. Chieffo, T. Kheoh, C. M. Haqq, and H. I. Scher. 2011. "Abiraterone and increased survival in metastatic prostate cancer." *N Engl J Med* 364 (21):1995–2005. doi: 10.1056/NEJMoa1014618.

Dillard, P. R., M.-F. Lin, and S. A. Khan. 2008. "Androgen-independent prostate cancer cells acquire the complete steroidogenic potential of synthesizing testosterone from cholesterol." *Mol Cell Endocrinol* 295 (1):115–120. doi: 10.1016/j.mce.2008.08.013.

Fan, L., C. V. Pepicelli, C. C. Dibble, W. Catbagan, J. L. Zarycki, R. Laciak, J. Gipp, A. Shaw, M. L. G. Lamm, A. Munoz, R. Lipinski, J. Brantley Thrasher, and W. Bushman. 2004. "Hedgehog signaling promotes prostate xenograft tumor growth." *Endocrinology* 145 (8):3961–3970. doi: 10.1210/en.2004-0079.

Farwell, W. R., L. W. D'Avolio, R. E. Scranton, E. V. Lawler, and J. Michael Gaziano. 2011. "Statins and prostate cancer diagnosis and grade in a veterans population." *J Natl Cancer Inst* 103 (11):885–892. doi: 10.1093/jnci/djr108.

Feldman, B. J., and D. Feldman. 2001. "The development of androgen-independent prostate cancer." *Nat Rev Cancer* 1 (1):34–45. doi: 10.1038/35094009.

Fernández, C., M. Martín, D. Gómez-Coronado, and M. A. Lasunción. 2005. "Effects of distal cholesterol biosynthesis inhibitors on cell proliferation and cell cycle progression." *J Lipid Res* 46 (5):920–929. doi: 10.1194/jlr.M400407-JLR200.

Freeman, M. R., and K. R. Solomon. 2004. "Cholesterol and prostate cancer." *J Cell Biochem* 91 (1):54–69. doi: 10.1002/jcb.10724.

Fulcher, J., R. O'Connell, M. Voysey, J. Emberson, L. Blackwell, B. Mihaylova, J. Simes, R. Collins, A. Kirby, H. Colhoun, E. Braunwald, J. La Rosa, T. R. Pedersen, A. Tonkin, B. Davis, P. Sleight, M. G. Franzosi, C. Baigent, and A. Keech. 2015. "Efficacy and safety of LDL-lowering therapy among men and women: meta-analysis of individual data from 174,000 participants in 27 randomised trials." *Lancet* 385 (9976):1397–1405. doi: 10.1016/s0140-6736(14)61368-4.

Gao, B., H. W. Lue, J. Podolak, S. Fan, Y. Zhang, A. Serawat, J. J. Alumkal, O. Fiehn, and G. V. Thomas. 2019. "Multi-omics analyses detail metabolic reprogramming in lipids, carnitines, and use of glycolytic intermediates between prostate small cell neuroendocrine carcinoma and prostate adenocarcinoma." *Metabolites* 9 (5):82. doi: 10.3390/metabo9050082.

Gobel, A., M. Rauner, L. C. Hofbauer, and T. D. Rachner. 2020. "Cholesterol and beyond - the role of the mevalonate pathway in cancer biology." *Biochim Biophys Acta Rev Cancer* 1873 (2):188351. doi: 10.1016/j.bbcan.2020.188351.

Goldstein, J. L., and M. S. Brown. 2009. "The LDL receptor." *Arterioscler Thromb Vasc Biol* 29 (4):431–438. doi: 10.1161/ATVBAHA.108.179564.

Gould, R. G., C. B. Taylor, J. S. Hagerman, I. Warner, and D. J. Campbell. 1953. "Cholesterol metabolism. I. Effect of dietary cholesterol on the synthesis of cholesterol in dog tissue in vitro." *J Biol Chem* 201 (2):519–528.

Grolez, G. P., D. V. Gordiendko, M. Clarisse, M. Hammadi, E. Desruelles, G. Fromont, N. Prevarskaya, C. Slomianny, and D. Gkika. 2019. "TRPM8-androgen receptor association within lipid rafts promotes prostate cancer cell migration." *Cell Death Dis* 10 (9):652. doi: 10.1038/s41419-019-1891-8.

Gruenbacher, G., and M. Thurnher. 2015. "Mevalonate metabolism in cancer." *Cancer Lett* 356 (2, Part A):192–196. doi: 10.1016/j.canlet.2014.01.013.

Gruenbacher, G., and M. Thurnher. 2018. "Mevalonate metabolism in cancer stemness and trained immunity." *Front Oncol* 8:394.

Grytli, H. H., M. W. Fagerland, S. D. Fosså, and K. A. Taskén. 2014. "Association between use of β-blockers and prostate cancer–specific survival: a cohort study of 3561 prostate cancer patients with high-risk or metastatic disease." *Eur Urol* 65 (3):635–641. doi: 10.1016/j.eururo.2013.01.007.

Gurel, B., T. Iwata, C. M. Koh, S. Yegnasubramanian, W. G. Nelson, and A. M. De Marzo. 2008. "Molecular alterations in prostate cancer as diagnostic, prognostic, and therapeutic targets." *Adv Anat Pathol* 15 (6):319–331. doi: 10.1097/PAP.0b013e31818a5c19.

Hager, M. H., K. R. Solomon, and M. R. Freeman. 2006. "The role of cholesterol in prostate cancer." *Curr Opin Clin Nutr Metab Care* 9 (4):379–385. doi: 10.1097/01.mco.0000232896.66791.62.

Haka, A., Z. Volynskaya, J. Gardecki, J. Nazemi, R. Shenk, N. Wang, R. Dasari, M. Fitzmaurice, and M. Feld. 2009. "Diagnosing breast cancer using Raman spectroscopy: prospective analysis." *J Biomed Opt* 14 (5):054023.

Han, H. H., J. W. Park, J. C. Na, B. H. Chung, C.-S. Kim, and W. J. Ko. 2015. "Epidemiology of prostate cancer in South Korea." *Prostate Int* 3 (3):99–102. doi: 10.1016/j.prnil.2015.06.003.

Hinson, D. D., K. L. Chambliss, M. J. Toth, R. D. Tanaka, and K. M. Gibson. 1997. "Post-translational regulation of mevalonate kinase by intermediates of the cholesterol and nonsterol isoprene biosynthetic pathways." *J Lipid Res* 38 (11):2216–2223.

Horton, J. D., J. L. Goldstein, and M. S. Brown. 2002. "SREBPs: activators of the complete program of cholesterol and fatty acid synthesis in the liver." *J Clin Investig* 109 (9):1125–1131. doi: 10.1172/JCI15593.

Hsu, J. L., W. J. Leu, L. C. Hsu, S. P. Liu, N. S. Zhong, and J. H. Guh. 2018. "Para-toluenesulfonamide induces anti-tumor activity through Akt-dependent and -independent mTOR/p70S6K pathway: roles of lipid raft and cholesterol contents." *Front Pharmacol* 9:1223. doi: 10.3389/fphar.2018.01223.

Hua, X., A. Nohturfft, J. L. Goldstein, and M. S. Brown. 1996. "Sterol resistance in CHO cells traced to point mutation in SREBP cleavage-activating protein." *Cell* 87 (3):415–426. doi: 10.1016/s0092-8674(00)81362-8.

Huang, B., B.-L. Song, and C. Xu. 2020. "Cholesterol metabolism in cancer: mechanisms and therapeutic opportunities." *Nat Metab* 2 (2):132–141. doi: 10.1038/s42255-020-0174-0.

Hughes-Fulford, M., Y. Chen, and R. R. Tjandrawinata. 2001. "Fatty acid regulates gene expression and growth of human prostate cancer PC-3 cells." *Carcinogenesis* 22 (5):701–707. doi: 10.1093/carcin/22.5.701.

Inoue, N., H. Shimano, M. Nakakuki, T. Matsuzaka, Y. Nakagawa, T. Yamamoto, R. Sato, A. Takahashi, H. Sone, N. Yahagi, H. Suzuki, H. Toyoshima, and N. Yamada. 2005. "Lipid synthetic transcription factor SREBP-1a Activates p21[WAF1/CIP1], a universal cyclin-dependent kinase inhibitor." *Mol Cell Biol* 25 (20):8938–8947. doi: 10.1128/mcb.25.20.8938-8947.2005.

Jacobs, E. J., C. Rodriguez, E. B. Bain, Y. Wang, M. J. Thun, and E. E. Calle. 2007. "Cholesterol-lowering drugs and advanced prostate cancer incidence in a large U.S. cohort." *Cancer Epidemiol Biomarkers Prev* 16 (11):2213–2217. doi: 10.1158/1055-9965.Epi-07-0448.

Jeong, A., K. F. Suazo, W. G. Wood, M. D. Distefano, and L. Li. 2018. "Isoprenoids and protein prenylation: implications in the pathogenesis and therapeutic intervention of Alzheimer's disease." *Crit Rev Biochem Mol Biol* 53 (3):279–310. doi: 10.1080/10409238.2018.1458070.

Kamibeppu, T., K. Yamasaki, K. Nakahara, T. Nagai, N. Terada, H. Tsukino, S. Mukai, and T. Kamoto. 2018. "Caveolin-1 and -2 regulate cell motility in castration-resistant prostate cancer." *Res Rep Urol* 10:135–144 doi: 10.2147/rru.S173377.

Karpen, H. E., J. T. Bukowski, T. Hughes, J. P. Gratton, W. C. Sessa, and M. R. Gailani. 2001. "The sonic hedgehog receptor patched associates with caveolin-1 in cholesterol-rich microdomains of the plasma membrane." *J Biol Chem* 276 (22):19503–19511. doi: 10.1074/jbc.M010832200.

Kim, J., R. M. Adam, K. R. Solomon, and M. R. Freeman. 2004. "Involvement of cholesterol-rich lipid rafts in interleukin-6-induced neuroendocrine differentiation of LNCaP prostate cancer cells." *Endocrinology* 145 (2):613–619. doi: 10.1210/en.2003-0772.

Kollmeier, M. A., M. S. Katz, K. Mak, Y. Yamada, D. J. Feder, Z. Zhang, X. Jia, W. Shi, and M. J. Zelefsky. 2011. "Improved biochemical outcomes with statin use in patients with high-risk localized prostate cancer treated with radiotherapy." *Int J Radiat Oncol Biol Phys* 79 (3):713–718. doi: 10.1016/j.ijrobp.2009.12.006.

Krycer, J. R., and A. J. Brown. 2013. "Cholesterol accumulation in prostate cancer: a classic observation from a modern perspective." *Biochim Biophys Acta* 1835 (2):219–229. doi: 10.1016/j.bbcan.2013.01.002.

Krycer, J. R., I. Kristiana, and A. J. Brown. 2010. "Cholesterol homeostasis in two commonly used human prostate cancer cell-lines, LNCaP and PC-3." *PLoS One* 4 (12):e8496. doi: 10.1371/journal.pone.0008496.

Kuo, S. R., S. A. Tahir, S. Park, T. C. Thompson, S. Coffield, A. E. Frankel, and J. S. Liu. 2012. "Anti-caveolin-1 antibodies as anti-prostate cancer therapeutics." *Hybridoma (Larchmt)* 31 (2):77–86. doi: 10.1089/hyb.2011.0100.

Lee, S. J., M. J. Ha, J. Lee, P. Nguyen, Y. H. Choi, F. Pirnia, W. K. Kang, X. F. Wang, S. J. Kim, and J. B. Trepel. 1998. "Inhibition of the 3-hydroxy-3-methylglutaryl-coenzyme A reductase pathway induces p53-independent transcriptional regulation of p21(WAF1/CIP1) in human prostate carcinoma cells." *J Biol Chem* 273 (17):10618–10623. doi: 10.1074/jbc.273.17.10618.

Leichner, G. S., R. Avner, D. Harats, and J. Roitelman. 2009. "Dislocation of HMG-CoA reductase and Insig-1, two polytopic endoplasmic reticulum proteins, en route to proteasomal degradation." *Mol Biol Cell* 20 (14):3330–3341. doi: 10.1091/mbc.e08-09-0953.

Leon, C. G., J. A. Locke, H. H. Adomat, S. L. Etinger, A. L. Twiddy, R. D. Neumann, C. C. Nelson, E. S. Guns, and K. M. Wasan. 2010. "Alterations in cholesterol regulation contribute to the production of intratumoral androgens during progression to castration-resistant prostate cancer in a mouse xenograft model." *Prostate* 70 (4):390–400. doi: 10.1002/pros.21072.

Li, X., Y.-T. Chen, S. Josson, N. K. Mukhopadhyay, J. Kim, M. R. Freeman, and W.-C. Huang. 2013. "MicroRNA-185 and 342 inhibit tumorigenicity and induce apoptosis through blockade of the SREBP metabolic pathway in prostate cancer cells." *PLoS One* 8 (8):e70987. doi: 10.1371/journal.pone.0070987.

Lin, C. J., E. J. Yun, U. G. Lo, Y. L. Tai, S. Deng, E. Hernandez, A. Dang, Y. A. Chen, D. Saha, P. Mu, H. Lin, T. K. Li, T. L. Shen, C. H. Lai, and J. T. Hsieh. 2019. "The paracrine induction of prostate cancer progression by caveolin-1." *Cell Death Dis* 10 (11):834. doi: 10.1038/s41419-019-2066-3.

Liu, X., C. Yu, Y. Bi, and Z. J. Zhang. 2019. "Trends and age-period-cohort effect on incidence and mortality of prostate cancer from 1990 to 2017 in China." *Public Health* 172:70–80 doi: 10.1016/j.puhe.2019.04.016.

Liu, Y., L. Chen, Z. Gong, L. Shen, C. Kao, J. M. Hock, L. Sun, and X. Li. 2015. "Lovastatin enhances adenovirus-mediated TRAIL induced apoptosis by depleting cholesterol of lipid rafts and affecting CAR and death receptor expression of prostate cancer cells." *Oncotarget* 6 (5):3055–3070. doi: 10.18632/oncotarget.3073.

Locke, J. A., E. S. Guns, A. A. Lubik, H. H. Adomat, S. C. Hendy, C. A. Wood, S. L. Ettinger, M. E. Gleave, and C. C. Nelson. 2008. "Androgen levels increase by intratumoral de novo steroidogenesis during progression of castration-resistant prostate cancer." *Cancer Res* 68 (15):6407–6415. doi: 10.1158/0008-5472.Can-07-5997.

Locke, J. A., C. C. Nelson, H. H. Adomat, S. C. Hendy, M. E. Gleave, and E. S. Tomlinson Guns. 2009. "Steroidogenesis inhibitors alter but do not eliminate androgen synthesis mechanisms during progression to castration-resistance in LNCaP prostate xenografts." *J Steroid Biochem Mol Biol* 115 (3):126–136. doi: 10.1016/j.jsbmb.2009.03.011.

Marcelli, M., G. R. Cunningham, S. J. Haidacher, S. J. Padayatty, L. Sturgis, C. Kagan, and L. Denner. 1998. "Caspase-7 is activated during lovastatin-induced apoptosis of the prostate cancer cell line LNCaP." *Cancer Res* 58 (1):76–83.

Martínez-Botas, J., A. J. Ferruelo, Y. Suárez, C. Fernández, D. Gómez-Coronado, and M. A. Lasunción. 2001. "Dose-dependent effects of lovastatin on cell cycle progression. Distinct requirement of cholesterol and non-sterol mevalonate derivatives." *Biochim Biophys Acta* 1532 (3):185–194. doi: 10.1016/S1388-1981(01)00125-1.

Martínez-Botas, J., Y. Suárez, A. J. Ferruelo, D. Gómez-Coronado, and M. A Lasunció. 1999. "Cholesterol starvation decreases P34cdc2 kinase activity and arrests the cell cycle at G2." *FASEB J* 13 (11):1359–1370. doi: 10.1096/fasebj.13.11.1359.

Maxfield, F. R., and G. van Meer. 2010. "Cholesterol, the central lipid of mammalian cells." *Curr Opin Cell Biol* 22 (4):422–429. doi: 10.1016/j.ceb.2010.05.004.

Mollinedo, F., and C. Gajate. 2015. "Lipid rafts as major platforms for signaling regulation in cancer." *Adv Biol Regul* 57:130–146 doi: 10.1016/j.jbior.2014.10.003.

Montgomery, R. Bruce, E. A. Mostaghel, R. Vessella, D. L. Hess, T. F. Kalhorn, C. S. Higano, L. D. True, and P. S. Nelson. 2008. "Maintenance of intratumoral androgens in metastatic prostate cancer: a mechanism for castration-resistant tumor growth." *Cancer Res* 68 (11):4447–4454. doi: 10.1158/0008-5472.Can-08-0249.

Morote, J., A. Celma, J. Planas, J. Placer, I. de Torres, M. Olivan, J. Carles, J. Reventós, and A. Doll. 2014. "Role of serum cholesterol and statin use in the risk of prostate cancer detection and tumor aggressiveness." *Int J Mol Sci* 15 (8):13615–13623. doi: 10.3390/ijms150813615.

Mostaghel, E. A., K. R. Solomon, K. Pelton, M. R. Freeman, and R. Bruce Montgomery. 2012. "Impact of circulating cholesterol levels on growth and intratumoral androgen concentration of prostate tumors." *PLoS One* 7 (1):e30062. doi: 10.1371/journal.pone.0030062.

Moyad, M., G. Merrick, W. Butler, K. Wallner, R. Galbreath, E. Butler, Z. Allen, and E. Adamovich. 2006. "Statins, especially atorvastatin, may improve survival following brachytherapy for clinically localized prostate cancer." *Urol Nurs* 26 4:298–303.

Mullen, P. J., R. Yu, J. Longo, M. C. Archer, and L. Z. Penn. 2016. "The interplay between cell signalling and the mevalonate pathway in cancer." *Nat Rev Cancer* 16 (11):718–731. doi: 10.1038/nrc.2016.76.

Narwal, V., R. Deswal, B. Batra, V. Kalra, R. Hooda, M. Sharma, and J. S. Rana. 2019. "Cholesterol biosensors: a review." *Steroids* 143:6–17 doi: 10.1016/j.steroids.2018.12.003.

Nassar, Z. D., and M.-O. Parat. 2020. "Caveola-forming proteins and prostate cancer." *Cancer Metastasis Rev* 39 (2):415–433. doi: 10.1007/s10555-020-09874-x.

Nasu, Y., T. L. Timme, G. Yang, C. H. Bangma, L. Li, C. Ren, S. H. Park, M. DeLeon, J. Wang, and T. C. Thompson. 1998. "Suppression of caveolin expression induces androgen sensitivity in metastatic androgen-insensitive mouse prostate cancer cells." *Nat Med* 4 (9):1062–1064. doi: 10.1038/2048.

Nielsen, S. F., B. G. Nordestgaard, and S. E. Bojesen. 2013. "Statin use and reduced cancer-related mortality." *N Engl J Med* 368 (6):576–577. doi: 10.1056/NEJMc1214827.

Oh, D. S., B. Koontz, S. J. Freedland, L. Gerber, P. Patel, S. Lewis, D. S. Yoo, J. Oleson, and J. K. Salama. 2015. "Statin use is associated with decreased prostate cancer recurrence in men treated with brachytherapy." *World J Urol* 33 (1):93–97. doi: 10.1007/s00345-014-1281-x.

Oh, H. Y., E. J. Lee, S. Yoon, B. H. Chung, K. S. Cho, and S. J. Hong. 2007. "Cholesterol level of lipid raft microdomains regulates apoptotic cell death in prostate cancer cells through EGFR-mediated Akt and ERK signal transduction." *Prostate* 67 (10):1061–1069. doi: 10.1002/pros.20593.

Papadopoulos, V., H. Amri, H. Li, N. Boujrad, B. Vidic, and M. Garnier. 1997. "Targeted disruption of the peripheral-type benzodiazepine receptor gene inhibits steroidogenesis in the R2C Leydig tumor cell line." *J Biol Chem* 272 (51):32129–32135. doi: 10.1074/jbc.272.51.32129.

Park, H. S., J. D. Schoenfeld, R. B. Mailhot, M. Shive, R. I. Hartman, R. Ogembo, and L. A. Mucci. 2013. "Statins and prostate cancer recurrence following radical prostatectomy or radiotherapy: a systematic review and meta-analysis." *Ann Oncol* 24 (6):1427–1434. doi: 10.1093/annonc/mdt077.

Payne, A. H., and D. B. Hales. 2004. "Overview of steroidogenic enzymes in the pathway from cholesterol to active steroid hormones." *Endocr Rev* 25 (6):947–970. doi: 10.1210/er.2003-0030.

Pellinen, T., S. Blom, S. Sánchez, K. Välimäki, J.-P. Mpindi, H. Azegrouz, R. Strippoli, R. Nieto, M. Vitón, I. Palacios, R. Turkki, Y. Wang, M. Sánchez-Alvarez, S. Nordling, A. Bützow, T. Mirtti, A. Rannikko, M. C. Montoya, O. Kallioniemi, and M. A. Del Pozo. 2018. "ITGB1-dependent upregulation of caveolin-1 switches TGFβ signalling from tumour-suppressive to oncogenic in prostate cancer." *Sci Rep* 8 (1):2338–2338. doi: 10.1038/s41598-018-20161-2.

Phillips, M. C. 2014. "Molecular mechanisms of cellular cholesterol efflux." *J Biol Chem* 289 (35):24020–24029. doi: 10.1074/jbc.R114.583658.

Platz, E. A., M. F. Leitzmann, K. Visvanathan, E. B. Rimm, M. J. Stampfer, W. C. Willett, and E. Giovannucci. 2006. "Statin drugs and risk of advanced prostate cancer." *J Natl Cancer Inst* 98 (24):1819–1825. doi: 10.1093/jnci/djj499.

Pommier, A. J. C., G. Alves, E. Viennois, S. Bernard, Y. Communal, B. Sion, G. Marceau, C. Damon, K. Mouzat, F. Caira, S. Baron, and J. M. A. Lobaccaro. 2010. "Liver X receptor activation downregulates AKT survival signaling in lipid rafts and induces apoptosis of prostate cancer cells." *Oncogene* 29 (18):2712–2723. doi: 10.1038/onc.2010.30.

Pu, Y. S., H. S. Chiang, C. C. Lin, C. Y. Huang, K. H. Huang, and J. Chen. 2004. "Changing trends of prostate cancer in Asia." *Aging Male* 7 (2):120–132. doi: 10.1080/13685530412331284687.

Rice, M. A., S. V. Malhotra, and T. Stoyanova. 2019. "Second-generation antiandrogens: from discovery to standard of care in castration resistant prostate cancer." *Front Oncol* 9 (801). doi: 10.3389/fonc.2019.00801.

Riobo, N. A. 2012. "Cholesterol and its derivatives in Sonic Hedgehog signaling and cancer." *Curr Opin Pharmacol* 12 (6):736–741. doi: 10.1016/j.coph.2012.07.002.

Schaffner, C. P. 1981. "Prostatic cholesterol metabolism: regulation and alteration." *Prog Clin Biol Res* 75a:279–324.

Scher, H. I., K. Fizazi, F. Saad, M. E. Taplin, C. N. Sternberg, K. Miller, R. de Wit, P. Mulders, K. N. Chi, N. D. Shore, A. J. Armstrong, T. W. Flaig, A. Fléchon, P. Mainwaring, M. Fleming, J. D. Hainsworth, M. Hirmand, B. Selby, L. Seely, and J. S. de Bono. 2012. "Increased survival with enzalutamide in prostate cancer after chemotherapy." *N Engl J Med* 367 (13):1187–1197. doi: 10.1056/NEJMoa1207506.

Shafi, A. A., A. E. Yen, and N. L. Weigel. 2013. "Androgen receptors in hormone-dependent and castration-resistant prostate cancer." *Pharmacol Ther* 140 (3):223–238. doi: 10.1016/j.pharmthera.2013.07.003.

Sharpe, L. J., and A. J. Brown. 2013. "Controlling cholesterol synthesis beyond 3-hydroxy-3-methylglutaryl-CoA reductase (HMGCR)." *J Biol Chem* 288 (26):18707–18715. doi: 10.1074/jbc.R113.479808.

Siegel, R. L., K. D. Miller, and A. Jemal. 2020. "Cancer statistics, 2020." *CA* 70 (1):7–30. doi: 10.3322/caac.21590.

Simons, K., and R. Ehehalt. 2002. "Cholesterol, lipid rafts, and disease." *J Clin Investig* 110 (5):597–603. doi: 10.1172/JCI16390.

Simons, K., and E. Ikonen. 2000. "How cells handle cholesterol." *Science* 290 (5497):1721–1726. doi: 10.1126/science.290.5497.1721.

Singh, G., S. Sankanagoudar, P. Dogra, and N. Chandra. 2017. "Interlink between cholesterol & cell cycle in prostate carcinoma." *Indian J Med Res* 146:38.

Sivaprasad, U., T. Abbas, and A. Dutta. 2006. "Differential efficacy of 3-hydroxy-3-methylglutaryl CoA reductase inhibitors on the cell cycle of prostate cancer cells." *Mol Cancer Ther* 5 (9):2310–2316. doi: 10.1158/1535-7163.Mct-06-0175.

Stoykova, G. E., and I. R. Schlaepfer. 2019. "Lipid metabolism and endocrine resistance in prostate cancer, and new opportunities for therapy." *Int J Mol Sci* 20 (11). doi: 10.3390/ijms20112626.

Suárez, Y., C. Fernández, B. Ledo, A. J. Ferruelo, M. Martín, M. A. Vega, D. Gómez-Coronado, and M. A. Lasunción. 2002. "Differential effects of ergosterol and cholesterol on Cdk1 activation and SRE-driven transcription." *Eur J Biochem* 269 (6):1761–1771. doi: 10.1046/j.1432-1327.2002.02822.x.

Swyer, G. I. M. 1942. "The cholesterol content of normal and enlarged prostates." *Cancer Res* 2 (5):372–375.

Thurnher, M., G. Gruenbacher, and O. Nussbaumer. 2013. "Regulation of mevalonate metabolism in cancer and immune cells." *Biochim Biophys Acta* 1831 (6):1009–1015. doi: 10.1016/j.bbalip.2013.03.003.

Thurnher, M., O. Nussbaumer, and G. Gruenbacher. 2012. "Novel aspects of mevalonate pathway inhibitors as antitumor agents." *Clin Cancer Res* 18 (13):3524–3531. doi: 10.1158/1078-0432.Ccr-12-0489.

Wang, M., and P. J. Casey. 2016. "Protein prenylation: unique fats make their mark on biology." *Nat Rev Mol Cell Biol* 17 (2):110–122. doi: 10.1038/nrm.2015.11.

Whitaker, B. D., and D. L. Nelson. 1988. "Sterol synergism in Paramecium tetraurelia." *Microbiology* 134 (6):1441–1447. doi: 10.1099/00221287-134-6-1441.

Yap, T. A., A. D. Smith, R. Ferraldeschi, B. Al-Lazikani, P. Workman, and J. S. de Bono. 2016. "Drug discovery in advanced prostate cancer: translating biology into therapy." *Nat Rev Drug Discov* 15 (10):699–718. doi: 10.1038/nrd.2016.120.

Yu, O., M. Eberg, S. Benayoun, A. Aprikian, G. Batist, S. Suissa, and L. Azoulay. 2014. "Use of statins and the risk of death in patients with prostate cancer." *J Clin Oncol* 32 (1):5–11. doi: 10.1200/jco.2013.49.4757.

Zhuang, L., J. Kim, R. M. Adam, K. R. Solomon, and M. R. Freeman. 2005. "Cholesterol targeting alters lipid raft composition and cell survival in prostate cancer cells and xenografts." *J Clin Investig* 115 (4):959–968. doi: 10.1172/JCI19935.

Zhuang, L., J. Lin, M. L. Lu, K. R. Solomon, and M. R. Freeman. 2002. "Cholesterol-rich lipid rafts mediate Akt-regulated survival in prostate cancer cells." *Cancer Res* 62 (8):2227–2231.

11 The Microbiome and Cancer

David Heber and Zhaoping Li
UCLA Center for Human Nutrition

CONTENTS

INTRODUCTION

The microbiome has been called the "forgotten organ" as its discovery required application of advanced genomic technologies not available until the last 30 years. Prior to that time, there was an awareness of gut microbes, but their anaerobic metabolism made it difficult to study them using cell culture. Nonetheless, many gut bacteria were identified using anaerobic culture methods including some associated with severe gastrointestinal diseases including *Helicobacter pylori* and *Clostridia perfringens* (Guilhot et al. 2018). The microbiome evolves from birth with maternal bacteria which help to establish the gut-associated immune system through specific bacteria in breast milk and then the microbiome gets more diverse with the introduction of a variety of foods (Underwood et al. 2015).

The microbiome appears to be stable within an individual over time, but varies between individuals due to the interaction of host factors, bacteria, and environmental exposures (Berg et al. 2020, Dominguez-Bello et al. 2019). The complex communities of bacteria in the microbiome interact by sharing nutrients and genetic material. The bacterial families and species have been defined using sequencing of 16S ribosomal RNA (rRNA) bacterial genes which are conserved within species. The impact of the microbiome goes beyond its bacterial taxonomy to include the genes and genomes of bacteria, as well as their metabolic products. The complete microbial environment includes plasmid DNA, viruses, archaea, and fungi, but the focus of the studies to be reviewed here on microbiota and cancer has focused on gut bacteria and bacteria associated with tumors, adjacent tissues, and organs (Whiteside et al. 2015).

There is exciting and emerging science supporting the notion that the microbiome can affect the immunotherapy of advanced cancers with checkpoint inhibitors. In patients with metastatic melanoma treated with the anti-CTLA-4 antibody ipilimumab, treatment with broad spectrum antibiotics impacted the gut microbiome. The use of antibiotics by patients during immunotherapy was associated with poorer responses while particular bacterial populations within patient microbiomes were associated with longer progression-free survival and greater overall survival (Vetizou et al. 2015). The gut microbiome profile in melanoma patients was also associated with response to treatment with antiprogrammed cell death protein-I (anti-PD-I) antibodies (Gopalakrishnan et al. 2018). In patients with advanced cancers treated with immunotherapy, resistance was associated with an abnormal gut microbiome and with antibiotic therapy (Routy et al. 2018). In support of these observations, fecal transplants from responders into germ-free mice enhanced antitumor immunity to xenograft tumors compared to patients who received broad spectrum antibiotics.

Antibiotic treatment in patients with advanced renal cell carcinoma and nonsmall-cell lung cancer decreased the effectiveness of anti-PDLI monoclonal antibody treatment. Patients who had recent antibiotic treatment had a higher risk of primary progressive disease, shorter progression-free survival, and shorter overall survival from renal cell carcinoma and nonsmall-cell lung cancer (Derosa et al. 2018).

Prior exposure to broad-spectrum antibiotics has been observed to increase the risk of other cancers as well including lung, gastric, prostate, and breast cancers suggesting that the microbiome may play a role in the risk for cancer development (Boursi et al. 2015) (see Figure 11.1).

Bacteria have also been found within tumors. The blood vessels within the poorly perfused areas of tumors are leaky and permit bacteria to settle where immune cells cannot clear them easily enabling bacterial growth (Syed Khaja et al. 2017). Anaerobic and necrotic areas of tumor tissue promote the growth of anaerobic bacteria (Wei et al. 2007). Each tumor type has a distinct microbiome composition. The intratumor bacteria are mostly intracellular and are present in both cancer and immune cells (Nejman et al. 2020). The bacteria persist both in metastatic lesions and in tumor xenografts in mice. Treatment of mice bearing colorectal cancer xenografts with metronidazole decreases tumor bacterial load and tumor growth, suggesting that the bacteria may have a role in tumor proliferation (Bullman et al. 2017).

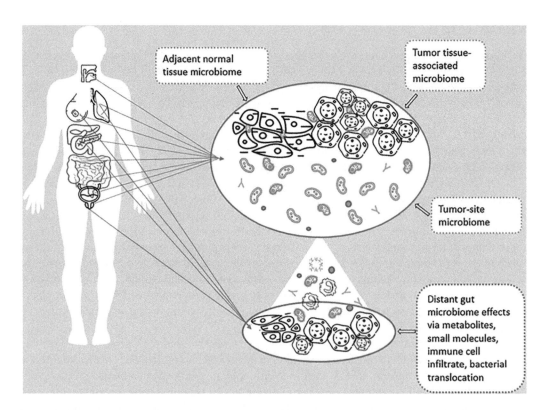

FIGURE 11.1 The relationship of microbiome to cancer. Tumor tissue has its own microbiome. Adjacent "normal" tissue also contains microbiota which may resemble the microbiome of the tumor, which suggests that alterations in bacterial species may play a causative role in tumor formation. Sites adjacent to the tumor such as feces and urine contain microbes, metabolites, and inflammatory molecules which may promote tumorigenesis, tumor progression, and response to treatment. Finally, bacteria in the gut as well as associated immune cells, cytokines, bacterial metabolites, and other molecules may affect systemic immunity which could influence tumor formation and treatment response. (Adapted from Picardo, Coburn, and Hansen 2019.)

This above series of exciting observations on the role of the microbiome in cancer suggests a new pathway through which nutrition including prebiotics and probiotics may be used to enhance immunotherapy by modifying the microbiome.

THE MICROBIOME

The microbiota of the gut and their collective genomes constitutes the microbiome. The microbiome can be studied using metagenomics by combining next-generation sequencing platforms with the computational analysis and assembly of targeted (16S ribosomal RNA hypervariable region) and random (whole genome shotgun) DNA sequences (Heintz-Buschart and Wilmes 2018).

The communities of bacteria that live within the gut benefit from nutrients provided from foods in the diet especially carbohydrate foods. Gut bacteria digest glycans into disaccharides and monosaccharides for the human host as well as for their own energy utilization. To carry out this function, the gut microbiome is highly enriched for genes involved in carbohydrate metabolism including over 115 families of glycoside hydrolases and over 21 families of polysaccharide lyases (Ley et al. 2006, Gill et al. 2006). In contrast, the human genome has relatively few genes that encode carbohydrate-metabolizing enzymes, presumably because mammals (and their genomes) coevolved with gut microbiota (and the gut microbiome). As a result of the symbiotic while the higher taxa of the bacterial populations are conserved in humans (Costea et al. 2018), metagenomic studies have demonstrated substantial variation at the genus and species levels among different individuals (Costello et al. 2009, Qin et al. 2010). This individual variation is the result of interactions of the gut bacteria with both host genetics and environmental factors. The effects of host genetics on the microbiome were demonstrated in a genome-wide association study combined with 16S ribosomal RNA metagenomics data on a large (n = 645) panel of mouse lines identified a number of quantitative trait loci that influence the relative abundance of specific microbial taxa (Leamy et al. 2014). The impact of environmental factors is illustrated by the variations in microbiota within a human individual in response to diet, stress, circadian rhythm, household pets, antibiotics, chemotherapy, and environmental toxins (Claesson et al. 2011, Song et al. 2013, Albenberg and Wu 2014, Zwielehner et al. 2011, Antonopoulos et al. 2009, Voigt et al. 2016).

GERM-FREE MICE

After obtaining an association of genomic and metagenomic information on the microbiome with regard to cancer promotion or cancer immunotherapy, researchers have proceeded to studies with germ-free (gnotobiotic) mouse models to further substantiate and explore the role of diet and the microbiome in cancer treatment. Tumor-bearing mice can be raised in a completely germ-free state in specialized gnotobiotic facilities which are kept sterile through sterilization of the environment and the use of germ-free diets which are autoclaved and also fortified with certain essential vitamins that are normally synthesized by the gut bacteria (Wostmann 1981).

It is important to realize that like other mouse models, this model is not comparable to a wild mouse or even a laboratory mouse in some respects. Compared to mice raised in a typical vivarium, germ-free mice consume more food but have about 35% less body fat (Backhed et al. 2007). This clearly observed difference emphasizes the role of the microbiota in extracting nutrients and calories from the diet. Germ-free mice have decreased levels of glucose, insulin, and glycogen and are somewhat resistant to obesity when provided a high-fat diet (Backhed et al. 2007).

Germ-free mice have been used in experiments demonstrating the role of the microbiota in immunity and inflammation (Nagao-Kitamoto et al. 2016). For example, interleukin (IL)-10 is a potent, immunosuppressive cytokine, and IL-10 knockout mice are used to study the effects of eliminating this control on immunity and its influence on inflammatory diseases. IL-10 knockout mice exhibit a colitis phenotype that is rescued by maintaining them in a germ-free state consistent with a primary function of IL-10 as preventing an inappropriate inflammatory response against normal gut microbiota. In other experiments, Inflammatory Bowel Disease (IBD)-associated microbiota transferred into IL-10 knockout gnotobiotic mice induced a proinflammatory gene expression profile in the gut that resembled the immunologic responses found in Crohn's disease patients. Furthermore, microbiota from Crohn's disease patients triggered more severe colitis than healthy control microbiota when colonized in germ-free IL-10-deficient mice (Nagao-Kitamoto et al. 2016).

These observations support the notion that changes in the microbiome can potentially contribute to the pathogenesis of IBD and other inflammatory conditions including cancer by increasing host proinflammatory immune responses. Obesity is also associated with inflammation and changes in the microbiome may explain in part the association of obesity and cancer (Henao-Mejia et al. 2012, Netto Candido, Bressan, and Alfenas 2018). Transforming growth factor-$\beta1$ knockout mice exhibit colorectal inflammation and cancer, and the inflammation and cancer observed under normal laboratory conditions are prevented in germ-free mice (Engle et al. 2002). Germ-free mice also have fewer proinflammatory T helper 17 cells in the gut-associated immune system of the gut-associated immune cells in the lamina propria than pathogen-free controls (Atarashi et al. 2015).

The interaction of the microbiome and the immune system allows for the tolerance of healthy gut bacteria and the elimination of potentially harmful bacteria that cause infection, inflammation, and even cancer. The microbiota can also contribute to innate and adaptive immune responses more broadly. Germ-free mice have altered IgA secretion and a reduced size of Peyer's patches and draining mesenteric lymph nodes (Johansson et al. 2015, Spiljar, Merkler, and Trajkovski 2017). There is extensive evidence supporting the notion that the gut microbiota establishes and supports overall immune function (Honda and Littman 2016). The role of microbiome in cancer could relate to its effects on energy balance and immunity. In studies of nutrition and cancer, alterations in the microbiome can be defined and then tested in specific strains of germ-free mice to assess their role in carcinogenesis or the response to immunotherapy.

CANCER TREATMENT

The immune system is critical to mostly all forms of cancer treatment through effects on tumor development, progression, and in mediating the cellular responses which kill or clear cancer cells. Aging is a risk factor for most forms of cancer and senescence of the immune system in association with reduced diversity of gut bacteria has been proposed to account in part for this enhanced susceptibility to cancer with age (Biragyn and Ferrucci 2018) (see Figure 11.2).

The gut-associated lymphoid tissue is the largest element of the immune system and strongly impacts immune responses systemically (Ahluwalia, Magnusson, and Ohman 2017), and recent research on immunotherapy demonstrated that intact systemic immunity is essential to durable responses (Chen and Mellman 2013, 2017, Spitzer et al. 2017).

Research on immunotherapy using checkpoint inhibitors changed the focus of precision oncology from the genetic and protein markers of tumor cells (Snyder et al. 2014), their particular cancer metabolism, and tumor sensitivity to immune destruction (Snyder et al. 2014) to a recognition that gut associated-lymphoid tissue, the microbiome, and diet contribute to overall immune status and the durability of tumor responses to immunotherapy (Blank et al. 2016). This insight also highlighted again the importance of the tumor microenvironment including other cells such as infiltrating immune cells that either stimulate or inhibit an immune response to the tumor cells (Blank et al. 2016, Sharma et al. 2017).

As already discussed in the introduction, the revolutionary discovery of immunotherapy utilizing immune checkpoint inhibitors for metastatic disease has garnered greater interest on the potential impact of nutrition on the microbiome and gut-associated immune system. The drugs that are used target immunoinhibitory proteins generated by tumor cells which act on the surface receptor of T cells or their ligands to enhance antitumor immune responses. It has been observed that a significant proportion of patients do not experience objective or durable responses, and differences in the gut microbiota may be responsible for this observation (Cogdill et al. 2018, Sharma et al. 2017).

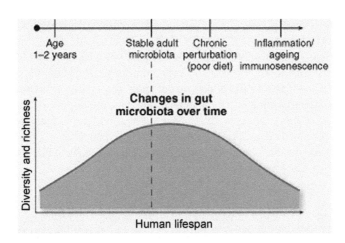

FIGURE 11.2 The gut microbiota during the human life span. Over the first 2–3`years of life, the gut micro-biota undergoes dynamic changes wherein highly adapted communities are established resulting in a healthy microbiome in a state of homeostasis. Environmental factors such as sustained intake of a high-fat, high-carbohydrate diet may drive the gut microbiota into a state of dysbiosis that may influence human diseases such as obesity, diabetes, and colorectal cancer. With aging, the gut microbiota may degenerate into a state of dysbiosis resulting in chronic inflammation (inflammaging) and reduced immune function (immunose-nescence) accounting in part for aging as a major risk factor for cancer. (Adapted from Peterson et al. 2015.)

Studies have also demonstrated the impact of the gut microbiota on responses to several other types of cancer therapies as well (Kroemer and Zitvogel 2018).

The use of antibiotics affects the microbiota in cancer patients and has been shown to reduce the response to immune checkpoint blockade in a large cohort of patients with nonsmall-cell lung cancer, renal cell carcinoma, and urological cancers. Patients treated with antibiotics for routine indications shortly before, during, or shortly after treatment with antiPD1/PD-L1 monoclonal antibodies had significantly lower progression-free survival and overall survival rates compared to patients who had not received antibiotics. These findings suggest that antibiotics can impact the gut microbiota and impair antitumor immune responses as well as responses to immune checkpoint blockade (Routy et al. 2017).

Further support for the concept that the microbiome is integral to responses to immunotherapy comes from the whole metagenomic sequencing of fecal samples from patients treated with immunotherapy. Responders to PD-I blockade had different gut bacteria populations than nonresponders. Furthermore, when fecal transplants were performed into germ-free mice using feces from either responder or nonresponder patients prior to treatment with PD1 blockade, the germ-free mice receiving responder fecal transplants demonstrated enhanced anti-PD1 blockade responses compared to animals transplanted with feces from nonresponders. Furthermore, the reduced efficacy of anti-PD-1 in mice receiving nonresponder fecal transplants could be restored with some strains of bacteria found in the responder feces (Routy et al. 2018). In studies of patients with metastatic melanoma receiving anti-PD-1 therapy, responders were found to have greater diversity of bacteria in their gut microbiome than nonresponders along with specific differences in bacterial genera (Gopalakrishnan et al. 2018, Matson et al. 2018).

A significant number of patients receiving immunotherapy experience toxicities. Sixteen percent of patients receiving anti-PD-I and 27% of patients receiving anti-CTLA-4 therapy suffer toxicities severe enough to limit treatment (Larkin et al. 2015). A third of patients undergoing anti-CTLA-4 therapy develop intestinal inflammation due to mucosal immune dysregulation (Berman et al. 2010, Weber et al. 2015). Studies in animals demonstrated an improvement in toxicity scores in anti-CTLA-4-treated mice with oral gavage of two species of bacteria (*Bacteroides fragilis* and

Burkholderia cepacia) (Vetizou et al. 2015). The influence of the gut microbiota on toxicity has also been demonstrated in human cohorts (Chaput et al. 2017, Dubin et al. 2016, Frankel et al. 2017).

While there are clearly bacterial taxa that are associated with response and toxicity, there is also significant overlap in the bacterial populations observed in responders compared to nonresponders. Broad generalizations applicable to all patients do not apply at this time. More research is needed on how communities of bacteria influence the metabolomic environment of the microbiome to affect systemic immunity. Despite these issues, the impact of the gut microbiota on therapeutic responses to immunotherapy is established, and emerging science suggests that the gut microbiota can impact both anti-tumor immune responses and responses to immune checkpoint blockade.

DIET

The gut microbiota aid in extraction of calories and nutrients from foods through a host–microbiome interaction that results in digestion and metabolism of compounds that humans cannot process without the help of bacteria (Backhed et al. 2005). In this dynamic process, foods and nutrients digested by bacteria also promote the growth of some bacteria over others altering the composition of the microbiome. While individual microbiomes are relatively stable due to the communal nature of the bacteria in the gut through the actions of the immune system and bacterial community sharing of nutrients and genetic material, intensive changes in dietary intake can change the microbiome.

A key insight in the understanding of the physiological role of the microbiome is that it can adapt metabolically to changes in the diet. In the research literature in this field to date, gut microbiota has been classified into enterotypes based on the dominant phyla found. The three major enterotypes identified in the literature are *Bacteroides*, *Prevotella*, and *Ruminococcus* (Arumugam et al. 2011). Dietary patterns have been associated with these enterotypes providing insights into the effects of diet on the microbiome. *Bacteroides* is associated with a diet high in fat, while Prevotella is associated with a high carbohydrate diet (Wu et al. 2011). A typical Western diet which is high both in fat and sugar results in reduction of Bacteroidetes and an increase in Firmicutes (Hildebrandt et al. 2009, Zimmer et al. 2012). Vegetarian and vegan diets by comparison to omnivores demonstrate a reduced abundance of *Bacteroides*, *Bifidobacterium*, *E. coli*, and Enterobactericieae species (Zimmer et al. 2012, Kabeerdoss et al. 2012). With a shift from animal-based to plant-based diets, the gut microbiota undergoes rapid changes in composition (David et al. 2014). The changes in microbial populations observed due to this rapid change in dietary pattern were larger than the interpersonal differences distinguishing individual stable gut microbiota, indicating the potential of diet to modulate the microbiome.

The potential to modify immune responses through modulation of gut bacterial composition and function has focused on nutrition intervention, probiotics supplementation, and bacterial transplantation. If it could be proven to affect immune function, nutrition intervention through prebiotics and probiotics would be practical and secure. We may be able to reduce cancer risk and improve the safety and effectiveness of cancer therapy. Obviously, additional clinical research is necessary in this field.

Considering that the intestine is the shared site of nutrient digestion, microbe habitat, and immune cell location, this geographic proximity has led to extensive research on their interaction. The responsiveness of specific bacterial groups and their downstream metabolites to a variety of nutrients and immune parameters have provided some preliminary insights into how dietary modulation could be used as a strategy to enrich the gut microbiome and immune health (Ma et al. 2018, Shortt et al. 2018). While not yet clinically tested, there are parallel questions that could be explored in the context of cancer treatment.

While dietary interventions may seem relatively simple to design and implement, the effects on the microbiota can be modest, and patient compliance is difficult to enforce and monitor. Nonetheless, instituting a dietary pattern involves eating a variety of fruits and vegetables with prebiotic polyphenols and fiber as well as an adequate amount of high-quality protein to help maintain intestinal barrier integrity and a healthy diverse microbiome. Additionally, a multivitamin/multimineral supplement and other selected dietary supplements may be used with the knowledge of the patient's healthcare team.

Probiotics or fermented foods have also been proposed as a direct way to affect the microbiome and immune function. In patients with colorectal cancer given preoperative probiotic therapy, mucosal immunity was assessed. Altered cytokine profiles were noted at the time of colonic resection with those patients receiving probiotics having lower levels of IL-13, IL-10, and IL-23A mRNA levels compared to controls who received no probiotics. In the healthy colonic mucosa of these patients, there was decreased production of both proinflammatory and anti-inflammatory cytokines noted (Consoli et al. 2016). While it is difficult to interpret what these cytokine changes mean in terms of colorectal cancer development and progression or response to therapy, the study is a proof of principle that probiotic therapy can alter some aspects of local immunity in the colonic mucosa.

A number of studies are currently in development, and it is important to highlight that the assessment of relevant antitumor immune responses in association with changes in the microbiome is critical to understanding the adjunctive value of nutritional and probiotic interventions. Probiotic formulations are available with regard to their composition, stability, and authenticity (Huys et al. 2013). At the current state of knowledge, it is premature to recommend probiotics to all patients undergoing immunotherapy. However, future research may establish clinical guidelines for their use along with dietary patterns and other supplements that increase the diversity of the microbiota and have specific metabolic effects that enhance the efficacy, safety, and tolerability of immunotherapy.

FECAL MICROBIOTA TRANSPLANT

The administration of feces for the treatment of food poisoning or severe diarrhea was recorded in China about 1,700 years ago (Zhang et al. 2018). The fecal microbiota transplant (FMT) was used to treat severe pseudomembranous enterocolitis 1958 (Eiseman et al. 1958), but became more widely known by gastroenterologists after the use of FMT to treat Clostridium difficile infection in 1983 (Schwan et al. 1983). At the present time, FMT is approved for the treatment of recurrent Clostridium difficile infection, and its clinical effectiveness for this condition is about 90% (Surawicz et al. 2013, Konturek et al. 2015). Emerging data suggest that FMT is beneficial for the treatment of inflammatory bowel diseases and intractable functional constipation (Xu et al. 2015, Costello et al. 2017). Following the observation of dysbiosis in cancer, there has been increasing interest in the potential of FMT for the management of cancer.

FMT has been designated as a biological drug by the U.S. Food and Drug Administration, and an investigational new drug application must be submitted in order to obtain permission to implement FMT for any disease other than recurrent Clostridia difficile infection. Due to the potential pathogenicity of fecal bacteria, the safety of FMT is still under study (Olesen et al. 2018) and has not been approved for cancer treatment. A systematic review including 1,089 patients receiving FMT in a total of 50 publications found that serious side effects, such as death and virus infections, were not rare (Wang et al. 2016). Although there are some encouraging case studies, the quality of evidence of FMT in cancer management remains generally low. Much more high-quality research is needed before FMT can be recommended for any form of cancer therapy including immunotherapy.

CONCLUSION

The discovery of the microbiome and the potential modulation of immune function through nutrition have led to new directions of research on diet, microbiota, and cancer. Both preclinical and clinical studies on the role of microbiota in cancer progression, treatment, and prevention of relapse have led to the possibility that nutrition could be used to enhance immune function in cancer patients as an integral component of Precision Oncology linked to Precision Nutrition. There are many exciting observations in animals and humans that link the potential influence of the microbiome on immunity and cancer, but the role of nutrition has yet to be established in well-designed clinical trials.

The optimal strategies to modulate the gut microbiome to enhance responses to cancer immunotherapy may be the best place to start these research efforts as the preliminary observations in humans and in germ-free mice are intriguing and suggest the potential of nutrition, dietary supplements, and probiotics to alter the gut-associated immune response to cancer immunotherapy. Metagenomic studies have pointed out the complex nature of the communities of bacteria and their interactions metabolically and in modulating immune function. In addition to methodological issues with the metagenomic study of the microbiome, the influence of other factors impacting the gut microbiome such as medications, stress, and environmental factors will need to be considered in the design of these clinical trials to establish a beneficial role for nutrition in immunotherapy and other forms of cancer treatment.

REFERENCES

Ahluwalia, B., M. K. Magnusson, and L. Ohman. 2017. "Mucosal immune system of the gastrointestinal tract: maintaining balance between the good and the bad." *Scand J Gastroenterol* 52 (11):1185–1193. doi: 10.1080/00365521.2017.1349173.

Albenberg, L. G., and G. D. Wu. 2014. "Diet and the intestinal microbiome: associations, functions, and implications for health and disease." *Gastroenterology* 146 (6):1564–1572. doi: 10.1053/j.gastro.2014.01.058.

Antonopoulos, D. A., S. M. Huse, H. G. Morrison, T. M. Schmidt, M. L. Sogin, and V. B. Young. 2009. "Reproducible community dynamics of the gastrointestinal microbiota following antibiotic perturbation." *Infect Immun* 77 (6):2367–2375. doi: 10.1128/IAI.01520-08.

Arumugam, M., J. Raes, E. Pelletier, D. Le Paslier, T. Yamada, D. R. Mende, G. R. Fernandes, J. Tap, T. Bruls, J. M. Batto, M. Bertalan, N. Borruel, F. Casellas, L. Fernandez, L. Gautier, T. Hansen, M. Hattori, T. Hayashi, M. Kleerebezem, K. Kurokawa, M. Leclerc, F. Levenez, C. Manichanh, H. B. Nielsen, T. Nielsen, N. Pons, J. Poulain, J. Qin, T. Sicheritz-Ponten, S. Tims, D. Torrents, E. Ugarte, E. G. Zoetendal, J. Wang, F. Guarner, O. Pedersen, W. M. de Vos, S. Brunak, J. Dore, H. I. T. Consortium Meta, M. Antolin, F. Artiguenave, H. M. Blottiere, M. Almeida, C. Brechot, C. Cara, C. Chervaux, A. Cultrone, C. Delorme, G. Denariaz, R. Dervyn, K. U. Foerstner, C. Friss, M. van de Guchte, E. Guedon, F. Haimet, W. Huber, J. van Hylckama-Vlieg, A. Jamet, C. Juste, G. Kaci, J. Knol, O. Lakhdari, S. Layec, K. Le Roux, E. Maguin, A. Merieux, R. Melo Minardi, C. M'Rini, J. Muller, R. Oozeer, J. Parkhill, P. Renault, M. Rescigno, N. Sanchez, S. Sunagawa, A. Torrejon, K. Turner, G. Vandemeulebrouck, E. Varela, Y. Winogradsky, G. Zeller, J. Weissenbach, S. D. Ehrlich, and P. Bork. 2011. "Enterotypes of the human gut microbiome." *Nature* 473 (7346):174–180. doi: 10.1038/nature09944.

Atarashi, K., T. Tanoue, M. Ando, N. Kamada, Y. Nagano, S. Narushima, W. Suda, A. Imaoka, H. Setoyama, T. Nagamori, E. Ishikawa, T. Shima, T. Hara, S. Kado, T. Jinnohara, H. Ohno, T. Kondo, K. Toyooka, E. Watanabe, S. Yokoyama, S. Tokoro, H. Mori, Y. Noguchi, H. Morita, Ivanov, II, T. Sugiyama, G. Nunez, J. G. Camp, M. Hattori, Y. Umesaki, and K. Honda. 2015. "Th17 cell induction by adhesion of microbes to intestinal epithelial cells." *Cell* 163 (2):367–380. doi: 10.1016/j.cell.2015.08.058.

Backhed, F., R. E. Ley, J. L. Sonnenburg, D. A. Peterson, and J. I. Gordon. 2005. "Host-bacterial mutualism in the human intestine." *Science* 307 (5717):1915–1920. doi: 10.1126/science.1104816.

Backhed, F., J. K. Manchester, C. F. Semenkovich, and J. I. Gordon. 2007. "Mechanisms underlying the resistance to diet-induced obesity in germ-free mice." *Proc Natl Acad Sci U S A* 104 (3):979–984. doi: 10.1073/pnas.0605374104.

Berg, G., D. Rybakova, D. Fischer, T. Cernava, M. C. Verges, T. Charles, X. Chen, L. Cocolin, K. Eversole, G. H. Corral, M. Kazou, L. Kinkel, L. Lange, N. Lima, A. Loy, J. A. Macklin, E. Maguin, T. Mauchline, R. McClure, B. Mitter, M. Ryan, I. Sarand, H. Smidt, B. Schelkle, H. Roume, G. S. Kiran, J. Selvin, R. S. C. Souza, L. van Overbeek, B. K. Singh, M. Wagner, A. Walsh, A. Sessitsch, and M. Schloter. 2020. "Microbiome definition re-visited: old concepts and new challenges." *Microbiome* 8 (1):103. doi: 10.1186/s40168-020-00875-0.

Berman, D., S. M. Parker, J. Siegel, S. D. Chasalow, J. Weber, S. Galbraith, S. R. Targan, and H. L. Wang. 2010. "Blockade of cytotoxic T-lymphocyte antigen-4 by ipilimumab results in dysregulation of gastrointestinal immunity in patients with advanced melanoma." *Cancer Immun* 10:11.

Biragyn, A., and L. Ferrucci. 2018. "Gut dysbiosis: a potential link between increased cancer risk in ageing and inflammaging." *Lancet Oncol* 19 (6):e295–e304. doi: 10.1016/S1470-2045(18)30095-0.

Blank, C. U., J. B. Haanen, A. Ribas, and T. N. Schumacher. 2016. "Cancer immunology. The "cancer immunogram"." *Science* 352 (6286):658–660. doi: 10.1126/science.aaf2834.

Boursi, B., R. Mamtani, K. Haynes, and Y. X. Yang. 2015. "Recurrent antibiotic exposure may promote cancer formation--another step in understanding the role of the human microbiota?" *Eur J Cancer* 51 (17):2655–2664. doi: 10.1016/j.ejca.2015.08.015.

Bullman, S., C. S. Pedamallu, E. Sicinska, T. E. Clancy, X. Zhang, D. Cai, D. Neuberg, K. Huang, F. Guevara, T. Nelson, O. Chipashvili, T. Hagan, M. Walker, A. Ramachandran, B. Diosdado, G. Serna, N. Mulet, S. Landolfi, Y. Cajal S. Ramon, R. Fasani, A. J. Aguirre, K. Ng, E. Elez, S. Ogino, J. Tabernero, C. S. Fuchs, W. C. Hahn, P. Nuciforo, and M. Meyerson. 2017. "Analysis of Fusobacterium persistence and antibiotic response in colorectal cancer." *Science* 358 (6369):1443–1448. doi: 10.1126/science.aal5240.

Chaput, N., P. Lepage, C. Coutzac, E. Soularue, K. Le Roux, C. Monot, L. Boselli, E. Routier, L. Cassard, M. Collins, T. Vaysse, L. Marthey, A. Eggermont, V. Asvatourian, E. Lanoy, C. Mateus, C. Robert, and F. Carbonnel. 2017. "Baseline gut microbiota predicts clinical response and colitis in metastatic melanoma patients treated with ipilimumab." *Ann Oncol* 28 (6):1368–1379. doi: 10.1093/annonc/mdx108.

Chen, D. S., and I. Mellman. 2013. "Oncology meets immunology: the cancer-immunity cycle." *Immunity* 39 (1):1–10. doi: 10.1016/j.immuni.2013.07.012.

Chen, D. S., and I. Mellman. 2017. "Elements of cancer immunity and the cancer-immune set point." *Nature* 541 (7637):321–330. doi: 10.1038/nature21349.

Claesson, M. J., S. Cusack, O. O'Sullivan, R. Greene-Diniz, H. de Weerd, E. Flannery, J. R. Marchesi, D. Falush, T. Dinan, G. Fitzgerald, C. Stanton, D. van Sinderen, M. O'Connor, N. Harnedy, K. O'Connor, C. Henry, D. O'Mahony, A. P. Fitzgerald, F. Shanahan, C. Twomey, C. Hill, R. P. Ross, and P. W. O'Toole. 2011. "Composition, variability, and temporal stability of the intestinal microbiota of the elderly." *Proc Natl Acad Sci U S A* 108 (Suppl 1):4586–4591. doi: 10.1073/pnas.1000097107.

Cogdill, A. P., P. O. Gaudreau, R. Arora, V. Gopalakrishnan, and J. A. Wargo. 2018. "The impact of intratumoral and gastrointestinal microbiota on systemic cancer therapy." *Trends Immunol* 39 (11):900–920. doi: 10.1016/j.it.2018.09.007.

Consoli SG, Consoli SM. Countertransference in Dermatology. *Acta Derm Venereol.* 2016 Aug 23;96(217): 18-21. doi: 10.2340/00015555-2414. PMID: 27282987.

Costea, P. I., F. Hildebrand, M. Arumugam, F. Backhed, M. J. Blaser, F. D. Bushman, W. M. de Vos, S. D. Ehrlich, C. M. Fraser, M. Hattori, C. Huttenhower, I. B. Jeffery, D. Knights, J. D. Lewis, R. E. Ley, H. Ochman, P. W. O'Toole, C. Quince, D. A. Relman, F. Shanahan, S. Sunagawa, J. Wang, G. M. Weinstock, G. D. Wu, G. Zeller, L. Zhao, J. Raes, R. Knight, and P. Bork. 2018. "Enterotypes in the landscape of gut microbial community composition." *Nat Microbiol* 3 (1):8–16. doi: 10.1038/s41564-017-0072-8.

Costello, E. K., C. L. Lauber, M. Hamady, N. Fierer, J. I. Gordon, and R. Knight. 2009. "Bacterial community variation in human body habitats across space and time." *Science* 326 (5960):1694–1697. doi: 10.1126/science.1177486.

Costello, S. P., W. Soo, R. V. Bryant, V. Jairath, A. L. Hart, and J. M. Andrews. 2017. "Systematic review with meta-analysis: faecal microbiota transplantation for the induction of remission for active ulcerative colitis." *Aliment Pharmacol Ther* 46 (3):213–224. doi: 10.1111/apt.14173.

David, L. A., C. F. Maurice, R. N. Carmody, D. B. Gootenberg, J. E. Button, B. E. Wolfe, A. V. Ling, A. S. Devlin, Y. Varma, M. A. Fischbach, S. B. Biddinger, R. J. Dutton, and P. J. Turnbaugh. 2014. "Diet rapidly and reproducibly alters the human gut microbiome." *Nature* 505 (7484):559–563. doi: 10.1038/nature12820.

Derosa, L., M. D. Hellmann, M. Spaziano, D. Halpenny, M. Fidelle, H. Rizvi, N. Long, A. J. Plodkowski, K. C. Arbour, J. E. Chaft, J. A. Rouche, L. Zitvogel, G. Zalcman, L. Albiges, B. Escudier, and B. Routy. 2018. "Negative association of antibiotics on clinical activity of immune checkpoint inhibitors in patients with advanced renal cell and non-small-cell lung cancer." *Ann Oncol* 29 (6):1437–1444. doi: 10.1093/annonc/mdy103.

Dominguez-Bello, M. G., F. Godoy-Vitorino, R. Knight, and M. J. Blaser. 2019. "Role of the microbiome in human development." *Gut* 68 (6):1108–1114. doi: 10.1136/gutjnl-2018-317503.

Dubin, K., M. K. Callahan, B. Ren, R. Khanin, A. Viale, L. Ling, D. No, A. Gobourne, E. Littmann, C. Huttenhower, E. G. Pamer, and J. D. Wolchok. 2016. "Intestinal microbiome analyses identify melanoma patients at risk for checkpoint-blockade-induced colitis." *Nat Commun* 7:10391. doi: 10.1038/ncomms10391.

Eiseman, B., W. Silen, G. S. Bascom, and A. J. Kauvar. 1958. "Fecal enema as an adjunct in the treatment of pseudomembranous enterocolitis." *Surgery* 44 (5):854–859.

Engle, S. J., I. Ormsby, S. Pawlowski, G. P. Boivin, J. Croft, E. Balish, and T. Doetschman. 2002. "Elimination of colon cancer in germ-free transforming growth factor beta 1-deficient mice." *Cancer Res* 62 (22):6362–6366.

Frankel, A. E., L. A. Coughlin, J. Kim, T. W. Froehlich, Y. Xie, E. P. Frenkel, and A. Y. Koh. 2017. "Metagenomic shotgun sequencing and unbiased metabolomic profiling identify specific human gut microbiota and metabolites associated with immune checkpoint therapy efficacy in melanoma patients." *Neoplasia* 19 (10):848–855. doi: 10.1016/j.neo.2017.08.004.

Gill, S. R., M. Pop, R. T. Deboy, P. B. Eckburg, P. J. Turnbaugh, B. S. Samuel, J. I. Gordon, D. A. Relman, C. M. Fraser-Liggett, and K. E. Nelson. 2006. "Metagenomic analysis of the human distal gut microbiome." *Science* 312 (5778):1355–1359. doi: 10.1126/science.1124234.

Gopalakrishnan, V., C. N. Spencer, L. Nezi, A. Reuben, M. C. Andrews, T. V. Karpinets, P. A. Prieto, D. Vicente, K. Hoffman, S. C. Wei, A. P. Cogdill, L. Zhao, C. W. Hudgens, D. S. Hutchinson, T. Manzo, M. Petaccia de Macedo, T. Cotechini, T. Kumar, W. S. Chen, S. M. Reddy, R. Szczepaniak Sloane, J. Galloway-Pena, H. Jiang, P. L. Chen, E. J. Shpall, K. Rezvani, A. M. Alousi, R. F. Chemaly, S. Shelburne, L. M. Vence, P. C. Okhuysen, V. B. Jensen, A. G. Swennes, F. McAllister, E. Marcelo Riquelme Sanchez, Y. Zhang, E. Le Chatelier, L. Zitvogel, N. Pons, J. L. Austin-Breneman, L. E. Haydu, E. M. Burton, J. M. Gardner, E. Sirmans, J. Hu, A. J. Lazar, T. Tsujikawa, A. Diab, H. Tawbi, I. C. Glitza, W. J. Hwu, S. P. Patel, S. E. Woodman, R. N. Amaria, M. A. Davies, J. E. Gershenwald, P. Hwu, J. E. Lee, J. Zhang, L. M. Coussens, Z. A. Cooper, P. A. Futreal, C. R. Daniel, N. J. Ajami, J. F. Petrosino, M. T. Tetzlaff, P. Sharma, J. P. Allison, R. R. Jenq, and J. A. Wargo. 2018. "Gut microbiome modulates response to anti-PD-1 immunotherapy in melanoma patients." *Science* 359 (6371):97–103. doi: 10.1126/science.aan4236.

Guilhot, E., S. Khelaifia, B. La Scola, D. Raoult, and G. Dubourg. 2018. "Methods for culturing anaerobes from human specimen." *Future Microbiol* 13:369–381. doi: 10.2217/fmb-2017-0170.

Heintz-Buschart, A., and P. Wilmes. 2018. "Human gut microbiome: function matters." *Trends Microbiol* 26 (7):563–574. doi: 10.1016/j.tim.2017.11.002.

Henao-Mejia, J., E. Elinav, C. Jin, L. Hao, W. Z. Mehal, T. Strowig, C. A. Thaiss, A. L. Kau, S. C. Eisenbarth, M. J. Jurczak, J. P. Camporez, G. I. Shulman, J. I. Gordon, H. M. Hoffman, and R. A. Flavell. 2012. "Inflammasome-mediated dysbiosis regulates progression of NAFLD and obesity." *Nature* 482 (7384):179–185. doi: 10.1038/nature10809.

Hildebrandt, M. A., C. Hoffmann, S. A. Sherrill-Mix, S. A. Keilbaugh, M. Hamady, Y. Y. Chen, R. Knight, R. S. Ahima, F. Bushman, and G. D. Wu. 2009. "High-fat diet determines the composition of the murine gut microbiome independently of obesity." *Gastroenterology* 137 (5):1716–1724.e1–e2. doi: 10.1053/j. gastro.2009.08.042.

Honda, K., and D. R. Littman. 2016. "The microbiota in adaptive immune homeostasis and disease." *Nature* 535 (7610):75–84. doi: 10.1038/nature18848.

Huys, G., N. Botteldoorn, F. Delvigne, L. De Vuyst, M. Heyndrickx, B. Pot, J. J. Dubois, and G. Daube. 2013. "Microbial characterization of probiotics--advisory report of the Working Group "8651 Probiotics" of the Belgian Superior Health Council (SHC)." *Mol Nutr Food Res* 57 (8):1479–504. doi: 10.1002/ mnfr.201300065.

Johansson, M. E., H. E. Jakobsson, J. Holmen-Larsson, A. Schutte, A. Ermund, A. M. Rodriguez-Pineiro, L. Arike, C. Wising, F. Svensson, F. Backhed, and G. C. Hansson. 2015. "Normalization of host intestinal mucus layers requires long-term microbial colonization." *Cell Host Microbe* 18 (5):582–592. doi: 10.1016/j.chom.2015.10.007.

Kabeerdoss, J., R. S. Devi, R. R. Mary, and B. S. Ramakrishna. 2012. "Faecal microbiota composition in vegetarians: comparison with omnivores in a cohort of young women in southern India." *Br J Nutr* 108 (6):953–957. doi: 10.1017/S0007114511006362.

Konturek, P. C., D. Haziri, T. Brzozowski, T. Hess, S. Heyman, S. Kwiecien, S. J. Konturek, and J. Koziel. 2015. "Emerging role of fecal microbiota therapy in the treatment of gastrointestinal and extra-gastrointestinal diseases." *J Physiol Pharmacol* 66 (4):483–491.

Kroemer, G., and L. Zitvogel. 2018. "Cancer immunotherapy in 2017: The breakthrough of the microbiota." *Nat Rev Immunol* 18 (2):87–88. doi: 10.1038/nri.2018.4.

Larkin, J., V. Chiarion-Sileni, R. Gonzalez, J. J. Grob, C. L. Cowey, C. D. Lao, D. Schadendorf, R. Dummer, M. Smylie, P. Rutkowski, P. F. Ferrucci, A. Hill, J. Wagstaff, M. S. Carlino, J. B. Haanen, M. Maio, I. Marquez-Rodas, G. A. McArthur, P. A. Ascierto, G. V. Long, M. K. Callahan, M. A. Postow, K. Grossmann, M. Sznol, B. Dreno, L. Bastholt, A. Yang, L. M. Rollin, C. Horak, F. S. Hodi, and J. D. Wolchok. 2015. "Combined nivolumab and ipilimumab or monotherapy in untreated melanoma." *N Engl J Med* 373 (1):23–34. doi: 10.1056/NEJMoa1504030.

Leamy, L. J., S. A. Kelly, J. Nietfeldt, R. M. Legge, F. Ma, K. Hua, R. Sinha, D. A. Peterson, J. Walter, A. K. Benson, and D. Pomp. 2014. "Host genetics and diet, but not immunoglobulin A expression, converge to shape compositional features of the gut microbiome in an advanced intercross population of mice." *Genome Biol* 15 (12):552. doi: 10.1186/s13059-014-0552-6.

Ley, R. E., P. J. Turnbaugh, S. Klein, and J. I. Gordon. 2006. "Microbial ecology: human gut microbes associated with obesity." *Nature* 444 (7122):1022–1023. doi: 10.1038/4441022a.

Ma, N., P. Guo, J. Zhang, T. He, S. W. Kim, G. Zhang, and X. Ma. 2018. "Nutrients mediate intestinal bacteria-mucosal immune crosstalk." *Front Immunol* 9:5. doi: 10.3389/fimmu.2018.00005.

Matson, V., J. Fessler, R. Bao, T. Chongsuwat, Y. Zha, M. L. Alegre, J. J. Luke, and T. F. Gajewski. 2018. "The commensal microbiome is associated with anti-PD-1 efficacy in metastatic melanoma patients." *Science* 359 (6371):104–108. doi: 10.1126/science.aao3290.

Nagao-Kitamoto, H., A. B. Shreiner, M. G. Gillilland, 3rd, S. Kitamoto, C. Ishii, A. Hirayama, P. Kuffa, M. El-Zaatari, H. Grasberger, A. M. Seekatz, P. D. Higgins, V. B. Young, S. Fukuda, J. Y. Kao, and N. Kamada. 2016. "Functional characterization of inflammatory bowel disease-associated gut dysbiosis in gnotobiotic mice." *Cell Mol Gastroenterol Hepatol* 2 (4):468–481. doi: 10.1016/j.jcmgh.2016.02.003.

Nejman, D., I. Livyatan, G. Fuks, N. Gavert, Y. Zwang, L. T. Geller, A. Rotter-Maskowitz, R. Weiser, G. Mallel, E. Gigi, A. Meltser, G. M. Douglas, I. Kamer, V. Gopalakrishnan, T. Dadosh, S. Levin-Zaidman, S. Avnet, T. Atlan, Z. A. Cooper, R. Arora, A. P. Cogdill, M. A. W. Khan, G. Ologun, Y. Bussi, A. Weinberger, M. Lotan-Pompan, O. Golani, G. Perry, M. Rokah, K. Bahar-Shany, E. A. Rozeman, C. U. Blank, A. Ronai, R. Shaoul, A. Amit, T. Dorfman, R. Kremer, Z. R. Cohen, S. Harnof, T. Siegal, E. Yehuda-Shnaidman, E. N. Gal-Yam, H. Shapira, N. Baldini, M. G. I. Langille, A. Ben-Nun, B. Kaufman, A. Nissan, T. Golan, M. Dadiani, K. Levanon, J. Bar, S. Yust-Katz, I. Barshack, D. S. Peeper, D. J. Raz, E. Segal, J. A. Wargo, J. Sandbank, N. Shental, and R. Straussman. 2020. "The human tumor microbiome is composed of tumor type-specific intracellular bacteria." *Science* 368 (6494):973–980. doi: 10.1126/science.aay9189.

Netto Candido, T. L., J. Bressan, and R. C. G. Alfenas. 2018. "Dysbiosis and metabolic endotoxemia induced by high-fat diet." *Nutr Hosp* 35 (6):1432–1440. doi: 10.20960/nh.1792.

Olesen, S. W., M. M. Leier, E. J. Alm, and S. A. Kahn. 2018. "Searching for superstool: maximizing the therapeutic potential of FMT." *Nat Rev Gastroenterol Hepatol* 15 (7):387–388. doi: 10.1038/s41575-018-0019-4.

Peterson, C. T., V. Sharma, L. Elmen, and S. N. Peterson. 2015. "Immune homeostasis, dysbiosis and therapeutic modulation of the gut microbiota." *Clin Exp Immunol* 179 (3):363–377. doi: 10.1111/cei.12474.

Picardo, S. L., B. Coburn, and A. R. Hansen. 2019. "The microbiome and cancer for clinicians." *Crit Rev Oncol Hematol* 141:1–12. doi: 10.1016/j.critrevonc.2019.06.004.

Qin, J., R. Li, J. Raes, M. Arumugam, K. S. Burgdorf, C. Manichanh, T. Nielsen, N. Pons, F. Levenez, T. Yamada, D. R. Mende, J. Li, J. Xu, S. Li, D. Li, J. Cao, B. Wang, H. Liang, H. Zheng, Y. Xie, J. Tap, P. Lepage, M. Bertalan, J. M. Batto, T. Hansen, D. Le Paslier, A. Linneberg, H. B. Nielsen, E. Pelletier, P. Renault, T. Sicheritz-Ponten, K. Turner, H. Zhu, C. Yu, S. Li, M. Jian, Y. Zhou, Y. Li, X. Zhang, S. Li, N. Qin, H. Yang, J. Wang, S. Brunak, J. Dore, F. Guarner, K. Kristiansen, O. Pedersen, J. Parkhill, J. Weissenbach, H. I. T. Consortium Meta, P. Bork, S. D. Ehrlich, and J. Wang. 2010. "A human gut microbial gene catalogue established by metagenomic sequencing." *Nature* 464 (7285):59–65. doi: 10.1038/nature08821.

Routy, B., E. Le Chatelier, L. Derosa, C. P. M. Duong, M. T. Alou, R. Daillere, A. Fluckiger, M. Messaoudene, C. Rauber, M. P. Roberti, M. Fidelle, C. Flament, V. Poirier-Colame, P. Opolon, C. Klein, K. Iribarren, L. Mondragon, N. Jacquelot, B. Qu, G. Ferrere, C. Clemenson, L. Mezquita, J. R. Masip, C. Naltet, S. Brosseau, C. Kaderbhai, C. Richard, H. Rizvi, F. Levenez, N. Galleron, B. Quinquis, N. Pons, B. Ryffel, V. Minard-Colin, P. Gonin, J. C. Soria, E. Deutsch, Y. Loriot, F. Ghiringhelli, G. Zalcman, F. Goldwasser, B. Escudier, M. D. Hellmann, A. Eggermont, D. Raoult, L. Albiges, G. Kroemer, and L. Zitvogel. 2018. "Gut microbiome influences efficacy of PD-1-based immunotherapy against epithelial tumors." *Science* 359 (6371):91–97. doi: 10.1126/science.aan3706.

Routy, B., C. Letendre, D. Enot, M. Chenard-Poirier, V. Mehraj, N. C. Seguin, K. Guenda, K. Gagnon, P. L. Woerther, D. Ghez, and S. Lachance. 2017. "The influence of gut-decontamination prophylactic antibiotics on acute graft-versus-host disease and survival following allogeneic hematopoietic stem cell transplantation." *Oncoimmunology* 6 (1):e1258506. doi: 10.1080/2162402X.2016.1258506.

Schwan, A., S. Sjolin, U. Trottestam, and B. Aronsson. 1983. "Relapsing Clostridium difficile enterocolitis cured by rectal infusion of homologous faeces." *Lancet* 2 (8354):845. doi: 10.1016/s0140-6736(83)90753-5.

Sharma, P., S. Hu-Lieskovan, J. A. Wargo, and A. Ribas. 2017. "Primary, adaptive, and acquired resistance to cancer immunotherapy." *Cell* 168 (4):707–723. doi: 10.1016/j.cell.2017.01.017.

Shortt, C., O. Hasselwander, A. Meynier, A. Nauta, E. N. Fernandez, P. Putz, I. Rowland, J. Swann, J. Turk, J. Vermeiren, and J. M. Antoine. 2018. "Systematic review of the effects of the intestinal microbiota on selected nutrients and non-nutrients." *Eur J Nutr* 57 (1):25–49. doi: 10.1007/s00394-017-1546-4.

Snyder, A., V. Makarov, T. Merghoub, J. Yuan, J. M. Zaretsky, A. Desrichard, L. A. Walsh, M. A. Postow, P. Wong, T. S. Ho, T. J. Hollmann, C. Bruggeman, K. Kannan, Y. Li, C. Elipenahli, C. Liu, C. T. Harbison, L. Wang, A. Ribas, J. D. Wolchok, and T. A. Chan. 2014. "Genetic basis for clinical response to CTLA-4 blockade in melanoma." *N Engl J Med* 371 (23):2189–2199. doi: 10.1056/NEJMoa1406498.

Song, S. J., C. Lauber, E. K. Costello, C. A. Lozupone, G. Humphrey, D. Berg-Lyons, J. G. Caporaso, D. Knights, J. C. Clemente, S. Nakielny, J. I. Gordon, N. Fierer, and R. Knight. 2013. "Cohabiting family members share microbiota with one another and with their dogs." *Elife* 2:e00458. doi: 10.7554/eLife.00458.

Spiljar, M., D. Merkler, and M. Trajkovski. 2017. "The immune system bridges the gut microbiota with systemic energy homeostasis: focus on TLRs, mucosal barrier, and SCFAs." *Front Immunol* 8:1353. doi: 10.3389/fimmu.2017.01353.

Spitzer, M. H., Y. Carmi, N. E. Reticker-Flynn, S. S. Kwek, D. Madhireddy, M. M. Martins, P. F. Gherardini, T. R. Prestwood, J. Chabon, S. C. Bendall, L. Fong, G. P. Nolan, and E. G. Engleman. 2017. "Systemic immunity is required for effective cancer immunotherapy." *Cell* 168 (3):487–502.e15. doi: 10.1016/j.cell.2016.12.022.

Surawicz, C. M., L. J. Brandt, D. G. Binion, A. N. Ananthakrishnan, S. R. Curry, P. H. Gilligan, L. V. McFarland, M. Mellow, and B. S. Zuckerbraun. 2013. "Guidelines for diagnosis, treatment, and prevention of Clostridium difficile infections." *Am J Gastroenterol* 108 (4):478–498; quiz 499. doi: 10.1038/ajg.2013.4.

Syed Khaja, A. S., S. M. Toor, H. El Salhat, I. Faour, N. Ul Haq, B. R. Ali, and E. Elkord. 2017. "Preferential accumulation of regulatory T cells with highly immunosuppressive characteristics in breast tumor microenvironment." *Oncotarget* 8 (20):33159–33171. doi: 10.18632/oncotarget.16565.

Underwood, M. A., J. B. German, C. B. Lebrilla, and D. A. Mills. 2015. "Bifidobacterium longum subspecies infantis: champion colonizer of the infant gut." *Pediatr Res* 77 (1–2):229–235. doi: 10.1038/pr.2014.156.

Vetizou, M., J. M. Pitt, R. Daillere, P. Lepage, N. Waldschmitt, C. Flament, S. Rusakiewicz, B. Routy, M. P. Roberti, C. P. Duong, V. Poirier-Colame, A. Roux, S. Becharef, S. Formenti, E. Golden, S. Cording, G. Eberl, A. Schlitzer, F. Ginhoux, S. Mani, T. Yamazaki, N. Jacquelot, D. P. Enot, M. Berard, J. Nigou, P. Opolon, A. Eggermont, P. L. Woerther, E. Chachaty, N. Chaput, C. Robert, C. Mateus, G. Kroemer, D. Raoult, I. G. Boneca, F. Carbonnel, M. Chamaillard, and L. Zitvogel. 2015. "Anticancer immunotherapy by CTLA-4 blockade relies on the gut microbiota." *Science* 350 (6264):1079–1084. doi: 10.1126/science.aad1329.

Voigt, R. M., C. B. Forsyth, S. J. Green, P. A. Engen, and A. Keshavarzian. 2016. "Circadian rhythm and the gut microbiome." *Int Rev Neurobiol* 131:193–205. doi: 10.1016/bs.irn.2016.07.002.

Wang, S., M. Xu, W. Wang, X. Cao, M. Piao, S. Khan, F. Yan, H. Cao, and B. Wang. 2016. "Systematic review: adverse events of fecal microbiota transplantation." *PLoS One* 11 (8):e0161174. doi: 10.1371/journal.pone.0161174.

Weber, D., P. J. Oefner, A. Hiergeist, J. Koestler, A. Gessner, M. Weber, J. Hahn, D. Wolff, F. Stammler, R. Spang, W. Herr, K. Dettmer, and E. Holler. 2015. "Low urinary indoxyl sulfate levels early after transplantation reflect a disrupted microbiome and are associated with poor outcome." *Blood* 126 (14):1723–1728. doi: 10.1182/blood-2015-04-638858.

Whiteside, S. A., H. Razvi, S. Dave, G. Reid, and J. P. Burton. 2015. "The microbiome of the urinary tract--a role beyond infection." *Nat Rev Urol* 12 (2):81–90. doi: 10.1038/nrurol.2014.361.

Wostmann, B. S. 1981. "The germfree animal in nutritional studies." *Annu Rev Nutr* 1:257–279. doi: 10.1146/annurev.nu.01.070181.001353.

Wu, G. D., J. Chen, C. Hoffmann, K. Bittinger, Y. Y. Chen, S. A. Keilbaugh, M. Bewtra, D. Knights, W. A. Walters, R. Knight, R. Sinha, E. Gilroy, K. Gupta, R. Baldassano, L. Nessel, H. Li, F. D. Bushman, and J. D. Lewis. 2011. "Linking long-term dietary patterns with gut microbial enterotypes." *Science* 334 (6052):105–108. doi: 10.1126/science.1208344.

Xu, M. Q., H. L. Cao, W. Q. Wang, S. Wang, X. C. Cao, F. Yan, and B. M. Wang. 2015. "Fecal microbiota transplantation broadening its application beyond intestinal disorders." *World J Gastroenterol* 21 (1):102–111. doi: 10.3748/wjg.v21.i1.102.

Zhang, F., B. Cui, X. He, Y. Nie, K. Wu, D. Fan, and FMT-Standardization Study Group. 2018. "Microbiota transplantation: concept, methodology and strategy for its modernization." *Protein Cell* 9 (5):462–473. doi: 10.1007/s13238-018-0541-8.

Zimmer, J., B. Lange, J. S. Frick, H. Sauer, K. Zimmermann, A. Schwiertz, K. Rusch, S. Klosterhalfen, and P. Enck. 2012. "A vegan or vegetarian diet substantially alters the human colonic faecal microbiota." *Eur J Clin Nutr* 66 (1):53–60. doi: 10.1038/ejcn.2011.141.

Zwielehner, J., C. Lassl, B. Hippe, A. Pointner, O. J. Switzeny, M. Remely, E. Kitzweger, R. Ruckser, and A. G. Haslberger. 2011. "Changes in human fecal microbiota due to chemotherapy analyzed by TaqMan-PCR, 454 sequencing and PCR-DGGE fingerprinting." *PLoS One* 6 (12):e28654. doi: 10.1371/journal.pone.0028654.

12 Exercise, Energy Balance, Body Composition, and Cancer Risk

Catherine L. Carpenter
UCLA Center for Human Nutrition
Schools of Nursing, Medicine and Public Health

CONTENTS

INTRODUCTION

Evidence from numerous population studies, prevention trials, clinical trials, clinical studies, and experimental research has consistently demonstrated the protective role that exercise plays in risk reduction and improved recovery from cancers that occur at multiple sites. Physiologic changes resulting from exercise are differently associated with risk of multiple cancers depending on disease etiology and underlying mechanisms. These physiologic changes include adipose tissue reduction, increase in muscle mass, improved cardiovascular and respiratory function, changed inflammatory response, increased metabolic rate, modified energy balance, and altered hormonal levels. This chapter provides a description of physiologic changes that occur as a function of exercise, describes how exercise functions to maintain energy balance, outlines evidence for exercise and cancer-site specific risk, and examines the potential causative associations among exercise, physiologic mechanisms, energy balance, and body composition in relationship to cancer risk and prognosis.

PHYSIOLOGIC CHANGES RESULTING FROM EXERCISE

Physical activity occupies a central role in the maintenance of good health, and people of all ages benefit from regular exercise. Physical activity is defined as bodily movement produced by skeletal muscle contractions that increase energy expenditure above basal metabolism (U. S. Department of

Health and Human Services 1996). Physical activity is a complex set of behaviors that has spawned a myriad of measurement approaches, and descriptions of physical activity vary according to several criteria. Studies of exercise and cancer risk generally classify physical activity into three types: total physical activity, recreational physical activity, and occupational physical activity (World Cancer Research Fund/American Institute for Cancer Research 2018a). Other parameters of physical activity include intensity (vigorous, moderate, or light), with the total volume of exercise summarized by the combination of frequency, intensity, and duration of different types of physical activity (World Cancer Research Fund/American Institute for Cancer Research 2018a). Physical activity influences several physiologic systems, including circulation, metabolism, adipose tissue, skeletal muscle, endocrine system, and immunity. The effect of exercise activity on these systems, in turn, can modify the risk of cancer.

EXERCISE AND ADIPOSE TISSUE

Excess adipose tissue cells, a regulator of metabolism in both health and disease, increases the risk of several different forms of cancer (Hursting et al. 2012, Bhaskaran et al. 2014). Adipocytes primarily function to store fatty acids as triglycerides during energy excess and release fatty acids via lipolysis during energy demand (Tsiloulis and Watt 2015). This metabolically rich tissue also provides critical signaling molecules for appetite regulation and metabolic feedback.

Because obesity increases the risk for multiple cancers, the effect of physical activity on adipose tissue provides an important pathway for cancer risk reduction. Exercise training affects lipolysis, or the breakdown of fat, differently depending on intensity and duration as well as type of exercise. In the "crossover concept" theory, substrate metabolism during endurance exercise changes as exercise intensity increases beyond 45%–65% of VO_{2max}. Glycogen and glucose become the primary fuels during high-intensity exercise, and prior to reaching that threshold of exercise intensity, lipid utilization is more predominant (Brooks and Mercier 1985). Athletes experiencing prolonged endurance running will switch to fat stores for fuel if their glycogen stores are exhausted (Rapoport 2010). To avoid this, many endurance athletes including cyclists and runners consume simple carbohydrates during exercise to maintain their glycogen stores.

Carbohydrate oxidation is a more critical and efficient component for high-intensity aerobic exercise, whereas fatty acid oxidation is better suited for moderate exercise (Rapoport 2010). Further evidence demonstrated fat oxidation differences in a carefully controlled equal-caloric exercise study of severely obese adolescent boys (Lazzer et al. 2010b). The investigators compared substrate oxidation rates during and after low- or high-intensity exercise on a graded treadmill with oxidation rates measured by VO_{2max}. Figure 12.1 demonstrates dramatically different patterns of carbohydrate and fat oxidation, with fat oxidation primarily occurring at low intensity and carbohydrate oxidation occurring at high-intensity exercise (Lazzer et al. 2010b).

Variations in type of exercise may also influence fat distribution differently. In a small controlled study of obese postmenopausal women with type 2 diabetes, comparisons were drawn between high-intensity interval training and moderate intensity training for 16 weeks, in relationship to whole body and abdominal fat mass changes. With isocaloric conditions maintained throughout the intervention period, both groups decreased in overall fat mass, with the high intensity group experiencing a significantly greater loss of total abdominal and visceral fat compared to moderate intensity, suggesting that high-intensity exercise may be more effective at reducing abdominal fat (Maillard et al. 2016). In a larger randomized controlled trial of sedentary overweight postmenopausal women, a moderate exercise intensity intervention compared to a stretching control group found moderate exercise led to a significant reduction in total fat and intraabdominal fat with a greater response found with increasing duration of exercise (Irwin et al. 2003).

A small pilot study was conducted in seven obese postmenopausal women who underwent a controlled diet and exercise intervention with a high protein, low fat, and high fiber diet and combined aerobic and resistance training over 3 months. All participants lost weight, lost fat mass, and

(a)

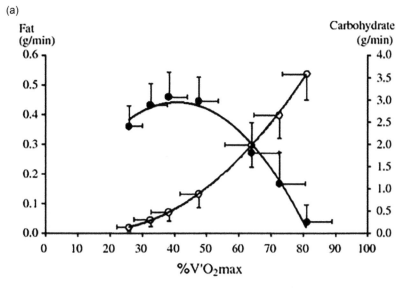

(b)

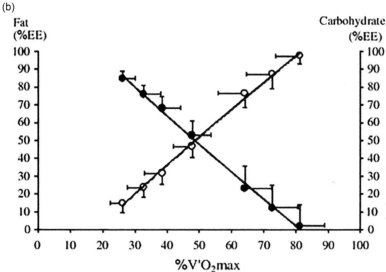

FIGURE 12.1 Fat (filled circle) and carbohydrate (open circle) oxidation rates expressed in absolute values (g/min, a) and as percent of total energy expenditure (%EE, b) as a function of exercise intensity expressed as percent of maximal oxygen uptake (VO_{2max}). (Adapted from Lazzer et al. (2010a).)

gained muscle strength and aerobic fitness (Carpenter et al. 2012). Most participants also lost muscle mass, although a small proportion gained in muscle mass while simultaneously losing fat mass.

In summary, exercise results in lipolysis, and depending on the type, intensity, and duration of exercise, fat loss may be greater with lower intensity exercise, with the exception of visceral fat. Visceral fat loss, in particular, may depend on higher intensity exercise over longer durations.

EXERCISE AND SKELETAL MUSCLE

Skeletal muscle occupies ~40% of body mass and accounts for over 70% of energy expenditure during exercise (Pant, Bal, and Periasamy 2016, Egan and Zierath 2013). At rest skeletal muscle accounts for ~30% of the resting metabolic rate in adults (Zurlo et al. 1990). Skeletal muscle tissue has several major functions including movement, whole body metabolism, thermogenesis and is considered an important metabolic and endocrine organ (Pant, Bal, and Periasamy 2016, Egan and Zierath 2013, Marieb, Brady, and Mallet 2020). Muscle undergoes constant metabolic change and, therefore, serves as a key determinant of the basal metabolic rate and metabolic homeostasis. Because the major substrate for muscle function is glucose and glycogen, skeletal muscle energy stores are subject to regulation by both the liver and the pancreas. Metabolic flexibility enables muscle to utilize fatty acids for fuel at low and moderate rates of exertion sparing limited stores of glycogen in muscle and liver (Rapoport 2010, Pant, Bal, and Periasamy 2016). Moreover, during starvation, the skeletal muscle tissue breaks down protein to provide glucogenic amino acids for obligate glucose consumption by the brain and the red blood cells. The liver converts these amino acids into glucose through the energy-requiring process of gluconeogenesis (Pant, Bal, and Periasamy 2016).

Skeletal muscle responds to exercise in several different ways. The size of human skeletal muscle mass is dependent on the relationship between synthesis of muscle protein and muscle protein breakdown with resistance exercise promoting muscle cell hypertrophy. With adequate dietary protein intake, resistance training stimulates an increase in muscle size where muscle cells in the trained muscle take up amino acids to synthesize protein which enlarges and strengthens muscle fibers (McGlory and Phillips 2015). Skeletal muscle also responds to endurance exercise with an increase in numbers and quality of mitochondria with improved efficiency in fatty acid and glucose metabolism (Booth et al. 2015). The increase in mitochondria results in a greater capacity for metabolism of glucose and fatty acids to provide energy for ongoing muscle function. At the same time, the cardiovascular and respiratory systems increase gas exchange efficiency as well as gas delivery to the muscle resulting in increased oxygen consumption and carbon dioxide production by developing increased vasculature and surface areas in the respiratory system and by strengthening the cardiac muscle.

SKELETAL MUSCLE AND GLUCOSE REGULATION

Skeletal muscle plays a critical role in glycemic regulation and metabolic stability. Muscle is a major site for glucose metabolism under insulin stimulation. Muscle stores glycogen and can take up glucose through insulin action and independent of insulin (DiMeo, Iossa, and Venditt 2017).

Experimental studies have shown a potential for glucose uptake by skeletal muscle to occur both by insulin facilitation and through an independent mechanism (Mul et al. 2015). The independent mechanism triggered by exercise occurs through intramolecular signaling which enables the glucose transporter (GLUT4) to reach the muscle cell surface and create a channel for glucose entry. Regular physical activity greatly improves insulin resistance through insulin-independent glucose uptake. Insulin resistance, in turn, is an important determinant of type 2 diabetes, and while exercise stimulates entry of glucose into the muscle cell independent of insulin, exercise also facilitates a more efficient response to insulin (DiMeo, Iossa, and Venditt 2017, Mul et al. 2015).

SKELETAL MUSCLE AND LIPID METABOLISM

To provide readily available fuel to muscle in addition to glycogen deposits, lipid droplets are stored in close proximity to skeletal muscle cells. In normal weighted individuals, these myocellular lipid droplets are readily oxidized to energy. Under conditions of obesity and excess body fat, fatty acids are stored in skeletal muscle and not sufficiently metabolized (Horowitz 2007). These excess fatty acid deposits in muscle have been found to induce insulin resistance. Studies using magnetic resonance spectroscopy (MRS) to image glycogen, glucose, and fatty acid distribution within skeletal muscle cells found that excess fatty acids were inhibiting glucose uptake into skeletal muscle by inhibiting the activity of the insulin receptors present on the cell membranes of muscle cells (Petersen and Schulman 2006). Prolonged insulin resistance exhibited by skeletal muscle can promote the onset of type 2 diabetes as insulin secretion at the pancreatic beta-cells is exhausted over time. In a recent study in our laboratory, MRS imaged both intramyocellular lipid (IMCL) and extramyocellular lipid (EMCL) among a cross-sectional sample of obese and nonobese adults (Nagarajan et al. 2017). The IMCLs measured in our study were comparable to the amounts of IMCLs observed in other MRS studies (Petersen and Schulman 2006). We conducted MRS scans of the calf muscles, gastrocnemius, tibialis, and soleus muscles. The levels of IMCL were compared in obese subjects and nonobese controls. IMCL content was elevated in the obese subjects only in the soleus muscle condition, while higher lipid levels were found among obese subjects compared to nonobese subjects in the gastrocnemius and tibialis muscles for both IMCL and EMCL. The soleus muscle has predominantly type 1 fibers and principally engages in aerobic respiration, while gastrocnemius and tibialis have type 1 and type 2 fibers, and engage in a mixture of aerobic and anaerobic respiration. We compared insulin sensitivity among the obese subjects for the three muscle groups and found an association with IMCL and insulin sensitivity for the gastrocnemius muscle (Nagarajan et al. 2017).

In summary, exercise can reduce cancer risk through lipolysis of adipose tissue stores, through the increase in skeletal muscle causing elevation in basal metabolism and by improving insulin sensitivity.

ENERGY BALANCE

Exercise serves an important role in the prevention of weight gain as well as functioning to promote weight loss among individuals with excess body fat. The maintenance of energy balance requires energy intake to be equivalent to energy expenditure with the achievement of stable body weight contingent upon energy balance being in dynamic equilibrium (see Figure 12.2). Under normal circumstances, balance is achieved through complex regulation by the brain, hormonal signaling, and metabolism (World Cancer Research Fund/American Institute for Cancer Research 2018a).

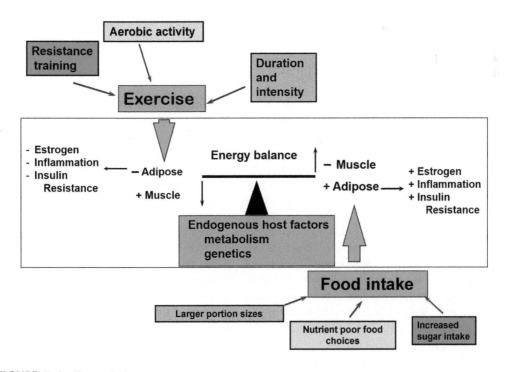

FIGURE 12.2 Energy balance.

In addition to the balancing role played by the brain, adipose tissue and skeletal muscle are important substrates that work to store and oxidize excess energy with the liver and pancreas organs functioning in a regulatory fashion.

Many studies have evaluated the weight loss effects from exercise with the presumption that less exercise is required to maintain weight and prevent weight gain. Exercise is regarded as a critical component to weight management. However, its main benefit is weight maintenance after weight loss rather than accelerating weight loss during dieting. During dieting, caloric restriction plays a predominant role in weight loss. Nonetheless, combining exercise and diet during weight loss is beneficial in establishing exercise habits that will help to maintain weight in the long-term (Miller, Koceja, and Hamilton 1997, Shaw et al. 2006). Exercise has a major benefit in leading to a reduction of fat mass together with retention of or increase of fat-free mass (Quist et al. 2018).

Maintenance of energy balance however appears to be a more complicated endeavor to study than evaluation of weight loss. Energy balance achieved through exercise is a function of multiple factors including fitness level (sedentary or athletic), body composition, and type and duration of exercise performed.

EXERCISE AND WEIGHT MAINTENANCE

Maintenance of a stable weight in adulthood depends on closely matching energy intake from food and drink with the energy expended in basal metabolism and physical activity (World Cancer Research Fund/American Institute for Cancer Research 2018b). Over the past two decades, the concurrent decline in physical activity coupled with rise in obesity prevalence points to the important role that exercise plays in the prevention of weight gain. There is lack of agreement however about how much exercise is required to maintain weight and/or prevent weight gain. In a consensus statement from the International Association for the Study of Obesity, the suggested Surgeon General's guideline for 30 minutes of moderate intensity exercise per day was determined to be insufficient for preventing weight gain. Moreover, "prevention of weight regain in formerly obese individuals requires 60–90 minutes of moderate intensity activity per day or lesser amounts of vigorous intensity activity" (Saris et al. 2003). The 2020 American Cancer Society's Guidelines for Physical Activity recommend that "adults should engage in 150–300 minutes of moderate physical activity (30–60 minutes per day for 5 days a week) or 75–150 minutes of vigorous intensity activity" (Rock et al. 2020).

Fitness level and presence of excess body fat may influence exercise effects on energy balance and weight maintenance. In a controlled dietary and exercise studies of obese, overweight, and lean individuals, the rate of fat oxidation compared to lean individuals, given the same exercise challenge, was measured (Bergouignan et al. 2014). Subjects were evaluated over a 24-hour period in a controlled chamber where caloric intake and expenditure were carefully assessed and blood drawn every 30 minutes. Exercise consisted of step exercises during two 20-minute intervals over the 24-hour period with speeds meant to approximate a moderate walk. Contrary to expectations, the obese and overweight individuals oxidized the same amount of fat as the lean individuals, with all groups demonstrating fat oxidation as a function of exercise. All participants engaged in the same level and type of exercise, and all subjects equally oxidized fat (Bergouignan et al. 2014). It is important to consider, however, that in naturalistic settings, lean individuals generally engage in higher intensity exercise due to their increased fitness levels, and therefore could potentially oxidize greater amounts of fat, than less fit obese individuals.

Fitness level and degree of body fat may jointly influence fat metabolism resulting from exercise. In a controlled study of individuals varying in fitness and body fat but maintained in the same state of energy balance, the acute effects of exercise on fat oxidation were evaluated (Melanson et al. 2009). Lean sedentary, lean endurance-trained, and obese sedentary men and women were studied over a 24-hour period of at-rest control condition versus a 24-hour period of 1-hour moderate stationary cycling (55% of aerobic fitness capacity). Subjects were measured in a metabolic ward setting where meals were calibrated to energy expenditure so that energy balance was maintained for each subject. Fat oxidation did not vary between the groups and fat oxidation during exercise did not increase for each of the three groups compared to at-rest control as long as energy balance was maintained (Melanson et al. 2009). This study pointed out the importance of caloric restriction in addition to exercise to mobilize body fat and reduce excess body fat so that a period of daily exercise cannot make up for excessive caloric intake during the day unless overall energy balance is changed.

Cross-sectional assessments of individuals in energy balance who varied in fitness and obesity levels did not show differences in fat oxidation effects from acute exercise (Bergouignan et al. 2014, Melanson et al. 2009). Exercise training over time however may improve fat oxidation especially among sedentary individuals. In a controlled study of sedentary lean and overweight men, 2 months of controlled training for a 1-hour session on a cycle ergometer four times per week resulted in a significantly greater amount of fat oxidation for overweight compared to lean individuals (Lefai et al. 2017).

In summary, acute exercise does not appear to influence energy balance in the short term for individuals that vary in fitness and levels of obesity. However, consistent and frequent moderate exercise over time does appear to result in negative energy balance for overweight individuals, particularly when dietary intake is relatively constant (e.g., does not increase during training). Maintenance of a stable weight through exercise necessitates regular intervals of moderate exercise that should exceed 30 minutes per day for most days of the week.

EXERCISE AND CANCER RISK

The Continuous Update Project from the World Cancer Research Fund has concluded that there is strong evidence for physical activity decreasing the risk of cancers of the colon, postmenopausal breast, and endometrium. Furthermore, there is strong evidence that undertaking vigorous physical activity reduces the risk of both pre- and postmenopausal breast cancer (World Cancer Research Fund/American Institute for Cancer Research 2018a). Other cancers have also shown reduced risk due to physical activity, although there is lack of consensus about which cancers. The American Cancer Society lists breast, colorectal, endometrial, gall bladder, kidney, liver, lung, ovary, pancreas, stomach, and upper aerodigestive tract as demonstrating risk reduction due to physical activity (Rock et al. 2020). The 2018 Physical Activity Guidelines Committee from Health and Human Services, on the other hand, notes risk reduction for breast, kidney, colon, endometrial, bladder, esophageal, and stomach with limited evidence for brain, ovarian, head and neck, pancreas, and prostate (U. S. Department of Health and Human Services 2018). A further update to the Guidelines confirmed the strong evidence for bladder, breast, colon, endometrial, esophageal adenocarcinoma, renal (kidney) and gastric cancer; moderate evidence for lung, with limited evidence for head and neck, ovary, pancreas, prostate, thyroid, and rectal (McTiernan et al. 2019). As further evidence accumulates there may be additional cancers identified that are positively influenced by exercise, as well as further clarifications of existing associations.

Several biological mechanisms link physical activity to cancer risk reduction (McTiernan 2008, Hojman et al. 2018, Rock et al. 2020). These mechanisms include effects of exercise on metabolism immunity, inflammation, steroid hormones, oxidative stress, genomic instability, and myokines. Exercise can directly reduce serum estrogen levels in premenopausal women and can indirectly reduce estrogen levels by reducing adipose tissue stores resulting in reduced aromatization of adrenal androgen estrogen precursors (Rock et al. 2020, McTiernan 2008, Hojman et al. 2018).

BREAST CANCER

Evidence from multiple pooled analyses, meta-analyses, and systematic reviews has demonstrated a "probable" inverse association between increased levels of physical activity and reduced breast cancer risk in postmenopausal women (World Cancer Research Fund/American Institute for Cancer Research 2018a,b Hursting et al. 2012, Bhaskaran et al. 2014, Rock et al. 2020, U. S. Department of Health and Human Services 2018, McTiernan et al. 2019, Neilson et al. 2016). Evidence for breast-cancer risk reduction in premenopausal women is considered "probable" for vigorous physical activity (World Cancer Research Fund/American Institute for Cancer Research 2018a). Several important factors modify the association between physical activity and breast cancer risk including reproductive interval (premenopause, postmenopause), body mass index (BMI), family history, and use of hormone therapy (Neilson et al. 2016).

Development of premenopausal breast cancer is different from postmenopausal breast cancer, particularly with regard to obesity and physical activity. While hormone production in each menstrual cycle during the premenopausal years affects proliferation of ductal cells and their differentiation (Pike et al. 1993), after menopause, production of ovarian estrogen greatly diminishes and there is an involution of the ducts and alveoli in the breast (Allred, Mohan, and Fuqua 2001). After menopause, surrounding fibrous connective tissue change in density and breast tissues is replaced by adipose tissue. In addition, after ovarian hormone production ceases, adipose tissue becomes the primary source of estrogen production through activity by the aromatase enzyme (Cleary and Grossmann 2009).

Estrogen targets the breast ductal epithelium and causes cell replication during the follicular phase of the menstrual cycle prior to ovulation. Moreover, the breast environment can be affected by circulating endocrine and paracrine hormones as well as inflammatory cytokines (Carpenter et al. 2012). Fat tissue surrounding the stroma and ductal epithelium, for instance, has particularly high levels of aromatase enzyme activity (Bulun et al. 2007, Miller 2006). Enhanced localized aromatase activity coupled with estradiol levels in the circulating plasma can potentially deliver a more potent dose of estradiol to the localized breast than the rest of the body (Carpenter et al. 2012). Prior to menopause, cyclical variations in estrogen levels influence both cell replication and apoptosis.

In general, associations between physical activity and premenopausal breast cancer are less consistent and weaker in magnitude (Neilson et al. 2016). During the menstrual years, excess body fat and obesity cause anovulation with a subsequent decline in production of ovarian estrogen (Silvestris et al. 2018). Because exercise promotes weight loss and reduction in body fat, there may be a potentially muted association with premenopausal breast cancer, due to the influence of adipose tissue, particularly among obese women.

After menopause, biologic mechanisms that explain exercise and breast-cancer prevention are more direct than mechanisms to explain risk reduction prior to menopause. The decrease in adipose tissue and associated reductions in estrogen, inflammation, and cytokine production that occurs with moderate to vigorous activity appears to explain most of the association between exercise and reduced risk of breast cancer after menopause (Neilson et al. 2016).

COLON CANCER

Evidence from multiple cohort and case control studies has demonstrated an inverse association between physical activity and colon cancer risk. According to the World Cancer Research Fund, physical activity strongly and convincingly reduces the risk of colon cancer, with several large meta-analyses finding up to a 20% reduction among men (World Cancer Research Fund/American Institute for Cancer Research 2018a, Harriss et al. 2009) and an overall reduction in colon cancer risk of 24% in men and women (Wolin et al. 2009).

Chronic inflammation associated with excess adipose tissue mass appears to be a mediating influence on increased colon cancer risk (Ulrich et al. 2018). Evidence suggests obesity-related pro-inflammatory markers such as IL-6 and TNF-α (Tumor Necrosis Factor-alpha) are the link between obesity, inflammation, and colon cancer development (Kern et al. 2018). In a randomized dietary and exercise weight loss trial of healthy overweight to obese postmenopausal women, the combination of dietary intake designed for weight loss and exercise was most effective in reducing percent body fat and markers of inflammation associated with obesity such as IL-6 and C-reactive protein (Imayama et al. 2012). As discussed earlier, estrogen synthesis occurs in adipose tissue through aromatase enzymatic activity. Estrogen is protective for colon cancer development and therefore the excess estrogen associated with obesity is not likely to be an explanation for the association between obesity and colon cancer, nor is the reduction of estrogen levels due to aerobic exercise likely to be an explanation for risk reduction due to exercise (Ulrich et al. 2018). Exercise reduces body fat and inflammatory markers associated with body fat, and therefore, the link between exercise and prevention of colon cancer may be largely due to diminishing adipose tissue stores. Other obesity-related factors such as insulin, leptin, insulin growth factors (IGF-1), and insulin-binding proteins (IGF-BP3) are also associated with increased colon cancer risk (Ulrich et al. 2018, Kern et al. 2018, Otani et al. 2007, Stattin et al. 2004), and exercise has been shown to reduce levels of these markers as well (Imayama et al. 2012).

In summary, colon cancer prevention due to exercise is driven largely by reduction in adipose tissue stores. Evidence from multiple studies has shown exercise decreases associated cytokines, inflammatory and metabolic factors that occur in conjunction with excess body fat.

ENDOMETRIAL CANCER

The pathogenesis of endometrial cancer, similar to breast cancer, has a close link to estrogen (Bulun et al. 2007). There is strong evidence that being physically active decreases the risk of endometrial cancer (World Cancer Research Fund/American Institute for Cancer Research 2018a), with further evidence that the reduction in risk is independent of BMI in studies which adjusted for BMI (Hursting et al. 2012). A large meta-analysis of cohort and case-control studies has determined that the protective association between exercise and endometrial cancer was limited to postmenopausal women, with all three types of exercise, recreational, occupational, and home-based activity demonstrating a reduction in risk. Associations were protective and marginally significant among premenopausal women (Schmid et al. 2015). In studies that stratified for BMI, the protective association was limited to overweight women whose BMI equaled or exceeded 25.0 kg/m^2 (Schmid et al. 2015). There is not complete consistency however with another review concluding that effect modification by BMI and effect modification by menopausal status were not evident (Brown et al. 2012). In a detailed examination of underlying mechanisms, steroid and metabolic hormones associated with elevated adipose tissue that are influenced by physical activity appear to mechanistically explain the reduction in endometrial cancer risk (McTiernan 2008). An earlier synthetic review noted an excess of estrogen in conjunction with reduced progesterone among obese premenopausal women that may explain an increased endometrial cancer risk among obese premenopausal women (Kaaks 2002). The effect of exercise on reduction of adipose tissue, may, according to Kaaks et al., explain the slightly protective association among premenopausal women observed in the large meta-analysis conducted by Schmid et al. (Schmid et al. 2015, Kaaks 2002). Similar to breast cancer, the exercise effect on endometrial cancer risk appears muted in premenopausal women.

In summary, endometrial-cancer risk is moderately and consistently associated with physical activity. Increased levels of different types of exercise reduce endometrial cancer risk among postmenopausal women with some evidence for risk reduction among premenopausal women. Obesity appears to be an important mediator between exercise and endometrial cancer.

OTHER CANCER SITES (LUNG, KIDNEY, PROSTATE, PANCREATIC)

Apart from endometrial cancer, which has a similar etiology to postmenopausal breast cancer, there is a lack of consistency about exercise and risk reduction of other cancer sites. Exercise appears to lower the risk of mortality among prostate cancer survivors (Kenfield 2011), but evidence for reduction in risk of prostate cancer due to exercise is weak (Liu et al. 2011). A few studies have shown a reduction in risk for advanced prostate cancer (Nilsen, Romundstad, and Vatten 2006, Hrafnkelsdottir et al. 2015), but consistent evidence appears to be lacking for earlier stage prostate cancer. While it is plausible that exercise could reduce prostate cancer risk through the effects of exercise on reduction in testosterone level, unfortunately associations remain inconsistent in relationship to hormone level, exercise, and risk (Lee et al. 2001).

The relationship between exercise and lung cancer risk is challenging to measure due to the interdependence of exercise and smoking. Evidence is suggestive for exercise and reduction in lung-cancer risk but the sizeable confounding by cigarette smoking cannot be dismissed (World Cancer Research Fund/American Institute for Cancer Research 2018a). A recent large meta-analysis noted a mildly protective association between exercise and risk of pancreatic cancer (Farris et al. 2015), although the result could have been influenced by study design with stronger associations observed in case–control studies. Evidence exists for associations between a previous history of type 2 diabetes and increased pancreatic cancer risk with some evidence that insulin and insulin resistance could affect development of pancreatic cancer (McTiernan 2008, Kaaks and Lukanova 2001). The Physical Activity Guidelines Committee concluded "limited evidence" for exercise associations with pancreatic risk reduction, because no dose–response relationship could be determined (U. S. Department of Health and Human Services 2018).

Kidney or renal cell cancer has a more consistent association with exercise where greater amounts of physical activity have resulted in reduced risks of renal cancer (World Cancer Research Fund/American Institute for Cancer Research 2015). A large pooled analysis that evaluated leisure time physical activity and risk of multiple types of cancers found a 23% reduction in risk of kidney cancer that changed to a 16% reduction when adjusting for BMI, with the adjusted estimate remaining significant (Moore et al. 2016). A large meta-analysis of exercise and risk of renal cancer found similar estimates to the pooled analysis with a 12% overall reduction in risk that was significant (Behrens and Leitzmann 2013).

In summary, physical activity primarily functions to reduce postmenopausal breast, endometrial, colon, pancreatic, and kidney cancers through reduction in body fat and subsequent decreases in obesity-related hormonal, inflammatory, and metabolic factors. Changes in skeletal muscle metabolism, while receiving little study, may also play an indirect role in cancer risk reduction by facilitating increases in basal metabolic rate, improving insulin sensitivity and increasing the rate of lipolysis.

REFERENCES

Allred, D. C., S. K. Mohan, and S. A. Fuqua. 2001. "Histological and biological evolution of human premalignant breast disease." *Endocr Relat Cancer* 8:47–61.

Behrens, G., and M. F. Leitzmann. 2013. "The association between physical activity and renal cancer: Systematic review and meta-analysis." *Br J Cancer* 108:798–811.

Bergouignan, A., E. H. Kealey, S. L. Schmidt, M. R. Jackman, and D. H. Bessesen. 2014. "Twenty-four hour total and dietary fat oxidation in lean, obese and reduced-obese adults with and without a bout of exercise." *PLoS One* 9 (4):94181.

Bhaskaran, K., I. Douglas, H. Forbes, I. dos-Santos, D. A. Leon, and L. Smeeth. 2014. "Body-mass index and risk of 22 specific cancers: A population based cohort study of 5.24 million UK adults." *Lancet* 384:755–65.

Booth, F.W., G. N. Ruegsegger, R. G. Toedebusch, and Z. Yan. 2015. "Endurance exercise and the regulation of skeletal muscle metabolism." *Prog Mol. Biol Transl Sci* 135:129–51.

Brooks, G. A., and J. Mercier. 1985. "Balance of carbohydrate and lipid utilization during exercise: The "crossover" concept." *J Appl Physiol* 76 (6):2253–61.

Brown, J. C., K. Winters-Stone, A. Lee, and K. H. Schmitz. 2012. "Cancer, physical activity, and exercise." *Compr Physiol* 2:2775–809.

Bulun, S. E., D. Chen, M. Lu, et al. 2007. "Aromatase excess in cancers of breast, endometrium and ovary." *J Steroid Biochem Mol Biol* 106:81–96.

Carpenter, C. L., K. Kuvall, P. Jardack, L. Li, S. M. Henning, Z. Li, and D. Heber. 2012. "Weight loss reduces breast ductal fluid estrogens in obese postmenopausal women: A single arm intervention pilot study." *Nutr J* 11. http://www.nutritionj.com/content/11/1/102.

Cleary, M. P., and M. E. Grossmann. 2009. "Minireview: Obesity and breast cancer: The estrogen connection." *Endocrinology* 150:2537–42.

DiMeo, S., S. Iossa, and P. Vendittl. 2017. "Improvement of obesity-linked skeletal muscle insulin resistance by strength and endurance training." *J Endocrin* 234(3):R139–81.

Egan, B., and J. B. Zierath. 2013. "Exercise metabolism and the molecular regulation of skeletal muscle adaptation." *Cell Metab* 17:162–84.

Farris, M. S., M. H. Mosli, A. A. McFadden, C. M. Friedenreich, and D. R. Brenner. 2015. "The association between leisure time physical activity and pancreatic cancer risk in adults: A systematic review and meta-analysis." *Cancer Epidemiol Biomarkers Prev* 24 (10):1462.

Harriss, D. J., G. Atkinson, A. Batterham, K. George, N. T. Cable, T. Reilly, N. Haboubi, A. G. Renehan, and Colorectal Cancer, Exercise Lifestyle, and Research Group. 2009. "Lifestyle factors and colorectal cancer risk (2): A systematic review and meta-analysis of associations with leisure-time physical activity." *Colorectal Dis* 11:689–704.

Hojman, P., J. Gehl, J. F. Christensen, and B. K. Pedersen. 2018. "Molecular mechanisms linking exercise to cancer prevention and treatment." *Cell Metab* 27:10–21.

Horowitz, J. F. 2007. "Exercise-induced alterations in muscle lipid metabolism improves insulin sensitivity." *Exercise Sport Sci Rev* 35 (4):192–6.

Hrafnkelsdottir, S. M., J. E. Torfadottie, T. Aspelund, K. T. Magnusson, L. Tyggvadottir, V. Gudnason, L. A. Mucci, M. Stampfer, and U. A. Valdimarsdottir. 2015. "Physical activity from early adulthood and risk of prostate cancer: A 24-year follow-up study among Icelandic men." *Cancer Prev Res* 8 (10):905–11.

Hursting, S. D., J. Digiovanni, A. J. Dannenberg, M. Azrad, D. Leroth, W. Demark-Wahnefried, M. Kakarala, A. Brode, and N. A. Berger. 2012. "Obesity, energy balance, and cancer: New opportunities for prevention." *Cancer Prev Res* 5:1260–72.

Imayama, I., C. M. Ulrich, C. M. Alfano, C. Wang, L. Xiao, M. H. Wener, K. L. Campbell, C. Duggan, K. E. Foster-Schubert, A. Kong, C. E. Mason, C. Y. Want, G. L. Blackburn, C. E. Bain, H. J. Thompson, and A. McTiernan. 2012. "Effects of a caloric restriction weight loss diet and exercise on inflammatory biomarkers in overweight/obese postmenopausal women: A randomized controlled trial." *Cancer Res* 72 (9):2314–26.

Irwin, M. I., Y. Yasui, C. M. Ulrich, and D. Bowen. 2003. "Effect of exercise on total and intra-abdominal body fat in postmenopausal women: A randomized controlled trial." *JAMA* 289 (3):323–30.

Kaaks, R., and A. Lukanova. 2001. "Energy balance and cancer: The role of insulin and insulin-like growth factor-I." *Proc Nut Soc* 60:91–106.

Kaaks, R., A. Lukanova, and M. S. Kurzer. 2002. "Obesity, endogenous hormones, and endometrial cancer risk: A synthetic review." *Cancer Epidemiol Biomarkers Prev* 11 (12):1531–43.

Kenfield, S. A., M. J. Stampfer, E. Giovannucci, and J. M. Chan. 2011. "Physical actvity and survival after prostate cancer diagnosis in the Health Professionals Follow-Up Study." *J Clin Oncol* 29:726–32.

Kern, L., M. J. Mittenbuhler, A. J. Vesting, A. L. Ostermann, C. M. Wunderlich, and F. T. Wunderlich. 2018. "Obesity-induced TNFα and Il-6 signaling: The missing link between obesity and inflammation: Driven liver and colorectal cancers." *Cancers* 11. doi: 10.3390/cancers11010024.

Lazzer, S., C. Lafortuna, C. Busti, R. Galli, T. Tinozzi, F. Agosti, and A. Sartorio. 2010a. "Fat oxidation rate during and after a low- or high-intensity exercise in severely obese Caucasian adolescents." *Eur J Appl Physiol* 108 (2):383–91. doi: 10.1007/s00421-009-1234-z.

Lazzer, S., C. Lafortuna, C. Busti, R. Galli, T. Tinozzi, F. Agosti, and A. Sartorio. 2010b. "Fat oxidation rate during and after a low- or high-intensity exercise in severely obese Caucasian adolescents." *Eur J Appl Physiol* 108:383–91.

Lee, I. M., H. D. Sesso, J. J. Chen, and R. S. Paffenbarger. 2001. "Does physical activity play a role in the prevention of prostate cancer." *Epidemiol Rev* 23:132–7.

Lefai, E., S. Blanc, I. Momken, E. Antoun, I. Cherry, A. Zahariev, L. Gabert, A. Bergouignan, and C. Simon. 2017. "Exercise training improves fat metabolism independent of total energy expenditure in sedentary overweight men, but does not restore lean metabolic phenotype." *Int J Obesity* 41:1728–36.

Liu, Y., F. Hu, D. Li, F. Wang, L. Zhu, W. Y. Chen, J. Ge, R. H. An, and Y. S. Zhao. 2011. "Does physical activity reduce the risk of prostate cancer? A systematic review and meta-analysis." *Eur Urol* 60:1029–44.

Maillard, F., S. Rousset, B. Pereira, A. Traore, and P. De Pradel Del Amaze. 2016. "High-intensity interval training reduces abdominal fat mass in postmenopausal women with type 2 diabetes." *Diabetes Metab* 42:433–41.

Marieb, E. N., P. M. Brady, and J. Mallet. 2020. *Human Anatomy*. Hoboken, NJ: Pearson Publishing.

McGlory, C., and S. M. Phillips. 2015. "Exercise and the regulation of skeletal muscle hypertrophy." *Prog Mol Biol Transl Sci* 135:153–73.

McTiernan, A. M. 2008. "Mechanisms linking physical activity with cancer." *Nat Rev Cancer* 8:205–211.

McTiernan, A. M., C. M. Friedenreich, P. T. Katzmarzyk, et al. 2019. "Physical activity in cancer prevention and survival: A systematic review." *Med Sci Sports Exerc* 51 (6):1252–61.

Melanson, E. L., W. S. Gozansky, D. W. Barry, P. S. MacLean, G. K. Grunwald, and J. O. Hill. 2009. "When energy balance is maintained, exercise does not induce negative fat balance in lean sedentary, obese sedentary, or lean endurance-trained individuals." *J Appl Physiol* 107:1847–1856.

Miller, W. R. 2006. "Aromatase and the breast: Regulation and clinical aspects." *Maturitas* 54:335–41.

Miller, W. C., D. M. Koceja, and E. J. Hamilton. 1997. "A meta-analysis of the past 25 years of weight loss research using diet, exercise or diet plus exercise intervention." *Int J Obes Relat Metab Disord* 21:941–7.

Moore, S. C., I. M. Weiderpass Lee, E. Campbell, P. T. Sampson, J. N. Kitahara, C. M. Keadle, S. K. Arem, A. B. H. de Gonzalez, and P. Hartge. 2016. "Leisure-time physical activity and risk of 26 types of cancer in 1.44 million adults." *JAMA Intern Med* 176 (6):816–825.

Mul, J. D., K. L. Stanford, M. F. Hirshman, and L. J. Goodyear. 2015. "Exercise and regulation of carbohydrate metabolism." *Prog Mol Biol Transl Sci* 135:17–37.

Nagarajan, R., C. L. Carpenter, C. C. Lee, N. Michael, M. K. Sarma, R. Souza, E. Xu, S. S. Velan, T.J. Hahn, and V. L. Go. 2017. "Assessment of lipid and metabolite changes in obese calf muscle using Multi-Echo Echo-planar correlated spectroscopic imaging." *Sci Rep* 7 (1):17338.

Neilson, H. K., M. S. Farris, C. R. Stone, M. M. Vaska, D. R. Brenner, and C. M. Friedenreich. 2016. "Moderate-vigorous recreational physical activity and breast cancer risk, stratified by menopause status: A systematic review and meta-analysis." *Menopause* 24:322–44.

Nilsen, T. I. I., P. R. Romundstad, and L. J. Vatten. 2006. "Recreational physical activity and risk of prostate cancer: A prospective population-based study in Norway (the HUNT study)." *Int J Cancer* 119:2943–7.

Otani, T., S. Iwasaki, S. Isasazuki, M. Inoue, S. Tsugane, and Japan Public Health Center-Based Prospective Study Group. 2007. "Dietary fiber intake and subsequent risk of colorectal cancer: the Japan Public Health Center-based prospective study." *Int J Cancer* 119(6):1475–80.

Pant, M., N. C. Bal, and M. Periasamy. 2016. "Sarcolipin: A key thermogenic and metabolic ragulator in skeletal muscle." *Trends Endocrinol Metab* 27 (2):881–92.

Petersen, K. F., and G. I. Schulman. 2006. "New insights into the pathogenesis of insulin resistance in humans using magnetic resonance spectroscopy." *Obesity* 14 (Supplement):40.

Pike, M. C., D. V. Spicer, L. Dahmouh, and M. F. Press. 1993. "Estrogens, progestogens, normal breast cenn proliferation, and breast cancer risk." *Epidemiol Rev* 15:17–35.

Quist, J. S., S. Rosenkilde, M. B. Petersen, A. S. Gram, A. Sjodin, and B. Stalknecht. 2018. "Effects of active commuting and leisure-time exercise on fat loss in women and men with overweight and obesity: A randomized controlled trial." *Int J Obes Relat Metab Disord* 42:469–78.

Rapoport, B. I. 2010. "Metabolic factors limiting performance in marathon runners." *PLoS Comput Biol* 6 (10):100960.

Rock, C. L., C. Thomson, T. Gansler, et al. 2020. "American cancer society guideline for diet and physical activity for cancer prevention." *CA Cancer J Clin* 0:1–27.

Saris, W. H. M., S. N. Blair, M. A. vanBaak, et al. 2003. "How much physical activity is enough to prevent unhealthy weight gain? Outcome of the IASO 1st Stock conference and consensus statement." *Obesity Rev* 4:101–14.

Schmid, D., G. Gehrens, M. Keimling, C. Jochem, C. Ricci, and M. Leitzmann. 2015. "A systematic review and meta-analysis of physical activity and endometrial cancer risk." *Eur J Epidemiol* 30:397–412.

Shaw, K. A., H. C. Gennat, P. O'Rourke, and C. Del Mar. 2006. "Exercise for overweight or obesity (review." *Cochrane Database Syst Rev* 4:CD003817.

Silvestris, E., G. Pergola, R. Rosania, and G. Loverro. 2018. "Obesity as disruptor of the female fertility." *Reprod Biol Endocrinol* 16 (22). doi: 10.1186/s12958-018-0336-z.

Stattin, P., A. Lukanova, C. Biessy, S. Soderberg, R. Palmqvist, R. Kaaks, T. Olsson, and E. Jillim. 2004. "Obesity and colon cancer: Does leptin provide a link?" *Int J Cancer* 109:149–52.

Tsiloulis, T., and M. J. Watt. 2015. "Exercise and the regulation of adipose tissue metabolism." *Prog Mol Biol Transl Sci* 135:175–201.

U. S. Department of Health and Human Services. 1996. "Physical activity and health: A report of the surgeon general." *U.S. Department of Health and Human Services, Centers for Disease Control and Prevention, National Center for Chronic Disease Prevention and Health Promotion*, Atlanta, GA.

U. S. Department of Health and Human Services. 2018. "Physical activity guidelines advisory committee scientific report." U.S. Department of Health and Human Services.

Ulrich, C. M., C. Himbert, A. N. Holowatyj, and S. D. Hursting. 2018. "Energy balance and gastrointestinal cancer: Risk, interventions, outcomes and mechanisms." *Nat Rev Gastroenterol Hepatol* 15:683–98.

Wolin, K. Y., Y. Yan, G. A. Colditz, and I. M. Lee. 2009. "Physical activity and colon cancer prevention: A meta-analysis." *Br J Cancer* 100:611–6.

World Cancer Research Fund/American Institute for Cancer Research. 2015. "Physical activity and Kidney Cancer "World Cancer Research Fund/American Institute for Cancer Research" http://www.wcrf.org/kidney-cancer-2015.

World Cancer Research Fund/American Institute for Cancer Research. 2018a. Continuous Update Project Expert Report 2018. Physical Activity and the Risk of Cancer.

World Cancer Research Fund/American Institute for Cancer Research. 2018b. "Diet, nutrition and physical activity: Energy balance and body fatness: Continuous update project expert report." World Cancer Research Fund/American Institute for Cancer Research.

Zurlo, F., K. Larson, C. Bogardus, and E. Ravussin. 1990. "Skeletal muscle metabolism is a major determinant of resting energy expenditure." *J Clin Invest* 86:1423–7.

13 Nutrition, Hormones, Cancer Risk, and Progression

David Heber and Zhaoping Li
UCLA Center for Human Nutrition

CONTENTS

OBESITY AND CANCER

Obesity is the most common endocrine disorder globally. When properly defined not as excess body weight or Body Mass Index (BMI) but as excess body fat, the impact of obesity on both peptides and steroid hormones implicated in the multistep process of carcinogenesis can be fully appreciated. Increases in the incidence of obesity-related malignancies over the past decades emphasize the importance of obesity as a global public health priority in the fight against cancer. Worldwide, the percentage of total cancers on a population basis attributable to obesity is 11.9% in men and 13.1% in women (Avgerinos et al. 2019). There is convincing evidence that excess body weight is associated with an increased risk of at least 13 different cancer diagnoses, including endometrial, esophageal, renal, and pancreatic adenocarcinomas; hepatocellular carcinoma; gastric cancer; meningioma; multiple myeloma; colorectal cancer, postmenopausal breast cancer, ovarian cancer, gallbladder cancer, and thyroid cancers (Avgerinos et al. 2019).

Obesity affects steroid and peptide hormones and cytokines including adipocytokines secreted by fat cells which affect mechanisms at both the cancer cell, its microenvironment, and in the blood that promote carcinogenesis. In this sense, obesity establishes both a unique local adipose tissue microenvironment and a concomitant systemic endocrine environment favoring both tumor initiation and progression (Iyengar et al. 2016a, Park et al. 2014) (see Figure 13.1).

Obesity develops as a result of chronic caloric excess relative to energy expenditure. Hidden fat and sugar in the modern diet in combination with a sedentary lifestyle have made this condition prevalent around the world. Excess energy is stored as triglycerides in adipose tissue, and the endocrine and metabolic properties of obese adipocytes are altered as their fat stores increase leading to the production of inflammatory cytokines especially in visceral/abdominal adipocytes but also in fat adjacent to breast and prostate epithelium. As reviewed below, adipocytes produce estrogens

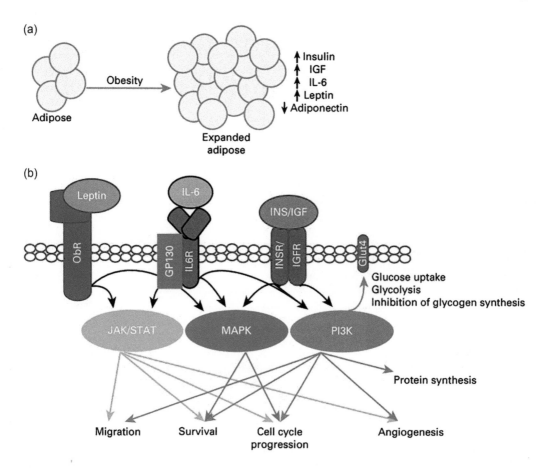

FIGURE 13.1   Obesity-related hormonal and cytokine factors promoting carcinogenesis. (a) Expansion of adipose tissue with obesity and resulting changes in hormones. The changes in the size of adipose depots affect systemic homeostasis and lead to increases in insulin (INS), insulin-like growth factor (IGF), leptin, inflammatory cytokines, and result in decreased levels of adiponectin. IL-6, interleukin 6. (b) These signaling molecules activate cell surface receptors and drive signaling through the Janus kinase (JAK)/signal transducers and activators of transcription (STAT), mitogen-activated protein kinase (MAPK), and PI3K signaling pathways, all of which are frequently altered in cancer. By chronically activating metabolic signaling cascades, the obese state lowers the barrier for oncogenic transformation by driving cell growth and proliferation, and resisting apoptosis. Glut4, glucose transporter type 4; GP130, glycoprotein 130; IGFR, insulin-like growth factor receptor; IL6R, interleukin 6 receptor; INSR, insulin receptor; ObR, leptin receptor. (Adapted from Hopkins, Goncalves, and Cantley (2016) with permission.)

through aromatization of adrenal androgens and become a primary source of estrogens in men and postmenopausal women. Obesity is also associated with lower levels of sex hormone–binding globulin, which increases the free estradiol that is associated with a greater cancer risk (Kaaks et al. 2002).

Excess fat may also accumulate in other metabolic organs including the liver, bone marrow, and skeletal muscle contributing to systemic changes in metabolism such as insulin resistance (IR) and hyperinsulinemia. In this way, common everyday obesity and overweight create an overall hormonal environment that chronically transmits a signal of nutrient excess to normal cells, stem cells, and cancer cells (Hopkins, Goncalves, and Cantley 2016).

As a result, signaling cascades that drive glucose uptake, cell growth, cell proliferation, and angiogenesis are activated and lower the barrier for oncogenic transformation. For example, rodents and humans that have increased circulating insulin and insulin-like growth factor 1 (IGF-1) levels are predisposed to developing multiple types of cancer (Ferguson et al. 2012, Hammarsten and Hogstedt 2005, Yoon et al. 2015, Hernandez et al. 2015).

In addition to the extracellular signals driving cells to grow, specific mutations in metabolically important genes that stimulate proliferation and growth present in tumors are likely to play a role in the tumor response to the obese state. For example, tumors with alterations in the phosphatidylinositol 3-kinase (PI3K) pathway have been shown to be more resistant to caloric restriction, whereas those without alterations in this pathway maintain sensitivity (Kalaany and Sabatini 2009).

Major metabolic differences in cancer cells compared to normal cells have been extensively reviewed elsewhere in this text. Altered cancer metabolism distinguishes tumor cells and their stroma from nontransformed healthy cells and tissues. Importantly, these metabolic differences may be specifically induced by cancer cells and then affect the stroma and blood vessels that surrounds the tumor cells constituting the tumor microenvironment. As a result, some hormones and other factors from the tumor and its stromal vascular compartment reach the systemic circulation as well including steroid hormones, insulin, and insulin-like growth factors, and cytokines that can contribute to tumor progression and metastasis.

ESTROGENS

Estrogens are produced by the ovary in premenopausal women through the aromatization of testosterone and androstenedione by aromatase, a cytochrome P450 enzyme. Adipose tissue and skin produce aromatase through aromatization of adrenal androgens. Aromatase conversion of adrenal androgens is the primary source of estrogens in men and postmenopausal women (Cleland, Mendelson, and Simpson 1983). Excess body fat even in the absence of excess body weight is characterized by increased estrogen production which impacts breast cancer risk (Dieli-Conwright et al. 2018).

Adipose tissue expansion is characterized by adipocyte hypertrophy and the development of adipose tissue inflammation which is histologically demonstrated by the detection of crown-like structures, composed of dead or dying adipocytes enveloped by macrophages (Iyengar et al. 2016b, Cinti et al. 2005, Morris et al. 2011). Ninety percent of Caucasian women with BMI of 30 kg/m^2 or greater have adipose tissue inflammation in the breast (Iyengar et al. 2015). Unlike premenopausal breast cancer in the US, luminal A breast cancer driven by estrogen with estrogen receptor (ER)-positive tumors is more common in Asian women who have a different body fat distribution with more abdominal fat (Bernstein et al. 1990). Moreover, adipose tissue inflammation is found in both pre- and postmenopausal Taiwanese women. While in American Caucasian women, adipose tissue inflammation is associated with menopause (Iyengar et al. 2015). Taiwanese women with the highest body fat percentages are more likely to have ER+ tumors than other subtypes, suggesting that increased local production of estrogen occurring within inflamed breast tissue in women with increased body fat drives tumorigenesis even in the absence of increased body weight.

Breast adipose tissue inflammation is associated with increased breast tissue levels of aromatase, which could locally drive the growth of ER-positive tumors (Brown et al. 2017). Adipose tissue inflammation may also promote breast tumor growth through systemic effects by producing increased circulating levels of insulin and C-reactive protein (Iyengar et al. 2016b). These systemic factors deriving from excess body fat are associated with greater breast cancer risk including in normal weight women who may have sarcopenic obesity (Dieli-Conwright et al. 2018). For women with established breast tumors, adipose tissue inflammation is associated with reduced recurrence free- and overall survival independent of BMI (Koru-Sengul et al. 2016). The presence of breast adipose tissue inflammation in cancer-free women could contribute to the development of tumors via similar mechanisms (Iyengar et al. 2018), supporting the public health promotion of diet and exercise for weight management in women to prevent breast cancer.

Breast cancer is the most common cancer among women in the United States (other than skin cancer). It can be divided into four main molecular subtypes based on the presence or absence of routinely evaluated biological markers: hormone (estrogen or progesterone) receptors (HR+/HR−) and excess levels of human epidermal growth factor receptor 2 (HER2+/HER2−), a protein promoting breast epithelial cell growth (Perou et al. 2000, Cancer Genome Atlas 2012). These four subtypes are luminal A (HR+/HER2−, 74%); luminal B (HR+/HER2+, 10%); HER2-enriched (HR−/HER2+, 4%); and triple negative (HR−/HER2−, 12%) (Anderson et al. 2014, Kohler et al. 2015). The majority of breast cancers (84%) express estrogen and progesterone receptors, supporting the view that estrogen has an essential role in breast cancer development (Zhao et al. 2016).

The luminal subtype of breast tumors accounts for ~70% of all breast tumors and is primarily driven by the ER. ER signaling, which in normal breast tissue drives differentiation, is altered to become a key oncogenic driver of luminal breast cancers through multiple effects that are thought to promote tumor growth. Normal ER signaling is lost and tumor-specific ER signaling is gained during breast tumorigenesis. Activation of aromatase and abnormal estrogen receptor signaling together stimulate cellular proliferation, inhibit apoptosis, and induce angiogenesis (Chi et al. 2019, Zahid, Simpson, and Brown 2016).

There are three sources of estrogen that support the development and growth of breast cancers (Zhao et al. 2016). Estrogen synthesized in the ovaries by granulosa cells can reach the breast tissue via the systemic circulation to act in an endocrine manner. In addition, estrogen can be synthesized by aromatase in extraovarian body sites such as subcutaneous adipose tissue and skin which can then act on the breast in an endocrine manner. Finally, aromatase overexpression within the tumor tissue or in the surrounding stroma can increase local levels of estrogen, which then act at the site of synthesis in a paracrine and/or intracrine manner (Gerard and Brown 2018).

Estrogens also have critical functions in extragonadal tissues including liver, heart, muscle, bone, and brain via two cytoplasmic receptors labeled as the alpha- and beta-estrogen receptors. Estrogenic potency refers to the affinity for binding and action through the ER-α involved in breast tumorigenesis. There are three major forms of physiological estrogens in women: estrone (E1), estradiol (E2, or 17 β-estradiol), and estriol (E3) (Cui, Shen, and Li 2013). Estrone or E1 is synthesized in skin and adipose tissues from circulating androstenedione of adrenal origin and is the major form of estrogen produced in postmenopausal women (Bulun et al. 2003). E2 commonly called estradiol is the most potent estrogen and is the major estrogen product synthesized in the premenopausal ovaries. As in premenopausal women, E2 is also the most biologically active estrogen in postmenopausal women even if the circulating E2 levels are low. It is synthesized either by reduction of E1 in extragonadal sites including skin and adipose tissue or alternatively by direct aromatization of circulating testosterone. E3 is the least potent estrogen and is formed from E1 through 16α-hydroxylation. It plays a larger role during pregnancy when it is produced in large quantities by the placenta.

Estrogen deactivation is regulated via estrogen metabolism. The first metabolic pathway of estrogen inactivation involves the conversion of E2 to the less active Estrone by 17β-hydroxysteroid dehydrogenase and subsequently conversion by estrogen sulfotransferase to estrone sulfate, which is a storage form of estrogen that does not interact with estrogen receptors. The sulfated estrone can also be reverted to E2 first through deconjugation by steroid sulfatase and then further reduction. The ability to form estrone sulfate and store large amounts is critical in the smooth regulation of the activation of the ER in estrogen-responsive cells (Suzuki et al. 2005, Cos et al. 2014). Conjugation of lipophilic estrogens with sulfate is a main pathway for estrogen inactivation in estrogen target tissues.

AROMATASE

Aromatase is a member of the cytochrome P450 superfamily denoted as CYP19 and is widely expressed in many sites, including brain, gonads, blood vessels, liver, bone, skin, adipose tissue, and endometrium (Blakemore and Naftolin 2016). Tissue-specific expression of aromatase depends on three major factors: alternative splicing mechanisms, tissue-specific promoters, and different transcription factors (Chen et al. 2009). The human aromatase gene CYP19 comprises a 93 kb 5′-regulatory region and a 30 kb 3′-coding region. The regulatory region contains ten tissue-specific promoters for local estrogen biosynthesis under normal physiological or pathological conditions such as breast cancer and endometriosis. Activation of each promoter gives rise to alternatively spliced forms of mature mRNA with the first exon a tissue-specific, untranslated region (5′-UTR) upstream of the coding region. The coding region spans nine exons (exon II-X), which are identical in all mRNA species and encode the same protein and 3′-UTR of the mRNA regardless of the tissue or the promoter used.

In breast adipose tissue, most aromatase (80%–90%) expression is found in adipose fibroblasts rather than in mature adipocytes (Price et al. 1992). Normal breast adipose tissue maintains low levels of aromatase expression. In breast cancer, malignant epithelial cells enrich the population of adipose fibroblasts by secreting large amounts of cytokines such as tumor necrosis factor alpha, and interleukin-1 (IL-1) to inhibit differentiation of preadipocytes into mature adipocytes creating a dense fibroblast layer surrounding malignant epithelial cells in a process called the desmoplastic reaction (Meng et al. 2001). Malignant breast epithelial cells secrete prostaglandin E2 (PGE2) and other factors to cause increased production of aromatase (Zhao et al. 1996, Zhou et al. 2001, Diaz-Cruz et al. 2005). In addition to breast adipose fibroblasts, breast tumors produce high levels of aromatase (Avvaru et al. 2018). Finally, breast endothelial cells, which proliferate in the proangiogenic environment of breast cancer, appear to be a significant site of aromatase expression (Zahid, Simpson, and Brown 2016). The balance between estrogen synthesis and deactivation maintains physiological estrogen homeostasis. Aromatase catalyzes the last and rate-limiting step in E2 synthesis, and aromatase regulation is a major mechanism for controlling estrogen synthesis. The regulation of aromatase in the breast adipose stromal cell in response to inflammatory mediators is under the control of complex signaling pathways, including metabolic pathways involving LKB1/AMPK, p53, HIF1α, and PKM2.

Overweight or obese postmenopausal women exhibit a three-fold higher risk for developing breast cancer compared with normal-weight postmenopausal women (Ziegler 1997, Maas et al. 2016) suggesting that estrogen produced in skin and adipose tissue reaches breast tissue via the circulation to stimulate tumor growth. Interventions aimed at weight management, including diet and exercise, are associated with reductions in adipose tissue inflammation and estrogen production that are likely to impact breast cancer risk (Zahid, Simpson, and Brown 2016).

In a 12-week controlled dietary and exercise intervention in seven healthy obese postmenopausal women (average BMI 33.6), serum and breast ductal fluid samples were collected before and after the intervention in order to examine the changes in systemic and localized biomarkers relevant to breast cancer risk. Breast ductal fluid was collected by nipple aspiration and biomarker changes resulting from weight loss secondary to the diet and exercise intervention included reductions in estradiol (−24%) and IL-6 (−20%) while serum biomarker reductions observed from baseline included leptin (−36%), estrone sulfate (−10%), estradiol (−25%), and Il-6 (−33%) (Carpenter et al. 2012).

METABOLIC SYNDROME

Metabolic syndrome (MS) is defined by the presence of at least three of the following: abdominal obesity, high blood triglycerides, low high-density lipoprotein cholesterol, high blood pressure, and high fasting glucose (Alberti et al. 2009). These metabolic abnormalities have been linked to impaired insulin sensitivity and hyperinsulinemia (Riccardi and Rivellese 2000). MS has been demonstrated to be a risk factor for prostate, pancreatic, breast, and colorectal cancers. MS could influence risk in hormone-dependent forms of cancer through obesity-related and nutrition-related effects of interrelated signals in pathways involving insulin, estrogens, growth factors, and cytokines (Vona-Davis, Howard-McNatt, and Rose 2007, Xue and Michels 2007).

Over the past 30 years, a significant increase in the prevalence of IR and MS has been observed in parallel to the increased in the global prevalence of obesity and overweight.

IR, which is the key metabolic abnormality in MS, is associated with the more frequent occurrence of impaired glucose tolerance, diabetes, excessive weight, heart disease, and common forms of cancer. Recent studies have emphasized the importance of reducing IR both through weight management and change in the diet including reducing the intake of simple sugars, especially from sweetened beverages, cakes, candies, and pastries to reduce obesity and the impact of IR.

INSULIN AND IGF-1

IR, hyperinsulinemia due to IR or exogenously administered insulin, and elevated levels of IGF-1 or IGF-2 reduce apoptosis and increase cell proliferation in target cells, leading to tumor development in experiments in cells and animals (Samani et al. 2007). Epidemiological studies, studies in animals, and studies in cell culture indicate that high levels of circulating IGF-1 are associated with increased risk and progression of several common cancers, including breast, prostate, colorectal, and ovarian cancer among others (Anisimov and Bartke 2013).

Insulin itself is also known to have mitogenic properties, and in particular, both the liver and the pancreas are exposed to a high level of endogenously produced insulin. The effects of insulin and hyperinsulinemia on tumorigenesis are thought to be mediated by the insulin receptor, which is expressed in both normal tissues and tumors. Activation of insulin receptor signaling pathways leads to proliferative and antiapoptotic changes in cells (Vigneri, Goldfine, and Frittitta 2016).

Insulin/IGF signaling has been highly conserved during evolution. DAF-2, an insulin receptor-like protein, has been shown to regulate metabolism, development, and aging in *Caenorhabditis elegans* worms (Kimura et al. 1997). In humans, insulin is produced in pancreatic beta cells, which secrete insulin in response to increases in blood glucose levels and the increases in some amino acids such as leucine after meals (Layman and Walker 2006).

Once secreted, insulin enters the blood stream and circulates throughout the body, where it can bind to IR on cell membranes. This extracellular interaction activates the tyrosine kinase domain of IR, allowing it to catalyze the phosphorylation of the IR substrate proteins 1 and 2, which propagate the signal to multiple signaling pathways within cells including both the PI3K and MAPK signaling pathways (Gallagher and LeRoith 2011).

IR has been shown to be elevated in breast cancer, which may explain this tumor's sensitivity to hyperinsulinemia (Chan, Hackel, and Yee 2017). Insulin receptor (IR) and the type I insulin-like growth factor (IGF1R) are homologous receptors necessary for signal transduction by their cognate ligands insulin, IGF-I and IGF-II.

IGF-1 is secreted by the liver in response to growth hormone and is nutritionally modulated. The circulating levels of IGF-1 in the blood are regulated by IGF binding proteins (IGFBPs), which bind free IGF-1 and inhibit binding to the IGF-1 receptor (IGF1R). In this manner, the ratio of IGF-1 to IGFBPs is critical to determining the bioactive levels of IGF-1 in circulation. Increased IGF-1 levels are associated with an elevated risk of cancer including prostate and breast cancer (Rowlands et al. 2009, Papadakis et al. 2017).

Insulin-like growth factor-2 (IGF-2) is a small peptide, produced mainly by the liver, that circulates at levels in the blood that are 3-fold higher than IGF-1 (Livingstone 2013). IGF-2 concentrations are increased with obesity as estimated by increased BMI and are elevated in patients with type 2 diabetes (Livingstone 2013). IGF-2 is able to act either through IGF1R or IR-A to promote tumorigenesis (Alvino et al. 2011). Loss of epigenetic control of IGF-2 gene expression is found in Wilm's tumor, mesenchymal tumors, and colon cancer where stromal IGF2 promotes colon cancer progression in a paracrine and autocrine manner (Bharathavikru and Hastie 2018, Unger et al. 2017). The expression of IGF-2 in some mesenchymal tumors can be so high that IGF-2 induces a refractory hypoglycemia. Hepatomas, fibromas, and fibrosarcomas are the most common tumors that can release enough IGF-2-related peptides into the circulation to mimic the fasting hypoglycemia characteristic of patients with insulin-producing islet-cell tumors (Unger et al. 2017).

In adipose tissue, the main role of insulin is controlling fat storage by inhibiting lipolysis. When glucose and insulin levels are high for prolonged periods of time as the result of overeating and lack of exercise, insulin can stimulate fat storage in ectopic locations including skeletal muscle. The ectopic accumulation of intramuscular fatty acids is the most well-accepted concept of the mechanism of obesity-associated insulin resistance. Muscle insulin resistance, due to fat deposits in muscle, precedes liver insulin resistance and diverts glucose to the liver, resulting in increased hepatic de novo lipogenesis and hyperlipidemia (Samuel and Shulman 2016).

IGF-1 signaling through the PI3K/AKT/mTORC1 signaling pathway has a well-documented role in cell growth and also in oncogenic transformation and cancer progression. IGF-1 signaling is strongly linked with glycolysis (Elstrom et al. 2004) and the expression of glucose transporters, but the IGF signaling pathway is also linked with enhanced mitochondrial respiration in normal tissues, including the liver, and with PGC-1β expression in breast cancer cells (Lyons et al. 2017, Sadaba et al. 2016). Moreover, the antitumorigenic activity of metformin has been linked to reduced IGF-1 signaling (Cao et al. 2016).

Insulin and IGF-1 underlie the mechanisms by which IR and hyperinsulinemia increase the risk of many tumor types including endometrial, breast, kidney, colorectal, and pancreatic cancer. In cancer cells, an increased uptake of glucose stimulated by insulin or IGFs can provide nutrients to meet the increased metabolic demand for both energy and biomass that is created by the tumor cell's hyperproliferative state (Zhu and Thompson 2019, Boroughs and DeBerardinis 2015). Insulin increases hepatic production of IGF-1 and downregulates the production of IGFBP-1, which leads to increased bioavailable IGF-1 levels in the circulation (Moschos and Mantzoros 2002).

Production of the estrogen can also be modulated by insulin and hyperinsulinemia, and as reviewed above, estrogens play an important role in tumorigenesis. Several mechanisms combine to provide an understanding of the association between breast cancer and diabetes, including activation of the insulin pathway, activation of the IGF pathway, and altered regulation of sex hormones (Kang, LeRoith, and Gallagher 2018).

ANDROGENS

Androgens play a key role in prostate cancer. Most prostate cancers express androgen receptors (AR). In the early 1940s, Huggins reported that removal of the testes promoted prostate tumor regression (Huggins 1942). Androgen Deprivation Therapy (ADT) using synthetic gonadotrophin-releasing hormone (GnRH) long-acting agonists or antagonists are used to cause tumor regression or stabilization in the majority of prostate cancer patients. Long-acting GnRH agonists and antagonists achieve medical castration by suppressing luteinizing hormone (LH) release and ablating testicular androgen synthesis. Long-acting GnRH agonists such as leuprolide acetate produce an initial surge in LH and testosterone, then disrupt the pulsatile stimulation of pituitary gonadotropin receptors, resulting in receptor desensitization leading to reduced LH secretion. GnRH antagonists such as degarelix competitively inhibit GnRH binding and do not produce an initial hormone surge. Both treatments decrease LH and testosterone concentrations to castrate levels. GnRH analogs are the cornerstone of ADT in prostate cancer.

However, many patients experience disease relapse months to years later. Originally, prostate-cancer recurrences ADT were assumed to be "androgen-independent". However, androgen-dependent genes are found in both relapsing tumors and their metastases (Mohler et al. 2004). Therefore, this clinical condition has been renamed "castration-resistant prostate cancer" (CRPC), and most prostate cancer deaths are due to CRPC (Scher and Sawyers 2005). The mechanisms of castration resistance include amplification or overexpression of AR, which makes the receptor more sensitive to lower levels of circulating androgens (Visakorpi et al. 1995). The AR can also acquire gain-of-function mutations, which enable the receptor to be activated by other steroids including AR antagonists (Veldscholte et al. 1990). Some prostate cancers develop the mechanisms to produce androgens either de novo or by metabolism of circulating precursor steroids (Chang et al. 2013).

Beyond suppressing LH secretion and blocking AR, a third strategy to treat CRPC is to inhibit the synthesis of testosterone. Considerable efforts were made to develop selective CYP17A1 inhibitors to treat CRPC by inhibiting androgen synthesis at an early step. As a result of these efforts, abiraterone, an irreversible inhibitor of both the 17α-hydroxylase and 17,20-lyase activities of CYP17A1 was able to significantly reduce circulating concentrations of dehydroepiandrosterone, androstenedione, and testosterone (Garrido et al. 2014). However, the simultaneous inhibition of 17α-hydroxylase activity prevents the conversion of pregnenolone into cortisol, leading to a rise ACTH as cortisol feedback is reduced, with the accumulation of cortisol precursors. Some precursors with mineralocorticoid activity, primarily 11-deoxycorticosterone, and corticosterone (Attard et al. 2012) accumulation causes hypertension and hypokalemia similar to genetic 17-hydroxylase deficiency (Costa-Santos et al. 2004). The administration of mineralocorticoid antagonist or glucocorticoid normalizes these side effects (Attard et al. 2012). During abiraterone treatment, administration of a glucocorticoid (such as prednisolone 5 mg BID) is done to avoid these side effects.

Androgens are vital for growth and maintenance of the prostate. On the other hand, the concept that pathologic prostate growth, benign or malignant, can be stimulated by androgens is a commonly held belief without scientific basis (Laurent et al. 2016). Serum androgen levels, within a broad range, are not associated with prostate cancer risk. Conversely, at time of diagnosis of prostate cancer, low rather than high serum testosterone levels have been found to be associated with advanced or high-grade disease. The available evidence indicates that testosterone replacement therapy (TRT) neither increases the risk of prostate cancer nor affects the natural history of cancer recurrence in men who have undergone definitive treatment without residual disease. Furthermore, exogenous testosterone administration does not significantly increase intraprostatic androgen levels in hypogonadal men (Marks et al. 2006).

Testosterone plays a major role in the regulation of muscle mass, adipose tissue, inflammation, and insulin sensitivity and is therefore indirectly regulating several metabolic pathways relevant to prostate cancer. TRT is widely used in patients with symptoms of hypogonadism; however, it is not commonly used as preventive intervention or treatment in men treated for prostate cancer with no evidence of residual disease. Hypogonadism and obesity share many common characteristics which could promote prostate carcinogenesis (Fink, Matsumoto, and Tamura 2018). Excess adiposity common in hypogonadism has been proposed to be involved in the pathogenesis of prostate cancer through different biological mechanisms that include deregulation of the insulin axis, sex hormone secretion, adipokine signaling, inflammation, and oxidative stress. Hypertrophic peritumoral adipocytes have been demonstrated to secrete chemokines which facilitate the local spread of prostate cancer by attracting cancer cells and stimulating migration locally into periprostatic fat.

Local spread of prostate cancer outside the gland is a widely acknowledged adverse factor in prostate cancer and an important determinant of prostate cancer recurrence after treatment. The periprostatic adipose tissue is mainly composed of adipocytes, although other cell types contained in the so-called stromal vascular fraction contribute to its growth and function, including adipocyte-derived stem cells, preadipocytes, lymphocytes, macrophages, fibroblasts, and vascular endothelial cells. Mature adipocytes secrete hormones, growth factors, chemokines, and adipokines implicated in the multistep process of prostate carcinogenesis (Bandini, Gandaglia, and Briganti 2017, Laurent et al. 2016).

In addition to the above obesity-associated conditions, polycystic ovary syndrome (PCOS) is the most common endocrine disorder of women during reproductive age. PCOS is characterized by hyperandrogenemia, hyperinsulinemia, and inflammatory adipokine secretion. Androgen excess is associated with obesity due to changes in the pattern of secretion or metabolism of androgens and in their actions at the level of target tissues including adipocytes. Androgens play a key role in the expansion of visceral fat and abdominal obesity. The combination of androgen excess and obesity promotes the development of metabolic disorders including MS and type 2 diabetes already discussed above.

In addition to reduced insulin sensitivity and hyperinsulinemia, PCOS is characterized by β-cell dysfunction (Patel 2018, Ajmal, Khan, and Shaikh 2019). While infertile when obese, women with PCOS become fertile and reduce circulating androgen levels after weight loss (Jiskoot et al. 2017). Metformin has also resulted in return of fertility implicating the role of hyperinsulinemia in the infertility of PCOS patients (Xu, Wu, and Huang 2017). This obesity-associated condition increases the risk of hormone-dependent cancers (Dumesic and Lobo 2013).

Obesity can also develop after chronic stress and anxiety, which is characterized by increased activity of the hypothalamic-pituitary-adrenal axis and the sympathetic system combined with higher than normal androgen production rates in women. A study of hirsute and PCOS adolescent and young women demonstrated increased salivary glucocorticoid measurements in response to stressful stimuli compared to controls. These observations indicated that the higher the hypothalamic pituitary-adrenal–axis activity, the higher the adrenal androgen output and the worse the metabolic profile (Mezzullo et al. 2018). The presence of a hyperandrogenic state can also be detected in menopausal women, secondary to changes in sex hormone balance which, in turn, may play some role in determining the development of visceral adiposity, obesity, and metabolic disorders (Pasquali and Oriolo 2019). The potential negative effects of androgen excess in obese women at all ages may provide additional rationale for weight management as an integral aspect of cancer prevention in women.

DIETARY FIBER

Higher intakes of dietary fiber can reduce the levels of circulating estrogen which could theoretically reduce breast and endometrial cancer risk. The Fiber Hypothesis which had its origins in the work of Burkitt and others in the early 1970s focused largely on fiber's beneficial effects on colon cancer and disorders of the gastric intestinal tract (O'Keefe 2019, Burkitt 1969).

In the 1980s it was proposed that fiber may also have beneficial effects on breast cancer and a rational for this was proposed involving modulation, by fiber, of the enterohepatic recirculation of estrogens. Urinary and fecal excretion and plasma levels of estrogens were measured in pre- and postmenopausal women eating different diets (Gorbach and Goldin 1987). When premenopausal U.S. women eating a "Western diet," comprising high fat (40% of calories) and low fiber, were compared with age-matched vegetarians eating a moderate-fat (30%), high-fiber diet, it was found that the vegetarians excreted threefold more estrogen in their feces, had lower urinary excretion, and had 15%–20% lower plasma estrogen levels. When U.S. pre- and postmenopausal women eating a Western diet were compared with recent Asian immigrants eating a very low-fat diet (20%–25% of calories), similar results were obtained except that plasma estrogen levels were 30% lower among Asians compared with those among Western omnivore women. Correlation analysis of dietary components and plasma estrogen showed that plasma estrogen was positively associated with fat and was negatively associated with fiber. The results indicated that diet can alter the route of excretion of estrogen by influencing the enterohepatic circulation and that this, in turn, influences plasma estrogen levels.

A significant reduction in serum estrone and estradiol levels during the early follicular and late luteal phases was observed in 12 premenopausal women carefully followed for 3 months in a metabolic ward to determine the effects of a diet providing 30% of their energy from fat and 15–25 g of dietary fiber per day for 1 month, and they consumed a very low fat, high fiber, and libitum diet providing 10% of their energy from fat and 25–35 g of dietary fiber per day for 2 months (Bagga et al. 1995). Despite a significant decrease in serum estradiol and estrone levels after 2 months of a very low fat, high fiber diet, there was no interference with ovulation or the magnitude of the mid-cycle luteinizing hormone surge. Small changes in menstrual cycle length of up to 3 days were not ruled out due to the small sample size of the study. Asian women consuming their traditional low fat, high fiber diets have lower blood estrogen levels before and after menopause and lower rates of breast cancer compared with Western women. This controlled feeding study of premenopausal women demonstrated that a low-fat, high-fiber diet in Western women could achieve a similar reduction in estradiol levels without adverse effects on menstrual function.

MICROBIOME

The major substrates for growth of gut bacteria include 100–200 g wet weight per day of sloughed intestinal cells, plant polysaccharides, starch, and cellulose as well as bile components. From these substrates, gut bacteria produce short-chain fatty acids (acetate, propionate, butyrate) that can account for up to 10% of the total caloric intake/day (Donohoe et al. 2011). Butyrate is an important energy source and regulatory molecule for colonocyte (Christl et al. 1996). Gut bacteria also produce metabolites from the fermentation of amino acids which have been called postbiotics (e.g., cresol, phenyl acetate, indole).

The human microbiome can potentially influence prostate cancer initiation and/or progression through both direct and indirect interactions (Porter et al. 2018). To date, the majority of studies have focused on direct interactions including the influence of prostate infections on prostate cancer risk and, more recently, on the composition of the urinary microbiome in relation to prostate cancer. Less well understood are indirect interactions of the microbiome with prostate cancer, such as the influence of the gastrointestinal or oral microbiota on pro- or anticarcinogenic xenobiotic metabolism, and treatment response.

The gut microbiota regulates estrogen levels in the circulation through secretion of β-glucuronidase, an enzyme that deconjugates estrogens into their active forms for absorption. When this process is impaired through dysbiosis of gut microbiota, characterized by lower microbial diversity, the decrease in deconjugation results in a reduction of circulating estrogens. The alteration in circulating estrogens may contribute to the development of conditions already discussed including obesity, MS, PCOS which could influence cancer risk (Baker, Al-Nakkash, and Herbst-Kralovetz 2017). Hepatically conjugated estrogens excreted in the bile can be deconjugated by bacterial species with β-glucuronidase activity in the gut, leading to their reabsorption into the circulation. Especially relevant are gut bacteria possessing β-glucuronidases and β-glucosidases, hydrolytic enzymes involved in the deconjugation of estrogens (Kwa et al. 2016). β-glucuronidase activity can be modulated by diet and by changes in the microbiota. Increased fecal β-glucuronidase activity has been reported in healthy humans consuming diets high in fat or protein whereas fiber consumption decreases the amount of this enzyme.

Dietary fiber was originally defined as including only polysaccharides, but more recent definitions have included oligosaccharides as dietary fiber, not based on their chemical measurement as dietary fiber by the accepted total dietary fiber method, but on their physiological effects. Inulin, fructo-oligosaccharides, xylooligosachharides, and other oligosaccharides are the best known prebiotics causing changes in the gastrointestinal microflora that confer benefits upon host well-bring and health (Yang et al. 2015). Prebiotics are carbohydrate compounds known to resist digestion in the human small intestine and reach the colon where they are fermented by the gut microflora. Recently, some polyphenols form fruits, vegetables, and spices have also demonstrated prebiotic effects (Lu et al. 2019). Other isolated carbohydrates and carbohydrate-containing foods, including galactooligosaccharides, polydextrose, wheat dextrin, acacia gum, psyllium, banana, whole grain wheat, and whole grain corn, also have prebiotic effects (Slavin 2013).

Bile acid pool size has recently been shown to be a function of microbial metabolism of bile acids in the intestines. Recent studies have shown potential mechanisms explaining how perturbations in the microbiome affect bile acid pool size and composition. Bile acids are emerging as regulators of the gut microbiome. The role of bile acids as hormones and potentiators of liver cancer is also emerging.

GI HORMONES

Gut and adipose hormones interact with the reproductive axis as well as with each other. While leptin and insulin have stimulatory effects and ghrelin has inhibitory effects on hypothalamic GnRH secretion, there is increasing evidence for their roles in other sites of the reproductive axis as well as evidence for the roles of other gut and adipose hormones in the complex interplay between nutrition and reproduction. As our understanding improves, so will our ability to identify and design novel therapeutic options for reproductive disorders and accompanying metabolic disorders (Comninos, Jayasena, and Dhillo 2014).

Circadian rhythm rotation of the earth around the sun every 24 hours results in daily fluctuations of light and dark which affect endogenously generated rhythms that result from biological clocks in the brain and peripheral organs that play a fundamental role in physiology and behavior. Circadian rhythms enable optimal energy utilization and reproduction through sleep-wake cycles, body temperature regulation, and hormone secretion. The proper functioning of the gut microbiome in metabolism is affected by light-dark cycles (Di Marzo and Silvestri 2019). Modern life styles frequently disrupt circadian rhythm leading to dysfunctions of hormonal secretion and dysbiosis of the microbiome which may contribute to increased cancer risk. There is a demonstrated link between disruptions of the molecular clock machinery and aspects of carcinogenesis including angiogenesis, cell proliferation, apoptosis, and DNA repair (Duboc, Coffin, and Siproudhis 2020).

CONCLUSION

The levels of hormones and cytokines relevant to cancer prevention, treatment and relapse prevention reflect systemic factors related to diet and lifestyle including epigenetics and the microbiome. Many of the interactions of hormones, cytokines, and inflammation relevant to nutrition have been described in relationship to obesity, overweight, and the effects of excess body fat especially visceral abdominal fat which leads to IR. Individual variations in the reproductive hormonal axis are among the most varied in evolutionary biology. For example, many variants of estrogen metabolism are relevant to breast cancer risk (Dierssen-Sotos et al. 2018, Warren Andersen et al. 2013). Research on the impact of nutrition on hormones, cytokines, and inflammation relevant to cancer will benefit greatly in the future from the application of personalized nutrition to phenotype, genotype, and provide personalized diets to optimize the systemic hormonal milieu and minimize the risk of cancer development and progression. In the meantime, the information on nutritional impacts on hormones that we have currently clearly support effort to optimize diet and lifestyle through personalized nutrition to reduce cancer risk, cancer progression, and relapse in cancer survivors.

REFERENCES

Ajmal, N., S. Z. Khan, and R. Shaikh. 2019. "Polycystic ovary syndrome (PCOS) and genetic predisposition: A review article." *Eur J Obstet Gynecol Reprod Biol X* 3:100060. doi: 10.1016/j.eurox.2019.100060.

Alberti, K. G., R. H. Eckel, S. M. Grundy, P. Z. Zimmet, J. I. Cleeman, K. A. Donato, J. C. Fruchart, W. P. James, C. M. Loria, S. C. Smith, Jr., Epidemiology International Diabetes Federation Task Force on, Prevention, Lung Hational Heart, Institute Blood, Association American Heart, Federation World Heart, Society International Atherosclerosis, and Obesity International Association for the Study of. 2009. "Harmonizing the metabolic syndrome: A joint interim statement of the International Diabetes Federation Task Force on Epidemiology and Prevention; National Heart, Lung, and Blood Institute; American Heart Association; World Heart Federation; International Atherosclerosis Society; and International Association for the Study of Obesity." *Circulation* 120(16):1640–5. doi: 10.1161/CIRCULATIONAHA.109.192644.

Alvino, C. L., S. C. Ong, K. A. McNeil, C. Delaine, G. W. Booker, J. C. Wallace, and B. E. Forbes. 2011. "Understanding the mechanism of insulin and insulin-like growth factor (IGF) receptor activation by IGF-II." *PLoS One* 6(11):e27488. doi: 10.1371/journal.pone.0027488.

Anderson, W. F., P. S. Rosenberg, A. Prat, C. M. Perou, and M. E. Sherman. 2014. "How many etiological subtypes of breast cancer: Two, three, four, or more?" *J Natl Cancer Inst* 106(8). doi: 10.1093/jnci/dju165.

Anisimov, V. N., and A. Bartke. 2013. "The key role of growth hormone-insulin-IGF-1 signaling in aging and cancer." *Crit Rev Oncol Hematol* 87(3):201–23. doi: 10.1016/j.critrevonc.2013.01.005.

Attard, G., A. H. Reid, R. J. Auchus, B. A. Hughes, A. M. Cassidy, E. Thompson, N. B. Oommen, E. Folkerd, M. Dowsett, W. Arlt, and J. S. de Bono. 2012. "Clinical and biochemical consequences of CYP17A1 inhibition with abiraterone given with and without exogenous glucocorticoids in castrate men with advanced prostate cancer." *J Clin Endocrinol Metab* 97(2):507–16. doi: 10.1210/jc.2011-2189.

Avgerinos, K. I., N. Spyrou, C. S. Mantzoros, and M. Dalamaga. 2019. "Obesity and cancer risk: Emerging biological mechanisms and perspectives." *Metabolism* 92:121–135. doi: 10.1016/j.metabol.2018.11.001.

Avvaru, S. P., M. N. Noolvi, T. M. Aminbhavi, S. Chkraborty, A. Dash, and S. S. Shukla. 2018. "Aromatase inhibitors evolution as potential class of drugs in the treatment of postmenopausal breast cancer women." *Mini Rev Med Chem* 18(7):609–21. doi: 10.2174/1389557517666171101100902.

Bagga, D., J. M. Ashley, S. P. Geffrey, H. J. Wang, R. J. Barnard, S. Korenman, and D. Heber. 1995. "Effects of a very low fat, high fiber diet on serum hormones and menstrual function: Implications for breast cancer prevention." *Cancer* 76(12):2491–6. doi: 10.1002/1097-0142(19951215)76:12<2491::aid-cncr2820761213>3.0.co;2-r.

Baker, J. M., L. Al-Nakkash, and M. M. Herbst-Kralovetz. 2017. "Estrogen-gut microbiome axis: Physiological and clinical implications." *Maturitas* 103:45–53. doi: 10.1016/j.maturitas.2017.06.025.

Bandini, M., G. Gandaglia, and A. Briganti. 2017. "Obesity and prostate cancer." *Curr Opin Urol* 27(5):-415–21. doi: 10.1097/MOU.0000000000000424.

Bernstein, L., J. M. Yuan, R. K. Ross, M. C. Pike, R. Hanisch, R. Lobo, F. Stanczyk, Y. T. Gao, and B. E. Henderson. 1990. "Serum hormone levels in pre-menopausal Chinese women in Shanghai and white women in Los Angeles: Results from two breast cancer case-control studies." *Cancer Causes Control* 1(1):51–8. doi: 10.1007/BF00053183.

Bharathavikru, R., and N. D. Hastie. 2018. "Overgrowth syndromes and pediatric cancers: How many roads lead to IGF2?" *Genes Dev* 32(15–16):993–5. doi: 10.1101/gad.317792.118.

Blakemore, J., and F. Naftolin. 2016. "Aromatase: Contributions to physiology and disease in women and men." *Physiology (Bethesda)* 31(4):258–69. doi: 10.1152/physiol.00054.2015.

Boroughs, L. K., and R. J. DeBerardinis. 2015. "Metabolic pathways promoting cancer cell survival and growth." *Nat Cell Biol* 17(4):351–9. doi: 10.1038/ncb3124.

Brown, K. A., N. M. Iyengar, X. K. Zhou, A. Gucalp, K. Subbaramaiah, H. Wang, D. D. Giri, M. Morrow, D. J. Falcone, N. K. Wendel, L. A. Winston, M. Pollak, A. Dierickx, C. A. Hudis, and A. J. Dannenberg. 2017. "Menopause is a determinant of breast aromatase expression and its associations with BMI, inflammation, and systemic markers." *J Clin Endocrinol Metab* 102(5):1692–701. doi: 10.1210/jc.2016-3606.

Bulun, S. E., S. Sebastian, K. Takayama, T. Suzuki, H. Sasano, and M. Shozu. 2003. "The human CYP19 (aromatase P450) gene: Update on physiologic roles and genomic organization of promoters." *J Steroid Biochem Mol Biol* 86(3–5):219–24. doi: 10.1016/s0960-0760(03)00359-5.

Burkitt, D. P. 1969. "Related disease--related cause?" *Lancet* 2(7632):1229–31. doi: 10.1016/s0140-6736(69)90757-0.

Cancer Genome Atlas, Network. 2012. "Comprehensive molecular portraits of human breast tumours." *Nature* 490(7418):61–70. doi: 10.1038/nature11412.

Cao, H., W. Dong, X. Qu, H. Shen, J. Xu, L. Zhu, Q. Liu, and J. Du. 2016. "Metformin enhances the therapy effects of anti-IGF-1R mAb Figitumumab to NSCLC." *Sci Rep* 6:31072. doi: 10.1038/srep31072.

Carpenter, C. L., K. Duvall, P. Jardack, L. Li, S. M. Henning, Z. Li, and D. Heber. 2012. "Weight loss reduces breast ductal fluid estrogens in obese postmenopausal women: A single arm intervention pilot study." *Nutr J* 11:102. doi: 10.1186/1475-2891-11-102.

Chan, J. Y., B. J. Hackel, and D. Yee. 2017. "Targeting insulin receptor in breast cancer using small engineered protein scaffolds." *Mol Cancer Ther* 16(7):1324–34. doi: 10.1158/1535-7163.MCT-16-0685.

Chang, K. H., R. Li, B. Kuri, Y. Lotan, C. G. Roehrborn, J. Liu, R. Vessella, P. S. Nelson, P. Kapur, X. Guo, H. Mirzaei, R. J. Auchus, and N. Sharifi. 2013. "A gain-of-function mutation in DHT synthesis in castration-resistant prostate cancer." *Cell* 154(5):1074–84. doi: 10.1016/j.cell.2013.07.029.

Chen, D., S. Reierstad, M. Lu, Z. Lin, H. Ishikawa, and S. E. Bulun. 2009. "Regulation of breast cancer-associated aromatase promoters." *Cancer Lett* 273(1):15–27. doi: 10.1016/j.canlet.2008.05.038.

Chi, D., H. Singhal, L. Li, T. Xiao, W. Liu, M. Pun, R. Jeselsohn, H. He, E. Lim, R. Vadhi, P. Rao, H. Long, J. Garber, and M. Brown. 2019. "Estrogen receptor signaling is reprogrammed during breast tumorigenesis." *Proc Natl Acad Sci U S A* 116(23):11437–43. doi: 10.1073/pnas.1819155116.

Christl, S. U., H. D. Eisner, G. Dusel, H. Kasper, and W. Scheppach. 1996. "Antagonistic effects of sulfide and butyrate on proliferation of colonic mucosa: A potential role for these agents in the pathogenesis of ulcerative colitis." *Dig Dis Sci* 41(12):2477–81. doi: 10.1007/BF02100146.

Cinti, S., G. Mitchell, G. Barbatelli, I. Murano, E. Ceresi, E. Faloia, S. Wang, M. Fortier, A. S. Greenberg, and M. S. Obin. 2005. "Adipocyte death defines macrophage localization and function in adipose tissue of obese mice and humans." *J Lipid Res* 46(11):2347–55. doi: 10.1194/jlr.M500294-JLR200.

Cleland, W. H., C. R. Mendelson, and E. R. Simpson. 1983. "Aromatase activity of membrane fractions of human adipose tissue stromal cells and adipocytes." *Endocrinology* 113(6):2155–60. doi: 10.1210/endo-113-6-2155.

Comninos, A. N., C. N. Jayasena, and W. S. Dhillo. 2014. "The relationship between gut and adipose hormones, and reproduction." *Hum Reprod Update* 20(2):153–74. doi: 10.1093/humupd/dmt033.

Cos, S., V. Alvarez-Garcia, A. Gonzalez, C. Alonso-Gonzalez, and C. Martinez-Campa. 2014. "Melatonin modulation of crosstalk among malignant epithelial, endothelial and adipose cells in breast cancer (review)." *Oncol Lett* 8(2):487–92. doi: 10.3892/ol.2014.2203.

Costa-Santos, M., C. E. Kater, R. J. Auchus, and Group Brazilian Congenital Adrenal Hyperplasia Multicenter Study. 2004. "Two prevalent CYP17 mutations and genotype-phenotype correlations in 24 Brazilian patients with 17-hydroxylase deficiency." *J Clin Endocrinol Metab* 89(1):49–60. doi: 10.1210/jc.2003-031021.

Cui, J., Y. Shen, and R. Li. 2013. "Estrogen synthesis and signaling pathways during aging: From periphery to brain." *Trends Mol Med* 19(3):197–209. doi: 10.1016/j.molmed.2012.12.007.

Díaz-Cruz ES, Shapiro CL, Brueggemeier RW. Cyclooxygenase inhibitors suppress aromatase expression and activity in breast cancer cells. *J Clin Endocrinol Metab*. 2005 May;90(5):2563–70. doi: 10.1210/jc.2004-2029. Epub 2005 Feb 1. PMID: 15687328.

Di Marzo, V., and C. Silvestri. 2019. "Lifestyle and metabolic syndrome: Contribution of the endocannabinoidome." *Nutrients* 11(8). doi: 10.3390/nu11081956.

Dieli-Conwright, C. M., K. S. Courneya, W. Demark-Wahnefried, N. Sami, K. Lee, T. A. Buchanan, D. V. Spicer, D. Tripathy, L. Bernstein, and J. E. Mortimer. 2018. "Effects of aerobic and resistance exercise on metabolic syndrome, sarcopenic obesity, and circulating biomarkers in overweight or obese survivors of breast cancer: A randomized controlled trial." *J Clin Oncol* 36(9):875–83. doi: 10.1200/JCO.2017.75.7526.

Dierssen-Sotos, T., C. Palazuelos-Calderon, J. J. Jimenez-Moleon, N. Aragones, J. M. Altzibar, G. Castano-Vinyals, V. Martin-Sanchez, I. Gomez-Acebo, M. Guevara, A. Tardon, B. Perez-Gomez, P. Amiano, V. Moreno, A. J. Molina, J. Alonso-Molero, C. Moreno-Iribas, M. Kogevinas, M. Pollan, and J. Llorca. 2018. "Reproductive risk factors in breast cancer and genetic hormonal pathways: A gene-environment interaction in the MCC-Spain project." *BMC Cancer* 18(1):280. doi: 10.1186/s12885-018-4182-3.

Donohoe, D. R., N. Garge, X. Zhang, W. Sun, T. M. O'Connell, M. K. Bunger, and S. J. Bultman. 2011. "The microbiome and butyrate regulate energy metabolism and autophagy in the mammalian colon." *Cell Metab* 13(5):517–26. doi: 10.1016/j.cmet.2011.02.018.

Duboc, H., B. Coffin, and L. Siproudhis. 2020. "Disruption of circadian rhythms and gut motility: An overview of underlying mechanisms and associated pathologies." *J Clin Gastroenterol* 54(5):405–14. doi: 10.1097/MCG.0000000000001333.

Dumesic, D. A., and R. A. Lobo. 2013. "Cancer risk and PCOS." *Steroids* 78(8):782–5. doi: 10.1016/j.steroids.2013.04.004.

Elstrom, R. L., D. E. Bauer, M. Buzzai, R. Karnauskas, M. H. Harris, D. R. Plas, H. Zhuang, R. M. Cinalli, A. Alavi, C. M. Rudin, and C. B. Thompson. 2004. "Akt stimulates aerobic glycolysis in cancer cells." *Cancer Res* 64(11):3892–9. doi: 10.1158/0008-5472.CAN-03-2904.

Ferguson, R. D., R. Novosyadlyy, Y. Fierz, N. Alikhani, H. Sun, S. Yakar, and D. Leroith. 2012. "Hyperinsulinemia enhances c-Myc-mediated mammary tumor development and advances metastatic progression to the lung in a mouse model of type 2 diabetes." *Breast Cancer Res* 14(1):R8. doi: 10.1186/bcr3089.

Fink, J., M. Matsumoto, and Y. Tamura. 2018. "Potential application of testosterone replacement therapy as treatment for obesity and type 2 diabetes in men." *Steroids* 138:161–6. doi: 10.1016/j.steroids.2018.08.002.

Gallagher, E. J., and D. LeRoith. 2011. "Minireview: IGF, insulin, and cancer." *Endocrinology* 152(7):2546–51. doi: 10.1210/en.2011-0231.

Garrido, M., H. M. Peng, F. K. Yoshimoto, S. K. Upadhyay, E. Bratoeff, and R. J. Auchus. 2014. "A-ring modified steroidal azoles retaining similar potent and slowly reversible CYP17A1 inhibition as abiraterone." *J Steroid Biochem Mol Biol* 143:1–10. doi: 10.1016/j.jsbmb.2014.01.013.

Gerard, C., and K. A. Brown. 2018. "Obesity and breast cancer: Role of estrogens and the molecular underpinnings of aromatase regulation in breast adipose tissue." *Mol Cell Endocrinol* 466:15–30. doi: 10.1016/j.mce.2017.09.014.

Gorbach, S. L., and B. R. Goldin. 1987. "Diet and the excretion and enterohepatic cycling of estrogens." *Prev Med* 16(4):525–31. doi: 10.1016/0091-7435(87)90067-3.

Hammarsten, J., and B. Hogstedt. 2005. "Hyperinsulinaemia: A prospective risk factor for lethal clinical prostate cancer." *Eur J Cancer* 41(18):2887–95. doi: 10.1016/j.ejca.2005.09.003.

Hernandez, A. V., V. Pasupuleti, V. A. Benites-Zapata, P. Thota, A. Deshpande, and F. R. Perez-Lopez. 2015. "Insulin resistance and endometrial cancer risk: A systematic review and meta-analysis." *Eur J Cancer* 51(18):2747–58. doi: 10.1016/j.ejca.2015.08.031.

Hopkins, B. D., M. D. Goncalves, and L. C. Cantley. 2016. "Obesity and cancer mechanisms: Cancer metabolism." *J Clin Oncol* 34(35):4277–83. doi: 10.1200/JCO.2016.67.9712.

Huggins, C. 1942. "Effect of orchiectomy and irradiation on cancer of the prostate." *Ann Surg* 115(6):1192–200. doi: 10.1097/00000658-194206000-00030.

Iyengar, N. M., P. G. Morris, X. K. Zhou, A. Gucalp, D. Giri, M. D. Harbus, D. J. Falcone, M. D. Krasne, L. T. Vahdat, K. Subbaramaiah, M. Morrow, C. A. Hudis, and A. J. Dannenberg. 2015. "Menopause is a determinant of breast adipose inflammation." *Cancer Prev Res (Phila)* 8(5):349–58. doi: 10.1158/1940-6207.CAPR-14-0243.

Iyengar, N. M., A. Gucalp, A. J. Dannenberg, and C. A. Hudis. 2016a. "Obesity and cancer mechanisms: Tumor microenvironment and inflammation." *J Clin Oncol* 34(35):4270–6. doi: 10.1200/JCO.2016.67.4283.

Iyengar, N. M., X. K. Zhou, A. Gucalp, P. G. Morris, L. R. Howe, D. D. Giri, M. Morrow, H. Wang, M. Pollak, L. W. Jones, C. A. Hudis, and A. J. Dannenberg. 2016b. "Systemic correlates of white adipose tissue inflammation in early-stage breast cancer." *Clin Cancer Res* 22(9):2283–9. doi: 10.1158/1078-0432.CCR-15-2239.

Iyengar, N. M., I. C. Chen, X. K. Zhou, D. D. Giri, D. J. Falcone, L. A. Winston, H. Wang, S. Williams, Y. S. Lu, T. H. Hsueh, A. L. Cheng, C. A. Hudis, C. H. Lin, and A. J. Dannenberg. 2018. "Adiposity, inflammation, and breast cancer pathogenesis in Asian women." *Cancer Prev Res (Phila)* 11(4):227–36. doi: 10.1158/1940-6207.CAPR-17-0283.

Jiskoot, G., S. H. Benneheij, A. Beerthuizen, J. E. de Niet, C. de Klerk, R. Timman, J. J. Busschbach, and J. S. Laven. 2017. "A three-component cognitive behavioural lifestyle program for preconceptional weight-loss in women with polycystic ovary syndrome (PCOS): A protocol for a randomized controlled trial." *Reprod Health* 14(1):34. doi: 10.1186/s12978-017-0295-4.

Kaaks R, Lukanova A, Kurzer MS. Obesity, endogenous hormones, and endometrial cancer risk: a synthetic review. *Cancer Epidemiol Biomarkers Prev.* 2002 Dec;11(12):1531–43. PMID: 12496040.

Kalaany, N. Y., and D. M. Sabatini. 2009. "Tumours with PI3K activation are resistant to dietary restriction." *Nature* 458(7239):725–31. doi: 10.1038/nature07782.

Kang, C., D. LeRoith, and E. J. Gallagher. 2018. "Diabetes, obesity, and breast cancer." *Endocrinology* 159(11):3801–12. doi: 10.1210/en.2018-00574.

Kimura, K. D., H. A. Tissenbaum, Y. Liu, and G. Ruvkun. 1997. "daf-2, an insulin receptor-like gene that regulates longevity and diapause in Caenorhabditis elegans." *Science* 277(5328):942–6. doi: 10.1126/science.277.5328.942.

Kohler, B. A., R. L. Sherman, N. Howlader, A. Jemal, A. B. Ryerson, K. A. Henry, F. P. Boscoe, K. A. Cronin, A. Lake, A. M. Noone, S. J. Henley, C. R. Eheman, R. N. Anderson, and L. Penberthy. 2015. "Annual report to the nation on the status of cancer, 1975-2011, featuring incidence of breast cancer subtypes by race/ethnicity, poverty, and state." *J Natl Cancer Inst* 107(6):djv048. doi: 10.1093/jnci/djv048.

Koru-Sengul, T., A. M. Santander, F. Miao, L. G. Sanchez, M. Jorda, S. Gluck, T. A. Ince, M. Nadji, Z. Chen, M. L. Penichet, M. P. Cleary, and M. Torroella-Kouri. 2016. "Breast cancers from black women exhibit higher numbers of immunosuppressive macrophages with proliferative activity and of crown-like structures associated with lower survival compared to non-black Latinas and Caucasians." *Breast Cancer Res Treat* 158(1):113–26. doi: 10.1007/s10549-016-3847-3.

Kwa, M., C. S. Plottel, M. J. Blaser, and S. Adams. 2016. "The intestinal microbiome and estrogen receptor-positive female breast cancer." *J Natl Cancer Inst* 108(8). doi: 10.1093/jnci/djw029.

Laurent, V., A. Guerard, C. Mazerolles, S. Le Gonidec, A. Toulet, L. Nieto, F. Zaidi, B. Majed, D. Garandeau, Y. Socrier, M. Golzio, T. Cadoudal, K. Chaoui, C. Dray, B. Monsarrat, O. Schiltz, Y. Y. Wang, B. Couderc, P. Valet, B. Malavaud, and C. Muller. 2016. "Periprostatic adipocytes act as a driving force for prostate cancer progression in obesity." *Nat Commun* 7:10230. doi: 10.1038/ncomms10230.

Layman, D. K., and D. A. Walker. 2006. "Potential importance of leucine in treatment of obesity and the metabolic syndrome." *J Nutr* 136(1 Suppl):319S–23S. doi: 10.1093/jn/136.1.319S.

Livingstone, C. 2013. "IGF2 and cancer." *Endocr Relat Cancer* 20(6):R321–39. doi: 10.1530/ERC-13-0231.

Lu, Q. Y., A. M. Rasmussen, J. Yang, R. P. Lee, J. Huang, P. Shao, C. L. Carpenter, I. Gilbuena, G. Thames, S. M. Henning, D. Heber, and Z. Li. 2019. "Mixed spices at culinary doses have prebiotic effects in healthy adults: A pilot study." *Nutrients* 11(6). doi: 10.3390/nu11061425.

Lyons, A., M. Coleman, S. Riis, C. Favre, C. H. O'Flanagan, A. V. Zhdanov, D. B. Papkovsky, S. D. Hursting, and R. O'Connor. 2017. "Insulin-like growth factor 1 signaling is essential for mitochondrial biogenesis and mitophagy in cancer cells." *J Biol Chem* 292(41):16983–98. doi: 10.1074/jbc.M117.792838.

Maas, P., M. Barrdahl, A. D. Joshi, P. L. Auer, M. M. Gaudet, R. L. Milne, F. R. Schumacher, W. F. Anderson, D. Check, S. Chattopadhyay, L. Baglietto, C. D. Berg, S. J. Chanock, D. G. Cox, J. D. Figueroa, M. H. Gail, B. I. Graubard, C. A. Haiman, S. E. Hankinson, R. N. Hoover, C. Isaacs, L. N. Kolonel, L. Le Marchand, I. M. Lee, S. Lindstrom, K. Overvad, I. Romieu, M. J. Sanchez, M. C. Southey, D. O. Stram, R. Tumino, T. J. VanderWeele, W. C. Willett, S. Zhang, J. E. Buring, F. Canzian, S. M. Gapstur, B. E. Henderson, D. J. Hunter, G. G. Giles, R. L. Prentice, R. G. Ziegler, P. Kraft, M. Garcia-Closas, and N. Chatterjee. 2016. "Breast cancer risk from modifiable and nonmodifiable risk factors among white women in the united states." *JAMA Oncol* 2(10):1295–302. doi: 10.1001/jamaoncol.2016.1025.

Marks, L. S., N. A. Mazer, E. Mostaghel, D. L. Hess, F. J. Dorey, J. I. Epstein, R. W. Veltri, D. V. Makarov, A. W. Partin, D. G. Bostwick, M. L. Macairan, and P. S. Nelson. 2006. "Effect of testosterone replacement therapy on prostate tissue in men with late-onset hypogonadism: A randomized controlled trial." *JAMA* 296(19):2351–61. doi: 10.1001/jama.296.19.2351.

Meng, L., J. Zhou, H. Sasano, T. Suzuki, K. M. Zeitoun, and S. E. Bulun. 2001. "Tumor necrosis factor alpha and interleukin 11 secreted by malignant breast epithelial cells inhibit adipocyte differentiation by selectively down-regulating CCAAT/enhancer binding protein alpha and peroxisome proliferator-activated receptor gamma: Mechanism of desmoplastic reaction." *Cancer Res* 61(5):2250–5.

Mezzullo, M., F. Fanelli, A. Di Dalmazi, A. Fazzini, D. Ibarra-Gasparini, M. Mastroroberto, J. Guidi, A. M. Morselli-Labate, R. Pasquali, U. Pagotto, and A. Gambineri. 2018. "Salivary cortisol and cortisone responses to short-term psychological stress challenge in late adolescent and young women with different hyperandrogenic states." *Psychoneuroendocrinology* 91:31–40. doi: 10.1016/j.psyneuen.2018.02.022.

Mohler, J. L., C. W. Gregory, O. H. Ford, 3rd, D. Kim, C. M. Weaver, P. Petrusz, E. M. Wilson, and F. S. French. 2004. "The androgen axis in recurrent prostate cancer." *Clin Cancer Res* 10(2):440–8. doi: 10.1158/1078-0432.ccr-1146-03.

Morris, P. G., C. A. Hudis, D. Giri, M. Morrow, D. J. Falcone, X. K. Zhou, B. Du, E. Brogi, C. B. Crawford, L. Kopelovich, K. Subbaramaiah, and A. J. Dannenberg. 2011. "Inflammation and increased aromatase expression occur in the breast tissue of obese women with breast cancer." *Cancer Prev Res (Phila)* 4(7):1021–9. doi: 10.1158/1940-6207.CAPR-11-0110.

Moschos, S. J., and C. S. Mantzoros. 2002. "The role of the IGF system in cancer: From basic to clinical studies and clinical applications." *Oncology* 63(4):317–32. doi: 10.1159/000066230.

O'Keefe, S. J. 2019. "The association between dietary fibre deficiency and high-income lifestyle-associated diseases: Burkitt's hypothesis revisited." *Lancet Gastroenterol Hepatol* 4(12):984–96. doi: 10.1016/S2468-1253(19)30257-2.

Papadakis, G. Z., D. Mavroudis, V. Georgoulias, J. Souglakos, A. K. Alegakis, G. Samonis, U. Bagci, A. Makrigiannakis, and O. Zoras. 2017. "Serum IGF-1, IGFBP-3 levels and circulating tumor cells (CTCs) in early breast cancer patients." *Growth Horm IGF Res* 33:28–34. doi: 10.1016/j.ghir.2017.02.001.

Park, J., T. S. Morley, M. Kim, D. J. Clegg, and P. E. Scherer. 2014. "Obesity and cancer--mechanisms underlying tumour progression and recurrence." *Nat Rev Endocrinol* 10(8):455–65. doi: 10.1038/nrendo.2014.94.

Pasquali, R., and C. Oriolo. 2019. "Obesity and androgens in women." *Front Horm Res* 53:120–34. doi: 10.1159/000494908.

Patel, S. 2018. "Polycystic ovary syndrome (PCOS), an inflammatory, systemic, lifestyle endocrinopathy." *J Steroid Biochem Mol Biol* 182:27–36. doi: 10.1016/j.jsbmb.2018.04.008.

Perou, C. M., T. Sorlie, M. B. Eisen, M. van de Rijn, S. S. Jeffrey, C. A. Rees, J. R. Pollack, D. T. Ross, H. Johnsen, L. A. Akslen, O. Fluge, A. Pergamenschikov, C. Williams, S. X. Zhu, P. E. Lonning, A. L. Borresen-Dale, P. O. Brown, and D. Botstein. 2000. "Molecular portraits of human breast tumours." *Nature* 406(6797):747–52. doi: 10.1038/35021093.

Porter, C. M., E. Shrestha, L. B. Peiffer, and K. S. Sfanos. 2018. "The microbiome in prostate inflammation and prostate cancer." *Prostate Cancer Prostatic Dis* 21(3):345–54. doi: 10.1038/s41391-018-0041-1.

Price, T., J. Aitken, J. Head, M. Mahendroo, G. Means, and E. Simpson. 1992. "Determination of aromatase cytochrome P450 messenger ribonucleic acid in human breast tissue by competitive polymerase chain reaction amplification." *J Clin Endocrinol Metab* 74(6):1247–52. doi: 10.1210/jcem.74.6.1592866.

Riccardi, G., and A. A. Rivellese. 2000. "Dietary treatment of the metabolic syndrome--the optimal diet." *Br J Nutr* 83(suppl 1):S143–8. doi: 10.1017/s0007114500001082.

Rowlands, M. A., D. Gunnell, R. Harris, L. J. Vatten, J. M. Holly, and R. M. Martin. 2009. "Circulating insulin-like growth factor peptides and prostate cancer risk: A systematic review and meta-analysis." *Int J Cancer* 124(10):2416–29. doi: 10.1002/ijc.24202.

Sadaba, M. C., I. Martin-Estal, J. E. Puche, and I. Castilla-Cortazar. 2016. "Insulin-like growth factor 1 (IGF-1) therapy: Mitochondrial dysfunction and diseases." *Biochim Biophys Acta* 1862(7):1267–78. doi: 10.1016/j.bbadis.2016.03.010.

Samani, A. A., S. Yakar, D. LeRoith, and P. Brodt. 2007. "The role of the IGF system in cancer growth and metastasis: Overview and recent insights." *Endocr Rev* 28(1):20–47. doi: 10.1210/er.2006-0001.

Samuel, V. T., and G. I. Shulman. 2016. "The pathogenesis of insulin resistance: Integrating signaling pathways and substrate flux." *J Clin Invest* 126(1):12–22. doi: 10.1172/JCI77812.

Scher, H. I., and C. L. Sawyers. 2005. "Biology of progressive, castration-resistant prostate cancer: Directed therapies targeting the androgen-receptor signaling axis." *J Clin Oncol* 23(32):8253–61. doi: 10.1200/JCO.2005.03.4777.

Slavin, J. 2013. "Fiber and prebiotics: Mechanisms and health benefits." *Nutrients* 5(4):1417–35. doi: 10.3390/nu5041417.

Suzuki, T., Y. Miki, Y. Nakamura, T. Moriya, K. Ito, N. Ohuchi, and H. Sasano. 2005. "Sex steroid-producing enzymes in human breast cancer." *Endocr Relat Cancer* 12(4):701–20. doi: 10.1677/erc.1.00834.

Unger, C., N. Kramer, D. Unterleuthner, M. Scherzer, A. Burian, A. Rudisch, M. Stadler, M. Schlederer, D. Lenhardt, A. Riedl, S. Walter, A. Wernitznig, L. Kenner, M. Hengstschlager, J. Schuler, W. Sommergruber, and H. Dolznig. 2017. "Stromal-derived IGF2 promotes colon cancer progression via paracrine and autocrine mechanisms." *Oncogene* 36(38):5341–55. doi: 10.1038/onc.2017.116.

Veldscholte, J., C. Ris-Stalpers, G. G. Kuiper, G. Jenster, C. Berrevoets, E. Claassen, H. C. van Rooij, J. Trapman, A. O. Brinkmann, and E. Mulder. 1990. "A mutation in the ligand binding domain of the androgen receptor of human LNCaP cells affects steroid binding characteristics and response to anti-androgens." *Biochem Biophys Res Commun* 173(2):534–40. doi: 10.1016/s0006-291x(05)80067-1.

Vigneri, R., I. D. Goldfine, and L. Frittitta. 2016. "Insulin, insulin receptors, and cancer." *J Endocrinol Invest* 39(12):1365–76. doi: 10.1007/s40618-016-0508-7.

Visakorpi, T., E. Hyytinen, P. Koivisto, M. Tanner, R. Keinanen, C. Palmberg, A. Palotie, T. Tammela, J. Isola, and O. P. Kallioniemi. 1995. "In vivo amplification of the androgen receptor gene and progression of human prostate cancer." *Nat Genet* 9(4):401–6. doi: 10.1038/ng0495-401.

Vona-Davis, L., M. Howard-McNatt, and D. P. Rose. 2007. "Adiposity, type 2 diabetes and the metabolic syndrome in breast cancer." *Obes Rev* 8(5):395–408. doi: 10.1111/j.1467-789X.2007.00396.x.

Warren Andersen, S., A. Trentham-Dietz, R. E. Gangnon, J. M. Hampton, J. D. Figueroa, H. G. Skinner, C. D. Engelman, B. E. Klein, L. J. Titus, and P. A. Newcomb. 2013. "The associations between a polygenic score, reproductive and menstrual risk factors and breast cancer risk." *Breast Cancer Res Treat* 140(2):427–34. doi: 10.1007/s10549-013-2646-3.

Xu, Y., Y. Wu, and Q. Huang. 2017. "Comparison of the effect between pioglitazone and metformin in treating patients with PCOS:a meta-analysis." *Arch Gynecol Obstet* 296(4):661–77. doi: 10.1007/s00404-017-4480-z.

Xue, F., and K. B. Michels. 2007. "Diabetes, metabolic syndrome, and breast cancer: A review of the current evidence." *Am J Clin Nutr* 86(3):S823–35. doi: 10.1093/ajcn/86.3.823S.

Yang, J., P. H. Summanen, S. M. Henning, M. Hsu, H. Lam, J. Huang, C. H. Tseng, S. E. Dowd, S. M. Finegold, D. Heber, and Z. Li. 2015. "Xylooligosaccharide supplementation alters gut bacteria in both healthy and prediabetic adults: A pilot study." *Front Physiol* 6:216. doi: 10.3389/fphys.2015.00216.

Yoon, Y. S., N. Keum, X. Zhang, E. Cho, and E. L. Giovannucci. 2015. "Hyperinsulinemia, insulin resistance and colorectal adenomas: A meta-analysis." *Metabolism* 64(10):1324–33. doi: 10.1016/j.metabol.2015.06.013.

Zahid, H., E. R. Simpson, and K. A. Brown. 2016. "Inflammation, dysregulated metabolism and aromatase in obesity and breast cancer." *Curr Opin Pharmacol* 31:90–6. doi: 10.1016/j.coph.2016.11.003.

Zhao, H., L. Zhou, A. J. Shangguan, and S. E. Bulun. 2016. "Aromatase expression and regulation in breast and endometrial cancer." *J Mol Endocrinol* 57(1):R19–33. doi: 10.1530/JME-15-0310.

Zhu, J., and C. B. Thompson. 2019. "Metabolic regulation of cell growth and proliferation." *Nat Rev Mol Cell Biol* 20(7):436–50. doi: 10.1038/s41580-019-0123-5.

Ziegler, R. G. 1997. "Anthropometry and breast cancer." *J Nutr* 127(5 Suppl):924S–8S. doi: 10.1093/jn/127.5.924S.

14 Nutrition Support for Cancer Patients throughout the Continuum of Care

Refaat Hegazi
Abbott Nutrition Research & Development
Mansoura University

Katie N. Robinson, Bridget A. Cassady, and Sara Thomas
Abbott Nutrition Research & Development

Mohamed El-Gamal
Mansoura University

David G.A. Williams
Duke University

Michael D. Bastasch, MD
University of Texas East Health

CONTENTS

ABBREVIATIONS

American College of Surgeons (ACS) Strong for Surgery
American Society of Anesthesiologists (ASA)
American Society for Enhanced Recovery (ASER)
American Society for Parenteral and Enteral Nutrition (ASPEN)
Body Mass Index (BMI)
C-reactive protein-to-albumin (CRP/Alb)
Enhanced Recovery After Surgery (ERAS)
ERAS® Interactive Audit System (EIAS)
ERAS® Implementation Program (EIP)
Enteral Nutrition (EN)
European Society for Clinical Nutrition and Metabolism (ESPEN)
Global Leadership Initiative on Malnutrition (GLIM)
Immunonutrition (IMN)
Malnutrition Screening Tool (MST)
Nutrition-Focused Physical Exam (NFPE)
Oral nutrition supplements (ONS)
Perioperative Quality Initiate (POQI)
Parenteral Nutrition (PN)
Patient-Generated Subjective Global Assessment (PG-SGA)
Prevalence of Malnutrition in Oncology (PreMiO)
Registered Dietitian Nutritionist (RDN)
Society of Critical Care Medicine (SCCM)

NUTRITIONAL NEEDS OF PATIENTS WITH CANCER

Currently, patients newly diagnosed with cancer are expected to live longer and go through multiple types of treatment modalities and rounds of treatment during their course of care. However, they are also at high risk for many nutritional challenges, including weight loss, malnutrition and loss of muscle mass. In fact, half of the cancer patients have already lost critical muscle mass and are malnourished at diagnosis, impacting their recovery and overall health status (Halpern-Silveira et al. 2010, Ottery 1994). Additionally, research shows that up to 85% of these patients experience weight loss or malnutrition during their treatment and up to 79% of cancer patients experience significant loss of muscle mass (Dewyse et al. 1980). Muscle mass loss can range from 25% in metastatic breast cancer to as high as 71% in metastatic colorectal cancer (CRC) (Ryan et al. 2016). Some of the most prevalent cancers have the greatest risk for muscle loss; pancreatic, gastroesophageal, and head and neck cancers are very prevalent and more than 65% of patients with gastroesophageal or pancreatic cancers have muscle mass loss (Baracos et al. 2018, Muscaritoli et al. 2017). However, identifying patients with muscle loss may be difficult in patients with cancer as 40%–60% are overweight or obese (Ryan et al. 2016).

Nutrition decline is a common occurrence among patients with cancer during the progression of the disease and its treatment. Malnutrition is highly prevalent in oncology patients due to increased nutrition demands on the body stemming from the disease process. Malnutrition in patients with cancer is associated with poor prognosis, and weight loss is considered a predictor of mortality (Bosaeus et al. 2008, Vigano et al. 2004). In fact, it is estimated that about 20% of patients with cancer die because of malnutrition rather than the malignant disease (Ottery et al. 1994). Cancer-related weight loss is known to reduce the immune response to infection and increase the chances of post-surgical complications (van Bokhorst et al. 1997, Jagoe et al. 2001). Many patients experience weight loss even prior to cancer diagnosis. In a prospective observational study (Prevalence of Malnutrition in Oncology (PreMiO) study) of 22 oncology centers with 1952 enrolled patients making their first medical oncology visit after initial diagnosis, 51% of patients were nutritionally impaired, including risk for malnutrition and overt malnutrition (Muscaritoli et al. 2017) (Figure 14.1). During the 6 months prior to the initial visit, 64% of patients lost 1–10 kg. In addition to cancer itself,

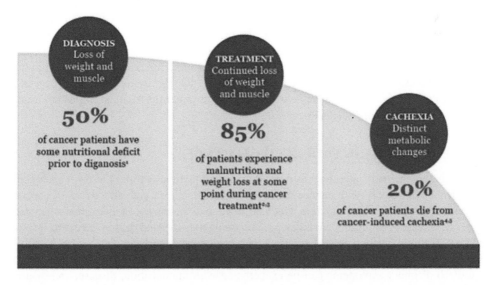

FIGURE 14.1 Weight loss and malnutrition experienced by patients during cancer treatment (Muscaritoli et al. 2017, Dewys et al. 1980, Laviano and Meguid 1996, Tisdale 2002, Davidson et al. 2012).

cancer treatments, including surgery, can have a significant impact on the nutrition status of a patient. Malnutrition and weight loss affect 30%–85% of cancer patients during treatment depending on the stage of the disease and site of the tumor (Bachmann et al. 2008, Martin et al. 2015).

The causes of nutritional deterioration are multifactorial, mostly determined by the type and stage of cancer, anatomic location, duration of disease, protein and energy intake, and cancer treatment(s) (Ravasco et al. 2003). Systemic and local effects of the tumor, in addition to the side effects of cancer treatment, contribute to malnutrition (Rivadeneira et al. 1998, Shils et al. 1979). Cancer, as a general condition, exerts a systemic effect by causing inflammation which alters metabolism generally, whereas a tumor, as a local process, can lead to malabsorption, obstruction, nausea, vomiting, and diarrhea, from local mass effect (Bloch et al. 1990). The side effects of cancer treatment often cause decreased appetite, early satiety, swallowing difficulties, dry mouth, taste changes, mouth sores, odor sensitivities and nausea, all of which could reduce dietary intake (Grosvenor et al. 1989).

Anorexia is often a presenting symptom of cancer and is seen in approximately half of newly diagnosed patients with cancer leading to an involuntary decline of food intake (Grosvenor et al. 1989). The mechanisms causing anorexia are not completely understood. Changes in the perception of food taste, learned food aversions, delayed gastric emptying, decreased muscle strength, and neurochemical changes such as increased hypothalamic serotonergic activity have all been proposed to cause anorexia (Laviano et al. 1996).

When the diagnosis of cancer is delivered to the patient, the psychological reaction can lead to depression and grief which both can contribute to inanition (Watson et al. 1999, Giannousi et al. 2012). Additional abscopal effects of the cancer stem from a multifactorial foundation and contribute to a systemic inflammatory state which leads to anorexia and cachexia (Roxburgh et al. 2014). Adverse effects on survival are a consequence of this prevalent malnutrition. Consistently, nutrition status has been reported to be a strong prognostic marker in ovarian cancer patients' overall survival before chemotherapy, with moderately to severely malnourished patients' survival being only 48 months compared to 80 months for normal or mildly malnourished patients ($p = 0.014$) (Yoon et al. 2014).

The anorexic state may facilitate the development of cachexia in certain patients, which is a complex metabolic syndrome characterized by an ongoing inflammation-associated loss of skeletal muscle mass leading to severe weight loss and progressive functional impairment (Fearon et al. 2011).Cancer cachexia is characterized by weight loss that includes loss of fat and/or muscle mass that cannot be reversed by traditional nutrition support. Cachexia is thought to result from a combination of various factors including inadequate energy intake, tumor induced increase in energy expenditure, altered metabolism, and an imbalance of proinflammatory and anti-inflammatory cytokines (Nitenberg et al. 2000). Cachexia additionally predisposes patients to a symptom triad of pain, depression, and fatigue that adversely impact their physical function, an important aspect of quality of life (QOL) (Laird et al. 2011).

THE ROLE OF MUSCLE IN PATIENTS WITH CANCER

Sarcopenia is the age associated loss of muscle mass and/or function and the term sarcopenia is often used interchangeably with cancer cachexia. Cancer cachexia and sarcopenia in cancer are closely related to systemic inflammation which occurs due to the release of inflammatory cytokines by cancer cells leading to muscle breakdown. Sarcopenia may develop during cancer as a result of a combination of malnutrition, muscle disuse, and systemic inflammation.

The loss of muscle mass and function begins at the age of 40 and sharply progresses after the age of 70. Primary sarcopenia can be exacerbated with malnutrition, disease, and disuse, all these factors being common in patients with cancer. The important role of low muscle mass on the prognosis of patients with cancer has been illustrated in multiple clinical studies. In a study of 137 patients with locally advanced head and neck squamous cell carcinoma patients treated with chemoradiotherapy/bioradiotherapy, baseline muscle wasting was an independent prognostic factor of decreased overall survival, increased treatment toxicity, and decreased tolerance (Willemsen et al. 2019). Additionally, Prado et al (2016) had shown that dose-limiting toxicity is significantly higher among patients with low muscle mass. It was also concluded that while current therapeutic regimes attenuate weight loss, they do not address the loss of muscle mass and function during therapy and called for nutrition and additional strategies targeting cancer associated loss of muscle mass, and function (Willemsen et al. 2019).

In 2012, the term "Malnutrition Sarcopenia Syndrome (MSS)" was proposed to indicate the inherent association between the two conditions (Vandewoude et al., 2012). Both malnutrition and sarcopenia are independent factors of disease-associated clinical and functional adverse outcomes. MSS could be diagnosed in both underweight and obese patients. Patients are at risk of MSS when four or more of these clinical findings are present:

1. Recent history of reduced appetite that resulted in poor food intake
2. Unintentional weight loss of 3 kg or more over the last 3 months
3. Low muscle mass (as measured by dual-energy x-ray absorptiometry (DEXA), Computed Tomography (CT), Magnetic Resonance Imaging (MRI) or Bioelectrical Impedance Analysis (BIA)
4. Decreased gait speed (<0.8 m/s)
5. Reduced hand grip strength for age and gender.

This MSS concept of assessing muscle mass and function as criteria to diagnose malnutrition was consistent with the 2012 Academy of Nutrition and Dietetics (AND) and the American Society for Parenteral and Enteral Nutrition (ASPEN) diagnostic criteria (Jensen et al. 2012) and the GLIM (Global Leadership In Malnutrition) consensus diagnosis of malnutrition (Jensen et al. 2018). Both consensus statements of diagnosis of malnutrition addressed an important factor: the importance of assessing muscle mass and function. With growing prevalence rates of obesity and overweight globally, using low Body Mass Index (BMI) as a sole criterion to diagnose malnutrition could lead to missing many cases of malnourished patients with cancer. Patients with malnutrition are not always frail and underweight. According to GLIM, the presence of one etiologic criterion (of either decreased food intake or the presence of disease) and one phenotypic criterion (of either weight loss, low BMI, and low muscle mass and/or function) are required to make the diagnosis of malnutrition (Jensen et al. 2018). The inclusion of low muscle mass/function in the diagnosis of malnutrition is also consistent with the previously published diagnostic criteria of adult undernutrition by a consensus of ASPEN and AND experts (Jensen et al. 2012). Both GLIM and AND/ASPEN diagnostic criteria have been shown to correctly identify malnourished patients and those with an increased risk for mortality, extended length of stay (LOS), and higher likelihood for readmission (Mogensen et al. 2019).

An overweight or obese patient with cancer can have substantial muscle depletion at the time of diagnosis. This is called "sarcopenic obesity" and is an independent predictor of functional status and survival among patients with cancer (Prado et al. 2008). Increasing evidence indicates that sarcopenia is present in 20%–70% of patients with cancer regardless of BMI (Ryan et al. 2016) and is associated with negative outcomes, including surgical complications and shortened survival (Carneiro, Mazurak, and Prado 2016, Antoun et al. 2013). Indeed, sarcopenia was found to be prevalent across all levels of nutrition risk in overweight and obese, newly diagnosed patients with head, neck, lung, and gastrointestinal cancer (Martin et al. 2020). The presence of sarcopenic obesity can be challenging to identify due to the lack of uniform standards for diagnosis. One way to identify sarcopenic obesity is by using image-based methods such as CT or MRI scans. Fearon et al. (2011) described that the loss of lean body mass (LBM) can be determined by employing the following methods of assessment—"mid-upper-arm muscle area by anthropometry (men <32 cm^2, women <18 cm^2), appendicular skeletal muscle index determined by dual-energy X-ray absorptiometry (men <7.26 kg/m^2, women <5.45 kg/m^2), lumbar skeletal-muscle index determined from oncology CT imaging (men <55 cm^2/m^2, women <39 cm^2/m^2), and whole-body fat-free mass index without bone determined by bioelectrical impedance (men <14.6 kg/m^2, women <11.4 kg/m^2)."

Such image analyses can reveal significant loss of muscle mass, equivalent to that of a patient with frank cachexia, in obese and overweight patients (Prado et al. 2008, Tan et al. 2009). Using these imaging techniques, the prevalence of sarcopenic obesity was found to range from 9% to 14% in patients with esophageal cancer (Anandavadivelan et al. 2016, Grotenhuis et al. 2016); 12.7% in prostatic cancer (Cushen et al. 2016); and 16.2% in pancreatic cancer (Tan et al. 2009); up to 28.7% among patients undergoing partial hepatectomy due to colorectal liver metastases (Lodewick et al. 2015).

Sarcopenic obesity is consistently associated with increased risk of poor prognosis among cancer patients. For instance, the C-SCANS study investigated association between body composition and CRC survival and body composition as an explanation of the obesity paradox (decreased mortality among obese patients). In this study of 3,262 early stage (I-III) male (50%) and female (50%) patients with CRC, sarcopenic patients had a 27% (HR 1.27; 95% CI 1.09, 1.48) higher risk of overall mortality than those who were not sarcopenic. Females with both low muscle and high adiposity had a 64% higher risk of overall motality (OM) (HR 1.64; 95% CI 1.05, 2.57) when compared to females with adequate muscle and lower adiposity. The lowest risk of overall mortality was seen in patients with a BMI between 25 and <30 kg/m^2, a range associated with the greatest number of patients (58.6%) who were not at increased risk of OM due to either low muscle or high levels of total adipose tissue. The study concluded that sarcopenia along with adiposity should be a standard oncologic marker to screen for in cancer patients (Caan et al. 2016).

It is recommended that overweight and obese patients with cancer also be included in the initial nutrition screen plan. The use of imaging methods such as CT scans to assess body composition helps predict the prognosis and potentially improve cancer treatment.

NUTRITION SUPPORT FOR PATIENTS WITH CANCER

Screening, Assessment, and Diagnosis of Malnutrition in Patients with Cancer

Malnutrition is defined as "a state of nutrition in which a deficiency, excess, or imbalance of energy, protein, and other nutrients causes measurable adverse effects on body function and clinical outcome" (Elia et al. 2000). This definition of malnutrition encompasses any imbalance between nutrient intake and needs independent of body weight or BMI. Body weight and BMI are false indicators of the loss of muscle mass and/or function, which is a critical prognostic factor of poor outcome in cancer patients. Consistently, one study found that 79% of patients identified as malnourished were normal weight, overweight or obese (Davidson et al. 2012).

Clinical evidence supports that appropriate and timely nutrition screening and support is beneficial in improving patient outcomes. The goals of nutrition support are in line with the goals of cancer treatment, which include providing effective treatment that is well tolerated by the patients, minimizing complications, improving QOL and ensuring proper recovery. In fact, numerous studies have shown that early nutrition intervention improves patient outcomes including improvements in nutrition status, performance status, tolerance to treatment, and QOL (Caro et al. 2007). It also contributes to decreased rate of complications, and reduced morbidity and mortality. Several modes of nutrition support such as nutrition counseling, oral nutrition supplements (ONS), enteral nutrition, parental nutrition, and immune modulating nutrients have been used to achieve this goal.

It is vital that nutrition specialists (e.g., physician nutrition specialists and Registered Dietitian Nutritionists (RDNs)) are active members of the multidisciplinary cancer care team. The nutrition care process for cancer patients begins with nutrition screening. Patients found to be at-risk for malnutrition based on a validated nutrition screen should be referred to nutrition specialists for

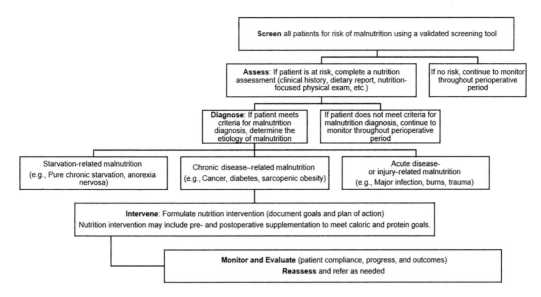

Screen all patients for risk of malnutrition using a validated screening tool

Assess: If patient is at risk, complete a nutrition assessment (clinical history, dietary report, nutrition-focused physical exam, etc.)

If no risk, continue to monitor throughout perioperative period

Diagnose: If patient meets criteria for malnutrition diagnosis, determine the etiology of malnutrition

If patient does not meet criteria for malnutrition diagnosis, continue to monitor throughout perioperative period

Starvation-related malnutrition (e.g., Pure chronic starvation, anorexia nervosa)

Chronic disease–related malnutrition (e.g., Cancer, diabetes, sarcopenic obesity)

Acute disease- or injury-related malnutrition (e.g., Major infection, burns, trauma)

Intervene: Formulate nutrition intervention (document goals and plan of action)
Nutrition intervention may include pre- and postoperative supplementation to meet caloric and protein goals.

Monitor and Evaluate (patient compliance, progress, and outcomes)
Reassess and refer as needed

FIGURE 14.2 Preoperative nutrition care process for surgical patients with cancer.

nutrition assessment, diagnosis, intervention, monitoring, and evaluation. The nutrition care process is reviewed in Figure 14.2. Nutrition specialists trained to implement evidence-based nutrition and provide practical guidance are crucial for patients to meet calorie, protein, and other nutrient needs.

One of the challenges that could hinder prompt and adequate nutrition support is the difficulty in diagnosing malnutrition in cancer patients. Diagnostic markers such as serum albumin, which were historically employed for detecting nutritional status, are imperfect because they could be negatively associated with the malignancy-associated inflammation. Rather, validated nutrition screening and assessment tools should be used for the early detection and risk stratification of malnutrition. Some of the validated screening tools are Malnutrition Screening Tool (MST), Malnutrition Universal Screening Tool, and Nutrition Risk Screening (NRS-2002). Validated assessment tools include the Subjective Global Assessment (SGA) (Paccagnella et al. 2011). It is recommended that nutrition screening should be part of the initial evaluation of the patient at the time of diagnosis. Expert guidelines emphasize the need to identify malnutrition early and intervene early and throughout cancer care. A study showed that early and regular nutrition assessment, followed by intervention, and a multidisciplinary approach to nutrition care results in improved treatment tolerance for patients with esophageal cancer receiving chemoradiation (Odelli et al. 2005). However, despite ample evidence, there is lack of sufficient effort and expertise in health systems to detect malnutrition early and provide sustained support throughout the course of cancer treatment.

One of the myths due to which nutrition support is not initiated in patients with cancer by clinicians is the perception of nutrition (especially carbohydrates and fats) potentially stimulating tumor growth. However, this has never been demonstrated in clinical studies (Bozzetti et al. 1999). The evaluation of tumor growth in vivo is challenging, and although a few studies have been performed, the results did not consistently support this myth (Nitenberg et al. 2000, Bozzetti et al. 1989). On the contrary, nutrition intervention studies reviewed in detail in the current chapter not only never showed any adverse events on tumor growth but also showed gain of weight and reversal of the loss of muscle mass and improved clinical outcomes.

Moreover, it is hypothesized that tumor growth could be inhibited by including nutrients that cannot be metabolized by the tumor such as modified carbohydrates or medium-chain triglycerides and omega-3 fatty acids (Nitenberg et al. 2000). Another immunomodulatory nutrient that could potentially inhibit tumor growth is arginine. The antitumor effects of arginine have been widely recognized in animal models (Daly et al. 1992, Ye et al. 1992, Ma et al. 1996). These effects of arginine are related to its positive effects on the immune system, such as increase in T-lymphocyte count and increase in the natural killer cell activity (Ye et al. 1992). A randomized study reported that perioperative enteral supplementation with an arginine-enriched mixture in malnourished patients with head and neck cancer significantly increased long-term survival in these patients (Buijs et al. 2010). Other studies have shown that the use of arginine in the post-operative period reduced complications and improved wound healing in patients with cancer (Farreras et al. 2005, Casas-Rodera et al. 2008). Furthermore, early supplementation of parenteral nutrition had been shown to have positive effects on outcome in patients with advanced cancer (Shang et al. 2006). Patients who received intensified enteral nutrition supplemented with parenteral nutrition showed a significant improvement in body composition and QOL. The cumulative survival rate was also significantly greater in this group ($p < 0.0001$), compared to the control group. These data stand to falsify the myth that "feeding the patient feeds the tumor". Therefore, appropriate nutrition could be utilized to facilitate cancer treatment by either enhancing the immune response or potentiating therapy.

GUIDELINES FOR IMPLEMENTING NUTRITION SUPPORT FOR PATIENTS WITH CANCER

American, European, and Australian guidelines all recommend and support early and continuous nutrition support in patients with cancer (Table 14.1). These guidelines emphasize the need to identify and address malnutrition in patients and recommend intervention soon after diagnosis and throughout cancer care. The American Society of Clinical Oncology 2020 Guideline recommends that "dietary counseling may be offered with the goals of providing patients and caregivers with advice for the management of cachexia". The American College of Surgeons (ACS) Commission on Cancer 2012 Program Standards considers nutrition management as an integral component of comprehensive cancer care and recommends nutrition care including screening, assessment, counseling, and education across the cancer continuum (Cancer ACoSCo, 2014). The Association of Community Cancer Centers 2012 Cancer Program guidelines recommend individualized, patient specific nutrition care plan developed by a nutrition professional through screening, assessment, intervention, and education throughout the cancer treatment process (Cancer Program Guidelines, 2012).

TABLE 14.1
Guidelines for the Nutritional Management of Patients with Cancer

Society	Guidelines
American Society of Clinical Oncology 2020 Guideline	Dietary counseling may be offered with the goals of providing patients and caregivers with advice for the management of cachexia
AND 2017 Oncology Evidence-Based Nutrition Practice Guideline for Adults	Adult oncology patients should be screened using a MST validated in the setting in which the tool is intended for use. The following tools have been shown to be valid and reliable in identifying malnutrition risk in adult oncology patients
American Society of Parenteral and Enteral Nutrition (ASPEN) 2012 clinical guidelines	Screening and assessment of patients, followed by implementation of a nutrition care plan, is recommended
ESPEN 2017 guidelines on nutrition in cancer patients	All cancer patients should be screened regularly for the risk or the presence of malnutrition. In all patients with the exception of end-of-life-care energy and substrate requirements should be met by offering in a stepwise manner nutritional interventions from counseling to parenteral nutrition

Consistently, the AND 2017 Oncology Evidence-Based Nutrition Practice Guideline for Adults and the European Society for Clinical Nutrition and Metabolism (ESPEN) 2017 guidelines on nutrition in cancer patients recommend early screening of nutritional risk (Table 14.1).

While major societies agree on the need for early screening cancer patients for nutritional risk, they do not provide specifics on how to optimize nutrition intervention, reflecting perhaps the novelty of integrating nutrition as a component of a scientifically grounded yet holistic cancer treatment paradigm. This hesitancy of being too prescriptive of specific nutritional care plans might be driven from a perception of healthcare providers that nutrition interventions, aside from enteral/parenteral feedings for obvious needs, are of the plethora of fad "cancer diets" and specious "supplements" found in the media and on line. Nearly every physician in practice has been confronted frequently by diet quackery presented in good faith from desperate patients and families.

METHODS OF NUTRITION SUPPORT FOR PATIENTS WITH CANCER

Individuals with cancer often have a reduced overall food intake and need extra calories and nutrients, especially protein. Resting energy expenditure (REE) is often increased during cancer and its treatment and can make it difficult for patients to gain or maintain weight and muscle mass. For many patients, intervention with nutrition support is necessary to maintain weight and muscle mass, and help the patient maintain their strength and energy and tolerate treatment.

There are various effective options for nutrition intervention following the diagnosis of malnutrition. Nutrition intervention in cancer patients can involve many strategies including dietary counseling, fortified foods, ONS, and enteral and parenteral nutrition. Nutrition intervention, including oral nutrition supplementation, started as early as possible can result in a reduction in malnutrition or improvement in nutrition status (Bauer et al. 2005), improvement in QOL (Bauer et al. 2005, Ravasco et al. 2004, Davidson et al. 2004, Read et al. 2006), improved performance score (Bauer et al. 2005), strength (Glare, Jongs, and Zafiropoulos 2010, von Meyenfeldt 2002), and physical activity (Moses et al. 2004, Ryan et al. 2009, van der Meij et al. 2012), increased tolerance to treatment (Odelli et al. 2005), and treatment outcomes (Nayel et al. 1992).

When oral intake of food is preserved, the first step of the intervention process is nutrition counseling to improve diet quality and quantity for patients who are at risk of malnutrition. It has been shown that individualized nutrition counseling improves the nutrition status of patients, improves outcomes and QOL, and reduces morbidity (Ravasco et al. 2005). The modifications to the diet include choice of high energy/high-protein food, fortifying existing food, and providing information on healthful eating choices.

If these measures do not meet the nutrition needs of the patient, ONS especially these containing high ratios of protein to nonprotein calories are recommended. ONS are ready to use and convenient in a variety of forms such as liquids, puddings and nutrient bars. In terms of ONS, many studies have been conducted on standard ONS in various cancer diagnoses. ONS are shown to improve physical function and increase body weight in patients with chronic illnesses. These beneficial effects were more pronounced in malnourished patients (Stratton 2000). In a meta-analysis, high-protein ONS (with 20% of energy from protein) have been shown to reduce complications, hospital readmissions, improved muscle function, and protein and calorie intake (Cawood 2012). To shed light on the cancer patient population using standard ONS, some of these studies are highlighted below.

Nayel et al assessed the effect of oral nutrition supplementation for 10–15 days in patients with head and neck tumors prior to treatment with irradiation (Nayel et al. 1992). Twelve patients were randomly assigned to radiotherapy only and 11 to supplementation plus radiotherapy. All 11 patients who received nutrition supplementation gained weight, whereas 7 of the 12 patients treated with radiotherapy alone lost weight, a significant difference ($p = 0.001$) (Nayel et al. 1992). Radiotherapy had to be discontinued in 5 of the 12 patients who received no nutrition support due to severe mucositis or poor performance status, while all 11 who received supplementation received a course of irradiation without interruption (Nayel et al. 1992).

A study of 60 patients with head and neck cancer or lower gastrointestinal cancer undergoing radiation therapy by Bauer et al compared usual care to a program of nutrition intervention of dietary counseling including provision of ONS. Patients in the nutrition intervention group compared to the usual care group had better weight maintenance ($p = 0.001$), less deterioration in nutrition status ($p = 0.02$), and a smaller decrease and faster recovery in global QOL and physical function ($p = 0.009$) measured by European Organization for the Research and Treatment of Cancer (EORTC) (Bauer et al. 2005).

Davidson et al. studied patients with pancreatic cancer experiencing on average 17% weight loss prior to entering the study (Davidson et al. 2004). Those patients who reached weight stabilization had improved QOL scores (EORTC) ($p = 0.037$) and longer survival ($p = 0.019$) (Davidson et al. 2004). In a small study of CRC patients receiving ONS prior to and during treatment with combination chemotherapy of folinic acid, 5 fluoruracil, and irinotecan (FOLFIRI) showed not only improved QOL ($p = 0.05$) but also increases in weight ($p = 0.03$) and preservation of LBM (Read et al. 2006). In another study in patients receiving chemotherapy for nonsmall cell lung or pancreatic cancer, intense dietary counseling and oral nutrition supplementation showed improvement in nutrition status ($p = 0.019$), QOL ($p = 0.01$), and performance status ($p = 0.019$) (Bauer et al. 2005).

Odelli et al showed that patients undergoing chemo/radiotherapy for esophageal cancer in a nutrition intervention program experienced better outcomes than those who had received usual care. The patients receiving nutrition intervention had greater treatment completion rates (92% vs. 50%; $p = 0.001$), fewer unplanned hospital admissions (46 vs 75; $p = 0.04$), and those who were admitted to hospital had shorter LOS (3.2 days vs. 13.5 days; $p = 0.002$) compared to the patients receiving usual care (Odelli et al. 2005).

Nutrition intervention can result in improvements in performance status. Glare showed improvement in hand grip strength, weight maintenance, and symptom control in an intervention study with intense dietary counseling and ONS in patients undergoing treatment for lung or gastrointestinal (GI) tract cancer (Glare, Jongs, and Zafiropoulos 2010). Patients with pancreatic cancer receiving ONS also showed an improvement in hand grip strength ($p = 0.009$) (von Meyenfeldt 2002). Improvement in patients' physical activity is associated with improvement in performance score and nutrition intervention with ONS or enteral feeding has been shown to improve physical activity in patients undergoing chemoradiation for nonsmall cell lung cancer (NSCLC) (van der Meij et al. 2012), surgery for esophageal cancer (Ryan et al. 2009), and patients with pancreatic cancer (Moses et al. 2004).

Additionally, a 2012 systematic review and meta-analysis by Baldwin et al. evaluated the effect of oral nutrition interventions in this population on nutrition and clinical outcomes and QOL in 13 studies with 1,414 patients (Baldwin et al. 2012). The results showed that nutrition intervention was associated with:

- Statistically significant improvements in weight and energy intake compared with routine care (mean difference in weight = 1.86 kg, 95% CI = 0.25–3.47, $p = 0.02$; and mean difference in energy intake = 432 kcal/d, 95% CI = 172–693, $p = 0.001$).
- Beneficial effect on some aspects of QOL (emotional functioning, dyspnea, loss of appetite, and global QOL).
- No effect on mortality (relative risk = 1.06, 95% CI = 0.92–1.22, $p = 0.43$; I(2) = 0%; p (heterogeneity) = 0.56).

If oral intake does not satisfy the nutrient needs or if it is contraindicated, other methods of nutrition support are employed. These include enteral and parenteral nutrition. The decision to advance nutrition therapy beyond oral nutrition supplementation to Enteral Nutrition (EN) or Parenteral Nutrition (PN) depends on multiple factors which are summarized in Table 14.2. If the gastrointestinal function is intact, international guidelines recommend the use of enteral nutrition over parenteral nutrition, since the former is more physiological, less prone to complications, less expensive,

TABLE 14.2

Questions to Ask When Considering Advancing to Enteral or Parenteral Nutrition in Patients with Cancer

- Is food intake anticipated to be inadequate (<50% of energy requirements) for more than 10 days due to surgery, chemotherapy, or radiotherapy?
- Has food intake been inadequate (<50% of energy requirements) for more than 2 weeks?
- Is my patient undernourished and expected not to be able to eat or absorb nutrients for a long period of time due to antineoplastic treatments?
- Does my patient have a tumor which impairs oral intake or movement of food through the GI tract?

and easier to monitor (August et al. 2001, Braunschweig et al. 2001). In addition, enteral nutrition helps maintain the absorptive and immune functions of the gut (The Veterans Affairs Total Parenteral Nutrition Cooperative Study Group, 1991).

PN is only recommended in specific situations when the gastrointestinal tract cannot be used or accessed, such as cases of severe mucositis or enteritis in malnourished patients or those who are at risk of malnutrition and treated for definitive cure. Numerous studies have examined the role of PN in patients with cancer and the results are conflicting. Early supplementation of PN had been shown to have positive effects on outcome in malnourished patients with advanced cancer (Shang et al. 2006). Patients who received intensified EN supplemented with PN showed a significant improvement in body composition and QOL. The cumulative survival rate was also significantly greater in this group ($p < 0.0001$), compared to the control group. These data stand to falsify the myth that "feeding the patient feeds the tumor". Therefore, appropriate nutrition could be utilized to facilitate cancer treatment by either enhancing the immune response or potentiating therapy. Some of the early studies raised concerns over the benefit of intravenous feeding and showed that PN is associated with an increased rate of septic complications (The Veterans Affairs Total Parenteral Nutrition Cooperative Study Group, 1991). Advances in the knowledge of the proper amounts and types of macronutrients have minimized the complications associated with PN. A meta-analysis of 28 prospective randomized controlled clinical trials evaluating the use of PN in patients with cancer showed no significant benefit from PN on survival, treatment tolerance, treatment toxicity, or tumor response in patients receiving chemotherapy or radiotherapy (Klein et al. 1986). The only instance where PN appeared to be beneficial was in decreasing surgical complications and operative mortality when used preoperatively in patients with gastrointestinal tract cancer (Klein et al. 1986). Another instance where PN is the only route of nutrition support is in patients with solid tumors or hematologic malignancies receiving bone marrow transplantation (BMT) (Stratton et al. 2000). In these patients, the use of PN is warranted due to the severe mucositis associated with BMT related therapies. In addition, studies that investigated the use of home parenteral nutrition (HPN) in severely malnourished patients with advanced cancer have reported an improvement in the QOL for patients who survived for more than 3 months (Bozzetti et al. 2013). Hence, not all patients will benefit from HPN, and it should be tailored only to the cases where all other routes of nutrition support are exhausted.

NUTRITION CONSIDERATION IN THE MANAGEMENT OF CANCER CACHEXIA

For the oncology patient, there are many nutrition challenges, including maintaining a good nutrition status and avoiding weight loss, muscle loss, malnutrition, and cachexia. Research demonstrates that the majority of patients with cancer suffer from various nutrition deficits and up to 85% of patients experience some form of weight loss or malnutrition during their cancer treatment (von Haehling and Anker 2010, Dewys et al. 1980). For some patients, the nutrition deficits can proceed to cancer cachexia, a specific form of malnutrition characterized by loss of lean mass, muscle wasting, and impaired immune, physical, and mental function (Fearon et al. 2011, Ryan et al. 2016). Furthermore, a poor nutrition status, weight loss, and malnutrition lead to poor outcomes for patients including decreased QOL, decreased functional status, increased complication rates, treatment disruptions, increased risk of cancer recurrence, and reduced cancer survival (Dewys et al. 1980, Andreyev et al. 1998, Caro, Laviano, and Pichard 2007). Conversely, research shows that providing early nutrition intervention for patients can improve patients' nutrition status and help patients to maintain body weight, maintain LBM, better tolerate treatment, and improve QOL (Caro, Laviano, and Pichard 2007, Nayel et al. 1992, Isenring, Capra, and Bauer 2004, Bauer et al. 2005, Odelli et al. 2005, Ravasco 2005, CL 2005). ONS enriched with omega-3 fatty acids have been demonstrated in extensive research to benefit patients with cancer cachexia in terms of improvements in muscle mass and outcomes. Expert oncology associations recognize the importance of identifying and treating nutrition deficits and recommend nutrition screening and specific nutrition intervention in practice guidelines to improve care and outcomes for oncology patients (ACSs Commission on Cancer. Cancer Program Standards 2012: Ensuring Patient Centered Care. Chicago, 2012).

NUTRITION CHALLENGES FOR PATIENTS WITH CANCER CACHEXIA

Cancer systemically leads to malnutrition and muscle loss in multiple ways, including declined ability for proper muscle contraction due to altered protein production; altered metabolism as a result of impaired glucose, lipid, and protein metabolism; increased energy requirements secondary to tumor growth, infection/fever, inflammatory status, surgery, and cancer treatments; and decreased food intake resulting from side effects such as nausea, vomiting, constipation, diarrhea, and anorexia (Argilés et al. 2014). Some patients develop cancer cachexia, a devastating and multifactorial syndrome that affects 50%–80% of cancer patients, depending on tumor type (Argilés et al. 2014, Ryan et al. 2016). A 2011 consensus by Fearon et al. established the definition and classification of different stages of cachexia with distinct differences in weight and muscle loss (see Figure 14.3) (Fearon et al. 2011). Cancer cachexia results in significant weight loss, which is primarily from loss of skeletal muscle and body fat; is associated with poorer outcomes including fatigue, impaired physical function, decreased QOL, reduced tolerance to treatment, and decreased survival; and may account for up to 20% of cancer deaths (Ryan et al. 2016, Argilés et al. 2014). Once cancer cachexia is present, it cannot be reversed by conventional nutrition intervention, ultimately leading to progressive functional impairment (Andreyev et al. 1998).

Cancer-associated weight loss does not respond to simply increasing dietary intake as the metabolic alterations secondary to the tumor itself constitute a complex mechanism of muscle wasting

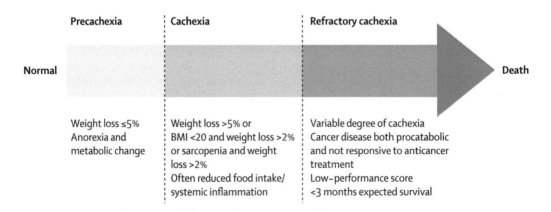

FIGURE 14.3   Stages of cancer cachexia. (Adapted from Fearon et al. 2011.)

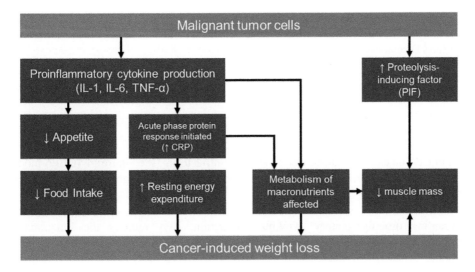

FIGURE 14.4 Metabolic changes leading to cancer-induced weight loss. (Adapted from Giacosa and Rondanelli 2008.)

and weight loss (Giacosa and Rondanelli 2008). Proinflammatory cytokines plan a central role in cancer-induced weight loss by (see Figure 14.4) (Giacosa and Rondanelli 2008):

1. They initiate the acute-phase protein response, in which acute-phase proteins are produced and resting energy expenditure is increased. They alter macronutrient metabolism.
2. Depressed appetite which in turn leads to reduced food intake.

Both of these metabolic responses affect the metabolism of macronutrients driving catabolism of muscle mass to provide substrates for gluconeogenesis and protein biosynthesis. In cancer, the metabolic needs in the body increase but the food intake is severely reduced; this results in a negative energy and protein balance, leading to ongoing involuntary muscle wasting (Fearon, Arends, and Baracos 2013).

Cancer-induced weight loss is a complex metabolic syndrome in which patients experience anorexia, fatigue, and early satiety; is characterized by significant weight loss; and is different than weight loss due to caloric deficiency (Kotler 2000). In caloric deficiency, metabolic adaptations conserve lean mass and favor fat metabolism, thereby fat tissue is metabolized preferentially over lean mass, which leads to a preservation of lean mass (Kotler 2000). In contrast, patients with the cancer-induced weight loss lose equal amounts of fat and lean mass, mostly skeletal muscle. Protein turnover increases and synthesis of muscle protein decreases; thus, protein degradation is increased. REE is increased, the acute phase response is initiated, and proteolysis-inducing factor (PIF) is produced (Kotler 2000).

CLINICAL EFFECTS OF OMEGA-3 ENRICHED ONS FOR CANCER CACHEXIA

Patients with cancer cachexia, severe muscle mass loss, and/or inflammation may not respond to standard oral nutrition supplementation and may need more specialized nutrition support. Much research over the past 20 years has highlighted the benefit of omega-3 fatty acids, particularly eicosapentaenoic acid (EPA), on outcomes in patients with cancer-induced weight loss compared to conventional nutrition support. EPA is a long-chain polyunsaturated fatty acid (PUFA) of the omega-3 (n-3) family and is found naturally in deep-sea oily fish such as salmon, mackerel, herring, sardines, and tuna. EPA has been introduced as a nutrition supplement for people with cancer because it attenuated metabolic changes due to cancer-induced weight loss and has been shown to improve outcomes. Dietary EPA (as fish oil or pure EPA) exerts beneficial effects including (August, Huhmann, and Directors 2009):

- Down-regulating the inflammatory response
- Decreasing cytokine production
- Reducing the level and activity of PIF
- Stabilizing weight in patients with solid tumors

The effect of EPA on cancer-induced weight loss is multifactorial (see Figure 14.4). EPA moderates some of the metabolic abnormalities associated with cancer-induced weight loss including (Colomer et al. 2007):

1. Decreasing proinflammatory cytokine production, EPA reduces the inflammatory response and helps improve appetite and food intake. EPA moderates the acute phase response evidenced by decreased C-reactive protein levels and helps normalize resting energy expenditure.
2. Reducing the activity and production of proteolysis-inducing factor, and as a result, weight and lean muscle mass stabilizes.

In animal and human studies, dietary EPA (as fish oil or pure EPA) has been linked with a wide range of beneficial effects in conditions of excessive inflammation, including:

- Decreases proinflammatory cytokine production (Wigmore et al. 1996, 1997, Barber et al. 2001, Endres et al. 1989)
- Down-regulates the inflammatory response (Wigmore et al. 1996, 1997, Barber et al. 2001, Jho et al. 2003)
- Down-regulates level/activity of PIF (Barber et al. 2001, Lorite, Cariuk, and Tisdale 1997)

Nutrition intervention with EPA-enriched ONS has been shown to improve clinical outcomes in patients with cancer in various clinical trials as well as systematic reviews and meta-analysis. Several of those studies and reviews are highlighted below.

CLINICAL TRIALS OF OMEGA-3 ENRICHED ONS FOR CANCER CACHEXIA

In 2020, Laviano et al. conducted a pilot, double-blind, comparator-controlled trial to evaluate the safety and tolerability of an oral targeted medical nutrition (TMN) supplement for the management of cachexia in patients with NSCLC (Laviano et al. 2020). Patients were randomized to receive either a juice-based TMN (~200 kcal; 10 g whey protein; ≥2.0 g EPA/DHA in fish oil; and 10 µg 25-hydroxy-vitamin D3) or a milk-based isocaloric comparator twice daily for 12 weeks. The study results showed that the TMN group ($n = 26$; mean 64.4 years) experienced fewer adverse events (64 vs. 87) than the comparator group ($n = 29$; mean 66.0 years), including fewer cases of neutropenia (0 vs. 4). Compliance was slightly lower in the TMN (58.5%) vs. comparator group (73.6%). There were no statistically significant between-group differences in efficacy endpoints. Fewer (4 vs. 10) patients who received TMN than comparator had died by 1-year post.

Another recent study by Schmidt et al. (2020) investigated the acceptability and compliance to a nutrition drink with fish oil compared to an equivalent dose of fish oil administered as capsules in patients receiving chemotherapy for GI tract cancers (Schmidt et al. 2020). The study included 41 patients who received either 10 capsules/day for 4 weeks or 400 mL/day of a nutrition drink with same dose of n-3 LC PUFA dose. At the end of the study, compliance and daily consumption of n-3 LC PUFAs were 96.4% (94.1–99.3) and 4.8 (4.7–4.9) g/day in the capsule group and 80.8

(55.4–93.6) % and 4.0 (2.8–4.7) g/day in the nutrition drink group, respectively ($p \leq 0.02$). No differences were found between the groups with respect to changes in whole blood n-3 LC PUFAs, weight, nutrition status, acceptability, or side effects. Overall, this study concluded that fish oil capsules resulted in better compliance compared to a nutrition drink with an equivalent dose of n-3 LC PUFAs, but that capsules and the drink did not differ with respect to the effect on nutrition status or side effects.

A 2019 study by Mizumachi et al. examined the effect of a nutrition supplement with a high blend ratio of ω-3 fatty acids on body weight loss, oral mucositis, and the completion rate of chemoradiotherapy in patients with oropharyngeal and hypopharyngeal cancer (Mizumachi et al. 2019). The study included 17 patients who received 2 servings of the supplement per day during chemoradiation. The results showed the reduction in body weight was significantly improved compared with that in the historical control group that did not receive the supplement (7.3% vs 10.3%, $p < 0.01$), and the rate of Grade 3–4 oral mucositis was significantly reduced for the patient groups that received the supplement (CTCAE v3.0 Grade B3; 24% vs 58%, $p < 0.05$). Additionally, the completion rate of chemoradiotherapy was not significantly different between both groups (77% vs 60%, NS).

A 2018 study by Hanai et al evaluated whether a nutrition supplement with a high blend ratio of ω-3 fatty acids can minimize weight loss and attenuate increases in inflammatory marker levels during the perioperative period in patients undergoing surgery for head and neck carcinoma (Hanai et al. 2018). Patients were randomized into two groups: the "nutrition supplementation group" and the "nonintervention group", with the nutrition supplementation group receiving two servings of an EPA-enriched ONS per day for 28 days during the perioperative period. The results showed that compliance with the supplement dosage was very good at 6,277/6,720 mL (average) before surgery (93%) and 5,229/6,720 mL after surgery (78%), and a significant increase in EPA concentration was shown in the group that received the supplement ($p < 0.0001$). However, 28 days of nutrition supplementation did not lead to further weight change or changes in the inflammatory marker levels of patients who were already showing cachexia (based on weight loss); no further change in the mean weight was noted in these patients; and the incidence of postoperative complications did not differ between the two groups.

In 2014 de Luis et al. investigated the influence of a hypercaloric and hyperproteic oral supplement enriched with ω-3 fatty acids and fiber on clinical parameters in head and neck tumor postsurgical ambulatory patients with or without radiotherapy (de Luis et al. 2014). The study consisted of 37 ambulatory patients who consumed 2 servings of the supplement for a 12-week period. Results showed a significant increase of albumin and transferrin levels in total group and in patients undergoing radiotherapy and without it. No differences were detected in weight and other anthropometric parameters in total group and in patients with radiotherapy during the protocol. Patients without radiotherapy showed a significant improvement of BMI; weight, fat free mass, and fat mass.

A 2014 study by Sanchez-Lara et al. compared the effect of an oral EPA-enriched supplement with an isocaloric diet on nutrition, clinical, and inflammatory parameters and health-related quality of life in advanced NSCLC patients (Sánchez-Lara et al. 2014). Ninety-two patients we randomized to receive diet plus ONS containing EPA (ONS-EPA) or only isocaloric diet (C). At the end of the study, the ONS-EPA group had significantly greater energy ($p < 0.001$) and protein ($p < 0.001$) intake compared with control. Compared with baseline, patients receiving the ONS-EPA gained 1.6±5 kg of LBM compared with a loss of −2.0±6 kg in the control ($p = 0.01$). Fatigue, loss of appetite, and neuropathy decreased in the ONS-EPA group ($p \leq 0.05$). There was no difference in response rate or overall survival between groups.

In 2012 van der Meij et al. investigated the effects of an ONS containing n-3 PUFA on QOL, performance status, handgrip strength, and physical activity in patients with NSCLC undergoing multimodality treatment (van der Meij et al. 2012). Forty subjects were randomized to either 2 servings per day of a protein- and energy-dense ONS containing n-3 PUFAs (2.02 g EPA acid

+0.92 g DHA/day) or an isocaloric control supplement. Results showed that the intervention group reported significantly higher on the QOL parameters, physical and cognitive function ($B = 11.6$ and $B = 20.7$, $P < 0.01$), global health status ($B = 12.2$, $p = 0.04$), and social function ($B = 22.1$, $p = 0.04$) than the control group after 5 weeks. The intervention group also had a higher Karnofsky Performance Status ($B = 5.3$, $p = 0.04$) than the control group after 3 weeks. However, handgrip strength did not significantly differ between groups over time. The intervention group also tended to have a higher physical activity than the control group after 3 and 5 weeks ($B = 6.6$, $p = 0.04$ and $B = 2.5$, $p = 0.05$).

Trabal et al. in 2010 assessed the effect of an intervention with an EPA-enriched ONS on chemotherapy tolerability in patients with advanced CRC (Trabal et al. 2010). The study included 13 patients who received either 2 servings per day of an EPA-enriched supplement or dietary counseling for 12 weeks. At the end of the trial, patients in the supplemented group significantly increased their weight after the intervention and had better scores in important domains of HRQOL, compared to controls. Although not statistically significant, the supplemented group did not experience interruptions in their chemotherapy treatment compared to the control group, with more interruptions due to toxicity.

In 2008 de Luis et al. investigated whether oral ambulatory nutrition of postsurgical head and neck cancer patients with recent weight loss, using two different omega-3 fatty acids enhanced diets could improve nutrition variables as well as clinical outcome (de Luis et al. 2008). A sample of 65 ambulatory postsurgical patients with oral and laryngeal cancer and recent weight loss was enrolled. At hospital discharge postsurgical head and neck cancer patients were asked to consume two cans per day of either a specially designed omega-3 fatty acid enhanced supplement with a high ratio of omega3/omega6 (I) or an omega-3 fatty acid enhanced supplement with a low ratio of omega3/omega6 (II). Serum albumin, prealbumin, and transferrin concentrations improved with both enhanced formulas. Weight stabilization was reached with both formulas. Gastrointestinal tolerance (diarrhea episodes) with both formulas was good (6.45% vs 5.88%: ns). The postoperative infectious complications were similar in both groups (29 group I vs 15.7% group II: ns). No local complications were detected in surgery wound. In conclusion, at dose taken, omega-3 enhanced formulas with different omega-3/omega-6 ratios improved serum protein concentrations in ambulatory postoperative head and neck cancer patients with good tolerance.

A 2007 study by Read et al. assessed the impact of an eicosapentanoic acid-containing protein and energy dense oral nutrition supplement (EPA-ONS) on nutrition and inflammatory status, QOL, plasma phospholipids (PPL) and cytokine profile, tolerance of irinotecan-containing chemotherapy and EPA-ONS in patients with advanced CRC receiving chemotherapy (Read et al. 2007). Twenty-three patients were enrolled in the study and received 480 mL of the EPA-ONS for 3 weeks. The mean EPA-ONS intake was 1.7 servings per day (408 mL). There was a significant increase in mean weight (2.5 kg) at 3 weeks ($p = 0.03$). LBM was maintained. Protein and energy intake significantly decreased after the commencement of chemotherapy (protein $p = 0.003$, energy $p = 0.02$). There was a significant increase in energy levels ($p = 0.03$), but all other QOL measures were maintained. PPL EPA levels increased significantly over the first 3 weeks. Mean C-reactive protein (CRP) increased by 14.9 mg/L over the first 3 weeks ($p = 0.004$), but decreased to baseline levels by the end of the study. There was a significant correlation between plasma IL-6 and IL-10 concentrations and survival, and between IL-12 and toxicity.

Bauer et al. in 2005 conducted a study to examine the effect of dietary compliance on intake and body composition in patients with unresectable pancreatic cancer (Bauer et al. 2005). The study included 200 patients who were randomized to receive 2 cans/day of a protein and energy dense, ONS ± n-3 fatty acids over 8 weeks. After the study period, there were significant differences in energy intake (501 kcal), protein intake (25.4 g), and weight (1.7 kg) between patients who were compliant with the nutrition prescription compared to noncompliant patients controlling for n-3 fatty acid randomization, baseline weight, and QOL. Over the 8-week period, there was significant improvement in weight only. There was no significant difference in the energy intake from meals of the total group over the 8 weeks.

In 2004 Moses et al. conducted a study to assess an EPA-enriched ONS in home-living cachectic patients with advanced pancreatic cancer (Moses et al. 2004). Twenty-four patients received an energy and protein dense oral supplement either enriched with or without the n-3 fatty acid EPA over an 8-week period. At baseline, REE was increased compared with predicted values for healthy individuals (1,387(42) vs 1,268(32) kcal day(−1), $p = 0.001$), but TEE (1,732(82) vs 1,903(48) kcal day(−1), $p = 0.023$) and PAL (1.24(0.04) vs 1.50) were reduced. After 8 weeks, the REE, TEE, and PAL of patients who received the control supplement did not change significantly. In contrast, although REE did not change, TEE and PAL increased significantly in those who received the n-3 (EPA) enriched supplement. In summary, patients with advanced pancreatic cancer were hypermetabolic. However, TEE was reduced, and this was secondary to a reduction in physical activity. The control energy and protein dense oral supplement did not influence the physical activity component of TEE. In contrast, administration of the supplement enriched with EPA was associated with an increase in physical activity, which may reflect improved QOL.

In 1999, Barber et al. conducted a study to determine if a combination of EPA with a conventional ONS could result in weight gain in patients with advanced pancreatic cancer (Barber et al. 1999). Twenty patients with unresectable pancreatic adenocarcinoma were provided with two servings of a fish oil-enriched nutrition supplement per day in addition to their normal food intake. Patients consumed a median of 1.9 servings per day (−1). After administration of the fish oil-enriched supplement, patients had significant weight-gain at both 3 (median 1 kg, $p = 0.024$) and 7 weeks (median 2 kg, $p = 0.033$). Dietary intake increased significantly by almost 400 kcal day(−1) ($p = 0.002$). REE per kg body weight and per kg LBM fell significantly. Performance status and appetite were significantly improved at 3 weeks.

SYSTEMATIC REVIEWS AND META-ANALYSES OF OMEGA-3 ENRICHED ONS FOR CANCER CACHEXIA

A 2020 systematic review by Ukovic and Porter aimed to systematically determine nutrition interventions that improve appetite and nutrition-related outcomes of adults with cancer undergoing cancer treatments, and to identify appetite assessment tools used to measure appetite (Ukovic and Porter 2020). This review included 24 studies and showed that the use of ONS and dietary counselling and increases in EPA from fish oil supplementation improved the appetite and nutrition outcomes of patients with cancer undergoing cancer treatments.

A 2018 systematic review by de van der Schueren et al. examined the evidence for oral nutrition interventions during chemo(radiotherapy) (de van der Schueren et al. 2018). This review included 11 studies and showed overall benefit of interventions on body weight during chemo(radio)therapy (+1.31 kg, 95% CI 0.24–2.38, $p = 0.02$, heterogeneity $Q = 21.1$, $p = 0.007$). Subgroup analysis showed no effect of dietary counseling and/or high-energy ONS (+0.80 kg, 95% CI −1.14 to 2.74, $p = 0.32$; $Q = 10.5$, $p = 0.03$). A significant effect was observed for high-protein n-3 PUFA-enriched intervention compared with isocaloric controls (+1.89 kg, 95% CI 0.51–3.27, $p = 0.02$; $Q = 3.1$ $p = 0.37$). High-protein, n-3 PUFA-enriched ONS studies showed attenuation of LBM loss ($N = 2$ studies) and improvement of some QOL domains ($N = 3$ studies).

In 2011 van der Meij et al. systematically reviewed the effects of oral or enteral and parenteral n-3 fatty acids supplementation on clinical outcomes and to describe the incorporation of n-3 fatty acids into phospholipids of plasma, blood cells, and mucosal tissue and the subsequent washout in these patients (van der Meij et al. 2011). Results demonstrated that oral or enteral supplementation of n-3 fatty acids contributed to the maintenance of body weight and QOL but not to survival in cancer patients.

Paccagnella et al. in 2011 conducted a review to assess various types of nutrition intervention for improving treatment tolerance in patients with malnutrition related to the cancer anorexia-cachexia syndrome (Paccagnella, Morassutti, and Rosti 2011). Results showed that supplementation with n-3 fatty acids appears to offer benefits that are verifiable at a biochemical, clinical, and functional level.

In 2007 Colomer et al. conducted a systematic review on n-3 fatty acids, cancer, and cachexia (Colomer et al. 2007). This review included seventeen studies and demonstrated that oral supplements with n-3 fatty acids benefit patients with advanced cancer and weight loss, and are indicated in tumors of the upper digestive tract and pancreas; the advantages observed were: increased weight and appetite, improved QoL, and reduced postsurgical morbidity; there is no defined pattern for combining different n-3 fatty acids, and it is recommended to administer >1.5 g/day of n-3 fatty acids; and better tolerance is obtained administering low-fat formulas for a period of at least 8 weeks.

A 2006 systematic review by Elia et al. aimed to determine the efficacy and potential benefits of enteral nutrition support (ONS or enteral tube feeding (ETF)), and EPA, free acid, ethyl esters, or fish oil; provided as capsules or enriched ONS or ETF in patients with cancer (Elia et al. 2006). Individual studies of EPA supplementation as capsules showed improvements in survival, complications, and inflammatory markers in patients undergoing BMT. In palliative care patients receiving EPA-enriched ONS or capsules, there were inconsistent positive effects on survival and QOL. In those undergoing surgery, EPA-enriched ETF had no effect.

EXPERT RECOMMENDATIONS AND GUIDELINES ON OMEGA-3 ENRICHED ONS FOR CANCER CACHEXIA

Based on the amount of evidence, several expert nutrition organizations have included recommendations for the use of EPA-enriched ONS in their guidelines. These guidelines include those from the AND, the ASPEN, and the ESPEN. Table 14.3 summarizes the current recommendations from each of these organizations for use of EPA-enriched ONS.

Nutrition challenges such as weight loss, malnutrition, loss of muscle mass, and cachexia are all evident in patients with cancer. These nutrition issues can result in numerous adverse effects on the patient and the healthcare system. Nutrition intervention, particularly with ONS, has been shown to improve outcomes in patients with cancer. In addition, ONS enriched with EPA, an omega-3 fatty acid, have been shown to be particularly beneficial in patients with muscle mass loss and cachexia. The use of supplements with EPA has also been recommended by various expert nutrition organizations to help improve outcomes in patients with muscle loss and cachexia.

OTHER NUTRIENTS/INGREDIENTS TO INHIBIT MUSCLE PROTEIN DEGRADATION

In addition to the immune modulating effect of fish oils (FO) in cancer patients, few other nutrients or ingredients possess anticatabolic effects could have a potentially important role in mitigating the extent of muscle loss associated with cancer cachexia. One example of such ingredients is β-hydroxy-β-methylbutyrate (HMB). HMB is a bioactive metabolite of the essential amino acid leucine and had been shown to stimulate muscle protein synthesis and inhibits muscle protein breakdown. A recent meta-analysis showed that HMB increased muscle mass and strength in a variety of clinical conditions (Bear et al. 2019). Consistently, Ritch et al. (2019) randomized elderly patients with bladder cancer undergoing surgery into two groups. The intervention group ($n = 31$) received standard diet plus an oral nutrition shake supplemented with 1.5 g of HMB while the control group was provided standard diet plus a multivitamin supplement ($n = 30$). Both groups received their dietary intervention for 4 weeks before and after surgery. At the end of the study duration, there was

TABLE 14.3

Society Guidelines on the Use of EPA-Enriched Oral Nutritional Supplements in Cancer Patients

Society	Recommendation(s)	Grading
AND (AND) (Thompson et al. 2017)	Dietary supplements or Medical Food Supplement (MFS) containing fish oil	Strong; imperative
	If suboptimal symptom control or inadequate dietary intake has been addressed and the adult	
	Oncology patient is still experiencing loss of weight and LBM, an RDN may consider use of dietary supplements containing EPA as a component of nutrition intervention	
	Dietary supplements or MFS containing fish oil	Strong; imperative
	If suboptimal symptom control or inadequate dietary intake has been addressed and the Adult oncology patient is still experiencing loss of weight and LBM, an RDN may consider use of MFS	
	Containing EPA as a component of nutrition intervention	
ASPEN (August, Huhmann, and Directors 2009)	ω-3 fatty acid supplementation may help stabilize weight in cancer patients on oral diets experiencing progressive, unintentional weight loss	B
ESPEN (Arends, et al. 2017a)	In patients with advanced cancer undergoing chemotherapy and at risk of weight loss or malnourished, we suggest to use supplementation with long-chain N-3 fatty acids or fish oil to stabilize or improve appetite, food intake, LBM, and body weight	Weak
ESPEN (Arends, et al. 2017b)	While studies are still needed to confirm improvement in clinical outcomes, fish oil remains promising as an important part of overall nutrition management	N/A

20% increase in sarcopenic patients ($p = 0.01$) in the control group and 16.7% increase in sarcopenic obese patients ($p = 0.01$) while there was a 33% decrease in the number of sarcopenic obese patients ($p = 0.01$). The study also showed a significant increase in lean mass in the intervention group as compared to controls.

PERIOPERATIVE NUTRITION NEEDS AND THE IMPACT OF MALNUTRITION ON THE SURGICAL ONCOLOGY PATIENT

PREVALENCE OF MALNUTRITION IN THE SURGICAL ONCOLOGY PATIENT

Malnutrition is a potentially modifiable risk factor for cancer patients though continues to be underdiagnosed in surgical populations (Williams et al. 2020). Malnutrition is especially prevalent among patients with gastrointestinal cancers, including pancreatic, liver, intestinal, and head and neck cancers. In the PreMiO study, patients with gastrointestinal tumors had the highest frequency of malnutrition compared to other tumor types at the first medical oncology visit (Muscaritoli et al. 2017). Surgery is often part of the treatment regimen in patients with gastrointestinal cancer and there is an especially high prevalence of malnutrition in this patient population. In a prospective study of 694 surgical patients, the prevalence of preoperative malnutrition was 65.3% for all surgical patients compared to 84.9% of gastrointestinal cancer patients (Shpata et al. 2014).

IMPACT OF MALNUTRITION ON THE SURGICAL PATIENT AND
EFFECT OF SARCOPENIA ON SURGICAL OUTCOMES

Malnutrition has a significant impact on surgical patients and is an independent predictor of poor outcomes after surgery (Figure 14.5). It is common during cancer due to increased metabolic needs, insufficient nutrient intake, and nutrient loss which can lead to weight loss, sarcopenia, and cancer cachexia. Patients with cancer are especially vulnerable when malnutrition, sarcopenia, and/ or cancer cachexia are present before surgery since surgery evokes a catabolic response resulting in further inflammation, muscle breakdown, and nitrogen losses leading to worse postsurgical outcomes.

As demonstrated in several studies, sarcopenia can significantly impact postoperative outcomes and overall survival in many cancer types, including gastric, esophageal, and CRC. According to a systematic review and meta-analysis of literature assessing body composition, sarcopenic gastric cancer patients had significantly higher rates of postoperative major complications, pulmonary complications, and worse survival after gastrectomy (Kamarajah, Bundred, and Tan 2018). In patients with esophageal cancer, Matsunaga et al. (2019) found a relationship between sarcopenia and the systemic inflammatory response before esophagectomy that was significantly associated with overall survival (Matsunaga et al. 2019).

Sarcopenia was significantly associated with a high C-reactive protein-to-albumin (CRP/Alb) ratio while the latter was an independent prognostic factor for recurrence-free survival. In patients receiving CRC resection, sarcopenia was associated with postoperative complications with longer postoperative hospital stays compared to nonsarcopenic patients (Nakanishi et al. 2018). Among postoperative complications, sarcopenia was associated with nonsurgical site infections (SSIs). Several studies report more patients with sarcopenia experiencing anticancer drug dose limiting toxicities in a variety of cancers including breast, colon, renal, liver, and thyroid compared to patients without sarcopenia (Antoun et al. 2013, Huillard et al. 2013, Massicotte et al. 2013, Mir et al. 2012,

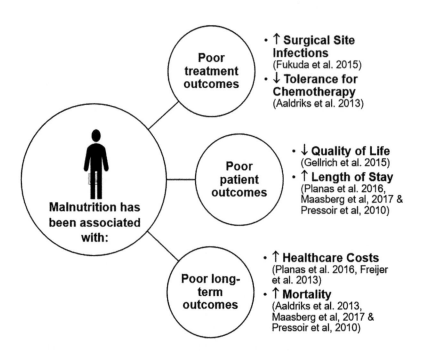

FIGURE 14.5 Patients with cancer and malnutrition have a higher risk for poor outcomes throughout cancer care (Fukuda et al. 2015, Aaldriks et al. 2013, Freijer et al. 2013, Gellrich et al. 2015, Maasberg et al. 2017, Planas et al. 2016, Pressoir et al. 2010).

Prado et al. 2007, Prado et al. 2009). Thirty to as high as 80% of oncology patients with sarcopenia experienced a dose-limiting toxicity compared to 2%–30% of patients without sarcopenia.

Controversy exists on whether obesity is protective for postsurgical outcomes based on the "obesity paradox" where the presence of obesity is protective in certain chronic diseases (Valentijn et al. 2013). However, the concomitant presence of obesity and sarcopenia is detrimental. Several studies demonstrate poorer postsurgical outcomes and survival in patients with pancreatic, liver, colorectal, and gastric cancer and sarcopenic obesity. In 2,297 patients with pancreatic ductal adenocarcinoma, a systematic review and meta-analysis reports that both sarcopenia and sarcopenic obesity are associated with a poorer overall survival (HR 1.49, $p < 0.001$ and HR 2.01, $p < 0.001$) (Mintziras et al. 2018). In a retrospective analysis of 465 patients undergoing surgical resection for hepatocellular carcinoma, Kobayashi et al. showed that preoperative sarcopenic obesity was an independent risk factor for death and recurrence of hepatocellular carcinoma posthepatectomy (Kobayashi et al. 2019). Sarcopenic obesity is also recognized as a strong risk factor for poor short- and long-term outcomes following gastrectomy. In a retrospective study of patients with gastric cancer who underwent laparoscopic total gastrectomy, sarcopenic obesity was found to be an independent risk factor for development of SSIs postsurgery (Nishigori et al. 2016). Zhang et al. (2018) found that sarcopenic obesity is an independent predictor of severe postoperative complications while Lou et al. 2017 found that sarcopenia in overweight and obese gastric cancer patients is predictive of postsurgical complications (Zhang et al. 2018, Lou et al. 2017). Thus, these publications support that sarcopenic obesity is an important risk factor for poor postsurgical outcomes and survival in the oncology population.

Preoperative Malnutrition Screening and Assessment in Surgical Oncology

For surgical oncology patients, early preoperative nutrition screening and assessment is recommended to allow for early integration of nutrition intervention prior to surgery. Screening and assessment tools must be able to detect malnutrition based on nutrition intake, as well as severity and duration of a disease, which can contribute to differing malnutrition pathophysiology. ESPEN recommends preoperative nutrition support in patients who meet at least one of the following criteria: severe weight loss (>10%–15% in 6 months), low BMI (BMI <18.5 kg/m^2), SGA Grade C, or serum albumin <30 g/L (in the absence of hepatic or renal failure) (see Table 14.4) (Weimann et al. 2017).

Monitoring and Evaluation: Nutrition Challenges of the GI Surgical Patient

GI cancers, including pancreatic, esophageal, gastric, and CRC, are among the most frequent cancers associated with malnutrition, weight loss, and cachexia (Baracos et al. 2018, Muscaritoli et al. 2017). The prevalence of weight loss in colorectal, head and neck, gastroesophageal, and

TABLE 14.4
ESPEN Clinical Guidelines Recommend Preoperative Nutrition Support in Patients Meeting at Least One of the Following Criteria

Criteria	Value
Weight loss	>10%–15% within 6 months
BMI	<18.5 kg/m^2
SGA	Grade C or NRS >5
Preoperative serum albumin	<30 g/L (with no evidence of hepatic or renal dysfunction)

Source: Weimann et al. (2017).

pancreatic ranges from 45% to 65% of patients. The prevalence of cachexia varies by cancer site and stage with muscle loss occurring in 65% (stages 1–3) versus 85% (stage 4) of patients with gastroesophageal cancer and in 30% (stages 1–3) versus 45% (stage 4) head and neck cancer.

Meeting the nutrition needs of the surgical patient with GI cancer is especially challenging due to the location of the tumor and/or its impact on the digestive process or side effects from cancer treatments. Many cancer treatment-related side effects may impact appetite including diarrhea, fatigue, abdominal cramps, dry mouth, taste changes, and nausea (Aslam 2014, Gamper et al. 2012). Appetite suppression can be exacerbated in the GI patient due to bowel obstruction from the mechanical effects of the tumor, which can cause nausea, vomiting, early satiety, and abdominal pain. Smaller, more frequent meals and including nutrient dense ONS can help improve nutrition intake. Chemotherapy and radiation therapy can cause several complications that may impact appetite such as altered taste perceptions including an intolerance to meat or a metallic taste (Jensen et al. 2008) and depression of sweet, bitter, and salty taste (Deshpande et al. 2018), respectively. Both chemotherapy and radiation treatments can lead to nausea and/or diarrhea and oral mucositis which commonly occurs in the tongue, cheeks, and lips, making eating and swallowing painful. Additionally, poor absorption of nutrients after surgery can worsen or lead to malnutrition. If weight loss occurs due to inability to meet nutrition needs or oral intake is insufficient then nutrition support such as high-calorie, high-protein ONS should be prescribed. If weight loss becomes severe or the patient is unable to orally consume foods, then EN (if the digestive tract is functional) or PN should be implemented.

Nutrition and pharmacological interventions may attenuate the hypermetabolic response to surgery resulting in improved patient outcomes. Therefore, the main goals of nutrition therapy in surgical patients are to provide adequate nutrition intake to maintain and prevent muscle loss, modulate inflammation and the immune response, control glucose levels, attenuate the hypermetabolic response, and provide nutrition to help with the healing and recovery process (Weimann et al. 2017). These goals will be discussed in more detail in the following sections and are summarized in Table 14.5.

PERIOPERATIVE NUTRITION CARE OF THE SURGICAL ONCOLOGY PATIENT

Due to the challenges of caring for surgical oncology patients, a large body of research has focused on optimizing nutrition-related protocols to improve outcomes in this group. Multiple professional societies have authored evidence-based guidelines informed by these data. Guidance from the following societies will be discussed in this section: American Society for Enhanced Recovery (ASER) and Perioperative Quality Initiate (POQI), American Society of Anesthesiologists (ASA), the ESPEN, Enhanced Recovery After Surgery (ERAS), ASPEN and Society of Critical Care Medicine (ASPEN/SCCM), and ACS Strong for Surgery. These recommendations vary in the timing of interventions with some focusing primarily on the preoperative preparation of patients for surgery, while others, such as ERAS, discuss protocols which span the entire perioperative period. Figure 14.6 summarizes evidence-based perioperative nutrition protocols which will be discussed in more detail in the following sections.

TABLE 14.5

Medical Nutrition Therapy Goals in Surgical Oncology Patients

- Provide adequate nutritional intake to maintain and prevent muscle loss
- Modulate inflammation and the immune response
- Manage perioperative glucose levels
- Attenuate the hypermetabolic response
- Provide nutrition to assist with healing and recovery

Protocol	Preoperative				Day of Surgery	Postoperative			
	Initial Visit	–15d	–10d	–5d		5d	10d	15d	+20d
Screen all patients for risk of malnutrition	●								
Encourage preoperative nutrition support in high-risk patients	◄———————								
Suggest perioperative immunonutrition support				●———		——●			
Minimize preoperative fasting period (allow clears until 2h preop)					●				
Recommend preoperative carbohydrate loading					●				
Allow intake on postoperative day one						●			
Encourage continued postoperative nutrition support						——————————————►			

FIGURE 14.6 Example protocol for perioperative nutrition care of oncology patients predicated on evidence-based guidelines and recommendations.

Prehabilitation care refers to attempts made to optimize modifiable lifestyle factors prior to surgery. For example, the ACS Strong for Surgery program recommends preoperative interventions such as improving glycemic control and screening for malnutrition. Prehabilitation may take place during routine cancer care once the decision for surgery has been made or patients may be referred to a preoperative clinic if available within the institution. Patients found to be at increased risk after malnutrition screening are referred to an Registered Dietitian Nutritionist (RDN). During nutrition counseling, the RDN may address barriers to consuming appropriate nutrient needs, strategies to improve intake prior to surgery, and suggestions for supplementation including fortified foods and/ or ONS if the patient is unable to meet calorie needs through traditional diet. Preoperative clinics may also make other needed referrals beyond the RDN (such as endocrinology, physical therapy, social work) to prepare patients for elective procedures.

Although the optimal timing of prehabilitation is not clear, Fukuda et al. analyzed a cohort of 152 patients with gastric cancer and malnutrition and found that a longer duration of preoperative nutrition support (including ONS) was associated with a significant reduction in postoperative SSIs. SSIs occurred in 50.8% of patients who received no nutrition intervention, 37.5% of patients receiving nutrition intervention for 1–9 days, 18.2% of those receiving nutrition intervention for 10–13 days, and 16.1% of those receiving nutrition intervention for >14 days (Fukuda et al. 2015). During the preoperative period, patients may also begin to consume supplements containing immune-modulating nutrients (see "immunonutrition" section) to prepare for surgery.

Additional nutrition strategies which may be employed prior to surgery include a minimized preoperative fasting period which is supported by multiple organizations including the ASA, ASER/ POQI, and ERAS. Although these recommendations are not new, it is still common for patients to be asked to fast from midnight the day before surgery regardless of their malnutrition status or scheduled operation time. This request may be based on the misconception that intake of fluids prior to surgery will increase aspiration risk during surgery. In fact, multiple studies have reported that clear liquids can be consumed up to 2 hours prior to surgery without complication (Ljungqvist and Soreide 2003). Based on these and subsequent findings, the ASA recommends that patients be allowed to eat solids up to 6 hours preoperatively and to consume clear liquids until 2 hours prior to anesthesia. The ASA describes clear liquids as water, tea, coffee, carbonated beverages, fruit juice with no pulp, and carbohydrate-containing nutrition drinks (Ljungqvist and Soreide 2003).

Preoperative Carbohydrate Loading for Surgical Oncology

Preoperative carbohydrates may offer a unique advantage with regard to surgical outcomes as they have been associated with significant improvements in preoperative patient reported outcomes and postoperative insulin resistance (Wang et al. 2010). Surgery elicits a stress response, driven by counter-regulatory hormones and circulating cytokines which stimulates mobilization of fuels through glycogenolysis, proteolysis, and lipolysis. Although this is thought to be an adaptive response to trauma to provide fuel for healing and support the immune response, in the setting of a controlled operating room, this contributes to hyperglycemia and insulin resistance.

Hyperglycemia and fluctuations in blood glucose have been associated with negative outcomes such as SSIs (Ambiru et al. 2008), postoperative complications (Fiorillo et al. 2017), and mortality (Li et al. 2012, Awad et al. 2013, Jackson et al. 2012) in surgical oncology patients. Therefore, attempts to manage blood glucose levels and minimize glucose excursions should be pursued.

Multiple meta-analyses have reported that intake of preoperative carbohydrate-containing drinks decreases postoperative insulin resistance. Some have even reported a small but significant reduction in LOS by 0.7–1.1 days in those consuming a preoperative carbohydrate load versus fasting or placebo in patients undergoing major surgeries (Awad et al. 2013, Amer et al. 2017). Of significance to surgical patients, multiple trials have also reported improved patient-reported outcomes including a reduction in preoperative thirst, hunger, and anxiety (Hausel et al. 2001, Canbay et al. 2014). Another study in colorectal surgery patients reported a significant reduction in nausea and requests for antiemetic medications in those receiving carbohydrates 2 hours preoperatively compared to those advised to fast for 8 hours preoperatively (Rizvanovic et al. 2019). An example carbohydrate loading regimen commonly used in the literature is 100 g of carbohydrates the night before surgery and 50 g 2–3 hours before induction of anesthesia. Preoperative carbohydrate loading is supported by multiple societies including ERAS, ASA, and ASER/POQI. The ASER/POQI recommendations suggest that ingestion of complex carbohydrates is preferable to drinks containing simple sugars.

Currently, carbohydrate loading is not recommended in patients with type 1 diabetes. Additionally, there is limited data to support strong recommendations in patients with type 2 diabetes. Surgical patients with diabetes are at an increased risk of postoperative impaired glycemic control. Due to concerns of delayed gastric emptying, risk of aspiration, and poor perioperative glycemic control, many surgical patients with diabetes do not receive preoperative carbohydrate loading (Gustafsson et al. 2008). However, limited data suggest that type 2 diabetic patients may safely receive preoperative carbohydrate loading 3 hours before anesthesia. A 2008 study examined gastric emptying rates and postprandial glucose rates in subjects with well-controlled type 2 diabetic compared to nondiabetic subjects and found no signs of delayed gastric emptying (Gustafsson et al. 2008). Ultimately, clinical judgement based on individual patient's needs should guide implementation of preoperative carbohydrate loading in patients with type 2 diabetes at this time.

Immunonutrition for Surgical Oncology

Beyond hyperglycemia, surgical stress may also encourage inflammation and a resultant arginine-deficient state by stimulating arginase-releasing myeloid-derived suppressor cells, thus decreasing the availability of arginine (Makarenkova et al. 2006, Marik and Flemmer 2012). Additionally, the concentration of circulating arginine has been reported to be lower in individuals with cancer than healthy individuals matched for age and sex (Vissers et al. 2005). Arginine is an important precursor for the production of nitric oxide through endothelial nitric-oxide synthase and also contributes to optimal T-regulatory cell function and collagen formation (Zhu et al. 2014, Makarenkova et al. 2006). Following surgical stress, inflammatory cytokines are transiently increased which has been associated with greater risk for complications (Baker et al. 2006). Therefore, nutrients that modulate inflammation may also be of benefit such as omega-3 fatty acids (DHA and EPA).

Preclinical studies suggest that omega-3 fatty acids modulate the inflammatory response by displacing arachidonic acid in the cell membrane of immune cells creating a more fluid membrane and reducing the production of proinflammatory prostaglandins and leukotrienes (Calder 2008, 2013). Additionally, DHA and EPA serve as precursors for specialized proresolving mediators (resolvins and protectins) which act to modulate the inflammatory response. Finally, omega-3 fatty acids can reduce the action of tumor necrosis factor alpha via peroxisome proliferator-activated receptor gamma, thus reducing the transcription of proinflammatory cytokines. The combination of arginine and omega-3 fatty acids has been suggested to have a synergistic effect in improving surgical outcomes such as wound healing and infectious complications. Additionally, the combination of arginine and omega-3 fatty acids has been found to increase immune cell populations and decrease proinflammatory cytokines (Wu, Zhang, and Wu 2001, Gianotti et al. 1999, Chen et al. 2005,

Liu et al. 2012). Although other nutrients such as nucleotides have been incorporated into commercially available immunonutrition supplements, the unique contribution of their presence remains to be elucidated in trials with surgical patients.

A consistent stream of literature on immunonutrition has been published over the last three decades. A recent meta-analysis identified 61 randomized control trials (RCTs) and reported that immunonutrition as compared to standard enteral formula, significantly reduced the risk of wound infections, risk of respiratory tract infections, risk of anastomotic leak, and the length of hospital stay by 2.1 days in patients with cancer (Yu et al. 2020). Even well-nourished patients with cancer appear to benefit from immunonutrition by means of reduced postoperative infectious complications (Zhang et al. 2020). Importantly, the patients in these meta-analyses included a variety of surgery types including colorectal, liver, pancreatic, and head/neck. To more specifically review the evidence, the following sections will organize available data based on surgical subsets of the oncology surgery population.

It is worth noting that in addition to surgical cancer patients, immunonutrition is also utilized in chemoradiation therapy. While the role of immunonutrition in reducing inflammation in chemoradiation is debated (Leung and Chan 2016), data show that glutamine may improve the severity and incidence of oral mucositis caused by radiotherapy (Cao et al. 2017). A 2020 systematic review and meta-analysis of the effects of immunonutrition, including glutamine, on 1,478 chemoradiotherapy patients from 27 studies (Zheng et al. 2020) observed that immunonutrition reduced grade >3 oral mucositis, grade >3 diarrhea, grade >3 esophagitis, and reducing the rate of >5% body weight loss. No significant effects of immunonutrition on incidence rates of oral mucositis, diarrhea, or esophagitis were observed.

Gastrointestinal Cancer

The use of immunonutrition has been extensively studied in patients undergoing surgeries of the upper and lower GI tract. Common oncology GI surgeries include esophagectomy, gastrectomy, and colorectal surgery. Meta-analyses data of 16 trials including gastrectomy patients reported a significant reduction in SSIs, a shorter length of hospital stay (−1.3 days) and reduced C-reactive protein and white blood cell counts in those receiving immunonutrition rather than standard nutrition (Niu et al. 2020). In colorectal surgery patients, a meta-analysis of nine RCTs reported that immunonutrition significantly reduced the length of hospital stay by 2.5 days and reduced infectious complications (Xu et al. 2018). Moya and colleagues reported that the use of immunonutrition also yields benefits within the context of an ERAS program (Moya et al. 2016). Specifically, infectious complications were 23.8% in the control group versus 10.7% in the group receiving immunonutrition ($p = 0.0007$).

Mingliang conducted a meta-analysis of 7 RCTs comparing perioperative use of immunonutrition versus standard nutrition in 606 esophagectomy patients (Mingliang et al. 2020). Although a trend toward a reduction in anastomotic leakage was reported (5.4% vs 9.4%, $p = 0.07$), the authors found no difference in postoperative complications, wound infection, sepsis, or urinary tract infections.

Taken together, these findings suggest that the use of immunonutrition is beneficial in patients receiving GI oncology surgery, specifically, those receiving colorectal surgery. In fact, use of immunonutrition is supported by ERAS guidelines for CRC patients with malnutrition (Gustafsson et al. 2019).

The use of perioperative oral immunonutrition was not supported in the 2016 ERAS guidelines for liver surgery due to limited evidence. Subsequent studies have found that immunonutrition may be beneficial for patients receiving hepatectomy. Zhang et al. conducted a meta-analysis of eight studies and found that immunonutrition use, compared with an isocaloric control diet, significantly reduced the relative risk of infectious complications, total postoperative complication, and LOS (−0.49 days) in hepatectomy patients (Zhang et al. 2017). No significant difference in mortality was reported in this study.

In 2019, a meta-analysis of 4 RCTs including 299 pancreaticoduodenectomy patients receiving immunonutrition reported beneficial outcomes (Guan, Chen, and Huang 2019). Specifically, postoperative infectious complications were significantly lower in the group receiving immunonutrition and LOS was also reduced by 1.8 days compared to standard enteral nutrition formulas. Risk of noninfectious complications and mortality were not significantly different between groups. Despite these positive findings and a lack of data suggesting that immunonutrition is inferior to standard enteral nutrition formulas, the 2020 ERAS guidelines for pancreatoduodenectomy do not support the routine use of immunonutrition citing study heterogeneity as a significant barrier.

Head and Neck Cancers

The use of immunonutrition was evaluated in 96 patients receiving salvage surgery for recurrent head and neck squamous cell carcinoma. Compared to historic controls which did not receive immunonutrition, those who received preoperative immunonutrition had a lower rate of overall complications (35% versus 58%, $p = 0.034$). The control group in this study also had a hospital LOS of 17 days versus 6 days in the immunonutrition group ($p < 0.001$) (Mueller et al. 2019). Similar results were reported in a larger study of 411 patients with head and neck squamous cell carcinoma (Aeberhard et al. 2018). Hospital LOS was 5.65 days shorter in the group receiving perioperative immunonutrition ($p < 0.001$) and infections were reduced from 15.3% in the control group to 7.4% in the immunonutrition group ($p = 0.006$). These findings align with a previously published meta-analysis which found that arginine-enriched enteral formulas were superior to nonarginine containing formulas when given peri- or postoperatively to surgical patients with head and neck cancer (Vidal-Casariego et al. 2014). Specifically, the meta-analysis included six studies and concluded that arginine-containing formulas were associated with a reduced risk of fistulas and a 6.8-day reduction in length of hospital stay.

Overall, these studies reveal multiple benefits associated with the use of immunonutrition in patients with cancer of the head and neck; however, available guidelines from the ERAS society state, "there are insufficient data to provide a recommendation on the use of IMN" for head and neck cancer patients at this time (Dort et al. 2017).

Timing of Immunonutrition for Surgical Oncology

The use of immunonutrition (IMN) is supported by multiple guidelines including ESPEN (Arends et al. 2017a), ASPEN/SCCM (McClave et al. 2016), ASER/POQI (Wischmeyer et al. 2018), and specific surgery subsets within ERAS as shown in the sections above and in Table 14.6. Noticeably, the guidelines vary on the recommended timing of immunonutrition intervention. Perioperative administration of immunonutrition extends 5–7 days before surgery and is continued for 5–7 days postoperatively. Perioperative immunonutrition is supported in the ERAS guidelines for CRC surgery and ASER/POQI guidelines for patients receiving major abdominal (Gustafsson et al. 2019, Wischmeyer et al. 2018). The ESPEN guidelines suggest that immunonutrition should be provided perioperatively or at minimum postoperatively and the ASPEN guidelines suggest routine use of immunonutrition in the postoperative surgical ICU patient. Finally, the ACS Strong for Surgery Toolkit suggests that immunonutrition be provided 5 days preoperatively (Thornblade et al. 2017).

Due to inconsistencies in the existing guidelines, questions remain about the most ideal timing for immunonutrition. At least three meta-analyses and a systematic review have sought to answer this question (Marimuthu et al. 2012, Drover et al. 2011, Osland et al. 2014, Song et al. 2015). In 2011, Drover and colleagues conducted a systematic review and reported that the relative risk for infectious complications and hospital LOS were lower in patients receiving arginine-enriched formula perioperatively than patients receiving arginine-enriched formula only in the pre- or postoperative setting (Drover et al. 2011). Studies included in this systematic review primarily recruited patients with various forms of cancer (head and neck, gastric, colorectal, pancreatic, etc.). The following year, a meta-analysis of 26 RCTs including patients with open GI surgery, found infectious

TABLE 14.6
Selected Immunonutrition Recommendations

Society	Immunonutrition Guideline
SCCM and ASPEN (McClave et al. 2016)	We suggest the routine use of an immune-modulating formula (containing arginine and fish oils) in the SICU for the postoperative patient who requires EN therapy
ESPEN (Weimann et al. 2017)	Peri- or at least postoperative administration of specific formula enriched with immunonutrients (arginine, omega-3-fatty acids, ribonucleotides) should be given in malnourished patients undergoing major cancer surgery.
	There is currently no clear evidence for the use of these formulae enriched with immunonutrients vs. standard oral nutritional supplements exclusively in the preoperative period
ESPEN (Arends et al. 2017a)	In upper GI cancer patients undergoing surgical resection in the context of traditional perioperative care we recommend oral/enteral immunonutrition
ASER and POQI (Wischmeyer et al. 2018)	Preoperative IMN should be considered for all patients undergoing elective major abdominal surgery
	IMN should be considered in all postoperative major abdominal surgical patients for at least 7 days
ERAS society: elective colorectal surgery (Gustafsson et al. 2019)	Perioperative IMN in malnourished patients is beneficial in CRC surgery

complication risk to be reduced regardless of the timing of immunonutrition. However, reductions in LOS and noninfectious complications were most pronounced in those receiving peri- and postoperative immunonutrition administration (Marimuthu et al. 2012).

This finding was replicated in a later meta-analysis of 20 studies by Osland et al. (2014). Notably, this group also reported that perioperative immunonutrition yielded an additional advantage; lower risk for anastomotic dehiscence. Finally, results from a Bayesian network meta-analysis provide even further data concerning the optimal timing of immunonutrition intervention (Song et al. 2015). After analysis of 27 RCTs, the authors conclude that "perioperative enteral immunonutrition regime is the optimum option" for patients receiving surgical treatment for gastrointestinal cancer. To summarize, these studies provide strong scientific support for the provision of immunonutrition both before and after surgery to ensure optimal patient outcomes.

Postoperative Nutrition Care for Surgical Oncology

Following surgery, it is important that cancer patients, especially those with pre-existing malnutrition, are allowed early access to nutrition within 24–48 hours of surgery. Early enteral nutrition is supported by ASPEN/SCCM, ESPEN, and ASER/POQI. Traditionally, oral nutrition intake began with clear liquids and continued through a transitional diet until the patient was allowed full solid food. Unfortunately, this transitional diet may unnecessarily restrict the dietary intake of postsurgical patients and provide inadequate amounts of protein and calories, thus exacerbating the patients risk for malnutrition. Therefore, this protocol has been challenged. In fact, the 2016 ASPEN/SCCM critical care guidelines state that clear liquids may not be needed as the first meal following surgery and advocate that solid food be allowed as tolerated. This recommendation was based on expert consensus and the findings that when compared to clear-liquids, standard meals on postoperative day one did not increase complications or nausea (Pearl et al. 2002, Jeffery et al. 1996, Lassen et al. 2008). Yet, if clear liquids are still used in the early preoperative period, attempts should be made to provide high-protein clear liquids. ASER/POQI suggest that, in the postoperative period, clear and full liquids diets should not be used and that meeting protein goals should be prioritized over meeting calorie goals (Wischmeyer et al. 2018).

Following discharge, oncology surgery patients may continue to have elevated nutrition needs that are exacerbated by the surgical recovery process. Therefore, patients may struggle to meet recommended intake through diet alone leading to weight loss and postoperative complications. Postoperative patients should be routinely assessed for ability to meet dietary recommendations and weight loss. If dietary intake is found to be inadequate, the use of ONS may be beneficial. Oral nutrition supplementation for 12 weeks following total gastrectomy was associated with significantly less weight loss compared to usual care (-6.9 vs -9.1 kg; $p = 0.03$) (Hatao et al. 2017). In another RCT, postsurgical oncology patients receiving ONS for 90 days had significantly greater weight gain of 1.35 ± 0.53 kg and 1.35 ± 0.73 kg at 60- and 90-day follow-up compared to standard care (-1.01 ± 0.54 kg, and -1.60 ± 0.81 kg at 60 and 90 days) (Zhu et al. 2019). Beyond general weight loss, postoperative oncology patients may experience an accelerated loss of LBM placing them at risk for sarcopenia or cachexia.

The use of ONS during recovery has been found to reduce the prevalence of sarcopenia. Over the 3-month postoperative period, oncology patients were randomized to either standard dietary advice or dietary advice with ONS. At follow-up, sarcopenia prevalence was 28.6% in CRC surgery patients receiving ONS and dietary advice versus 42.1% in the group only receiving dietary advice ($p = 0.04$) (Tan et al. 2020). This study design was also repeated in 337 gastric cancer surgery patients with a similar reduction in sarcopenia prevalence reported as well as other benefits in the dietary advice and ONS group such as lower perceived fatigue and a reduction in appetite loss (Meng et al. 2021).

In line with these findings, ASER/POQI suggest that high protein-ONS be consumed for a minimum of 4–8 weeks after major surgeries (Wischmeyer et al. 2018). They suggest that ONS use may be needed for 3–6 months in higher risk patients such as those with severe malnutrition or who required longer lengths of stay following surgery.

Finally, depending on the type of procedure, patients may need on-going monitoring for nutrition complications. For example, gastrectomy patients may experience loss of intrinsic factor and stomach acidity which may increase risk for long-term deficiencies of vitamin B12, calcium, and iron. At 48-month follow-up, anemia was reported in 60.7% of total gastrectomy patients and 31.3% of those receiving partial gastrectomy (Lim et al. 2012, Lee et al. 2019). Gastrectomy as well as pancreatic resection may increase risk of dumping syndrome and steatorrhea, thus challenging the absorption and availability of fat-soluble vitamins (Gilliland et al. 2017). Finally, because nutrients are absorbed at various locations within the intestine, surgical alteration at these sites may lead to nutrition deficiencies and weight loss overtime.

Implementing Perioperative Protocols in Surgical Oncology

Given the strong scientific support for the perioperative nutrition care of cancer patients and programs such as ERAS, many institutions are seeking to implement these protocols. Yet, implementation may be a challenge. For example, in a national survey of colorectal and GI surgical oncology programs, only 38% of programs had a formal nutrition screening process and 43% of patients received nutrition screening preoperatively (Williams and Wischmeyer 2017). Of surveyed surgeons, 83% of surgeons agreed that preop ONS may reduce complication rate, yet, only 21% of patients received ONS preoperatively. Postoperative use of ONS may be even lower. Of 2.8 million surgical encounters across 172 hospitals, only 15% of malnourished patients received postoperative ONS (Williams et al. 2020). Another challenge may be access to allied health professionals such as an RDN within cancer care settings. It has been reported that there is 1 RDN for every 2,308 oncology patients (Trujillo et al. 2019). Given these barriers, multiple organizations have created toolkits to assist with implementation and monitoring of perioperative protocols (see Table 14.7).

TABLE 14.7
Implementation Toolkits and Resources

ASER enhanced recovery implementation guide	https://aserhq.org
ERAS® implementation program (EIP)	https://erassociety.org/implementation/
ERAS® interactive audit system	https://erassociety.org/interactive-audit/
ACS strong for surgery toolkit	https://www.facs.org/quality-programs/strong-for-surgery/access

The protocols detailed above promote patient-centered care by considering factors such as the presence of malnutrition and how nutrition needs may vary based on treatment. These protocols also represent opportunities to engage the patient and their family members or caretakers in pre-/postsurgical care.

Perioperative protocols promote patient-centered care by considering factors such as the presence of malnutrition and how nutrition needs may vary based on treatment. These protocols also represent opportunities to engage the patient and their family members or caretakers in pre-/post-surgical care.

TRANSITIONS OF CARE AND LONG-TERM NUTRITION SUPPORT OF THE SURGICAL ONCOLOGY PATIENT

Cancer patients, particularly patients with gastrointestinal cancer, may still be malnourished or at high risk for malnutrition following surgery due to postoperative complications, reduced postoperative dietary intake, chronic comorbidities, involuntary weight loss prior to surgery (Wischmeyer et al. 2018), or the decline in nutritional status that frequently results with chemoradiotherapy (Lin et al. 2016). Even if nutritional support occurs while inpatient, this nutritional risk may continue following hospital discharge. Therefore, following discharge, oncology surgery patients may continue to have elevated nutrition needs that are exacerbated by the surgical recovery process. Patients may struggle to meet recommended intake through diet alone leading to weight loss and postoperative complications. A compromised nutritional status, without adequate support at home is, associated with a downward spiral in health that often results in an increased risk of readmission to hospital and a longer length of hospital stay (Deutz et al. 2016, Barker, Gout, and Crowe 2011), resulting in overall higher healthcare costs (Buitrago et al. 2019). The deleterious impact of malnutrition may be enhanced in the cancer patient. Therefore, appropriate discharge planning should include a long-term nutrition optimization strategy to ensure that nutrition resources are available when transitioned from the hospital setting back into the community.

Postdischarge Dietitian Counseling

Strategies to improve postdischarge nutrition care may include individualized dietary counselling following discharge, which can improve long term nutritional status of patients at nutritional risk. A meta-analysis by Munk et al. demonstrated that individualized dietary counselling by dietitians following discharge from acute hospital to home significantly improved body weight [mean difference (MD) = 1.01 kg, 95% CI = 0.08–1.95, $p = 0.03$], energy intake (MD = 1.10 MJ day(−1), 95% confidence interval (CI) = 0.66–1.54, $P < 0.001$), and protein intake (MD = 10.13 g day(−1), 95% CI = 5.14–15.13, $P < 0.001$) (Munk et al. 2016). Similarly, a study Hamirudin et al. aimed to determine if a model of home-based dietetic care could improve dietary intake and weight status in older adults posthospitalization. Dietetic intervention resulted in significantly higher mean protein intake per body weight (1.7 ± 0.4 g/kg) in the underweight group (BMI < 23 kg/m^2) compared to those who were a desirable weight (BMI 23–27 kg/m^2) (1.4 ± 0.3 g/kg) or overweight (BMI > 27 kg m^2)

$(1.1 \pm 0.3$ g/kg$)$ $(p < 0.001)$ 3 months after hospital discharge in older adults living in the community (Hamirudin et al. 2017). These findings are echoed by Beck et al. who randomized geriatric patients at nutritional risk to receive dietitian counseling at hospital discharge. The authors conclude that adding a dietitian to the discharge team could improve the nutritional status of geriatric patients through increased body weight, energy and protein intake, and reduce hospital readmission rates at 6 months (Beck et al. 2015). Collectively, these studies support the potential benefit in nutrition care by including dietitian counseling in the postdischarge planning of cancer patients.

ORAL NUTRITION SUPPLEMENTS

The use of various types of ONS after hospital discharge is another common strategy to continue postdischarge nutritional support in the community setting if dietary intake is found to be inadequate, as these products have been shown to reduce readmissions (Cawood, Elia, and Stratton 2012, Stratton, Hebuterne, and Elia 2013) and increase dietary intake (Milne et al. 2009), while remaining cost-effective (Barker, Gout, and Crowe 2011, Buitrago et al. 2019, Curtis et al. 2017, Elia et al. 2016). A recent RCT assessed the impact of consuming ONS on postoperative health outcomes in postdischarge patients at nutritional risk based on the Nutritional Risk Screening 2002 following CRC surgery (Tan et al. 2020). In this study, patient were randomized to receive either dietary advice alone (control group) or dietary advice in combination with daily ONS (ONS group) for 3 months (Tan et al. 2020). The ONS group had a significantly lower sarcopenia prevalence (28.6% vs 42.1%, $p = 0.040$). This study also showed that chemotherapy modifications, such as delay, dose reduction, or termination, were significantly reduced in the ONS group (21.2% vs 36.8%, $p = 0.024$). While no significant difference between the two groups was found in the 90-day readmission rate $(p > 0.05)$ or in QOL $(p > 0.05)$, this study suggests the long-term use of ONS in postdischarge patients at nutritional risk following CRC surgery may reduce skeletal muscle loss, and improve chemotherapy tolerance, compared with dietary advice alone. Moreover, oral nutrition supplementation for 12 weeks following total gastrectomy was associated with significantly less weight loss compared to usual care (-6.9 kg vs -9.1 kg; $p = 0.03$) (Hatao et al. 2017). In another RCT, postsurgical oncology patients receiving ONS for 90 days had significantly greater weight gain of 1.35 ± 0.53 kg and 1.35 ± 0.73 kg at 60- and 90-day follow-up compared to standard care (-1.01 ± 0.54 kg, and -1.60 ± 0.81 kg at 60 and 90 days) (Zhu et al. 2019).

DILIGENT POSTDISCHARGE MALNUTRITION SURVEILLANCE

The ESPEN recommend the use of appropriate nutritional support therapy for surgical cancer patients at risk of malnutrition after discharge from the hospital to improve their nutritional status and prognosis (Arends et al. 2017a). Postdischarge nutrition support plans for all cancer patients should include regular screening for the risk or the presence of malnutrition. Nutrition risk screening aims to increase awareness and allow early recognition and treatment. Protein catabolism resulting inflammation is associated with altered protein turnover, loss of fat and muscle mass, and an increase in the production of acute phase proteins. Skeletal muscle loss, with or without fat loss, is the main characteristic of cancer-associated malnutrition that predicts risk of physical impairment, postoperative complications, chemotherapy toxicity, and mortality (Baracos and Kazemi-Bajestani 2013, Martin et al. 2013). Moreover, weight loss (Dewys et al. 1980), impaired physical performance (Jang et al. 2014), and systemic inflammation in patients with cancer are all independent risk factors for increased toxicity of anticancer treatments that may lead to reductions or interruptions of treatment, reduced QOL, and poor prognosis (Arends et al. 2017a). With the exception of end of life care, all cancer patients with an inability to achieve their energy substrate requirements should receive a step-wise nutritional intervention from counseling by a nutrition professional to advanced nutrition therapy throughout the continuum of care.

ONCOLOGY NUTRITION ECONOMICS AND QUALITY IMPROVEMENT PROGRAMS

Cancer diagnoses are among the costliest diseases in the US. Each year more than 1.6 million Americans are diagnosed with cancer (Centers for Medicare & Medicaid Services, 2020b) and this is predicted to rise to 1.91 million by 2026 (Thompson, 2018). Medical advances have helped to significantly increase survival, with cancer mortality falling 23% in a single generation (Siegel et al., 2016). However, the same innovations and developments that have increased survival rates have also increased healthcare costs. Medical expenditures for cancer are projected to reach over $158 billion in 2020, a 27% increase from 2010, with a significant proportion of those costs paid by Medicare (Centers for Medicare & Medicaid Services Innovation Center, 2020a).

It is believed that the US healthcare system—led by reforms in Medicare payments—has reached a tipping point in moving toward value-based care (Harpaz, 2019). The transition away from fee-for-service to value-based care models is in part driven by concerns that the continued rising cost of healthcare limits access to care. Certainly, rising cancer incidence and costs of care are part of this equation, particularly as some patients and families face "financial toxicity" where they become unable to continue paying for expensive cancer treatments (Zafar and Abernethy, 2013).

Other major areas of focus in today's evolving healthcare models are patient centeredness and telehealth. In this section, we discuss how quality oncology nutrition care can support value-based care and quality programs as well as support patient-centered care and the developments in telehealth.

Opportunities in Value-Based Care and Nutrition-Focused Quality Improvement Programs for Cancer Patients

In the United States, the Centers for Medicare & Medicaid Services (CMS) healthcare payment and delivery models are structured to reinforce its three-part aim of better care for individuals, better health for populations, and lower costs. To achieve this, Medicare value-based care and quality programs link payments to specific quality measure reporting and targeted outcomes. Many of these measures and outcomes can be improved by good nutrition care. Malnutrition interventions, including nutrition support through dietary counseling, diet fortification, ONS, and enteral and parenteral nutrition, can help impact quality measures and improve health outcomes (Arends et al. 2017a). A formal way to introduce nutrition interventions to healthcare systems is through Quality Improvement Programs (QIPs). A nutrition-focused QIP can enhance identification and management of patients who are malnourished or at risk for malnutrition and yield significant improvements in health and economic outcomes throughout the continuum of care. Addressing malnutrition across different care settings has been well documented to improve patient outcomes and reduce costs of care in patients with cancer and nutrition-focused QIPs are one way to help achieve this (Arensberg et al. 2020). Key steps or interventions of a comprehensive nutrition-focused QIP are outlined in Table 14.8, and examples of QIPs utilizing these steps in the hospital, home health, and outpatient space are listed below.

Nutrition-Focused QIP in the Hospital Setting

A large health system in Illinois tested the effectiveness of a comprehensive nutrition-focused QIP in four hospitals and looked at patients with a variety of primary diagnoses (Sriram et al. 2017). Of those diagnoses, the largest subpopulation was oncology patients. The QIP included malnutrition risk screening at admission, prompt initiation of ONS for at-risk patients, and nutrition support during the hospital stay. Patients were also followed up over the 30-days posthospital discharge via phone calls by a healthcare professional or a research team member. The primary outcome measure was unplanned 30-day readmission to any system hospital while the secondary outcome was hospital LOS. Researchers found hospitalized oncology/cancer patients at risk for malnutrition

TABLE 14.8
Nutrition Focus Quality Improvement Program Example

Identify Risk	Intervention	Education	Follow-up
Systematically screen and assess patients for poor nutritional status (undernutrition or overnutrition) using nutrition screening tools	Provide recommendation and instructions for disease-specific ONS use in addition to regular meals (for undernourished patient population) or as a meal/snack replacement (for overnourished patient population)	Educate patients and caregivers on the importance of proper nutrition and ONS compliance	Follow-up calls/visits with patient to ensure compliance and reinforce education

showed a 42.7% or 3.5-day reduction in hospital LOS with implementation of the nutrition focused QIP. The study also found that the nutrition focused QIP was associated with a 37.6% reduction in 30-day readmissions (Arensberg et al. 2020). As a result of improved health outcomes for the treated patients, reduction in readmission rates, and reduced LOS, the nutrition focused QIP led to a total cost savings of $4,896,758 over the 6-month time period resulting in a per patient net savings of $3,858 (Sulo et al. 2017).

In a separate premier academic medical center, the QIP model and ONS were utilized and associated with reduced readmissions and LOS among oncology patients. The impact of ONS provided to hospitalized patients with a variety of primary diagnoses was again studied in a retrospective cohort analysis. Within the data set, ONS was used in 274 of 8,713 (3.1%) adult (18+) inpatient encounters. Additional analysis compared malnourished oncology patients who received ONS vs the malnourished oncology patients who did not. ONS usage and early ONS initiation among malnourished oncology patients were associated with 46% reduction in all-cause 30-day readmissions and 10% reduction in length of hospital stay (Mullin et al. 2019). Such results could impact acute care measures, including those in the Hospital Inpatient Quality Reporting (IQR) Program and the Hospital Acquired Condition (HAC) Reduction Program.

Nutrition-Focused QIP in the Postacute Setting

There are also opportunities for quality improvement to address perioperative nutrition in oncology surgery patients as part of the Home Health Quality Reporting Program. For example, the same researchers that studied the hospital-based QIP that included cancer patients also investigated the impact of a similar QIP on home health patients post institutional discharge or outpatient visit. A large percentage of these patients had a cancer diagnosis and the study documented significant reductions in 90-day hospitalizations, overall healthcare resource utilization (hospitalization, emergency department (ED), and outpatient visits), and cost savings of $1,500 per patient treated (Riley et al. 2020). Table 14.9 identifies some of the measures in CMS institutional and home care value-based and quality programs that could potentially be impacted by nutrition.

Nutrition-Focused QIP in the Outpatient Setting

To date, to our knowledge, there have been no QIPs implemented in the outpatient setting focusing on the dietary needs of the cancer population. QIPs thus far have been intended to include patients of all diagnoses and have showcased positive results (Arensberg et al. 2020). There is a critical need for QIPs strictly focusing on the cancer population to determine the benefits of nutrition interventions across the care continuum, especially in the outpatient setting. In the US, at some point, nearly

TABLE 14.9

Examples of CMS Value-Based Care and Quality Program Measures Potentially Impacted by Nutrition That May Be Important for Oncology Care

CMS Program	Examples of Measures Potentially Impacted by Nutrition
Hospital IQR program	• Hospital-wide all-cause unplanned readmission
HAC reduction program	**CMS Patient Safety Indicators** • Pressure ulcer rate • Postoperative wound dehiscence rate **CDC National Healthcare Safety Network Healthcare-Associated Infection Measures** • SSI (colon and hysterectomy)
Hospital outpatient quality reporting program	• Hospital visits after hospital outpatient surgery • ED visits or inpatient admission for any of ten specific conditions within 30 days of chemotherapy
OCM	• ED visits/observation stays within 6-month chemotherapy episode
Home health quality reporting program	**Potentially Avoidable Events Quality Measures** • Increase in number of pressure ulcers/injuries • Discharged to the community needing wound care or medication assistance • Discharged to the community with an unhealed stage 2 pressure ulcer **Outcome Quality Measures** • Changes in skin integrity postacute care: pressure ulcer/injury • Acute care hospitalization during the first 60 days of home health • Emergency department use without hospitalization during the first 60 days of home health • Medicare spending per beneficiary • Potentially preventable 30-day postdischarge readmission measure • Discharge to community **Process Quality Measures** • Diabetic foot care and patient/caregiver education implemented during all episodes of care
Quality Payment Program (QPP) MIPS	**MIPS Quality Measures** • SSI • Patient-centered surgical risk assessment and communication • Unplanned reoperation within the 30-day postoperative period • Unplanned hospital readmission within 30 days of principal procedure • All-cause hospital readmission **Improvement Activity Measures** • Appropriate documentation of a malnutrition diagnosis (premier clinician performance registry) • Obtaining preoperative nutritional recommendations from an RDN in nutritionally at-risk surgical patients (U.S. wound registry) • Promotion of use of patient-reported outcome tools • Implementation of a falls screening and assessment program • Implementation of practices/processes for developing regular individual care plans • Implementation of condition-specific chronic disease self-management support programs

all oncology patients will receive treatment in an outpatient setting. Unfortunately, in addition to the lack of QIP or clinical studies examining outpatient nutritional interventions, outpatient nutritional care standards and interventions for cancer are unclear and inconsistently applied (Trujillo et al. 2018). Therefore, implementation and successful evaluation of nutrition interventions are needed in the outpatient setting to optimize overall patient care as well as prevent ED visits that may or may not lead to hospitalizations.

The ED for example remains a critical access point for acute illness issues and the continuum of cancer management and over 4.5 million US ED visits are accounted for by patients with cancer. The estimate, derived from ED diagnostic codes, likely underestimates the true annual incidence of cancer-related ED visits among the 15.5 million US residents with cancer (Caterino et al. 2019). Based on this population, 29% of US residents with cancer will visit the ED. Cancer patients are at particular risk of malnutrition and evidence suggests malnutrition is currently diagnosed at a low rate in US EDs, even though the economic burden of malnutrition is substantial in this care setting (Lanctin et al. 2019). The study analyzed 238 million ED visits between 2006 and 2014; the overall population had a malnutrition diagnosis prevalence of 0.7% in 2006 compared to 1.15% in 2014. A malnutrition diagnosis in the ED was associated with 4.23 times higher odds of hospitalization and $21,892 higher mean total charges (Lanctin et al. 2019).

The ED and outpatient clinics are the first line of defense in screening for malnutrition and implementing effective nutrition interventions via comprehensive nutrition focused QIPs. Many outpatient settings and EDs do not have the resources to efficiently screen and implement early nutrition interventions. In the outpatient setting, the registered dietitian to patient ratio was 1:2,308 while the desirable ratio is 1:120 (Trujillo et al. 2018). In the ED setting, a registered dietician may be more available but nutritional deficiencies are rarely the reason why patients will present to the ED. Also, due to competing priorities, EDs may rarely have dedicated resources including registered dietitians to screen for and address malnutrition in the ED setting. Registered nurses, however, are usually the first clinician a patient will interact with during any medical visit at an ED or outpatient facility. Registered nurses in the inpatient and postacute care settings have proven the ability to adequately screen for malnutrition and its risk as well as initiate nutrition interventions (Sriram et al. 2017) (Riley et al. 2017); therefore, we believe that they can be educated to address malnutrition screen in the outpatient and ED settings.

With 90% of US cancer care delivered outside the hospital (Halpern and Yabroff 2008), there is a critical need for nutrition-focused QIPs focused on cancer patients across the care continuum and in the outpatient clinics and EDs across US. The current evidence highlights the need for implementing and assessing the impact of outpatient and ED initiated malnutrition screening and nutrition intervention programs on oncology patient health and economic outcomes. While nutrition interventions can alleviate the economic burden of disease-associated malnutrition, they also offer a great opportunity to potentially reduce the overall economic burden of cancer care for patients receiving care in different healthcare facilities.

CMS is piloting new healthcare payment and delivery models in specialty care to improve care effectiveness and efficiency. One such model is the Oncology Care Model (OCM), developed as an episode-based model and targeting chemotherapy and related care during a 6-month patient care period (beginning with the patient's receipt of chemotherapy treatment). Physician practices participating in the OCM are in part incentivized by performance-based payments. These payments are calculated retrospectively, based on an OCM physician practice's performance against specific quality measures and reductions in Medicare expenditures. The OCM quality measure specific to ED visits/observation stays (Table 14.9) has important implications for nutrition, because some of the more common reasons that chemotherapy patients may visit an ED—such as nausea and vomiting (Bayrak and Kitis 2018)—may be impacted by nutrition. In addition, since poor nutrition can lead to increased complications (Tujillo et al. 2018), postoperative malnourished oncology patients may have more prolonged, expensive recoveries that could impact an OCM physician practice's expenditures against CMS established targets.

Similarly, the CMS Outpatient Quality Reporting Program now requires reporting on a chemotherapy-specific measure (Table 14.9). In an effort to reduce the frequency and cost of unnecessary ED visits, the measure reports the number of oncology patients who have an ED visit or inpatient admission for anemia, nausea, dehydration, neutropenia, diarrhea, pain, emesis, pneumonia, fever, or sepsis within 30 days after chemotherapy. Again, some of these conditions could be impacted by quality nutrition care.

Physicians and other practitioners are also required to report quality measure performance as part of CMS' Merit-based Incentive Payment System (MIPS). Quality measures in MIPS focus on acute care, surgical care, and preventive care, which can provide an opportunity for quality nutrition care. Specific MIPS quality and improvement activity measures that could be impacted by nutrition are identified in Table 14.9.

While there are many different quality measures across the various programs, there are no CMS-required nutrition quality measures—although malnutrition electronic clinical quality measures have been developed and submitted for CMS consideration (AND n.d.). The development of value-based metrics in clinical areas such as cancer surgical procedures is said to still be in its infancy (Schwartz and Margenthaler 2019) and represents an opportunity for further development.

Oncology Nutrition Care Alignment with Patient-Centered Care

CMS defines value-based care as paying for health care services in a way that directly links performance on cost, quality, and the patient's experience of care. And patient-reported outcomes have been identified by payers as the next frontier in value-based care (Higgins et al. 2019). However, Lievens et al. (2019) identified that in oncology the lack of emphasis on patient perspectives and continued reliance on traditional, trial-based endpoints (such as survival, disease-free survival, and safety) supports the need for a new framework focused on the whole spectrum of patient-centered endpoints. These endpoints could include perioperative and postoperative complications and functional outcomes (Lievens et al. 2019) and such endpoints are where quality nutrition care could have an impact.

Relatedly, surgeons have been called on to take an active role in both assessing and optimizing patient-reported outcomes. Some surgeons are using initiatives such as the American College of Surgeons National Surgical Quality Improvement Program (ACS NSQIP®), which is a risk-adjusted and validated outcomes registry, to drive uptake of patient-reported outcome measures (Kadakia et al. 2020). This comes at a time when patients with cancer are starting to act much more like consumers (Thompson 2018) and aided by technology, and are taking their health into their own hands (Harpaz 2019).

Patient engagement is crucial for the effectiveness of nutrition care pathways. The level of patient nutrition education affects adherence to nutrition recommendations and can enhance the positive effects of nutrition interventions. For example, Tian et al divided a cohort of 172 patients with lung cancer into two groups: patients in the intervention group ($n = 62$) were provided with educational information regarding their diet, treatment, and rehabilitation during chemotherapy and compared to the control group ($n = 110$) who were not provided such information. The study showed that educated group had a significantly higher daily protein intake (54.84% vs. 70.00%, $p = 0.046$) and higher rates of performance status and lower rates of depression and side effects of treatment. The need for a more patient-centered approach is further underscored by recent research using NSQIP data that found common definitions of malnutrition do not apply equally to all cancers in assessment of preoperative risk and depend on cancer type (McKenna et al. 2020).

One of the ways CMS value-based care and quality programs assess the patient experience is through the Consumer Assessment of Healthcare Providers and Systems (CAHPS) program of the US Agency for Health Research and Quality. The main purpose of the CAHPS Cancer Care Survey is to help providers improve the patient-centeredness of their cancer care (CAHPS ahrq.gov).

TABLE 14.10

Medicare CAHPS[a] Cancer Care Survey Questions Related to Energy and Diet

CAHPS Cancer Care Survey Question

In the past 6 months, did you and your drug therapy team talk about any changes in your energy levels related to your cancer or drug therapy?

In the past 6 months, were you bothered by changes in your energy levels related to your cancer or drug therapy?

In the past 6 months, did your drug therapy team advise you about or help you deal with these changes in your energy levels?

In the past 6 months, did you and your drug therapy team talk about things you can do to maintain your health during cancer treatment, such as what to eat and what exercises to do?

[a] CAHPS survey of the US Agency for Health Research and Quality.

This survey is also a mandatory quality measure component of CMS' OCM model. The CAHPS Cancer Care Survey includes multiple questions on energy and one question on diet (Table 14.10), which underscores that nutrition is indeed important to patients receiving cancer treatment.

DEVELOPMENTS IN TELEHEALTH AND ONCOLOGY NUTRITION

A patient engagement area that has certainly been at the fore of healthcare innovation is telehealth. Prior to 2020, telemedicine was already one of the most rapidly expanding components of the healthcare system (Huang et al. 2019). Patient willingness to use telemedicine in the postoperative setting has been high and postoperative telemedicine has been implemented across multiple modalities, including short message services text messaging, smart-phone applications, automated calls, and wearable devices (Williams et al. 2018). There have also been reports of successful telehealth models for the nutrition management of patients with cancer (Collins et al. 2017).

Many advantages of telemedicine have been documented—including excellent clinical outcomes and patient satisfaction, time and cost savings, revenue generation, and improved care access. Yet state and federal barriers for practitioners (including licensure and practice laws) and CMS and other payer coverage restrictions have continued to thwart widespread adoption (Williams et al. 2018). The COVID-19 pandemic broke through these barriers and CMS has already issued its first proposed regulatory changes for telecommunications technology use in care provided under the Medicare home health benefit (CMS 2020). It is expected that CMS will issue similar proposals to reduce the regulatory roadblocks in other care settings as well. Thus, in the coming decade, telemedicine and telesurgery are predicted to mature, aided by the reduction in restrictions and an explosion of interconnected consumer health devices and high-speed 5G connectivity (Contreras et al. 2020).

To be supportive of all patients with cancer, proactive efforts are needed to ensure equity. While widespread expansion of telemedicine is a positive, it could further increase rather than reduce healthcare disparities, particularly for those with limited digital literacy or access (including rural populations), racial/ethnic minorities, older adults, lower income populations, and those with limited English proficiency or low health literacy (Nouri et al. 2020). There is also the potential for discrimination and mistrust to be magnified during virtual encounters, when patients may feel more limited in their ability to communicate and providers may be less mindful of guarding against implicit bias. Another concern is the potential for bias to be encoded into telehealth algorithms, particularly if certain groups are underrepresented in the algorithmic data. And patients' uninformed use of such algorithms—in leu of seeking professional medical advice—could be detrimental to their health (Clair et al. 2020).

The Health and Human Services (HHS) specifically targeted health disparities when it funded several different programs to expand telehealth availability and increase telehealth access and infrastructure in response to the COVID-19 pandemic (HHS, 2020), but a more lasting investment and a much broader approach are necessary. Recommended actions oncology clinicians can take to help ensure widescale telemedicine adoption that does not exacerbate health disparities include: being proactive to explore potential disparities, developing solutions to mitigate the barriers for digital literacy and healthcare systems' ability to provide video visits, and advocating for the policies and infrastructure needed to ensure equitable telemedicine access (Nouri et al. 2020).

CONCLUSIONS AND FUTURE DIRECTIONS OF ONCOLOGY NUTRITION SUPPORT

The current review highlights the key role nutrition and muscle health plays in the overall care of cancer patient. Both dietary inadequacy and inflammation predisposed cancer patients to significant nutritional deficiency and muscle loss, which warrants early identification and proper nutritional intervention. Medical nutritional therapy including ONS, enteral, and parenteral nutrition could be helpful tools to address cancer-associated protein-calorie undernutrition, muscle loss, and micronutrient deficiencies. Based on this literature review, early nutrition intervention could help improve clinical and patient-reported outcomes. Immunonutrition which are oral nutrition shakes supplemented with immune-modulating nutrients, especially fish oil and arginine have been shown to preserve muscle mass and improve clinical outcomes like decrease chemotherapy disruptions and associated side effects, postoperative infections, and improve patient-reported outcomes and QOL.

The research detailed in previous sections considers how malnutrition and nutrition needs may vary and represents opportunities to engage patients and family members in quality cancer care. Future research should emphasize the interaction of nutrition and genotypes of different cancer types. The concept of personalized nutrition will help select the best nutrition therapy for the individual patient based on age, metabolic profile, microbiome profile, pathological type, and comorbid conditions.

Another area discussed for future advances in the field of nutrition therapy of cancer is the role of telehealth. The integration of digital health into the implementation of the nutrition care pathway will help connect patients with providers. The use of electronic devices to monitor responses to diet and nutrition therapy (e.g., continuous glucose monitoring devices) will allow providers and patients to track the glycemic responses to nutrition interventions and better manage them. Digital health could significantly help track the effects of early medical nutrition therapy. Measuring muscle mass and function using electronic devices could also facilitate choosing the best nutrition intervention to promote muscle accretion by optimizing the amount of dietary protein, allowing patients at high-risk of sarcopenia being early diagnosed and properly managed. Integrating these technologies to improve muscle mass and function will enhance the QOL allowing patients to be fully engaged in their management plan.

The use of nutrition focused digital applications could help track their lifestyle activities and responses to nutrition therapy. Patients could also gain access to millions of recipes accessible to accommodate the taste changes during chemotherapy and radiation therapy along with the journey of treatment. It will allow multidisciplinary teams to care for the same patient at one time.

The future of clinical nutrition care for patients with cancer will tremendously focus on the role of muscle health and how to maximize the prevention of muscle protein breakdown. Researching specialized nutrients that improve muscle protein synthesis and inhibit protein degradation (e.g., HMB and fish oil) will provide value to the management of cancer patients. Future research will also stress the importance of insulin sensitivity and ways to prevent the pro inflammatory effects of cytokines secreted by cancer cells. Addressing the unique nutrition needs of patients with sarcopenic obesity will be highlighted as therapies aiming to increase muscle mass and decrease fat mass will be mandated. Consequently, the important role of multimodal therapy combining exercise, anti-inflammatory drugs, and dietary protein is key to the success of nutrition therapy.

In addition to advances in nutrition solutions to address cancer-associated nutrition diseases, the keystone to their implementation lies on the physicians' leadership and support. Clearly most of the work would be performed by ancillary staff and physician extenders; however, they take direction from the physicians and rely on their support to secure resources such as institutional acceptance, resource allocation, placement in work-flow, and inclusion in quality assurance study. Dedicated educational time devoted to nutrition and cancer has not traditionally been a part of residency or fellowship; however, with the advent of systematic practice resources quick reading of crucial aspects of cancer nutrition and intervention is now possible. Of interest, is the imbalance in the National Comprehensive Cancer Network (NCCN) guidelines which contain information dedicated to the patient on symptoms of cancer and its treatments in which diet and weight changes are reviewed in lay man's terms (NCCN); however, no counterpart for physicians exists except in palliative care (NCCN). While palliative care interventions yield important benefits, nutrition should be front and center at the time of the initial diagnosis. The American Society of Clinical Oncology (ASCO) has initiated a series of guidelines which address patient related problems including cancer cachexia (Roeland et al. 2020). It provides an evidence-based framework to review various interventions indicating generally limited evidence to guide physicians when confronted with cachexia. Dietary counseling and oral nutritional supplements have evidence to support their use to reverse cachexia as measured by body weight. Ideally a registered dietician would be available for a referral for cachexia and, in fact, that may be case in large centers. Most cancer patients, however, are treated in community practices where resources are less robust. The responsibility falls on the shoulders of the physician as a result. The swath of benefits merits integration from day one as it is likely the single most cost-effective measure to improve outcomes in curable patients available to physicians.

Interdisciplinary care has evolved over the past 50 years to coordinate care and to improve treatment plans for increasingly complex medical and surgical interventions from specialties that evolved into knowledge silos (Thenappan et al. 2017, Wright et al. 2007). No one can now keep abreast of all the necessary let alone esoteric diagnostic and interventional options for the care of even the "straight forward" cancer patient (Newman et al. 2006). That idea may be consigned to history's dust bin. Including nutrition at the tumor board conference would be an optimal first step to broadening the knowledge base of all the physicians and staff while easing pain points in programmatic development (Keating et al. 2013). Such has occurred with the inclusion of multiple physician subspecialties, nurse navigators (Rocque et al. 2017, Muñoz et al. 2018), psychologists, and social workers (Miller et al. 2018, Pillay et al. 2016, Wright et al. 2007). The format of the tumor board allows for a disposition for an individual patient at the initial presentation and eases follow-up reports.

Outcomes of positive interventions accrue across various interests in the healthcare arena; health-related outcome measures, improved QOL, higher patient satisfaction, and function increased communication between the patient and his healthcare team, higher compliance to the prescribed course of therapy, and improved completion of planned surgery, chemotherapy, and radiotherapy. The role of nutrition on the function of the immune system (Bourke, Berkley, and Prendergast 2016) and interactions with biologic agents operating on those pathways are attracting increased attention (Brocco, Di Marino, and Grassandonia 2019) as the response can be characterized as capricious on occasion (Huang et al. 2018). Host-mediated factors may contain the explanation (Cortellini et al. 2019). Until those phenomena have an explanation, it would make sense to optimize the host's nutrition.

As cancer therapeutics proliferates, pharmacy costs rise and other care costs are affected by inflationary pressures in the healthcare system, thereby, straining the hope of balancing the budget. Pocketbook concerns now increasingly extend to patients who find themselves on the hook for more.

As a result, hard questions will press providers who ultimately dictate care and thus cost. Increased emphasis on value-based care, such as 30-day readmission penalties, demands that all resources are on deck (Caterino et al. 2019). Quality of medicine is what will be reimbursed. Models may emerge whereby payment is tied to completion rates as well as toxicity, most obviously assessed by emergency room visits and hospitalizations (Medicare). Marshalling all tools to assess and to optimize the patient prior to embarking on costly therapy would seem a basic improvement. Nutritional evaluation and intervention are important factors in an oncology patient's prospects. It is time for nutrition to come out of the kitchen and to the table.

These outcomes carry importance above successful individual results as mandated public reporting of various end points will only increase in time and lead to more comparisons among healthcare facilities with explicit goal of allowing patients to determine where they go based on quality metrics. Aligned goals across all parts of the healthcare team will foster a successful initiative which can be as simple as leaving samples of oral nutritional supplements on the front desk instead of breath mints. Opportunities for computerized assessments in the clinic or at home would allow for tracking of weight, energy, and other metrics associated with cachexia. Patient empowerment is a powerful tool to enhance compliance and to infer a true team approach to care with the patient, family, physician, dietician, and nurse all participating (Fringer et al. 2020). After all, the inanition may be a direct consequence of the treatment prescribed, i.e., radiation or chemotherapy, thus making physicians responsible to manage iatrogenic adverse effects, ideally with nutrition counseling and oral nutritional supplements (Lee, Leong, and Lim 2016).

Challenges to successful implementation of nutrition interventions; lack of knowledge, lack of coordination, lack of time are mimicked in tumor board participation rates and other widely accepted interventions designated nowadays as standard. In the resource constrained circumstance, nutrition evaluation and intervention can be successfully conducted with primary oncologists at the initial visit (Muscaritoli et al. 2017). As the features of nutrition evaluation and intervention grow more robust in hard data, programmatic description, and reported outcomes, many of these foregoing points can be assembled by practitioners without fanfare and only in a few minutes of conversation which certainly are appreciated by the patient and caregiver alike. After all, food is fundamental (van der Riet et al. 2008) and laden with emotional charge across cultures with changes in weight and eating habits causing distress for the patient, spouse, and family (Hopkinson 2016). Talking about nutrition is an opportunity to establish a rapport that communicates care about the patient as a human being as opposed to a diagnosis (Poole and Froggatt 2002).

ACKNOWLEDGMENTS

The authors acknowledge the great contributions by Abby Sauer, MPH, RD, Cory Brunton, MS, BSN, RN and Mary Beth Arensberg, PhD, RDN throughout the process of developing this book chapter.

REFERENCES

Academy of Nutrition and Dietetics. 2012. Electronic Clinical Quality Measures (eCQMs). Available at: https://www.eatrightpro.org/practice/quality-management/quality-improvement/malnutrition-quality-improvement-initiative.

Achilli, P., M. Mazzola, C. L. Bertoglio, C. Magistro, M. Origi, P. Carnevali, F. Gervasi, C. Mastellone, N. Guanziroli, E. Corradi, and G. Ferrari. 2020. "Preoperative immunonutrition in frail patients with colorectal cancer: An intervention to improve postoperative outcomes." *Int J Colorectal Dis* 35 (1): 19–27. doi: 10.1007/s00384-019-03438-4.

Aeberhard, C., C. Mayer, S. Meyer, S. A. Mueller, P. Schuetz, Z. Stanga, and R. Giger. 2018. "Effect of preoperative immunonutrition on postoperative short-term outcomes of patients with head and neck squamous cell carcinoma." *Head Neck* 40 (5):1057–67. doi: 10.1002/hed.25072.

Ambiru, S., A. Kato, F. Kimura, H. Shimizu, H. Yoshidome, M. Otsuka, and M. Miyazaki. 2008. "Poor postoperative blood glucose control increases surgical site infections after surgery for hepato-biliary-pancreatic cancer: A prospective study in a high-volume institute in Japan." *J Hosp Infect* 68 (3):230–3. doi: 10.1016/j.jhin.2007.12.002.

Amer, M. A., M. D. Smith, G. P. Herbison, L. D. Plank, and J. L. McCall. 2017. "Network meta-analysis of the effect of preoperative carbohydrate loading on recovery after elective surgery." *Br J Surg* 104 (3):187–97. doi: 10.1002/bjs.10408.

American College of Surgeons Commission on Cancer. 2011. *Cancer Program Standards 2012: Ensuring Patient Centered Care.* Chicago, IL: American College of Surgeons.

Anandavadivelan, P., T. B. Brismar, M. Nilsson, A. M. Johar, and L. Martin. 2016. "Sarcopenic obesity: A probable risk factor for dose limiting toxicity during neo-adjuvant chemotherapy in oesophageal cancer patients". *Clin Nutr*, Elsevier Ltd 35(3):724–30. doi: 10.1016/j.clnu.2015.05.011.

Andreyev, J. H. N., A. R. Norman, J. Oates, and D. Cunningham. 1998. "Why do patients with weight loss have a worse outcome when undergoing chemotherapy for gastrointestinal malignancies?" *Eur J Cancer* 34:503–9.

Antoun, S., E. Lanoy, R. Iacovelli, L. Albiges-Sauvin, Y. Loriot, M. Merad-Taoufik, K. Fizazi, M. di Palma, V. E. Baracos, and B. Escudier. 2013. "Skeletal muscle density predicts prognosis in patients with metastatic renal cell carcinoma treated with targeted therapies." *Cancer* 119 (18):3377–84. doi: 10.1002/cncr.28218.

Arends J., G. Bodoky, F. Bozzetti, K. Fearon, M. Muscaritoli, G. Selga, M. A. van Bokhorst-de van der Schueren, M. von Meyenfeldt, G. Zurcher, R. Fietkau, E. Aulbert, B. Frick , M. Holm, M. Kneba, H. J. Mestrom, and A. Zander. 2006. "ESPEN guidelines on enteral nutrition: Non-surgical oncology." *Clin Nutr* 25:245–59.

Arends, J., P. Bachmann, V. Baracos, N. Barthelemy, H. Bertz, F. Bozzetti, K. Fearon, E. Hutterer, E. Isenring, S. Kaasa, Z. Krznaric, B. Laird, M. Larsson, A. Laviano, S. Muhlebach, M. Muscaritoli, L. Oldervoll, P. Ravasco, T. Solheim, F. Strasser, M. de van der Schueren, and J. C. Preiser. 2017a. "ESPEN guidelines on nutrition in cancer patients." *Clin Nutr* 36 (1):11–48. doi: 10.1016/j.clnu.2016.07.015.

Arends, J., V. Baracos, H. Bertz, F. Bozzetti, P. C. Calder, N. E. P. Deutz, N. Erickson, A. Laviano, M. P. Lisanti, D. N. Lobo, D. C. McMillan, M. Muscaritoli, J. Ockenga, M. Pirlich, F. Strasser, M. de van der Schueren, A. Van Gossum, P. Vaupel, and A. Weimann. 2017b. "ESPEN expert group recommendations for action against cancer-related malnutrition." *Clin Nutr* 36 (5):1187–96. doi: 10.1016/j.clnu.2017.06.017.

Argilés, J. M., S. Busquets, B. Stemmler, and F. L. López-Soriano. 2014. "Cancer cachexia: Understanding the molecular basis". *Nat Rev Cancer* 14 (11):754–62.

Aslam, M., S. Naveed, A. Ahmed, Z. Abbas, I. Gull, and M. Athar. 2014. "Side effects of chemotherapy in cancer patients and evaluation of patients opinion about starvation based differential chemotherapy." *J Cancer Ther* 5:817–22.

August, D. A., M. B. Huhmann, and American Society for Parenteral and Enteral Nutrition (A.S.P.E.N.). 2009. "A.S.P.E.N. clinical guidelines: Nutrition support therapy during adult anticancer treatment and in hematopoietic cell transplantation." *JPEN J Parenter Enteral Nutr* 33 (5):472–500.

Awad, S., K. K. Varadhan, O. Ljungqvist, and D. N. Lobo. 2013. "A meta-analysis of randomised controlled trials on preoperative oral carbohydrate treatment in elective surgery." *Clin Nutr* 32 (1):34–44. doi: 10.1016/j.clnu.2012.10.011.

Bachmann, J., M. Heiligensetzer, H. Krakowski-Roosen, M. W. Buchler, H. Friess, and M. E. Martignoni. 2008. "Cachexia worsens prognosis in patients with resectable pancreatic cancer." *J Gastrointest Surg* 12 (7):1193–201. doi: 10.1007/s11605-008-0505-z.

Baker, E. A., S. El-Gaddal, L. Williams, and D. J. Leaper. 2006. "Profiles of inflammatory cytokines following colorectal surgery: Relationship with wound healing and outcome." *Wound Repair Regen* 14 (5):566–72. doi: 10.1111/j.1743-6109.2006.00163.x.

Baldwin, C., A. Spiro, R. Ahern, and P. W. Emery. 2012. "Oral nutritional interventions in malnourished patients with cancer: A systematic review and meta-analysis." *Review J Natl Cancer Inst* 104 (5):371–85. doi: 10.1093/jnci/djr556.

Baracos, V., and S. M. R. Kazemi-Bajestani. 2013. "Clinical outcomes related to muscle mass in humans with cancer and catabolic illnesses." *Int J Biochem Cell Biol* 45(10):2302–8.

Baracos, V. E., L. Martin, M. Korc, D. C. Guttridge, and K. C. H. Fearon. 2018. "Cancer-associated cachexia." *Nat Rev Dis Primers* 4:17105. doi: 10.1038/nrdp.2017.105.

Barber, M. D., J. A. Ross, A. C. Voss, M. J. Tisdale, and K. C. Fearon. 1999. "The effect of an oral nutritional supplement enriched with fish oil on weight-loss in patients with pancreatic cancer." *Br J Cancer* 81 (1):80–6. doi: 10.1038/sj.bjc.6690654.

Barber, M. D., K. C. Fearon, M. J. Tisdale, D. C. McMillan, and J. A. Ross. 2001. "Effect of a fish oil-enriched nutritional supplement on metabolic mediators in patients with pancreatic cancer cachexia." *Nutr Cancer* 40 (2):118–24. doi: 10.1207/S15327914NC402_7.

Barker, L. A., B. S. Gout, and T. C. Crowe. 2011. "Hospital malnutrition: Prevalence, identification and impact on patients and the healthcare system." *Int J Environ Res Public Health* 8 (2):514–27. doi: 10.3390/ijerph8020514.

Bauer, J., S. Capra, D. Battistutta, W. Davidson, and S. Ash. 2005. "Compliance with nutrition prescription improves outcomes in patients with unresectable pancreatic cancer." *Clin Nutr* 24 (6):998–1004. doi: 10.1016/j.clnu.2005.07.002.

Bauer J., S. Ash, W. Davidson, J. Hill, T. Brown, E. Isenring, and M. Reeves. 2006. "Evidencebased practice guidelines for the nutritional management of cancer cachexia and chronic kidney disease." *Nutr Dietetics.* 63:S35–S45.

Bayrak, E., and Y. Kitis. 2018. "The main reasons for emergency department visits in cancer patients." *Med Bull Haseki* 56:6–13. doi: 10.4274/haseki.83997

Beck, A., U. T. Andersen, E. Leedo, et al. 2015. "Does adding a dietician to the liaison team after discharge of geriatric patients improve nutritional outcome: A randomised controlled trial." *Clin Rehabil* 29 (11):1117–28.

Bloch, A. S. 1990. *Nutrition Management of the Cancer Patient.* Rockville, MD: Aspen Publishers.

Bosaeus, I. 2008. "Nutritional support in multimodal therapy for cancer cachexia." *Support Care Cancer* 16:447–51.

Bourke, C. D., J. A. Berkley, and A. J. Prendergast. 2016. "Immune dysfunction as a cause and consequence of malnutrition." *Trends Immunol* 37 (6):386–98. doi: 10.1016/j.it.2016.04.003.

Bozzetti, F. 2013. "Nutritional support of the oncology patient." *Crit Rev Oncol Hematol.* 87:172–200.

Bozzetti, F., C. Gavazzi, L. Mariani, and F. Crippa. 1999. "Artificial nutrition in cancer patients: Which route, what composition?" *World J Surg* 23:577–83.

Braunschweig, C. L., P. Levy, P. M. Sheean, and X. Wang. 2001. "Enteral compared with parenteral nutrition: A meta-analysis." *Am J Clin Nutr.* 74:534–42.

Brocco, D., P. Di Marino, and A. Grassandonia. 2019. "From cachexia to obesity: The role of host metabolism in cancer immunotherapy." *Curr Opin Support Palliat Care* 13 (4):305–10. doi: 10.1097/SPC.0000000000000457.

Buchman, A. L., A. A. Moukarzel, S. Bhuta, M. Belle, M. E. Ament, C. D. Eckhert, D. Hollander, J. Gornbein, J. D. Kopple, and S. R. Vijayaroghavan. 1995. "Parenteral nutrition is associated with intestinal morphologic and functional changes in humans." *JPEN J Parenter Enteral Nutr* 19:453–60.

Buijs, N., M. A. van Bokhorst-de van der Schueren, J. A. Langius, C. R. Leemans, D. J. Kuik, M. A. Vermeulen, and P. A. van Leeuwen. 2010. "Perioperative arginine-supplemented nutrition in malnourished patients with head and neck cancer improves longterm survival." *Am J Clin Nutr.* 92:1151–6.

Buitrago, G., J. Vargas, S. Sulo, J. S. Partridge, M. Guevara-Nieto, G. Gomez, J. D. Misas, and M. Correia. 2019. "Targeting malnutrition: Nutrition programs yield cost savings for hospitalized patients." *Clin Nutr.* doi: 10.1016/j.clnu.2019.12.025.

Calder, P. C. 2008. "The relationship between the fatty acid composition of immune cells and their function." *Prostaglandins Leukot Essent Fatty Acids* 79 (3–5):101–8. doi: 10.1016/j.plefa.2008.09.016.

Calder, P. C. 2013. "Omega-3 polyunsaturated fatty acids and inflammatory processes: Nutrition or pharmacology?" *Br J Clin Pharmacol* 75 (3):645–62. doi: 10.1111/j.1365-2125.2012.04374.x.

Canbay, O., S. Adar, A. H. Karagoz, N. Celebi, and C. Y. Bilen. 2014. "Effect of preoperative consumption of high carbohydrate drink (Pre-Op) on postoperative metabolic stress reaction in patients undergoing radical prostatectomy." *Int Urol Nephrol* 46 (7):1329–33. doi: 10.1007/s11255-013-0612-y.

Cancer ACoSCo. 2014. *Cancer Program Standards 2012: Ensuring Patient Centered Care.* Chicago, IL: American College of Surgeons.

Cao, D. D., H. L. Xu, M. Xu, X. Y. Qian, Z. C. Yin, and W. Ge. 2017. "Therapeutic role of glutamine in management of radiation enteritis: A meta-analysis of 13 randomized controlled trials." *Oncotarget* 8 (18):30595–605. doi: 10.18632/oncotarget.15741.

Carneiro, I. P., V. C. Mazurak, and C. M. Prado. 2016. "Clinical implications of sarcopenic obesity in cancer." *Curr Oncol Rep* 18 (10):62. doi: 10.1007/s11912-016-0546-5.

Caro, M. M., A. Laviano, and C. Pichard. 2007. "Nutritional intervention and quality of life in adult oncology patients." *Clin Nutr* 26 (3):289–301. doi: 10.1016/j.clnu.2007.01.005.

Caro, M. M., A. Laviano, C. Pichard, and C. G. Candela. 2007. "Relationship between nutritional intervention and quality of life in cancer patients." *Nutr Hosp* 22:337–50.

Casas-Rodera, P., C. Gomez-Candela, S. Benitez, R. Mateo, M. Armero, R. Castillo, and J. M. Culebras. 2008. "Immunoenhanced enteral nutrition formulas in head and neck cancer surgery: A prospective, randomized clinical trial." *Nutr Hosp.* 23:105–10.

Caterino, J. M., D. Adler, D. D. Durham, S. J. Yeung, M. F. Hudson, A. Bastani, S. L. Bernstein, C. W. Baugh, C. J. Coyne, C. R. Grudzen, D. J. Henning, A. Klotz, T. E. Madsen, D. J. Pallin, C. C. Reyes-Gibby, J. F. Rico, R. J. Ryan, N. I. Shapiro, R. Swor, A. Venkat, J. Wilson, C. R. Thomas, J. J. Bischof, and G. H. Lyman. 2019. "Analysis of diagnoses, symptoms, medications, and admissions among patients with cancer presenting to emergency departments." *JAMA Netw Open* 2 (3):e190979. doi: 10.1001/jamanetworkopen.2019.0979.

Cawood, A. L., M. Elia, and R. J. Stratton. 2012. "Systematic review and meta-analysis of the effects of high protein oral nutritional supplements." *Ageing Res Rev* 11 (2):278–96. doi: 10.1016/j.arr.2011.12.008.

CDC. "Health care associated infections."** https://www.cdc.gov/hai/index.html.

Cederholm, T., G. L. Jensen, Mitd Correia, M. C. Gonzalez, R. Fukushima, T. Higashiguchi, G. Baptista, R. Barazzoni, R. Blaauw, A. Coats, A. Crivelli, D. C. Evans, L. Gramlich, V. Fuchs-Tarlovsky, H. Keller, L. Llido, A. Malone, K. M. Mogensen, J. E. Morley, M. Muscaritoli, I. Nyulasi, M. Pirlich, V. Pisprasert, M. A. E. de van der Schueren, S. Siltharm, P. Singer, K. Tappenden, N. Velasco, D. Waitzberg, P. Yamwong, J. Yu, A. Van Gossum, C. Compher, and Glim Core Leadership Committee, and Glim Working Group. 2019. "GLIM criteria for the diagnosis of malnutrition: A consensus report from the global clinical nutrition community." *Clin Nutr* 38 (1):1–9. doi: 10.1016/j.clnu.2018.08.002.

Centers for Medicare & Medicaid Services. 2020a. Medicare and Medicaid Programs; CY 2021 Home Health Prospective Payment System Rate Update; Home Health Quality Reporting Requirements; and Home Infusion Therapy Services Requirements A Proposed Rule by the Centers for Medicare & Medicaid Services on 06/30/2020.

Centers for Medicare & Medicaid Services. 2020b, June 22. Oncology Care Model. Innovation.cms.gov. https://innovation.cms.gov/innovation-models/oncology-care

Chen, D. W., Z. Wei Fei, Y. C. Zhang, J. M. Ou, and J. Xu. 2005. "Role of enteral immunonutrition in patients with gastric carcinoma undergoing major surgery." *Asian J Surg* 28 (2):121–4. doi: 10.1016/s1015-9584(09)60275-x.

Clair, M., B. W. Clair, and W. K. Clair. June 26, 2020. Unless it's done carefully, the rise of telehealth could widen health disparities. First Opinion, STAT. https://www.statnews.com/2020/06/26/unless-its-done-carefully-the-rise-of-telehealth-could-widen-health-disparities/.

Collins, A., C. L. Burns, E. C. Ward, T. Comans, C. Blake, L. Kenny, P. Greenup, D. Best. 2017. "Home-based telehealth service for swallowing and nutrition management following head and neck cancer treatment." *J Telemed Telecare* 23(10):866–72. doi: 10.1177/1357633X17733020.

Colomer, R., J. M. Moreno-Nogueira, P. P. García-Luna, P. García-Peris, A. García-de-Lorenzo, A. Zarazaga, L. Quecedo, J. del Llano, L. Usán, and C. Casimiro. 2007. "N-3 fatty acids, cancer and cachexia: A systematic review of the literature." *Br J Nutr* 97 (5):823–31. doi: 10.1017/S000711450765795X.

Contreras, C. M., G. A. Metzger, J. D. Beane, P. H. Dedhia, A. Ejaz, and T. M. Pawlik. 2020. "Telemedicine: Patient-provoider clinical engagement during the COVID-19 pandemic and beyond." *J Gastrointestinal Surgery.* https://link.springer.com/article/10.1007/s11605-020-04623-5.

Cortellini, A., L. Verna, G. Porzio, F. Bozzetti, P. Palumbo, C. Masciocchi, K. Cannita, A. Parisi, D. Brocco, N. Tinari, and C. Ficorella. 2019. "Predictive value of skeletal muscle mass for immunotherapy with nivolumab in non-small cell lung cancer patients: A "hypothesis-generator" preliminary report." *Thorac Cancer* 10 (2):347–51. doi: 10.1111/1759-7714.12965.

Curtis, L. J., P. Bernier, K. Jeejeebhoy, J. Allard, D. Duerksen, L. Gramlich, M. Laporte, and H. H. Keller. 2017. "Costs of hospital malnutrition." *Clin Nutr* 36 (5):1391–6. doi: 10.1016/j.clnu.2016.09.009.

Cushen, S. J., D. G. Power, K. P. Murphy, R. McDermott, B. T. Griffin, M. Lim, L. Daly, P. MacEneaney, K. O' Sullivan, C. M. Prado, and A. M. Ryan. 2016. "Impact of body composition parameters on clinical outcomes in patients with metastatic castrate-resistant prostate cancer treated with docetaxel." *Clin Nutr ESPEN*, Elsevier, 13:e39–45. doi: 10.1016/j.clnesp.2016.04.001.

Daly, J. M., M. D. Lieberman, J. Goldfine, J. Shou, F. Weintraub, E. F. Rosato, and P. Lavin. 1992. "Enteral nutrition with supplemental arginine, RNA, and omega-3 fatty acids in patients after operation: Immunologic, metabolic, and clinical outcome." *Surgery* 112:56–67.

Danis, K., M. Kline, M. Munson, et al. 2019. "Identifying and managing malnourished hospitalized patients utilizing the Malnutrition Quality Improvement Initiative: The UPMC experience." *J Acad Nutr Diet* 119(9S2): S40–3. doi: 10.1016/j.jand.2019.05.020.

Davidson, W., S. Ash, S. Capra, and J. Bauer. 2004. "Weight stabilisation is associated with improved survival duration and quality of life in unresectable pancreatic cancer." *Clin Nutr* 23 (2):239–47. doi: 10.1016/j.clnu.2003.07.001.

Davidson, W., L. Teleni, J. Muller, M. Ferguson, A. L. McCarthy, J. Vick, and E. Isenring. 2012. "Malnutrition and chemotherapy-induced nausea and vomiting: Implications for practice." *Oncol Nurs Forum* 39 (4):E340–5. doi: 10.1188/12.ONF.E340-E345.

de Luis, D. A., O. Izaola, A. Aller, L. Cuellar, MC. Terroba, and T. Martin. 2008. "A randomized clinical trial with two omega 3 fatty acid enhanced oral supplements in head and neck cancer ambulatory patients." *Eur Rev Med Pharmacol Sci* 12 (3):177–81.

de Luis, D. A., B. de la Fuente, O. Izaola, T. Martin, L. Cuellar, and M. C. Terroba. 2014. "Clinical effects of a hypercaloric and hyperproteic oral suplemment enhanced with W3 fatty acids and dietary fiber in postsurgical ambulatory head and neck cancer patients." *Nutr Hosp* 31 (2):759–63.

de van der Schueren, M. A. E., A. Laviano, H. Blanchard, M. Jourdan, J. Arends, and V. E. Baracos. 2018. "Systematic review and meta-analysis of the evidence for oral nutritional intervention on nutritional and clinical outcomes during chemo(radio)therapy: Current evidence and guidance for design of future trials." *Ann Oncol* 29 (5):1141–53. doi: 10.1093/annonc/mdy114.

Deshpande, T. S., P. Blanchard, L. Wang, R. L. Foote, X. Zhang, and S. J. Frank. 2018. "Radiation-related alterations of taste function in patients with head and neck cancer: A systematic review." *Curr Treat Options Oncol* 19 (12):72. doi: 10.1007/s11864-018-0580-7.

Deutz, N. E., E. M. Matheson, L. E. Matarese, M. Luo, G. E. Baggs, J. L. Nelson, R. A. Hegazi, K. A. Tappenden, T. R. Ziegler, and Nourish Study Group. 2016. "Readmission and mortality in malnourished, older, hospitalized adults treated with a specialized oral nutritional supplement: A randomized clinical trial." *Clin Nutr* 35 (1):18–26. doi: 10.1016/j.clnu.2015.12.010.

Dewys, W. D., C. Begg, P. T. Lavin, P. R. Band, J. M. Bennett, J. R. Bertino, M. H. Cohen, H. O. Douglass, Jr., P. F. Engstrom, E. Z. Ezdinli, J. Horton, G. J. Johnson, C. G. Moertel, M. M. Oken, C. Perlia, C. Rosenbaum, M. N. Silverstein, R. T. Skeel, R. W. Sponzo, and D. C. Tormey. 1980. "Prognostic effect of weight loss prior to chemotherapy in cancer patients: Eastern Cooperative Oncology Group." *Am J Med* 69 (4):491–7. doi: 10.1016/s0149-2918(05)80001-3.

Dort, J. C., D. G. Farwell, M. Findlay, G. F. Huber, P. Kerr, M. A. Shea-Budgell, C. Simon, J. Uppington, D. Zygun, O. Ljungqvist, and J. Harris. 2017. "Optimal perioperative care in major head and neck cancer surgery with free flap reconstruction: A consensus review and recommendations from the enhanced recovery after surgery society." *JAMA Otolaryngol Head Neck Surg* 143 (3):292–303. doi: 10.1001/jamaoto.2016.2981.

Drover, J. W., R. Dhaliwal, L. Weitzel, P. E. Wischmeyer, J. B. Ochoa, and D. K. Heyland. 2011. "Perioperative use of arginine-supplemented diets: A systematic review of the evidence." *J Am Coll Surg* 212 (3):385–99, 399 e1. doi: 10.1016/j.jamcollsurg.2010.10.016.

Elia, M. 2000. *Guidelines for the Detection and Management of Malnutrition: A Report of the Malnutrition Advisory Group.* Maidenhead, UK: British Association for Parenteral and Enteral Nutrition (BAPEN).

Elia, M., M. A. E. vann Bokhorst-de van der Schueren, J. Garvey, A. Goedhart, K. Lundholm, G. Nitenberg, and R. J. Stratton. 2006. "Enteral (oral or tube administration) nutritional support and eicosapentaenoic acid in patients with cancer: A systematic review." *Int J Oncol* 28 (1):5–23. doi: 10.3892/ijo.28.1.5.

Elia, M., C. Normand, K. Norman, and A. Laviano. 2016. "A systematic review of the cost and cost effectiveness of using standard oral nutritional supplements in the hospital setting." *Clin Nutr* 35 (2):370–80. doi: 10.1016/j.clnu.2015.05.010.

Endres, S., R. Ghorbani, V. E. Kelley, K. Georgilis, G. Lonnemann, J. W. van der Meer, J. G. Cannon, T. S. Rogers, M. S. Klempner, and P. C. Weber. 1989. "The effect of dietary supplementation with N-3 polyunsaturated fatty acids on the synthesis of interleukin-1 and tumor necrosis factor by mononuclear cells." *N Engl J Med* 320 (5):265–71. doi: 10.1056/NEJM198902023200501.

Farreras, N., V. Artigas, D. Cardona, X. Rius, M. Trias, and J. A. Gonzalez. 2005. "Effect of early postoperative enteral immunonutrition on wound healing in patients undergoing surgery for gastric cancer." *Clin Nutr* 24:55–65.

Fearon, K., J. Arends, and V. Baracos. 2013. "Understanding the mechanisms and treatment options in cancer cachexia." *Nat Rev Clin Oncol* 10 (2):90–99. doi: 10.1038/nrclinonc.2012.209.

Fearon, K., F. Strasser, S. D. Anker, I. Bosaeus, E. Bruera, R. L. Fainsinger, A. Jatoi, C. Loprinzi, N. MacDonald, G. Mantovani, M. Davis, M. Muscaritoli, F. Ottery, L. Radbruch, P. Ravasco, D. Walsh, A. Wilcock, S. Kaasa, and V. E. Baracos. 2011. "Definition and classification of cancer cachexia: An international consensus." *Review Lancet Oncol* 12 (5):489–95. doi: 10.1016/S1470-2045(10)70218-7.

Federal Register. https://www.federalregister.gov/documents/2020/06/30/2020-13792/medicare-and-medicaid-programs-cy-2021-home-health-prospective-payment-system-rate-update-home.

Fiorillo, C., F. Rosa, G. Quero, R. Menghi, G. B. Doglietto, and S. Alfieri. 2017. "Postoperative hyperglycemia in nondiabetic patients after gastric surgery for cancer: Perioperative outcomes." *Gastric Cancer* 20 (3):536–42. doi: 10.1007/s10120-016-0621-5.

Fringer, A., S. Stängle, D. Büche, S. C. Ott, and W. Schnepp. 2020. "The associations of palliative care experts regarding food refusal: A cross-sectional study with an open question evaluated by triangulation analysis." *PLoS One* 15 (4):e0231312. doi: 10.1371/journal.pone.0231312.

Fukuda, Y., K. Yamamoto, M. Hirao, K. Nishikawa, S. Maeda, N. Haraguchi, M. Miyake, N. Hama, A. Miyamoto, M. Ikeda, S. Nakamori, M. Sekimoto, K. Fujitani, and T. Tsujinaka. 2015. "Prevalence of malnutrition among gastric cancer patients undergoing gastrectomy and optimal preoperative nutritional support for preventing surgical site infections." *Ann Surg Oncol* 22 (Suppl 3):S778–85. doi: 10.1245/s10434-015-4820-9.

Gamper, E. M., A. Zabernigg, L. M. Wintner, J. M. Giesinger, A. Oberguggenberger, G. Kemmler, B. Sperner-Unterweger, and B. Holzner. 2012. "Coming to your senses: Detecting taste and smell alterations in chemotherapy patients: A systematic review." *J Pain Symptom Manage* 44 (6):880–95. doi: 10.1016/j.jpainsymman.2011.11.011.

Giacosa, A., and M. Rondanelli. 2008. "Fish oil and treatment of cancer cachexia." *Genes Nutr* 3 (1):25–8. doi: 10.1007/s12263-008-0078-1.

Giannousi, Z, I. Gioulbasanis, A. G. Pallis, A. Xyrafas, D. Dalliani, K. Kalbakis, V. Papadopoulos, D. Mavroudis, V. Georgoulias, and C. N. Papandreou. 2012. "Nutritional status, acute phase response and depression in metastatic lung cancer patients: Correlations and association prognosis." *Support Care Cancer* 20:1823–9.

Gianotti, L., M. Braga, C. Fortis, L. Soldini, A. Vignali, S. Colombo, G. Radaelli, and V. Di Carlo. 1999. "A prospective, randomized clinical trial on perioperative feeding with an arginine-, omega-3 fatty acid-, and RNA-enriched enteral diet: Effect on host response and nutritional status." *JPEN J Parenter Enteral Nutr* 23 (6):314–20. doi: 10.1177/0148607199023006314.

Gilliland, T. M., N. Villafane-Ferriol, K. P. Shah, R. M. Shah, H. S. Tran Cao, N. N. Massarweh, E. J. Silberfein, E. A. Choi, C. Hsu, A. L. McElhany, O. Barakat, W. Fisher, and G. Van Buren. 2017. "Nutritional and metabolic derangements in pancreatic cancer and pancreatic resection." *Nutrients* 9 (3). doi: 10.3390/nu9030243.

Glare, P., W. Jongs, and B. Zafiropoulos. 2010. "Establishing a cancer nutrition rehabilitation program (CNRP) for ambulatory patients attending an Australian cancer center." *Supportive Care in Cancer* 19 (4):445–54. doi: 10.1007/s00520-010-0834-9.

Grosvenor, M., L. Bulcavage, and R. T. Chlebowski. 1989. "Symptoms potentially influencing weight loss in a cancer population: Correlations with primary site, nutritional status, and chemotherapy administration." *Cancer* 63:330–4.

Grotenhuis, B. A., J. Shapiro, S. van Adrichem, M. de Vries, M. Koek, B. P. L. Wijnhoven, and J. J. B. van Lanschot. 2016. "Sarcopenia/muscle mass is not a prognostic factor for short- and long-term outcome after esophagectomy for cancer." *World J Surg* 40(11):2698–704. doi: 10.1007/s00268-016-3603-1.

Guan, H., S. Chen, and Q. Huang. 2019. "Effects of enteral immunonutrition in patients undergoing pancreaticoduodenectomy: A meta-analysis of randomized controlled trials." *Ann Nutr Metab* 74 (1):53–61. doi: 10.1159/000495468.

Gustafsson, U. O., J. Nygren, A. Thorell, M. Soop, P. M. Hellstrom, O. Ljungqvist, and E. Hagstrom-Toft. 2008. "Pre-operative carbohydrate loading may be used in type 2 diabetes patients." *Acta Anaesthesiol Scand* 52 (7):946–51. doi: 10.1111/j.1399-6576.2008.01599.x.

Gustafsson, U. O., M. J. Scott, M. Hubner, J. Nygren, N. Demartines, N. Francis, T. A. Rockall, T. M. Young-Fadok, A. G. Hill, M. Soop, H. D. de Boer, R. D. Urman, G. J. Chang, A. Fichera, H. Kessler, F. Grass, E. E. Whang, W. J. Fawcett, F. Carli, D. N. Lobo, K. E. Rollins, A. Balfour, G. Baldini, B. Riedel, and O. Ljungqvist. 2019. "Guidelines for perioperative care in elective colorectal surgery: Enhanced recovery after surgery (ERAS(R)) society recommendations: 2018." *World J Surg* 43 (3):659–95. doi: 10.1007/s00268-018-4844-y.

Halpern, M. T., and K. R. Yabroff. 2008. "Prevalence of outpatient cancer treatment in the United States: Estimates from the Medical Panel Expenditures Survey (MEPS)." *Cancer Invest* 26 (6):647–51. doi: 10.1080/07357900801905519.

Halpern-Silveira, D., L. R. O. Susin, L. R. Borges, S. I. Paiva, M. C. F. Assunção, and M. C. Gonzalez. 2010. "Body weight and fat-free mass changes in a cohort of patients receiving chemotherapy." *Support Care Cancer* 18 (5):617–25. doi: 10.1007/s00520-009-0703-6.

Hamirudin, A. H, K. Walton, K. Charlton, et al. 2017. "Feasibility of home-based dietetic intervention to improve the nutritional status of older adults post-hospital discharge." *Nutr Diet* 74 (3):217–23.

Hanai, N., H. Terada, H. Hirakawa, H. Suzuki, D. Nishikawa, S. Beppu, and Y. Hasegawa. 2018. "Prospective randomized investigation implementing immunonutritional therapy using a nutritional supplement with a high blend ratio of ω-3 fatty acids during the perioperative period for head and neck carcinomas." *Jpn J Clin Oncol* 48 (4):356–61. doi: 10.1093/jjco/hyy008.

Harpaz, J. 2019, December 9. 5 Ways technology will enable value-based care in 2020 and beyond. Forbes. com. https://www.forbes.com/sites/joeharpaz/2019/12/09/5-ways-technology-will-enable-value-based-care-in-2020/#39f5c6413511.

Hatao, F., K. Y. Chen, J. M. Wu, M. Y. Wang, S. Aikou, H. Onoyama, N. Shimizu, K. Fukatsu, Y. Seto, and M. T. Lin. 2017. "Randomized controlled clinical trial assessing the effects of oral nutritional supplements in postoperative gastric cancer patients." *Langenbecks Arch Surg* 402 (2):203–11. doi: 10.1007/s00423-016-1527-8.

Hausel, J., J. Nygren, M. Lagerkranser, P. M. Hellstrom, F. Hammarqvist, C. Almstrom, A. Lindh, A. Thorell, and O. Ljungqvist. 2001. "A carbohydrate-rich drink reduces preoperative discomfort in elective surgery patients." *Anesth Analg* 93 (5):1344–50. doi: 10.1097/00000539-200111000-00063.

HHS. 2020. HHS initiatives to address the disparate impact of COVID-19 on African Americans and other racial and ethnic minorities. https://www.hhs.gov/sites/default/files/hhs-fact-sheet-addressing-disparities-in-covid-19-impact-on-minorities.pdf.

Higgins, A., et al. 2019, Septembere 12. Measurement for value-based payment: Harnessing patient-centered outcomes to define quality. Duke-Margolis Center for Health Policy. Avaliable at: https://healthpolicy.duke.edu/publications/measurement-value-based-payment-harnessing-patient-centered-outcomes-define-quality.

Hong, K., W. Wang, S. Sulo, L. Huettner, R. Taroyan, and C. Kaloostian. 2020. "Nutrition program reduces healthcare use of adult outpatients with poor nutrition status" *Clin Nutr ESPEN* 40:412e690.

Hopkinson, J. B. 2016. "Food connections: A qualitative exploratory study of weight- and eating-related distress in families affected by advanced cancer." *Eur J Oncol Nurs* 20:87–96. doi: 10.1016/j.ejon.2015.06.002.

Huang, Q., H. Zhang, J. Hai, M. A. Socinski, E. Lim, H. Chen, and J. Stebbing. 2018. "Impact of PD-L1 expression, driver mutations and clinical characteristics on survival after anti-PD-1/PD-L1 immunotherapy versus chemotherapy in non-small-cell lung cancer: A meta-analysis of randomized trials." *Oncoimmunology* 7 (12):e1396403. doi: 10.1080/2162402X.2017.1396403.

Huang, E. Y., S. Knight, C. R. Guetter, C. H. Davis, M. Moller, E. Slama, and M. Crandall. 2019. "Telemedicine and telementoring in the surgical specialties: A narrative review." *Am J Surg* 218(4): 760–66. doi: 10.1016/j.amjsurg.2019.07.018 TeO.

Huhmann, M. B., and D. A. August. 2008. "Review of American Society for Parenteral and Enteral Nutrition (ASPEN) clinical guidelines for nutrition support in cancer patients: Nutrition screening and assessment." *Nutr Clin Pract* 23 (2):182–8. doi: 10.1177/0884533608314530.

Huillard, O., O. Mir, M. Peyromaure, C. Tlemsani, J. Giroux, P. Boudou-Rouquette, S. Ropert, N. B. Delongchamps, M. Zerbib, and F. Goldwasser. 2013. "Sarcopenia and body mass index predict sunitinib-induced early dose-limiting toxicities in renal cancer patients." *Br J Cancer* 108 (5):1034–41. doi: 10.1038/bjc.2013.58.

Isenring, E. A., S. Capra, and J. D. Bauer. 2004. "Nutrition intervention is beneficial in oncology outpatients receiving radiotherapy to the gastrointestinal or head and neck area." *Br J Cancer* 91 (3):447–52. doi: 10.1038/sj.bjc.6601962.

Jackson, R. S., R. L. Amdur, J. C. White, and R. A. Macsata. 2012. "Hyperglycemia is associated with increased risk of morbidity and mortality after colectomy for cancer." *J Am Coll Surg* 214 (1):68–80. doi: 10.1016/j.jamcollsurg.2011.09.016.

Jagoe, R. T., T. H. Goodship, and G. J. Gibson. 2001. "The influence of nutritional status on complications after operations for lung cancer." *Ann Thorac Surg* 71:936–43.

Jang, R. W., V. B. Caraiscos, N. Swami, S. Banerjee, E. Mak, E. Kaya, G. Rodin, J. Bryson, J. Z. Ridley, L. W. Le, and C. Zimmermann. 2014. "Simple prognostic model for patients with advanced cancer based on performance status." *J Oncol Pract* 10 (5):e335–41. doi: 10.1200/jop.2014.001457.

Jeffery, K. M., B. Harkins, G. A. Cresci, and R. G. Martindale. 1996. "The clear liquid diet is no longer a necessity in the routine postoperative management of surgical patients." *Am Surg* 62 (3):167–70.

Jensen, S. B., H. T. Mouridsen, O. J. Bergmann, J. Reibel, N. Brunner, and B. Nauntofte. 2008. "Oral mucosal lesions, microbial changes, and taste disturbances induced by adjuvant chemotherapy in breast cancer patients." *Oral Surg Oral Med Oral Pathol Oral Radiol Endod* 106 (2):217–26. doi: 10.1016/j.tripleo.2008.04.003.

Jensen, G. L., J. Mirtallo, C. Compher, R. Dhaliwal, A. Forbes, R. F. Grijalba, G. Hardy, J. Kondrup, D. Labadarios, I. Nyulasi, J. C. Castillo Pineda, D. Waitzberg, and Committee International Consensus Guideline. 2010. "Adult starvation and disease-related malnutrition: A proposal for etiology-based diagnosis in the clinical practice setting from the International Consensus Guideline Committee." *JPEN J Parenter Enteral Nutr* 34 (2):156–9. doi: 10.1177/0148607110361910.

Jho, D., T. A. Babcock, W. S. Helton, and N. J. Espat. 2003. "Omega-3 fatty acids: Implications for the treatment of tumor-associated inflammation." *Am Surg* 69 (1):32–6.

Joint Commission on Accreditation of Healthcare Organizations. 2007. *Comprehensive Accreditation Manual for Hospitals.* Chicago, IL: Joint Commission on Accreditation of Healthcare Organizations.

Kadakia, K., L. A. Fleisher, C. J. Stimson, T. Aloia, and A. C. Offodile. 2020. "Charting a roadmap for value-based surgery in the post-pandemic era." *Ann Surg* 272(2):e43–e4.

Kamarajah, S. K., J. Bundred, and B. Tan. 2018. "Body composition assessment and sarcopenia in patients with gastric cancer: A systematic review and meta-analysis." *Gastric Cancer* 22:10–22.

Keating, N. L., M. B. Landrum, E. B. Lamont, S. R. Bozeman, L. N. Shulman, and B. J. McNeil. 2013. "Tumor boards and the quality of cancer care." *J Natl Cancer Inst* 105 (2):113–21. doi: 10.1093/jnci/djs502.

Klein, S., J. Simes, and G. L. Blackburn. 1986. "Total parenteral nutrition and cancer clinical trials." *Cancer* 58:1378–86.

Kobayashi, A., T. Kaido, Y. Hamaguchi, S. Okumura, H. Shirai, S. Yao, N. Kamo, S. Yagi, K. Taura, H. Okajima, and S. Uemoto. 2019. "Impact of sarcopenic obesity on outcomes in patients undergoing hepatectomy for hepatocellular carcinoma." *Ann Surg* 269 (5):924–31. doi: 10.1097/SLA.0000000000002555.

Kotler, D. P. 2000. "Cachexia." *Ann Intern Med* 133(8):622–34. doi: 10.7326/0003-4819-133-8-200010170-00015.

Laird, B. J., A. C. Scott, L. A. Colvin, A. L. McKeon, G. D. Murray, K. C. Fearon, M. T. Fallon. 2011. "Pain, depression, and fatigue as a symptom cluster in advanced cancer." *J Pain Symptom Manage* 42:1–11.

Lanctin, D. P., F. Merced-Nieves, R. M. Mallett, M. B. Arensberg, P. Guenter, S. Sulo, and T. F. Platts-Mills. 2019. "Prevalence and economic burden of malnutrition diagnosis among patients presenting to United States emergency departments." *Acad Emerg Med.* doi: 10.1111/acem.13887.

Lassen, K., J. Kjaeve, T. Fetveit, G. Trano, H. K. Sigurdsson, A. Horn, and A. Revhaug. 2008. "Allowing normal food at will after major upper gastrointestinal surgery does not increase morbidity: A randomized multicenter trial." *Ann Surg* 247 (5):721–9. doi: 10.1097/SLA.0b013e31815cca68.

Laviano, A., and M. M. Meguid. 1996. "Nutritional issues in cancer management." *Nutrition* 12 (5):358–71. doi: 10.1016/s0899-9007(96)80061-x.

Laviano, A., P. C. Calder, A. M. W. J. Schols, F. Lonnqvist, M. Bech, and M. Muscaritoli. 2020. "Safety and tolerability of targeted medical nutrition for cachexia in non-small-cell lung cancer: A randomized, double-blind, controlled pilot trial." *Nutr Cancer* 72 (3):439–50. doi: 10.1080/01635581.2019.1634746.

Lee, J. L. C., L. P. Leong, and S. L. Lim. 2016. "Nutrition intervention approaches to reduce malnutrition in oncology patients: A systematic review." *Support Care Cancer* 24 (1):469–80. doi: 10.1007/s00520-015-2958-4.

Lee, S. M., J. Oh, M. R. Chun, and S. Y. Lee. 2019. "Methylmalonic acid and homocysteine as indicators of vitamin B12 deficiency in patients with gastric cancer after gastrectomy." *Nutrients* 11 (2). doi: 10.3390/nu11020450.

Lees, J. 1999. "Incidence of weight loss in head and neck patients with cancer on commencing radiotherapy treatment at a regional oncology centre." *Eur J Cancer Care (Engl).* 8:133–6.

Leung, H. W., and A. L. Chan. 2016. "Glutamine in alleviation of radiation-induced severe oral mucositis: A meta-analysis." *Nutr Cancer* 68 (5):734–42. doi: 10.1080/01635581.2016.1159700.

Li, L., Z. Wang, X. Ying, J. Tian, T. Sun, K. Yi, P. Zhang, Z. Jing, and K. Yang. 2012. "Preoperative carbohydrate loading for elective surgery: A systematic review and meta-analysis." *Surg Today* 42 (7):613–24. doi: 10.1007/s00595-012-0188-7.

Lievens, Y., R. Audisio, I. Banks, L. Collette, C. Grau, and K. Oliver. 2019. "Towards an evidence-informed vaule scale for surgical and radiation oncology: A multi-stakeholder perspective." *Lancet Oncol* 20(2):E112–23. doi: 10.1016/S1470-2045(18)30917-3.

Lim, C. H., S. W. Kim, W. C. Kim, J. S. Kim, Y. K. Cho, J. M. Park, I. S. Lee, M. G. Choi, K. Y. Song, H. M. Jeon, and C. H. Park. 2012. "Anemia after gastrectomy for early gastric cancer: Long-term follow-up observational study." *World J Gastroenterol* 18 (42):6114–9. doi: 10.3748/wjg.v18.i42.6114.

Lin, J., J. Peng, A. Qdaisat, L. Li, G. Chen, Z. Lu, X. Wu, Y. Gao, Z. Zeng, P. Ding, and Z. Pan. 2016. "Severe weight loss during preoperative chemoradiotherapy compromises survival outcome for patients with locally advanced rectal cancer." *J Cancer Res Clin Oncol* 142 (12):2551–60. doi: 10.1007/s00432-016-2225-1.

Liu, H., W. Ling, Z. Y. Shen, X. Jin, and H. Cao. 2012. "Clinical application of immune-enhanced enteral nutrition in patients with advanced gastric cancer after total gastrectomy." *J Dig Dis* 13 (8):401–6. doi: 10.1111/j.1751-2980.2012.00596.x.

Ljungqvist, O., and E. Soreide. 2003. "Preoperative fasting." *Br J Surg* 90 (4):400–6. doi: 10.1002/bjs.4066.

Ljungqvist, O., N. X. Thanh, and G. Nelson. 2017. "ERAS-value based surgery." *J Surg Oncol* 116(5). doi: 10.1002/jso.24820.

Lodewick, T. M., van Nijnatten, T. J. A., van Dam, R. M., van Mierlo, K., Dello, S. A. W. G., Neumann, U. P., Olde Damink, S. W. M. and Dejong, C. H. C. 2015 "Are sarcopenia, obesity and sarcopenic obesity predictive of outcome in patients with colorectal liver metastases?" *HPB*, Elsevier, 17(5):438–46. doi: 10.1111/HPB.12373.

Loprinzi, C., N. MacDonald, G. Mantovani, M. Davis, M. Muscaritoli, F. Ottery, L. Radbruch, P. Ravasco, D. Walsh, A. Wilcock, S. Kaasa, and V. E. Baracos. 2011. "Definition and classification of cancer cachexia: An international consensus. *Lancet Oncol* 12:489–95.

Lorite, M.J., P. Cariuk, and M. J. Tisdale. 1997. "Induction of muscle protein degradation by a tumour factor." *Br J Cancer* 76 (8):1035–40. doi: 10.1038/bjc.1997.504.

Lou, N., C. H. Chi, X. D. Chen, C. J. Zhou, S. L. Wang, C. L. Zhuang, and X. Shen. 2017. "Sarcopenia in overweight and obese patients is a predictive factor for postoperative complication in gastric cancer: A prospective study." *Eur J Surg Oncol* 43 (1):188–95. doi: 10.1016/j.ejso.2016.09.006.

Ma, Q., M. Hoper, N. Anderson, and B. J. Rowlands. 1996. "Effect of supplemental L-arginine in a chemical-induced model of colorectal cancer." *World J Surg* 20:1087–91.

Makarenkova, V. P., V. Bansal, B. M. Matta, L. A. Perez, and J. B. Ochoa. 2006. "CD11b+/Gr-1+ myeloid suppressor cells cause T cell dysfunction after traumatic stress." *J Immunol* 176 (4):2085–94. doi: 10.4049/jimmunol.176.4.2085.

Marik, P. E., and M. Flemmer. 2012. "The immune response to surgery and trauma: Implications for treatment." *J Trauma Acute Care Surg* 73 (4):801–8. doi: 10.1097/TA.0b013e318265cf87.

Marimuthu, K., K. K. Varadhan, O. Ljungqvist, and D. N. Lobo. 2012. "A meta-analysis of the effect of combinations of immune modulating nutrients on outcome in patients undergoing major open gastrointestinal surgery." *Ann Surg* 255 (6):1060–8. doi: 10.1097/SLA.0b013e318252edf8.

Martin, L., L. Birdsell, N. Macdonald, T. Reiman, M. T. Clandinin, L. J. McCargar, R. Murphy, S. Ghosh, M. B. Sawyer, and V. E. Baracos. 2013. "Cancer cachexia in the age of obesity: Skeletal muscle depletion is a powerful prognostic factor, independent of body mass index." *J Clin Oncol* 31 (12):1539–47. doi: 10.1200/jco.2012.45.2722.

Martin, L., P. Senesse, I. Gioulbasanis, S. Antoun, F. Bozzetti, C. Deans, F. Strasser, L. Thoresen, R. T. Jagoe, M. Chasen, K. Lundholm, I. Bosaeus, K. H. Fearon, and V. E. Baracos. 2015. "Diagnostic criteria for the classification of cancer-associated weight loss." *J Clin Oncol* 33 (1):90–9. doi: 10.1200/JCO.2014.56.1894.

Martin, L., I. Gioulbasanis, P. Senesse, and V. E. Baracos. 2020. "Cancer-associated malnutrition and CT-defined sarcopenia and myosteatosis are endemic in overweight and obese patients." *JPEN J Parenter Enteral Nutr* 44 (2):227–38. doi: 10.1002/jpen.1597.

Massicotte, M. H., I. Borget, S. Broutin, V. E. Baracos, S. Leboulleux, E. Baudin, A. Paci, A. Deroussent, M. Schlumberger, and S. Antoun. 2013. "Body composition variation and impact of low skeletal muscle mass in patients with advanced medullary thyroid carcinoma treated with vandetanib: Results from a placebo-controlled study." *J Clin Endocrinol Metab* 98 (6):2401–8. doi: 10.1210/jc.2013-1115.

Matsunaga, T., H. Miyata, K. Sugimura, M. Motoori, K. Asukai, Y. Yanagimoto, Y. Takahashi, A. Tomokuni, K. Yamamoto, H. Akita, J. Nishimura, H. Wada, H. Takahashi, M. Yasui, T. Omori, M. Oue, and M. Yano. 2019. "Prognostic significance of sarcopenia and systemic inflammatory response in patients with esophageal cancer." *Anticancer Res* 39 (1):449–58. doi: 10.21873/anticanres.13133.

McClave, S. A., B. E. Taylor, R. G. Martindale, M. M. Warren, D. R. Johnson, C. Braunschweig, M. S. McCarthy, E. Davanos, T. W. Rice, G. A. Cresci, J. M. Gervasio, G. S. Sacks, P. R. Roberts, and C. Compher. 2016. "Guidelines for the provision and assessment of nutrition support therapy in the adult critically Ill patient: Society of Critical Care Medicine (SCCM) and American Society for Parenteral and Enteral Nutrition (A.S.P.E.N.)." *JPEN J Parenter Enteral Nutr* 40 (2):159–211. doi: 10.1177/0148607115621863.

McKenna, N. P., K. A. Bews, W. B. Al-Refaie, J. H. Pemberton, R. R. Cima, and E.B. Habermann. 2020. "Assessming malnutrition before major oncologic surgery: One size does not fit all." *J Am Coll Surgeons* 230(4):451–60. 10.1016/j.jamcolllsurg.2019.12.034.

Medicare. "Hospital comparison." https://www.medicare.gov/hospitalcompare/search.html.

Medicare. "Medicare." https://www.medicare.gov/hospitalcompare/linking-quality-to-payment.html.

Mendes, N. P., T. A. Barros, C. O. B. Rosa, and S. Franceschini. 2019. "Nutritional screening tools used and validated for cancer patients: A systematic review." *Nutr Cancer* 71 (6):898–907. doi: 10.1080/01635581.2019.1595045.

Meng, Q., S. Tan, Y. Jiang, J. Han, Q. Xi, Q. Zhuang, and G. Wu. 2021. "Post-discharge oral nutritional supplements with dietary advice in patients at nutritional risk after surgery for gastric cancer: A randomized clinical trial." *Clin Nutr.* doi: 10.1016/j.clnu.2020.04.043.

Miller, C. J., B. Kim, A. Silverman, and M. S. Bauer. 2018. "A systematic review of team-building interventions in non-acute healthcare settings." *BMC Health Serv Res* 18 (1):146. doi: 10.1186/s12913-018-2961-9.

Milne, A. C., J. Potter, A. Vivanti, and A. Avenell. 2009. "Protein and energy supplementation in elderly people at risk from malnutrition." *Cochrane Database Syst Rev* 2009 (2):Cd003288. doi: 10.1002/14651858.CD003288.pub3.

Mingliang, W., K. Zhangyan, F. Fangfang, W. Huizhen, and L. Yongxiang. 2020. "Perioperative immunonutrition in esophageal cancer patients undergoing esophagectomy: The first meta-analysis of randomized clinical trials." *Dis Esophagus* 33 (4). doi: 10.1093/dote/doz111.

Mintziras, I., M. Miligkos, S. Wachter, J. Manoharan, E. Maurer, and D. K. Bartsch. 2018. "Sarcopenia and sarcopenic obesity are significantly associated with poorer overall survival in patients with pancreatic cancer: Systematic review and meta-analysis." *Int J Surg* 59:19–26. doi: 10.1016/j.ijsu.2018.09.014.

Mir, O., R. Coriat, B. Blanchet, J. P. Durand, P. Boudou-Rouquette, J. Michels, S. Ropert, M. Vidal, S. Pol, S. Chaussade, and F. Goldwasser. 2012. "Sarcopenia predicts early dose-limiting toxicities and pharmacokinetics of sorafenib in patients with hepatocellular carcinoma." *PLoS One* 7 (5):e37563. doi: 10.1371/journal.pone.0037563.

Mizumachi, T., S. Kano, A. Homma, M. Akazawa, C. Hasegawa, Y. Shiroishi, C. Okamoto, S. Kumagai, M. Nishimura, H. Takasaki, H. Takeda, K. Yasuda, H. Minatogawa, Y. Dekura, R. Onimaru, H. Shirato, and S. Fukuda. 2019. "A nutritional supplement with a high blend ratio of ω-3 fatty acids(Prosure®) reduces severe oral mucositis and body weight loss for head and neck cancer patients treated with chemoradiotherapy." *Gan To Kagaku Ryoho* 46 (4):685–9.

Mogensen, K. M., A. Malone, P. Becker, S. Cutrell, L. Frank, K. Gonzales, L. Hudson, S. Miller, and P. Guenter. 2019. "Academy of Nutrition and Dietetics/American Society for Parenteral and Enteral Nutrition Consensus Malnutrition Characteristics: Usability and association with outcomes." *Nutr Clin Pract* 34 (5):657–65. doi: 10.1002/ncp.10310.

Moses, A. W. G., C. Slater, T. Preston, M. D. Barber, and K. C. H. Fearon. 2004. "Reduced total energy expenditure and physical activity in cachectic patients with pancreatic cancer can be modulated by an energy and protein dense oral supplement enriched with n-3 fatty acids." *Br J Cancer* 90 (5):996–1002. doi: 10.1038/sj.bjc.6601620.

Moya, P., L. Soriano-Irigaray, J. M. Ramirez, A. Garcea, O. Blasco, F. J. Blanco, C. Brugiotti, E. Miranda, and A. Arroyo. 2016. "Perioperative standard oral nutrition supplements versus immunonutrition in patients undergoing colorectal resection in an enhanced recovery (ERAS) protocol: A multicenter randomized clinical trial (SONVI Study)." *Medicine (Baltimore)* 95 (21):e3704. doi: 10.1097/MD.0000000000003704.

Mueller, C., C. Compher, and D. M. Ellen. 2011. "A.S.P.E.N. clinical guidelines: Nutrition screening, assessment, and intervention in adults." *JPEN J Parenter Enteral Nutr* 35 (1):16–24. doi: 10.1177/0148607110389335.

Mueller, S. A., C. Mayer, B. Bojaxhiu, C. Aeberhard, P. Schuetz, Z. Stanga, and R. Giger. 2019. "Effect of preoperative immunonutrition on complications after salvage surgery in head and neck cancer." *J Otolaryngol Head Neck Surg* 48 (1):25. doi: 10.1186/s40463-019-0345-8.

Mullin, G. E., L. Fan, S. Sulo, and J. Partridge. 2019. "The association between oral nutritional supplements and 30-day hospital readmissions of malnourished patients at a US Academic Medical Center." *J Acad Nutr Diet* 119 (7):1168–75. doi: 10.1016/j.jand.2019.01.014.

Munk, T., U. Tolstrup, A. M. Beck, et al. 2016. "Individualised dietary counselling for nutritionally at-risk older patients following discharge from acute hospital to home: A systematic review and meta-analysis." *J Hum Nutr Diet* 29(2):196–208.

Muñoz, R., L. Farshidpour, U. B. Chaudhary, and A. H. Fathi. 2018. "Multidisciplinary cancer care model: A positive association between oncology nurse navigation and improved outcomes for patients with cancer." *Clin J Oncol Nurs* 22 (5):E141–5. doi: 10.1188/18.CJON.E141-E145.

Muscaritoli, M., S. Lucia, A. Farcomeni, V. Lorusso, V. Saracino, C. Barone, F. Plastino, S. Gori, R. Magarotto, G. Carteni, B. Chiurazzi, I. Pavese, L. Marchetti, V. Zagonel, E. Bergo, G. Tonini, M. Imperatori, C. Iacono, L. Maiorana, C. Pinto, D. Rubino, L. Cavanna, R. Di Cicilia, T. Gamucci, S. Quadrini, S.

Palazzo, S. Minardi, M. Merlano, G. Colucci, P. Marchetti, and PreMi Study Group. 2017. "Prevalence of malnutrition in patients at first medical oncology visit: The PreMiO study." *Oncotarget* 8 (45):79884–96. doi: 10.18632/oncotarget.20168.

Nakanishi, R., E. Oki, S. Sasaki, K. Hirose, T. Jogo, K. Edahiro, S. Korehisa, D. Taniguchi, K. Kudo, J. Kurashige, M. Sugiyama, Y. Nakashima, K. Ohgaki, H. Saeki, and Y. Maehara. 2018. "Sarcopenia is an independent predictor of complications after colorectal cancer surgery." *Surg Today* 48 (2):151–7. doi: 10.1007/s00595-017-1564-0.

National Cancer Institute. NCI dictionary of cancer terms. http://www.cancer.gov.

Nayel, H., E. El-Ghonelmy, and S. El-Haddad. 1992. "Impact of nutritional supplementation on treatment delay and morbidity in patients with head and neck tumors treated with irradiation." *Nutrition* 8:13–8.

NCCN. "Palliative care." https://www.nccn.org/professionals/physician_gls/pdf/palliative.pdf.

NCCN. https://www.nccn.org/patients/resources/life_with_cancer/managing_symptoms/impact_on_diet.aspx

NCCN. symptom management.

NCI. "NCI dictionary." National Cancer Institute. NCI dictionary of cancer terms. http://www.cancer.gov.

Newman, E. A., A. B. Guest, M. A. Helvie, M. A. Roubidoux, A. E. Chang, C. G. Kleer, K. M. Diehl, V. M. Cimmino, L. Pierce, D. Hayes, L. A. Newman, and M. S. Sabel. 2006. "Changes in surgical management resulting from case review at a breast cancer multidisciplinary tumor board." *Cancer* 107 (10):2346–51. doi: 10.1002/cncr.22266.

Nishigori, T., S. Tsunoda, H. Okabe, E. Tanaka, S. Hisamori, H. Hosogi, H. Shinohara, and Y. Sakai. 2016. "Impact of sarcopenic obesity on surgical site infection after laparoscopic total gastrectomy." *Ann Surg Oncol* 23 (Suppl 4):524–31. doi: 10.1245/s10434-016-5385-y.

Nitenberg, G., and B. Raynard. 2000. "Nutritional support of the cancer patient: Issues and dilemmas." *Crit Rev Oncol Hematol* 34:137–68.

Niu, J. W., L. Zhou, Z. Z. Liu, D. P. Pei, W. Q. Fan, and W. Ning. 2020. "A systematic review and meta-analysis of the effects of perioperative immunonutrition in gastrointestinal cancer patients." *Nutr Cancer*:1–10. doi: 10.1080/01635581.2020.1749291.

Nouri, S., E. C. Khoong, C. R. Lyles, and L. Karliner. 2020. "Addressing equity in telemedicine for chronic disease management during the COVID-19 pandemic." *NEJM Catalyst, Innovations in Care Delivery*. https://catalyst.nejm.org/doi/full/10.1056/CAT.20.0123.

Odelli, C., D. Burgess, L. Bateman, A. Hughes, S. Ackland, J. Gillies, and C. E. Collins. 2005. "Nutrition support improves patient outcomes, treatment tolerance and admission characteristics in oesophageal cancer." *Clin Oncol* 17 (8):639–45. doi: 10.1016/j.clon.2005.03.015.

Osland, E., M. B. Hossain, S. Khan, and M. A. Memon. 2014. "Effect of timing of pharmaconutrition (immuno-nutrition) administration on outcomes of elective surgery for gastrointestinal malignancies: A systematic review and meta-analysis." *JPEN J Parenter Enteral Nutr* 38 (1):53–69. doi: 10.1177/0148607112474825.

Ottery, F. D. 1994. "Cancer cachexia: Prevention, early diagnosis, and management." *Cancer Pract* 2 (2):123–31.

Paccagnella, A., I. Morassutti, and G. Rosti. 2011. "Nutritional intervention for improving treatment tolerance in cancer patients." *Curr Opin Oncol* 23 (4):322–30. doi: 10.1097/CCO.0b013e3283479c66.

Pearl, M. L., M. Frandina, L. Mahler, F. A. Valea, P. A. DiSilvestro, and E. Chalas. 2002. "A randomized controlled trial of a regular diet as the first meal in gynecologic oncology patients undergoing intraabdominal surgery." *Obstet Gynecol* 100 (2):230–4. doi: 10.1016/s0029-7844(02)02067-7.

Perioperative Total Parenteral Nutrition in Surgical Patients. 1991. "The veterans affairs total parenteral nutrition cooperative study group." *N Engl J Med* 325:525–32.

Persson, C., P. O. Sjoden, and B. Glimelius. 1999. "The Swedish version of the patientgenerated subjective global assessment of nutritional status: Gastrointestinal vs urological cancers. *Clin Nutr.* 18:71–77.

Pillay, B., A. C. Wootten, H. Crowe, N. Corcoran, B. Tran, P. Bowden, J. Crowe, and A. J. Costello. 2016. "The impact of multidisciplinary team meetings on patient assessment, management and outcomes in oncology settings: A systematic review of the literature." *Cancer Treat Rev* 42:56–72 doi: 10.1016/j.ctrv.2015.11.007.

Poole, K. and K. Froggatt. 2002. "Loss of weight and loss of appetite in advanced cancer: A problem for the patient, the carer, or the health professional?" *Palliat Med* 16 (6):499–506. doi: 10.1191/0269216302pm593oa.

Prado, C. M., V. E. Baracos, L. J. McCargar, M. Mourtzakis, K. E. Mulder, T. Reiman, C. A. Butts, A. G. Scarfe, and M. B. Sawyer. 2007. "Body composition as an independent determinant of 5-fluorouracil-based chemotherapy toxicity." *Clin Cancer Res* 13 (11):3264–8. doi: 10.1158/1078-0432.CCR-06-3067.

Prado, C. M., J. R. Lieffers, L. J. McCargar, T. Reiman, M. B. Sawyer, L. Martin, and V. E. Baracos. 2008. "Prevalence and clinical implications of sarcopenic obesity in patients with solid tumours of the respiratory and gastrointestinal tracts: A population-based study." *Lancet Oncol* 9:629–35.

Prado, C. M., V. E. Baracos, L. J. McCargar, T. Reiman, M. Mourtzakis, K. Tonkin, J. R. Mackey, S. Koski, E. Pituskin, and M. B. Sawyer. 2009. "Sarcopenia as a determinant of chemotherapy toxicity and time to tumor progression in metastatic breast cancer patients receiving capecitabine treatment." *Clin Cancer Res* 15 (8):2920–6. doi: 10.1158/1078-0432.CCR-08-2242.

Ravasco, P. 2005. "Dietary counseling improves patient outcomes: A prospective, randomized, controlled trial in colorectal cancer patients undergoing radiotherapy." *J Clin Oncol* 23 (7):1431–8. doi: 10.1200/jco.2005.02.054.

Ravasco, P. 2019. "Nutrition in cancer patients." *J Clin Med* 8 (8). doi: 10.3390/jcm8081211.

Ravasco, P, I. Monteiro-Grillo, P. M. Vidal, and M. E. Camilo. 2003. "Nutritional deterioration in cancer: The role of disease and diet." *Clin Oncol (R Coll Radiol)* 15:443–50.

Ravasco, P., I. Monteiro-Grillo, P. M. Vidal, and M. E. Camilo. 2004. "Cancer: Disease and nutrition are key determinants of patients' quality of life." *Support Care Cancer* 12 (4):246–52. doi: 10.1007/s00520-003-0568-z.

Ravasco, P., I. Monteiro-Grillo, P. M. Vidal, and M. E. Camilo. 2005. "Dietary counseling improves patient outcomes: A prospective, randomized, controlled trial in colorectal patients with cancer undergoing radiotherapy." *J Clin Oncol* 23:1431–8.

Read, J. A., P. J. Beale, D. H. Volker, N. Smith, A. Childs, and S. J. Clarke. 2006. "Nutrition intervention using an eicosapentaenoic acid (EPA)-containing supplement in patients with advanced colorectal cancer: Effects on nutritional and inflammatory status: A phase II trial." *Supportive Care Cancer* 15 (3):301–7. doi: 10.1007/s00520-006-0153-3.

Riley, K., S. Sulo, F. Dabbous, et al. 2020. "Reducing hospitalizations and costs: A home health nutrition-focused quality improvement program." *JPEN J Parenter Enteral Nutr* 44 (1): 58–68. doi: 10.1002/jpen.1606

Rivadeneira, D. E., D. Evoy, T. J. Fahey, 3rd, M. D. Lieberman, and J. M. Daly. 1998. "Nutritional support of the cancer patient." *CA Cancer J Clin* 48:69–80.

Rizvanovic, N., V. Nesek Adam, S. Causevic, S. Dervisevic, and S. Delibegovic. 2019. "A randomised controlled study of preoperative oral carbohydrate loading versus fasting in patients undergoing colorectal surgery." *Int J Colorectal Dis* 34 (9):1551–61. doi: 10.1007/s00384-019-03349-4.

Rock, C. L. 2005. "Dietary counseling is beneficial for the patient with cancer." *J Clin Oncol* 23 (7): 1348–9.

Rocque, G. B., M. Pisu, B. E. Jackson, E. A. Kvale, W. Demark-Wahnfried, M. Y. Martin, K. Meneses, Y. Li, R. A. Taylor, A. Acemgil, C. P. Williams, N. Lisovicz, M. Fouad, K. M. Kenzik, and Partridge, and Patient Care Connect Group. 2017. "Resource use and medicare costs during lay navigation for geriatric patients with cancer." *JAMA Oncol* 3 (6):817–25. doi: 10.1001/jamaoncol.2016.6307.

Roeland, E. J., K. Bohlke, V. E. Baracos, E. Bruera, E. Del Fabbro, S. Dixon, M. Fallon, J. Herrstedt, H. Lau, M. Platek, H. S. Rugo, H. H. Schnipper, T. J. Smith, W. Tan, and C. L. Loprinzi. 2020. "Management of cancer cachexia: ASCO guideline." *J Clin Oncol* 38 (21):2438–53. doi: 10.1200/JCO.20.00611.

Roxburgh, C. S., and D. C. McMillan. 2014. "Cancer and systemic inflammation: Treat the tumour and treat the host." *Br J Cancer* 110:1409–12.

Ryan, A. M., J. V. Reynolds, L. Healy, M. Byrne, J. Moore, N. Brannelly, A. McHugh, D. McCormack, and P. Flood. 2009. "Enteral nutrition enriched with eicosapentaenoic acid (EPA) preserves lean body mass following esophageal cancer surgery: Results of a double-blinded randomized controlled trial." *Ann Surg* 249 (3):355–63. doi: 10.1097/SLA.0b013e31819a4789.

Ryan, A. M., D. G. Power, L. Daly, S. J. Cushen, E. N. Bhuachalla, and C. M. Prado. 2016. "Cancer-associated malnutrition, cachexia and sarcopenia: The skeleton in the hospital closet 40 years later." *Proc Nutr Soc* 75 (2):199–211. doi: 10.1017/S002966511500419X.

Sánchez-Lara, K., J. G. Turcott, E. Juárez-Hernández, C. Nuñez-Valencia, G. Villanueva, P. Guevara, M. De la Torre-Vallejo, A. Mohar, and O. Arrieta. 2014. "Effects of an oral nutritional supplement containing eicosapentaenoic acid on nutritional and clinical outcomes in patients with advanced non-small cell lung cancer: Randomised trial." *Clin Nutr* 33 (6):1017–23. doi: 10.1016/j.clnu.2014.03.006.

Schmidt, N., G. Møller, L. Bæksgaard, K. Østerlind, KD. Stark, L. Lauritzen, and J. R. Andersen. 2020. "Fish oil supplementation in cancer patients: Capsules or nutritional drink supplements? A controlled study of compliance." *Clin Nutr ESPEN* 35:63–8. doi: 10.1016/j.clnesp.2019.12.004.

Schwwartz, T. L., and J. A. Margenthaler. 2019. "Value-based analysis for breast cancer treatment: We don't know what we don't know." *Ann Surg Oncol* 26:1167–69 https://link.springer.com/article/10.1245/s10434-019-07170-9.

Shang, E., C. Weiss, S. Post, and G. Kaehler. 2006. "The influence of early supplementation of parenteral nutrition on quality of life and body composition in patients with advanced cancer." *JPEN J Parenter Enteral Nutr* 30:222–30.

Shils, M. E. 1979. "Principles of nutritional therapy." *Cancer* 43:2093–102.

Shpata, V., X. Prendushi, M. Kreka, I. Kola, F. Kurti, and I. Ohri. 2014. "Malnutrition at the time of surgery affects negatively the clinical outcome of critically ill patients with gastrointestinal cancer." *Med Arch* 68 (4):263–7. doi: 10.5455/medarh.2014.68.263-267.

Siegel, R. L., K. D. Miller, and A. Jemal. 2016. "Cancer statistics, 2016." *CA Cancer J Clin* 66(1), 7–30. doi: 10.3322/caac.21332.

Skipper, A., A. Coltman, J. Tomesko, P. Charney, J. Porcari, T. A. Piemonte, D. Handu, and F. W. Cheng. 2020. "Position of the academy of nutrition and dietetics: Malnutrition (undernutrition) screening tools for all adults." *J Acad Nutr Diet* 120 (4):709–13. doi: 10.1016/j.jand.2019.09.011.

Song, G. M., X. Tian, H. Liang, L. J. Yi, J. G. Zhou, Z. Zeng, T. Shuai, Y. X. Ou, L. Zhang, and Y. Wang. 2015. "Role of enteral immunonutrition in patients undergoing surgery for gastric cancer: A systematic review and meta-analysis of randomized controlled trials." *Medicine (Baltimore)* 94 (31):e1311. doi: 10.1097/MD.0000000000001311.

Sriram, K., S. Sulo, G. VanDerBosch, J. Partridge, J. Feldstein, R. A. Hegazi, and W. T. Summerfelt. 2017. "A comprehensive nutrition-focused quality improvement program reduces 30-day readmissions and length of stay in hospitalized patients." *JPEN J Parenter Enteral Nutr* 41 (3):384–91. doi: 10.1177/0148607116681468.

Stratton, R. J. 2000. "Summary of a systematic review on oral nutritional supplement use in the community." *Proc Nutr Soc* 59:469–76.

Stratton, R. J., C. J. Green, and M. Elia. 2003. *Disease-Related Malnutrition: An Evidence-Based Approach to Treatment*. Wallingford: CABI Publishing.

Stratton, R. J., X. Hebuterne, and M. Elia. 2013. "A systematic review and meta-analysis of the impact of oral nutritional supplements on hospital readmissions." *Ageing Res Rev* 12(4):884–97.

Sulo, S., S. Kozmic, W. T. Summerfelt, J. Partridge, R. Hegazi, and K. Sriram. 2017. "Nutrition based interventions decrease readmission rates and length of stay among malnourished hospitalized adult patients with cardiovascular, oncological, and gastrointestinal diagnoses." Hospital Medicine 2017, May 1–4, 2017, Las Vegas, NV.

Tan, B. H. L., Birdsell, L. A., Martin, L., Baracos, V. E. and Fearon, K. C. H. 2009. 'Sarcopenia in an overweight or obese patient is an adverse prognostic factor in pancreatic cancer.' *Clin Cancer Res Off J Am Assoc Cancer Res* 15(22):6973–9. doi: 10.1158/1078-0432.CCR-09-1525.

Tan, S., Q. Meng, Y. Jiang, Q. Zhuang, Q. Xi, J. Xu, J. Zhao, X. Sui, and G. Wu. 2020. "Impact of oral nutritional supplements in post-discharge patients at nutritional risk following colorectal cancer surgery: A randomised clinical trial." *Clin Nutr*. doi: 10.1016/j.clnu.2020.05.038.

The Association of Community Cancer Centers Cancer Nutrition Services. 2012. A Practical Guide for Cancer Programs.

The Association of Community Cancer Centers. 2012. Cancer program guidelines.

Thenappan, A., I. Halaweish, R. J. Mody, E. A. Smith, J. D. Geiger, P. F. Ehrlich, R. Jasty Rao, R. Hutchinson, G. Yanik, R. M. Rabah, A. Heider, T. Stoll, and E. A. Newman. 2017. "Review at a multidisciplinary tumor board impacts critical management decisions of pediatric patients with cancer." *Pediatr Blood Cancer* 64 (2):254–8. doi: 10.1002/pbc.26201.

Thompson, G. 2018. "Top 4 trends that are changing oncology practices." *Oncol Pract Manage* 8(8). Available at: http://oncpracticemanagement.com/issues/2018/august-2018-vol-8-no-8/623-top-4-trends-that-are-changing-oncology-practices.

Thompson, K. L., L. Elliott, V. Fuchs-Tarlovsky, R. M. Levin, A. C. Voss, and T. Piemonte. 2017. "Oncology evidence-based nutrition practice guideline for adults." *J Acad Nutr Diet* 117 (2):297–310 e47. doi: 10.1016/j.jand.2016.05.010.

Thornblade, L. W., T. K. Varghese, Jr., X. Shi, E. K. Johnson, A. Bastawrous, R. P. Billingham, R. Thirlby, A. Fichera, and D. R. Flum. 2017. "Preoperative immunonutrition and elective colorectal resection outcomes." *Dis Colon Rectum* 60 (1):68–75. doi: 10.1097/DCR.0000000000000740.

Tisdale, M. J. 2002. "Cachexia in cancer patients." *Nat Rev Cancer* 2 (11):862–71. doi: 10.1038/nrc927.

Trabal, J., P. Leyes, M. Forga, and J. Maurel. 2010. "Potential usefulness of an EPA-enriched nutritional supplement on chemotherapy tolerability in cancer patients without overt malnutrition." *Nutr Hosp* 25:736–40.

Trujillo, E. B., S. W. Dixon, K. Claghorn, R. M. Levin, J. B. Mills, and C. K. Spees. 2018. "Closgin the gap in nutrition care at outpatient cancer centers: Ongoing intiatives of the Onclogy Nutrition Dietetic Practice Group." *J Acad Nutr Diet*, 118(4): 749–60.

Trujillo, E. B., K. Claghorn, S. W. Dixon, E. B. Hill, A. Braun, E. Lipinski, M. E. Platek, M. T. Vergo, and C. Spees. 2019. "Inadequate Nutrition Coverage in Outpatient Cancer Centers: Results of a National Survey." *J Oncol* 2019:7462940. doi: 10.1155/2019/7462940.

Ukovic, B., and J. Porter. 2020. "Nutrition interventions to improve the appetite of adults undergoing cancer treatment: A systematic review." *Support Care Cancer*. doi: 10.1007/s00520-020-05475-0.

Valentijn, T. M., W. Galal, E. K. Tjeertes, S. E. Hoeks, H. J. Verhagen, and R. J. Stolker. 2013. "The obesity paradox in the surgical population." *Surgeon* 11 (3):169–76. doi: 10.1016/j.surge.2013.02.003.

van Bokhorst-de van der Schueren, M. A., P. A. van Leeuwen, H. P. Sauerwein, D. J. Kuik, G. B. Snow, and J. J. Quak. 1997. "Assessment of malnutrition parameters in head and neck cancer and their relation to postoperative complications." *Head Neck* 19:419–25.

van der Meij, B. S., M. A. E. van Bokhorst-de van der Schueren, J. A. E. Langius, I. A. Brouwer, and P. A. M. van Leeuwen. 2011. "n-3 PUFAs in cancer, surgery, and critical care: A systematic review on clinical effects, incorporation, and washout of oral or enteral compared with parenteral supplementation." *Am J Clin Nutr* 94:1248–65 doi: 10.3945/ajcn.110.007377.

van der Meij, B. S., J. A. E. Langius, M. D. Spreeuwenberg, S. M. Slootmaker, M. A. Paul, E. F. Smit, and P. A. M. van Leeuwen. 2012. "Oral nutritional supplements containing N-3 polyunsaturated fatty acids affect quality of life and functional status in lung cancer patients during multimodality treatment: An RCT." *Eur J Clin Nutr* 66 (3):399–404. doi: 10.1038/ejcn.2011.214.

van der Riet, P., P. Good, I. Higgins, and L. Sneesby. 2008. "Palliative care professionals' perceptions of nutrition and hydration at the end of life." *Int J Palliat Nurs* 14 (3):145–51. doi: 10.12968/ijpn.2008.14.3.28895.

Vandewoude, M. F., C. J. Alish, A. C. Sauer, and R. A. Hegazi. 2012. "Malnutrition-sarcopenia syndrome: Is this the future of nutrition screening and assessment for older adults? *J Aging Res*. 2012:651570.

Vidal-Casariego, A., A. Calleja-Fernandez, R. Villar-Taibo, G. Kyriakos, and M. D. Ballesteros-Pomar. 2014. "Efficacy of arginine-enriched enteral formulas in the reduction of surgical complications in head and neck cancer: A systematic review and meta-analysis." *Clin Nutr* 33 (6):951–7. doi: 10.1016/j.clnu.2014.04.020.

Vigano, A., N. Donaldson, I. J. Higginson, E. Bruera, S. Mahmud, and M. Suarez-Almazor. 2004. "Quality of life and survival prediction in terminal cancer patients: A multicenter study." *Cancer*. 101:1090–8.

Vissers, Y. L., C. H. Dejong, Y. C. Luiking, K. C. Fearon, M. F. von Meyenfeldt, and N. E. Deutz. 2005. "Plasma arginine concentrations are reduced in cancer patients: Evidence for arginine deficiency?" *Am J Clin Nutr* 81 (5):1142–6. doi: 10.1093/ajcn/81.5.1142.

von Haehling, S., and S. D. Anker. 2010. "Cachexia as a major underestimated and unmet medical need: Facts and numbers." *J Cachexia Sarcopenia Muscle* 1 (1):1–5. doi: 10.1007/s13539-010-0002-6.

von Meyenfeldt, M., K. Fearon, K. Moses, et al. 2002. "Weight gain is associated with improved quality of life in patients with cancer cachexia consuming an energy and protein dense, high n-3 fatty acid oral supplement." *Proc Am Soc Clin Oncol* 21:385A.

Wang, Z. G., Q. Wang, W. J. Wang, and H. L. Qin. 2010. "Randomized clinical trial to compare the effects of preoperative oral carbohydrate versus placebo on insulin resistance after colorectal surgery." *Br J Surg* 97 (3):317–27. doi: 10.1002/bjs.6963.

Watson, M., J. S. Haviland, S. Greer, J. Davidson, and J. M. Bliss. 1999. "Influence of psychological response on survival in breast cancer: A population-based cohort study." *Lancet*. 354:1331–1336.

Weimann, A., M. Braga, F. Carli, T. Higashiguchi, M. Hubner, S. Klek, A. Laviano, O. Ljungqvist, D. N. Lobo, R. Martindale, D. L. Waitzberg, S. C. Bischoff, and P. Singer. 2017. "ESPEN guideline: Clinical nutrition in surgery." *Clin Nutr* 36 (3):623–50. doi: 10.1016/j.clnu.2017.02.013.

Wigmore, S. J., J. A. Ross, J. S. Falconer, C. E. Plester, M. J. Tisdale, D. C. Carter, and K. C. Fearon. 1996. "The effect of polyunsaturated fatty acids on the progress of cachexia in patients with pancreatic cancer." *Nutrition* 12:S27–30. doi: 10.1016/0899-9007(96)90014-3.

Wigmore, S. J., K. C. Fearon, J. P. Maingay, and J. A. Ross. 1997. "Down-regulation of the acute-phase response in patients with pancreatic cancer cachexia receiving oral eicosapentaenoic acid is mediated via suppression of interleukin-6." *Clin Sci (Lond)* 92 (2):215–21. doi: 10.1042/cs0920215.

Willemsen, A. C. H, A. Hoeben, R. I. Lalisang, A. van Helvoort, F. Wesseling, F. Hoebers, L. Baijens, A. Schols. 2020. "Disease-induced and treatment-induced alterations in body composition in locally advanced head and neck squamous cell carcinoma." *J Cachexia Sarcopenia Muscle* 11(1):145–59.

Williams, J. D., and P. E. Wischmeyer. 2017. "Assessment of perioperative nutrition practices and attitudes-A national survey of colorectal and GI surgical oncology programs." *Am J Surg* 213 (6):1010–18. doi: 10.1016/j.amjsurg.2016.10.008.

Williams, A. M., U. F. Bhatti, H. B. Alam, and V. C. Nikolian. 2018. "The role of telemedicine in postoperative care." *Mhealth* 4:11. doi: 10.21037/mhealth.2018.04.03.

Williams, D. G. A., T. Ohnuma, V. Krishnamoorthy, K. Raghunathan, S. Sulo, B. A. Cassady, R. Hegazi, and P. E. Wischmeyer. 2020. "Postoperative utilization of oral nutritional supplements in surgical patients in US hospitals." *JPEN J Parenter Enteral Nutr.* doi: 10.1002/jpen.1862.

Wischmeyer, P. E., F. Carli, D. C. Evans, S. Guilbert, R. Kozar, A. Pryor, R. H. Thiele, S. Everett, M. Grocott, T. J. Gan, A. D. Shaw, J. K. M. Thacker, T. E. Miller, T. L. Hedrick, M. D. McEvoy, M. G. Mythen, R. Bergamaschi, R. Gupta, S. D. Holubar, A. J. Senagore, R. E. Abola, E. Bennett-Guerrero, M. L. Kent, L. S. Feldman, J. F. Fiore, Jr., and Workgroup Perioperative Quality Initiative. 2018. "American society for enhanced recovery and perioperative quality initiative joint consensus statement on nutrition screening and therapy within a surgical enhanced recovery pathway." *Anesth Analg* 126 (6):1883–95. doi: 10.1213/ANE.0000000000002743.

Wright, F. C., C. De Vito, B. Langer, A. Hunter, and Expert Panel on Multidisciplinary Cancer Conference Standards. 2007. "Multidisciplinary cancer conferences: A systematic review and development of practice standards." *Eur J Cancer* 43 (6):1002–10. doi: 10.1016/j.ejca.2007.01.025.

Wu, G. H., Y. W. Zhang, and Z. H. Wu. 2001. "Modulation of postoperative immune and inflammatory response by immune-enhancing enteral diet in gastrointestinal cancer patients." *World J Gastroenterol* 7 (3):357–62. doi: 10.3748/wjg.v7.i3.357.

Xu, J., X. Sun, Q. Xin, Y. Cheng, Z. Zhan, J. Zhang, and J. Wu. 2018. "Effect of immunonutrition on colorectal cancer patients undergoing surgery: A meta-analysis." *Int J Colorectal Dis* 33 (3):273–83. doi: 10.1007/s00384-017-2958-6.

Ye, S. L., N. W. Istfan, D. F. Driscoll, and B. R. Bistrian. 1992. "Tumor and host response to arginine and branched chain amino acid-enriched total parenteral nutrition: A study involving Walker 256 carcinosarcoma-bearing rats." *Cancer* 69:261–70.

Yoon, J., G. Yim, S. Kim, E. Nam, S. Kim, J. Kim, and Y. Kim. 2014. Nutritional risk index as a significant prognostic factor in advanced-stage epithelial ovarian cancer patients. *Society of Gynecologic Oncology 45th Annual Meeting on Women's Cancer*, Tampa, FL.

Yu, K., X. Zheng, G. Wang, M. Liu, Y. Li, P. Yu, M. Yang, N. Guo, X. Ma, Y. Bu, Y. Peng, C. Han, K. Yu, and C. Wang. 2020. "Immunonutrition vs standard nutrition for cancer patients: A systematic review and meta-analysis (Part 1)." *JPEN J Parenter Enteral Nutr* 44 (5):742–67. doi: 10.1002/jpen.1736.

Zafar, S. Y., and A. P. Abernethy. 2013. "Financial toxicity, part 1: A new name for a growing problem." *Oncology (Williston Park)* 27(23), 80–81, 149.

Zhang, C., B. Chen, A. Jiao, F. Li, B. Wang, N. Sun, and J. Zhang. 2017. "The benefit of immunonutrition in patients undergoing hepatectomy: A systematic review and meta-analysis." *Oncotarget* 8 (49): 86843–52. doi: 10.18632/oncotarget.20045.

Zhang, W. T., J. Lin, W. S. Chen, Y. S. Huang, R. S. Wu, X. D. Chen, N. Lou, C. H. Chi, C. Y. Hu, and X. Shen. 2018. "Sarcopenic obesity is associated with severe postoperative complications in gastric cancer patients undergoing gastrectomy: A prospective study." *J Gastrointest Surg* 22 (11):1861–69. doi: 10.1007/s11605-018-3835-5.

Zhang, X., X. Chen, J. Yang, Y. Hu, and K. Li. 2020. "Effects of nutritional support on the clinical outcomes of well-nourished patients with cancer: A meta-analysis." *Eur J Clin Nutr.* doi: 10.1038/s41430-020-0595-6.

Zheng, X., K. Yu, G. Wang, M. Liu, Y. Li, P. Yu, M. Yang, N. Guo, X. Ma, Y. Bu, Y. Peng, C. Han, K. Yu, and C. Wang. 2020. "Effects of immunonutrition on chemoradiotherapy patients: A systematic review and meta-analysis." *JPEN J Parenter Enteral Nutr* 44 (5):768–78. doi: 10.1002/jpen.1735.

Zhu, X., J. P. Pribis, P. C. Rodriguez, S. M. Morris, Jr., Y. Vodovotz, T. R. Billiar, and J. B. Ochoa. 2014. "The central role of arginine catabolism in T-cell dysfunction and increased susceptibility to infection after physical injury." *Ann Surg* 259 (1):171–8. doi: 10.1097/SLA.0b013e31828611f8.

Zhu, M. W., X. Yang, D. R. Xiu, Y. Yang, G. X. Li, W. G. Hu, Z. G. Wang, H. Y. Cui, and J. M. Wei. 2019. "Effect of oral nutritional supplementation on the post-discharge nutritional status and quality of life of gastrointestinal cancer patients after surgery: A multi-center study." *Asia Pac J Clin Nutr* 28 (3):450–6. doi: 10.6133/apjcn.201909_28(3).0004.

15 Malnutrition and Cancer Cachexia

David Heber, Zhaoping Li, and Vijaya Surampudi
UCLA Center for Human Nutrition

CONTENTS

INTRODUCTION

Malnutrition is an often unrecognized complication of cancer affecting the majority of cancer patients. Studies indicate that up to 80% of cancer patients experience involuntary weight loss at some point (Laviano et al. 2005). The effects of reduced food intake are often complicated by the syndrome of cancer cachexia with muscle loss with or without fat loss and an inability to respond adequately to nutritional support (Fearon et al. 2011, Martin et al. 2015). Cancer cachexia is typically due in large part to the effects of cancer itself with factors promoting appetite suppression leading to decreased protein and overall caloric intake with resultant losses in skeletal muscle mass (Ryan et al. 2016). Associated weakness may lead to loss of the ability to undertake activities of daily living and regular exercise.

Weight loss and muscle mass losses may also contribute to fatigue, sleep disturbances, depression, and psychological distress related to the fear of cancer progression (Grutsch et al. 2011, Nipp et al. 2018). Studies suggest that malnutrition and sarcopenia are associated with a greater risk of potentially avoidable negative treatment outcomes, decreased treatment tolerance (Bozzetti 2017, Arrieta et al. 2010), lower response rates to chemotherapy (Di Fiore et al. 2014, Davis and Panikkar 2019), and reduced survival (Deng et al. 2018, Kuwada et al. 2019, Yang et al. 2019). Patients advanced nonsmall-cell lung cancer (NSCLC) with sarcopenia treated with immunotherapy have shorter disease-free survival than patients without sarcopenia (Nishioka et al. 2019).

The pathophysiology of cancer cachexia differs from the normal physiological adaptations to starvation or malnutrition (Suzuki et al. 2013). In the normal adaptation to starvation there is a shift to a fat fuel economy utilizing ketone bodies formed in the liver from fatty acids released from body fat to spare muscle protein breakdown by reducing the release of glucogenic amino acids. In 1970, Dr. George Cahill summarized what had been discovered in the 1940s about the metabolic adaptations to starvation including the above switch to a fat-fuel economy and a decrease in resting metabolic rate (Cahill 1970). The complex adaptations at a central nervous system level including the discovery of a series of interacting hormones integrated in the arcuate nucleus of the hypothalamus which mediated the adaptations to starvation underlying these metabolic shifts were defined during the 1980s including the discovery of leptin.

Leptin while discovered for its impact on obesity actually defends the body from the risks associated with being too thin during starvation through a negative feedback loop that maintains homeostatic control of adipose tissue mass. (Friedman 2016). Leptin levels fall during starvation and elicit adaptive responses in many other physiologic systems, the net effect of which is to reduce energy expenditure. These effects include cessation of menstruation, insulin resistance, alterations of immune function, and neuroendocrine dysfunction, among others. Starvation or a loss of body fat normally leads to a decrease in leptin. As a result, during starvation there is a compensatory response mediated by the increased production of ghrelin, neuropeptide Y (NPY), and other appetite-stimulating neuropeptides, and decreased activity of anorexigenic neuropeptides such as corticotropin-releasing factor and melanocortin (See Figure 15.1). When an energy deficit occurs during starvation or malnutrition, adaptation occurs with increased activity of the orexigenic NPY/ agouti-related protein (AgRP) neurons inhibition of the anorexigenic proopiomelanocortin (POMC)/ cocaine- and amphetamine-related transcript (CART) neurons, resulting in increased energy intake secondary to increased appetite when food is available. Hunger is characteristic of normal starvation while loss of appetite is characteristic of cancer cachexia. This negative effect of cachexia on the normal appetite-stimulating mechanisms is thought to result from the effects of inflammatory cytokines at both central and peripheral levels leading to anorexia and unopposed weight loss.

CYTOKINES

The cytokines are proteins synthesized and released by lymphocytes, macrophages, and adipocytes that mediate and regulate immunity, inflammation, and hematopoiesis (Fridman et al. 2012, Candido and Hagemann 2013, Daas, Rizeq, and Nasrallah 2018). Cytokines that are released into the circulation can be transported to the brain through the blood–brain barrier (Almutairi et al. 2016). Cytokines may influence the brain via neural pathways or second messengers such as nitric oxide and eicosanoids (Qu, Tang, and Hua 2018, Dennis and Norris 2015, Wang et al. 2005). Cytokines are also produced within the brain by neurons and glial cells (Ojo et al. 2015). As described above, neurons in the arcuate nucleus of the hypothalamus are centrally involved in the neuroendocrine regulation of feeding and receive input from leptin and insulin in the periphery. Increased brain cytokine expression disrupts this normal hypothalamic neurochemistry in the arcuate nucleus of the hypothalamus (Buchanan and Johnson 2007). Cytokines activate the POMC/CART neurons, while inactivating the NPY/AgRP neurons (Paulsen et al. 2017). Cytokines are also able to induce muscle wasting directly through inhibition of protein synthesis, increases in protein degradation, or a combination of both (Peterson, Bakkar, and Guttridge 2011, Schiaffino et al. 2013).

The pathophysiological role of cytokines in cancer cachexia has been studied in animals and in human subjects. Interleukin-1 (IL-I), tumor necrosis factor (TNF)-alpha, and IL-6 have been linked to the development of weight loss, skeletal muscle catabolism, and adipose tissue depletion in rodents (Argiles, Busquets, and Lopez-Soriano 2019). On the other hand, blocking the same mediators with the administration of anticytokine antibodies was able to attenuate cachexia in animal tumor models (Zaki, Nemeth, and Trikha 2004). In clinical studies of patients with different cancer types, high levels of peripheral inflammatory cytokines (i.e., IL-6, TNF-alpha) have been associated with clinical and biochemical markers of cachexia including weight loss, high resting metabolism, and decreased levels of serum albumin, total protein, and hemoglobin (Kuroda et al. 2007,

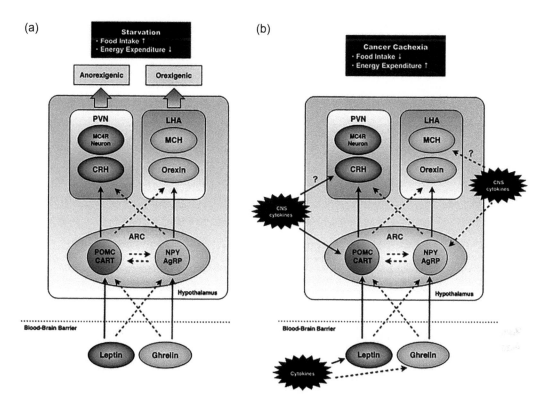

FIGURE 15.1 A simplified model of the hypothalamic neuropeptide circuitry contrasting the response to starvation or protein malnutrition (a) and the effects on this system during cancer cachexia (b). The arcuate nucleus (ARC) of the hypothalamus according to the information from the periphery conveyed to the brain by leptin and other hormones may activate or inhibit POMC/CART and NPY/AgRP neurons. During malnutrition or starvation without cachexia, leptin falls and orexigenic NPY/AgRP neurons are activated while anorexigenic POMC/CART neurons are inhibited, resulting in increased desire for energy intake. During cancer, cachectic factors such as cytokines elicit effects on energy homeostasis that mimic leptin in some respects and suppress orexigenic Ghrelin-NPY/AgRP signaling. The anorexia and unopposed weight loss in cachexia are the result of cytokine disruption of these central mechanisms regulating energy intake and expenditure. AgRP, Agouti-related peptide; MCH, melanin-concentrating hormone; CART, cocaine- and amphetamine-related transcript; NPY, neuropeptide Y; POMC, proopiomelanocortin; CRH, c0lticotropin-releasing hormone; MC4R, melanocortin-4 receptor; PVN, paraventricular nucleus; LHA, lateral hypothalamic area. (From Suzuki et al. (2013) with permission.)

Gerber et al. 2018, Ryan et al. 2016). Whether cytokine production is primarily from tumor or host inflammatory cells is not established, but it has been proposed that tumor cell cytokine production directly or as a result of the host inflammatory cell response to tumor cells can be the source of elevated cytokine levels observed in cachexia (Donohoe, Ryan, and Reynolds 2011).

Cancer cachexia is characterized by an upregulation of muscle proteolysis and lipolysis that is often attributed to an increased inflammatory response mediated by cytokines, such as IL-6 and IL-1 and TNF (see Figure 15.2). These inflammatory cytokines activate the ubiquitin-proteasome pathway via nuclear factor kappa B (NF-κB), resulting in a protein degradation pathway in the myocytes. An important role for inflammatory cytokines such as TNF-α, mediated by the generation of reactive oxygen species (ROS) has been demonstrated in muscle wasting. Moreover, activation of the transcription factor NF-κB is a key factor in the overall processes that mediate muscle atrophy. The significance of NF-κB as a key regulator of muscle atrophy has been demonstrated in several in vivo studies in which NF-κB-targeted therapies can prevent muscle atrophy (Thoma and Lightfoot 2018).

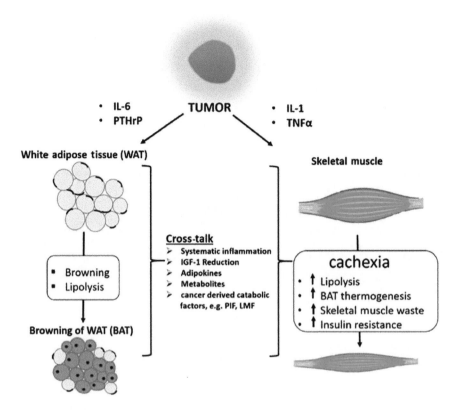

FIGURE 15.2 Effects of tumor cytokines on muscle and fat physiology. Lipolysis leads to loss of body fat, and cross-talk with muscle promotes muscle wasting while browning of WAT increases energy expenditure. (From Daas, Rizeq, and Nasrallah (2018) with permission.)

MUSCLE WASTING

Muscle wasting contributes the most to a decrease in function in cancer patients and is associated with an increased risk of chemotherapy-induced toxicity and poor outcome (Prado et al. 2007, Damrauer et al. 2018). Cancer- and chemotherapy-induced muscle atrophy is incompletely understood (Damrauer et al. 2018). Nutritional supplements alone do not reverse muscle wasting associated with cancer cachexia (Fearon et al. 2011). Resistance training may improve muscle strength and lean body mass, but it is not commonly prescribed to patients with cancer cachexia (Little and Phillips 2009). As reviewed above, progesterone-like drugs have been shown to increase only fat mass but not lean body mass (Loprinzi et al. 1999).

The gastric hormone ghrelin causes weight gain by increasing food intake and by food intake-independent mechanisms (Garcia et al. 2013, Sugiyama et al. 2012), and ghrelin or ghrelin receptor agonists have been proposed as potential therapies for cancer cachexia as they may improve anorexia, muscle mass and strength, and weight loss in patients with cancer, particularly those receiving cisplatin-based chemotherapy (Hiura et al. 2012, Garcia, Friend, and Allen 2013). However, the mechanisms of action of ghrelin in muscle remain to be fully elucidated.

An increase in muscle proteolysis and a decrease in protein synthesis driven by activation of the ubiquitin-proteasome (Lecker et al. 1999), mitogen-activated protein kinases (Cai et al. 2004), and myostatin pathways (Little and Phillips 2009) have been identified as key processes in tumor-induced muscle wasting. However, there is heterogeneity of mediators, signaling, and metabolic pathways within and between model systems, so that the pathways leading to muscle wasting in cancer cachexia have not been fully characterized (Fearon, Glass, and Guttridge 2012).

LIPID MOBILIZATION

The loss of body fat energy stores as well as metabolic transformations of fat cell function contributes to the metabolic imbalance and clinical impact of cachexia (Tsoli, Swarbrick, and Robertson 2016). In some cases, the depletion of body fat in cancer patients can be more visibly pronounced than loss of muscle (Zuijdgeest-van Leeuwen et al. 2000). Rapid mobilization of fatty acids as an energy source from triglycerides stored within adipocytes is normally mediated through balanced homeostatic control of lipolysis by lipase enzymes in adipose tissue including adipose triglyceride lipase (ATGL), hormone-sensitive lipase, and monoglyceride lipase. Studies of fat loss in animal models of cancer cachexia have demonstrated a prominent role for ATGL in initiating fat loss through links of tumor-derived factors and the signaling pathways that within fat cells controlling lipid metabolism (Dahlman et al. 2010).

The primary mechanism of fat loss in cancer cachexia in humans and animals is related to increases in lipolytic activity and lipid utilization (Dahlman et al. 2010). A longitudinal body composition study using dual-energy X-ray absorptiometry (DEXA) study was carried out in 311 cancer patients with the following tumor types: 84 colorectal tumors; 74 pancreatic tumors; 73 upper gastrointestinal tumors; 51 liver-biliary tumors; 3 breast tumors; 5 melanomas; and 21 other tumor types (Fouladiun et al. 2005). A loss in body fat was demonstrated which occurred more rapidly and earlier than the loss of lean tissue. Fat was lost preferentially from the trunk, followed by the legs and arms. A separate study in advanced cancer patients with various solid tumors demonstrated accelerated fat loss which began 7 months prior to death, with an average loss of 29% at 2 months before death (Murphy et al. 2010). In that study, the adipose tissue losses occurred together with losses in plasma phospholipid fatty acids and were predictive of survival. Studies also suggest that the shrinkage in size of adipose tissue depots results from depletion of lipid reserves with significantly smaller adipocyte cell size, but not a decrease in the number of fat cells secondary to cell death (Agustsson et al. 2007).

While studies of adipose tissue suggest lipolysis and increased fatty acid oxidation from adipocytes, studies of liver and muscle tissue in more advanced stages of cachexia suggest that there is a concomitant reduction in fatty acid oxidation in liver (Kazantzis and Seelaender 2005, Silverio et al. 2012, Siddiqui and Williams 1989) and muscle (Julienne et al. 2012) with lipid deposition in these tissues. Studies of lipid metabolism in adipose, liver, and muscle tissues have not been reported for early stages of cachexia when weight loss is <10% of initial body weight, but based on animal studies, it is likely that these metabolic adaptations occur early in the course of cancer cachexia before major loss of fat depots is evident (Kliewer et al. 2015). A gene expression profile of subcutaneous adipose tissue comparing cachectic cancer patients with about 10% weight loss to weight-stable cancer patients demonstrated upregulation of genes linked to fatty acid degradation and oxidation in association with increased whole body levels of fatty acid oxidation (Dahlman et al. 2010).

Increased thermogenesis in brown fat during cancer cachexia has also been shown suggesting an additional factor promoting energy imbalance in cancer cachexia (Dalal 2019). An association between brown fat in cancer patients and increased energy expenditure in cancer cachexia has been proposed for many years (Shellock, Riedinger, and Fishbein 1986, Tisdale 2009). Brown adipose tissue (BAT) plays an important role in nonshivering thermogenesis and maintains body temperature in infants. Small amounts of BAT have also been found in adults. Positron Emission Tomography studies identified increased BAT in cancer patients as compared to healthy age-matched controls in one study (Shellock, Riedinger, and Fishbein 1986), while another study found that a majority of adults had BAT, with no difference between cancer patients and controls (Lee et al. 2010). Well-designed studies are needed to clarify the role of BAT in human cancer cachexia.

Emerging evidence suggests that, during cancer cachexia, white adipose tissue (WAT) undergoes a browning process forming so-called beige or white-beige adipocytes with uncoupled oxidative phosphorylation, resulting in increased lipid mobilization and energy expenditure. Beige adipocytes have demonstrated increased thermogenic activity contributing to accelerated energy expenditure and propagation of cachexia in experimental tumor mouse models and cancer patients (Kir et al. 2014, Petruzzelli et al. 2014). Independent studies in various cancer cachexia rodent models further demonstrate mechanistic links between the tumor and WAT browning in cancer cachexia. These studies confirm the generation of beige adipocytes in WAT, demonstrated by increased expression of uncoupling protein 1 (UCP1) mRNA and protein, increased thermogenic activity, as an early event in the development and progression of adipose tissue and skeletal muscle wasting in cancer (Petruzzelli et al. 2014).

Parathyroid hormone (PTH) and parathyroid hormone-related peptide (PTHrP) cause "browning" of white adipose tissue plus energy production via activation of uncoupling protein-1. In mice bearing Lewis Lung Carcinoma (LLC) cells, browning was associated with muscle wasting. The pathway to browning included PTH/PTHrP activation of protein kinase A and muscle wasting via the ubiquitin proteasome proteolytic system. The injection of antiPTHrP antibody in LLC-bearing mice significantly decreased UCP1 expression in adipocytes, decreased energy expenditure, and decreased the severity of fat and muscle loss (Thomas and Mitch 2017). However, fat and muscle losses were not completely prevented, suggesting the involvement of other factors in fat cell browning. As further evidence of this phenomenon, 17 of 47 lung and colon cancer patients in the study had detectable PTHrP levels that were associated with lower lean body mass and increased resting energy expenditure (REE) (Thomas and Mitch 2017).

In a second study, higher UCP1 expression in WAT was demonstrated along with increased IL-6 expression in several cancer cachexia murine models (Petruzzelli et al. 2014). As compared to mice transplanted with tumor cells that did not express IL-6, mice transplanted with IL-6 expressing tumor cells developed substantial weight loss, and administration of an IL-6 blocking antibody reduced but did not fully suppress cachexia. Blockade of beta-adrenergic receptors using antagonists also significantly reduced the onset of cachexia in mice, which was associated with reduced expression levels of UCP1 in beige fat cells. In addition, UCP1 expression was found in seven of eight samples of human adipose tissue from patients with colon cancer and cachexia, and none from 20 patients without cachexia (Petruzzelli et al. 2014).

These findings are consistent with a catabolic pathway in cancer cachexia that results in losses of both adipose tissue and muscle mass. Utilization of fatty acids liberated from adipose tissue to generate heat represents an additional factor that may promote the progression of cachexia independent of reduced food intake.

ANOREXIA

Therapeutic approaches to the anorexia associated with cancer cachexia acknowledge the complexity of the pathophysiology of anorexia in cancer patients (Mantovani, Madeddu, and Maccio 2013). The comprehensive assessment and treatment of anorexia includes pharmacologic treatment of depression, impaired gastric motility, impaired digestion, and consideration of nutrition consultation and support along with exercise recommendations as well as pharmacologic appetite stimulation (Zhang et al. 2018). Some single-center clinical studies have shown the benefit of combination approaches including progestins, anti-inflammatory and antioxidant agents, and immunomodulation (Mantovani et al. 2008).

High-dose megestrol acetate has been shown to increase appetite and body weight in advanced cancer. The effects of high-dose megestrol acetate in the treatment of anorexia and weight loss in patients with advanced hormone-insensitive malignant lesions were examined in a randomized double-blind placebo-controlled trial (Ruiz-Garcia et al. 2018). Patients receiving megestrol acetate for 1 month reported a significant improvement in appetite and adequacy of food intake compared with those receiving placebo. A three-item scale measuring appetite, adequacy of food intake, and concern about weight revealed a higher improvement with megestrol acetate than with placebo. Patients who worsened while receiving placebo had similar favorable changes after the cross over to megestrol acetate. Another study was conducted to investigate the effects of medroxyprogesterone acetate (MPA) on food intake, body composition, and REE (Simons et al. 1998). In a double-blind study, 54 patients with nonhormone-sensitive cancer, complicated by substantial weight loss and hypermetabolism, received either MPA, 500 mg, or placebo twice daily for 12 weeks. Food intake was measured by dietary history, body composition was assessed by deuterium dilution to estimate both fat mass and fat-free mass, and REE was measured by indirect calorimetry. Compared with placebo, 12 weeks of MPA led to an increase in energy intake (between-group difference, 426 kcal/day; $P=0.01$). This increase in energy intake was significantly associated with an increase in fat mass ($r=0.68$, $P=0.003$) with a between-group difference of 2.5 kg ($P=0.009$). Fat-free mass was not significantly influenced indicating a potential lack of effect on muscle mass over the period of study. REE increased during MPA treatment at 6 weeks with a between-group difference of 135 kcal/day ($P=0.009$). After 12 weeks, this difference in REE was 93 kcal/day ($P=0.07$). The authors concluded that MPA was able to stimulate increased food intake significantly and to reverse fat loss concomitantly in patients with nonhormone-sensitive cancer. The observations in these studies indicate that megestrol acetate may improve appetite and food intake in patients with advanced cancer. However, this approach has not been validated in larger placebo-controlled studies, and no treatment is currently U.S. Food and Drug Administration (FDA) approved for the prevention or treatment of anorexia associated with cancer cachexia.

Anorexia can also be related to physical obstruction of the gastrointestinal tract, pain, depression, constipation, malabsorption, cancer-associated hypercalcemia, debility or the side effects of treatment such as opiates, radiotherapy, or chemotherapy (Simons et al. 1998). Nonetheless, for a number of patients with cancer, no obvious clinical cause of reduced food intake can be identified as a factor of cancer cachexia compared to normal starvation.

TASTE AND SMELL

Taste and smell changes (TSCs) occur in 40%–50% of those with cancer cachexia (Spotten et al. 2017, Yavuzsen et al. 2009). Cancer and its therapy, including chemotherapy and radiation therapy, can directly alter and damage taste and smell. These alterations affect the daily QoL of patients and may lead to malnutrition and, in severe cases, significant morbidity. Cancer patients experience decreases in sensitivity to taste and odor, as well as unpleasant metallic and bitter sensations (Hong et al. 2009).

Both increased and decreased detection and recognition thresholds for basic tastes have been noted (Belqaid et al. 2018, Steinbach et al. 2010). Bitter, chemical, metallic, or nauseating tastes are also common post-chemotherapy (CT) and radiation therapy (RT) (McGreevy et al. 2014). For example, metallic taste has been reported in 32% of individuals with breast, colorectal, head and neck, lung, stomach, and other cancers following CT and/or RT in one study (Newell et al. 1998) and in 16% of those with lung cancer in another (Sarhill et al. 2003). Objectively and subjectively elevated salt thresholds have also been documented.

A recent study found a high prevalence of TSCs in newly diagnosed cancer patients before treatment (Ui Dhuibhir et al. 2020). This suggests that TSCs may sometimes originate from the tumor itself or its systemic effects in newly diagnosed cancer patients before treatment. In consecutive, newly diagnosed, treatment-naïve patients with solid tumors at a Radiation Oncology outpatient center, self-reported TSCs since becoming ill were evaluated using a modified Taste and Smell Survey, and objective taste and smell tests were conducted. Nutritional status was assessed with an abridged Patient-Generated Subjective Global Assessment (PG-SGA). Over two-thirds had at least one TSC and almost half were at malnutrition risk based on global assessment before any treatment. Self-reported TSCs included changes in taste and smell perception, and most commonly persistent bad taste.

TSCs are common side effects in cancer patients undergoing chemotherapy and radiation treatments. Although taste and smell receptor cells are renewed regularly, chemotherapy and radiation treatments may cause permanent damage to these cells due to alterations in receptor cell structure, reduction in number, nerve damage, or damage to salivary glands causing reduced saliva production (Hong et al. 2009). This can lead to inadequate food and supplement intakes and more rapid development of malnutrition and cachexia.

A study of taste and smell was conducted with 151 patients undergoing chemotherapy at an outpatient oncology unit in Spain (Amezaga et al. 2018). Seventy-six percent of the patients reported taste disorders and 45% reported smell changes. Xerostomia was the most frequent symptom reported by patients receiving chemotherapy affecting 63.6% of the patients and it was strongly associated to a bad taste in the mouth and loss of taste perception (OR = 5.96). Anthracyclines, paclitaxel, carboplatin, and docetaxel were the CT agents producing the highest taste disturbance rates. Cisplatin and 5-fluorouracil are the CT resulting in the lowest complaints.

Self-reported taste and smell perception were significantly lower in 135 newly diagnosed breast cancer patients shortly after completing chemotherapy compared to the comparison group of 114 women without cancer (De Vries et al. 2018). Most patients recovered their taste 6 months after chemotherapy, although patients who were still receiving trastuzumab then reported a lower taste and smell perception compared to patients who were not. A lower self-reported taste and smell were statistically significantly associated with a worse QoL, social, emotional, and role functioning shortly after chemotherapy. Six months after chemotherapy, taste and smell were statistically significantly associated with QoL, social, and role functioning, but only in patients receiving trastuzumab.

Intensified nutritional counseling with taste and smell training may improve taste perception of patients undergoing chemotherapy. Sixty two patients (48 women and 14 men) who had gastrointestinal ($n=29$), breast ($n=31$), or lung cancer ($n=2$) were studied (von Grundherr et al. 2019). Taste disorders were more frequent in gastrointestinal than in breast cancer patients. Of 62 patients screened, 30 patients showed taste disorders. Patients were allocated based on the detection of taste disorders (≤8 taste strips points) to an intervention group with a taste and smell training at baseline and weeks 3–5 or were only followed up, if no taste disorder was detected (≥9 taste strips points) (nonintervention group). At baseline, all patients received a nutritional counseling. The primary endpoint was the minimal clinically relevant improvement of taste strips score by 2 taste strips points in at least 50% of the patients with taste disorders. In 23 of 25 patients completing the intervention, taste significantly improved from baseline to week 12 ($P \leq 0.001$). Patients of the nonintervention group who completed the reassessment ($n=27$ of 32) experienced no change in taste perception in the 3-month follow-up ($P=0.897$). This study supports the idea that intensified nutritional counseling with taste and smell training may improve the taste perception of patients undergoing chemotherapy, but larger randomized confirmatory trials are needed.

PREVALENCE

The prevalence of cancer cachexia is relatively low in the general population, compared to many common diseases and can be considered an orphan disease (Anker et al. 2019). This is a relevant consideration in advancing research efforts on cancer cachexia, because both the United States (US) and the European Union (EU) have implemented special clinical development rules to promote research into orphan diseases and supported the development of new therapies for rare diseases.

In order to examine whether cancer cachexia can be considered an orphan disease, data were obtained from 21 original reports on a total of over 31,000 patients with 14 cancer diagnoses including the 10 most frequent cancer diagnoses and another 4 cancer types frequently associated with cancer cachexia (Anker et al. 2019) (See Figure 15.3).

The prevalence of cancer cachexia as an actual number of patients estimated to be affected was calculated in the individual tumor types by organ of origin including the following three factors quantitatively: (1) the prevalence of each cancer type; (2) the percentage of such patients at risk to develop cachexia; and (3) the prevalence of cachexia among the patients at risk. Based on prior clinical experience that the intensity and progression of the cancer disease process is directly related to metabolic disorders responsible for cachexia, it was assumed that patients with lower 5-year

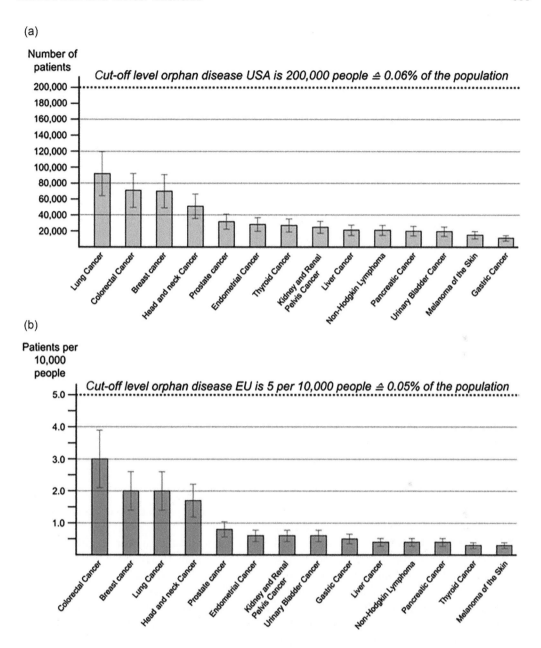

FIGURE 15.3 Prevalence of cancer cachexia (a) in the USA (2014) and (b) in the EU 2013 with ±30% error bars to indicate the estimated uncertainty of the estimates. (From Anker et al. (2019) with permission.)

survival rates would be more prone to develop cachexia, and therefore, they were classified as having a higher risk for cachexia development (see Table 15.1). For calculation of the patients at risk in each diagnosis, four groups of very high, high, middle, and lower risk of cancer cachexia were separated by taking into account the respective 5-year survival rates of each tumor class. In the very high risk group with 5-year survival rates up to 30% including liver, pancreatic, and lung cancer, between 80% and 90% of patients are at risk to develop cancer cachexia. In the high-risk group with 5-year survival rates of 31%–66% including head and neck, gastric and colorectal cancer, the risk of developing cancer cachexia is 50%–70%. In the middle-risk group with 5-year survival rates of 67%–90%, the risk of developing cancer cachexia is 30%–40%. In the lower risk group with 5-year

TABLE 15.1

Frequency of Cancer Cachexia and of Patients at Risk to Develop Cachexia

Cancer Type (*n*, 5-Year Survival Rate)	Estimated Cancer Cachexia Prevalence in Patients at Risk (%)	Patients at Risk to Develop Cachexia (%)
Very high risk group—5-year survival rate 0%–30%		
Liver cancer (1,678, 19%)	50.1	90
Pancreatic cancer (755, 9%)	45.6	90
Lung cancer (4,929, 20%)	37.2	80
High risk group—5-year survival rate 31%–66%		
Head and neck cancer (856, 66%)	42.3	70
Gastric cancer (2,638, 31%)	33.3	70
Colorectal cancer (3,716, 66%)	31.8	50
Middle-risk group—5-year survival rate 67%–90%		
Endometrial cancer (1,280, 83%)	32.2	40
Kidney and renal pelvis cancer (1,549, 75%)	31.6	40
Non-Hodgkin lymphoma (1,220, 73%)	28.4	30
Urinary bladder cancer (3,329, 78%)	25.2	30
Lower risk group—5-year survival rate 91%–100%		
Thyroid cancer (534, 98%)	39.9	30
Breast cancer (4,565, 91%)	23.5	30
Melanoma of the skin (<500, 94%)	22.1	20

Source: From Anker et al. (2019) with permission.

survival rates of 91%–100% including thyroid cancer, breast cancer, prostate cancer, and melanoma, the risk of developing cancer cachexia is 20%–30%.

The extensive analysis of the data set enabled the estimation of the number of cancer patients likely to be suffering from cancer cachexia in the US (See Figure 15.3a) and in the EU (Figure 15.3b) by tumor type. In 2014, in the US, it was estimated that 527,100 patients suffered from cancer cachexia amounting to 16.5 individuals per 10,000 of the total population given a population at the time of about 319 million. In 2013, in the EU, a total of 800,300 patients suffered from cancer cachexia amounting to 15.8 subjects per 10,000 in the population of about 505 million people in 28 countries. For each specific cancer type, the absolute numbers of patients suffering of cachexia were lower than 200,000 patients in the US, or <5 per 10,000 people in the EU, and for most types, substantially below the threshold prevalence defining an orphan disease. Even if a high margin of error of ±30% is applied to the final results, cancer cachexia remains an orphan disease if each cancer type is considered separately, and this was true for all the specific cancer types studied.

The estimates of cancer cachexia prevalence made are simply averages, and within each tumor type, there can be patients where cancer cachexia is a prominent factor in the course of their disease. It has been estimated that cachexia is the immediate or primary cause of death in ~30% of cancer patients (Hui, Dev, and Bruera 2015, Arthur et al. 2016). Cancer cachexia is also associated with increased length of hospital stay as well as increased overall treatment costs (Arthur et al. 2014, 2014). The mechanism through which cancer cachexia can cause death has been the subject of investigations which have concluded that in addition to cachexia interfering in the treatment of the cancer itself, cachexia can act as a contributor to mortality (Muscaritoli et al. 2015). Treatments for cachexia can be considered as either addressing symptoms and QoL or contributing to the adjunctive treatment of the tumor itself to impact mortality.

Cancer cachexia is not a single disease but has different characteristics in each of the cancer types described below. The estimation of the prevalence of cachexia in cancer requires both epidemiological determination of numbers of cases and a clinical analysis of the actual clinical development of cachexia in multiple cancer types. The pathophysiology, genetics, and biochemistry of each cancer as well as the symptoms and prognostic importance of malnutrition are distinct in their impact on disease progression to cachexia which is relevant for the development of novel treatment and prevention strategies. Research on the treatment of cachexia remains in its infancy. As discussed elsewhere in this text each type of cancer is distinct in its genetic origins regardless of organ site and develops unique characteristics requiring individualized management strategies. However, there are some commonalities by cancer type discussed below. What follows is a brief summary of observed course of cachexia for each of the most common cancers affected by anorexia and cachexia.

LUNG CANCER

A study by Dewys and colleagues in 1980 reported the frequency of weight loss in patients with newly diagnosed non-small cell lung cancer (NSCLC) to be 61%. A more recent study in 2004 reported the same incidence of weight loss for lung cancer patients on diagnosis. Both studies demonstrated convincingly that weight loss was an independent negative prognostic factor for survival of patients with NSCLC, Small Cell Lung Cancer (SCLC), and mesothelioma.

To determine whether metabolic abnormalities occur as part of the process of malnutrition in lung cancer before the development of cachexia, 12 patients with non-oat cell lung cancer and 6 age-matched healthy controls were studied under metabolic ward conditions (Heber et al. 1982). Under conditions of constant caloric and nitrogen intake, total body protein turnover was measured by the continuous infusion of [^{14}C]lysine. Total body protein turnover was significantly increased ($P<0.05$) in lung cancer patients [3.15 ± 0.51 (SD) g/kg/day] compared to that of controls [1.87 ± 0.32 g/kg/day]. Increased protein recycling characterized by both increased synthesis and breakdown of body proteins in the lung cancer patients was inversely correlated with percentage of ideal body weight at the time of study ($r=-0.69$; $P<0.05$). Muscle catabolism rates determined by quantitating urinary 3-methylhistidine-creatinine excretion rates were increased in lung cancer patients (106 ± 11 μmol/g creatinine) compared to those of controls (71 ± 8 μmol/creatinine; $P<0.05$). Glucose production rates assessed by the continuous infusion of [6-^{3}H]glucose were increased in lung cancer patients (2.84 ± 0.16 mg/kg/min) compared to those of controls (2.18 ± 0.06 mg/kg/min; $P<0.05$). There was no evidence of ectopic adrenocorticotropic hormone production in these patients, and 24-hours, urinary-free cortisol excretion in these patients was not increased compared to that of controls. Serum insulin and plasma glucose levels measured before and 2 hours after a standard oral glucose load were not different in patients and controls. Thus, increases in protein turnover, glucose production, and muscle catabolism were evident metabolic abnormalities in patients with non-oat cell lung cancer. The identification of these metabolic abnormalities as an integral part of the nonoat cell lung cancer disease process led to the evaluation of therapies designed to prevent cancer cachexia by interrupting the cycle of increased glucose turnover leading to increased protein breakdown. Hydrazine sulfate blocks gluconeogenesis through inhibition of the enzyme phosphoenolpyruvate carboxykinase. In a prospective double-blind trial, 12 malnourished patients with lung cancer were randomized to receive either placebo or hydrazine sulfate (60 mg three times daily) for 30 days (Tayek, Heber, and Chlebowski 1987). Fasting lysine flux was determined by a primed 4-hour continuous infusion of ^{14}C-lysine before and after 1 month of hydrazine treatment. Baseline plasma lysine flux was 2,580 (SD 580) μmol/h for the placebo group and 2,510 (440) μmol/h for the hydrazine group. After 1 month the placebo group showed a slight rise to 2,920 (450) μmol/h ($P=0.08$) and the hydrazine group showed a significant fall to 1,840 (750) μmol/h $P<0.05$. Serum albumin fell in the placebo group and was unchanged in the hydrazine group. Administration of hydrazine sulfate to reduce amino acid flux was shown to favorably influence the metabolic abnormalities linking increased glucose turnover to protein breakdown in these early studies of lung cancer cachexia. Of course, these studies were carried out before the role of cytokines in cancer cachexia was known.

As already discussed, cytokines and inflammation are central to the pathogenesis of cancer cachexia. In lung cancer, chronic lung inflammation and systemic inflammation are proposed as one of the main factors promoting carcinogenesis and cachexia. Cigarette smoking is the main behavior promoting the generation of ROS in the lungs and thus inducing inflammatory-related injuries and metabolic changes in lung cancer (Lee, Walser, and Dubinett 2009). Several studies have also indicated that lung carcinogenesis is directly linked with redox imbalance, both systemically and in the lungs (Zablocka-Slowinska et al. 2018a, Jaruga et al. 1994). Although the link between cigarette smoking and redox imbalance in lung cancer has been extensively studied and is widely known, factors other than tobacco smoke may also contribute to systemic oxidative stress in lung cancer patients, since prevalence of the disease is systematically increasing also among nonsmokers (Lin et al. 2017b). Carotenoids including lycopene, beta- and alpha-carotene, and cryptoxanthin may have anticancer properties, but findings from population-based and interventional research have been inconsistent (Holick et al. 2002, Mannisto et al. 2004). Alterations in redox balance in lung cancer may also be influenced by alterations in glucose metabolism (Zablocka-Slowinska et al. 2018a) as well as trace element status (Zablocka-Slowinska et al. 2018b). Alterations of lipid metabolism in lung cancer patients have been demonstrated and have even been considered as potential risk factors (Lin et al. 2017a, Chi et al. 2014, Kucharska-Newton et al. 2008, Zhou et al. 2017). High density lipoprotein cholesterol (HDL)-C may exert direct antioxidant activity (Karabacak et al. 2014), while the level of modification of others, e.g., Low density lipoprotein cholesterol (LDL)-C and triglycerides (TG), may indirectly protect from oxidative stress and inflammation (Jurek et al. 2006, Rodriguez-Carrio et al. 2017).

HEAD AND NECK CANCER

Head and neck cancer is frequently associated with cancer cachexia (Willemsen et al. 2020) and its localized growth provides insights into the remote effects of tumor and cancer therapy on cancer cachexia including both anorexia and muscle wasting. The prevalence of cachexia is between 3% and 52% at diagnosis in squamous cell carcinoma of the head and neck, depending on tumor location and stage (Gorenc, Kozjek, and Strojan 2015, Couch et al. 2015). Surgical resection of head and neck tumors can be truly mutilating, preventing sufficient oral intake, which can lead to increased weight loss. Preparatory procedures for radiotherapy, such as tooth extractions also impair eating (Irie et al. 2018). During postoperative radiation, chemoradiation (CRT) or primary CRT of locally advanced head and neck squamous cell carcinoma, weight loss with reductions in fat mass, fat-free mass, or both, is common due to therapy-related toxicity including mucositis, loss of taste, and dysphagia (Farhangfar et al. 2014). Low skeletal muscle mass in head and neck cancer patients is associated with increased radiotherapy-induced toxicity including mucositis, radiation dermatitis, neutropenia, and nephrotoxicity. These complications cause treatment interruptions leading to decreased treatment efficacy and cure rates (Couch et al. 2015, Wendrich et al. 2017). Furthermore, skeletal muscle mass loss during the course of radiation therapy has been associated with higher mortality rates (Pai et al. 2018).

The assessment of body composition prior to and during treatment of head and neck patients undergoing surgery and radiation therapy can be used to individually tailor nutritional interventions that optimize weight in general and muscle mass in particular. Body mass index (BMI) measurement alone does not reveal low muscle mass. Ideally, a rapid screening method for muscle mass such as bioelectrical impedance is suitable for clinical assessment. Newer methods for directly measuring muscle mass utilizing deuterated creatine may be used in research and clinical practice in the future. A study of patients with locally advanced head and neck cancer undergoing concurrent CRT characterized changes in total psoas muscle area, lean psoas area, and psoas muscle density by CT scan before and after CRT (Wang et al. 2016). Fifty patients who underwent CRT were selected for body composition analyses by either availability of pre-/post-treatment DEXA scans or a novel CT-based approach of body morphomics analysis (BMA). BMA changes (lean psoas and total psoas area) were compared to total lean body mass changes by DEXA scans using two-sample t tests. The study also examined the association between these changes in muscle with patient-reported QoL and tumor-related outcomes. Clinically significant declines in total psoas area and lean body mass of similar magnitude were observed in both BMA and DEXA cohorts after CRT. Loss of psoas area ($P <0.05$) was associated with greater frailty and mobility issues. Total psoas area was more sensitive for local recurrence than weight changes and T-stage on multivariate analyses. In this study, total psoas area predicted mortality in oropharyngeal cancer patients emphasizing the importance of muscle wasting on outcomes. The standard nutritional intervention for all head and neck cancer patients includes the administration of tube feeding to stabilize weight loss when oral intake is impaired throughout the total course of therapy (Bishop and Reed 2015).

PANCREATIC CANCER

Cachexia has been shown to be present in up to 70%–80% of patients with Pancreatic Ductal Adenocarcinoma (Uomo, Gallucci, and Rabitti 2006) and is associated with reduced survival, more progressive disease, and higher rates of metastatic disease (Bachmann et al. 2009, 2009). The presence of cachexia was shown to worsen the postoperative outcome of patients with pancreatic cancer (Bachmann et al. 2008, Pausch et al. 2012). The only hope for cure of pancreatic cancer at present is the complete surgical resection of the tumor, which is only possible in nonmetastatic and localized stages of this aggressive cancer.

Unfortunately, <15% of patients are eligible for surgery when they are diagnosed (Stathis and Moore 2010), and only about 70% of tumors are fully resectable at surgery (Bachmann et al. 2009). Palliative treatment of nonresectable pancreatic cancer includes options of chemotherapy, radiotherapy, and supportive care. An essential element of supportive care is the preservation of QoL. Cachexia substantially reduces QoL in pancreatic cancer patients.

Nutrition support is an important aspect of supportive care for cachectic patients with pancreatic cancer (Bachmann et al. 2009). Whenever possible, nutrition should be delivered via the enteral route to avoid the side effects of parenteral nutrition (Bozzetti et al. 2009). Cachectic patients should be supplemented with a balanced essential amino-acid mixture, given between meals (Bozzetti et al. 2009, Morley 2009). To assure adequate intestinal function, vitamin D and exocrine pancreatic insufficiency must be treated via supplementation (Morley 2009). Generally, 2000 lipase units (IE) of pancreatic enzymes are needed per 1 g of fat, and restriction of high fat foods is recommended. Concomitant symptoms that affect appetite and food intake, including mechanical or functional gastrointestinal disorders, depression, and fatigue should be addressed.

GASTRIC CANCER

Gastrectomy followed by chemotherapy is the standard treatment for gastric cancer. The majority of gastric cancer patients suffer weight loss and malnutrition (Seo et al. 2016). Partial or full gastrectomy leads to reduced food intake per serving and induces anastomotic and vagal nerve blocks causing abdominal distension, and frequent bowel movements. Chemotherapy following gastrectomy induces anorexia, sore throat, dry mouth, taste change, nausea, diarrhea, constipation, and fatigue all of which eventually lead to weight loss and malnutrition. The complication of malnutrition among gastrectomy patients was shown to delay the rate of recovery and increase cancer deaths (Santarpia, Contaldo, and Pasanisi 2011). In a study of the medical records of 234 gastric cancer patients who underwent gastrectomy and received adjuvant chemotherapy with extended lymph node dissection, nutritional status assessment included PG-SGA, body weight, BMI, serum albumin concentration, and Nutrition Risk Index. PG-SGA indicated 59% of the patients were malnourished and 27.8% of the patients revealed serious malnutrition with a high PG-SGA score of ≥9. About 15%

of patients lost ≥10% of their initial body weight, and14.5% of the patients had hypoalbuminemia (<3.5 g/dL). Overall, these patients were suffering from moderate to severe malnutrition (Seo et al. 2016).

COLORECTAL CANCER

Colorectal cancer is the third most common cancer in both males and females in the US and the second leading cause of cancer deaths with the estimated new cases of nearly 133,000 and deaths of 50,000 in 2015.

Cachexia is associated with poorer outcomes in colorectal cancer (van der Werf et al. 2018). In a study of 69 patients with colorectal cancer, 52% were identified as cachectic according to established diagnostic criteria including weight loss and sarcopenia determined on CT scan. Clinically cachectic patients had a shorter progression-free survival than clinically noncachectic patients ($P=0.016$).

Emerging evidence now suggests that dysbiosis with an imbalance in the normal intestinal microbiota can promote chronic inflammatory conditions and the production of carcinogenic metabolites, leading to tumor formation and progression (De Hertogh et al. 2012, Marchesi et al. 2011). Cancer incidence in the large intestine is known to be ~12-fold higher than that of the small intestine, which has been attributed to several magnitude greater bacterial density in the large intestine (10^{12} cells/mL) compared with that in the small intestine (10^2 cells/mL) (Sun and Kato 2016).

Compromised gut barrier function because of dysbiosis or intestinal inflammation can lead to translocation of microbial substances and the development of systemic inflammation with potential consequences for patients prone to cachexia. Preserving the integrity of the gut epithelial barrier to limit intestinal inflammation in colorectal cancer patients may help avoid the serious metabolic alterations associated with cachexia. More research is needed to clarify the role of gut microbiota and systemic inflammation in the pathogenesis of cancer cachexia in colorectal cancer patients. Multimodal treatment strategies that include interventions aimed at maintaining gut barrier function and correcting dysbiosis may be used to in controlling cachexia. Microbiota-based cancer prevention, diagnosis, and therapy are beginning to emerge as researchers learn to "decode" the meaning of human microbiota composition at different stages in colorectal cancer.

LIVER CANCER

Hepatocellular carcinoma (HCC) is the most common form of liver cancer. The prevalence of this cancer is steadily growing because obesity, type 2 diabetes, and nonalcoholic fatty liver disease (NAFLD) are replacing viral- and alcohol-related liver disease as major pre-existing conditions favoring hepatocarcinogenesis. HCC may be the presenting feature of an asymptomatic nonalcoholic steatohepatitis, the progressive form of NAFLD in the absence of cirrhosis. The HCC risk connected to metabolic factors has been underestimated. Systemic and hepatic molecular mechanisms involved in obesity- and NAFLD-induced hepatocarcinogenesis as well as potential early markers of HCC are being extensively investigated (Marengo, Rosso, and Bugianesi 2016).

Cachexia is induced by proinflammatory cytokines, responsible for a wide number of metabolic disorders including increased oxidation of lipids and increased overall oxidative metabolism. Oxidized LDL has been implicated in the actions of some cytokines in hepatocellular carcinogenesis (Motta et al. 2003). The removal of ox-LDL from the blood is performed by the liver and in a small study the levels of ox-LDL were lower in the serum of patients with hepatocellular cancer compared to controls. It was proposed that the increased clearance of ox-LDL by the reticuloendothelial system in the liver led to greater amounts of ox-LDL in liver cells. The intracellular amount of ox-LDL, through various cytokines, has been proposed to induce HCC through reduction of normal homeostasis via apoptotic mechanisms. It has been proposed that the cytokine action within the liver may account for the high incidence of cachexia documented in patients with HCC.

In the largest study of liver cancer patients, nutritional status was assessed in 8,895 patients admitted to the National Cancer Center in Korea (Wie et al. 2010). The nutritional status of each subject was assessed using BMI, serum albumin, total lymphocyte count, and diet and classified into three groups: high risk, moderate risk, and low risk of malnutrition. The prevalence of malnutrition among liver cancer patients was 86.6%.

PROSTATE CANCER

Androgen deprivation therapy (ADT) is used in the course of treating prostate cancer both in the neoadjuvant setting to reduce tumor mass prior to surgery and as primary therapy in men who are not surgical candidates. In many instances, long-term ADT leads to changes in body composition which have been documented in the first year of ADT (Griffin et al. 2019). Increases in fat mass and decreases in lean mass and muscle strength have been documented (Galvao et al. 2008, 2009, Nguyen et al. 2015). Following ADT for prostate cancer, fat mass has been shown to increase by about 10%, while lean mass decreased by about 3% (Smith et al. 2002, Tayek et al. 1990). The net result is often sarcopenic obesity (Heber 2010) which can lead to diabetes and cardiovascular disease (Tzortzis et al. 2017, Keating et al. 2010, Krahn et al. 2016).

An examination of the database developed by the Shared Equal Access Regional Cancer Hospital (Kim et al. 2011) found the above changes in body fat and lean already described but also indicated that nearly a third of men experienced weight loss on ADT. Given the evidence that obesity or excess body fat at ADT-initiation is associated with early development of castrate-resistant prostate cancer (CRPC), an increase in the risk of PC progression might also be expected with ADT-induced fat gain and muscle loss (Keto et al. 2012).

Men on ADT randomized to a 12-week lifestyle program comprising aerobic and resistance exercise showed improvements in muscle strength (Bourke et al. 2011). The improvement in strength observed with resistance and aerobic exercise interventions also increased lean body mass in men with PC on ADT which may have additional metabolic benefits (Segal et al. 2003, Owen et al. 2017).

Immediate initiation of ADT is supported by proven clinical benefits for men with symptomatic skeletal metastases, established lymphatic metastases and when combined with radiotherapy in locally advanced disease. However, as a result of PSA testing, men outside these groups are now started on ADT much earlier and remain on therapy for many years. ADST is associated with a number of adverse effects, such as reduced bone mineral density, increased fracture risk, decreased skeletal muscle function and fatigue. In addition, there is an increased risk of cardiovascular disease in association with ADT. Although AST clearly improves prostate cancer specific mortality (RR reduction of 17%), it does so at the expense of a 15% increase in the RR of nondisease specific mortality. Although CVD is of course highly prevalent in the population of older men receiving ADT evidence accruing from observational data now suggests ADT may significantly increase CVD morbidity and mortality (Bourke et al. 2012, Saylor et al. 2011).

Localized prostate cancer treated via definitive local therapy becomes metastatic in 30% of cases. Despite a temporary response to ADT, a CRPC requiring further therapy can then develop. Management of metastatic CRPC can include chemotherapeutic and nonchemotherapeutic agents, depending on disease burden and patient comorbidities. During prostate cancer progression, antineoplastic treatment and tumor–host interactions may result in anemia, anorexia, and cachexia, which severely compromise patient QoL (Maccio, Gramignano, and Madeddu 2015).

A study of 197 patients diagnosed with metastatic hormone-sensitive prostate cancer in demonstrated that 163 patients (82.7%) had sarcopenia (Ikeda et al. 2020). Cancer-specific survival and overall survival were significantly shorter in sarcopenic patients than in nonsarcopenic patients ($P=0.0099$ and $P=0.0465$, respectively) whereas castration-resistance prostate cancer-free survival did not significantly differ between the groups ($P=0.6063$).

CONCLUSION

Cancer is an increasing cause of morbidity and mortality around the world. On the other hand, new types of cancer diagnosis and treatment through Precision Oncology are more sophisticated and powerful than ever before in targeting specific forms of cancer. In many instances, cancers are not cured, but are put into long-term remission as they are converted into chronic diseases. However, the future success of Precision Oncology is clouded by the frequent development of malnutrition and metabolic derangements induced by tumors leading to anorexia and cachexia in cancer patients (Arends et al. 2017).

Cancer cachexia as reviewed above has a multifactorial pathogenesis which is associated with increased mortality and decreased well-being of patients. Therapies to reduce or reverse the loss of body weight and muscle mass in cancer cachexia are still lacking after many years of research (Ebner et al. 2013). Effective treatments for cancer cachexia and the associated anorexia and wasting are needed to improve cancer patients' QoL and their survival (Ebner, Anker, and von Haehling 2020).

Clinical trials are testing combination protocols of dietary supplements and pharmaceutical interventions. In a clinical trial comparing four different treatments including MPA, eicosapentanoic acid, L-carnitine, thalidomide over 4 months alone, and in combination in patients with advanced stage solid tumors, the most effective treatment in terms of lean body mass gain, REE, fatigue, appetite, IL-6 levels, and Eastern Cooperative Oncology Group performance status score was a combination regimen that included all four agents (Mantovani et al. 2010).

In a nonrandomized trial over 16 weeks, a diet with high polyphenol content, oral nutritional support enriched with $n-3$ fatty acids (eicosapentanoic acid [EPA] and docosahexanoic acid [DHA]), MPA, antioxidant treatment with alpha-lipoic acid and carbocysteine lysine salt, vitamins E, A, and C, and celecoxib resulted in a positive response with increase of lean body mass (LBM) and quality of in patients with advanced stage solid tumors. There was also a decrease of proinflammatory cytokines, and no adverse effects were noted (Mantovani et al. 2004).

In a randomized controlled study of 32 patients with cachexia and advanced stage colon, ovarian, lung, pancreatic, and other tumor types, a combination of β-hydroxy-β-methylbutyrate (HMB), arginine, and glutamine was administered over 4 weeks and compared to placebo demonstrated some overall benefit with an increase in lean body mass, improved mood, and improved hematological parameters (May et al. 2002). However, in a larger study of 472 advanced lung cancer patients along with other types of advanced cancer, a combination of HMB, glutamine, and arginine over 8 weeks demonstrated no additional benefits beyond those seen with administration of an isonitrogenous and isocaloric control intervention (Berk et al. 2008).

A group of nine malnourished patients with intra-abdominal cancer, received both conventional total parenteral nutrition (TPN) containing 19% branched-chain amino acids (BCAA) and isocaloric, isonitrogenous TPN containing 50% BCAA (BCAA-TPN) (Hunter et al. 1989). The patients receiving the daily BCAA-enriched TPN demonstrated an increase in the fractional albumin synthesis rate. A study of ten malnourished patients with intra-abdominal metastatic adenocarcinoma who were given either conventional TPN with 19% BCAA or a BCAA-enriched TPN formula with 50% of amino acids as BCAA demonstrated an increase in whole body protein synthesis and leucine balance.

Another randomized trial studied 104 advanced-stage gynecological cancer patients and assigned to receive either a combination of megestrol acetate (MA) with L-carnitine, celecoxib, and antioxidants or MA alone over 4 months. The combination treatment arm demonstrated more benefit with respect to REE, lean body mass, appetite, fatigue, and global QoL. The inflammation and oxidative stress parameters IL-6, TNF-α, C-reactive protein, and ROS decreased significantly in the combination arm, while no significant change was observed in the MA only arm (Madeddu et al. 2009). Another combination therapy trial compared two combination treatment arms, with or without MA, and found no superiority of additional MA administration (Madeddu et al. 2012).

Considering the multidimensional pathogenesis of cancer cachexia, it is being recognized that multimodal approaches, including exercise, nutrient supplementation, appetite stimulation, and pharmacological intervention, have been more successful when implemented and individually adjusted for patients at different stages of cachexia (Fearon, Arends, and Baracos 2013, Tsoli and Robertson 2013).

Even though a substantial amount of experimental, preclinical and clinical research has been carried out, there is still no effective treatment for cancer cachexia. A multimodal treatment approach including nutritional support and pharmacological intervention as well as the management of symptoms exacerbating weight loss such as chronic pain, gastrointestinal disorders, fatigue and depression are essential given the current state of knowledge and clinical options. Combination protocols using anti-inflammatory, antioxidative nutrients and drugs while promising are not yet proven in large prospective randomized trials. We know that treatment with single agents such as MPA or TNF-α inhibitors has been less successful. The challenge of treating cancer cachexia is to integrate nutritional support as early as possible into the care of the cancer patient. The tumor itself often promotes metabolic derangements which advance malnutrition so that any reduction in food quality and nutrient intakes early in the course of diagnosed tumors can cause simple malnutrition. The depletion of body muscle and fat stores then makes patients less able to withstand surgery, chemotherapy, radiation. Newer forms of therapy including immunotherapy and hormonal therapies are not associated with malnutrition and cachexia, but these patients can become malnourished due to other factors including depression. Multimodal interventions can be implemented in a stepwise manner in all cancer patients, starting with oral nutritional support and dietary counseling from the time of diagnosis. Individualized screening and monitoring of the progress of malnutrition, anorexia, cachexia and response to therapies can be performed regularly through the course of treatment of cancer patients.

Combination treatments as described in this review hold the greatest promise for reducing cachexia morbidity to provide patients with improved QoL. The heterogeneity of presentations is a challenge to meaningful research on cancer cachexia. Future clinical trials should use standardized diagnostic criteria and study designs as much as possible to make analyses and comparisons of future intervention trials useful to advance modes of treatment. New targeted therapies derived from a combination of animal models and clinical trial research promise new therapeutic approaches to this complex, devastating, and unfortunately common disorder in the future.

REFERENCES

Agustsson, T., M. Ryden, J. Hoffstedt, V. van Harmelen, A. Dicker, J. Laurencikiene, B. Isaksson, J. Permert, and P. Arner. 2007. "Mechanism of increased lipolysis in cancer cachexia." *Cancer Res* 67(11):5531–7. doi: 10.1158/0008-5472.CAN-06-4585.

Almutairi, M. M., C. Gong, Y. G. Xu, Y. Chang, and H. Shi. 2016. "Factors controlling permeability of the blood-brain barrier." *Cell Mol Life Sci* 73(1):57–77. doi: 10.1007/s00018-015-2050-8.

Amezaga, J., B. Alfaro, Y. Rios, A. Larraioz, G. Ugartemendia, A. Urruticoechea, and I. Tueros. 2018. "Assessing taste and smell alterations in cancer patients undergoing chemotherapy according to treatment." *Support Care Cancer* 26(12):4077–86. doi: 10.1007/s00520-018-4277-z.

Anker, M. S., R. Holcomb, M. Muscaritoli, S. von Haehling, W. Haverkamp, A. Jatoi, J. E. Morley, F. Strasser, U. Landmesser, A. J. S. Coats, and S. D. Anker. 2019. "Orphan disease status of cancer cachexia in the USA and in the European Union: A systematic review." *J Cachexia Sarcopenia Muscle* 10(1):22–34. doi: 10.1002/jcsm.12402.

Arends, J., P. Bachmann, V. Baracos, N. Barthelemy, H. Bertz, F. Bozzetti, K. Fearon, E. Hutterer, E. Isenring, S. Kaasa, Z. Krznaric, B. Laird, M. Larsson, A. Laviano, S. Muhlebach, M. Muscaritoli, L. Oldervoll, P. Ravasco, T. Solheim, F. Strasser, M. de van der Schueren, and J. C. Preiser. 2017. "ESPEN guidelines on nutrition in cancer patients." *Clin Nutr* 36(1):11–48. doi: 10.1016/j.clnu.2016.07.015.

Argiles, J. M., S. Busquets, and F. J. Lopez-Soriano. 2019. "Cancer cachexia, a clinical challenge." *Curr Opin Oncol* 31(4):286–90. doi: 10.1097/CCO.0000000000000517.

Arrieta, O., R. M. Michel Ortega, G. Villanueva-Rodriguez, M. G. Serna-Thome, D. Flores-Estrada, C. Diaz-Romero, C. M. Rodriguez, L. Martinez, and K. Sanchez-Lara. 2010. "Association of nutritional status and serum albumin levels with development of toxicity in patients with advanced non-small cell lung cancer treated with paclitaxel-cisplatin chemotherapy: A prospective study." *BMC Cancer* 10:50. doi: 10.1186/1471-2407-10-50.

Arthur, S. T., J. M. Noone, B. A. Van Doren, D. Roy, and C. M. Blanchette. 2014. "One-year prevalence, comorbidities and cost of cachexia-related inpatient admissions in the USA." *Drugs Context* 3:212265. doi: 10.7573/dic.212265.

Arthur, S. T., B. A. Van Doren, D. Roy, J. M. Noone, E. Zacherle, and C. M. Blanchette. 2016. "Cachexia among US cancer patients." *J Med Econ* 19(9):874–80. doi: 10.1080/13696998.2016.1181640.

Bachmann, J., M. Heiligensetzer, H. Krakowski-Roosen, M. W. Buchler, H. Friess, and M. E. Martignoni. 2008. "Cachexia worsens prognosis in patients with resectable pancreatic cancer." *J Gastrointest Surg* 12(7):1193–201. doi: 10.1007/s11605-008-0505-z.

Bachmann, J., K. Ketterer, C. Marsch, K. Fechtner, H. Krakowski-Roosen, M. W. Buchler, H. Friess, and M. E. Martignoni. 2009. "Pancreatic cancer related cachexia: Influence on metabolism and correlation to weight loss and pulmonary function." *BMC Cancer* 9:255. doi: 10.1186/1471-2407-9-255.

Bachmann, J., M. W. Buchler, H. Friess, and M. E. Martignoni. 2013. "Cachexia in patients with chronic pancreatitis and pancreatic cancer: Impact on survival and outcome." *Nutr Cancer* 65(6):827–33. doi: 10.1080/01635581.2013.804580.

Belqaid, K., C. Tishelman, Y. Orrevall, E. Mansson-Brahme, and B. M. Bernhardson. 2018. "Dealing with taste and smell alterations-A qualitative interview study of people treated for lung cancer." *PLoS One* 13(1):e0191117. doi: 10.1371/journal.pone.0191117.

Berk, L., J. James, A. Schwartz, E. Hug, A. Mahadevan, M. Samuels, L. Kachnic, and Rtog. 2008. "A randomized, double-blind, placebo-controlled trial of a beta-hydroxyl beta-methyl butyrate, glutamine, and arginine mixture for the treatment of cancer cachexia (RTOG 0122)." *Support Care Cancer* 16(10):1179–88. doi: 10.1007/s00520-008-0403-7.

Bishop, S., and W. M. Reed. 2015. "The provision of enteral nutritional support during definitive chemoradiotherapy in head and neck cancer patients." *J Med Radiat Sci* 62(4):267–76. doi: 10.1002/jmrs.132.

Bourke, L., H. Doll, H. Crank, A. Daley, D. Rosario, and J. M. Saxton. 2011. "Lifestyle intervention in men with advanced prostate cancer receiving androgen suppression therapy: A feasibility study." *Cancer Epidemiol Biomarkers Prev* 20(4):647–57. doi: 10.1158/1055-9965.EPI-10-1143.

Bourke, L., T. J. Chico, P. C. Albertsen, F. C. Hamdy, and D. J. Rosario. 2012. "Cardiovascular risk in androgen suppression: Underappreciated, under-researched and unresolved." *Heart* 98(5):345–8. doi: 10.1136/heartjnl-2011-300893.

Bozzetti, F. 2017. "Forcing the vicious circle: Sarcopenia increases toxicity, decreases response to chemotherapy and worsens with chemotherapy." *Ann Oncol* 28(9):2107–18. doi: 10.1093/annonc/mdx271.

Bozzetti, F., J. Arends, K. Lundholm, A. Micklewright, G. Zurcher, M. Muscaritoli, and Espen. 2009. "ESPEN Guidelines on Parenteral Nutrition: Non-surgical oncology." *Clin Nutr* 28(4):445–54. doi: 10.1016/j.clnu.2009.04.011.

Buchanan, J. B., and R. W. Johnson. 2007. "Regulation of food intake by inflammatory cytokines in the brain." *Neuroendocrinology* 86(3):183–90. doi: 10.1159/000108280.

Cahill, G. F., Jr. 1970. "Starvation in man." *N Engl J Med* 282(12):668–75. doi: 10.1056/NEJM197003192821209.

Cai, D., J. D. Frantz, N. E. Tawa, Jr., P. A. Melendez, B. C. Oh, H. G. Lidov, P. O. Hasselgren, W. R. Frontera, J. Lee, D. J. Glass, and S. E. Shoelson. 2004. "IKKbeta/NF-kappaB activation causes severe muscle wasting in mice." *Cell* 119(2):285–98. doi: 10.1016/j.cell.2004.09.027.

Candido, J., and T. Hagemann. 2013. "Cancer-related inflammation." *J Clin Immunol* 33(Suppl 1):S79–84. doi: 10.1007/s10875-012-9847-0.

Chi, P. D., W. Liu, H. Chen, J. P. Zhang, Y. Lin, X. Zheng, W. Liu, and S. Dai. 2014. "High-density lipoprotein cholesterol is a favorable prognostic factor and negatively correlated with C-reactive protein level in non-small cell lung carcinoma." *PLoS One* 9(3):e91080. doi: 10.1371/journal.pone.0091080.

Couch, M. E., K. Dittus, M. J. Toth, M. S. Willis, D. C. Guttridge, J. R. George, C. A. Barnes, C. G. Gourin, and H. Der-Torossian. 2015. "Cancer cachexia update in head and neck cancer: Definitions and diagnostic features." *Head Neck* 37(4):594–604. doi: 10.1002/hed.23599.

Daas, S. I., B. R. Rizeq, and G. K. Nasrallah. 2018. "Adipose tissue dysfunction in cancer cachexia." *J Cell Physiol* 234(1):13–22. doi: 10.1002/jcp.26811.

Dahlman, I., N. Mejhert, K. Linder, T. Agustsson, D. M. Mutch, A. Kulyte, B. Isaksson, J. Permert, N. Petrovic, J. Nedergaard, E. Sjolin, D. Brodin, K. Clement, K. Dahlman-Wright, M. Ryden, and P. Arner. 2010. "Adipose tissue pathways involved in weight loss of cancer cachexia." *Br J Cancer* 102(10):1541–8. doi: 10.1038/sj.bjc.6605665.

Dalal, S. 2019. "Lipid metabolism in cancer cachexia." *Ann Palliat Med* 8(1):13–23. doi: 10.21037/apm.2018.10.01.

Damrauer, J. S., M. E. Stadler, S. Acharyya, A. S. Baldwin, M. E. Couch, and D. C. Guttridge. 2018. "Chemotherapy-induced muscle wasting: Association with NF-kappaB and cancer cachexia." *Eur J Transl Myol* 28(2):7590. doi: 10.4081/ejtm.2018.7590.

Davis, M. P., and R. Panikkar. 2019. "Sarcopenia associated with chemotherapy and targeted agents for cancer therapy." *Ann Palliat Med* 8(1):86–101. doi: 10.21037/apm.2018.08.02.

De Hertogh, G., B. Lemmens, P. Verhasselt, R. de Hoogt, X. Sagaert, M. Joossens, G. Van Assche, P. Rutgeerts, S. Vermeire, and J. Aerssens. 2012. "Assessment of the microbiota in microdissected tissues of Crohn's disease patients." *Int J Inflam* 2012:505674. doi: 10.1155/2012/505674.

De Vries, Y. C., S. Boesveldt, C. S. Kelfkens, E. E. Posthuma, Mmga van den Berg, Jtcm de Kruif, A. Haringhuizen, D. W. Sommeijer, N. Buist, S. Grosfeld, C. de Graaf, H. W. M. van Laarhoven, E. Kampman, and R. M. Winkels. 2018. "Taste and smell perception and quality of life during and after systemic therapy for breast cancer." *Breast Cancer Res Treat* 170(1):27–34. doi: 10.1007/s10549-018-4720-3.

Deng, C. Y., Y. C. Lin, J. S. Wu, Y. C. Cheung, C. W. Fan, K. Y. Yeh, and C. J. McMahon. 2018. "Progressive Sarcopenia in Patients With Colorectal Cancer Predicts Survival." *Am J Roentgenol* 210(3):526–32. doi: 10.2214/AJR.17.18020.

Dennis, E. A., and P. C. Norris. 2015. "Eicosanoid storm in infection and inflammation." *Nat Rev Immunol* 15(8):511–23. doi: 10.1038/nri3859.

Di Fiore, A., S. Lecleire, A. Gangloff, O. Rigal, A. Benyoucef, V. Blondin, D. Sefrioui, M. Quiesse, I. Iwanicki-Caron, P. Michel, and F. Di Fiore. 2014. "Impact of nutritional parameter variations during definitive chemoradiotherapy in locally advanced oesophageal cancer." *Dig Liver Dis* 46(3):270–5. doi: 10.1016/j.dld.2013.10.016.

Donohoe, C. L., A. M. Ryan, and J. V. Reynolds. 2011. "Cancer cachexia: Mechanisms and clinical implications." *Gastroenterol Res Pract* 2011:601434. doi: 10.1155/2011/601434.

Ebner, N., S. D. Anker, and S. von Haehling. 2020. "Recent developments in the field of cachexia, sarcopenia, and muscle wasting: Highlights from the 12th Cachexia Conference." *J Cachexia Sarcopenia Muscle* 11(1):274–85. doi: 10.1002/jcsm.12552.

Ebner, N., J. Springer, K. Kalantar-Zadeh, M. Lainscak, W. Doehner, S. D. Anker, and S. von Haehling. 2013. "Mechanism and novel therapeutic approaches to wasting in chronic disease." *Maturitas* 75(3):199–206. doi: 10.1016/j.maturitas.2013.03.014.

Farhangfar, A., M. Makarewicz, S. Ghosh, N. Jha, R. Scrimger, L. Gramlich, and V. Baracos. 2014. "Nutrition impact symptoms in a population cohort of head and neck cancer patients: Multivariate regression analysis of symptoms on oral intake, weight loss and survival." *Oral Oncol* 50(9):877–83. doi: 10.1016/j.oraloncology.2014.06.009.

Fearon, K., F. Strasser, S. D. Anker, I. Bosaeus, E. Bruera, R. L. Fainsinger, A. Jatoi, C. Loprinzi, N. MacDonald, G. Mantovani, M. Davis, M. Muscaritoli, F. Ottery, L. Radbruch, P. Ravasco, D. Walsh, A. Wilcock, S. Kaasa, and V. E. Baracos. 2011. "Definition and classification of cancer cachexia: An international consensus." *Lancet Oncol* 12(5):489–95. doi: 10.1016/S1470-2045(10)70218-7.

Fearon, K. C., D. J. Glass, and D. C. Guttridge. 2012. "Cancer cachexia: Mediators, signaling, and metabolic pathways." *Cell Metab* 16(2):153–66. doi: 10.1016/j.cmet.2012.06.011.

Fearon, K., J. Arends, and V. Baracos. 2013. "Understanding the mechanisms and treatment options in cancer cachexia." *Nat Rev Clin Oncol* 10(2):90–9. doi: 10.1038/nrclinonc.2012.209.

Fouladiun, M., U. Korner, I. Bosaeus, P. Daneryd, A. Hyltander, and K. G. Lundholm. 2005. "Body composition and time course changes in regional distribution of fat and lean tissue in unselected cancer patients on palliative care--correlations with food intake, metabolism, exercise capacity, and hormones." *Cancer* 103(10):2189–98. doi: 10.1002/cncr.21013.

Friedman, J. 2016. "The long road to leptin." *J Clin Invest* 126(12):4727–34. doi: 10.1172/JCI91578.

Fridman, W. H., F. Pages, C. Sautes-Fridman, and J. Galon. 2012. "The immune contexture in human tumours: Impact on clinical outcome." *Nat Rev Cancer* 12(4):298–306. doi: 10.1038/nrc3245.

Galvao, D. A., N. A. Spry, D. R. Taaffe, R. U. Newton, J. Stanley, T. Shannon, C. Rowling, and R. Prince. 2008. "Changes in muscle, fat and bone mass after 36 weeks of maximal androgen blockade for prostate cancer." *BJU Int* 102(1):44–7. doi: 10.1111/j.1464-410X.2008.07539.x.

Galvao, D. A., D. R. Taaffe, N. Spry, D. Joseph, D. Turner, and R. U. Newton. 2009. "Reduced muscle strength and functional performance in men with prostate cancer undergoing androgen suppression: A comprehensive cross-sectional investigation." *Prostate Cancer Prostatic Dis* 12(2):198–203. doi: 10.1038/pcan.2008.51.

Garcia, J. M., J. Friend, and S. Allen. 2013. "Therapeutic potential of anamorelin, a novel, oral ghrelin mimetic, in patients with cancer-related cachexia: A multicenter, randomized, double-blind, crossover, pilot study." *Support Care Cancer* 21(1):129–37. doi: 10.1007/s00520-012-1500-1.

Garcia, J. M., T. Scherer, J. A. Chen, B. Guillory, A. Nassif, V. Papusha, J. Smiechowska, M. Asnicar, C. Buettner, and R. G. Smith. 2013. "Inhibition of cisplatin-induced lipid catabolism and weight loss by ghrelin in male mice." *Endocrinology* 154(9):3118–29. doi: 10.1210/en.2013-1179.

Gerber, M. H., P. W. Underwood, S. M. Judge, D. Delitto, A. E. Delitto, R. L. Nosacka, B. B. DiVita, R. M. Thomas, J. B. Permuth, S. J. Hughes, S. M. Wallet, A. R. Judge, and J. G. Trevino. 2018. "Local and systemic cytokine profiling for pancreatic ductal adenocarcinoma to study cancer cachexia in an era of precision medicine." *Int J Mol Sci* 19(12). doi: 10.3390/ijms19123836.

Gorenc, M., N. R. Kozjek, and P. Strojan. 2015. "Malnutrition and cachexia in patients with head and neck cancer treated with (chemo)radiotherapy." *Rep Pract Oncol Radiother* 20(4):249–58. doi: 10.1016/j.rpor.2015.03.001.

Griffin, K., I. Csizmadi, L. E. Howard, G. M. Pomann, W. J. Aronson, C. J. Kane, C. L. Amling, M. R. Cooperberg, M. K. Terris, J. Beebe-Dimmer, and S. J. Freedland. 2019. "First-year weight loss with androgen-deprivation therapy increases risks of prostate cancer progression and prostate cancer-specific mortality: Results from SEARCH." *Cancer Causes Control* 30(3):259–69. doi: 10.1007/s10552-019-1133-5.

Grutsch, J. F., C. Ferrans, P. A. Wood, J. Du-Quiton, D. F. Quiton, J. L. Reynolds, C. M. Ansell, E. Y. Oh, M. A. Daehler, R. D. Levin, D. P. Braun, D. Gupta, C. G. Lis, and W. J. Hrushesky. 2011. "The association of quality of life with potentially remediable disruptions of circadian sleep/activity rhythms in patients with advanced lung cancer." *BMC Cancer* 11:193. doi: 10.1186/1471-2407-11-193.

Heber, D. 2010. "An integrative view of obesity." *Am J Clin Nutr* 91(1):280S–3S. doi: 10.3945/ajcn.2009.28473B.

Heber, D., R. T. Chlebowski, D. E. Ishibashi, J. N. Herrold, and J. B. Block. 1982. "Abnormalities in glucose and protein metabolism in noncachectic lung cancer patients." *Cancer Res* 42(11):4815–9.

Hiura, Y., S. Takiguchi, K. Yamamoto, Y. Kurokawa, M. Yamasaki, K. Nakajima, H. Miyata, Y. Fujiwara, M. Mori, and Y. Doki. 2012. "Fall in plasma ghrelin concentrations after cisplatin-based chemotherapy in esophageal cancer patients." *Int J Clin Oncol* 17(4):316–23. doi: 10.1007/s10147-011-0289-0.

Holick, C. N., D. S. Michaud, R. Stolzenberg-Solomon, S. T. Mayne, P. Pietinen, P. R. Taylor, J. Virtamo, and D. Albanes. 2002. "Dietary carotenoids, serum beta-carotene, and retinol and risk of lung cancer in the alpha-tocopherol, beta-carotene cohort study." *Am J Epidemiol* 156(6):536–47. doi: 10.1093/aje/kwf072.

Hong, J. H., P. Omur-Ozbek, B. T. Stanek, A. M. Dietrich, S. E. Duncan, Y. W. Lee, and G. Lesser. 2009. "Taste and odor abnormalities in cancer patients." *J Support Oncol* 7(2):58–65.

Hui, D., R. Dev, and E. Bruera. 2015. "The last days of life: Symptom burden and impact on nutrition and hydration in cancer patients." *Curr Opin Support Palliat Care* 9(4):346–54. doi: 10.1097/SPC.0000000000000171.

Hunter, D. C., M. Weintraub, G. L. Blackburn, and B. R. Bistrian. 1989. "Branched chain amino acids as the protein component of parenteral nutrition in cancer cachexia." *Br J Surg* 76(2):149–53. doi: 10.1002/bjs.1800760215.

Ikeda, T., H. Ishihara, J. Iizuka, Y. Hashimoto, K. Yoshida, Y. Kakuta, T. Takagi, M. Okumi, H. Ishida, T. Kondo, and K. Tanabe. 2020. "Prognostic impact of sarcopenia in patients with metastatic hormone-sensitive prostate cancer." *Jpn J Clin Oncol.* doi: 10.1093/jjco/hyaa045.

Irie, M. S., E. M. Mendes, J. S. Borges, L. G. Osuna, G. D. Rabelo, and P. B. Soares. 2018. "Periodontal therapy for patients before and after radiotherapy: A review of the literature and topics of interest for clinicians." *Med Oral Patol Oral Cir Bucal* 23(5):e524–30. doi: 10.4317/medoral.22474.

Jaruga, P., T. H. Zastawny, J. Skokowski, M. Dizdaroglu, and R. Olinski. 1994. "Oxidative DNA base damage and antioxidant enzyme activities in human lung cancer." *FEBS Lett* 341(1):59–64. doi: 10.1016/0014-5793(94)80240-8.

Julienne, C. M., J. F. Dumas, C. Goupille, M. Pinault, C. Berri, A. Collin, S. Tesseraud, C. Couet, and S. Servais. 2012. "Cancer cachexia is associated with a decrease in skeletal muscle mitochondrial oxidative capacities without alteration of ATP production efficiency." *J Cachexia Sarcopenia Muscle* 3(4):265–75. doi: 10.1007/s13539-012-0071-9.

Jurek, A., B. Turyna, P. Kubit, and A. Klein. 2006. "LDL susceptibility to oxidation and HDL antioxidant capacity in patients with renal failure." *Clin Biochem* 39(1):19–27. doi: 10.1016/j.clinbiochem.2005.08.009.

Karabacak, M., E. Varol, F. Kahraman, M. Ozaydin, A. K. Turkdogan, and I. H. Ersoy. 2014. "Low high-density lipoprotein cholesterol is characterized by elevated oxidative stress." *Angiology* 65(10):927–31. doi: 10.1177/0003319713512173.

Kazantzis, M., and M. C. Seelaender. 2005. "Cancer cachexia modifies the zonal distribution of lipid metabo-lism-related proteins in rat liver." *Cell Tissue Res* 321(3):419–27. doi: 10.1007/s00441-005-1138-0.

Keating, N. L., A. J. O'Malley, S. J. Freedland, and M. R. Smith. 2010. "Diabetes and cardiovascular disease during androgen deprivation therapy: Observational study of veterans with prostate cancer." *J Natl Cancer Inst* 102(1):39–46. doi: 10.1093/jnci/djp404.

Keto, C. J., W. J. Aronson, M. K. Terris, J. C. Presti, C. J. Kane, C. L. Amling, and S. J. Freedland. 2012. "Obesity is associated with castration-resistant disease and metastasis in men treated with andro-gen deprivation therapy after radical prostatectomy: Results from the SEARCH database." *BJU Int* 110(4):492–8. doi: 10.1111/j.1464-410X.2011.10754.x.

Kim, H. S., D. M. Moreira, M. R. Smith, J. C. Presti, Jr., W. J. Aronson, M. K. Terris, C. J. Kane, C. L. Amling, and S. J. Freedland. 2011. "A natural history of weight change in men with prostate cancer on androgen-deprivation therapy (ADT): Results from the Shared Equal Access Regional Cancer Hospital (SEARCH) database." *BJU Int* 107(6):924–8. doi: 10.1111/j.1464-410X.2010.09679.x.

Kir, S., J. P. White, S. Kleiner, L. Kazak, P. Cohen, V. E. Baracos, and B. M. Spiegelman. 2014. "Tumour-derived PTH-related protein triggers adipose tissue browning and cancer cachexia." *Nature* 513(7516):100–4. doi: 10.1038/nature13528.

Kliewer, K. L., J. Y. Ke, M. Tian, R. M. Cole, R. R. Andridge, and M. A. Belury. 2015. "Adipose tissue lipolysis and energy metabolism in early cancer cachexia in mice." *Cancer Biol Ther* 16(6):886–97. doi: 10.4161/15384047.2014.987075.

Krahn, M. D., K. E. Bremner, J. Luo, G. Tomlinson, and S. M. Alibhai. 2016. "Long-term health care costs for prostate cancer patients on androgen deprivation therapy." *Curr Oncol* 23(5):e443–53. doi: 10.3747/co.23.2953.

Kucharska-Newton, A. M., W. D. Rosamond, J. C. Schroeder, A. M. McNeill, J. Coresh, A. R. Folsom, and Study Members of the Atherosclerosis Risk in Communities. 2008. "HDL-cholesterol and the incidence of lung cancer in the Atherosclerosis Risk in Communities (ARIC) study." *Lung Cancer* 61(3):292–300. doi: 10.1016/j.lungcan.2008.01.015.

Kuroda, K., J. Nakashima, K. Kanao, E. Kikuchi, A. Miyajima, Y. Horiguchi, K. Nakagawa, M. Oya, T. Ohigashi, and M. Murai. 2007. "Interleukin 6 is associated with cachexia in patients with prostate can-cer." *Urology* 69(1):113–7. doi: 10.1016/j.urology.2006.09.039.

Kuwada, K., S. Kuroda, S. Kikuchi, R. Yoshida, M. Nishizaki, S. Kagawa, and T. Fujiwara. 2019. "Clinical impact of sarcopenia on gastric cancer." *Anticancer Res* 39(5):2241–9. doi: 10.21873/anticanres.13340.

Laviano, A., M. M. Meguid, A. Inui, M. Muscaritoli, and F. Rossi-Fanelli. 2005. "Therapy insight: Cancer anorexia-cachexia syndrome--when all you can eat is yourself." *Nat Clin Pract Oncol* 2(3):158–65. doi: 10.1038/ncponc0112.

Lecker, S. H., V. Solomon, W. E. Mitch, and A. L. Goldberg. 1999. "Muscle protein breakdown and the critical role of the ubiquitin-proteasome pathway in normal and disease states." *J Nutr* 129(1S Suppl):227S–37S. doi: 10.1093/jn/129.1.227S.

Lee, G., T. C. Walser, and S. M. Dubinett. 2009. "Chronic inflammation, chronic obstructive pulmonary dis-ease, and lung cancer." *Curr Opin Pulm Med* 15(4):303–7. doi: 10.1097/MCP.0b013e32832c975a.

Lee, P., J. R. Greenfield, K. K. Ho, and M. J. Fulham. 2010. "A critical appraisal of the prevalence and metabolic significance of brown adipose tissue in adult humans." *Am J Physiol Endocrinol Metab* 299(4):E601–6. doi: 10.1152/ajpendo.00298.2010.

Lin, X., L. Lu, L. Liu, S. Wei, Y. He, J. Chang, and X. Lian. 2017a. "Blood lipids profile and lung can-cer risk in a meta-analysis of prospective cohort studies." *J Clin Lipidol* 11(4):1073–81. doi: 10.1016/j.jacl.2017.05.004.

Lin, K. F., H. F. Wu, W. C. Huang, P. L. Tang, M. T. Wu, and F. Z. Wu. 2017b. "Propensity score analysis of lung cancer risk in a population with high prevalence of non-smoking related lung cancer." *BMC Pulm Med* 17(1):120. doi: 10.1186/s12890-017-0465-8.

Little, J. P., and S. M. Phillips. 2009. "Resistance exercise and nutrition to counteract muscle wasting." *Appl Physiol Nutr Metab* 34(5):817–28. doi: 10.1139/H09-093.

Loprinzi, C. L., J. W. Kugler, J. A. Sloan, J. A. Mailliard, J. E. Krook, M. B. Wilwerding, K. M. Rowland, Jr., J. K. Camoriano, P. J. Novotny, and B. J. Christensen. 1999. "Randomized comparison of megestrol acetate versus dexamethasone versus fluoxymesterone for the treatment of cancer anorexia/cachexia." *J Clin Oncol* 17(10):3299–306. doi: 10.1200/JCO.1999.17.10.3299.

Maccio, A., G. Gramignano, and C. Madeddu. 2015. "A multitargeted treatment approach for anemia and cachexia in metastatic castration-resistant prostate cancer." *J Pain Symptom Manage* 50(2):e1–4. doi: 10.1016/j.jpainsymman.2015.04.014.

Madeddu, C., A. Maccio, F. Panzone, F. M. Tanca, and G. Mantovani. 2009. "Medroxyprogesterone acetate in the management of cancer cachexia." *Expert Opin Pharmacother* 10(8):1359–66. doi: 10.1517/14656560902960162.

Madeddu, C., M. Dessi, F. Panzone, R. Serpe, G. Antoni, M. C. Cau, L. Montaldo, Q. Mela, M. Mura, G. Astara, F. M. Tanca, A. Maccio, and G. Mantovani. 2012. "Randomized phase III clinical trial of a combined treatment with carnitine + celecoxib +/– megestrol acetate for patients with cancer-related anorexia/cachexia syndrome." *Clin Nutr* 31(2):176–82. doi: 10.1016/j.clnu.2011.10.005.

Mannisto, S., S. A. Smith-Warner, D. Spiegelman, D. Albanes, K. Anderson, P. A. van den Brandt, J. R. Cerhan, G. Colditz, D. Feskanich, J. L. Freudenheim, E. Giovannucci, R. A. Goldbohm, S. Graham, A. B. Miller, T. E. Rohan, J. Virtamo, W. C. Willett, and D. J. Hunter. 2004. "Dietary carotenoids and risk of lung cancer in a pooled analysis of seven cohort studies." *Cancer Epidemiol Biomarkers Prev* 13(1):40–8. doi: 10.1158/1055-9965.epi-038-3.

Mantovani, G., C. Madeddu, A. Maccio, G. Gramignano, M. R. Lusso, E. Massa, G. Astara, and R. Serpe. 2004. "Cancer-related anorexia/cachexia syndrome and oxidative stress: An innovative approach beyond current treatment." *Cancer Epidemiol Biomarkers Prev* 13(10):1651–9.

Mantovani, G., A. Maccio, C. Madeddu, G. Gramignano, R. Serpe, E. Massa, M. Dessi, F. M. Tanca, E. Sanna, L. Deiana, F. Panzone, P. Contu, and C. Floris. 2008. "Randomized phase III clinical trial of five different arms of treatment for patients with cancer cachexia: Interim results." *Nutrition* 24(4):305–13. doi: 10.1016/j.nut.2007.12.010.

Mantovani, G., A. Maccio, C. Madeddu, R. Serpe, E. Massa, M. Dessi, F. Panzone, and P. Contu. 2010. "Randomized phase III clinical trial of five different arms of treatment in 332 patients with cancer cachexia." *Oncologist* 15(2):200–11. doi: 10.1634/theoncologist.2009-0153.

Mantovani, G., C. Madeddu, and A. Maccio. 2013. "Drugs in development for treatment of patients with cancer-related anorexia and cachexia syndrome." *Drug Des Devel Ther* 7:645–56 doi: 10.2147/DDDT. S39771.

Marchesi, J. R., B. E. Dutilh, N. Hall, W. H. Peters, R. Roelofs, A. Boleij, and H. Tjalsma. 2011. "Towards the human colorectal cancer microbiome." *PLoS One* 6(5):e20447. doi: 10.1371/journal.pone.0020447.

Marengo, A., C. Rosso, and E. Bugianesi. 2016. "Liver cancer: Connections with obesity, fatty liver, and cirrhosis." *Annu Rev Med* 67:103–17 doi: 10.1146/annurev-med-090514-013832.

Martin, L., P. Senesse, I. Gioulbasanis, S. Antoun, F. Bozzetti, C. Deans, F. Strasser, L. Thoresen, R. T. Jagoe, M. Chasen, K. Lundholm, I. Bosaeus, K. H. Fearon, and V. E. Baracos. 2015. "Diagnostic criteria for the classification of cancer-associated weight loss." *J Clin Oncol* 33(1):90–9. doi: 10.1200/ JCO.2014.56.1894.

May, P. E., A. Barber, J. T. D'Olimpio, A. Hourihane, and N. N. Abumrad. 2002. "Reversal of cancer-related wasting using oral supplementation with a combination of beta-hydroxy-beta-methylbutyrate, arginine, and glutamine." *Am J Surg* 183(4):471–9. doi: 10.1016/s0002-9610(02)00823-1.

McGreevy, J., Y. Orrevall, K. Belqaid, W. Wismer, C. Tishelman, and B. M. Bernhardson. 2014. "Characteristics of taste and smell alterations reported by patients after starting treatment for lung cancer." *Support Care Cancer* 22(10):2635–44. doi: 10.1007/s00520-014-2215-2.

Morley, J. E. 2009. "Calories and cachexia." *Curr Opin Clin Nutr Metab Care* 12(6):607–10. doi: 10.1097/ MCO.0b013e328331e9ce.

Motta, M., G. Pistone, A. M. Franzone, M. A. Romeo, S. Di Mauro, I. Giugno, P. Ruello, and M. Malaguarnera. 2003. "Antibodies against ox-LDL serum levels in patients with hepatocellular carcinoma." *Panminerva Med* 45(1):69–73.

Murphy, R. A., M. S. Wilke, M. Perrine, M. Pawlowicz, M. Mourtzakis, J. R. Lieffers, M. Maneshgar, E. Bruera, M. T. Clandinin, V. E. Baracos, and V. C. Mazurak. 2010. "Loss of adipose tissue and plasma phospholipids: Relationship to survival in advanced cancer patients." *Clin Nutr* 29(4):482–7. doi: 10.1016/j.clnu.2009.11.006.

Muscaritoli, M., A. Molfino, S. Lucia, and F. Rossi Fanelli. 2015. "Cachexia: A preventable comorbidity of cancer. A T.A.R.G.E.T. approach." *Crit Rev Oncol Hematol* 94(2):251–9. doi: 10.1016/j. critrevonc.2014.10.014.

Newell, S., R. W. Sanson-Fisher, A. Girgis, and A. Bonaventura. 1998. "How well do medical oncologists' perceptions reflect their patients' reported psychosocial problems? Data from a survey of five oncologists." *Cancer* 83(8):1640–51.

Nguyen, P. L., S. M. Alibhai, S. Basaria, A. V. D'Amico, P. W. Kantoff, N. L. Keating, D. F. Penson, D. J. Rosario, B. Tombal, and M. R. Smith. 2015. "Adverse effects of androgen deprivation therapy and strategies to mitigate them." *Eur Urol* 67(5):825–36. doi: 10.1016/j.eururo.2014.07.010.

Nipp, R. D., G. Fuchs, A. El-Jawahri, J. Mario, F. M. Troschel, J. A. Greer, E. R. Gallagher, V. A. Jackson, A. Kambadakone, T. S. Hong, J. S. Temel, and F. J. Fintelmann. 2018. "Sarcopenia is associated with quality of life and depression in patients with advanced cancer." *Oncologist* 23(1):97–104. doi: 10.1634/theoncologist.2017-0255.

Nishioka, N., J. Uchino, S. Hirai, Y. Katayama, A. Yoshimura, N. Okura, K. Tanimura, S. Harita, T. Imabayashi, Y. Chihara, N. Tamiya, Y. Kaneko, T. Yamada, and K. Takayama. 2019. "Association of sarcopenia with and efficacy of anti-PD-1/PD-L1 therapy in non-small-cell lung cancer." *J Clin Med* 8(4). doi: 10.3390/jcm8040450.

Ojo, J. O., P. Rezaie, P. L. Gabbott, and M. G. Stewart. 2015. "Impact of age-related neuroglial cell responses on hippocampal deterioration." *Front Aging Neurosci* 7:57. doi: 10.3389/fnagi.2015.00057.

Owen, P. J., R. M. Daly, P. M. Livingston, and S. F. Fraser. 2017. "Lifestyle guidelines for managing adverse effects on bone health and body composition in men treated with androgen deprivation therapy for prostate cancer: An update." *Prostate Cancer Prostatic Dis* 20(2):137–45. doi: 10.1038/pcan.2016.69.

Pai, P. C., C. C. Chuang, W. C. Chuang, N. M. Tsang, C. K. Tseng, K. H. Chen, T. C. Yen, C. Y. Lin, K. P. Chang, and K. F. Lei. 2018. "Pretreatment subcutaneous adipose tissue predicts the outcomes of patients with head and neck cancer receiving definitive radiation and chemoradiation in Taiwan." *Cancer Med* 7(5):1630–41. doi: 10.1002/cam4.1365.

Paulsen, O., B. Laird, N. Aass, T. Lea, P. Fayers, S. Kaasa, and P. Klepstad. 2017. "The relationship between pro-inflammatory cytokines and pain, appetite and fatigue in patients with advanced cancer." *PLoS One* 12(5):e0177620. doi: 10.1371/journal.pone.0177620.

Pausch, T., W. Hartwig, U. Hinz, T. Swolana, B. D. Bundy, T. Hackert, L. Grenacher, M. W. Buchler, and J. Werner. 2012. "Cachexia but not obesity worsens the postoperative outcome after pancreatoduodenectomy in pancreatic cancer." *Surgery* 152(3 Suppl 1):S81–8. doi: 10.1016/j.surg.2012.05.028.

Peterson, J. M., N. Bakkar, and D. C. Guttridge. 2011. "NF-kappa B signaling in skeletal muscle health and disease." *Curr Top Dev Biol* 96:85–119 doi: 10.1016/B978-0-12-385940-2.00004-8.

Petruzzelli, M., M. Schweiger, R. Schreiber, R. Campos-Olivas, M. Tsoli, J. Allen, J. Swarbrick, S. Rose-John, M. Rincon, G. Robertson, R. Zechner, and E. F. Wagner. 2014. "A switch from white to brown fat increases energy expenditure in cancer-associated cachexia." *Cell Metab* 20(3):433–47. doi: 10.1016/j.cmet.2014.06.011.

Prado, C. M., V. E. Baracos, L. J. McCargar, M. Mourtzakis, K. E. Mulder, T. Reiman, C. A. Butts, A. G. Scarfe, and M. B. Sawyer. 2007. "Body composition as an independent determinant of 5-fluorouracil-based chemotherapy toxicity." *Clin Cancer Res* 13(11):3264–8. doi: 10.1158/1078-0432. CCR-06-3067.

Qu, X., Y. Tang, and S. Hua. 2018. "Immunological approaches towards cancer and inflammation: A cross talk." *Front Immunol* 9:563. doi: 10.3389/fimmu.2018.00563.

Rodriguez-Carrio, J., M. Alperi-Lopez, P. Lopez, R. Lopez-Mejias, S. Alonso-Castro, F. Abal, F. J. Ballina-Garcia, M. A. Gonzalez-Gay, and A. Suarez. 2017. "High triglycerides and low high-density lipoprotein cholesterol lipid profile in rheumatoid arthritis: A potential link among inflammation, oxidative status, and dysfunctional high-density lipoprotein." *J Clin Lipidol* 11(4):1043–54 e2. doi: 10.1016/j.jacl.2017.05.009.

Ruiz-Garcia, V., E. Lopez-Briz, R. Carbonell-Sanchis, S. Bort-Marti, and J. L. Gonzalvez-Perales. 2018. "Megestrol acetate for cachexia-anorexia syndrome: A systematic review." *J Cachexia Sarcopenia Muscle* 9(3):444–452. doi: 10.1002/jcsm.12292.

Ryan, A. M., D. G. Power, L. Daly, S. J. Cushen, E. Ni Bhuachalla, and C. M. Prado. 2016. "Cancer-associated malnutrition, cachexia and sarcopenia: The skeleton in the hospital closet 40 years later." *Proc Nutr Soc* 75(2):199–211. doi: 10.1017/S002966511500419X.

Santarpia, L., F. Contaldo, and F. Pasanisi. 2011. "Nutritional screening and early treatment of malnutrition in cancer patients." *J Cachexia Sarcopenia Muscle* 2(1):27–35. doi: 10.1007/s13539-011-0022-x.

Sarhill, N., F. Mahmoud, D. Walsh, K. A. Nelson, S. Komurcu, M. Davis, S. LeGrand, O. Abdullah, and L. Rybicki. 2003. "Evaluation of nutritional status in advanced metastatic cancer." *Support Care Cancer* 11(10):652–9. doi: 10.1007/s00520-003-0486-0.

Saylor, P. J., N. L. Keating, S. J. Freedland, and M. R. Smith. 2011. "Gonadotropin-releasing hormone agonists and the risks of type 2 diabetes and cardiovascular disease in men with prostate cancer." *Drugs* 71(3):255–61. doi: 10.2165/11588930-000000000-00000.

Schiaffino, S., K. A. Dyar, S. Ciciliot, B. Blaauw, and M. Sandri. 2013. "Mechanisms regulating skeletal muscle growth and atrophy." *FEBS J* 280(17):4294–314. doi: 10.1111/febs.12253.

Segal, R. J., R. D. Reid, K. S. Courneya, S. C. Malone, M. B. Parliament, C. G. Scott, P. M. Venner, H. A. Quinney, L. W. Jones, M. E. D'Angelo, and G. A. Wells. 2003. "Resistance exercise in men receiving androgen deprivation therapy for prostate cancer." *J Clin Oncol* 21(9):1653–9. doi: 10.1200/JCO.2003.09.534.

Seo, S. H., S. E. Kim, Y. K. Kang, B. Y. Ryoo, M. H. Ryu, J. H. Jeong, S. S. Kang, M. Yang, J. E. Lee, and M. K. Sung. 2016. "Association of nutritional status-related indices and chemotherapy-induced adverse events in gastric cancer patients." *BMC Cancer* 16(1):900. doi: 10.1186/s12885-016-2934-5.

Shellock, F. G., M. S. Riedinger, and M. C. Fishbein. 1986. "Brown adipose tissue in cancer patients: Possible cause of cancer-induced cachexia." *J Cancer Res Clin Oncol* 111(1):82–5. doi: 10.1007/BF00402783.

Siddiqui, R. A., and J. F. Williams. 1989. "The regulation of fatty acid and branched-chain amino acid oxidation in cancer cachectic rats: A proposed role for a cytokine, eicosanoid, and hormone trilogy." *Biochem Med Metab Biol* 42(1):71–86. doi: 10.1016/0885-4505(89)90043-1.

Silverio, R., A. Laviano, F. Rossi Fanelli, and M. Seelaender. 2012. "L-Carnitine induces recovery of liver lipid metabolism in cancer cachexia." *Amino Acids* 42(5):1783–92. doi: 10.1007/s00726-011-0898-y.

Simons, J. P., A. M. Schols, J. M. Hoefnagels, K. R. Westerterp, G. P. ten Velde, and E. F. Wouters. 1998. "Effects of medroxyprogesterone acetate on food intake, body composition, and resting energy expenditure in patients with advanced, nonhormone-sensitive cancer: A randomized, placebo-controlled trial." *Cancer* 82(3):553–60.

Smith, M. R., J. S. Finkelstein, F. J. McGovern, A. L. Zietman, M. A. Fallon, D. A. Schoenfeld, and P. W. Kantoff. 2002. "Changes in body composition during androgen deprivation therapy for prostate cancer." *J Clin Endocrinol Metab* 87(2):599–603. doi: 10.1210/jcem.87.2.8299.

Spotten, L. E., C. A. Corish, C. M. Lorton, P. M. Ui Dhuibhir, N. C. O'Donoghue, B. O'Connor, and T. D. Walsh. 2017. "Subjective and objective taste and smell changes in cancer." *Ann Oncol* 28(5):969–84. doi: 10.1093/annonc/mdx018.

Stathis, A., and M. J. Moore. 2010. "Advanced pancreatic carcinoma: Current treatment and future challenges." *Nat Rev Clin Oncol* 7(3):163–72. doi: 10.1038/nrclinonc.2009.236.

Steinbach, S., W. Hundt, T. Zahnert, S. Berktold, C. Bohner, N. Gottschalk, M. Hamann, M. Kriner, P. Heinrich, B. Schmalfeldt, and N. Harbeck. 2010. "Gustatory and olfactory function in breast cancer patients." *Support Care Cancer* 18(6):707–13. doi: 10.1007/s00520-009-0672-9.

Sugiyama, M., A. Yamaki, M. Furuya, N. Inomata, Y. Minamitake, K. Ohsuye, and K. Kangawa. 2012. "Ghrelin improves body weight loss and skeletal muscle catabolism associated with angiotensin II-induced cachexia in mice." *Regul Pept* 178(1–3):21–8. doi: 10.1016/j.regpep.2012.06.003.

Sun, J., and I. Kato. 2016. "Gut microbiota, inflammation and colorectal cancer." *Genes Dis* 3(2):130–43. doi: 10.1016/j.gendis.2016.03.004.

Suzuki, H., A. Asakawa, H. Amitani, N. Nakamura, and A. Inui. 2013. "Cancer cachexia--pathophysiology and management." *J Gastroenterol* 48(5):574–94. doi: 10.1007/s00535-013-0787-0.

Tayek, J. A., D. Heber, and R. T. Chlebowski. 1987. "Effect of hydrazine sulphate on whole-body protein breakdown measured by 14C-lysine metabolism in lung cancer patients." *Lancet* 2(8553):241–4. doi: 10.1016/s0140-6736(87)90828-2.

Tayek, J. A., D. Heber, L. O. Byerley, B. Steiner, J. Rajfer, and R. S. Swerdloff. 1990. "Nutritional and metabolic effects of gonadotropin-releasing hormone agonist treatment for prostate cancer." *Metabolism* 39(12):1314–9. doi: 10.1016/0026-0495(90)90190-n.

Thoma, A., and A. P. Lightfoot. 2018. "NF-kB and inflammatory cytokine signalling: Role in skeletal muscle atrophy." *Adv Exp Med Biol* 1088:267–79. doi: 10.1007/978-981-13-1435-3_12.

Thomas, S. S., and W. E. Mitch. 2017. "Parathyroid hormone stimulates adipose tissue browning: A pathway to muscle wasting." *Curr Opin Clin Nutr Metab Care* 20(3):153–7. doi: 10.1097/MCO.0000000000000357.

Tisdale, M. J. 2009. "Mechanisms of cancer cachexia." *Physiol Rev* 89(2):381–410. doi: 10.1152/physrev.00016.2008.

Tsoli, M., and G. Robertson. 2013. "Cancer cachexia: Malignant inflammation, tumorkines, and metabolic mayhem." *Trends Endocrinol Metab* 24(4):174–83. doi: 10.1016/j.tem.2012.10.006.

Tsoli, M., M. M. Swarbrick, and G. R. Robertson. 2016. "Lipolytic and thermogenic depletion of adipose tissue in cancer cachexia." *Semin Cell Dev Biol* 54:68–81 doi: 10.1016/j.semcdb.2015.10.039.

Tzortzis, V., M. Samarinas, I. Zachos, A. Oeconomou, L. L. Pisters, and A. Bargiota. 2017. "Adverse effects of androgen deprivation therapy in patients with prostate cancer: Focus on metabolic complications." *Hormones (Athens)* 16(2):115–23. doi: 10.14310/horm.2002.1727.

Ui Dhuibhir, P., M. Barrett, N. O'Donoghue, C. Gillham, N. El Beltagi, and D. Walsh. 2020. "Self-reported and objective taste and smell evaluation in treatment-naive solid tumour patients." *Support Care Cancer* 28(5):2389–96. doi: 10.1007/s00520-019-05017-3.

Uomo, G., F. Gallucci, and P. G. Rabitti. 2006. "Anorexia-cachexia syndrome in pancreatic cancer: Recent development in research and management." *JOP* 7(2):157–62.

van der Werf, A., Q. N. E. van Bokhorst, M. A. E. de van der Schueren, H. M. W. Verheul, and J. A. E. Langius. 2018. "Cancer cachexia: Identification by clinical assessment versus international consensus criteria in patients with metastatic colorectal cancer." *Nutr Cancer* 70(8):1322–29. doi: 10.1080/01635581.2018.1504092.

von Grundherr, J., B. Koch, D. Grimm, J. Salchow, L. Valentini, T. Hummel, C. Bokemeyer, A. Stein, and J. Mann. 2019. "Impact of taste and smell training on taste disorders during chemotherapy: TASTE trial." *Cancer Manag Res* 11:4493–504 doi: 10.2147/CMAR.S188903.

Wang, W., M. Andersson, C. Lonnroth, E. Svanberg, and K. Lundholm. 2005. "Anorexia and cachexia in prostaglandin EP1 and EP3 subtype receptor knockout mice bearing a tumor with high intrinsic PGE2 production and prostaglandin related cachexia." *J Exp Clin Cancer Res* 24(1):99–107.

Wang, C., J. M. Vainshtein, M. Veksler, P. E. Rabban, J. A. Sullivan, S. C. Wang, A. Eisbruch, and S. Jolly. 2016. "Investigating the clinical significance of body composition changes in patients undergoing chemoradiation for oropharyngeal cancer using analytic morphomics." *Springerplus* 5:429. doi: 10.1186/s40064-016-2076-x.

Wendrich, A. W., J. E. Swartz, S. I. Bril, I. Wegner, A. de Graeff, E. J. Smid, R. de Bree, and A. J. Pothen. 2017. "Low skeletal muscle mass is a predictive factor for chemotherapy dose-limiting toxicity in patients with locally advanced head and neck cancer." *Oral Oncol* 71:26–33. doi: 10.1016/j.oraloncology.2017.05.012.

Wie, G. A., Y. A. Cho, S. Y. Kim, S. M. Kim, J. M. Bae, and H. Joung. 2010. "Prevalence and risk factors of malnutrition among cancer patients according to tumor location and stage in the National Cancer Center in Korea." *Nutrition* 26(3):263–8. doi: 10.1016/j.nut.2009.04.013.

Willemsen, A. C. H., A. Hoeben, R. I. Lalisang, A. Van Helvoort, F. W. R. Wesseling, F. Hoebers, L. W. J. Baijens, and Amwj Schols. 2020. "Disease-induced and treatment-induced alterations in body composition in locally advanced head and neck squamous cell carcinoma." *J Cachexia Sarcopenia Muscle* 11(1):145–159. doi: 10.1002/jcsm.12487.

Yang, M., Y. Shen, L. Tan, and W. Li. 2019. "Prognostic value of sarcopenia in lung cancer: A systematic review and meta-analysis." *Chest* 156(1):101–111. doi: 10.1016/j.chest.2019.04.115.

Yavuzsen, T., D. Walsh, M. P. Davis, J. Kirkova, T. Jin, S. LeGrand, R. Lagman, L. Bicanovsky, B. Estfan, B. Cheema, and A. Haddad. 2009. "Components of the anorexia-cachexia syndrome: Gastrointestinal symptom correlates of cancer anorexia." *Support Care Cancer* 17(12):1531–41. doi: 10.1007/s00520-009-0623-5.

Zablocka-Slowinska, K., S. Placzkowska, A. Prescha, K. Pawelczyk, M. Kosacka, I. Porebska, and H. Grajeta. 2018a. "Systemic redox status in lung cancer patients is related to altered glucose metabolism." *PLoS One* 13(9):e0204173. doi: 10.1371/journal.pone.0204173.

Zablocka-Slowinska, K., S. Placzkowska, A. Prescha, K. Pawelczyk, I. Porebska, M. Kosacka, L. Pawlik-Sobecka, and H. Grajeta. 2018b. "Serum and whole blood Zn, Cu and Mn profiles and their relation to redox status in lung cancer patients." *J Trace Elem Med Biol* 45:78–84 doi: 10.1016/j.jtemb.2017.09.024.

Zaki, M. H., J. A. Nemeth, and M. Trikha. 2004. "CNTO 328, a monoclonal antibody to IL-6, inhibits human tumor-induced cachexia in nude mice." *Int J Cancer* 111(4):592–5. doi: 10.1002/ijc.20270.

Zhang, F., A. Shen, Y. Jin, and W. Qiang. 2018. "The management strategies of cancer-associated anorexia: A critical appraisal of systematic reviews." *BMC Complement Altern Med* 18(1):236. doi: 10.1186/s12906-018-2304-8.

Zhou, T., J. Zhan, W. Fang, Y. Zhao, Y. Yang, X. Hou, Z. Zhang, X. He, Y. Zhang, Y. Huang, and L. Zhang. 2017. "Serum low-density lipoprotein and low-density lipoprotein expression level at diagnosis are favorable prognostic factors in patients with small-cell lung cancer (SCLC)." *BMC Cancer* 17(1):269. doi: 10.1186/s12885-017-3239-z.

Zuijdgeest-van Leeuwen, S. D., J. W. van den Berg, J. L. Wattimena, A. van der Gaast, G. R. Swart, J. H. Wilson, and P. C. Dagnelie. 2000. "Lipolysis and lipid oxidation in weight-losing cancer patients and healthy subjects." *Metabolism* 49(7):931–6. doi: 10.1053/meta.2000.6740.

16 Nutrition and Chemotherapy in the Epidemic of Obesity

Rebecca L. Paszkiewicz and Steven D. Mittelman
David Geffen School of Medicine at UCLA

CONTENTS

INTRODUCTION

Over the past century, the treatment efficacy of cancer has improved (Mittelman 2020). The 5-year survival rate from all cancers has increased from 49% to 70% over the past 40 years (2018b), with minimal sex differences. Early detection, advancements in treatment, and improved supportive care have all contributed to improved survival (Miller et al. 2016). Notably, the development of combination chemotherapy regimens and the cloning of oncogenes such as the Philadelphia chromosome, HER2, and BRCA1/2 have helped to bolster these outcomes (2015). Throughout this century, childhood acute lymphoblastic leukemia (ALL) has changed from a nearly uniformly fatal disease to a highly curable one (Silverman et al. 2010). Despite these advances, however, cancer diagnoses instill feelings of disbelief, shock, grief, and anger. In response, and in conjunction with fear of chemotherapy and its side effects, patients often seek alternative treatments outside of the clinic. These treatments range from the addition of vitamins and supplements as complements to prescribed therapies to use of homeopathic remedies and alternative medicine.

The role of diet has been a major topic of research in terms of overall health as well as an alternative or supplemental treatment for diseases such as diabetes, heart disease, and cancer. While it is well-established that obesity is associated with higher cancer incidence and mortality, there is sparse data linking this association to specific diets, macronutrients, or supplements. Further, very little data exist examining the role of diet and nutrition on chemotherapy efficacy and how interventions may impact outcomes, especially in patients who are at higher-risk of treatment failure or toxicity because of their obesity.

In the present chapter, we will examine the evidence from both preclinical and clinical studies on the effects of diet on cancer outcomes. Changes to diet are known to improve obesity and obesity-related comorbidities, at least temporarily. Herein, we will examine the evidence for the role of diet in improving prognosis and treatment outcome in various cancers. Weight loss *per se* may not be the trigger for such improvements; changes to hormones, inflammation, metabolic fuels, and other alterations to signaling pathways as a result of decreased adiposity or change in dietary intake will be explored. While we will discuss the role of diet in cancer incidence and progression, we will focus primarily on the state of the science evaluating treatment efficacy in patients who undergo dietary interventions as part of their treatment protocol.

EPIDEMIOLOGY AND PROGNOSIS OF CANCER IN THE FACE OF OBESITY

CANCER INCIDENCE

Effects of Obesity

The World Cancer Research Fund and American Institute of Cancer Research's (WCRF/AICR) Continuous Update Project concluded that there was *convincing* evidence that body fatness increases the risk of esophageal, pancreatic, liver, colorectal, postmenopausal breast, endometrial, and kidney cancer, and *probable* evidence that it increases oropharyngeal, stomach, gallbladder, ovarian, and advanced prostate cancers. Of note, the studies in the analysis defined body fatness by multiple measures, such as body mass index (BMI), waist circumference, or waist-to-hip ratio. Most epidemiological studies examining cancer incidence and mortality have focused on obesity based on the anthropomorphic definition, where obesity is defined by a BMI ≥ 30 kg/m^2 ($\geq$95th percentile of weight in youth) and overweight BMI ≥ 25 kg/m^2 ($\geq$85th percentile in youth). This measure is straightforward and easy to obtain, unlike most measures body composition measures, and is used to define overweight and obesity for clinical purposes. However, BMI is not the most accurate representation of body composition and can give fallacious results in some individuals. Treatments for some cancers are associated with large changes in body composition; children with leukemia, for example, develop sarcopenic obesity during their steroid-containing chemotherapy, involving decreased lean body mass and increased adiposity, which are not reflected by changes in BMI (Orgel et al. 2016b). Further, as reviewed by Lennon et al., the variability in the timing of BMI calculation compared to diagnosis and disease onset, the absence of true adiposity measures through imaging, and the possibility of detection bias have led to the "obesity paradox" whereby some studies have shown that overweight and early obesity confers protection from cancer outcome (Lennon et al. 2016). This has been shown for patients undergoing surgery for colorectal and renal cancers, patients with undergoing liver resection colorectal metastases, and patients with lymphoma undergoing autologous hematopoietic cell transplantation.

Given the evidence that BMI may not be the most appropriate measure of obesity at diagnosis or accurately reflect the effects of adiposity on cancer outcomes, others have examined the physiologic aspects of obesity. The combination of high blood pressure, insulin resistance, and abnormal cholesterol or triglyceride levels, known collectively as the metabolic syndrome, tends to cluster in the obese, particularly those with visceral obesity. In contrast, the term "metabolically healthy obese," or colloquially "fat fit," describes those who are physically obese but show no metabolic perturbations. In a prospective study of over 20,000 patients, metabolic health was the main contributor to cancer risk (Akinyemiju et al. 2018). Overweight and obesity status *per se* did not increase the risk of cancer mortality in metabolically healthy individuals. In fact, in metabolically unhealthy individuals, overweight and obesity appeared to offer somewhat of a protective effect. This study provides further evidence that BMI may not be the most precise measure to examine the link between increased adiposity and cancer, and that obesity, particularly defined by BMI, may just be a surrogate for metabolic syndrome, adiposity, or some other mechanistic link(s) in cancer outcome.

Type 2 diabetes (T2D) is associated with obesity and is often characterized under the umbrella of the metabolic syndrome. Increased risk of developing and dying from cancer has been shown in T2D, but the data are conflicting (Chen et al. 2017, Tsilidis et al. 2015). While T2D is associated with obesity, studies have found that after adjusting for BMI there is still an independent correlation between diabetes and cancer (Bao et al. 2013, Yuhara et al. 2011).

Effects of Diet

Diet composition has also been linked to cancer incidence. Worldwide leukemia incidence has been positively correlated with calorie intake (Hursting, Margolin, and Switzer 1993), and a 20% calorie reduction decreased breast cancer risk in premenopausal women (Lope et al. 2019). While high protein intake was associated with an increased risk of cancer mortality in people aged 50–65, red meat intake has only been specifically linked to breast (Wu et al. 2016) and not prostate, ovarian, colorectal, or renal cell cancer risk (Lai et al. 2017, Lee et al. 2008, Mao, Tie, and Du 2018, Pang and Wang 2018). In response to these studies and others, both the American Cancer Society and the WCRF/AICR have published dietary guidelines for cancer prevention (Kohler et al. 2016) in which they promote the maintenance of a healthy weight, being physically active, consuming fruits and vegetables, and limiting the consumption of red meat and alcohol. Adherence to these diets has been associated with a decreased risk of overall, breast, colorectal, and endometrial cancers (Kohler et al. 2016).

Effects of Weight Loss

With mounting evidence of the role of obesity in cancer incidence, the impact of weight loss on prevention of cancer has also been examined. Self-reported weight loss, including weight loss due to bariatric surgery, has been shown to decrease the risk of developing endometrial, breast, and pancreatic cancers (Luo et al. 2017, Hardefeldt et al. 2018, Xu et al. 2018). However, there is significant heterogeneity in studies following bariatric surgery (Casagrande et al. 2014) which may be related to weight cycling (Zhang et al. 2019a). A recent meta-analysis tie decreases in overall cancer incidence after bariatric surgery to weight loss, reduced inflammation, and decreased markers of proliferation; the contradictory increased risk of colorectal cancer may be tied to increased proliferation of colonic epithelial cells that has been seen following surgery in a minority of patients (Bruno and Berger 2020), or a decreased use of statins, which have been shown to be protective against development of colorectal cancer (Bardou, Barkun, and Martel 2010, Demierre et al. 2005).

CANCER OUTCOME

This link between obesity and cancer mortality was established by a prospective cohort of over 900,000 subjects in the United States (Calle et al. 2003). This landmark study showed increases in both specific tumor type and overall cancer mortality associated with obesity. Men with a BMI between 30.0 and 34.9 kg/m^2 (obese) had a 9% increased risk in cancer mortality, while BMI between 35.0 and 39.9 kg/m^2 (severe obesity) conferred a 20% increase and BMI $\geq$40 kg/m^2 (morbid obesity) a 52% increase. Obesity significantly increased mortality risk in males with cancers of the prostate, kidney, gallbladder, colon and rectum, esophagus, stomach, pancreas, and liver and non-Hodgkin's lymphoma and multiple myeloma. Results for the women in the study were even more striking, with females exhibiting a 23%, 32%, and 62% increased risk of dying from cancer in obese, severely obese, and morbidly obese women, respectively. Obese females had increased risk of death from multiple myeloma, colon and rectum cancer, ovary cancer, liver cancer, non-Hodgkin's lymphoma, breast cancer, cancer of the gallbladder, esophageal cancer, pancreatic cancer, cervical cancer, kidney cancer, and cancer of the uterus. Overall, the study estimated that overweight and obesity were responsibly for ~14% of cancer deaths in men and 20% of cancer deaths in women in the US. Since publication in 2003, many studies have confirmed these findings, in the US and worldwide (Renehan et al. 2008, Rapp et al. 2005).

Much of the association between obesity and cancer mortality is based on the higher risk of being diagnosed with cancer (i.e., higher incidence). There is also evidence that obese patients, once diagnosed with cancer, have a poorer outcome than nonobese patients. Since the Calle et al. study, poorer outcome and increased mortality have been observed in obese patients following diagnosis of breast (Conroy et al. 2011), colon (Sinicrope et al. 2010), prostate (Allott, Masko, and Freedland 2013), pancreatic (Yuan et al. 2013), ovarian (Yang et al. 2011), and hematologic (Orgel et al. 2016a) cancers. While many reports support this conclusion, a recent systematic review concluded that few studies were designed to examine this relationship, and so warned caution in interpreting these results (Parekh, Chandran, and Bandera 2012). Interestingly, obesity is associated with an *improved* outcome in patients with metastatic melanoma treated with targeted therapy or immunotherapy (McQuade et al. 2018); no significant effect was observed in patients treated with chemotherapy. Thus, current evidence suggests that obesity generally increases one's risk of both developing cancer and decreases survival for most, but not all cancers.

POTENTIAL MECHANISMS LINKING OBESITY TO CANCER OUTCOME

Obesity impacts a number of factors including physical, genetic, physiological, socioeconomic, and behavioral, many of which could contribute to the association with cancer. These interactions make unraveling the true cause of obesity's impact(s) on malignancy difficult and impede the ability to find causality among many associations. However, animal models provide evidence that the observed associations between obesity and cancer in humans are likely based on biology. Obesity increases the rate of cancer development and growth in most preclinical models of genetic cancer predisposition (Gravaghi et al. 2008, Hirose et al. 2004, Yun et al. 2010), carcinogen (Zhu et al. 2017, Sikalidis, Fitch, and Fleming 2013, Hirose et al. 2004), and cancer implantation (Zaytouni et al. 2017, Dong et al. 2017, Yakar et al. 2006). Furthermore, there is evidence that while African Americans and Hispanic Americans have comparable socioeconomic status (SES) and similar behavioral risk factors, an "Hispanic paradox" exists, with Hispanic American participants across 58 studies demonstrating a 17.5% lower risk of all-cause mortality compared to other groups, but a similar risk of cancer compared to Caucasian Americans (Ruiz, Steffen, and Smith 2013). Racial and ethnic differences in the genotypes and phenotypes related to obesity and inflammation may explain the differences in incidence and outcome at a biological, rather than at a specifically sociological level (Özdemir and Dotto 2017). Uncovering the biologic mechanisms linking obesity to cancer may provide some clues to how to reverse these links and to reduce their impact after diagnosis. Few studies, however, have looked at how obesity impairs cancer treatment in preclinical models (Incio et al. 2016, Behan et al. 2009, Ehsanipour et al. 2013, Tucci et al. 2018).

Genetics, Ethnicity, and Race

There could be a genetic component underlying the risk of both obesity and cancer. As a phenotypically complex disease, there is no one polymorphism or gene responsible for obesity. Fat mass and obesity-related (FTO) gene polymorphisms are fairly common in obese individual, with a 67% increased risk of adult obesity in people homozygous for the risk allele (Frayling et al. 2007). An increased risk of leukemia and glioblastoma has been linked to FTO polymorphisms (Deng et al. 2018). Pancreatic cancer risk has also been causally correlated with genes that drive increased BMI and fasting insulin (OR: 1.34 and 1.66, respectively) (Carreras-Torres et al. 2017a). Similarly, a group of polymorphisms related to increased fasting insulin were associated an increased risk of lung cancer (OR: 1.63), while polymorphisms related to increased low-density lipoprotein cholesterol was associated with decreased lung cancer risk (OR: 0.90) (Carreras-Torres et al. 2017b). As more studies are conducted, more genetic polymorphisms or groups of genes associated with obesity may be found which also play a direct or indirect role in cancer.

While some of the predisposition to obesity and cancer can be mediated by SES, and SES is associated with race and ethnicity, there is evidence that these factors may play independent roles in cancer risk. As discussed above, despite the higher risk of obesity and T2D, the incidence of cancer in Hispanics living in the US is lower than in African Americans and similar to non-Hispanic whites, with the exceptions of higher incidence for Hispanics for stomach, gall bladder, liver, and cervical cancers (Miller et al. 2018). The increased prevalence of childhood ALL in older Hispanic children has been the largest contributor to the overall increased prevalence of the disease (Barrington-Trimis et al. 2017). Further, Hispanic children have an overall worse survival from all hematologic malignancies (Kehm et al. 2018). While these associations may be linked to any number of factors, the label of Hispanic race encompasses many different groups of people from varying backgrounds, possibly making it difficult to pinpoint exact causes or associations between risk-factors and outcomes based on race or ethnicity.

Black males in the US are at a higher risk of developing and dying from cancer than non-Hispanic whites (Siegel, Miller, and Jemal 2017). While Black women have a lower risk of developing breast cancer, they are more likely to have more aggressive forms at diagnosis and poorer outcomes (Newman and Kaljee 2017). Even after adjusting for confounders such as advanced stage at diagnosis, disparate healthcare, and overall higher burden of other health issues, a modest cancer-specific survival difference by race still exists (Bach et al. 2002).

Socioeconomic Status

It is clear that lower SES contributes to cancer risk and mortality. This disparity may be linked to less access to preventative medicine and palliative care, decreases and delays in screening, increased risk behaviors, increased tumor burden at diagnosis, and barriers to timely and adequate treatment, among other factors (Ward et al. 2004). Poverty itself is considered a carcinogen (Broder 1991) and may be a mediating factor between obesity and cancer (Sheehan et al. 2017), independent of race or ethnicity (Brower 2008). While more work is needed to tease out the cultural, genetic, and SES differences in order to identify potential mechanisms behind these associations, it is clear that there are many opportunities to decrease health disparities and improve outcomes for all patients, regardless of background (Ward et al. 2004) (further commentary in (Freeman 2004)).

Behavior

There are a number of risk behaviors and lifestyle factors that are associated with both obesity and cancer. Obese individuals are more likely to be heavy drinkers (Sayon-Orea, Martinez-Gonzalez, and Bes-Rastrollo 2011) and to be exposed to air pollution (McConnell et al. 2016). They also tend to eat less fiber (Slavin 2005) and foods containing antioxidants (Hosseini, Saedisomeolia, and Allman-Farinelli 2017) and consume more red meat (Rouhani et al. 2014), all of which increase the risk of cancer. A Mendelian randomization analysis found increased risk of smoking as BMI increased (Carreras-Torres et al. 2018); again displaying the complexity of gene-environment-behavior analysis on incidence and outcomes. Former smokers have an increased risk of obesity compared to both current (OR: 1.33) or never smokers (OR: 1.14); however among current smokers, the risk of obesity increases with increased daily cigarette counts (OR: 1.60) (Dare, Mackay, and Pell 2015).

Screenings for some cancers are decreased in obese individuals (Seibert et al. 2017, Beeken et al. 2014), due to a number of factors including: decreased health visits by obese individuals who are dissatisfied with the previous focus on weight loss rather than the underlying reason for the visit, physician discomfort, and lack of proper training in performing physical assessments on obese patients (Ferrante et al. 2010). There are also size-induced barriers to effective self-detection and difficulty in imaging for the purpose of diagnosis (Fursevich et al. 2016). These factors may contribute to delayed detection of malignancies and lead to poorer outcomes and decreased survival. However, with proper equipment and training, these barriers may be overcome and outcomes can be improved (Ahmed, Lemkau, and Birt 2002).

PHARMACOKINETICS

Obesity can affect both the volume of distribution and clearance of chemotherapies (Powis et al. 1987), but obese subjects are often not included in early phases of drug pharmacokinetics (PK) testing. Based on this and the lack of scientific consensus, oncologists treating obese patients may face a dilemma regarding how much chemotherapy to use. In addition, obesity may alter PK differently in youth and adults (Kendrick, Carr, and Ensom 2015, van Rongen et al. 2018), highlighting the importance of studies in various populations. Obesity and excess adiposity could affect drug distribution and/or drug clearance. We have shown that adipocytes themselves metabolize and inactivate the chemotherapy daunorubicin (Sheng et al. 2017). Alone or in combination, decreased exposure to chemotherapeutics, through either capping or alterations in PK, could disproportionately affect obese patients, decreasing adverse events but, also, effective treatment (Hall et al. 2013). Despite the dearth of scientific data, the American Society of Clinical Oncology guidelines state that chemotherapy should be dosed in obese adult patients based on actual weight, rather than a modified body weight or an arbitrarily lowered dose (Griggs et al. 2012). However, clinicians may have reservations prescribing large doses of chemotherapies by actual body weight, particularly in obese patients who are already at higher risk of some toxicities.

INFLAMMATION

Inflammation is a hallmark of both cancer (Hanahan and Weinberg 2000) and obesity. Excess adipose tissue can give rise to an inflammatory environment that supports tumor initiation and progression (Deng et al. 2016). Normal adipose tissue functions as a mediator between metabolism and inflammation; immune cells, including macrophages, B and T lymphocytes, natural killer, and natural killer T (NKT) cells, infiltrate the adipose tissue can affect adipose storage, cytokine and adipokine secretion, and insulin sensitivity. With increasing adiposity, the immune profile switches from an anti- to a proinflammatory state. Expansion of breast and colon cancer into adjacent adipose tissue is associated with local adipose tissue inflammation (Koru-Sengul et al. 2016, Zoico et al. 2017) and potentially a poorer outcome (Koru-Sengul et al. 2016). Evidence has also demonstrated that some chemotherapy drugs induce inflammation, which may impair their ability to decrease tumor burden (Vyas, Laput, and Vyas 2014). Adiponectin, which is decreased in obesity, is secreted by adipocytes and acts an anti-inflammatory signal. In contrast, leptin stimulates T helper 1 cell expansion, inducing an increase in macrophages, resulting in an overall increase in tumor necrosis factor-α (TNF-α) and other proinflammatory cytokines. Inflammatory macrophages accumulate around necrotic adipocytes, forming the hallmark "crown-like" structures. Macrophages and crown-like structures in breast adipose tissue have been linked with breast cancer (Morris et al. 2011). CD8+ T cells, B cells, mast cells, NKT cells, and eosinophils, increase in adipose tissue in the obese state (Anderson, Gutierrez, and Hasty 2010) as do a number of proinflammatory cytokines, including TNFα, interleukin (IL)-6, IL-1β, and plasminogen activator inhibitor-1 (Berg and Scherer 2005). This inflammatory environment can promote cancer cell survival and proliferation and increase angiogenesis, another hallmark of cancer (Kiraly et al. 2015, Hermouet, Bigot-Corbel, and Gardie 2015).

HORMONES

Insulin-Like Growth Factor-1

Increased insulin-like growth factor-1 (IGF-1) activity represents a likely link between obesity and cancer. IGF-1 has similar effects on cells to insulin (see below), activating signaling pathways implicated in cancer, such as phosphoinositide 3-kinase/protein kinase B (PI3K/AKT), signal transducer and activator of transcription (STAT), and mitogen-activated protein kinase (MAPK)/extracellular signal-regulated kinase (ERK). IGF-1 has been shown to increase cellular proliferation, migration, and metastasis, and to decrease epithelial integrity. Increases in the hormone aggressively increase tumor burden (Gallagher and LeRoith 2011, Inoue and Tsugane 2012) and induce resistance to chemotherapy in a number of cancers (Gusscott et al. 2016, Li et al. 2013). Patients with growth hormone (GH) insensitivity, known as Laron Syndrome, have extremely low IGF-1 levels and are protected from cancer (Laron 2015), a finding recapitulated in animal models of low IGF-1 (Pinkston et al. 2006, Ramsey et al. 2002).

Insulin

Insulin resistance is associated with hyperinsulinemia, obesity, hyperlipidemia, and inflammation. While insulin resistance impacts glucose homeostasis and can lead to hyperglycemia, the downstream effects of insulin on protein synthesis and cell proliferation are maintained and, therefore, tend to be overactive in the insulin resistant, hyperinsulinemic state. Further, insulin increases the production of IGF-1 and the bioavailability of estrogen. Similar to IGF-1, insulin also increases tumor migration and metastasis and decreases epithelial integrity in a number of cancers (Gallagher and LeRoith 2011, Inoue and Tsugane 2012).

Leptin

Adipocytes secrete leptin in proportion to body fat, increasing as weight increases (Considine et al. 1996). However, evidence linking leptin and cancer incidence has not been consistent (Gupta et al. 2016, Yeung et al. 2013). In fact, leptin receptor expression has been associated with both improved outcomes in leukemia (Kong et al. 2019, Lu et al. 2017) and decreased survival in breast cancer (Uddin et al. 2009). Leptin binds to its receptor and signals through Janus kinase (JAK)/STAT, modulating PI3K, mammalian target of rapamycin (mTOR), and AKT signaling. This signaling could contribute to cancer cell progression through increases in cell proliferation, migration, and tissue invasion (Uddin et al. 2010, Ghasemi et al. 2019). Leptin signaling through the Notch pathway may be important for cancer stem cells, as blocking this pathway can improve outcomes of pancreatic (Harbuzariu et al. 2017) and breast cancer (Wang et al. 2018) in *in vivo* models.

Adiponectin

Adiponectin is secreted by adipocytes in inverse proportion to adiposity. Adiponectin's signaling through the AMP-activated protein kinase (AMPK) pathway may promote apoptosis in cancer cells (Leclerc et al. 2013) and has overall positive effects on local and whole-body metabolism and inflammation. As reviewed in Dalamaga et al. (Dalamaga, Diakopoulos, and Mantzoros 2012), adiponectin may decrease angiogenesis, and limit tumor growth, displaying antitumorigenic effects in most cell lines tested. An increased ratio of adiponectin to leptin has been associated with decreased endometrial cancer (Gong et al. 2015). Decreased circulating adiponectin in the obese state may minimize the anticancer effects of the hormone and, in conjunction with increased insulin and leptin, promote tumor development.

Osteopontin

Osteopontin is another adipocyte-derived protein that is increased with obesity. It plays roles in inflammation, cell migration, and the remodeling of tissue (Kiefer et al. 2008). While it is still unclear exactly how osteopontin promotes cancer progression, *in vitro* experiments have shown that it enhances growth of tumor cells in suspension and regulates migration toward some chemokines (Rittling and Chambers 2004). Increased expression of osteopontin has been seen in colon (Rohde et al. 2007), gastric (Lin et al. 2015), and ampullary cancers (Hsu et al. 2010).

Estrogen

Increased estrogen is known to increase the risk of cancer in estrogen-sensitive tissues, such as breast, endometrium, and ovaries. However, estrogen is also linked to increased incidence of other cancers, including lung (Hsu, Chu, and Kao 2017, Kawai et al. 2005). Outside of the ovaries in females, adipose tissue is the major source of estrogen due to its high aromatase expression. Therefore, obesity is associated with increased aromatase activity and systemic estrogen. Obesity confers a lower risk of premenopausal breast cancer, when most of the estrogen is derived from ovarian secretion, and a higher risk of postmenopausal breast cancer, when estrogen production occurs in mainly in the adipose tissue (2018a). However, menopausal status does not affect outcomes, with obesity decreasing survival in all women (Chan et al. 2014).

METABOLIC FUELS

Obesity is associated with increased availability of both stored and circulating fuels. Systemic glucose, triglycerides, and amino acids increase with increasing adiposity and the metabolic syndrome. Dietary intake can impact the nutrients available to cancer cells and affect their growth. In a mouse model of prostate cancer, dietary saturated fatty acids induced *MYC* overexpression, while MYC expression in patients was correlated with dietary intake of saturated fats, disease progression, and metastasis (Labbé et al. 2019). Increases in plasma glucose have been linked to an increased risk of pancreatic cancer (Liao et al. 2015), and glycosylation profiles associated with hyperglycemia have been shown to promote tumor growth (Slawson, Copeland, and Hart 2010, Nie et al. 2020). Given the increased metabolic demand of proliferating cells and the ability of cancer cells to alter their metabolism, increased fuel availability in obesity may contribute to an optimal environment to promote tumorigenesis and allow cancer cells to survive in the face of antitumor therapies.

The Warburg Effect, first described by Otto Warburg in 1925, describes the altered metabolism of cancer cells to preferentially use glycolysis rather than aerobic respiration for production of energy, increasing their uptake of glucose and reducing reliance on oxygen (Warburg 1925). The shift toward glycolysis rather than mitochondrial metabolism allows the cancer cells to continue proliferating quickly in a possibly hypoxic environment and to produce other metabolic intermediates, nucleic acids, and amino acids via anapleurosis.

However, a Reverse Warburg Effect has also been demonstrated, whereby cancer cells induce neighboring cells to increase glycolysis and secrete intermediates into the microenvironment for cancer cell uptake (Pavlides et al. 2009). This phenomenon may help explain why some tumors appear to have high respiratory rates (Xu et al. 2015) in contradiction to the Warburg Effect.

In addition, cells in the tumor microenvironment can be induced to secrete amino acids. It has been shown in our lab that adipocytes secrete glutamine which is taken up by leukemia, helping the cells to avoid cell death via L-asparaginase treatment and leading to worse survival in obese mice (Ehsanipour et al. 2013). Glutamine is also extremely important for other cancer cells, where it contributes to the synthesis of nucleotides, amino acids, and citric acid cycle intermediates (Zhang, Pavlova, and Thompson 2017). Cancer cells use branched chain amino acids (BCAA) for protein synthesis and energy metabolism and often overexpress branched chain aminotransferase enzymes needed for BCAA metabolism (Ananieva and Wilkinson 2018).

Cancer cells are also dependent on free fatty acids (FFA) to provide the acyl chains of phospholipids. Given the high rate of proliferation of cancer cells, they have an increasing demand of FFA to form plasma and organelle membranes. However, synthesis of FFA is energetically expensive. Cancer cell survival is increased in environments such as the adipose tissue, where abundant FFA can be taken up and also used as an energy source via FFA oxidation (Nieman et al. 2013, Tabe et al. 2017). Increases in uptake of FFA and *de novo* FFA synthesis have been linked to increased cancer aggressiveness and decreased survival (Kridel et al. 2004, Nieman et al. 2011, Oppezzo et al. 2005, Samudio et al. 2010). Thus, the unique metabolic needs of cancer cells may be met in adipose-rich environments.

MICROBIOME

The importance of the microbiome to human health has become increasingly clear over the past few decades. The gut microbiome is influenced by diet, whereby obesity is associated with a typical microbial shift, favoring firmicutes, and decreasing representation of bacteroides. However, recent consensus points to a decrease in microbial diversity in obesity, rather than a specific signature of microbes (Maruvada et al. 2017, Vallianou et al. 2019). Fecal transplant studies have demonstrated the role of microbiome diversity on host metabolism with some evidence suggesting that this loss of diversity may be causal or, at the least, reinforcing of the development and persistence of obesity. While not conclusive (Greathouse et al. 2019), evidence has linked the obesity-associated microbiome with colorectal (O'Keefe 2016) and liver (Yoshimoto et al. 2013) cancers.

Short-chain fatty acids are a link between diet, microbiome, metabolism, and inflammation (den Besten et al. 2013). Butyrate, one of the more-studied short-chain fatty acids, has been shown to decrease inflammation and colon cancer cell growth (Blouin et al. 2011). On the other hand, poor diet is linked to microbial byproducts that promote inflammation and carcinogenesis (O'Keefe 2016). The contribution of the microbiome to the inflammatory state seen in obesity may contribute significantly to the progression of tumor growth (Figure.16.1).

SPECIFIC CANCERS RELATED TO UNDERLYING OBESITY-RELATED CONDITIONS

In addition to systemic and overarching influences, obesity has effects on specific organs that can predispose them to cancer development and/or limit cancer treatment.

NONALCOHOLIC FATTY LIVER DISEASE

Lipid accumulation in the liver, or nonalcoholic fatty liver disease (NAFLD), is common in obesity and often associated with the metabolic syndrome. NAFLD can progress to nonalcoholic steatohepatitis (NASH) and both diseases increase the risk of developing hepatocellular carcinoma (HCC). Almost 60% of patients with HCC developed the disease in the context of underlying NAFLD, and HCC was the cause of 47% of deaths in NASH patients (Marengo, Rosso, and Bugianesi 2016). With a higher prevalence of NAFLD and NASH, Hispanic patients are at increased risk of developing HCC when other metabolic risk factors are present (Wong et al. 2018). Clearly the progression to NAFLD and NASH helps explain why obese men are ~4.5 times more likely to die from liver cancer (Calle et al. 2003).

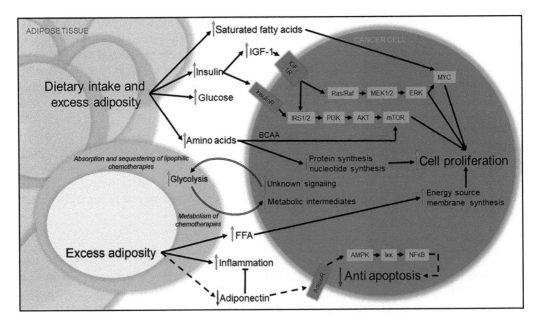

FIGURE 16.1 Proposed mechanisms of effects of overweight/obesity on cancer cell survival overweight and obesity may contribute to increased cancer growth through various mechanisms. Increased nutrient intake and excess adiposity increase circulating fatty acids, insulin, glucose, and amino acids that can be used for cancer cell survival and proliferation. Signals from tumors may also induce increased glycolysis in adipocytes of the microenvironment, which release intermediates for uptake by the tumor cells. Excess adipose tissue is associated with decreased adiponectin, which results in decreased antiapoptosis signaling in nearby cells and increases local and systemic inflammation. Adipose tissue itself can also metabolize or sequester chemotherapies, resulting in decreased availability for tumor killing and reduced efficacy. IGF-1, insulin-like growth factor-1; BCAA, branched-chain amino acid; FFA, free fatty acid.

Barrett's Esophagus

Esophageal adenocarcinoma is the most common form of esophageal cancer and has a high mortality rate, with a 5-year survival rate around 20% (Njei, McCarty, and Birk 2016). Progression often starts with chronic gastrointestinal reflux, with stomach acid damaging the esophageal columnar epithelium. Progression to low-grade dysplasia and then high-grade dysplasia (Barrett's esophagus) results in carcinoma (Thrift, Pandeya, and Whiteman 2012). Obesity places patients at higher risk of each stage in this progression (reflux OR: 1.73, Barrett's esophagus OR: 1.24, and esophageal adenocarcinoma OR: 2.45; see Richter and Rubenstein (2018)), likely due in part by increased abdominal pressure in obese subjects. However, obesity-related inflammation and dietary factors may also contribute to progression.

Interestingly, *Helicobacter pylori*, the main cause of gastric cancer (Amieva and Peek 2016), is protective against esophageal adenocarcinoma related to Barrett's esophagus (Fischbach et al. 2014). *H. pylori* is found to be increased in some overweight/obese populations (Arslan, Atilgan, and Yavaşoğlu 2009, Al-Zubaidi et al. 2018) and infection itself may promote obesity (Dhurandhar, Bailey, and Thomas 2015), so the role of *H. pylori* in obesity-related cancer could be a double-edged sword.

Pancreatitis

Despite advances in many cancer treatments, pancreatic cancer has a 5-year survival under 10%. Many of the risk factors for pancreatic cancer overlap with risk factors for obesity, such as low consumption of fruits and vegetables and excessive alcohol intake (Tsai and Chang 2019).

Obese patients have twice the mortality as lean patients (Calle et al. 2003), with BMI at diagnosis predicting survival (Yuan et al. 2013). Chronic pancreatitis, which is strongly associated with obesity, is a risk factor for developing pancreatic cancer, though it contributes to only a small percentage of pancreatic cancer cases (Duell et al. 2012). The increased pancreatitis seen in obese patients is mediated at least in part by the increased prevalence of diabetes, gallstones, and hypertriglyceridemia (Khatua, El-Kurdi, and Singh 2017).

WEIGHT CHANGES DURING CANCER TREATMENT

Changes in body weight and composition are common during both cancer development and treatment, making it difficult to accurately correlate BMI-associated effects on cancer incidence and prognosis. Recently, more research has been conducted on changes in body composition after cancer survival and the effects of cancer and chemotherapy on future metabolic health, raising questions about what can be done to prevent future metabolic abnormalities in patients who have already survived cancer.

The most common change to body composition that occurs around the time of a cancer diagnosis is the loss of lean body mass, known as cachexia. Despite weight loss, cachectic patients appear to mostly maintain fat mass by disproportionately losing lean muscle mass. While the exact mechanism relating malignancy to cachexia is unclear, inflammation seems to play a significant role (Rihacek et al. 2015). Weight loss that occurs due to cachexia is considered a poor prognostic sign, and perhaps a marker of aggressive growth or a toxic response to therapy (Dodson et al. 2011). The unhealthy loss of muscle can impair treatment and affect outcomes, in addition to the fatigue, disability, and diminished quality of life experienced by patients. Separately, the diagnosis itself and treatment of the cancer can lead to weight loss induced by pain, nausea, fatigue, and depression.

In contrast, significant weight gain can be seen in some cancers. Glucocorticoids, commonly used in hematologic cancers, have adipogenic effects and can lead to treatment-induced gain of fat mass. "Sarcopenic obesity" is the gain of fat mass and loss of muscle mass that may or may not be reflected by significant changes in body weight. During the first month of treatment, adolescent patients with ALL lost 6 kg of lean mass but gained ~1.5 kg of body fat (Orgel et al. 2016b), confirming that body weight and BMI are not accurate predictors of adiposity in these patients. Additionally, increased adiposity and obesity persist through treatment for patients with ALL. Adult survivors of childhood cancer are more likely to develop obesity, hypertension, dyslipidemia, and insulin resistance (Nottage et al. 2014), leading to four times the risk of developing the metabolic syndrome (Faienza et al. 2015).

A unique environment for adipocytes, the bone marrow is subject to dramatic changes during chemotherapy. Marrow adipocytes are increased in obesity (Ambrosi et al. 2017), but also paradoxically increased during times of calorie restriction or nutrient deprivation (Devlin 2011). As hematopoietic cells are killed during chemotherapy, they are replaced by bone marrow adipocytes, which have a different phenotype compared to either white or brown adipocytes. This unique microenvironment may also impact further treatment, promote disease progression, and/or attract circulating tumor cells, though these effects need to be studied more (Liu et al. 2019a, Templeton et al. 2015).

DIET INTERVENTIONS

A large number of patients are hesitant to undergo intensive chemotherapy or radiation, viewing these treatments as toxic and causing more harm than good. Alternative medicine has been on the rise in the past few decades, as exemplified by the creation of the Office of Alternative Medicine at the NIH in 1992. The office was renamed the National Center for Complementary and Integrative Health, as the focus has shifted from alternative to complementary therapies, used to supplement treatment. A study published in 2019 found that over half of physicians recommend complementary approaches, such as massage, herbs/nonvitamin supplements, and acupuncture to patients in their daily practices (Stussman et al. 2020). In one study, 40% of Hispanic patients with colorectal cancer used complementary therapy, while only 76% reported it to their physicians (Black et al. 2016). In a study of cancer survivors, 30% of patients reported using complementary therapy, but <50% disclosed their use to their physicians (Sohl et al. 2015). However, over 60% of physicians in the study recommended continuation of complementary treatments when informed by their patients, suggesting that supplementation with complementary approaches may be well-received when openly discussed as a part of the treatment plan.

Given this environment and the relationship between obesity and cancer, research into how changes to diet or the addition of supplements affects cancer is important. There is some evidence that changes to diet can decrease chemotherapy-induced toxicities and reduce the number or severity of side effects. The data presented below summarize much of the work that has been done, focusing on the benefits of such interventions on the efficacy of chemotherapy.

FASTING

The health benefits of fasting have been promoted for decades. Fasting is generally considered restriction from caloric intake for >24 hours. While this extreme protocol is tolerable to some (Wilhelmi de Toledo et al. 2019), other less restrictive forms of fasting such as intermittent fasting, timed-feeding, alternate day fasting, and a fasting mimicking diet (FMD) have shown health benefits as well. Epidemiological studies of people who fast for religious purposes have shown increased lifespan, improvements in overall health, and reduced incidence of cardiovascular disease, though to our knowledge this finding has not yet been extended to cancer (Trepanowski and Bloomer 2010).

Preclinical models of fasting to reduce cancer progression in the absence of treatment have produced mixed results. A meta-analysis of intermittent fasting and cancer found five studies showing benefit and three showing no change (Lv et al. 2014). Perhaps due to cancer-specific effects, studies have found decreased growth of tumors of some cell types (Marsh, Mukherjee, and Seyfried 2008, Lu et al. 2017, Saleh et al. 2013, Lee et al. 2012, Bianchi et al. 2015, Sun et al. 2017, Caffa et al. 2015) but not others (Lu et al. 2017, Lee et al. 2012, Kusuoka et al. 2018, Raffaghello et al. 2008, de la Cruz Bonilla et al. 2019, Buschemeyer et al. 2010, Thomas et al. 2010). Variability may also lie in the effects of the immune system; teasing apart these studies, 9 out of 14 immunocompetent mouse models demonstrated a benefit to fasting, as opposed to only 4 of 8 immunocompromised animal models. Further support of the role of the immune system in the benefits of fasting includes the reduction in autoimmunity (Choi, Lee, and Longo 2017) and tumor-associated macrophages following fasting (Sun et al. 2017). Studies have also shown a more consistent benefit of fasting in models of spontaneous tumor development, delaying tumor onset and progression (Berrigan et al. 2002, Shuang et al. 2017, Tomasi et al. 1999, Rocha et al. 2002).

Table 16.1 shows preclinical studies on the impact of fasting on cancer treatment outcomes. With some exceptions, most studies found synergistic effects between fasting and radiation or chemotherapies. Importantly, fasting decreased the toxicity of several treatments including etoposide (Raffaghello et al. 2008), irinotecan (Jongbloed et al. 2019), doxorubicin (Brandhorst et al. 2013), and abdominal radiation (de la Cruz Bonilla et al. 2019). Reduced toxicity and side effects could have large therapeutic benefits to patients, by improving quality of life, reducing treatment-related mortality, and preventing treatment interruptions and dose reductions.

Clinical studies of the impact of fasting on treatment outcomes, while small in number, show promising results. In a case series of complete fasting for 36–140 hours before and 8–56 hours after chemotherapy, patients tolerated the fast and demonstrated a subjective reduction in side effects from the chemotherapy without any obvious impact on efficacy (Safdie et al. 2009). In a study of "dosing" fasting windows, patients with colorectal cancer tolerated 24–48 hours of fasting pre- and 24 hours of fasting post-treatment (Sun et al. 2017), further confirming feasibility of fasting in patients with cancer. In a study of 34 women with breast or ovarian cancer, patients were randomized in a crossover design to receive short-term fasting, consisting of 36 hours before and 24 hours

TABLE 16.1

Preclinical Studies Examining the Role of Fasting on Cancer Outcome

Cancer (Cell Line)	Animal Model	Route	Fasting Scheme	Effect of Fasting Alone	Effect of Fasting with Treatment	References
			Immunocompetent			
Breast (67NR and 4T1)	Female BALB/c mice	Orthotopic	Alternate day fasting	Slowed tumor growth	Synergy with irradiation	Saleh et al. (2013)
Breast (4T1)	Female BALB/c mice	SQ	Two 48–60 hours fasting cycles	Slowed tumor growth	Synergy with cyclophosphamide	Lee et al. (2012)
Breast (4T1)	Female BALB/c mice	IV	One 48-hour fast	N/A	Synergy with cyclophosphamide to prolong survival	Lee et al. (2012)
Colorectal (CT26)	Female BALB/c	SQ	Two 48-hour fasting cycles	Slowed tumor growth	Synergy with oxaliplatin	Bianchi et al. (2015)
Melanoma (B16)	Male and female C57BL/6 mice	SQ	48–60 hours fasting cycles	Slowed tumor growth	Synergy with doxorubicin	Lee et al. (2012)
Melanoma (B16)	Male and female C57BL/6 mice	IV	One 48-hour fast	No sustained benefit	Synergy with doxorubicin to prolong survival	Lee et al. (2012)
Neuroblastoma (NXS2)	Female A/J mice	IV	One 48-hour fast	No benefit	Less treatment toxicity of one high dose of etoposide, but more rapid tumor progression	Raffaghello et al. (2008)
Neuroblastoma (NXS2)	Female A/J mice	IV	Two 48-hour fasting cycles	N/A	Synergy with doxorubicin to prolong survival	Lee et al. (2012)
Neuroblastoma (Neuro 2A)	Female A/J mice	IV	One 48-hour fast	N/A	Synergy with doxorubicin and cisplatin cocktail to prolong survival	Lee et al. (2012)
Pancreatic (KPC)	Male and female C57BL/6J mice	Orthotopic	One 24-hour fast	No benefit	Synergy with irradiation	de la Cruz Bonilla et al. (2019)
			Immunocompromised			
Breast (MDA-MB-231)	Female nude mice	SQ	Four 48-hour fasting cycles	No sustained benefit	No apparent synergy with doxorubicin	Lee et al. (2012)
Breast (H3122)	Female, athymic BALB/c mice	SQ	Three 48-hour fasting cycles	Slowed tumor growth	Synergy with crizotinib (tyrosine kinase inhibitor)	Caffa et al. (2015)
Colorectal (HCT116)	Female, athymic BALB/c mice	SQ	Three 48-hours fasting cycles	Slowed tumor growth	Synergy with regorafenib (tyrosine kinase inhibitor)	Caffa et al. (2015)
Glioma (GL26)	Female nude mice	SQ	48–60 hours fasting cycles	Slowed tumor growth	Synergy with doxorubicin	Lee et al. (2012)
Ovarian (OVCAR3)	Female nude mice	SQ	Two 48-hour fasting cycles	No sustained benefit	No apparent synergy with doxorubicin	Lee et al. (2012)

Source: **Adapted from Mittelman (2020).**

N/A, not assessed; ADF, alternate day feeding; IV, intravenous; SQ, subcutaneous.

after chemotherapy, during the first or second half of their planned treatment. Compared to the *ad libitum* period, fasting showed improved quality of life and reduced fatigue (Bauersfeld et al. 2018), but the effect on chemotherapy efficacy was again not evaluated. Another small study of 13 patients with breast cancer used short-term fasting in conjunction with neo-adjuvant treatment. Six patients fasted for 24 hours before and 24 hours after treatment, and had higher red and white cell counts compared to the nonfasted group (de Groot et al. 2015). Compared to patients receiving oral carbohydrate loads at 18 and 2–4 hours before surgery, fasting patients with ER-positive breast cancer showed significantly less proliferation and improved relapse-free survival (Lende et al. 2019). Interestingly, postoperative pain was significantly less in patients who received preoperative carbohydrates. A recent randomized control trial of 131 patients with HER2 negative early breast cancer showed that use of an FMD 3 days prior to and on the day of treatment improved response to chemotherapy, with an increased number of fasting cycles correlated with increased response (de Groot et al. 2020). The FMD group experienced the same number of adverse events as the control group and less DNA damage to T-lymphocytes, despite not receiving dexamethasone, which was given to the control group to mitigate side effects.

CALORIE RESTRICTION

The cellular and physiological changes that occur during fasting may provide the greatest effects on altering metabolism and decreasing inflammation; however, undertaking periods of complete fasting may be difficult or unappealing to patients. Calorie restriction, in contrast, may be more feasible to a larger number of patients. Restriction can be achieved in a number of ways including the reduction of carbohydrates, the most common, reduction in calories from protein, or a nondiscriminatory reduction in overall calories. Each of these strategies may have different effects in cancer models and could contribute to the high degree of variability between study outcomes. The variety of reported outcome measures also makes it difficult to make direct comparisons and establish a consensus on optimal diet or restriction with the given data. In chronic calorie restriction studies, animals on the restriction protocol are generally provided with 60%–85% of what was consumed on an *ad libitum* diet. More severe reductions of 50%–67% of *ad libitum* have been studied for shorter periods of 1–3 weeks, which alternate with periods of ad libitum feeding or intake matched to a control *ad libitum* group.

There is a strong body of evidence that calorie restriction can delay cancer in various types of animal models, including spontaneous and carcinogenesis models (Dunn et al. 1997, Cleary et al. 2007, Engelman, Day, and Good 1994, Dogan et al. 2010, Ma et al. 2018b, Jiang, Zhu, and Thompson 2008, Thompson et al. 2004, Mizuno et al. 2013, Rossi et al. 2017, Gillette et al. 1997, Tomita 2012, Mai et al. 2003, James and Muskhelishvili 1994, Duan et al. 2017, Ploeger et al. 2017, Molina-Aguilar et al. 2017, Grigura et al. 2018, Carver et al. 2011, Lanza-Jacoby et al. 2013, Lashinger et al. 2011, Blando et al. 2011, Suttie et al. 2005, Bonorden et al. 2009, Boileau et al. 2003, Moore et al. 2012, Stewart et al. 2005, Diaz-Ruiz et al. 2019, Shields et al. 1991, Berrigan et al. 2002, Hursting et al. 1997, Hursting, Perkins, and Phang 1994, Yamaza et al. 2010, von Tungeln et al. 1996), models of syngeneic transplants (Cadoni et al. 2017, Harvey et al. 2013, Dunlap et al. 2012, Nogueira et al. 2012, De Lorenzo et al. 2011, van Ginhoven et al. 2010, Shelton et al. 2010, Phoenix et al. 2010, Seyfried et al. 2003), and xenograft models (Ma et al. 2018a, Galet et al. 2013, Jiang and Wang 2013, Lashinger et al. 2011). Only a minority of studies found no or a negative effect of calorie restriction (Tagliaferro et al. 1996, Pape-Ansorge et al. 2002, Birt et al. 1997, Kandori et al. 2005, McCormick et al. 2007, Tsao et al. 2002, Kusuoka et al. 2018, Brandhorst et al. 2013).

As shown in Table 16.2, a few studies have investigated the effects of calorie restriction on treatment efficacy in preclinical models. Our group showed that switching mice from a high-fat to a low-fat diet improved the treatment efficacy of vincristine against syngeneic B-cell ALL; however, we observed no synergy with dexamethasone or L-asparaginase (Tucci et al. 2018). Further, as shown in fasting models, the effects of calorie restriction may also improve chemotherapy tolerance

TABLE 16.2
Preclinical Studies Examining the Role of Caloric Restriction on Cancer Outcome

Cancer (Cell Line)	Animal Model	Route	Diet Scheme	Effect of Diet Alone	Effect of Diet with Treatment	References
B-ALL (8093)	Male C57BL/6J mice	Retro-orbital	Switch from 60% to 10% fat diet	No benefit	Improved efficacy of vincristine, but no effect on dexamethasone or L-asparaginase	Tucci et al. (2018)
Breast (4T1)	Female BALB/c mice	Orthotopic	70% of ad libitum	Slowed tumor growth	Synergy with irradiation, cisplatin, and docetaxol	Simone et al. (2016, 2018) and Saleh et al. (2013)
Breast (4T1)	Female BALB/c mice	SQ	50% of ad libitum	N/A	No synergy with cisplatin	Brandhorst et al. (2013)

Source: **Adapted from Mittelman (2020).**
SQ, subcutaneous; N/A, not assessed.

by reducing side effects. Conducted in only healthy (noncancerous) animals, calorie restriction was shown to decrease intestinal damage from 5-fluorouracil (Murakami et al. 2009) and cyclophosphamide (Liu et al. 2019b) in rodent models. Given that mucosal barrier injury due to chemotherapy can cause interruptions to effective and timely treatment (van Vliet et al. 2010, Touchefeu et al. 2014), restriction of calories may be an effective means of reducing these treatment delays and ultimately improve outcomes.

KETOGENIC DIET

Restricting specific macronutrients without reducing calories or implementing fasting may be a good alternative to these more stringent interventions. Specifically, the ketogenic diet has gained traction for use in patients as an alternative to fasting and caloric restriction. With a long record of safety and efficacy in patients with epilepsy, restricting carbohydrates with a ketogenic diet may be better tolerated and accepted by patients with cancer.

A recent meta-analysis identified 12 studies which tested ad libitum ketogenic diet against standard diet in murine cancer models and concluded an overall tumor growth delay with the ketogenic diet (Klement et al. 2016). An *in vitro* experiment showed that the ketone body β-hydroxybutyrate enhanced cisplatin-induced apoptosis in HCC cells (Mikami et al. 2020). The few studies in rodents that were exposed to a ketogenic diet during anticancer treatment are shown in Table 16.3. They report mostly positive effects, showing synergy between the diet and irradiation, metformin, and chemotherapy.

A systematic review of nonrandomized, uncontrolled trials in pediatric and adult patients with glioma found that a ketogenic diet was well tolerated, produced few adverse events, and may have conferred some benefit to overall and progression-free survival (Martin-McGill et al. 2018).

UNSATURATED FATTY ACIDS AND FISH OIL SUPPLEMENTATION

Changes in dietary fat composition, namely, changes from saturated to unsaturated fatty acids, have been of long interest in weight-loss, longevity, heart-health, and cancer studies. In one study, consumption of fish, or the long-chain omega-3 polyunsaturated fatty acids (PUFA), which are a major component of fish oils, were associated with an overall decrease in cancer mortality (Song et al. 2016). Another study in humans found a U-shaped curve for cancer mortality based on total fish consumption (Engeset et al. 2015). A meta-analysis of prostate cancer risk and mortality found no association between fish consumption and incidence of prostate cancer, but did show a 63% decrease in prostate cancer–specific mortality (Szymanski, Wheeler, and Mucci 2010), and significantly longer disease-free survival was noted in colon cancer patients in the highest quartile of fish consumption compared to those in the lowest quartile (van Blarigan et al. 2018).

Mouse models also show some potential for benefit with unsaturated fatty acids. An isocaloric substitution of long-chain omega-3 PUFA for omega-6 PUFA showed a decrease in proliferation of mammary tumor cells in a mouse model (Khadge et al. 2018). In another study of mammary tumors in mice, supplementation with omega-3 PUFA combined with intermittent calorie restriction reduced the tumor incidence to 15% compared to 87% in the control *ad libitum* mice (Mizuno et al. 2013). Omega-3 supplementation or intermittent calorie restriction alone showed intermediate reduction of tumor incidence (63% and 59%, respectively). Interestingly, chronic calorie restriction only reduced incidence to 59% and chronic calorie restriction plus omega-3 supplementation reduced incidence to 40%.

The use of fish oil supplementation during chemotherapy, however, is somewhat controversial. Mouse studies have shown that supplementation with fish oil impaired the effects of the chemotherapy cisplatin on colon and lung tumors in mice (Roodhart et al. 2011) and similar supplementation in humans showed an increase in the chemo-neutralizing fatty acid $16:4(n-3)$ in healthy human volunteers (Daenen et al. 2015). However, no effect of chemotherapy efficacy in humans was tested

TABLE 16.3

Preclinical Trials of Ketogenic Diets on Cancer Outcome

Cancer (Cell Line)	Animal Model	Route	Diet Scheme	Effect of Diet Alone	Effect of Diet with Treatment	References
Breast (4T1)	Female BALB/C mice	SQ	70% of AL of 2% CHO and 93.4% fat calories diet	Reduced tumor growth	Enhanced antitumor effect of metformin	Zhuang et al. (2014)
Glioma (GL261 cells)	Male albino C57BL/6 mice	Orthotopic	AL 3% CHO and 72% fat calories diet	Prolonged survival	Synergy with irradiation	Lussier et al. (2016) and Abdelwahab et al. (2012)
Glioma (GL261)	Female albino C57BL/6 mice	Orthotopic	AL 3% CHO and 72% fat calories diet	Prolonged survival	Synergistic with whole brain irradiation	Woolf et al. (2015) and Abdelwahab et al. (2012)
Lung (NCI-H292 and A549 cells)	Female athymic-nu/nu mice	SQ	AL 1.6% CHO and 90% fat calories diet	No effect of KD alone on tumor volume or survival	Enhanced tumor response and survival with irradiation±carboplatin	Allen et al. (2013)
Medulloblastoma (allograft from Ptch1 +/− Trp53 −/− mice)	NOD/SCID mice	SQ	AL 6:1 3.2% CHO and 75.1% fat paste diet	No effect on tumor growth	No effect on SMO inhibitor GDC-0449 antitumor activity	Dang et al. (2015)
Neuroblastoma (SK-N-BE(2) and SH-SY5Y cells)	Female CD1-nu mice	SQ	AL or two-thirds ad libitum KD with 8% CHO and 78% fat calories	CR KD slowed tumor growth and prolonged survival of both tumors. ad libitum KD only slowed tumor growth and prolonged survival for SK-N-BE(2) tumors	Both diets slowed growth of KH-SY5Y tumors but not SK-N-BE(2) tumors during cyclophosphamide treatment	Morscher et al. (2016) and Morscher et al. (2015)

Source: **Adapted from Mittelman (2020).**

SQ, subcutaneous; AL, ad libitum; CHO, carbohydrates; KD, ketogenic diet; SMO, smoothened gene, a component of the sonic hedgehog pathway.

in the study. As reviewed in Corsetto et al (Corsetto et al. 2017), there is evidence to suggest that supplementation with omega-3 fatty acids improves efficacy of a number of different chemotherapeutics in various cancer models, including doxorubicin in a lung xenograft model, epirubicin in an *in vitro* model of bladder cancer, 5-fluorouracil in a colon cancer cell line, mitomycin C in human colorectal cancer stem-like cells, arabinosylcytosine in mice with leukemia, and tamoxifen in *in vitro* breast cancer cells with constitutively active AKT. In 1998, *in vitro* data showed that both omega-6 and omega-3 PUFA potentiated the cytotoxicity of vincristine, cis-platinum, and doxorubicin on human cervical carcinoma cells (Das et al. 1998). As can be seen in Table 16.4, more work needs to be done in preclinical models, especially in regard to looking at possible sex differences. The limited data currently available, however, suggest that fish oil supplementation may be beneficial or, at the very least, not harmful to outcomes, with the exception of the aforementioned studies on cisplatin.

In a review of clinical trials, the ten studies examined did not show a net benefit or worse outcome for patients receiving an omega-3 supplement on tumor size or survival (de Aguiar Pastore Silva, Emilia de Souza Fabre, and Waitzberg 2015). However, as was shown with calorie restriction, supplementation with omega-3 PUFA may also decrease mucositis and result in increased chemotherapy tolerance and better survival outcomes (Zhang et al. 2019b). Supplementation has also been shown to decrease other chemotherapy side effects, such as osteoporosis (Raghu Nadhanan et al. 2013) and aromatase inhibitor-associated arthralgia (Shen et al. 2018).

Olive oil, high in monounsaturated fatty acids, is a major component of Mediterranean diets. Strict adherence to such diets has been linked with a reduction in cancer mortality and was specifically found to reduce mortality of breast, colorectal, head and neck, gastric, prostate, liver, respiratory and pancreatic cancers (Schwingshackl and Hoffmann 2015). Compared to the lowest level of olive oil consumption, subjects who were in the highest group of consumption were found to have decreased incidence of overall cancer, specifically cancer of the breast or gastrointestinal tract (Psaltopoulou et al. 2011).

ANIMAL PROTEIN RESTRICTION

Restriction of protein has been shown to slow the growth of breast and prostate cancer in xenograft models of human disease (Fontana et al. 2013). In a study of British participants, fish eaters and vegetarians had similar incidence of cancer (~6%), and both had lower incidence compared to meat eaters (10%) (Key et al. 2014), suggested that the source of protein may be mitigating factor in protection from cancer. A meta-analysis of plant-based diets showed that cancer incidence was decreased by ~8% in vegetarian and 15% in vegan diets (Dinu et al. 2017) and patients with a higher intake of vegetable versus animal fats had improved survival after prostate cancer diagnosis (Richman et al. 2013). However, an analysis of one prospective study demonstrated that meat eaters consume one-third of their calories from protein and vegetarians consume one-fourth of their calories from protein (Papier et al. 2019). These data suggest that it may be the overall decrease in protein intake that leads to the decreased risk of cancer. However, the same study found that vegetarians also consume more vegetables and whole grains and less fried foods, refined grains, and sugary drinks than meat eaters, which may be mitigating factors for the effects of vegetarian and vegan diets on cancer. Low intake of animal protein consumption was not shown to affect cancer mortality, but substituting plant protein for egg protein was associated with a 21% reduction in cancer mortality (Song et al. 2016). Another study found that substitution of plant protein for red meat was associated with a decrease in all-cause (HR: 0.54) and cancer mortality (HR: 0.50) (Budhathoki et al. 2019). These data further suggest that it may be other macro- or micronutrients and fiber associated with plant-based proteins that induce the protective effect and not the change in protein source. Increased consumption of plant versus animal protein has been shown to decrease all-cause mortality but, interestingly, one study found this only in those with one or more risk factors such as smoking, heavy alcohol drinking, overweight or obesity, and physical inactivity (Song et al. 2016).

TABLE 16.4

Preclinical Trials of Omega-3 Supplementation on Cancer Outcome

Cancer (Cell Line)	Animal Model	Route	Supplement Scheme	Effect of Supplement Alone	Effect of Supplement with Treatment	References
Breast (MDA-MB 231)	Female athymic nu/nu mice	SQ	3% w/w fish oil concentrate	No effect	Increased efficacy of doxorubicin on tumor growth rate, no change in toxicity	Hardman et al. (2001)
Breast (MCF-7)	Female nu/nu mice	SQ	3% or 5% w/w antioxidant-free fish oil	N/A	Increased efficacy of CPT-11 to diminish tumor size	Hardman, Moyer, and Cameron (1999)
Lung (A549 and H1299)	Female nu/nu mice	SQ	618 mg/kg MAG-DHA fish oil concentrate	Tumor growth was inhibited compared to vehicle and carboplatin controls	No difference in between MAG-DHA and MAG-DHA+carboplatin	Morin and Fortin (2017)

SQ, subcutaneous; N/A, not assessed; MAG, monoacylglyceride; DHA, docosahexaenoic acid.

To our knowledge, there are no studies evaluating protein restriction or protein source on chemotherapy efficacy in preclinical models or patients.

POSSIBLE MECHANISMS OF IMPROVED EFFICACY WITH DIET INTERVENTIONS

The diets mentioned above may help prevent cancer when implemented prior to cancer initiation. Public health initiatives to encourage overall healthy habits are likely the best avenue to reduce incidence of cancer. However, given the large number of people with overweight and obesity, a cancer diagnosis may be an opportunity to implement specific dietary changes that could improve outcomes in these patients. Dietary interventions may further offer a host of metabolic benefits for patients during and following treatment.

Limiting the available fuels for cancer cells through fasting and calorie restriction can impact cell growth, with healthy cells theoretically able to withstand prolonged fuel restriction while rapidly proliferating cancer cells cannot. This "differential stress" hypothesis is centered on the decrease in growth factors, such as IGF-1, leptin, and insulin (Raffaghello et al. 2008). Healthy cells are able to respond to reduction in these growth factors, primarily via increased mTOR and decreased AKT, to slow growth and replication and shift to fuel conservation through autophagy. This slowed growth protects healthy cells from the cytotoxic effects of many chemotherapies. The hallmark uncontrolled cell replication of cancer cells may not be altered in states of fasting or calorie restriction, given their relative independence from local and systemic signals. Thus, chemotherapy efficacy may increase while side effects may decline. Further, reduced availability of metabolic fuels may induce oxidative stress in the face of uncontrolled, rapid proliferation. Increased stress due to metabolic inflexibility may lead to increased cancer cell death due to DNA replication errors and catastrophic mitotic events. Calorie restriction can also reduce vascularization, further limiting tumor access to circulating nutrients and oxygen (Thompson et al. 2004). Changes to the lipid profile during fasting, calorie restriction, or omega-3 PUFA supplementation may alter membrane organization and cell signaling (Corsetto et al. 2011), increasing the vulnerability of the rapidly growing cells. Ketones themselves are toxic to some cancer cells, though some tumors express ketone metabolizing enzymes (Zhang et al. 2018).

Evidence for the important role of these hormones in diet inventions has been shown in several studies. Decreased IGF-1 was found to be causal for the reduced tumor progression in a model of dietary restriction in p53-deficient mice given bladder cancer (Dunn et al. 1997). In a rat model, incidence and severity of leukemia was decreased by calorie restriction, but this effect was reversed when either IGF-1 or GH was infused via osmotic pump (Hursting et al. 1993). Lu et al. demonstrated in an obese mouse model of leukemia that fasting improved leukemia outcome by inducing leptin receptor expression, leading to differentiation of leukemia cells (Lu et al. 2017). Alternatively, reductions in adiposity or the implementation of fasting or calorie restriction may lead to increased activation of adiponectin pathways, such as AMPK, that inhibit tumor formation, progression, and metastasis (Parida, Siddharth, and Sharma 2019).

Decreased inflammation from dietary interventions may also impact the progression of cancer and patient sensitivity to treatment. Increased dietary antioxidants were associated with decreased infections in children and adolescents with leukemia (Ladas et al. 2020). Energy restriction can decrease the number of inflammatory monocytes (Kim et al. 2017). Increased antitumor immunity was regulated by increased CD4+ non-T-reg cells during a ketogenic diet and was reversed with CD8+ T-cell depletion (Lussier et al. 2016). Further, alterations in the microbiome following changes to the diet can result in beneficial effects such as decreased inflammation, improved metabolism, and increased rate of absorption and bioavailability of oral antitumor therapeutics (Roy and Trinchieri 2017).

WHICH IS THE BEST DIET?

In general, the diet interventions discussed above show benefits or, at least, a lack of detriment to outcomes in cancer models. With most studies using animal models, translation into human studies is required, with the major caveat that these models may not accurately recapitulate the clinical situation. The diet-induced obese C57BL/6 mouse is the most commonly used model of obesity. This model uses 45% or 60% of calories from fat to induce and maintain an obese animal, in stark contrast to human obesity, which is generally associated with excess carbohydrate intake. The extreme, morbid obesity of the mice may also not reflect the typical overweight or obese patient seen in the clinic.

Few studies compare multiple diet interventions in a head-to-head manner. While it was shown that 60% calorie restriction produced superior survival compared to fasting 1 day per week in p53 heterozygous mice (Berrigan et al. 2002), other fasting protocols or macronutrient restrictions were not tested. What if one of these modes of diet modulation produced better results? Or, what if they produced similar results in humans but were also accompanied by better tolerability and patient preference? Fasting for 60 hours was found to better protect mice from doxorubicin toxicity than 50% calorie restriction (Brandhorst et al. 2013). However, the effects on doxorubicin efficacy or on the antitumor activity of the chemotherapy combinations used in patients was not studied. Further complicating the translation from animals to humans, a recent meta-analysis found that intermittent calorie restriction more effectively reduced the incidence of cancer in genetically engineered animal models but chronic calorie restriction was superior in carcinogen models (Chen et al. 2016).

Given the paucity of data examining dietary intervention during cancer treatment, particularly in patients, more work will need to be done to test which interventions have the best efficacy against specific cancers. In a review of intermittent fasting, calorie restriction, and ketogenic diet effects on cancer initiation, progression, and metastasis, both calorie restriction and the ketogenic diet were determined to be highly effective but the data on intermittent fasting were inconclusive (Lv et al. 2014). Given the scope of research needed in this field, it is possible that databases and computation methods may be the best next step to assess interactions between various diets or specific nutrients and chemotherapy efficacy (Zheng et al. 2017, Veselkov et al. 2019). With the increased focus on personalized medicine, it is also likely that diet recommendations would need to be made on a patient-to-patient, rather than a strictly cancer-to-cancer basis. Given difficulties with dietary compliance, it is also possible that the best diet for a specific patient could be the one that they will do.

SUMMARY/CONCLUSIONS

It is clear that diet plays important roles in the initiation, progression, and outcome of many diseases, including cancer. Given the toll on human health taken by cancer and the complications to treatment that are induced in the obese state, further exploration of the role of diet interventions as an adjunct to treatment is vital. *In vitro* and *in vivo* models have shown the increased efficacy of chemotherapies in the context of fasting and other forms of dietary restriction or manipulation. These data need to be confirmed in human studies and compared side-by-side, to determine their relative merits in terms of efficacy and acceptability. This will require the involvement of multidisciplinary teams, and strong therapeutic alliances with patients.

REFERENCES

Abdelwahab, M. G., K. E. Fenton, M. C. Preul, J. M. Rho, A. Lynch, P. Stafford, and A. C. Scheck. 2012. "The ketogenic diet is an effective adjuvant to radiation therapy for the treatment of malignant glioma." *PLoS One* 7 (5):e36197. doi: 10.1371/journal.pone.0036197.

Ahmed, S. M., J. P. Lemkau, and S. L. Birt. 2002. "Toward sensitive treatment of obese patients." *Fam Pract Manag* 9 (1):25–8.

Akinyemiju, T., J. X. Moore, M. Pisu, S. E. Judd, M. Goodman, J. M. Shikany, V. J. Howard, M. Safford, and S. C. Gilchrist. 2018. "A prospective study of obesity, metabolic health, and cancer mortality." *Obesity (Silver Spring)* 26 (1):193–201. doi: 10.1002/oby.22067.

Allen, B. G., S. K. Bhatia, J. M. Buatti, K. E. Brandt, K. E. Lindholm, A. M. Button, L. I. Szweda, B. J. Smith, D. R. Spitz, and M. A. Fath. 2013. "Ketogenic diets enhance oxidative stress and radio-chemotherapy responses in lung cancer xenografts." *Clin Cancer Res* 19 (14):3905–13. doi: 10.1158/1078-0432. CCR-12-0287.

Allott, E. H., E. M. Masko, and S. J. Freedland. 2013. "Obesity and prostate cancer: weighing the evidence." *Eur Urol* 63 (5):800–9. doi: 10.1016/j.eururo.2012.11.013.

Al-Zubaidi, A. M., A. H. Alzobydi, S. A. Alsareii, A. Al-Shahrani, N. Alzaman, and S. Kassim. 2018. "Body mass index and." *Int J Environ Res Public Health* 15 (11). doi: 10.3390/ijerph15112586.

Ambrosi, T. H., A. Scialdone, A. Graja, S. Gohlke, A. M. Jank, C. Bocian, L. Woelk, H. Fan, D. W. Logan, A. Schürmann, L. R. Saraiva, and T. J. Schulz. 2017. "Adipocyte accumulation in the bone marrow during obesity and aging impairs stem cell-based hematopoietic and bone regeneration." *Cell Stem Cell* 20 (6):771–84.e6. doi: 10.1016/j.stem.2017.02.009.

Amieva, M., and R. M. Peek. 2016. "Pathobiology of helicobacter pylori-induced gastric cancer." *Gastroenterology* 150 (1):64–78. doi: 10.1053/j.gastro.2015.09.004.

Ananieva, E. A., and A. C. Wilkinson. 2018. "Branched-chain amino acid metabolism in cancer." *Curr Opin Clin Nutr Metab Care* 21 (1):64–70. doi: 10.1097/MCO.0000000000000430.

Anderson, E. K., D. A. Gutierrez, and A. H. Hasty. 2010. "Adipose tissue recruitment of leukocytes." *Curr Opin Lipidol* 21 (3):172–7. doi: 10.1097/MOL.0b013e3283393867.

Arslan, E., H. Atilgan, and I. Yavaşoğlu. 2009. "The prevalence of Helicobacter pylori in obese subjects." *Eur J Intern Med* 20 (7):695–7. doi: 10.1016/j.ejim.2009.07.013.

Bach, P. B., D. Schrag, O. W. Brawley, A. Galaznik, S. Yakren, and C. B. Begg. 2002. "Survival of blacks and whites after a cancer diagnosis." *JAMA* 287 (16):2106–13. doi: 10.1001/jama.287.16.2106.

Bao, C., X. Yang, W. Xu, H. Luo, Z. Xu, C. Su, and X. Qi. 2013. "Diabetes mellitus and incidence and mortality of kidney cancer: a meta-analysis." *J Diabetes Complications* 27 (4):357–64. doi: 10.1016/j. jdiacomp.2013.01.004.

Bardou, M., A. Barkun, and M. Martel. 2010. "Effect of statin therapy on colorectal cancer." *Gut* 59 (11):1572–85. doi: 10.1136/gut.2009.190900.

Barrington-Trimis, J. L., M. Cockburn, C. Metayer, W. J. Gauderman, J. Wiemels, and R. McKean-Cowdin. 2017. "Trends in childhood leukemia incidence over two decades from 1992 to 2013." *Int J Cancer* 140 (5):1000–8. doi: 10.1002/ijc.30487.

Bauersfeld, S. P., C. S. Kessler, M. Wischnewsky, A. Jaensch, N. Steckhan, R. Stange, B. Kunz, B. Bruckner, J. Sehouli, and A. Michalsen. 2018. "The effects of short-term fasting on quality of life and tolerance to chemotherapy in patients with breast and ovarian cancer: a randomized cross-over pilot study." *BMC Cancer* 18 (1):476. doi: 10.1186/s12885-018-4353-2.

Beeken, R. J., R. Wilson, L. McDonald, and J. Wardle. 2014. "Body mass index and cancer screening: findings from the English Longitudinal Study of Ageing." *J Med Screen* 21 (2):76–81. doi: 10.1177/0969141314531409.

Behan, J. W., J. P. Yun, M. P. Proektor, E. A. Ehsanipour, A. Arutyunyan, A. S. Moses, V. I. Avramis, S. G. Louie, A. Butturini, N. Heisterkamp, and S. D. Mittelman. 2009. "Adipocytes impair leukemia treatment in mice." *Cancer Res* 69 (19):7867–74. doi: 10.1158/0008-5472.CAN-09-0800.

Berg, A. H., and P. E. Scherer. 2005. "Adipose tissue, inflammation, and cardiovascular disease." *Circ Res* 96 (9):939–49. doi: 10.1161/01.RES.0000163635.62927.34.

Berrigan, D., S. N. Perkins, D. C. Haines, and S. D. Hursting. 2002. "Adult-onset calorie restriction and fasting delay spontaneous tumorigenesis in p53-deficient mice." *Carcinogenesis* 23 (5):817–22. doi: 10.1093/carcin/23.5.817.

Bianchi, G., R. Martella, S. Ravera, C. Marini, S. Capitanio, A. Orengo, L. Emionite, C. Lavarello, A. Amaro, A. Petretto, U. Pfeffer, G. Sambuceti, V. Pistoia, L. Raffaghello, and V. D. Longo. 2015. "Fasting induces anti-Warburg effect that increases respiration but reduces ATP-synthesis to promote apoptosis in colon cancer models." *Oncotarget* 6 (14):11806–19. doi: 10.18632/oncotarget.3688.

Birt, D. F., P. M. Pour, D. L. Nagel, T. Barnett, D. Blackwood, and E. Duysen. 1997. "Dietary energy restriction does not inhibit pancreatic carcinogenesis by N-nitrosobis-2-(oxopropyl)amine in the Syrian hamster." *Carcinogenesis* 18 (11):2107–11. doi: 10.1093/carcin/18.11.2107.

Black, D. S., C. N. Lam, N. T. Nguyen, U. Ihenacho, and J. C. Figueiredo. 2016. "Complementary and integrative health practices among hispanics diagnosed with colorectal cancer: Utilization and communication with physicians." *J Altern Complement Med* 22 (6):473–9. doi: 10.1089/acm.2015.0332.

Blando, J., T. Moore, S. Hursting, G. Jiang, A. Saha, L. Beltran, J. Shen, J. Repass, S. Strom, and J. DiGiovanni. 2011. "Dietary energy balance modulates prostate cancer progression in Hi-Myc mice." *Cancer Prev Res (Phila)* 4 (12):2002–14. doi: 10.1158/1940-6207.CAPR-11-0182.

Blouin, J. M., G. Penot, M. Collinet, M. Nacfer, C. Forest, P. Laurent-Puig, X. Coumoul, R. Barouki, C. Benelli, and S. Bortoli. 2011. "Butyrate elicits a metabolic switch in human colon cancer cells by targeting the pyruvate dehydrogenase complex." *Int J Cancer* 128 (11):2591–601. doi: 10.1002/ijc.25599.

Boileau, T. W., Z. Liao, S. Kim, S. Lemeshow, J. W. Erdman, Jr., and S. K. Clinton. 2003. "Prostate carcinogenesis in N-methyl-N-nitrosourea (NMU)-testosterone-treated rats fed tomato powder, lycopene, or energy-restricted diets." *J Natl Cancer Inst* 95 (21):1578–86. doi: 10.1093/jnci/djg081.

Bonorden, M. J., O. P. Rogozina, C. M. Kluczny, M. E. Grossmann, P. L. Grambsch, J. P. Grande, S. Perkins, A. Lokshin, and M. P. Cleary. 2009. "Intermittent calorie restriction delays prostate tumor detection and increases survival time in TRAMP mice." *Nutr Cancer* 61 (2):265–75. doi: 10.1080/01635580802419798.

Brandhorst, S., M. Wei, S. Hwang, T. E. Morgan, and V. D. Longo. 2013. "Short-term calorie and protein restriction provide partial protection from chemotoxicity but do not delay glioma progression." *Exp Gerontol* 48 (10):1120–8. doi: 10.1016/j.exger.2013.02.016.

Broder, S. 1991. Progress and challenges in the national cancer program. Edited by J. Brugge, T. Curran, E. Harlow and F. McCormick, *Origins of Human Cancer: A Comprehensive Review*, (pp. 27–33). New York: Cold Spring Harbar Laboratry.

Brower, V. 2008. "Cancer disparities: disentangling the effects of race and genetics." *J Natl Cancer Inst* 100 (16):1126–9. doi: 10.1093/jnci/djn302.

Bruno, D. S., and N. A. Berger. 2020. "Impact of bariatric surgery on cancer risk reduction." *Ann Transl Med* 8 (Suppl 1):S13. doi: 10.21037/atm.2019.09.26.

Budhathoki, S., N. Sawada, M. Iwasaki, T. Yamaji, A. Goto, A. Kotemori, J. Ishihara, R. Takachi, H. Charvat, T. Mizoue, H. Iso, S. Tsugane, and Japan Public Health Center–based Prospective Study Group. 2019. "Association of animal and plant protein intake with all-cause and cause-specific mortality." *JAMA Intern Med.* doi: 10.1001/jamainternmed.2019.2806.

Buschemeyer, W. C., 3rd, J. C. Klink, J. C. Mavropoulos, S. H. Poulton, W. Demark-Wahnefried, S. D. Hursting, P. Cohen, D. Hwang, T. L. Johnson, and S. J. Freedland. 2010. "Effect of intermittent fasting with or without caloric restriction on prostate cancer growth and survival in SCID mice." *Prostate* 70 (10):1037–43. doi: 10.1002/pros.21136.

Cadoni, E., F. Marongiu, M. Fanti, M. Serra, and E. Laconi. 2017. "Caloric restriction delays early phases of carcinogenesis via effects on the tissue microenvironment." *Oncotarget* 8 (22):36020–32. doi: 10.18632/oncotarget.16421.

Caffa, I., V. D'Agostino, P. Damonte, D. Soncini, M. Cea, F. Monacelli, P. Odetti, A. Ballestrero, A. Provenzani, V. D. Longo, and A. Nencioni. 2015. "Fasting potentiates the anticancer activity of tyrosine kinase inhibitors by strengthening MAPK signaling inhibition." *Oncotarget* 6 (14):11820–32. doi: 10.18632/oncotarget.3689.

Calle, E. E., C. Rodriguez, K. Walker-Thurmond, and M. J. Thun. 2003. "Overweight, obesity, and mortality from cancer in a prospectively studied cohort of U.S. adults." *N Engl J Med* 348 (17):1625–38. doi: 10.1056/NEJMoa021423.

Carreras-Torres, R., M. Johansson, V. Gaborieau, P. C. Haycock, K. H. Wade, C. L. Relton, R. M. Martin, G. Davey Smith, and P. Brennan. 2017a. "The role of obesity, type 2 diabetes, and metabolic factors in pancreatic cancer: A mendelian randomization study." *J Natl Cancer Inst* 109 (9). doi: 10.1093/jnci/djx012.

Carreras-Torres, R., M. Johansson, P. C. Haycock, K. H. Wade, C. L. Relton, R. M. Martin, G. Davey Smith, D. Albanes, M. C. Aldrich, A. Andrew, S. M. Arnold, H. Bickeböller, S. E. Bojesen, H. Brunnström, J. Manjer, I. Brüske, N. E. Caporaso, C. Chen, D. C. Christiani, W. J. Christian, J. A. Doherty, E. J. Duell, J. K. Field, M. P. A. Davies, M. W. Marcus, G. E. Goodman, K. Grankvist, A. Haugen, Y. C. Hong, L. A. Kiemeney, E. H. F.M van der Heijden, P. Kraft, M. B. Johansson, S. Lam, M. T. Landi, P. Lazarus, L. Le Marchand, G. Liu, O. Melander, S. L. Park, G. Rennert, A. Risch, E. B. Haura, G. Scelo, D. Zaridze, A. Mukeriya, M. Savić, J. Lissowska, B. Swiatkowska, V. Janout, I. Holcatova, D. Mates, M. B. Schabath, H. Shen, A. Tardon, M. D. Teare, P. Woll, M. S. Tsao, X. Wu, J. M. Yuan, R. J. Hung, C. I. Amos, J. McKay, and P. Brennan. 2017b. "Obesity, metabolic factors and risk of different histological types of lung cancer: a mendelian randomization study." *PLoS One* 12 (6):e0177875. doi: 10.1371/journal.pone.0177875.

Carreras-Torres, R., M. Johansson, P. C. Haycock, C. L. Relton, G. Davey Smith, P. Brennan, and R. M. Martin. 2018. "Role of obesity in smoking behaviour: mendelian randomisation study in UK Biobank." *BMJ* 361:k1767. doi: 10.1136/bmj.k1767.

Carver, D. K., H. J. Barnes, K. E. Anderson, J. N. Petitte, R. Whitaker, A. Berchuck, and G. C. Rodriguez. 2011. "Reduction of ovarian and oviductal cancers in calorie-restricted laying chickens." *Cancer Prev Res (Phila)* 4 (4):562–7. doi: 10.1158/1940-6207.CAPR-10-0294.

Casagrande, D. S., D. D. Rosa, D. Umpierre, R. A. Sarmento, C. G. Rodrigues, and B. D. Schaan. 2014. "Incidence of cancer following bariatric surgery: systematic review and meta-analysis." *Obes Surg* 24 (9):1499–509. doi: 10.1007/s11695-014-1276-0.

Chan, D. S., A. R. Vieira, D. Aune, E. V. Bandera, D. C. Greenwood, A. McTiernan, D. Navarro Rosenblatt, I. Thune, R. Vieira, and T. Norat. 2014. "Body mass index and survival in women with breast cancer-systematic literature review and meta-analysis of 82 follow-up studies." *Ann Oncol* 25 (10):1901–14. doi: 10.1093/annonc/mdu042.

Chen, Y., L. Ling, G. Su, M. Han, X. Fan, P. Xun, and G. Xu. 2016. "Effect of intermittent versus chronic calorie restriction on tumor incidence: a systematic review and meta-analysis of animal studies." *Sci Rep* 6:33739. doi: 10.1038/srep33739.

Chen, Y., F. Wu, E. Saito, Y. Lin, M. Song, H. N. Luu, P. C. Gupta, N. Sawada, A. Tamakoshi, X. O. Shu, W. P. Koh, Y. B. Xiang, Y. Tomata, K. Sugiyama, S. K. Park, K. Matsuo, C. Nagata, Y. Sugawara, Y. L. Qiao, S. L. You, R. Wang, M. H. Shin, W. H. Pan, M. S. Pednekar, S. Tsugane, H. Cai, J. M. Yuan, Y. T. Gao, I. Tsuji, S. Kanemura, H. Ito, K. Wada, Y. O. Ahn, K. Y. Yoo, H. Ahsan, K. S. Chia, P. Boffetta, W. Zheng, M. Inoue, D. Kang, and J. D. Potter. 2017. "Association between type 2 diabetes and risk of cancer mortality: a pooled analysis of over 771,000 individuals in the Asia Cohort Consortium." *Diabetologia* 60 (6):1022–32. doi: 10.1007/s00125-017-4229-z.

Choi, I. Y., C. Lee, and V. D. Longo. 2017. "Nutrition and fasting mimicking diets in the prevention and treatment of autoimmune diseases and immunosenescence." *Mol Cell Endocrinol* 455:4–12. doi: 10.1016/j.mce.2017.01.042.

Cleary, M. P., X. Hu, M. E. Grossmann, S. C. Juneja, S. Dogan, J. P. Grande, and N. J. Maihle. 2007. "Prevention of mammary tumorigenesis by intermittent caloric restriction: does caloric intake during refeeding modulate the response?" *Exp Biol Med (Maywood)* 232 (1):70–80.

Conroy, S. M., G. Maskarinec, L. R. Wilkens, K. K. White, B. E. Henderson, and L. N. Kolonel. 2011. "Obesity and breast cancer survival in ethnically diverse postmenopausal women: the Multiethnic Cohort Study." *Breast Cancer Res Treat* 129 (2):565–74. doi: 10.1007/s10549-011-1468-4.

Considine, R. V., M. K. Sinha, M. L. Heiman, A. Kriauciunas, T. W. Stephens, M. R. Nyce, J. P. Ohannesian, C. C. Marco, L. J. McKee, T. L. Bauer, et al. 1996. "Serum immunoreactive-leptin concentrations in normal-weight and obese humans." *N Engl J Med* 334 (5):292–5. doi: 10.1056/NEJM199602013340503.

Corsetto, P. A., G. Montorfano, S. Zava, I. E. Jovenitti, A. Cremona, B. Berra, and A. M. Rizzo. 2011. "Effects of n-3 PUFAs on breast cancer cells through their incorporation in plasma membrane." *Lipids Health Dis* 10:73. doi: 10.1186/1476-511X-10-73.

Corsetto, P. A., I. Colombo, J. Kopecka, A. M. Rizzo, and C. Riganti. 2017. "ω-3 long chain polyunsaturated fatty acids as sensitizing agents and multidrug resistance revertants in cancer therapy." *Int J Mol Sci* 18 (12). doi: 10.3390/ijms18122770.

Daenen, L. G., G. A. Cirkel, J. M. Houthuijzen, J. Gerrits, I. Oosterom, J. M. Roodhart, H. van Tinteren, K. Ishihara, A. D. Huitema, N. M. Verhoeven-Duif, and E. E. Voest. 2015. "Increased plasma levels of chemoresistance-inducing fatty acid 16:4(n-3) after consumption of fish and fish oil." *JAMA Oncol* 1 (3):350–8. doi: 10.1001/jamaoncol.2015.0388.

Dalamaga, M., K. N. Diakopoulos, and C. S. Mantzoros. 2012. "The role of adiponectin in cancer: a review of current evidence." *Endocr Rev* 33 (4):547–94. doi: 10.1210/er.2011-1015.

Dang, M. T., S. Wehrli, C. V. Dang, and T. Curran. 2015. "The ketogenic diet does not affect growth of hedgehog pathway medulloblastoma in mice." *PLoS One* 10 (7):e0133633. doi: 10.1371/journal.pone.0133633.

Dare, S., D. F. Mackay, and J. P. Pell. 2015. "Relationship between smoking and obesity: a cross-sectional study of 499,504 middle-aged adults in the UK general population." *PLoS One* 10 (4):e0123579. doi: 10.1371/journal.pone.0123579.

Das, U. N., N. Madhavi, G. Sravan Kumar, M. Padma, and P. Sangeetha. 1998. "Can tumour cell drug resistance be reversed by essential fatty acids and their metabolites?" *Prostaglandins Leukot Essent Fatty Acids* 58 (1):39–54. doi: 10.1016/s0952-3278(98)90128-4.

de Aguiar Pastore Silva, J., M. Emilia de Souza Fabre, and D. L. Waitzberg. 2015. "Omega-3 supplements for patients in chemotherapy and/or radiotherapy: a systematic review." *Clin Nutr* 34 (3):359–66. doi: 10.1016/j.clnu.2014.11.005.

de Groot, S., M. P. Vreeswijk, M. J. Welters, G. Gravesteijn, J. J. Boei, A. Jochems, D. Houtsma, H. Putter, J. J. van der Hoeven, J. W. Nortier, H. Pijl, and J. R. Kroep. 2015. "The effects of short-term fasting on tolerance to (neo) adjuvant chemotherapy in HER2-negative breast cancer patients: a randomized pilot study." *BMC Cancer* 15:652. doi: 10.1186/s12885-015-1663-5.

de Groot, S., R. T. Lugtenberg, D. Cohen, M. J. P. Welters, I. Ehsan, M. P. G. Vreeswijk, V. T. H.BM Smit, H. de Graaf, J. B. Heijns, J. E. A. Portielje, A. J. van de Wouw, A. L. T. Imholz, L. W. Kessels, S. Vrijaldenhoven, A. Baars, E. M. Kranenbarg, M. D. Carpentier, H. Putter, J. J. M. van der Hoeven, J. W. R. Nortier, V. D. Longo, H. Pijl, J. R. Kroep, and Dutch Breast Cancer Research Group (BOOG). 2020. "Fasting mimicking diet as an adjunct to neoadjuvant chemotherapy for breast cancer in the multicentre randomized phase 2 DIRECT trial." *Nat Commun* 11 (1):3083. doi: 10.1038/s41467-020-16138-3.

de la Cruz Bonilla, M., K. M. Stemler, S. Jeter-Jones, T. N. Fujimoto, J. Molkentine, G. M. Asencio Torres, X. Zhang, R. R. Broaddus, C. M. Taniguchi, and H. Piwnica-Worms. 2019. "Fasting reduces intestinal radiotoxicity, enabling dose-escalated radiation therapy for pancreatic cancer." *Int J Radiat Oncol Biol Phys* 105 (3):537–47. doi: 10.1016/j.ijrobp.2019.06.2533.

De Lorenzo, M. S., E. Baljinnyam, D. E. Vatner, P. Abarzua, S. F. Vatner, and A. B. Rabson. 2011. "Caloric restriction reduces growth of mammary tumors and metastases." *Carcinogenesis* 32 (9):1381–7. doi: 10.1093/carcin/bgr107.

Demierre, M. F., P. D. Higgins, S. B. Gruber, E. Hawk, and S. M. Lippman. 2005. "Statins and cancer prevention." *Nat Rev Cancer* 5 (12):930–42. doi: 10.1038/nrc1751.

den Besten, G., K. van Eunen, A. K. Groen, K. Venema, D. J. Reijngoud, and B. M. Bakker. 2013. "The role of short-chain fatty acids in the interplay between diet, gut microbiota, and host energy metabolism." *J Lipid Res* 54 (9):2325–40. doi: 10.1194/jlr.R036012.

Deng, T., C. J. Lyon, S. Bergin, M. A. Caligiuri, and W. A. Hsueh. 2016. "Obesity, inflammation, and cancer." *Annu Rev Pathol* 11:421–49 doi: 10.1146/annurev-pathol-012615-044359.

Deng, X., R. Su, S. Stanford, and J. Chen. 2018. "Critical enzymatic functions of FTO in obesity and cancer." *Front Endocrinol (Lausanne)* 9:396. doi: 10.3389/fendo.2018.00396.

Devlin, M. J. 2011. "Why does starvation make bones fat?" *Am J Hum Biol* 23 (5):577–85. doi: 10.1002/ajhb.21202.

Dhurandhar, N. V., D. Bailey, and D. Thomas. 2015. "Interaction of obesity and infections." *Obes Rev* 16 (12):1017–29. doi: 10.1111/obr.12320.

Diaz-Ruiz, A., A. Di Francesco, B. A. Carboneau, S. R. Levan, K. J. Pearson, N. L. Price, T. M. Ward, M. Bernier, R. de Cabo, and E. M. Mercken. 2019. "Benefits of caloric restriction in longevity and chemical-induced tumorigenesis are transmitted independent of NQO1." *J Gerontol A Biol Sci Med Sci* 74 (2):155–62. doi: 10.1093/gerona/gly112.

Dinu, M., R. Abbate, G. F. Gensini, A. Casini, and F. Sofi. 2017. "Vegetarian, vegan diets and multiple health outcomes: a systematic review with meta-analysis of observational studies." *Crit Rev Food Sci Nutr* 57 (17):3640–49. doi: 10.1080/10408398.2016.1138447.

Dodson, S., V. E. Baracos, A. Jatoi, W. J. Evans, D. Cella, J. T. Dalton, and M. S. Steiner. 2011. "Muscle wasting in cancer cachexia: clinical implications, diagnosis, and emerging treatment strategies." *Annu Rev Med* 62:265–79 doi: 10.1146/annurev-med-061509-131248.

Dogan, S., O. P. Rogozina, A. E. Lokshin, J. P. Grande, and M. P. Cleary. 2010. "Effects of chronic vs. intermittent calorie restriction on mammary tumor incidence and serum adiponectin and leptin levels in MMTV-TGF-alpha mice at different ages." *Oncol Lett* 1 (1):167–76. doi: 10.3892/ol_00000031.

Dong, L., Y. Yuan, C. Opansky, Y. Chen, I. Aguilera-Barrantes, S. Wu, R. Yuan, Q. Cao, Y. C. Cheng, D. Sahoo, R. L. Silverstein, and B. Ren. 2017. "Diet-induced obesity links to ER positive breast cancer progression via LPA/PKD-1-CD36 signaling-mediated microvascular remodeling." *Oncotarget* 8 (14):22550–62. doi: 10.18632/oncotarget.15123.

Duan, T., W. Sun, M. Zhang, J. Ge, Y. He, J. Zhang, Y. Zheng, W. Yang, H. M. Shen, J. Yang, X. Zhu, and P. Yu. 2017. "Dietary restriction protects against diethylnitrosamine-induced hepatocellular tumorigenesis by restoring the disturbed gene expression profile." *Sci Rep* 7:43745. doi: 10.1038/srep43745.

Duell, E. J., E. Lucenteforte, S. H. Olson, P. M. Bracci, D. Li, H. A. Risch, D. T. Silverman, B. T. Ji, S. Gallinger, E. A. Holly, E. H. Fontham, P. Maisonneuve, H. B. Bueno-de-Mesquita, P. Ghadirian, R. C. Kurtz, E. Ludwig, H. Yu, A. B. Lowenfels, D. Seminara, G. M. Petersen, C. La Vecchia, and P. Boffetta. 2012. "Pancreatitis and pancreatic cancer risk: a pooled analysis in the International Pancreatic Cancer Case-Control Consortium (PanC4)." *Ann Oncol* 23 (11):2964–70. doi: 10.1093/annonc/mds140.

Dunlap, S. M., L. J. Chiao, L. Nogueira, J. Usary, C. M. Perou, L. Varticovski, and S. D. Hursting. 2012. "Dietary energy balance modulates epithelial-to-mesenchymal transition and tumor progression in murine claudin-low and basal-like mammary tumor models." *Cancer Prev Res (Phila)* 5 (7):930–42. doi: 10.1158/1940-6207.CAPR-12-0034.

Dunn, S. E., F. W. Kari, J. French, J. R. Leininger, G. Travlos, R. Wilson, and J. C. Barrett. 1997. "Dietary restriction reduces insulin-like growth factor I levels, which modulates apoptosis, cell proliferation, and tumor progression in p53-deficient mice." *Cancer Res* 57 (21):4667–72.

E, Shuang, K. Yamamoto, Y. Sakamoto, Y. Mizowaki, Y. Iwagaki, T. Kimura, K. Nakagawa, T. Miyazawa, and T. Tsuduki. 2017. "Intake of mulberry 1-deoxynojirimycin prevents colorectal cancer in mice." *J Clin Biochem Nutr* 61 (1):47–52. doi: 10.3164/jcbn.16-94.

Ehsanipour, E. A., X. Sheng, J. W. Behan, X. Wang, A. Butturini, V. I. Avramis, and S. D. Mittelman. 2013. "Adipocytes cause leukemia cell resistance to L-asparaginase via release of glutamine." *Cancer Res* 73 (10):2998–3006. doi: 10.1158/0008-5472.CAN-12-4402.

Engelman, R. W., N. K. Day, and R. A. Good. 1994. "Calorie intake during mammary development influences cancer risk: lasting inhibition of C3H/HeOu mammary tumorigenesis by peripubertal calorie restriction." *Cancer Res* 54 (21):5724–30.

Engeset, D., T. Braaten, B. Teucher, T. Kühn, H. B. Bueno-de-Mesquita, M. Leenders, A. Agudo, M. M. Bergmann, E. Valanou, A. Naska, A. Trichopoulou, T. J. Key, F. L. Crowe, K. Overvad, E. Sonestedt, A. Mattiello, P. H. Peeters, M. Wennberg, J. H. Jansson, M. C. Boutron-Ruault, L. Dossus, L. Dartois, K. Li, A. Barricarte, H. Ward, E. Riboli, C. Agnoli, J. M. Huerta, M. J. Sánchez, R. Tumino, J. M. Altzibar, P. Vineis, G. Masala, P. Ferrari, D. C. Muller, M. Johansson, M. Luisa Redondo, A. Tjønneland, A. Olsen, K. S. Olsen, M. Brustad, G. Skeie, and E. Lund. 2015. "Fish consumption and mortality in the European prospective investigation into cancer and nutrition cohort." *Eur J Epidemiol* 30 (1):57–70. doi: 10.1007/s10654-014-9966-4.

Faienza, M. F., M. Delvecchio, P. Giordano, L. Cavallo, M. Grano, G. Brunetti, and A. Ventura. 2015. "Metabolic syndrome in childhood leukemia survivors: a meta-analysis." *Endocrine* 49 (2):353–60. doi: 10.1007/s12020-014-0395-7.

Ferrante, J. M., D. C. Fyffe, M. L. Vega, A. K. Piasecki, P. A. Ohman-Strickland, and B. F. Crabtree. 2010. "Family physicians' barriers to cancer screening in extremely obese patients." *Obesity (Silver Spring)* 18 (6):1153–9. doi: 10.1038/oby.2009.481.

Fischbach, L. A., D. Y. Graham, J. R. Kramer, M. Rugge, G. Verstovsek, P. Parente, A. Alsarraj, S. Fitzgerald, Y. Shaib, N. S. Abraham, A. Kolpachi, S. Gupta, M. F. Vela, M. Velez, R. Cole, B. Anand, and H. B. El Serag. 2014. "Association between Helicobacter pylori and Barrett's esophagus: a case-control study." *Am J Gastroenterol* 109 (3):357–68. doi: 10.1038/ajg.2013.443.

Fontana, L., R. M. Adelaiye, A. L. Rastelli, K. M. Miles, E. Ciamporcero, V. D. Longo, H. Nguyen, R. Vessella, and R. Pili. 2013. "Dietary protein restriction inhibits tumor growth in human xenograft models." *Oncotarget* 4 (12):2451–61. doi: 10.18632/oncotarget.1586.

Frayling, T. M., N. J. Timpson, M. N. Weedon, E. Zeggini, R. M. Freathy, C. M. Lindgren, J. R. Perry, K. S. Elliott, H. Lango, N. W. Rayner, B. Shields, L. W. Harries, J. C. Barrett, S. Ellard, C. J. Groves, B. Knight, A. M. Patch, A. R. Ness, S. Ebrahim, D. A. Lawlor, S. M. Ring, Y. Ben-Shlomo, M. R. Jarvelin, U. Sovio, A. J. Bennett, D. Melzer, L. Ferrucci, R. J. Loos, I. Barroso, N. J. Wareham, F. Karpe, K. R. Owen, L. R. Cardon, M. Walker, G. A. Hitman, C. N. Palmer, A. S. Doney, A. D. Morris, G. D. Smith, A. T. Hattersley, and M. I. McCarthy. 2007. "A common variant in the FTO gene is associated with body mass index and predisposes to childhood and adult obesity." *Science* 316 (5826):889–94. doi: 10.1126/science.1141634.

Freeman, H. P. 2004. "Poverty, culture, and social injustice: determinants of cancer disparities." *CA Cancer J Clin* 54 (2):72–7. doi: 10.3322/canjclin.54.2.72.

Fursevich, D. M., G. M. LiMarzi, M. C. O'Dell, M. A. Hernandez, and W. F. Sensakovic. 2016. "Bariatric CT imaging: Challenges and solutions." *Radiographics* 36 (4):1076–86. doi: 10.1148/rg.2016150198.

Galet, C., A. Gray, J. W. Said, B. Castor, J. Wan, P. J. Beltran, F. J. Calzone, D. Elashoff, P. Cohen, and W. J. Aronson. 2013. "Effects of calorie restriction and IGF-1 receptor blockade on the progression of 22Rv1 prostate cancer xenografts." *Int J Mol Sci* 14 (7):13782–95. doi: 10.3390/ijms140713782.

Gallagher, E. J., and D. LeRoith. 2011. "Minireview: IGF, insulin, and cancer." *Endocrinology* 152 (7):2546–51. doi: 10.1210/en.2011-0231.

Ghasemi, A., J. Saeidi, M. Azimi-Nejad, and S. I. Hashemy. 2019. "Leptin-induced signaling pathways in cancer cell migration and invasion." *Cell Oncol (Dordr)* 42 (3):243–60. doi: 10.1007/s13402-019-00428-0.

Gillette, C. A., Z. Zhu, K. C. Westerlind, C. L. Melby, P. Wolfe, and H. J. Thompson. 1997. "Energy availability and mammary carcinogenesis: effects of calorie restriction and exercise." *Carcinogenesis* 18 (6):1183–8. doi: 10.1093/carcin/18.6.1183.

Gong, T. T., Q. J. Wu, Y. L. Wang, and X. X. Ma. 2015. "Circulating adiponectin, leptin and adiponectin-leptin ratio and endometrial cancer risk: evidence from a meta-analysis of epidemiologic studies." *Int J Cancer* 137 (8):1967–78. doi: 10.1002/ijc.29561.

Gravaghi, C., J. Bo, K. M. Laperle, F. Quimby, R. Kucherlapati, W. Edelmann, and S. A. Lamprecht. 2008. "Obesity enhances gastrointestinal tumorigenesis in Apc-mutant mice." *Int J Obes (Lond)* 32 (11):1716–9. doi: 10.1038/ijo.2008.149.

Greathouse, K. L., J. R. White, R. N. Padgett, B. G. Perrotta, G. D. Jenkins, N. Chia, and J. Chen. 2019. "Gut microbiome meta-analysis reveals dysbiosis is independent of body mass index in predicting risk of obesity-associated CRC." *BMJ Open Gastroenterol* 6 (1):e000247. doi: 10.1136/bmjgast-2018-000247.

Griggs, J. J., P. B. Mangu, H. Anderson, E. P. Balaban, J. J. Dignam, W. M. Hryniuk, V. A. Morrison, T. M. Pini, C. D. Runowicz, G. L. Rosner, M. Shayne, A. Sparreboom, L. E. Sucheston, G. H. Lyman, and Oncology American Society of Clinical. 2012. "Appropriate chemotherapy dosing for obese adult patients with cancer: American society of clinical oncology clinical practice guideline." *J Clin Oncol* 30 (13):1553–61. doi: 10.1200/JCO.2011.39.9436.

Grigura, V., M. Barbier, A. P. Zarov, and C. K. Kaufman. 2018. "Feeding amount significantly alters overt tumor onset rate in a zebrafish melanoma model." *Biol Open* 7 (1). doi: 10.1242/bio.030726.

Gupta, A., Y. Herman, C. Ayers, M. S. Beg, S. G. Lakoski, S. M. Abdullah, D. H. Johnson, and I. J. Neeland. 2016. "Plasma leptin levels and risk of incident cancer: Results from the dallas heart study." *PLoS One* 11 (9):e0162845. doi: 10.1371/journal.pone.0162845.

Gusscott, S., C. E. Jenkins, S. H. Lam, V. Giambra, M. Pollak, and A. P. Weng. 2016. "IGF1R derived PI3K/AKT signaling maintains growth in a subset of human T-cell acute lymphoblastic leukemias." *PLoS One* 11 (8):e0161158. doi: 10.1371/journal.pone.0161158.

Hall, R. G., G. W. Jean, M. Sigler, and S. Shah. 2013. "Dosing considerations for obese patients receiving cancer chemotherapeutic agents." *Ann Pharmacother* 47 (12):1666–74. doi: 10.1177/1060028013509789.

Hanahan, D., and R. A. Weinberg. 2000. "The hallmarks of cancer." *Cell* 100 (1):57–70. doi: 10.1016/S0092-8674(00)81683-9.

Harbuzariu, A., A. Rampoldi, D. S. Daley-Brown, P. Candelaria, T. L. Harmon, C. C. Lipsey, D. J. Beech, A. Quarshie, G. O. Ilies, and R. R. Gonzalez-Perez. 2017. "Leptin-notch signaling axis is involved in pancreatic cancer progression." *Oncotarget* 8 (5):7740–52. doi: 10.18632/oncotarget.13946.

Hardefeldt, P. J., R. Penninkilampi, S. Edirimanne, and G. D. Eslick. 2018. "Physical activity and weight loss reduce the risk of breast cancer: A meta-analysis of 139 prospective and retrospective studies." *Clin Breast Cancer* 18 (4):e601–12. doi: 10.1016/j.clbc.2017.10.010.

Hardman, W. E., M. P. Moyer, and I. L. Cameron. 1999. "Fish oil supplementation enhanced CPT-11 (irinotecan) efficacy against MCF7 breast carcinoma xenografts and ameliorated intestinal side-effects." *Br J Cancer* 81 (3):440–8. doi: 10.1038/sj.bjc.6690713.

Hardman, W. E., C. P. Avula, G. Fernandes, and I. L. Cameron. 2001. "Three percent dietary fish oil concentrate increased efficacy of doxorubicin against MDA-MB 231 breast cancer xenografts." *Clin Cancer Res* 7 (7):2041–9.

Harvey, A. E., L. M. Lashinger, G. Otto, N. P. Nunez, and S. D. Hursting. 2013. "Decreased systemic IGF-1 in response to calorie restriction modulates murine tumor cell growth, nuclear factor-kappaB activation, and inflammation-related gene expression." *Mol Carcinog* 52 (12):997–1006. doi: 10.1002/mc.21940.

Hermouet, S., E. Bigot-Corbel, and B. Gardie. 2015. "Pathogenesis of myeloproliferative neoplasms: Role and mechanisms of chronic inflammation." *Mediators Inflamm* 2015:145293. doi: 10.1155/2015/145293.

Hirose, Y., K. Hata, T. Kuno, K. Yoshida, K. Sakata, Y. Yamada, T. Tanaka, B. S. Reddy, and H. Mori. 2004. "Enhancement of development of azoxymethane-induced colonic premalignant lesions in C57BL/KsJ-db/db mice." *Carcinogenesis* 25 (5):821–5. doi: 10.1093/carcin/bgh059.

Hosseini, B., A. Saedisomeolia, and M. Allman-Farinelli. 2017. "Association between antioxidant intake/status and obesity: a systematic review of observational studies." *Biol Trace Elem Res* 175 (2):287–97. doi: 10.1007/s12011-016-0785-1.

Hsu, H. P., Y. S. Shan, M. D. Lai, and P. W. Lin. 2010. "Osteopontin-positive infiltrating tumor-associated macrophages in bulky ampullary cancer predict survival." *Cancer Biol Ther* 10 (2):144–54. doi: 10.4161/cbt.10.2.12160.

Hsu, L. H., N. M. Chu, and S. H. Kao. 2017. "Estrogen, estrogen receptor and lung cancer." *Int J Mol Sci* 18 (8). doi: 10.3390/ijms18081713.

Hursting, S. D., B. H. Margolin, and B. R. Switzer. 1993. "Diet and human leukemia: an analysis of international data." *Prev Med* 22 (3):409–22.

Hursting, S. D., B. R. Switzer, J. E. French, and F. W. Kari. 1993. "The growth hormone: insulin-like growth factor 1 axis is a mediator of diet restriction-induced inhibition of mononuclear cell leukemia in Fischer rats." *Cancer Res* 53 (12):2750–7.

Hursting, S. D., S. N. Perkins, and J. M. Phang. 1994. "Calorie restriction delays spontaneous tumorigenesis in p53-knockout transgenic mice." *Proc Natl Acad Sci U S A* 91 (15):7036–40. doi: 10.1073/pnas.91.15.7036.

Hursting, S. D., S. N. Perkins, C. C. Brown, D. C. Haines, and J. M. Phang. 1997. "Calorie restriction induces a p53-independent delay of spontaneous carcinogenesis in p53-deficient and wild-type mice." *Cancer Res* 57 (14):2843–6.

Incio, J., H. Liu, P. Suboj, S. M. Chin, I. X. Chen, M. Pinter, M. R. Ng, H. T. Nia, J. Grahovac, S. Kao, S. Babykutty, Y. Huang, K. Jung, N. N. Rahbari, X. Han, V. P. Chauhan, J. D. Martin, J. Kahn, P. Huang, V. Desphande, J. Michaelson, T. P. Michelakos, C. R. Ferrone, R. Soares, Y. Boucher, D. Fukumura, and R. K. Jain. 2016. "Obesity-induced inflammation and desmoplasia promote pancreatic cancer progression and resistance to chemotherapy." *Cancer Discov* 6 (8):852–69. doi: 10.1158/2159-8290.CD-15-1177.

Inoue, M., and S. Tsugane. 2012. "Insulin resistance and cancer: epidemiological evidence." *Endocr Relat Cancer* 19 (5):F1–8. doi: 10.1530/ERC-12-0142.

James, S. J., and L. Muskhelishvili. 1994. "Rates of apoptosis and proliferation vary with caloric intake and may influence incidence of spontaneous hepatoma in C57BL/6 x C3H F1 mice." *Cancer Res* 54 (21):5508–10.

Jiang, Y. S., and F. R. Wang. 2013. "Caloric restriction reduces edema and prolongs survival in a mouse glioma model." *J Neurooncol* 114 (1):25–32. doi: 10.1007/s11060-013-1154-y.

Jiang, W., Z. Zhu, and H. J. Thompson. 2008. "Dietary energy restriction modulates the activity of AMP-activated protein kinase, Akt, and mammalian target of rapamycin in mammary carcinomas, mammary gland, and liver." *Cancer Res* 68 (13):5492–9. doi: 10.1158/0008-5472.CAN-07-6721.

Jongbloed, F., S. A. Huisman, H. van Steeg, J. L. A. Pennings, I. Jzermans JNM, M. E. T. Dolle, and R. W. F. de Bruin. 2019. "The transcriptomic response to irinotecan in colon carcinoma bearing mice preconditioned by fasting." *Oncotarget* 10 (22):2224–34. doi: 10.18632/oncotarget.26776.

Kandori, H., S. Suzuki, M. Asamoto, T. Murasaki, T. Mingxi, K. Ogawa, and T. Shirai. 2005. "Influence of atrazine administration and reduction of calorie intake on prostate carcinogenesis in probasin/SV40 T antigen transgenic rats." *Cancer Sci* 96 (4):221–6. doi: 10.1111/j.1349-7006.2005.00041.x.

Kawai, H., A. Ishii, K. Washiya, T. Konno, H. Kon, C. Yamaya, I. Ono, Y. Minamiya, and J. Ogawa. 2005. "Estrogen receptor alpha and beta are prognostic factors in non-small cell lung cancer." *Clin Cancer Res* 11 (14):5084–9. doi: 10.1158/1078-0432.CCR-05-0200.

Kehm, R. D., L. G. Spector, J. N. Poynter, D. M. Vock, S. F. Altekruse, and T. L. Osypuk. 2018. "Does socioeconomic status account for racial and ethnic disparities in childhood cancer survival?" *Cancer* 124 (20):4090–7. doi: 10.1002/cncr.31560.

Kendrick, J. G., R. R. Carr, and M. H. Ensom. 2015. "Pediatric obesity: Pharmacokinetics and implications for drug dosing." *Clin Ther* 37 (9):1897–923. doi: 10.1016/j.clinthera.2015.05.495.

Key, T. J., P. N. Appleby, F. L. Crowe, K. E. Bradbury, J. A. Schmidt, and R. C. Travis. 2014. "Cancer in British vegetarians: updated analyses of 4998 incident cancers in a cohort of 32,491 meat eaters, 8612 fish eaters, 18,298 vegetarians, and 2246 vegans." *Am J Clin Nutr* 100 (Suppl 1):378S–85S. doi: 10.3945/ajcn.113.071266.

Khadge, S., G. M. Thiele, J. G. Sharp, T. R. McGuire, L. W. Klassen, P. N. Black, C. C. DiRusso, L. Cook, and J. E. Talmadge. 2018. "Long-chain omega-3 polyunsaturated fatty acids decrease mammary tumor growth, multiorgan metastasis and enhance survival." *Clin Exp Metastasis* 35 (8):797–818. doi: 10.1007/s10585-018-9941-7.

Khatua, B., B. El-Kurdi, and V. P. Singh. 2017. "Obesity and pancreatitis." *Curr Opin Gastroenterol* 33 (5):374–82. doi: 10.1097/MOG.0000000000000386.

Kiefer, F. W., M. Zeyda, J. Todoric, J. Huber, R. Geyeregger, T. Weichhart, O. Aszmann, B. Ludvik, G. R. Silberhumer, G. Prager, and T. M. Stulnig. 2008. "Osteopontin expression in human and murine obesity: extensive local up-regulation in adipose tissue but minimal systemic alterations." *Endocrinology* 149 (3):1350–7. doi: 10.1210/en.2007-1312.

Kim, J. E., G. Lin, J. Zhou, J. A. Mund, J. Case, and W. W. Campbell. 2017. "Weight loss achieved using an energy restriction diet with normal or higher dietary protein decreased the number of CD14(++)CD16(+) proinflammatory monocytes and plasma lipids and lipoproteins in middle-aged, overweight, and obese adults." *Nutr Res* 40:75–84 doi: 10.1016/j.nutres.2017.02.007.

Kiraly, O., G. Gong, W. Olipitz, S. Muthupalani, and B. P. Engelward. 2015. "Inflammation-induced cell proliferation potentiates DNA damage-induced mutations in vivo." *PLoS Genet* 11 (2):e1004901. doi: 10.1371/journal.pgen.1004901.

Klement, R. J., C. E. Champ, C. Otto, and U. Kammerer. 2016. "Anti-tumor effects of ketogenic diets in mice: A meta-analysis." *PLoS One* 11 (5):e0155050. doi: 10.1371/journal.pone.0155050.

Kohler, L. N., D. O. Garcia, R. B. Harris, E. Oren, D. J. Roe, and E. T. Jacobs. 2016. "Adherence to diet and physical activity cancer prevention guidelines and cancer outcomes: A systematic review." *Cancer Epidemiol Biomarkers Prev* 25 (7):1018–28. doi: 10.1158/1055-9965.EPI-16-0121.

Kong, Y., Q. Dong, H. Ji, M. Sang, Y. Ding, M. Zhao, H. Yang, and C. Geng. 2019. "The effect of the leptin and leptin receptor expression on the efficacy of neoadjuvant chemotherapy in breast cancer." *Med Sci Monit* 25:3005–13 doi: 10.12659/MSM.915368.

Koru-Sengul, T., A. M. Santander, F. Miao, L. G. Sanchez, M. Jorda, S. Gluck, T. A. Ince, M. Nadji, Z. Chen, M. L. Penichet, M. P. Cleary, and M. Torroella-Kouri. 2016. "Breast cancers from black women exhibit higher numbers of immunosuppressive macrophages with proliferative activity and of crown-like structures associated with lower survival compared to non-black Latinas and Caucasians." *Breast Cancer Res Treat* 158 (1):113–26. doi: 10.1007/s10549-016-3847-3.

Kridel, S.J., F. Axelrod, N. Rozenkrantz, and J.W. Smith. 2004. "Orlistat is a novel inhibitor of fatty acid synthase with antitumor activity." *Cancer Res* 64 (6):2070–75.

Kusuoka, O., R. Fujiwara-Tani, C. Nakashima, K. Fujii, H. Ohmori, T. Mori, S. Kishi, Y. Miyagawa, K. Goto, I. Kawahara, and H. Kuniyasu. 2018. "Intermittent calorie restriction enhances epithelial-mesenchymal transition through the alteration of energy metabolism in a mouse tumor model." *Int J Oncol* 52 (2):413–23. doi: 10.3892/ijo.2017.4229.

Labbé, D. P., G. Zadra, M. Yang, J. M. Reyes, C. Y. Lin, S. Cacciatore, E. M. Ebot, A. L. Creech, F. Giunchi, M. Fiorentino, H. Elfandy, S. Syamala, E. D. Karoly, M. Alshalalfa, N. Erho, A. Ross, E. M. Schaeffer, E. A. Gibb, M. Takhar, R. B. Den, J. Lehrer, R. J. Karnes, S. J. Freedland, E. Davicioni, D. E. Spratt, L. Ellis, J. D. Jaffe, A. V. D'Amico, P. W. Kantoff, J. E. Bradner, L. A. Mucci, J. E. Chavarro, M. Loda, and M. Brown. 2019. "High-fat diet fuels prostate cancer progression by rewiring the metabolome and amplifying the MYC program." *Nat Commun* 10 (1):4358. doi: 10.1038/s41467-019-12298-z.

Ladas, E. J., T. M. Blonquist, M. Puligandla, M. Orjuela, K. Stevenson, P. D. Cole, U. H. Athale, L. A. Clavell, J. M. Leclerc, C. Laverdiere, B. Michon, M. A. Schorin, J. Greene Welch, B. L. Asselin, S. E. Sallan, L. B. Silverman, and K. M. Kelly. 2020. "Protective effects of dietary intake of antioxidants and treatment-related toxicity in childhood leukemia: A report from the DALLT Cohort." *J Clin Oncol*:JCO1902555. doi: 10.1200/JCO.19.02555.

Lai, R., Z. Bian, H. Lin, J. Ren, H. Zhou, and H. Guo. 2017. "The association between dietary protein intake and colorectal cancer risk: a meta-analysis." *World J Surg Oncol* 15 (1):169. doi: 10.1186/s12957-017-1241-1.

Lanza-Jacoby, S., G. Yan, G. Radice, C. LePhong, J. Baliff, and R. Hess. 2013. "Calorie restriction delays the progression of lesions to pancreatic cancer in the LSL-KrasG12D; Pdx-1/Cre mouse model of pancreatic cancer." *Exp Biol Med (Maywood)* 238 (7):787–97. doi: 10.1177/1535370213493727.

Laron, Z. 2015. "Lessons from 50 years of study of laron syndrome." *Endocr Pract* 21 (12):1395–402. doi: 10.4158/EP15939.RA.

Lashinger, L. M., L. M. Malone, M. J. McArthur, J. A. Goldberg, E. A. Daniels, A. Pavone, J. K. Colby, N. C. Smith, S. N. Perkins, S. M. Fischer, and S. D. Hursting. 2011. "Genetic reduction of insulin-like growth factor-1 mimics the anticancer effects of calorie restriction on cyclooxygenase-2-driven pancreatic neoplasia." *Cancer Prev Res (Phila)* 4 (7):1030–40. doi: 10.1158/1940-6207.CAPR-11-0027.

Leclerc, G. M., G. J. Leclerc, J. N. Kuznetsov, J. DeSalvo, and J. C. Barredo. 2013. "Metformin induces apoptosis through AMPK-dependent inhibition of UPR signaling in ALL lymphoblasts." *PLoS One* 8 (8):e74420. doi: 10.1371/journal.pone.0074420.

Lee, J. E., D. Spiegelman, D. J. Hunter, D. Albanes, L. Bernstein, P. A. van den Brandt, J. E. Buring, E. Cho, D. R. English, J. L. Freudenheim, G. G. Giles, S. Graham, P. L. Horn-Ross, N. Hakansson, M. F. Leitzmann, S. Mannisto, M. L. McCullough, A. B. Miller, A. S. Parker, T. E. Rohan, A. Schatzkin, L. J. Schouten, C. Sweeney, W. C. Willett, A. Wolk, S. M. Zhang, and S. A. Smith-Warner. 2008. "Fat, protein, and meat consumption and renal cell cancer risk: a pooled analysis of 13 prospective studies." *J Natl Cancer Inst* 100 (23):1695–706. doi: 10.1093/jnci/djn386.

Lee, C., L. Raffaghello, S. Brandhorst, F. M. Safdie, G. Bianchi, A. Martin-Montalvo, V. Pistoia, M. Wei, S. Hwang, A. Merlino, L. Emionite, R. de Cabo, and V. D. Longo. 2012. "Fasting cycles retard growth of tumors and sensitize a range of cancer cell types to chemotherapy." *Sci Transl Med* 4 (124):124ra27. doi: 10.1126/scitranslmed.3003293.

Lende, T. H., M. Austdal, A. E. Varhaugvik, I. Skaland, E. Gudlaugsson, J. T. Kvaløy, L. A. Akslen, H. Søiland, E. A. M. Janssen, and J. P. A. Baak. 2019. "Influence of pre-operative oral carbohydrate loading vs. standard fasting on tumor proliferation and clinical outcome in breast cancer patients: a randomized trial." *BMC Cancer* 19 (1):1076. doi: 10.1186/s12885-019-6275-z.

Lennon, H., M. Sperrin, E. Badrick, and A. G. Renehan. 2016. "The obesity paradox in cancer: a review." *Curr Oncol Rep* 18 (9):56. doi: 10.1007/s11912-016-0539-4.

Li, X. J., X. Q. Luo, B. W. Han, F. T. Duan, P. P. Wei, and Y. Q. Chen. 2013. "MicroRNA-100/99a, deregulated in acute lymphoblastic leukaemia, suppress proliferation and promote apoptosis by regulating the FKBP51 and IGF1R/mTOR signalling pathways." *Br J Cancer* 109 (8):2189–98. doi: 10.1038/bjc.2013.562.

Liao, W. C., Y. K. Tu, M. S. Wu, J. T. Lin, H. P. Wang, and K. L. Chien. 2015. "Blood glucose concentration and risk of pancreatic cancer: systematic review and dose-response meta-analysis." *BMJ* 350:g7371. doi: 10.1136/bmj.g7371.

Lin, C. N., C. J. Wang, Y. J. Chao, M. D. Lai, and Y. S. Shan. 2015. "The significance of the co-existence of osteopontin and tumor-associated macrophages in gastric cancer progression." *BMC Cancer* 15:128. doi: 10.1186/s12885-015-1114-3.

Liu, H., J. He, S. P. Koh, Y. Zhong, Z. Liu, Z. Wang, Y. Zhang, Z. Li, B. T. Tam, P. Lin, M. Xiao, K. H. Young, B. Amini, M. W. Starbuck, H. C. Lee, N. M. Navone, R. E. Davis, Q. Tong, P. L. Bergsagel, J. Hou, Q. Yi, R. Z. Orlowski, R. F. Gagel, and J. Yang. 2019a. "Reprogrammed marrow adipocytes contribute to myeloma-induced bone disease." *Sci Transl Med* 11 (494). doi: 10.1126/scitranslmed.aau9087.

Liu, T., Y. Wu, L. Wang, X. Pang, L. Zhao, H. Yuan, and C. Zhang. 2019b. "A more robust gut microbiota in calorie-restricted mice is associated with attenuated intestinal injury caused by the chemotherapy drug cyclophosphamide." *mBio* 10 (2). doi: 10.1128/mBio.02903-18.

Lope, V., M. Martin, A. Castello, A. Ruiz, A. M. Casas, J. M. Baena-Canada, S. Antolin, M. Ramos-Vazquez, J. A. Garcia-Saenz, M. Munoz, A. Lluch, A. de Juan-Ferre, C. Jara, P. Sanchez-Rovira, A. Anton, J. I. Chacon, A. Arcusa, M. A. Jimeno, S. Bezares, J. Vioque, E. Carrasco, B. Perez-Gomez, and M. Pollan. 2019. "Overeating, caloric restriction and breast cancer risk by pathologic subtype: the EPIGEICAM study." *Sci Rep* 9 (1):3904. doi: 10.1038/s41598-019-39346-4.

Lu, Z., J. Xie, G. Wu, J. Shen, R. Collins, W. Chen, X. Kang, M. Luo, Y. Zou, L. J. Huang, J. F. Amatruda, T. Slone, N. Winick, P. E. Scherer, and C. C. Zhang. 2017. "Fasting selectively blocks development of acute lymphoblastic leukemia via leptin-receptor upregulation." *Nat Med* 23 (1):79–90. doi: 10.1038/nm.4252.

Luo, J., R. T. Chlebowski, M. Hendryx, T. Rohan, J. Wactawski-Wende, C. A. Thomson, A. S. Felix, C. Chen, W. Barrington, M. Coday, M. Stefanick, E. LeBlanc, and K. L. Margolis. 2017. "Intentional weight loss and endometrial cancer risk." *J Clin Oncol* 35 (11):1189–93. doi: 10.1200/JCO.2016.70.5822.

Lussier, D. M., E. C. Woolf, J. L. Johnson, K. S. Brooks, J. N. Blattman, and A. C. Scheck. 2016. "Enhanced immunity in a mouse model of malignant glioma is mediated by a therapeutic ketogenic diet." *BMC Cancer* 16:310. doi: 10.1186/s12885-016-2337-7.

Lv, M., X. Zhu, H. Wang, F. Wang, and W. Guan. 2014. "Roles of caloric restriction, ketogenic diet and intermittent fasting during initiation, progression and metastasis of cancer in animal models: a systematic review and meta-analysis." *PLoS One* 9 (12):e115147. doi: 10.1371/journal.pone.0115147.

Ma, D., X. Chen, P. Y. Zhang, H. Zhang, L. J. Wei, S. Hu, J. Z. Tang, M. T. Zhou, C. Xie, R. Ou, Y. Xu, and K. F. Tang. 2018a. "Upregulation of the ALDOA/DNA-PK/p53 pathway by dietary restriction suppresses tumor growth." *Oncogene* 37 (8):1041–48. doi: 10.1038/onc.2017.398.

Ma, Z., A. B. Parris, E. W. Howard, Y. Shi, S. Yang, Y. Jiang, L. Kong, and X. Yang. 2018b. "Caloric restriction inhibits mammary tumorigenesis in MMTV-ErbB2 transgenic mice through the suppression of ER and ErbB2 pathways and inhibition of epithelial cell stemness in premalignant mammary tissues." *Carcinogenesis* 39 (10):1264–73. doi: 10.1093/carcin/bgy096.

Mai, V., L. H. Colbert, D. Berrigan, S. N. Perkins, R. Pfeiffer, J. A. Lavigne, E. Lanza, D. C. Haines, A. Schatzkin, and S. D. Hursting. 2003. "Calorie restriction and diet composition modulate spontaneous intestinal tumorigenesis in Apc(Min) mice through different mechanisms." *Cancer Res* 63 (8):1752–5.

Mao, Y., Y. Tie, and J. Du. 2018. "Association between dietary protein intake and prostate cancer risk: evidence from a meta-analysis." *World J Surg Oncol* 16 (1):152. doi: 10.1186/s12957-018-1452-0.

Marengo, A., C. Rosso, and E. Bugianesi. 2016. "Liver cancer: Connections with Obesity, fatty liver, and cirrhosis." *Annu Rev Med* 67:103–17 doi: 10.1146/annurev-med-090514-013832.

Marsh, J., P. Mukherjee, and T. N. Seyfried. 2008. "Akt-dependent proapoptotic effects of dietary restriction on late-stage management of a phosphatase and tensin homologue/tuberous sclerosis complex 2-deficient mouse astrocytoma." *Clin Cancer Res* 14 (23):7751–62. doi: 10.1158/1078-0432.CCR-08-0213.

Martin-McGill, K. J., N. Srikandarajah, A. G. Marson, C. Tudur Smith, and M. D. Jenkinson. 2018. "The role of ketogenic diets in the therapeutic management of adult and paediatric gliomas: a systematic review." *CNS Oncol* 7 (2):CNS17. doi: 10.2217/cns-2017-0030.

Maruvada, P., V. Leone, L. M. Kaplan, and E. B. Chang. 2017. "The human microbiome and obesity: Moving beyond associations." *Cell Host Microbe* 22 (5):589–99. doi: 10.1016/j.chom.2017.10.005.

McConnell, R., F. D. Gilliland, M. Goran, H. Allayee, A. Hricko, and S. Mittelman. 2016. "Does near-roadway air pollution contribute to childhood obesity?" *Pediatr Obes* 11 (1):1–3. doi: 10.1111/ijpo.12016.

McCormick, D. L., W. D. Johnson, T. M. Haryu, M. C. Bosland, R. A. Lubet, and V. E. Steele. 2007. "Null effect of dietary restriction on prostate carcinogenesis in the Wistar-Unilever rat." *Nutr Cancer* 57 (2):194–200. doi: 10.1080/01635580701277494.

McQuade, J. L., C. R. Daniel, K. R. Hess, C. Mak, D. Y. Wang, R. R. Rai, J. J. Park, L. E. Haydu, C. Spencer, M. Wongchenko, S. Lane, D. Y. Lee, M. Kaper, M. McKean, K. E. Beckermann, S. M. Rubinstein, I. Rooney, L. Musib, N. Budha, J. Hsu, T. S. Nowicki, A. Avila, T. Haas, M. Puligandla, S. Lee, S. Fang, J. A. Wargo, J. E. Gershenwald, J. E. Lee, P. Hwu, P. B. Chapman, J. A. Sosman, D. Schadendorf, J. J. Grob, K. T. Flaherty, D. Walker, Y. Yan, E. McKenna, J. J. Legos, M. S. Carlino, A. Ribas, J. M. Kirkwood, G. V. Long, D. B. Johnson, A. M. Menzies, and M. A. Davies. 2018. "Association of body-mass index and outcomes in patients with metastatic melanoma treated with targeted therapy, immunotherapy, or chemotherapy: a retrospective, multicohort analysis." *Lancet Oncol* 19 (3):310–22. doi: 10.1016/S1470-2045(18)30078-0.

Mikami, D., M. Kobayashi, J. Uwada, T. Yazawa, K. Kamiyama, K. Nishimori, Y. Nishikawa, S. Nishikawa, S. Yokoi, T. Taniguchi, and M. Iwano. 2020. "β-Hydroxybutyrate enhances the cytotoxic effect of cisplatin via the inhibition of HDAC/survivin axis in human hepatocellular carcinoma cells." *J Pharmacol Sci* 142 (1):1–8. doi: 10.1016/j.jphs.2019.10.007.

Miller, K. D., R. L. Siegel, C. C. Lin, A. B. Mariotto, J. L. Kramer, J. H. Rowland, K. D. Stein, R. Alteri, and A. Jemal. 2016. "Cancer treatment and survivorship statistics, 2016." *CA Cancer J Clin* 66 (4):271–89. doi: 10.3322/caac.21349.

Miller, K. D., A. Goding Sauer, A. P. Ortiz, S. A. Fedewa, P. S. Pinheiro, G. Tortolero-Luna, D. Martinez-Tyson, A. Jemal, and R. L. Siegel. 2018. "Cancer statistics for hispanics/latinos, 2018." *CA Cancer J Clin* 68 (6):425–45. doi: 10.3322/caac.21494.

Mittelman, S. D. 2020. "The role of diet in cancer prevention and chemotherapy efficacy." *Annu Rev Nutr* 40:273–97 doi: 10.1146/annurev-nutr-013120-041149.

Mizuno, N. K., O. P. Rogozina, C. M. Seppanen, D. J. Liao, M. P. Cleary, and M. E. Grossmann. 2013. "Combination of intermittent calorie restriction and eicosapentaenoic acid for inhibition of mammary tumors." *Cancer Prev Res (Phila)* 6 (6):540–7. doi: 10.1158/1940-6207.CAPR-13-0033.

Molina-Aguilar, C., M. J. Guerrero-Carrillo, J. J. Espinosa-Aguirre, S. Olguin-Reyes, T. Castro-Belio, O. Vazquez-Martinez, J. B. Rivera-Zavala, and M. Diaz-Munoz. 2017. "Time-caloric restriction inhibits the neoplastic transformation of cirrhotic liver in rats treated with diethylnitrosamine." *Carcinogenesis* 38 (8):847–58. doi: 10.1093/carcin/bgx052.

Moore, T., L. Beltran, S. Carbajal, S. D. Hursting, and J. DiGiovanni. 2012. "Energy balance modulates mouse skin tumor promotion through altered IGF-1R and EGFR crosstalk." *Cancer Prev Res (Phila)* 5 (10):1236–46. doi: 10.1158/1940-6207.CAPR-12-0234.

Morin, C., and S. Fortin. 2017. "Docosahexaenoic acid monoglyceride increases carboplatin activity in lung cancer models by targeting EGFR." *Anticancer Res* 37 (11):6015–23. doi: 10.21873/anticanres. 12048.

Morris, P. G., C. A. Hudis, D. Giri, M. Morrow, D. J. Falcone, X. K. Zhou, B. Du, E. Brogi, C. B. Crawford, L. Kopelovich, K. Subbaramaiah, and A. J. Dannenberg. 2011. "Inflammation and increased aromatase expression occur in the breast tissue of obese women with breast cancer." *Cancer Prevention Research* 4 (7):1021–29. doi: 10.1158/1940-6207.Capr-11-0110.

Morscher, R. J., S. Aminzadeh-Gohari, R. G. Feichtinger, J. A. Mayr, R. Lang, D. Neureiter, W. Sperl, and B. Kofler. 2015. "Inhibition of neuroblastoma tumor growth by ketogenic diet and/or calorie restriction in a CD1-Nu mouse model." *PLoS One* 10 (6):e0129802. doi: 10.1371/journal.pone.0129802.

Morscher, R. J., S. Aminzadeh-Gohari, C. Hauser-Kronberger, R. G. Feichtinger, W. Sperl, and B. Kofler. 2016. "Combination of metronomic cyclophosphamide and dietary intervention inhibits neuroblastoma growth in a CD1-nu mouse model." *Oncotarget* 7 (13):17060–73. doi: 10.18632/oncotarget.7929.

Murakami, M., N. Sato, K. Tashiro, T. Nakamura, and H. Masunaga. 2009. "Effects of caloric intake on intestinal mucosal morphology and immune cells in rats treated with 5-Fluorouracil." *J Clin Biochem Nutr* 45 (1):74–81. doi: 10.3164/jcbn.08-264.

Newman, L. A., and L. M. Kaljee. 2017. "Health disparities and triple-negative breast cancer in African American women: A review." *JAMA Surg* 152 (5):485–93. doi: 10.1001/jamasurg.2017.0005.

Nie, H., H. Ju, J. Fan, X. Shi, Y. Cheng, X. Cang, Z. Zheng, X. Duan, and W. Yi. 2020. "O-GlcNAcylation of PGK1 coordinates glycolysis and TCA cycle to promote tumor growth." *Nat Commun* 11 (1):36. doi: 10.1038/s41467-019-13601-8.

Nieman, K.M., H.A. Kenny, C.V. Penicka, A. Ladanyi, R. Buell-Gutbrod, M.R. Zillhardt, I.L. Romero, M.S. Carey, G.B. Mills, G.S. Hotamisligil, S.D. Yamada, M.E. Peter, K. Gwin, and E. Lengyel. 2011. "Adipocytes promote ovarian cancer metastasis and provide energy for rapid tumor growth." *Nat.Med.* 17 (11):1498–503.

Nieman, K. M., I. L. Romero, B. Van Houten, and E. Lengyel. 2013. "Adipose tissue and adipocytes support tumorigenesis and metastasis." Biochim Biophys Acta 1831 (10):1533–41. doi: 10.1016/j.bbalip.2013.02.010.

Njei, B., T. R. McCarty, and J. W. Birk. 2016. "Trends in esophageal cancer survival in United States adults from 1973 to 2009: A SEER database analysis." *J Gastroenterol Hepatol* 31 (6):1141–6. doi: 10.1111/jgh.13289.

Nogueira, L. M., S. M. Dunlap, N. A. Ford, and S. D. Hursting. 2012. "Calorie restriction and rapamycin inhibit MMTV-Wnt-1 mammary tumor growth in a mouse model of postmenopausal obesity." *Endocr Relat Cancer* 19 (1):57–68. doi: 10.1530/ERC-11-0213.

Nottage, K. A., K. K. Ness, C. Li, D. Srivastava, L. L. Robison, and M. M. Hudson. 2014. "Metabolic syndrome and cardiovascular risk among long-term survivors of acute lymphoblastic leukaemia: from the St. Jude Lifetime Cohort." *Br J Haematol* 165 (3):364–74. doi: 10.1111/bjh.12754.

O'Keefe, S. J. 2016. "Diet, microorganisms and their metabolites, and colon cancer." *Nat Rev Gastroenterol Hepatol* 13 (12):691–706. doi: 10.1038/nrgastro.2016.165.

Oppezzo, P., Y. Vasconcelos, C. Settegrana, D. Jeannel, F. Vuillier, M. Legarff-Tavernier, E.Y. Kimura, S. Bechet, G. Dumas, M. Brissard, H. Merle-Beral, M. Yamamoto, G. Dighiero, and F. Davi. 2005. "The LPL/ADAM29 expression ratio is a novel prognosis indicator in chronic lymphocytic leukemia." *Blood* 106 (2):650–7.

Orgel, E., J. M. Genkinger, D. Aggarwal, L. Sung, M. Nieder, and E. J. Ladas. 2016a. "Association of body mass index and survival in pediatric leukemia: a meta-analysis." *Am J Clin Nutr* 103 (3):808–17. doi: 10.3945/ajcn.115.124586.

Orgel, E., N. M. Mueske, R. Sposto, V. Gilsanz, D. R. Freyer, and S. D. Mittelman. 2016b. "Limitations of body mass index to assess body composition due to sarcopenic obesity during leukemia therapy." *Leuk Lymphoma*:1–8. doi: 10.3109/10428194.2015.1136741.

Özdemir, B. C., and G. P. Dotto. 2017. "Racial differences in cancer susceptibility and survival: More than the color of the skin?" *Trends Cancer* 3 (3):181–97. doi: 10.1016/j.trecan.2017.02.002.

Pang, Y., and W. Wang. 2018. "Dietary protein intake and risk of ovarian cancer: evidence from a meta-analysis of observational studies." *Biosci Rep* 38 (6). doi: 10.1042/BSR20181857.

Pape-Ansorge, K. A., J. P. Grande, T. A. Christensen, N. J. Maihle, and M. P. Cleary. 2002. "Effect of moderate caloric restriction and/or weight cycling on mammary tumor incidence and latency in MMTV-Neu female mice." *Nutr Cancer* 44 (2):162–8. doi: 10.1207/S15327914NC4402_07.

Papier, K., T. Y. Tong, P. N. Appleby, K. E. Bradbury, G. K. Fensom, A. Knuppel, A. Perez-Cornago, J. A. Schmidt, R. C. Travis, and T. J. Key. 2019. "Comparison of major protein-source foods and other food groups in meat-eaters and non-meat-eaters in the EPIC-Oxford Cohort." *Nutrients* 11 (4). doi: 10.3390/nu11040824.

Parekh, N., U. Chandran, and E. V. Bandera. 2012. "Obesity in cancer survival." *Annu Rev Nutr* 32:311–42 doi: 10.1146/annurev-nutr-071811-150713.

Parida, S., S. Siddharth, and D. Sharma. 2019. "Adiponectin, obesity, and cancer: Clash of the bigwigs in health and disease." *Int J Mol Sci* 20 (10). doi: 10.3390/ijms20102519.

Pavlides, S., D. Whitaker-Menezes, R. Castello-Cros, N. Flomenberg, A. K. Witkiewicz, P. G. Frank, M. C. Casimiro, C. Wang, P. Fortina, S. Addya, R. G. Pestell, U. E. Martinez-Outschoorn, F. Sotgia, and M. P. Lisanti. 2009. "The reverse Warburg effect: Aerobic glycolysis in cancer associated fibroblasts and the tumor stroma." *Cell Cycle* 8 (23):3984–4001. doi: 10.4161/cc.8.23.10238.

Phoenix, K. N., F. Vumbaca, M. M. Fox, R. Evans, and K. P. Claffey. 2010. "Dietary energy availability affects primary and metastatic breast cancer and metformin efficacy." *Breast Cancer Res Treat* 123 (2):333–44. doi: 10.1007/s10549-009-0647-z.

Pinkston, J. M., D. Garigan, M. Hansen, and C. Kenyon. 2006. "Mutations that increase the life span of C. elegans inhibit tumor growth." *Science* 313 (5789):971–5. doi: 10.1126/science.1121908.

Ploeger, J. M., J. C. Manivel, L. N. Boatner, and D. G. Mashek. 2017. "Caloric restriction prevents carcinogen-initiated liver tumorigenesis in mice." *Cancer Prev Res (Phila)* 10 (11):660–70. doi: 10.1158/1940-6207. CAPR-17-0174.

Powis, G., P. Reece, D. L. Ahmann, and J. N. Ingle. 1987. "Effect of body weight on the pharmacokinetics of cyclophosphamide in breast cancer patients." *Cancer Chemother Pharmacol* 20 (3):219–22. doi: 10.1007/BF00570489.

Psaltopoulou, T., R. I. Kosti, D. Haidopoulos, M. Dimopoulos, and D. B. Panagiotakos. 2011. "Olive oil intake is inversely related to cancer prevalence: a systematic review and a meta-analysis of 13,800 patients and 23,340 controls in 19 observational studies." *Lipids Health Dis* 10:127. doi: 10.1186/1476-511X-10-127.

Raffaghello, L., C. Lee, F. M. Safdie, M. Wei, F. Madia, G. Bianchi, and V. D. Longo. 2008. "Starvation-dependent differential stress resistance protects normal but not cancer cells against high-dose chemotherapy." *Proc Natl Acad Sci U S A* 105 (24):8215–20. doi: 10.1073/pnas.0708100105.

Raghu Nadhanan, R., J. Skinner, R. Chung, Y. W. Su, P. R. Howe, and C. J. Xian. 2013. "Supplementation with fish oil and genistein, individually or in combination, protects bone against the adverse effects of methotrexate chemotherapy in rats." *PLoS One* 8 (8):e71592. doi: 10.1371/journal.pone.0071592.

Ramsey, M. M., R. L. Ingram, A. B. Cashion, A. H. Ng, J. M. Cline, A. F. Parlow, and W. E. Sonntag. 2002. "Growth hormone-deficient dwarf animals are resistant to dimethylbenzanthracine (DMBA)-induced mammary carcinogenesis." *Endocrinology* 143 (10):4139–42. doi: 10.1210/en.2002-220717.

Rapp, K., J. Schroeder, J. Klenk, S. Stoehr, H. Ulmer, H. Concin, G. Diem, W. Oberaigner, and S. K. Weiland. 2005. "Obesity and incidence of cancer: a large cohort study of over 145,000 adults in Austria." *Br J Cancer* 93 (9):1062–7. doi: 10.1038/sj.bjc.6602819.

Renehan, A. G., M. Tyson, M. Egger, R. F. Heller, and M. Zwahlen. 2008. "Body-mass index and incidence of cancer: a systematic review and meta-analysis of prospective observational studies." *Lancet* 371 (9612):569–78. doi: 10.1016/S0140-6736(08)60269-X.

Richman, E. L., S. A. Kenfield, J. E. Chavarro, M. J. Stampfer, E. L. Giovannucci, W. C. Willett, and J. M. Chan. 2013. "Fat intake after diagnosis and risk of lethal prostate cancer and all-cause mortality." *JAMA Intern Med* 173 (14):1318–26. doi: 10.1001/jamainternmed.2013.6536.

Richter, J. E., and J. H. Rubenstein. 2018. "Presentation and epidemiology of gastroesophageal reflux disease." *Gastroenterology* 154 (2):267–76. doi: 10.1053/j.gastro.2017.07.045.

Rihacek, M., J. Bienertova-Vasku, D. Valik, J. Sterba, K. Pilatova, and L. Zdrazilova-Dubska. 2015. "B-cell activating factor as a cancer biomarker and its implications in cancer-related cachexia." *Biomed Res Int* 2015:792187. doi: 10.1155/2015/792187.

Rittling, S. R., and A. F. Chambers. 2004. "Role of osteopontin in tumour progression." *Br J Cancer* 90 (10):1877–81. doi: 10.1038/sj.bjc.6601839.

Rocha, N. S., L. F. Barbisan, M. L. de Oliveira, and J. L. de Camargo. 2002. "Effects of fasting and intermittent fasting on rat hepatocarcinogenesis induced by diethylnitrosamine." *Teratog Carcinog Mutagen* 22 (2):129–38. doi: 10.1002/tcm.10005.

Rohde, F., C. Rimkus, J. Friederichs, R. Rosenberg, C. Marthen, D. Doll, B. Holzmann, J. R. Siewert, and K. P. Janssen. 2007. "Expression of osteopontin, a target gene of de-regulated Wnt signaling, predicts survival in colon cancer." *Int J Cancer* 121 (8):1717–23. doi: 10.1002/ijc.22868.

Roodhart, J. M., L. G. Daenen, E. C. Stigter, H. J. Prins, J. Gerrits, J. M. Houthuijzen, M. G. Gerritsen, H. S. Schipper, M. J. Backer, M. van Amersfoort, J. S. Vermaat, P. Moerer, K. Ishihara, E. Kalkhoven, J. H. Beijnen, P. W. Derksen, R. H. Medema, A. C. Martens, A. B. Brenkman, and E. E. Voest. 2011. "Mesenchymal stem cells induce resistance to chemotherapy through the release of platinum-induced fatty acids." *Cancer Cell* 20 (3):370–83. doi: 10.1016/j.ccr.2011.08.010.

Rossi, E. L., S. M. Dunlap, L. W. Bowers, S. A. Khatib, S. S. Doerstling, L. A. Smith, N. A. Ford, D. Holley, P. H. Brown, M. R. Estecio, D. F. Kusewitt, L. A. deGraffenried, S. J. Bultman, and S. D. Hursting. 2017. "Energy balance modulation impacts epigenetic reprogramming, ERalpha and ERbeta expression, and mammary tumor development in MMTV-neu transgenic mice." *Cancer Res* 77 (9):2500–11. doi: 10.1158/0008-5472.CAN-16-2795.

Rouhani, M. H., A. Salehi-Abargouei, P. J. Surkan, and L. Azadbakht. 2014. "Is there a relationship between red or processed meat intake and obesity? A systematic review and meta-analysis of observational studies." *Obes Rev* 15 (9):740–8. doi: 10.1111/obr.12172.

Roy, S., and G. Trinchieri. 2017. "Microbiota: a key orchestrator of cancer therapy." *Nat Rev Cancer* 17 (5):271–85. doi: 10.1038/nrc.2017.13.

Ruiz, J. M., P. Steffen, and T. B. Smith. 2013. "Hispanic mortality paradox: a systematic review and meta-analysis of the longitudinal literature." *Am J Public Health* 103 (3):e52–60. doi: 10.2105/AJPH.2012.301103.

Safdie, F. M., T. Dorff, D. Quinn, L. Fontana, M. Wei, C. Lee, P. Cohen, and V. D. Longo. 2009. "Fasting and cancer treatment in humans: a case series report." *Aging (Albany NY)* 1 (12):988–1007. doi: 10.18632/aging.100114.

Saleh, A. D., B. A. Simone, J. Palazzo, J. E. Savage, Y. Sano, T. Dan, L. Jin, C. E. Champ, S. Zhao, M. Lim, F. Sotgia, K. Camphausen, R. G. Pestell, J. B. Mitchell, M. P. Lisanti, and N. L. Simone. 2013. "Caloric restriction augments radiation efficacy in breast cancer." *Cell Cycle* 12 (12):1955–63. doi: 10.4161/cc.25016.

Samudio, I., R. Harmancey, M. Fiegl, H. Kantarjian, M. Konopleva, B. Korchin, K. Kaluarachchi, W. Bornmann, S. Duvvuri, H. Taegtmeyer, and M. Andreeff. 2010. "Pharmacologic inhibition of fatty acid oxidation sensitizes human leukemia cells to apoptosis induction." *J Clin.Invest* 120 (1):142–56.

Sayon-Orea, C., M. A. Martinez-Gonzalez, and M. Bes-Rastrollo. 2011. "Alcohol consumption and body weight: a systematic review." *Nutr Rev* 69 (8):419–31. doi: 10.1111/j.1753-4887.2011.00403.x.

Schwingshackl, L., and G. Hoffmann. 2015. "Adherence to mediterranean diet and risk of cancer: an updated systematic review and meta-analysis of observational studies." *Cancer Med* 4 (12):1933–47. doi: 10.1002/cam4.539.

Seibert, R. G., A. D. Hanchate, J. P. Berz, and P. C. Schroy, 3rd. 2017. "National disparities in colorectal cancer screening among obese adults." *Am J Prev Med* 53 (2):e41–9. doi: 10.1016/j.amepre.2017.01.006.

Seyfried, T. N., T. M. Sanderson, M. M. El-Abbadi, R. McGowan, and P. Mukherjee. 2003. "Role of glucose and ketone bodies in the metabolic control of experimental brain cancer." *Br J Cancer* 89 (7):1375–82. doi: 10.1038/sj.bjc.6601269.

Sheehan, C. M., P. A. Cantu, D. A. Powers, C. E. Margerison-Zilko, and C. Cubbin. 2017. "Long-term neighborhood poverty trajectories and obesity in a sample of california mothers." *Health Place* 46:49–57 doi: 10.1016/j.healthplace.2017.04.010.

Shelton, L. M., L. C. Huysentruyt, P. Mukherjee, and T. N. Seyfried. 2010. "Calorie restriction as an anti-invasive therapy for malignant brain cancer in the VM mouse." *ASN Neuro* 2 (3):e00038. doi: 10.1042/AN20100002.

Shen, S., J. M. Unger, K. D. Crew, C. Till, H. Greenlee, J. Gralow, S. R. Dakhil, L. M. Minasian, J. L. Wade, M. J. Fisch, N. L. Henry, and D. L. Hershman. 2018. "Omega-3 fatty acid use for obese breast cancer patients with aromatase inhibitor-related arthralgia (SWOG S0927)." *Breast Cancer Res Treat* 172 (3):603–10. doi: 10.1007/s10549-018-4946-0.

Sheng, X., J. H. Parmentier, J. Tucci, H. Pei, O. Cortez-Toledo, C. M. Dieli-Conwright, M. J. Oberley, M. Neely, E. Orgel, S. G. Louie, and S. D. Mittelman. 2017. "Adipocytes sequester and metabolize the chemotherapeutic daunorubicin." *Mol Cancer Res* 15 (12):1704–13. doi: 10.1158/1541-7786.MCR-17-0338.

Shields, B. A., R. W. Engelman, Y. Fukaura, R. A. Good, and N. K. Day. 1991. "Calorie restriction suppresses subgenomic mink cytopathic focus-forming murine leukemia virus transcription and frequency of genomic expression while impairing lymphoma formation." *Proc Natl Acad Sci U S A* 88 (24):11138–42. doi: 10.1073/pnas.88.24.11138.

Siegel, R. L., K. D. Miller, and A. Jemal. 2017. "Cancer statistics, 2017." *CA Cancer J Clin* 67 (1):7–30. doi: 10.3322/caac.21387.

Sikalidis, A. K., M. D. Fitch, and S. E. Fleming. 2013. "Diet induced obesity increases the risk of colonic tumorigenesis in mice." *Pathol Oncol Res* 19 (4):657–66. doi: 10.1007/s12253-013-9626-0.

Silverman, L. B., K. E. Stevenson, J. E. O'Brien, B. L. Asselin, R. D. Barr, L. Clavell, P. D. Cole, K. M. Kelly, C. Laverdiere, B. Michon, M. A. Schorin, C. L. Schwartz, E. W. O'Holleran, D. S. Neuberg, H. J. Cohen, and S. E. Sallan. 2010. "Long-term results of Dana-Farber Cancer Institute ALL Consortium protocols for children with newly diagnosed acute lymphoblastic leukemia (1985–2000)." *Leukemia* 24 (2):320–34. doi: 10.1038/leu.2009.253.

Simone, B. A., T. Dan, A. Palagani, L. Jin, S. Y. Han, C. Wright, J. E. Savage, R. Gitman, M. K. Lim, J. Palazzo, M. P. Mehta, and N. L. Simone. 2016. "Caloric restriction coupled with radiation decreases metastatic burden in triple negative breast cancer." *Cell Cycle* 15 (17):2265–74. doi: 10.1080/15384101.2016.1160982.

Simone, B. A., A. Palagani, K. Strickland, K. Ko, L. Jin, M. K. Lim, T. D. Dan, M. Sarich, D. A. Monti, M. Cristofanilli, and N. L. Simone. 2018. "Caloric restriction counteracts chemotherapy-induced inflammation and increases response to therapy in a triple negative breast cancer model." *Cell Cycle* 17 (13):1536–44. doi: 10.1080/15384101.2018.1471314.

Sinicrope, F. A., N. R. Foster, D. J. Sargent, M. J. O'Connell, and C. Rankin. 2010. "Obesity is an independent prognostic variable in colon cancer survivors." *Clin Cancer Res* 16 (6):1884–93. doi: 10.1158/1078-0432.CCR-09-2636.

Slavin, J. L. 2005. "Dietary fiber and body weight." *Nutrition* 21 (3):411–8. doi: 10.1016/j.nut.2004.08.018.

Slawson, C., R. J. Copeland, and G. W. Hart. 2010. "O-GlcNAc signaling: a metabolic link between diabetes and cancer?" *Trends Biochem Sci* 35 (10):547–55. doi: 10.1016/j.tibs.2010.04.005.

Sohl, S. J., L. A. Borowski, E. E. Kent, A. W. Smith, I. Oakley-Girvan, R. L. Rothman, and N. K. Arora. 2015. "Cancer survivors' disclosure of complementary health approaches to physicians: the role of patient-centered communication." *Cancer* 121 (6):900–7. doi: 10.1002/cncr.29138.

Song, M., T. T. Fung, F. B. Hu, W. C. Willett, V. D. Longo, A. T. Chan, and E. L. Giovannucci. 2016. "Association of animal and plant protein intake with all-cause and cause-specific mortality." *JAMA Intern Med* 176 (10):1453–63. doi: 10.1001/jamainternmed.2016.4182.

Stewart, J. W., K. Koehler, W. Jackson, J. Hawley, W. Wang, A. Au, R. Myers, and D. F. Birt. 2005. "Prevention of mouse skin tumor promotion by dietary energy restriction requires an intact adrenal gland and glucocorticoid supplementation restores inhibition." *Carcinogenesis* 26 (6):1077–84. doi: 10.1093/carcin/bgi051.

Stussman, B. J., R. R. Nahin, P. M. Barnes, and B. W. Ward. 2020. "U.S. physician recommendations to their patients about the use of complementary health approaches." *J Altern Complement Med* 26 (1):25–33. doi: 10.1089/acm.2019.0303.

Sun, P., H. Wang, Z. He, X. Chen, Q. Wu, W. Chen, Z. Sun, M. Weng, M. Zhu, D. Ma, and C. Miao. 2017. "Fasting inhibits colorectal cancer growth by reducing M2 polarization of tumor-associated macrophages." *Oncotarget* 8 (43):74649–60. doi: 10.18632/oncotarget.20301.

Surveillance, Epidemiology, and End Results (SEER) Program (www.seer.cancer.gov) SEER*Stat Database Research Data, 9 Registries, Nov 2019 Sub 1975-2017, National Cancer Institute, DCCPS, Surveillance Research Program, released April 2020, based on November 2019 submission.

Suttie, A. W., G. E. Dinse, A. Nyska, G. J. Moser, T. L. Goldsworthy, and R. R. Maronpot. 2005. "An investigation of the effects of late-onset dietary restriction on prostate cancer development in the TRAMP mouse." *Toxicol Pathol* 33 (3):386–97. doi: 10.1080/01926230590930272.

Szymanski, K. M., D. C. Wheeler, and L. A. Mucci. 2010. "Fish consumption and prostate cancer risk: a review and meta-analysis." *Am J Clin Nutr* 92 (5):1223–33. doi: 10.3945/ajcn.2010.29530.

Tabe, Y., S. Yamamoto, K. Saitoh, K. Sekihara, N. Monma, K. Ikeo, K. Mogushi, M. Shikami, V. Ruvolo, J. Ishizawa, N. Hail, Jr., S. Kazuno, M. Igarashi, H. Matsushita, Y. Yamanaka, H. Arai, I. Nagaoka, T. Miida, Y. Hayashizaki, M. Konopleva, and M. Andreeff. 2017. "Bone marrow adipocytes facilitate fatty acid oxidation activating AMPK and a transcriptional network supporting survival of acute monocytic leukemia cells." *Cancer Res* 77 (6):1453–64. doi: 10.1158/0008-5472.CAN-16-1645.

Tagliaferro, A. R., A. M. Ronan, L. D. Meeker, H. J. Thompson, A. L. Scott, and D. Sinha. 1996. "Cyclic food restriction alters substrate utilization and abolishes protection from mammary carcinogenesis female rats." *J Nutr* 126 (5):1398–405. doi: 10.1093/jn/126.5.1398.

Templeton, Z. S., W. R. Lie, W. Wang, Y. Rosenberg-Hasson, R. V. Alluri, J. S. Tamaresis, M. H. Bachmann, K. Lee, W. J. Maloney, C. H. Contag, and B. L. King. 2015. "Breast cancer cell colonization of the human bone marrow adipose tissue niche." *Neoplasia* 17 (12):849–61. doi: 10.1016/j.neo.2015.11.005.

Thomas, J. A., 2nd, J. A. Antonelli, J. C. Lloyd, E. M. Masko, S. H. Poulton, T. E. Phillips, M. Pollak, and S. J. Freedland. 2010. "Effect of intermittent fasting on prostate cancer tumor growth in a mouse model." *Prostate Cancer Prostatic Dis* 13 (4):350–5. doi: 10.1038/pcan.2010.24.

Thompson, H. J., J. N. McGinley, N. S. Spoelstra, W. Jiang, Z. Zhu, and P. Wolfe. 2004. "Effect of dietary energy restriction on vascular density during mammary carcinogenesis." *Cancer Res* 64 (16):5643–50. doi: 10.1158/0008-5472.CAN-04-0787.

Thrift, A. P., N. Pandeya, and D. C. Whiteman. 2012. "Current status and future perspectives on the etiology of esophageal adenocarcinoma." *Front Oncol* 2:11. doi: 10.3389/fonc.2012.00011.

Tomasi, C., E. Laconi, S. Laconi, M. Greco, D. S. Sarma, and P. Pani. 1999. "Effect of fasting/refeeding on the incidence of chemically induced hepatocellular carcinoma in the rat." *Carcinogenesis* 20 (10):1979–83. doi: 10.1093/carcin/20.10.1979.

Tomita, M. 2012. "Caloric restriction reduced 1, 2-dimethylhydrazine-induced aberrant crypt foci and induces the expression of Sirtuins in colonic mucosa of F344 rats." *J Carcinog* 11:10. doi: 10.4103/1477-3163.99176.

Touchefeu, Y., E. Montassier, K. Nieman, T. Gastinne, G. Potel, S. Bruley des Varannes, F. Le Vacon, and M. F. de La Cochetière. 2014. "Systematic review: the role of the gut microbiota in chemotherapy- or radiation-induced gastrointestinal mucositis - current evidence and potential clinical applications." *Aliment Pharmacol Ther* 40 (5):409–21. doi: 10.1111/apt.12878.

Trepanowski, J. F., and R. J. Bloomer. 2010. "The impact of religious fasting on human health." *Nutr J* 9:57. doi: 10.1186/1475-2891-9-57.

Tsai, H. J., and J. S. Chang. 2019. "Environmental risk factors of pancreatic cancer." *J Clin Med* 8 (9). doi: 10.3390/jcm8091427.

Tsao, J. L., S. Dudley, B. Kwok, A. E. Nickel, P. W. Laird, K. D. Siegmund, R. M. Liskay, and D. Shibata. 2002. "Diet, cancer and aging in DNA mismatch repair deficient mice." *Carcinogenesis* 23 (11):1807–10. doi: 10.1093/carcin/23.11.1807.

Tsilidis, K. K., J. C. Kasimis, D. S. Lopez, E. E. Ntzani, and J. P. Ioannidis. 2015. "Type 2 diabetes and cancer: umbrella review of meta-analyses of observational studies." *BMJ* 350:g7607. doi: 10.1136/bmj.g7607.

Tucci, J., W. Alhushki, T. Chen, X. Sheng, Y. M. Kim, and S. D. Mittelman. 2018. "Switch to low-fat diet improves outcome of acute lymphoblastic leukemia in obese mice." *Cancer Metab* 6:15. doi: 10.1186/s40170-018-0189-0.

Uddin, S., R. Bu, M. Ahmed, J. Abubaker, F. Al-Dayel, P. Bavi, and K. S. Al-Kuraya. 2009. "Overexpression of leptin receptor predicts an unfavorable outcome in Middle Eastern ovarian cancer." *Mol Cancer* 8:74. doi: 10.1186/1476-4598-8-74.

Uddin, S., P. Bavi, A. K. Siraj, M. Ahmed, M. Al-Rasheed, A. R. Hussain, T. Amin, A. Alzahrani, F. Al-Dayel, J. Abubaker, R. Bu, and K. S. Al-Kuraya. 2010. "Leptin-R and its association with PI3K/AKT signaling pathway in papillary thyroid carcinoma." *Endocr Relat Cancer* 17 (1):191–202. doi: 10.1677/ERC-09-0153.

Vallianou, N., T. Stratigou, G. S. Christodoulatos, and M. Dalamaga. 2019. "Understanding the role of the gut microbiome and microbial metabolites in obesity and obesity-associated metabolic disorders: Current evidence and perspectives." *Curr Obes Rep* 8 (3):317–332. doi: 10.1007/s13679-019-00352-2.

van Blarigan, E. L., C. S. Fuchs, D. Niedzwiecki, X. Ye, S. Zhang, M. Song, L. B. Saltz, R. J. Mayer, R. B. Mowat, R. Whittom, A. Hantel, A. Benson, D. Atienza, M. Messino, H. Kindler, A. Venook, S. Ogino, E. L. Giovannucci, and J. A. Meyerhardt. 2018. "Marine ω-3 polyunsaturated fatty acid and fish intake after colon cancer diagnosis and survival: CALGB 89803 (alliance)." *Cancer Epidemiol Biomarkers Prev* 27 (4):438–445. doi: 10.1158/1055-9965.EPI-17-0689.

van Ginhoven, T. M., J. W. van den Berg, W. A. Dik, J. N. Ijzermans, and R. W. de Bruin. 2010. "Preoperative dietary restriction reduces hepatic tumor load by reduced E-selectin-mediated adhesion in mice." *J Surg Oncol* 102 (4):348–53. doi: 10.1002/jso.21649.

van Rongen, A., M. J. E. Brill, J. D. Vaughns, P. A. J. Välitalo, E. P. A. van Dongen, B. van Ramshorst, J. S. Barrett, J. N. van den Anker, and C. A. J. Knibbe. 2018. "Higher midazolam clearance in obese adolescents compared with morbidly obese adults." *Clin Pharmacokinet* 57 (5):601–11. doi: 10.1007/s40262-017-0579-4.

van Vliet, M. J., H. J. Harmsen, E. S. de Bont, and W. J. Tissing. 2010. "The role of intestinal microbiota in the development and severity of chemotherapy-induced mucositis." *PLoS Pathog* 6 (5):e1000879. doi: 10.1371/journal.ppat.1000879.

Veselkov, K., G. Gonzalez, S. Aljifri, D. Galea, R. Mirnezami, J. Youssef, M. Bronstein, and I. Laponogov. 2019. "HyperFoods: Machine intelligent mapping of cancer-beating molecules in foods." *Sci Rep* 9 (1):9237. doi: 10.1038/s41598-019-45349-y.

von Tungeln, L. S., T. J. Bucci, R. W. Hart, F. F. Kadlubar, and P. P. Fu. 1996. "Inhibitory effect of caloric restriction on tumorigenicity induced by 4-aminobiphenyl and 2-amino-1-methyl-6-phenylimidazo-[4,5-b]pyridine (PhIP) in the CD1 newborn mouse bioassay." *Cancer Lett* 104 (2):133–6. doi: 10.1016/0304-3835(96)04232-2.

Vyas, D., G. Laput, and A. K. Vyas. 2014. "Chemotherapy-enhanced inflammation may lead to the failure of therapy and metastasis." *Onco Targets Ther* 7:1015–23 doi: 10.2147/OTT.S60114.

Wang, T., J. F. Fahrmann, H. Lee, Y. J. Li, S. C. Tripathi, C. Yue, C. Zhang, V. Lifshitz, J. Song, Y. Yuan, G. Somlo, R. Jandial, D. Ann, S. Hanash, R. Jove, and H. Yu. 2018. "JAK/STAT3-regulated fatty acid beta-oxidation is critical for breast cancer stem cell self-renewal and chemoresistance." *Cell Metab* 27 (1):136–50 e5. doi: 10.1016/j.cmet.2017.11.001.

Warburg, O. 1925. "The metabolism of carcinoma cells." *J. Cancer Res* 9 (1):148–63. doi: 10.1158/jcr.1925.148.

Ward, E., A. Jemal, V. Cokkinides, G. K. Singh, C. Cardinez, A. Ghafoor, and M. Thun. 2004. "Cancer disparities by race/ethnicity and socioeconomic status." *CA Cancer J Clin* 54 (2):78–93. doi: 10.3322/canjclin.54.2.78.

Wilhelmi de Toledo, F., F. Grundler, A. Bergouignan, S. Drinda, and A. Michalsen. 2019. "Safety, health improvement and well-being during a 4 to 21-day fasting period in an observational study including 1422 subjects." *PLoS One* 14 (1):e0209353. doi: 10.1371/journal.pone.0209353.

Wong, A., A. Le, M. H. Lee, Y. J. Lin, P. Nguyen, S. Trinh, H. Dang, and M. H. Nguyen. 2018. "Higher risk of hepatocellular carcinoma in Hispanic patients with hepatitis C cirrhosis and metabolic risk factors." *Sci Rep* 8 (1):7164. doi: 10.1038/s41598-018-25533-2.

Woolf, E. C., K. L. Curley, Q. Liu, G. H. Turner, J. A. Charlton, M. C. Preul, and A. C. Scheck. 2015. "The ketogenic diet alters the hypoxic response and affects expression of proteins associated with angiogenesis, invasive potential and vascular permeability in a mouse glioma model." *PLoS One* 10 (6):e0130357. doi: 10.1371/journal.pone.0130357.

World Cancer Research Fund/American Institute for Cancer Research. Diet, nutrition, physical activity and cancer: a global perspective. Continuous Update Project Expert Report 2018. Available at dietandcancerreport.org.

Wu, J., R. Zeng, J. Huang, X. Li, J. Zhang, J. C. Ho, and Y. Zheng. 2016. "Dietary protein sources and incidence of breast cancer: A dose-response meta-analysis of prospective studies." *Nutrients* 8 (11). doi: 10.3390/nu8110730.

Xu, X. D., S. X. Shao, H. P. Jiang, Y. W. Cao, Y. H. Wang, X. C. Yang, Y. L. Wang, X. S. Wang, and H. T. Niu. 2015. "Warburg effect or reverse warburg effect? A review of cancer metabolism." *Oncol Res Treat* 38 (3):117–22. doi: 10.1159/000375435.

Xu, M., X. Jung, O. J. Hines, G. Eibl, and Y. Chen. 2018. "Obesity and pancreatic cancer: Overview of epidemiology and potential prevention by weight loss." *Pancreas* 47 (2):158–62. doi: 10.1097/MPA.0000000000000974.

Yakar, S., N. P. Nunez, P. Pennisi, P. Brodt, H. Sun, L. Fallavollita, H. Zhao, L. Scavo, R. Novosyadlyy, N. Kurshan, B. Stannard, J. East-Palmer, N. C. Smith, S. N. Perkins, R. Fuchs-Young, J. C. Barrett, S. D. Hursting, and D. LeRoith. 2006. "Increased tumor growth in mice with diet-induced obesity: impact of ovarian hormones." *Endocrinology* 147 (12):5826–34. doi: 10.1210/en.2006-0311.

Yamaza, H., T. Komatsu, S. Wakita, C. Kijogi, S. Park, H. Hayashi, T. Chiba, R. Mori, T. Furuyama, N. Mori, and I. Shimokawa. 2010. "FoxO1 is involved in the antineoplastic effect of calorie restriction." *Aging Cell* 9 (3):372–82. doi: 10.1111/j.1474-9726.2010.00563.x.

Yang, H. S., C. Yoon, S. K. Myung, and S. M. Park. 2011. "Effect of obesity on survival of women with epithelial ovarian cancer: a systematic review and meta-analysis of observational studies." *Int J Gynecol Cancer* 21 (9):1525–32. doi: 10.1097/IGC.0b013e31822eb5f8.

Yeung, C. Y., A. W. Tso, A. Xu, Y. Wang, Y. C. Woo, T. H. Lam, S. V. Lo, C. H. Fong, N. M. Wat, J. Woo, B. M. Cheung, and K. S. Lam. 2013. "Pro-inflammatory adipokines as predictors of incident cancers in a Chinese cohort of low obesity prevalence in Hong Kong." *PLoS One* 8 (10):e78594. doi: 10.1371/journal.pone.0078594.

Yoshimoto, S., T. M. Loo, K. Atarashi, H. Kanda, S. Sato, S. Oyadomari, Y. Iwakura, K. Oshima, H. Morita, M. Hattori, K. Honda, Y. Ishikawa, E. Hara, and N. Ohtani. 2013. "Obesity-induced gut microbial metabolite promotes liver cancer through senescence secretome." *Nature* 499 (7456):97–101. doi: 10.1038/nature12347.

Yuan, C., Y. Bao, C. Wu, P. Kraft, S. Ogino, K. Ng, Z. R. Qian, D. A. Rubinson, M. J. Stampfer, E. L. Giovannucci, and B. M. Wolpin. 2013. "Prediagnostic body mass index and pancreatic cancer survival." *J Clin Oncol* 31 (33):4229–34. doi: 10.1200/JCO.2013.51.7532.

Yuhara, H., C. Steinmaus, S. E. Cohen, D. A. Corley, Y. Tei, and P. A. Buffler. 2011. "Is diabetes mellitus an independent risk factor for colon cancer and rectal cancer?" *Am J Gastroenterol* 106 (11):1911–21. doi: 10.1038/ajg.2011.301.

Yun, J. P., J. W. Behan, N. Heisterkamp, A. Butturini, L. Klemm, L. Ji, J. Groffen, M. Muschen, and S. D. Mittelman. 2010. "Diet-induced obesity accelerates acute lymphoblastic leukemia progression in two murine models." *Cancer Prev.Res (Phila Pa)* 3:1259–64.

Zaytouni, T., P. Y. Tsai, D. S. Hitchcock, C. D. DuBois, E. Freinkman, L. Lin, V. Morales-Oyarvide, P. J. Lenehan, B. M. Wolpin, M. Mino-Kenudson, E. M. Torres, N. Stylopoulos, C. B. Clish, and N. Y. Kalaany. 2017. "Critical role for arginase 2 in obesity-associated pancreatic cancer." *Nat Commun* 8 (1):242. doi: 10.1038/s41467-017-00331-y.

Zhang, J., N. N. Pavlova, and C. B. Thompson. 2017. "Cancer cell metabolism: the essential role of the nonessential amino acid, glutamine." *EMBO J* 36 (10):1302–15. doi: 10.15252/embj.201696151.

Zhang, J., P. P. Jia, Q. L. Liu, M. H. Cong, Y. Gao, H. P. Shi, W. N. Yu, and M. Y. Miao. 2018. "Low ketolytic enzyme levels in tumors predict ketogenic diet responses in cancer cell lines in vitro and in vivo." *J Lipid Res* 59 (4):625–34. doi: 10.1194/jlr.M082040.

Zhang, X., J. Rhoades, B. J. Caan, D. E. Cohn, R. Salani, S. Noria, A. A. Suarez, E. D. Paskett, and A. S. Felix. 2019a. "Intentional weight loss, weight cycling, and endometrial cancer risk: a systematic review and meta-analysis." *Int J Gynecol Cancer* 29 (9):1361–71. doi: 10.1136/ijgc-2019-000728.

Zhang, Y., B. Zhang, L. Dong, and P. Chang. 2019b. "Potential of omega-3 polyunsaturated fatty acids in managing chemotherapy- or radiotherapy-related intestinal microbial dysbiosis." *Adv Nutr* 10 (1):133–147. doi: 10.1093/advances/nmy076.

Zheng, T., Y. Ni, J. Li, B. K. C. Chow, and G. Panagiotou. 2017. "Designing dietary recommendations using system level interactomics analysis and network-based inference." *Front Physiol* 8:753. doi: 10.3389/fphys.2017.00753.

Zhu, Y., M. D. Aupperlee, S. Z. Haslam, and R. C. Schwartz. 2017. "Pubertally initiated high-fat diet promotes mammary tumorigenesis in obesity-prone FVB mice similarly to obesity-resistant BALB/c Mice." *Transl Oncol* 10 (6):928–35. doi: 10.1016/j.tranon.2017.09.004.

Zhuang, Y., D. K. Chan, A. B. Haugrud, and W. K. Miskimins. 2014. "Mechanisms by which low glucose enhances the cytotoxicity of metformin to cancer cells both in vitro and in vivo." *PLoS One* 9 (9):e108444. doi: 10.1371/journal.pone.0108444.

Zoico, E., V. Rizzatti, E. Darra, S. L. Budui, G. Franceschetti, F. Vinante, C. Pedrazzani, A. Guglielmi, G. De Manzoni, G. Mazzali, A. P. Rossi, F. Fantin, and M. Zamboni. 2017. "Morphological and functional changes in the peritumoral adipose tissue of colorectal cancer patients." *Obesity (Silver Spring)* 25 (Suppl 2):S87–S94. doi: 10.1002/oby.22008.

17 Integrative Oncology and Nutrition

David Heber and Zhaoping Li
UCLA Center for Human Nutrition

CONTENTS

INTRODUCTION

Integrative oncology uses a wide range of complementary medicine treatment modalities, which include nutritional guidance and advice on the use of botanical dietary supplements and medicinal herbs. A number of traditional medicine methods including acupuncture, meditation, music therapy, manual therapies, and various mind–body interventions. The National Center for Complementary and Integrative Health of the National Institutes of Health defines complementary health approaches as including dietary supplements, herbals, natural products, mind and body practices including meditation, yoga, massage, and acupuncture (Powell 2016). Complementary approaches also include other systems of care such as traditional Chinese medicine (TCM), Ayurvedic medicine, and naturopathy. Among adults in the United States, the most commonly used complementary approaches include dietary supplements other than vitamins and minerals, deep breathing, and practices such as yoga, tai chi, and qigong (Clarke et al. 2015).

Integrative oncology is the application of these complementary approaches alongside traditional methods of treatment for patients with cancer. Integrative oncology typically includes dietary supplements and personalized nutrition. Since personalized nutrition is discussed in detail elsewhere in this text, that information will not be repeated here. Instead there will be a review of dietary supplements and botanicals which have some overlap with personalized nutrition. This chapter will review the nature of evidence-based integrative oncology which is still a developing field in need of much more research. Increasingly, patients diagnosed with cancer are choosing to supplement their conventional oncology treatment with supportive complementary care provided by licensed complementary and alternative medicine (CAM) providers, psychologists, social workers, naturopaths, and doctors of TCM including licensed acupuncturists.

Integrative oncology as an evidence-informed approach to lifestyle and behavior modification in cancer is in its infancy. Due to the difficulty inherent in studying alternative modalities, many clinicians continue to rely on anecdotal evidence of benefits which cannot be verified scientifically. Much more research is needed on the efficacy and outcomes of the various modalities employed. Patients in these programs choose the therapies that they think will help them get some relief from cancer-related stress and cancer treatment-related symptoms. In the best situations, a partnership between the patient and caregiver may result in improvements in physical and psychosocial health. However, cancer patients represent a vulnerable population and it is important to recognize that they are sometimes exposed to unnecessary expense and even harm in some cases where unscrupulous individuals promise cures based on unscientific modalities. Therefore, it is vital to use an evidence-informed approach in recommending an integrative cancer plan that involves transparent communication between doctors and patients. It is likely that a significant subset of cancer patients will continue to seek out integrative oncology as part of their care and the nature of efforts to integrate integrative oncology and nutritional intervention will be reviewed in this chapter.

INTEGRATIVE ONCOLOGY

Integrative oncology applies a group of diverse medical and healthcare interventions, practices, products, and disciplines that are combined with conventional and experimental surgical and medical approaches to cancer care. Combining integrative oncology with a high standard of evidence-based personalized nutrition and oncology is particularly critical for cancer patients and survivors who represent a highly vulnerable population. Clearly the boundaries between integrative and conventional oncology are sometimes not clearly evident as integrative approaches have been shown to have some physiological benefits as reviewed below. In fact, many oncologists are supportive of meditation, stress reduction, and some nutritional supplementation in combination with conventional treatments as long as patients desire them.

Interest in and use of complementary health approaches is highest among individuals with cancer. While up to 38% of the general US population utilizes some complementary health approaches, up to 68% of cancer patients in some surveys utilize complementary approaches (Barnes, Bloom, and Nahin 2008). Patients who experience unmet needs from their oncology care providers (Mao et al. 2008) or who have a desire to engage in health-promoting behaviors often seek out integrative oncology (Richardson et al. 2000, Garland et al. 2013). Patients with cancer look to these approaches to improve wellness, enhance immune function, and to relieve symptoms of inflammation and pain.

The patterns of use of complementary health approaches were studied by examining data collected from a combined sample of 88,962 adults aged 18 and over as part of the 2002, 2007, and 2012 National Health Interview Survey. The prevalence of U.S. adults using selected complementary health approaches and selected sociodemographic characteristics of such users were characterized in this study (Clarke et al. 2015). Less than 5% of all U.S. adults are believed to use complementary health approaches as a substitute for conventional care which is particularly relevant in cancer patients where failure to use conventional approaches can be fatal (Nahin, Dahlhamer, and Stussman 2010). Nonvitamin, nonmineral dietary supplements are the most commonly used complementary health approach among U.S. adults, after vitamins and prayer (Frass et al. 2012). Among alternative approaches, yoga, tai chi, and qi gong showed an increase between 2002 and 2012, while deep-breathing exercises and chiropractic or osteopathic manipulation had no significant change. The frequency of use of integrative oncology by treatment is not yet available for cancer patients in integrative oncology programs, but would be of interest.

Many patients with cancer and their family members educate themselves about their disease and treatment options, including CAM and supportive care by searching the internet. A survey of 41 cancer centers in 2010 reported on the information included in websites and the quality of the information judged by two researchers using a four-point scale (Brauer et al. 2010). Twelve centers did not have functional websites with regard to information related to CAM. The most common approaches mentioned were as follows: acupuncture (59%), meditation/nutrition/spiritual support/yoga (56% for each), massage therapy (54%), and music therapy (51%). Twenty-three centers presented information on support groups, 19 centers (46%) provided information on patient seminars, and 17 centers (41%) provided information on survivorship and symptom management clinics. The median rating of the quality of websites was 50 of 100, with only 7 (17%) of centers receiving a composite score 80 (excellent) or better. This situation may have changed for the better in the last 10 years, but there is no further analysis of the frequency of information on the internet. Many centers discourage unsupervised searching of the internet as there is potentially alarming information on disease outcome which can lead to increased stress and anxiety for cancer patients.

In an attempt to meet patients' needs and guide the appropriate use of complementary approaches, an increasing number of cancer centers have developed, or are in the process of developing, integrative oncology programs (Lopez et al. 2017). These programs often incorporate integrative physician consultation, oncology massage, acupuncture, nutrition counseling, exercise or physical therapy consultation, and psychological support.

A cross-sectional descriptive survey of 123 integrative oncology centers in Europe was carried out between 2009 and 2013 (Rossi et al. 2015). Forty-seven out of 99 responding centers met inclusion criteria and provided information on integrative oncology treatments including 24 centers in Italy and 23 from other European countries. On average about 300 patients per year were seen in each center, and about 70% used fixed protocols and had research in progress or completed during the time of the survey. The complementary and alternative practices provided to cancer patients expressed as percent of the centers surveyed were acupuncture in 55%, homeopathy in 40%, herbal medicine in 38%, and TCM in 36%. Treatments were mainly directed to reduce adverse reactions to chemoradiotherapy (23.9%), in particular nausea and vomiting (13.4%), pain and fatigue (10.9%), side effects of iatrogenic menopause (8.8%) anxiety and depression (5.9%), gastrointestinal disorders (5%), sleep disturbances and neuropathy (3.8%), and leukopenia (5%).

Approximately 305,000 registered CAM providers can be identified in the including about 160,000 nonmedical and 45,000 medical practitioners (von Ammon et al. 2012). Acupuncture ($n = 96,380$) was the most utilized method for both medical (80,000) and nonmedical (16,380) practitioners, followed by homeopathy (45,000 medical and 5,800 nonmedical practitioners). Herbal medicine (29,000 practitioners) and reflexology (24,600 practitioners) were mainly provided by nonmedical practitioners. Naturopathy (22,300) was dominated by 15,000 mostly German doctors.

BOTANICAL DIETARY SUPPLEMENTS

In past decades, it was common for oncologists to issue a blanket direction to patients against the use of all nutritional supplements including botanicals during any cancer treatment. As a result, some patients sought alternative care including supplements without the knowledge of their oncologist. There are now many oncologists who discuss alternative treatments with their patients and consider each patient's goals of care in discussing the use of botanicals. If the goal is to cure the patient's cancer or treatment is being given adjunctively to decrease the risk of recurrence, delaying most botanicals until after active treatment is completed is a reasonable recommendation. It is important to point out those instances where there is a chance that there could be significant interference with therapy based on published observations. If treatment is palliative and cure is not likely, allowing the patient to experience some sense of control through judicious use of supplements during treatment is likely to be beneficial overall. The goal of this section is to provide some evidence on the safety and efficacy of dietary botanical supplements, so that clinicians can advise their patients on how to approach dietary supplements and botanicals. Most vitamins and minerals within the RDA and slightly above the RDA as found in over-the-counter multivitamin/multimineral supplements are considered safe in most cancer patients and will not be discussed here. There is more information on toxicities of vitamins and minerals in Chapter 6 on personalized nutrition.

Outside of active treatment, there are cases where patients take a large number of supplements that have been recommended to them. If some supplements and botanicals seem unsafe, ineffective, or excessively expensive, advising against their use may be helpful. Dietary supplements and herbal products can theoretically contribute to harm when combined with cancer therapies such as chemotherapy, targeted therapies, radiation, and surgery (Lawenda et al. 2008). The use of antioxidants during cancer therapy remains a concern because of an overall lack of clear research findings on whether antioxidants interfere with the efficacy of cancer therapy.

Herbal products and other antioxidant supplements could theoretically interfere with the efficacy of treatments such as radiation and chemotherapy which depend on generating reactive oxygen species (ROS) (Lawenda et al. 2008). Overall, examination of the evidence related to potential interactions between ROS and antioxidants has made this long-standing controversial topic a continuing area where more research is needed (Seifried et al. 2003). Some patients are advised to avoid all colorful fruits and vegetables due to their content of antioxidants. While the effects on radiation and chemotherapy of potent antioxidant supplements remain any area of ongoing research, eating antioxidant-rich fruits and vegetables is generally regarded as safe. The exception to this guideline exists for patients who have severely compromised immune function during bone marrow transplantation.

There is also concern that certain natural products use similar metabolic pathways to chemotherapeutic agents and, when combined with chemotherapy, may have inadvertent effects on the therapeutic dose or interfere with the pharmacokinetics or action of the drug (Yeung, Gubili, and Mao 2018). These possible interactions can be divided into pharmacokinetics, which describe how herbs can influence the absorption, distribution, metabolism, and excretion of other drugs, and pharmacodynamics, which defines how herbs can alter the actions of other drugs when they are administered concurrently. There are unsurprising pharmacokinetic effects of herbal supplements which utilize the same detoxifying enzyme systems as phytonutrients from plant foods.

Certain herbal products can increase bleeding risk, presenting a risk to patients with certain types of chemotherapy or recent surgical procedures (Abebe 2019). Most of these herbal products affect platelet function and can be safely consumed as long as there is vigilance around bleeding episodes. On the other hand, some chemotherapy is known to increase bleeding risk. For example, Ibrutinib is an irreversible inhibitor of Bruton's tyrosine kinase that has proven to be an effective therapeutic agent for multiple B-cell-mediated lymphoproliferative disorders. Ibrutinib, however, carries an increased bleeding risk compared with standard chemotherapy and patients are being cautioned against concomitant use of nonsteroidal anti-inflammatory drugs, fish oils, vitamin E, and aspirin (Shatzel et al. 2017).

Agents such as mushroom extracts have immune-modulatory properties and may have effects on the immune system, which have been touted based on in vitro evidence of anticancer activity. However, with the discovery of the microbiome, it is clear that mushrooms may have immune modulatory effects through interaction with gut bacteria as prebiotics. Mushrooms are rich in carbohydrates, like chitin, hemicellulose, β- and α-glucans, mannans, xylans, and galactans, which make them prebiotics that stimulate the growth of gut microbiota, conferring potential health benefits and research is needed on the potential interaction with immune-based therapies (Jayachandran, Xiao, and Xu 2017). Mushrooms may enhance or otherwise affect immune function, and it may be advisable to recommend against their use by patients with lymphoproliferative malignancies or those receiving immunotherapies. This caution is based on theoretical grounds, and there is a need to develop more information on this potential interaction.

The potential also exists for some of these herbals and natural products to rarely cause direct liver injury (Navarro et al. 2017). Idiosyncratic drug-induced liver injury (DILI) is a rare adverse drug reaction and it can lead to jaundice, liver failure, or even death. Antimicrobials, acetaminophen in combination with alcohol, and herbal and dietary supplements are among the common therapeutic classes to cause DILI in the Western world. DILI is a diagnosis of exclusion and thus careful history taking and thorough work-up for competing etiologies are essential for its timely diagnosis. The timing of the events, exclusion of alternative causes, and taking into account the clinical context should be systematically assessed and scored in a transparent manner. RUCAM (Roussel Uclaf Causality Assessment Method) is a well-established diagnostic algorithm and scale to assess causality in patients with suspected DILI. First published in 1993 and updated in 2016, RUCAM is now the most commonly used causality assessment method for DILI used internationally (Teschke 2019).

Gastroenterologists specializing in hepatology who are familiar with the above criteria should be consulted in case there is a suspected instance of herbal insult to the liver so that established diagnostic criteria can be followed in making decisions with regard to any suspected cause of liver toxicity due to an herbal dietary supplement (Teschke et al. 2013).

CURCUMIN

Turmeric spice, which is also called curry powder, has been used for centuries as a treatment for inflammatory diseases in Ayurveda and other traditional medical systems. Extensive research within the past two decades has shown that curcumin, diferuloylmethane, mediates its anti-inflammatory effects through the downregulation of inflammatory transcription factors, enzymes, and cytokines (Aggarwal and Sung 2009). The pharmacodynamics and pharmacokinetics of curcumin have been examined in animals and in humans. It is sometimes combined with black pepper extract containing piperine to increase its bioavailability by inhibiting methylation.

Preliminary data indicate that curcumin helps relieve adverse effects due to cancer treatments. A topical turmeric-based cream was reported to reduce radiotherapy-induced dermatitis (Palatty et al. 2014). Oral curcumin administration increased body weight, decreased serum TNF-α levels, increased apoptotic tumor cells, enhanced expression of p53 molecule in tumor tissue of patients with colorectal cancer, and modulated tumor cell apoptotic pathways (He et al. 2011). In a phase II trial involving 21 patients with advanced pancreatic cancer, curcumin demonstrated bioactivity by downregulating nuclear factor-κB and cyclooxygenase-2 (Dhillon et al. 2008).

Curcumin has been reported to be safe, but whether it interacts with any chemotherapy drugs is not known. It is known to interfere with CYP450 enzymes in healthy volunteers and could interact significantly with some drugs. Curcumin reduced the activities of CYP1A2 (28.6%) and increased the activity of CYP2A6 (+48.9%), using caffeine as a probe drug (Chen et al. 2010). Therefore, drug doses may have to be adjusted in some individuals given curcumin. Turmeric and curcumin are not mutagenic or genotoxic. Administration of oral curcumin in humans was safe at the dose of 6 g/day orally for 4–7 weeks, and it is generally regarded as safe for human consumption as it is eaten in large quantities in South Asian cuisine as a spice. However, some adverse effects such as gastrointestinal upsets may occur (Soleimani, Sahebkar, and Hosseinzadeh 2018).

GREEN TEA

The leaves of green tea (*Camellia sinensis*) are used to prepare tea by hot water extraction, and this method is safely used to prepare green tea extract capsules. This method of extraction maintains the normal ratios of the antioxidants in tea called catechins. The predominant catechin is epigallocatechin gallate or EGCG, but studies have shown that the full complement of catechins has more potent antioxidant activity than EGCG alone. A review of adverse event data from 159 human intervention studies found evidence of hepatic adverse events in a limited number of concentrated, catechin-rich green tea extracts in a dose-dependent manner when ingested in large doses as supplements, but not when consumed as brewed tea or extracts in beverages or as part of food. A safe intake level of 338 mg EGCG/day for adults was derived from toxicological and human safety data for tea preparations ingested as an extract preparation. An observed safe level of 704 mg EGCG/day was derived for tea preparations in beverage form based on human adverse event data (Hu et al. 2018). With origins in Asia and now consumed worldwide, green tea and its extracts have been used to prevent and treat hyperlipidemia, hypertension, atherosclerosis, and cancer.

Anticancer actions and the molecular mechanisms of green tea and EGCG have been found in various kinds of animal models and in vitro experiments using different types of cancer cells. In addition, findings in a number of epidemiological and interventional studies have indicated that green tea administration may play a role in cancer prevention. EGCG concentrations for exerting anticancer effects in cell culture experiments are much greater than those found in the tissue and plasma detected in human trials and animal experiments. In fact, typical tea consumption usually has catechins reach plasma levels only into the low micromolar range. Therefore, it still remains unclear whether the observations in in vitro studies with high concentrations of EGCG are able to be directly extrapolated to cancer chemoprevention in animals and humans (Shirakami and Shimizu 2018).

In an exploratory open label trial, 92 of 113 men diagnosed with prostate cancer were randomly assigned to consume six cups daily of brewed green tea, black tea, or water prior to radical prostatectomy (Henning et al. 2015). There was no significant difference in markers of proliferation, apoptosis, and oxidation in stromal prostate tissue obtained at prostatectomy in the groups consuming green tea, black tea, or water. The nuclear staining for NF-κB was significantly decreased in the prostate tissue of men consuming green tea ($P=0.013$) but not black tea ($P=0.931$) compared to the water control. Tea polyphenols were detected in the prostate tissue from 32 of 34 men consuming green tea but polyphenosl was not detected in the group consuming black tea compared to the control group. Evidence of a systemic antioxidant effect as reduced urinary 8-hydroxy-deoxyguanosine was observed only with green tea consumption ($P=0.03$). Green tea, but not black tea or water, also led to a small but statistically significant decrease in serum prostate-specific antigen levels ($P=0.04$) (Henning et al. 2015).

Topical application of green tea extract has been shown to be effective against external genital and perianal warts. One such extract, sinecatechins, is approved by the Food and Drug Administration (FDA) for the treatment of these conditions in one of the few successful applications to the FDA for botanical drugs (Tatti et al. 2008). Preclinical studies have shown that green tea polyphenols can block the action of bortezomib, a proteasome drug used in multiple myeloma (Golden et al. 2009). There is a need for clinical studies to assess the effects of these herb-drug pharmacodynamic interactions of green tea as well as the clinical significance of any pharmacokinetic effects on drugs used in cancer patients. In the absence of clear information, discontinuation during active therapy may be advisable.

GINGER

The root of the ginger plant (Zingiber officinale) is well known as a spice and flavoring. It has been used as a culinary spice and as a medicine in Asian and Arabic traditions to treat pregnancy-associated nausea, and joint inflammation. Clinical trials indicate that ginger can reduce nausea and vomiting following chemotherapy (Ryan et al. 2012). This is a totally safe adjunct as it is used to prevent or treat nausea during pregnancy and there are no reports of toxicity. It is available in the form of lozenges or candy that can be used effectively in mild nausea for this purpose.

However, there are well-developed drugs for nausea which can be employed for more severe postchemotherapy nausea as well if ginger is not effective. Palonosetron is a second-generation 5-HT3 receptor antagonist with proposed higher efficacy and sustained action for prophylaxis of postoperative nausea and vomiting than earlier drugs. In a large number of clinical trials for postoperative nausea and vomiting, palonosetron was as safe as and more effective than placebo, ramosetron, granisetron, and ondansetron in preventing delayed postoperative nausea and vomiting. For early onset nausea and vomiting, there was higher efficacy over placebo, granisetron, and ondansetron (Singh et al. 2016). When needed, these more potent drugs should be used together with avoidance of favorite foods on the day of chemotherapy or even fasting prior to chemotherapy to avoid acquired taste aversions due to nausea which can negatively impact nutrition support (Bernstein 1985, Chambers 2018).

Ashwaganda A shrub valued in Ayurveda for its medicinal effects; ashwagandha (*Withania somnifera*) is used to relieve stress, anxiety, and fatigue. The active constituents include alkaloids, saponins, and steroidal lactones known as withanolides. Clinical studies show its utility in relieving anxiety, and in mitigating chemotherapy-induced fatigue, along with improving quality of life in a small study of breast cancer patients. No serious adverse events or changes in hematological, biochemical, or vital parameters were reported in 30 clinical studies. Only mild and mainly transient type adverse events of somnolence, epigastric pain/discomfort, and loose stools were reported as most common (>5%); giddiness, drowsiness, hallucinogenic, vertigo, nasal congestion (rhinitis), cough, cold, decreased appetite, nausea, constipation, dry mouth, hyperactivity, nocturnal cramps, blurring of vision, hyperacidity, skin rash, and weight gain were reported as less common adverse events. There was no in vitro or in vivo inhibition seen for CYP3A4 and CYP2D6, the two major hepatic drug metabolizing enzymes (Tandon and Yadav 2020). An open-label prospective nonrandomized comparative trial on 100 patients with breast cancer undergoing either a combination of chemotherapy with oral *Withania somnifera* or chemotherapy alone demonstrated some positive effects on fatigue and quality of life. The root extract was administered to patients in the study group at a dose of 2 g every 8 hours, throughout the course of chemotherapy. The quality-of-life and fatigue scores were evaluated before, during, and on the last cycles of chemotherapy using the European Organisation for Research and Treatment of Cancer Quality of Life Questionnaires C-30 (EORTC QLQ-C30) (Version 3), Piper Fatigue Scale, and Schwartz Cancer Fatigue Scale (SCFS-6). Larger studies with placebo controls to evaluate efficacy are warranted because of the recent rise in the popularity of this herb.

Reishi mushroom

Reishi mushroom (*Ganoderma lucidum*) is commonly used by cancer patients. It is an important component of traditional medical systems in Asia and is used to strengthen the body, increase vitality, and to treat insomnia. Preliminary data in 34 cancer patients suggested that an aqueous polysaccharide fraction extracted from *G. lucidum* may be effective in enhancing immune responses in advanced-stage cancer patients (Gao et al. 2003). The anticancer properties of *G. lucidum* are primarily attributed to its polysaccharides and triterpenes. *G. lucidum* polysaccharides include $(1 \rightarrow 3)$, $(1 \rightarrow 6)$-α/β-glucans, glycoproteins, and water-soluble heteropolysaccharides. In vitro and in vivo studies have demonstrated that *Ganoderma lucidum* polysaccharides have potential anticancer activity through immunomodulatory, antiproliferative, proapoptotic, antimetastatic, and antiangiogenic effects (Sohretoglu and Huang 2018, Zhang et al. 2019, Kladar, Gavaric, and Bozin 2016). Extracts from the fruiting body as well as spores have been employed in clinical trials for cancer. Cultured human B lymphocytes and extract prepared from *G. lucidum* spores were demonstrated to reduce PD-1 protein suggesting a role for *G. lucidum* spore extracts in immunomodulation. PD-1 protein reduction was not caused by a transcriptional inhibition of the gene, and further in vivo studies are needed. Herbal supplements as Lingzhi have antioxidant effects in vivo and in vitro (Lin and Deng 2019, Wachtel-Galor et al. 2004). Antiplatelet effects touted as beneficial for cardiovascular risk are considered a potential toxic effect in cancer patients and must be considered in a clinical context (Poniedzialek et al. 2019). As with other botanicals, reishi has been reported to inhibit CYP450 enzymes, but pharmacokinetic studies have failed to define the clinical impact on chemotherapy (Yeung, Gubili, and Mao 2018).

Engaging the body's immune response against tumor cells by unmasking them through inhibition or blockade of checkpoint proteins has resulted in impressive durable clinical responses, and created the field of immunotherapy of cancer. The immune system can adapt and counter changes in the genetic landscape of cancer cells to prevent escape from the therapeutic effect. Immunomodulatory antibodies recently licensed in the United States include ipilimumab as well as nivolumab and pembrolizumab, neutralizing two different inhibitory pathways that block antitumor T cell responses. These agents have achieved some successes in treating late-stage cancers refractory to essentially any other treatments. Increased research on the interactions of botanical dietary supplements such as Ganoderma polysaccharides and the microbiome in modulation of anticancer immune responses is needed.

COMMUNICATING

Herbal product use by cancer patients has increased significantly over the last few decades. Many of these supplements are bioactive, with a potential for interactions with chemotherapy and other cancer drugs. It is important to communicate openly about herbal product use. Physicians should discuss patient expectations with their patients, clearly communicating the benefits and risks.

Some herbals act as food or spices in lesser doses for culinary use where they are not harmful and enhance taste promoting healthy nutrition. As regards nutritional consultation together with Integrative Oncology, the principles of Personalized Nutrition outlined in Chapter 6 should be followed but individualized to the situation of each cancer patient. While colorful fruits and vegetables, teas, spices, and healthy fats are organizing principles, there is a need to personalize each patient's program to their tastes and capabilities in regard to their stage of disease or recovery from cancer.

Some patients use a large number of supplement products simultaneously that have ingredients they may have seen in a study on the internet or heard about from friends. When they bring them to the oncologist or doctor seeking advice, it can be helpful to discuss the supplements, to look for interactions or higher than advisable doses based on known toxicities, and to simplify the regimen whenever possible.

When herbal supplements are not appropriate, you can recommend therapies such as acupuncture, yoga, and meditation. These have been effective in mitigating symptoms and improving quality of life for some patients. Patients are often receptive to these suggestions.

There are two sites where reliable and conservative information on herbals used by cancer patients can be found. First, the Integrative Medicine Service at Memorial Sloan Kettering Cancer Center has developed the "About Herbs" website: www.mskcc.org/aboutherbs. It contains objective information on dietary supplements used by cancer patients. Mechanisms of action underlying the effects of these products and the drugs with which they can potentially interact are listed. This site, which has both healthcare professional and consumer versions, is available free of charge to clinicians and patients. Other databases that provide reliable information include the National Institutes of Health's Office of Dietary Supplements (https://ods.od.nih.gov).

MIND–BODY PRACTICE

Mind–body practices include cognitive-behavioral therapy, meditation, yoga, tai chi, qigong, and expressive arts including art, music, and dance therapy. Meditation and relaxation therapies are contemplative practices that help cancer patients reduce worry by focusing attention on relaxing sounds and body sensations including the movement of the chest during normal breathing. These practices can reduce stress, fatigue, anxiety, and depression which often accompany the course of cancer treatment and recovery. Mindfulness and relaxation were effective at reducing fatigue severity in patients with cancer and recipients of bone marrow transplants (Duong et al. 2017). Meta-analyses of 170 trials of physical activity including aerobic, neuromotor, resistance, and combination exercises demonstrated reduced fatigue in cancer patients and recipients of bone marrow transplants (Oberoi et al. 2018). Cognitive-behavioral therapy and mind–body therapies including mindfulness meditation, yoga, and tai chi may benefit cancer patients who are fatigued secondary to sleep problems including difficulty initiating and maintaining quality sleep (Zhou, Gardiner, and Bertisch 2017). Music-based interventions may have a positive impact on pain, anxiety, mood disturbance, and quality of life in cancer patients, and research on the neurobiological effects of music may provide insight into the potential mechanisms by which music impacts these outcomes (Archie, Bruera, and Cohen 2013). As an important component of Integrative Oncology, mind–body practices can improve the quality of life for cancer patients, survivors, and those fearing relapse by reducing stress, anxiety, and depression, as well as reducing the impact of some physical symptoms such as pain, nausea, sleep disturbances, and mobility issues.

ACUPUNCTURE

Acupuncture has its origins in TCM (Deng, Bao, and Mao 2018). Classical acupuncture involves the insertion of needles at selected acupoints to a defined depth, followed by manipulation with physical forces, heat, or more recently, electrical stimuli. According to the theory behind acupuncture, vital energy called "chi" ("qi" in Chinese) flows through channels called meridian pathways. The interruption or obstruction of the flow of qi is believed to make one vulnerable to illness. The insertion of needles at specific meridian acupoints is thought to improve the flow of qi, thus producing a therapeutic benefit. The meridians and acupuncture points (or acupoints) on the body can be found in Zhenjiu jiayi jing ("Numbered book on acupuncture and moxibustion"), the oldest surviving writing on acupuncture and moxibustion (the application of heat to certain points on the body) published around 260 Century. Acupuncture is based on controlled irritation of particular active meridian points using special needles, heat (moxibustion), pressure (acupressure), suction (cupping), electricity (electroacupuncture), light (laser therapy), ultrasound (sonopuncture), static, or pulsating electromagnetic fields (magnetic therapy). The use of acupuncture as a method of pain relief has been studied in many clinical trials for both acute and chronic pain (Ondrejkovicova et al. 2016).

Pain signals are transmitted by peripheral afferent nerve endings to the central nervous system through modulation of various neurotransmitters and pathways (Cai et al. 2018). The discovery of endogenous opioids facilitated serious research on acupuncture in pain treatment (Chen et al. 2009). Other neuroscientific research is suggestive of the notion that acupuncture may provide clinical effects by modulating neurotransmitters and neuronal matrices that are activated or deactivated during acupuncture. These effects have been observed in functional magnetic resonance imaging (MRI) and positron emission tomography studies (Dougherty et al. 2008; Zhou et al. 2014). Therefore, qi and meridians can be seen as vehicles used by ancient people to explain clinical responses observed during acupuncture [18].

In a typical acupuncture session, a licensed therapist interviews the patient and performs a physical examination, including pulse and tongue appearance. A TCM diagnosis is made which describes syndrome patterns rather than a pathologic process. For example, presentation with insomnia, irritability, racing thoughts, dry mouth, and hot flashes are classified as a "heart fire" pattern (Ifrim Chen, Antochi, and Barbilian 2019).

Acupoints are selected based on the pattern diagnosis and single-use, sterile stainless steel needles are inserted. Acupuncture needles are filiform and very thin (28–40 gauge), similar to or thinner than insulin needles. In the United States, acupuncture needles are classified as medical devices. In a typical treatment, acupoints are located and the sites cleaned with alcohol swabs. The needle and its guide tube are placed at each site. A gentle tap applied to the top of the needle makes it penetrate the skin. The guide tube is then removed, and the needle advanced to the desired depth in a gentle twisting and pushing movement. The therapist may decide to apply heat or electrical stimuli to the needle. Traditionally, heat stimulation is provided by a heat lamp. In electroacupuncture, a small electric pulse–generating device connects to pairs of acupuncture needles to deliver electrical stimulation to the acupoints, in a manner akin to transcutaneous electrical nerve stimulation.

Acupuncture was judged to be effective in relieving cancer-related pain, particularly malignancy-related and surgery-induced pain in a meta-analysis of 29 randomized controlled trials (Chiu, Hsieh, and Tsai 2017). The Division of Cancer Treatment and Diagnosis, Office of Cancer Complementary and Alternative Medicine at the National Cancer Institute (NCI) held a symposium on "Acupuncture for Cancer Symptom Management" in 2017 (Zia et al. 2017). Oncology acupuncture is still a relatively new field. There is emerging research that has found some evidence in randomized controlled trials supporting a role in cancer patient care by relieving symptoms such as pain, fatigue, hot flashes, nausea/vomiting, and xerostomia (Garcia et al. 2013).

Acupuncture is an appropriate adjunctive treatment for chemotherapy-induced nausea/vomiting. Additional studies are needed to establish its efficacy in controlled trials for other cancer-related symptoms. These future studies should include standardized comparison groups and treatment methods using appropriate statistical measures and some biological endpoints.

MASSAGE

Oncology massage is the modification of massage techniques in the context of cancer care. A clinical oncology massage program was integrated into chemotherapy infusion units as a program to provide symptom control for patients with breast cancer (Mao et al. 2017). Among 692 breast cancer patients accepting an oncology massage after 1,090 massages were offered, there was a significant decrease in self-reported anxiety, nausea, pain, and fatigue after the massage in this self-selected population using self-report of symptom control. Reiki touch therapy is a Japanese traditional therapy designed to help the body's natural healing system through rebalancing of the energy fields of the body (Vitale 2007). As part of a study on the efficacy of a single session of massage or Reiki in a rural 396-bed hospital, patients requesting or referred to the healing arts team who received either a massage or reiki session and completed both a pre- and post-therapy symptom questionnaire were evaluated. Patients reported symptom relief with both reiki and massage therapy. Reiki improved fatigue and anxiety statistically more than massage in this study ($P < 0.01$). Pain, nausea, depression, and well-being changes were not statistically different between reiki and massage encounters. Immediate symptom relief was similar for cancer and noncancer patients for both reiki and massage therapy, and did not vary based on age, gender, length of session, and baseline symptoms. While evidence from multiple studies points to the benefits of massage for relieving symptoms such as pain, anxiety, fatigue, and general aspects of quality of life, the evidence is mostly based on self-report by necessity. While case report and expert opinion suggest a role for massage in the relief of overall common symptoms in patients undergoing chemotherapy or suffering from postchemotherapy side effects, more research is needed to better understand the symptoms that massage can help treat as well as the optimal length and frequency of treatments (Kinkead et al. 2018).

CONCLUSION

With increasing frequency over the last 20 years, cancer patients have been seeking integrative medicine approaches when experiencing greater symptom distress. Some patients evidence an increased desire for spiritual transformation, or express unfulfilled needs from their conventional treatment alone (Mao et al. 2007, 2008). Although limited, several types of integrative oncology approaches such as acupuncture, massage, and mind–body medicine have found to be beneficial for many patients in terms of symptom management and quality of life.

Patients use various approaches to reduce distress during and after cancer treatments, and integrative oncology has become a common coping strategy. One of the major challenges of integrative oncology deals with the incorporation of nutrition. The key questions requiring more research include determining the value of nutrition and various nutritional supplements, evaluating the role of physical therapy and exercise, investigating the mind–body connection, and determining as best as possible the benefit of incorporating integrative therapies such as spirituality, acupuncture, and massage.

Transparent communication between oncologists and their patients into the use of integrative oncology and nutrition approaches is essential. It increases the ability of healthcare providers to guide vulnerable cancer patients safely. At the same time, the role of nutrition in the patient's care should not be lumped in as an additional alternative medicine practice but should be included in the care of all oncology patients including those who choose to use integrative practices.

Many nutritional and natural products are safe for cancer patients to use with proper guidance on dose and time of administration. Integrative physicians in the future may be able to provide "bedside-to-bench" guidance on the safety of herbal products by testing for interference with chemotherapeutics or with drug metabolism (Ben-Arye and Samuels 2017).

In summary, while there is some emerging evidence supporting the use of integrative therapies, especially mind–body therapies, as effective supportive care strategies during cancer treatment, many integrative practices require more research in controlled settings beyond retrospective chart review and self-reported symptom control. Therefore, at present, there is insufficient evidence for some integrative approaches to be definitively recommended or avoided, and the patient and physician must decide together how to proceed as long as there is little risk of harm.

REFERENCES

Ernst, E (2008). "Anthroposophic medicine: A critical analysis". MMW Fortschritte der Medizin. 150 Suppl 1: 1–6. PMID 18540325.

Ades TB, ed. (2009). Mistletoe. American Cancer Society Complete Guide to Complementary and Alternative Cancer Therapies (2nd ed.). American Cancer Society. pp. 424–428. ISBN 9780944235713.

Horneber MA, Bueschel G, Huber R, Linde K, Rostock M (2008). "Mistletoe therapy in oncology". Cochrane Database Syst Rev (Systematic review) (2): CD003297. doi:10.1002/14651858.CD003297.pub2. PMC 7144832. PMID 18425885.

Ernst, E (2011). "Anthroposophy: A risk factor for noncompliance with measles immunization". The Pediatric Infectious Disease Journal. 30 (3): 187–9. doi:10.1097/INF.0b013e3182024274. PMID 21102363.

Kienle, Gunver S.; Kiene, Helmut; Albonico, Hans Ulrich (2006). "Anthroposophische Medizin: Health Technology Assessment Bericht – Kurzfassung". Forschende Komplementärmedizin. 13 (2): 7–18. doi:10.1159/000093481. PMID 16883076.

Ernst, E. (2006). "Mistletoe as a treatment for cancer". BMJ. 333 (7582): 1282–3. doi:10.1136/bmj.39055.493958.80. PMC 1761165. PMID 17185706.

Marinelli, R., Fuerst, B., et al. "The Heart is not a Pump: A refutation of the pressure propulsion premise of heart function", Frontier Perspectives 5(1), Fall-Winter 1995

Rawlings, Roger. "Rudolf Steiner's Quackery". QuackWatch. Retrieved 10 September 2012.

Offit, Paul A. (2011). Deadly Choices: How the Anti-Vaccine Movement Threatens Us All. Basic Books. p. 13. ISBN 978-0-465–02356–1.

Dougherty DD, Kong J, Webb M, Bonab AA, Fischman AJ, Gollub RL. A combined [11C]diprenorphine PET study and fMRI study of acupuncture analgesia. Behav Brain Res. 2008 Nov 3;193(1):63-8. doi: 10.1016/j.bbr.2008.04.020. Epub 2008 May 2. PMID: 18562019; PMCID: PMC2538486Fo.

Dugan, Dan (2002-01-01). Michael Shermer (ed.). Anthroposophy and Anthroposophical Medicine. The Skeptic Encyclopedia of Pseudoscience. ABC-CLIO. pp. 31–32. ISBN 978-1-57607-653–8.

Jump, Paul (11 May 2012). "Aberdeen decides against alternative medicine chair". Times Higher Education Supplement.

McKie, Robin; Hartmann, Laura (29 April 2012). "Holistic unit will 'tarnish' Aberdeen University reputation". The Observer.

Gorski, David (14 March 2011). "A University of Michigan Medical School alumnus confronts anthroposophic medicine at his alma mater". Science-Based Medicine. Retrieved 29 November 2018.

Shermer, Michael (2002). The Skeptic encyclopedia of pseudoscience. ABC-CLIO. p. 903. ISBN 1576076539. Retrieved 29 November 2018.

Singh, Simon (2009). Trick or treatment: the undeniable facts about alternative medicine (1st American ed.). W.W. Norton. ISBN 9780393337785.

Abebe, W. 2019. "Review of herbal medications with the potential to cause bleeding: dental implications, and risk prediction and prevention avenues." EPMA J 10 (1):51–64. doi: 10.1007/s13167-018-0158-2.

Aggarwal, B. B., and B. Sung. 2009. "Pharmacological basis for the role of curcumin in chronic diseases: an age-old spice with modern targets." Trends Pharmacol Sci 30 (2):85–94. doi: 10.1016/j.tips.2008.11.002.

Archie, P., E. Bruera, and L. Cohen. 2013. "Music-based interventions in palliative cancer care: a review of quantitative studies and neurobiological literature." Support Care Cancer 21 (9):2609–24. doi: 10.1007/s00520-013-1841-4.

Barnes, P. M., B. Bloom, and R. L. Nahin. 2008. "Complementary and alternative medicine use among adults and children: United States, 2007." Natl Health Stat Report 12:1–23.

Ben-Arye, E., and N. Samuels. 2017. "Integrative cancer care: crossing communication barriers." Oncotarget 8 (53):90634–5. doi: 10.18632/oncotarget.21890.

Bernstein, I. L. 1985. "Learned food aversions in the progression of cancer and its treatment." Ann N Y Acad Sci 443:365–80. doi: 10.1111/j.1749-6632.1985.tb27086.x.

Brauer, J. A., A. El Sehamy, J. M. Metz, and J. J. Mao. 2010. "Complementary and alternative medicine and supportive care at leading cancer centers: a systematic analysis of websites." *J Altern Complement Med* 16 (2):183–6. doi: 10.1089/acm.2009.0354.

Cai, R. L., G. M. Shen, H. Wang, and Y. Y. Guan. 2018. "Brain functional connectivity network studies of acupuncture: a systematic review on resting-state fMRI." *J Integr Med* 16 (1):26–33. doi: 10.1016/j.joim.2017.12.002.

Chambers, K. C. 2018. "Conditioned taste aversions." *World J Otorhinolaryngol Head Neck Surg* 4 (1):92–100. doi: 10.1016/j.wjorl.2018.02.003.

Chen, L., J. Zhang, F. Li, Y. Qiu, L. Wang, Y. H. Li, J. Shi, H. L. Pan, and M. Li. 2009. "Endogenous anandamide and cannabinoid receptor-2 contribute to electroacupuncture analgesia in rats." *J Pain* 10 (7):732–9. doi: 10.1016/j.jpain.2008.12.012.

Chen, Y., W. H. Liu, B. L. Chen, L. Fan, Y. Han, G. Wang, D. L. Hu, Z. R. Tan, G. Zhou, S. Cao, and H. H. Zhou. 2010. "Plant polyphenol curcumin significantly affects CYP1A2 and CYP2A6 activity in healthy, male Chinese volunteers." *Ann Pharmacother* 44 (6):1038–45. doi: 10.1345/aph.1M533.

Chiu, H. Y., Y. J. Hsieh, and P. S. Tsai. 2017. "Systematic review and meta-analysis of acupuncture to reduce cancer-related pain." *Eur J Cancer Care (Engl)* 26 (2). doi: 10.1111/ecc.12457.

Clarke, T. C., L. I. Black, B. J. Stussman, P. M. Barnes, and R. L. Nahin. 2015. "Trends in the use of complementary health approaches among adults: United States, 2002–2012." *Natl Health Stat Report* 79:1–16.

Deng, G., T. Bao, and J. J. Mao. 2018. "Understanding the benefits of acupuncture treatment for cancer pain management." *Oncology (Williston Park)* 32 (6):310–6.

Dhillon, N., B. B. Aggarwal, R. A. Newman, R. A. Wolff, A. B. Kunnumakkara, J. L. Abbruzzese, C. S. Ng, V. Badmaev, and R. Kurzrock. 2008. "Phase II trial of curcumin in patients with advanced pancreatic cancer." *Clin Cancer Res* 14 (14):4491–9. doi: 10.1158/1078-0432.CCR-08-0024.

Duong, N., H. Davis, P. D. Robinson, S. Oberoi, D. Cataudella, S. N. Culos-Reed, F. Gibson, M. Gotte, P. Hinds, S. L. Nijhof, D. Tomlinson, P. van der Torre, E. Ladas, S. Cabral, L. L. Dupuis, and L. Sung. 2017. "Mind and body practices for fatigue reduction in patients with cancer and hematopoietic stem cell transplant recipients: a systematic review and meta-analysis." *Crit Rev Oncol Hematol* 120:210–6. doi: 10.1016/j.critrevonc.2017.11.011.

Frass, M., R. P. Strassl, H. Friehs, M. Mullner, M. Kundi, and A. D. Kaye. 2012. "Use and acceptance of complementary and alternative medicine among the general population and medical personnel: a systematic review." *Ochsner J* 12 (1):45–56.

Gao, Y., S. Zhou, W. Jiang, M. Huang, and X. Dai. 2003. "Effects of ganopoly (a Ganoderma lucidum polysaccharide extract) on the immune functions in advanced-stage cancer patients." *Immunol Invest* 32 (3):201–15. doi: 10.1081/imm-120022979.

Garcia, M. K., J. McQuade, R. Haddad, S. Patel, R. Lee, P. Yang, J. L. Palmer, and L. Cohen. 2013. "Systematic review of acupuncture in cancer care: a synthesis of the evidence." *J Clin Oncol* 31 (7):952–60. doi: 10.1200/JCO.2012.43.5818.

Garland, S. N., D. Valentine, K. Desai, S. Li, C. Langer, T. Evans, and J. J. Mao. 2013. "Complementary and alternative medicine use and benefit finding among cancer patients." *J Altern Complement Med* 19 (11):876–81. doi: 10.1089/acm.2012.0964.

Golden, E. B., P. Y. Lam, A. Kardosh, K. J. Gaffney, E. Cadenas, S. G. Louie, N. A. Petasis, T. C. Chen, and A. H. Schonthal. 2009. "Green tea polyphenols block the anticancer effects of bortezomib and other boronic acid-based proteasome inhibitors." *Blood* 113 (23):5927–37. doi: 10.1182/blood-2008-07-171389.

He, Z. Y., C. B. Shi, H. Wen, F. L. Li, B. L. Wang, and J. Wang. 2011. "Upregulation of p53 expression in patients with colorectal cancer by administration of curcumin." *Cancer Invest* 29 (3):208–13. doi: 10.3109/07357907.2010.550592.

Henning, S. M., P. Wang, J. W. Said, M. Huang, T. Grogan, D. Elashoff, C. L. Carpenter, D. Heber, and W. J. Aronson. 2015. "Randomized clinical trial of brewed green and black tea in men with prostate cancer prior to prostatectomy." *Prostate* 75 (5):550–9. doi: 10.1002/pros.22943.

Hu, J., D. Webster, J. Cao, and A. Shao. 2018. "The safety of green tea and green tea extract consumption in adults: results of a systematic review." *Regul Toxicol Pharmacol* 95:412–33 doi: 10.1016/j.yrtph.2018.03.019.

Ifrim Chen, F., A. D. Antochi, and A. G. Barbilian. 2019. "Acupuncture and the retrospect of its modern research." *Rom J Morphol Embryol* 60 (2):411–8.

Jayachandran, M., J. Xiao, and B. Xu. 2017. "A critical review on health promoting benefits of edible mushrooms through gut microbiota." *Int J Mol Sci* 18 (9). doi: 10.3390/ijms18091934.

Kinkead, B., P. J. Schettler, E. R. Larson, D. Carroll, M. Sharenko, J. Nettles, S. A. Edwards, A. H. Miller, M. A. Torres, B. W. Dunlop, J. J. Rakofsky, and M. H. Rapaport. 2018. "Massage therapy decreases cancer-related fatigue: results from a randomized early phase trial." *Cancer* 124 (3):546–54. doi: 10.1002/cncr.31064.

Kladar, N. V., N. S. Gavaric, and B. N. Bozin. 2016. "Ganoderma: insights into anticancer effects." *Eur J Cancer Prev* 25 (5):462–71. doi: 10.1097/CEJ.0000000000000204.

Lawenda, B. D., K. M. Kelly, E. J. Ladas, S. M. Sagar, A. Vickers, and J. B. Blumberg. 2008. "Should supplemental antioxidant administration be avoided during chemotherapy and radiation therapy?" *J Natl Cancer Inst* 100 (11):773–83. doi: 10.1093/jnci/djn148.

Lin, Z., and A. Deng. 2019. "Antioxidative and free radical scavenging activity of Ganoderma (Lingzhi)." *Adv Exp Med Biol* 1182:271–97 doi: 10.1007/978-981-32-9421-9_12.

Lopez, G., W. Liu, J. McQuade, R. T. Lee, A. R. Spelman, B. Fellman, Y. Li, E. Bruera, and L. Cohen. 2017. "Integrative oncology outpatient consultations: Long-term effects on patient-reported symptoms and quality of life." *J Cancer* 8 (9):1640–6. doi: 10.7150/jca.18875.

Mao, J. J., J. T. Farrar, S. X. Xie, M. A. Bowman, and K. Armstrong. 2007. "Use of complementary and alternative medicine and prayer among a national sample of cancer survivors compared to other populations without cancer." *Complement Ther Med* 15 (1):21–9. doi: 10.1016/j.ctim.2006.07.006.

Mao, J. J., S. C. Palmer, J. B. Straton, P. F. Cronholm, S. Keddem, K. Knott, M. A. Bowman, and F. K. Barg. 2008. "Cancer survivors with unmet needs were more likely to use complementary and alternative medicine." *J Cancer Surviv* 2 (2):116–24. doi: 10.1007/s11764-008-0052-3.

Mao, J. J., K. E. Wagner, C. M. Seluzicki, A. Hugo, L. K. Galindez, H. Sheaffer, and K. R. Fox. 2017. "Integrating oncology massage into chemoinfusion suites: A program evaluation." *J Oncol Pract* 13 (3):e207–16. doi: 10.1200/JOP.2016.015081.

Nahin, R. L., J. M. Dahlhamer, and B. J. Stussman. 2010. "Health need and the use of alternative medicine among adults who do not use conventional medicine." *BMC Health Serv Res* 10:220. doi: 10.1186/1472-6963-10-220.

Navarro, V. J., I. Khan, E. Bjornsson, L. B. Seeff, J. Serrano, and J. H. Hoofnagle. 2017. "Liver injury from herbal and dietary supplements." *Hepatology* 65 (1):363–73. doi: 10.1002/hep.28813.

Oberoi, S., P. D. Robinson, D. Cataudella, S. N. Culos-Reed, H. Davis, N. Duong, F. Gibson, M. Gotte, P. Hinds, S. L. Nijhof, D. Tomlinson, P. van der Torre, S. Cabral, L. L. Dupuis, and L. Sung. 2018. "Physical activity reduces fatigue in patients with cancer and hematopoietic stem cell transplant recipients: a systematic review and meta-analysis of randomized trials." *Crit Rev Oncol Hematol* 122:52–9. doi: 10.1016/j.critrevonc.2017.12.011.

Ondrejkovicova, A., G. Petrovics, K. Svitkova, B. Bajtekova, and O. Bangha. 2016. "Why acupuncture in pain treatment?" *Neuro Endocrinol Lett* 37 (3):163–8.

Palatty, P. L., A. Azmidah, S. Rao, D. Jayachander, K. R. Thilakchand, M. P. Rai, R. Haniadka, P. Simon, R. Ravi, R. Jimmy, F. D'Souza P, R. Fayad, and M. S. Baliga. 2014. "Topical application of a sandal wood oil and turmeric based cream prevents radiodermatitis in head and neck cancer patients undergoing external beam radiotherapy: a pilot study." *Br J Radiol* 87 (1038):20130490. doi: 10.1259/bjr.20130490.

Poniedzialek, B., M. Siwulski, A. Wiater, I. Komaniecka, A. Komosa, M. Gasecka, Z. Magdziak, M. Mleczek, P. Niedzielski, J. Proch, M. Ropacka-Lesiak, M. Lesiak, E. Henao, and P. Rzymski. 2019. "The effect of mushroom extracts on human platelet and blood coagulation: In vitro screening of eight edible species." *Nutrients* 11 (12). doi: 10.3390/nu11123040.

Powell, S. K. 2016. "Integrative medicine and case management." *Prof Case Manag* 21 (3):111–3. doi: 10.1097/NCM.0000000000000152.

Richardson, M. A., T. Sanders, J. L. Palmer, A. Greisinger, and S. E. Singletary. 2000. "Complementary/alternative medicine use in a comprehensive cancer center and the implications for oncology." *J Clin Oncol* 18 (13):2505–14. doi: 10.1200/JCO.2000.18.13.2505.

Rossi, E., A. Vita, S. Baccetti, M. Di Stefano, F. Voller, and A. Zanobini. 2015. "Complementary and alternative medicine for cancer patients: results of the EPAAC survey on integrative oncology centres in Europe." *Support Care Cancer* 23 (6):1795–806. doi: 10.1007/s00520-014-2517-4.

Ryan, J. L., C. E. Heckler, J. A. Roscoe, S. R. Dakhil, J. Kirshner, P. J. Flynn, J. T. Hickok, and G. R. Morrow. 2012. "Ginger (Zingiber officinale) reduces acute chemotherapy-induced nausea: a URCC CCOP study of 576 patients." *Support Care Cancer* 20 (7):1479–89. doi: 10.1007/s00520-011-1236-3.

Seifried, H. E., S. S. McDonald, D. E. Anderson, P. Greenwald, and J. A. Milner. 2003. "The antioxidant conundrum in cancer." *Cancer Res* 63 (15):4295–8.

Shatzel, J. J., S. R. Olson, D. L. Tao, O. J. T. McCarty, A. V. Danilov, and T. G. DeLoughery. 2017. "Ibrutinib-associated bleeding: pathogenesis, management and risk reduction strategies." *J Thromb Haemost* 15 (5):835–47. doi: 10.1111/jth.13651.

Shirakami, Y., and M. Shimizu. 2018. "Possible mechanisms of green tea and its constituents against cancer." *Molecules* 23 (9). doi: 10.3390/molecules23092284.

Singh, P. M., A. Borle, D. Gouda, J. K. Makkar, M. K. Arora, A. Trikha, A. Sinha, and B. Goudra. 2016. "Efficacy of palonosetron in postoperative nausea and vomiting (PONV)-a meta-analysis." *J Clin Anesth* 34:459–82 doi: 10.1016/j.jclinane.2016.05.018.

Sohretoglu, D., and S. Huang. 2018. "Ganoderma lucidum polysaccharides as an anti-cancer agent." *Anticancer Agents Med Chem* 18 (5):667–74. doi: 10.2174/1871520617666171113121246.

Soleimani, V., A. Sahebkar, and H. Hosseinzadeh. 2018. "Turmeric (curcuma longa) and its major constituent (curcumin) as nontoxic and safe substances: review." *Phytother Res* 32 (6):985–95. doi: 10.1002/ptr.6054.

Tandon, N., and S. S. Yadav. 2020. "Safety and clinical effectiveness of Withania Somnifera (Linn.) Dunal root in human ailments." *J Ethnopharmacol* 255:112768. doi: 10.1016/j.jep.2020.112768.

Tatti, S., J. M. Swinehart, C. Thielert, H. Tawfik, A. Mescheder, and K. R. Beutner. 2008. "Sinecatechins, a defined green tea extract, in the treatment of external anogenital warts: a randomized controlled trial." *Obstet Gynecol* 111 (6):1371–9. doi: 10.1097/AOG.0b013e3181719b60.

Teschke, R. 2019. "Idiosyncratic DILI: analysis of 46,266 cases assessed for causality by RUCAM and published from 2014 to early 2019." *Front Pharmacol* 10:730. doi: 10.3389/fphar.2019.00730.

Teschke, R., C. Frenzel, J. Schulze, and A. Eickhoff. 2013. "Herbal hepatotoxicity: challenges and pitfalls of causality assessment methods." *World J Gastroenterol* 19 (19):2864–82. doi: 10.3748/wjg.v19.i19.2864.

Vitale, A. 2007. "An integrative review of Reiki touch therapy research." *Holist Nurs Pract* 21 (4):167–79. doi: 10.1097/01.HNP.0000280927.83506.f6.

von Ammon, K., M. Frei-Erb, F. Cardini, U. Daig, S. Dragan, G. Hegyi, P. Roberti di Sarsina, J. Sorensen, and G. Lewith. 2012. "Complementary and alternative medicine provision in Europe--first results approaching reality in an unclear field of practices." *Forsch Komplementmed* 19 (Suppl 2):37–43 doi: 10.1159/000343129.

Wachtel-Galor, S., Y. T. Szeto, B. Tomlinson, and I. F. Benzie. 2004. "Ganoderma lucidum ('Lingzhi'); acute and short-term biomarker response to supplementation." *Int J Food Sci Nutr* 55 (1):75–83. doi: 10.1080/09637480310001642510.

Yeung, K. S., J. Gubili, and J. J. Mao. 2018. "Herb-drug interactions in cancer care." *Oncology (Williston Park)* 32 (10):516–20.

Zhang, Y., Y. Jiang, M. Zhang, and L. Zhang. 2019. "Ganoderma sinense polysaccharide: an adjunctive drug used for cancer treatment." *Prog Mol Biol Transl Sci* 163:165–77. doi: 10.1016/bs.pmbts.2019.02.008.

Zhou, E. S., P. Gardiner, and S. M. Bertisch. 2017. "Integrative medicine for insomnia." *Med Clin North Am* 101 (5):865–79. doi: 10.1016/j.mcna.2017.04.005.

Zhou W, Benharash P. Effects and mechanisms of acupuncture based on the principle of meridians. *J Acupunct Meridian Stud.* 2014 Aug;7(4):190-3. doi: 10.1016/j.jams.2014.02.007. Epub 2014 Jun 24. PMID: 25151452.

Zia, F. Z., O. Olaku, T. Bao, A. Berger, G. Deng, A. Y. Fan, M. K. Garcia, P. M. Herman, T. J. Kaptchuk, E. J. Ladas, H. M. Langevin, L. Lao, W. Lu, V. Napadow, R. C. Niemtzow, A. J. Vickers, X. Shelley Wang, C. M. Witt, and J. J. Mao. 2017. "The National Cancer Institute's conference on acupuncture for symptom management in oncology: State of the science, evidence, and research gaps." *J Natl Cancer Inst Monogr* 2017 (52). doi: 10.1093/jncimonographs/lgx005.

18 Susceptibility to Common Age-Related Chronic Diseases

Lauren Lemieux and Zhaoping Li
UCLA Center for Human Nutrition

CONTENTS

INTRODUCTION

The prevention and management of chronic diseases are crucial aspects of comprehensive care for cancer survivors, especially as the number of cancer survivors continues to increase and people are living longer (Cohen 2006, Fosså, Vassilopoulou-Sellin, and Dahl 2008). The majority of cancer survivors (60%–78%) (Deckx et al. 2012, Janssen-Heijnen et al. 2005) have at least one chronic medical condition prior to being diagnosed with cancer; the most common pre-existing problems include cardiovascular disease (CVD), diabetes, and chronic obstructive pulmonary disease (COPD) (Deckx et al. 2012, Janssen-Heijnen et al. 2005). The Childhood Cancer Survivor Study, which looked a health outcome in adult survivors of childhood cancers such as brain tumors, leukemia, lymphoma, sarcomas, and bone tumors, found that up to 73.4% of adults by 30 years after their original cancer diagnoses had a chronic disease (Oeffinger et al. 2006). Other studies have found that the chronic diseases most commonly diagnosed in cancer survivors include second primary malignancies, CVD, diabetes, and osteoporosis (Deckx et al. 2012).

Overweight and obesity, which are increasing in prevalence in the United States, are commonly found in cancer survivors and increase the risk of developing other cancers and impact survival. In cancer survivors, a number of chronic diseases affect functional status, quality of life, and long-term survival (Cohen 2006, Hewitt, Rowland, and Yancik 2003). Furthermore, psychological problems such as depression and anxiety affect these patients. In this chapter, we will review the link between cancer survivorship and common chronic diseases including obesity, anxiety, depression, second malignancies, CVD, diabetes, and osteoporosis.

OBESITY

In 2018 it was estimated that 31.5% of cancer survivors (age 20 and older) were obese, similar to the observed prevalence of obesity in the US (Centers for Disease Control and Prevention). Obesity also increases the risk for developing a variety of different cancers. This is thought to be due to the connection between excess visceral adiposity, insulin resistance, and inflammation (Godsland 2009). Survivors of childhood acute lymphoblastic leukemia have an increased risk of obesity compared to the general population (females: odds ratio [OR], 1.5; 95% CI, 1.2–1.8; males: OR, 1.2; 95% CI, 1.0–1.5), and treatment with cranial radiotherapy is likely a contributing factor (Diller et al. 2009, Friedman, Tonorezos, and Cohen 2019). Additionally, certain cancer therapies including aromatase inhibitors, tamoxifen, gonadotropin-releasing hormone (GnRH) agonists, and glucocorticoids are known to cause weight gain.

A diagnosis of cancer can be a powerful motivator for behavior change to promote weight loss. In fact, in a study of patients with endometrial cancer, patients who were advised by their physician (primary care or oncologist) to lose weight followed through by attempting weight loss (Clark et al. 2016). Various lifestyle intervention studies (ENERGY, LEAN, RENEW) have demonstrated the efficacy of intensive dietary counseling for weight loss, prevention of physical decline, and reduction in inflammatory markers (Rock et al. 2015, Harrigan et al. 2016, Demark-Wahnefried et al. 2012). There are ongoing studies to evaluate the effects of weight on long-term survival.

ANXIETY AND DEPRESSION

Cancer survivors are at risk for developing emotional distress, and comprehensive care of these patients includes addressing mental health and well-being. While some may be diagnosed with anxiety or major depression, others may experience other forms of emotional distress such as feeling vulnerable or being afraid of cancer recurrence (Yi and Syrjala 2017). In the Childhood Cancer Survivor Study, emotional distress was more common in adult cancer survivors (11%) compared to sibling controls (5%) (D'Agostino et al. 2016). Another study examined the prevalence of depression in cancer survivors compared to a control population and found that five or more years after diagnosis the prevalence of depression and anxiety was similar to the control population; however, cancer survivors with <5 years since their diagnosis had a much higher prevalence compared to controls (23.3% vs. 7.6%) (Lee and Cartmell 2020). Ultimately, the prevalence of depression and anxiety varies depending on a variety of factors such as the type of cancer, time since diagnosis, comorbid conditions, sex (females at higher risk than males), and physical impairment, to name a few (Institute of Medicine Committee on Psychosocial Services to Cancer Patients/Families in a Community 2008, Yi and Syrjala 2017). Studies have also demonstrated that cancer survivors believe stress plays a role in their risk for cancer recurrence (Todd et al. 2014). Therefore, it is recommended that a combination of pharmacotherapy, psychotherapy, and behavioral changes be implemented in managing anxiety and depression in these patients in conjunction with a healthy diet and physical activity (Jacobsen 2009, Rock et al. 2012). Additionally, as depression (Luppino et al. 2010) and anxiety (Amiri and Behnezhad 2019) are commonly linked with obesity, maintaining a healthy body weight is important.

SECOND PRIMARY CANCERS

Adult cancer survivors are at risk for developing second malignancies and an estimated 15%–20% of all cancer diagnoses are due to second cancers (Demoor-Goldschmidt and de Vathaire 2019). The reasons for this increased risk range from genetic susceptibility to environmental factors to sequelae of cancer treatment (Fosså, Vassilopoulou-Sellin, and Dahl 2008, Travis 2006). For example, radiotherapy treatment for Hodgkin's disease increases the risk of solid tumors including breast, lung, and gastrointestinal cancers (Travis 2002) while certain chemotherapy treatments (e.g., alkylating agents, topoisomerases) can increase the risk for development of acute myelogenous leukemia (Travis 2006, Demoor-Goldschmidt and de Vathaire 2019). Tamoxifen, commonly used in the treatment of breast cancer, is known to increase the risk of endometrial cancer (Demoor-Goldschmidt and de Vathaire 2019). Additionally, the most common cause of death in childhood cancer survivors is subsequent malignancies (Armstrong et al. 2016). Obesity also increases the risk for the development of second cancers. Two large studies in Korea found that elevated body mass index (BMI) prior to the diagnosis of a primary cancer increased the risk for secondary cancers (Park et al. 2016, Jung et al. 2019).

CARDIOVASCULAR DISEASE

CVD in the context of cancer survivors broadly includes conditions such as atherosclerosis, myocardial infarction, cardiomyopathy, and valvular heart disease. In fact, heart disease was found to be the second most common cause of death in childhood cancer survivors (Armstrong et al. 2016). CVD risk is dependent on both the dose and duration of treatment as well as traditional cardiovascular risk factors (Wang et al. 2015). It is well known that certain chemotherapy drugs such as anthracyclines (e.g., doxorubicin, daunorubicin) are cardiotoxic and can lead to heart failure (Wang et al. 2015, Fosså, Vassilopoulou-Sellin, and Dahl 2008). However, there are a number of other chemotherapy agents, ranging from antimetabolites to alkylating agents and monoclonal antibodies that have also been implicated in the development of CVD, the details of which are beyond the scope of this overview (Floyd and Morgan 2020). Accelerated atherosclerosis, myocardial infarction, and cardiac insufficiency have also been reported in patients who have had mediastinal radiotherapy, and these findings may become clinically apparent between 5 and 20 years later (Fosså, Vassilopoulou-Sellin, and Dahl 2008). The cardiotoxic effects of cancer treatment may be related to the generation of free radicals which cause direct damage to cardiac myocytes (Wouters et al. 2005). Additionally, reactive oxygen species formation is thought to drive the oxidation of low-density lipoprotein cholesterol (LDL-C) leading to atherosclerosis (Torres et al. 2015). Importantly, a diet rich in colorful fruits and vegetables may be protective by providing antioxidants including phytonutrients and vitamins A, C, and E (Torres et al. 2015).

DIABETES

Type 2 diabetes mellitus increases the risk for cancer at eight different sites including liver, pancreatic, colorectal, renal, bladder, endometrial breast, and non-Hodgkin's lymphoma (Vigneri et al. 2009) and it is closely associated with overweight and obesity. It has been proposed that elevated levels of insulin and insulin-like growth factor 1 stimulate cancer cell division and proliferation (Vigneri et al. 2009). Furthermore, diabetes that is uncontrolled can lead to inflammation and the production of free radicals that can damage DNA (Vigneri et al. 2009). Meanwhile, new onset diabetes in an otherwise lean person without a family history of diabetes may be an early sign of underlying pancreatic cancer as the result of pancreatic dysfunction (Vigneri et al. 2009).

Cancer treatment can have downstream effects on insulin production, secretion, and sensitivity leading to hyperglycemia (Gallo et al. 2018). L-asparaginase inhibits insulin synthesis by depleting asparagine in pancreatic cell as well as by causing pancreatitis (Gallo et al. 2018). Similarly, immunotherapy (e.g., atezolizumab, avelumab, ipilimumab) can cause pancreatitis and subsequent pancreatic insufficiency leading to hyperglycemia. Diazoxide inhibits insulin secretion as a treatment for insulin-secreting pancreatic neuroendocrine tumors. Medications that promote insulin resistance include glucocorticoids (used for symptom management or treatment) and tyrosine kinase inhibitors (e.g., nilotinib, everolimus). The tyrosine kinase inhibitors disrupt insulin receptor signaling and thereby promote insulin resistance.

In studies of childhood cancer survivors, diabetes and dyslipidemia are commonly diagnosed later in life and further increase the risk of CVD (Friedman, Tonorezos, and Cohen 2019, Gallo et al. 2018). Specific risk factors that have been identified in these patients include a history of abdominal radiation, total body irradiation, and corticosteroid use (Friedman, Tonorezos, and Cohen 2019). As such, it is recommended that patients with a history of abdominal radiation or total body irradiation have a fasting blood glucose or glycosylated hemoglobin measured at least every 2 years (Friedman, Tonorezos, and Cohen 2019, Gallo et al. 2018).

In breast cancer survivors, use of hormone therapy such as tamoxifen (a selective estrogen receptor modulator) or aromatase inhibitors (which block estrogen synthesis) is associated with an increased risk of diabetes (hazard ratio 2.40; 95% CI, 1.26–4.55; $p=0.008$) (Hamood et al. 2018). Importantly, estrogen is thought to play a role in regulating insulin resistance, and decreased estrogen promotes weight gain, metabolic syndrome, and insulin resistance (Mauvais-Jarvis, Clegg, and Hevener 2013).

Compared to matched controls, survivors of colorectal cancer were found to have a 53% higher rate of developing diabetes 1 year after their cancer and this rate was still 19% higher compared to controls 5 years later regardless of cancer treatment (Singh et al. 2016). This may be due to the finding that conditions such as overweight and obesity, which increase the risk for colorectal cancer, also increase the risk for diabetes (Stürmer et al. 2006).

OSTEOPOROSIS

Osteoporosis, or decreased bone density, is a disease of aging, and cancer survivors may be at increased risk due to the treatments they have received that disrupt the balance between bone formation and resorption (Shapiro, Manola, and Leboff 2001, Khan and Khan 2008). Estrogen plays an important role in maintaining bone density by reducing bone resorption by osteoclasts (through effects on parathyroid hormone sensitivity, calcitonin production and induction of apoptosis), inhibiting osteoblast apoptosis, and altering dietary calcium absorption and excretion (Ji and Yu 2015, Khosla, Oursler, and Monroe 2012). Hypogonadism also increases the risk of osteoporosis, and in the context of cancer therapy can be due to ovarian failure, certain medications, castration, or radiation to the brain, ovaries, or testes (Rizzoli et al. 2013, Shapiro, Manola, and Leboff 2001, Khan and Khan 2008). Estrogen production is reduced by aromatase inhibitors GnRH analogues, commonly used in the treatment of breast and prostate cancer, respectively (VanderWalde and Hurria 2011). Meanwhile, tamoxifen, which acts as an estrogen agonist in bones, helps preserve bone density (Eastell et al. 2006, VanderWalde and Hurria 2011).

High-dose methotrexate, doxorubicin, and cyclophosphamide have been shown to reduce born formation and increase resorption in animal and/or human studies (VanderWalde and Hurria 2011). Long-term glucocorticoid use is known to promote bone resorption, reduce muscle strength, and decrease osteoblast activity. However, it appears that short courses of steroids, such as those used in certain chemotherapy regimens, may not affect the bone health long-term (VanderWalde and Hurria 2011, Ratcliffe et al. 1992). Finally, indirect effects of cancer such as decreased mobility, sarcopenia, and low vitamin D levels can lead to bone loss (Rizzoli et al. 2013).

ADDRESSING THE BEHAVIORAL AND NUTRITIONAL CONCERNS OF THE CANCER SURVIVOR

It is recommended that cancer survivors continue to maintain a healthy weight, stay physically active, and consume a healthy diet (Rock et al. 2012). These are also lifestyle interventions that can prevent and treat many of the common chronic diseases that affect this population. The following chapters will detail dietary and physical activity recommendations for cancer survivors. In general, a healthy diet should include a variety of colorful vegetables and fruits, legumes, whole grains, and adequate dietary protein. Furthermore, refined carbohydrates and processed foods should be minimized (Rock et al. 2012). Regular physical activity and stress reduction (Rock et al. 2012), through meditation, yoga, massage, and/or other interventions, are also recommended.

CONCLUSION

The development of certain chronic diseases in cancer survivors may be related to risk factors present prior to their cancer diagnosis and/or as a result of cancer treatment (Cohen 2006, Hewitt, Rowland, and Yancik 2003). Specifically, second primary cancers, CVD, diabetes osteoporosis, depression, and anxiety are some of the most commonly seen conditions in this population. Overweight and obesity are highlighted as they are exceedingly prevalent conditions and increase the risk for developing cancer. Fortunately, nutrition and lifestyle can play a crucial role in preventing as well as treating many of these conditions.

REFERENCES

Amiri, S., and S. Behnezhad. 2019. "Obesity and anxiety symptoms: a systematic review and meta-analysis." *Neuropsychiatrie* 33 (2):72–89. doi: 10.1007/s40211-019-0302-9.

Armstrong, G. T., Y. Chen, Y. Yasui, W. Leisenring, T. M. Gibson, A. C. Mertens, M. Stovall, K. C. Oeffinger, S. Bhatia, K. R. Krull, P. C. Nathan, J. P. Neglia, D. M. Green, M. M. Hudson, and L. L. Robison. 2016. "Reduction in late mortality among 5-year survivors of childhood cancer." *N Engl J Med* 374 (9):833–42. doi: 10.1056/NEJMoa1510795.

Centers for Disease Control and Prevention, National Center for Health Statistics. National Health Interview Survey, 1992–2018.

Clark, L. H., E. M. Ko, A. Kernodle, A. Harris, D. T. Moore, P. A. Gehrig, and V. Bae-Jump. 2016. "Endometrial cancer survivors' perceptions of provider obesity counseling and attempted behavior change: are we seizing the moment?" *Int J Gynecol Cancer* 26 (2):318–24. doi: 10.1097/igc.0000000000000596.

Cohen, H. J. 2006. "Keynote comment: cancer survivorship and ageing--a double whammy." *Lancet Oncol* 7 (11):882–3. doi: 10.1016/s1470-2045(06)70913-5.

D'Agostino, N., K. Edelstein, N. Zhang, C. Recklitis, T. Brinkman, D. Srivastava, W. Leisenring, L. Robison, G. Armstrong, and K. Krull. 2016. "Comorbid symptoms of emotional distress in adult survivors of childhood cancer." *Cancer* 122. doi: 10.1002/cncr.30171.

Deckx, L., M. van den Akker, J. Metsemakers, A. Knottnerus, F. Schellevis, and Frank Buntinx. 2012. "Chronic diseases among older cancer survivors." *J Cancer Epidemiol* 2012:206414. doi: 10.1155/2012/206414.

Demark-Wahnefried, W., M. C. Morey, R. Sloane, D. C. Snyder, P. E. Miller, T. J. Hartman, and H. J. Cohen. 2012. "Reach out to enhance wellness home-based diet-exercise intervention promotes reproducible and sustainable long-term improvements in health behaviors, body weight, and physical functioning in older, overweight/obese cancer survivors." *J Clin Oncol* 30 (19):2354–61. doi: 10.1200/jco.2011.40.0895.

Demoor-Goldschmidt, C., and F. de Vathaire. 2019. "Review of risk factors of secondary cancers among cancer survivors." *Br J Radiol* 92 (1093):20180390. doi: 10.1259/bjr.20180390.

Diller, L., E. J. Chow, J. G. Gurney, M. M. Hudson, N. S. Kadin-Lottick, T. I. Kawashima, W. M. Leisenring, L. R. Meacham, A. C. Mertens, D. A. Mulrooney, K. C. Oeffinger, R. J. Packer, L. L. Robison, and C. A. Sklar. 2009. "Chronic disease in the childhood cancer survivor study cohort: a review of published findings." *J. Clin Oncol Off J Am Soc Clin Oncol* 27 (14):2339–55. doi: 10.1200/JCO.2008.21.1953.

Eastell, R., R. A. Hannon, J. Cuzick, M. Dowsett, G. Clack, and J. E. Adams. 2006. "Effect of an aromatase inhibitor on bmd and bone turnover markers: 2-year results of the Anastrozole, Tamoxifen, Alone or in Combination (ATAC) trial (18233230)." *J Bone Miner Res* 21 (8):1215–23. doi: 10.1359/jbmr.060508.

Floyd, J. and P. J. Morgan. 2020. "Cardiotoxicity of non-anthracycline cancer chemotherapy agents." Last Modified May 28, 2020, accessed June 6, 2020. https://www.uptodate.com/contents/cardiotoxicity-of-non-anthra-cycline-cancer-chemotherapy-agents?search=cardiotoxicity%20chemotherapy&source=search_result&selectedTitle=1~150&usage_type=default&display_rank=1- references.

Fosså, S. D., R. Vassilopoulou-Sellin, and A. A. Dahl. 2008. "Long term physical sequelae after adult-onset cancer." *J Cancer Surviv* 2 (1):3–11. doi: 10.1007/s11764-007-0039-5.

Friedman, D. N., E. S. Tonorezos, and P. Cohen. 2019. "Diabetes and metabolic syndrome in survivors of childhood cancer." *Hormone Res Paediatrics* 91 (2):118–127. doi: 10.1159/000495698.

Gallo, M., G. Muscogiuri, F. Felicetti, A. Faggiano, F. Trimarchi, E. Arvat, R. Vigneri, and A. Colao. 2018. "Adverse glycaemic effects of cancer therapy: indications for a rational approach to cancer patients with diabetes." *Metabolism* 78:141–54. doi: 10.1016/j.metabol.2017.09.013.

Godsland, I. F. 2009. "Insulin resistance and hyperinsulinaemia in the development and progression of cancer." *Clin Sci* 118 (5):315–332. doi: 10.1042/cs20090399.

Hamood, R., H. Hamood, I. Merhasin, and L. Keinan-Boker. 2018. "Diabetes after hormone therapy in breast cancer survivors: a case-cohort study." *J Clin Oncol* 36 (20):2061–29. doi: 10.1200/jco.2017.76.3524.

Harrigan, M., B. Cartmel, E. Loftfield, T. Sanft, A. B. Chagpar, Y. Zhou, M. Playdon, F. Li, and M. L. Irwin. 2016. "Randomized trial comparing telephone versus in-person weight loss counseling on body composition and circulating biomarkers in women treated for breast cancer: The Lifestyle, Exercise, and Nutrition (LEAN) study." *J Clin Oncol* 34 (7):669–76. doi: 10.1200/jco.2015.61.6375.

Hewitt, M., J. H. Rowland, and R. Yancik. 2003. "Cancer survivors in the United States: age, health, and disability." *J Gerontol Ser A* 58 (1):M82–91. doi: 10.1093/gerona/58.1.M82.

Institute of Medicine Committee on Psychosocial Services to Cancer Patients/Families in a Community, Setting. 2008. "The national academies collection: Reports funded by National Institutes of Health." In *Cancer Care for the Whole Patient: Meeting Psychosocial Health Needs*, edited by N. E. Adler and A. E. K. Page. Washington (DC): National Academies Press (US).

Jacobsen, P. B. 2009. "Clinical practice guidelines for the psychosocial care of cancer survivors: current status and future prospects." *Cancer* 115 (18 Suppl):4419–29. doi: 10.1002/cncr.24589.

Janssen-Heijnen, M. L., S. Houterman, V. E. Lemmens, M. W. Louwman, H. A. Maas, and J. W. Coebergh. 2005. "Prognostic impact of increasing age and co-morbidity in cancer patients: a population-based approach." *Crit Rev Oncol Hematol* 55 (3):231–40. doi: 10.1016/j.critrevonc.2005.04.008.

Ji, M.-X., and Q. Yu. 2015. "Primary osteoporosis in postmenopausal women." *Chron Dis Transl Med* 1 (1):9–13. doi: 10.1016/j.cdtm.2015.02.006.

Jung, S.-Y., Y. A. Kim, M. Jo, S. M. Park, Y.-J. Won, H. Ghang, S.-Y. Kong, K.-W. Jung, and E. S. Lee. 2019. "Prediagnosis obesity and secondary primary cancer risk in female cancer survivors: a national cohort study." *Cancer Med* 8 (2):824–38. doi: 10.1002/cam4.1959.

Khan, M. N., and A. A. Khan. 2008. "Cancer treatment-related bone loss: a review and synthesis of the literature." *Curr Oncol* 15 (Suppl 1):S30–40. doi: 10.3747/co.2008.174.

Khosla, S., M. J. Oursler, and D. G. Monroe. 2012. "Estrogen and the skeleton." *Trends Endocrinol Metab TEM* 23 (11):576–81. doi: 10.1016/j.tem.2012.03.008.

Lee, S. J., and K. B. Cartmell. 2020. "Self-reported depression in cancer survivors versus the general population: a population-based propensity score-matching analysis." *Qual Life Res* 29 (2):483–94. doi: 10.1007/s11136-019-02339-x.

Luppino, F. S., L. M. de Wit, P. F. Bouvy, T. Stijnen, P. Cuijpers, B. W. Penninx, and F. G. Zitman. 2010. "Overweight, obesity, and depression: a systematic review and meta-analysis of longitudinal studies." *Arch Gen Psychiatry* 67 (3):220–9. doi: 10.1001/archgenpsychiatry.2010.2.

Mauvais-Jarvis, F., D. J. Clegg, and A. L. Hevener. 2013. "The role of estrogens in control of energy balance and glucose homeostasis." *Endocr Rev* 34 (3):309–38. doi: 10.1210/er.2012-1055.

Oeffinger, K. C., A. C. Mertens, C. A. Sklar, T. Kawashima, M. M. Hudson, A. T. Meadows, D. L. Friedman, N. Marina, W. Hobbie, N. S. Kadan-Lottick, C. L. Schwartz, W. Leisenring, and L. L. Robison. 2006. "Chronic health conditions in adult survivors of childhood cancer." *N Engl J Med* 355 (15):1572–82. doi: 10.1056/NEJMsa060185.

Park, S. M., Y. H. Yun, Y. A. Kim, M. Jo, Y. J. Won, J. H. Back, and E. S. Lee. 2016. "Prediagnosis body mass index and risk of secondary primary cancer in male cancer survivors: A large cohort study." *J Clin Oncol* 34 (34):4116–24. doi: 10.1200/jco.2016.66.4920.

Ratcliffe, M. A., S. A. Lanham, D. M. Reid, and A. A. Dawson. 1992. "Bone mineral density (BMD) in patients with lymphoma: the effects of chemotherapy, intermittent corticosteroids and premature menopause." *Hematol Oncol* 10 (3–4):181–7. doi: 10.1002/hon.2900100308.

Rizzoli, R., J. J. Body, M. L. Brandi, J. Cannata-Andia, D. Chappard, A. El Maghraoui, C. C. Glüer, D. Kendler, N. Napoli, A. Papaioannou, D. D. Pierroz, M. Rahme, C. H. Van Poznak, T. J. de Villiers, G. El Hajj Fuleihan, and Disease International Osteoporosis Foundation Committee of Scientific Advisors Working Group on Cancer-Induced Bone. 2013. "Cancer-associated bone disease." *Osteoporosis Int J Established Result Cooper Eur Found Osteoporosis Nat Osteoporosis Found USA* 24 (12):2929–53. doi: 10.1007/s00198-013-2530-3.

Rock, C. L., C. Doyle, W. Demark-Wahnefried, J. Meyerhardt, K. S. Courneya, A. L. Schwartz, E. V. Bandera, K. K. Hamilton, B. Grant, M. McCullough, T. Byers, and T. Gansler. 2012. "Nutrition and physical activity guidelines for cancer survivors." *CA Cancer J Clin* 62 (4):243–74. doi: 10.3322/caac.21142.

Rock, C. L., S. W. Flatt, T. E. Byers, G. A. Colditz, W. Demark-Wahnefried, P. A. Ganz, K. Y. Wolin, A. Elias, H. Krontiras, J. Liu, M. Naughton, B. Pakiz, B. A. Parker, R. L. Sedjo, and H. Wyatt. 2015. "Results of the Exercise and Nutrition to Enhance Recovery and Good Health for You (ENERGY) trial: a behavioral weight loss intervention in overweight or obese breast cancer survivors." *J Clin Oncol* 33 (28):3169–76. doi: 10.1200/jco.2015.61.1095.

Shapiro, C. L., J. Manola, and M. Leboff. 2001. "Ovarian failure after adjuvant chemotherapy is associated with rapid bone loss in women with early-stage breast cancer." *J Clin Oncol* 19 (14):3306–11. doi: 10.1200/jco.2001.19.14.3306.

Singh, S., C. C. Earle, S. J. Bae, H. D. Fischer, L. Yun, P. C. Austin, P. A. Rochon, G. M. Anderson, and L. Lipscombe. 2016. "Incidence of diabetes in colorectal cancer survivors." *J Natl Cancer Inst* 108 (6):djv402. doi: 10.1093/jnci/djv402.

Stürmer, T., J. E. Buring, I.-M. Lee, J. M. Gaziano, and R. J. Glynn. 2006. "Metabolic abnormalities and risk for colorectal cancer in the physicians' health study." *Cancer Epidemiol Biomarkers Prev* 15 (12):2391–7. doi: 10.1158/1055-9965.Epi-06-0391.

Todd, B. L., M. C. Moskowitz, A. Ottati, and M. Feuerstein. 2014. "Stressors, stress response, and cancer recurrence: a systematic review." *Cancer Nurs* 37 (2):114–25. doi: 10.1097/NCC.0b013e318289a6e2.

Torres, N., M. Guevara-Cruz, L. A. Velázquez-Villegas, and A. R. Tovar. 2015. "Nutrition and atherosclerosis." *Arch Med Res* 46 (5):408–26. doi: 10.1016/j.arcmed.2015.05.010.

Travis, L. B. 2002. "Therapy-associated solid tumors." *Acta Oncol* 41 (4):323–33. doi: 10.1080/028418602760169361.

Travis, L. B. 2006. "The epidemiology of second primary cancers." *Cancer Epidemiol Biomarkers Prev* 15 (11):2020–6. doi: 10.1158/1055-9965.Epi-06-0414.

VanderWalde, A., and A. Hurria. 2011. "Aging and osteoporosis in breast and prostate cancer." *CA Cancer J Clin* 61 (3):139–156. doi: 10.3322/caac.20103.

Vigneri, P., F. Frasca, L. Sciacca, G. Pandini, and R. Vigneri. 2009. "Diabetes and cancer." *Endocr Relat Cancer* 16 (4):1103–23. doi: 10.1677/erc-09-0087.

Wang, L., T. C. Tan, E. F. Halpern, T. G. Neilan, S. A. Francis, M. H. Picard, H. Fei, E. P. Hochberg, J. S. Abramson, A. E. Weyman, I. Kuter, and M. Scherrer-Crosbie. 2015. "Major cardiac events and the value of echocardiographic evaluation in patients receiving anthracycline-based chemotherapy." *Am J Cardiol* 116 (3):442–6. doi: 10.1016/j.amjcard.2015.04.064.

Wouters, K. A., L. C. Kremer, T. L. Miller, E. H. Herman, and S. E. Lipshultz. 2005. "Protecting against anthracycline-induced myocardial damage: a review of the most promising strategies." *Br J Haematol* 131 (5):561–78. doi: 10.1111/j.1365-2141.2005.05759.x.

Yi, J. C., and K. L. Syrjala. 2017. "Anxiety and depression in cancer survivors." *Med Clin North Am* 101 (6):1099–113. doi: 10.1016/j.mcna.2017.06.005.

19 Nutritional Advice and Dietary Supplements for the Cancer Survivor

Michael Garcia and David Heber
UCLA Center for Human Nutrition

CONTENTS

INTRODUCTION

A cancer survivor is any individual that has been diagnosed with cancer, and survivorship includes the time period from diagnosis through the remainder of life (Marzorati, Riva, and Pravettoni 2017, Berry et al. 2019). Survivors encompass a heterogeneous group of individuals with different cancer types at various stages of disease and treatment, who have unique medical and nonmedical experiences during the course of their lives. We will use the term "survivor" in this chapter. However, because of their unique experiences, not all individuals diagnosed with cancer consider themselves cancer survivors.

The trajectory following diagnosis includes all stages of treatment, transition to extended survival, and ensuing long-term survival (Miller et al. 2019). Due to continuous advances in early detection and treatment of cancer and the aging population, the number of living individuals diagnosed with cancer in the United States and Europe continues to grow (Rowland et al. 2013). In the United States, survivors include more than 16.9 million individuals as of 2019, with projections of more than 22.1 million by 2030 (Miller et al. 2019). Nearly 68% of Americans diagnosed with cancer live more than 5 years, and 18% live more than 20 years (Miller et al. 2019).

As you read in previous chapters, nutrition requirements can change at the time of diagnosis or even prior to a cancer diagnosis. Following treatment, numerous questions arise regarding nutrition and lifestyle factors that can be implemented to maintain a healthy diet, weight, and active lifestyle, and to help prevent cancer recurrence, development of second primary cancers, and other chronic diseases (Rock et al. 2012). These concerns include understanding the benefits of different nutrients and dietary patterns, as well as the potential role for dietary supplements in supporting the goals of cancer survivors. Current information and guidance on these aspects of survivorship are useful in promoting informed decision-making by individuals and their medical providers.

POST-TREATMENT TRANSITION

As individuals complete their cancer treatment, they transition to the period of long-term survival. Several challenges arise during this time. These challenges include managing the effects of treatment and the desire to optimize health status. Some effects from treatment may be short-term, while others might persist for extended periods of time, including fatigue, neuropathy, change in sense of taste, pain, difficulty chewing or swallowing, and bowel or bladder changes (Rock et al. 2012). While some may be cured of their cancer, it is important to remember that many patients in the period of long-term survival have stable or even advanced disease, and each person will have a unique nutritional status, which may include malnutrition or weight loss. Individuals living in these different disease states may need to permanently adjust their dietary patterns in order to adapt to ongoing symptoms or lasting treatment effects.

For those whose disease and treatment lead to underweight status, loss of lean body mass, or risk of nutritional inadequacy, nutritional guidance from medical providers is important (Rock et al. 2012, Ravasco et al. 2004, Gupta et al. 2006, Guo et al. 2020). We know that suboptimal nutritional intake and malnutrition, especially in advanced stages of cancer, can significantly affect quality of life (Capuano et al. 2010).

For those with difficulty obtaining adequate nutrition orally, the use of intensive nutrition support, including enteral and parenteral nutrition, should be considered for each on an individual basis. The American Society for Parenteral and Enteral Nutrition recommends that a patient receiving active treatment may be considered for nutrition support if they are unable to adequately absorb nutrients for a prolonged period of time that could lead to malnutrition and worsened outcomes, though they note that no survival benefit has been demonstrated (August et al. 2009). The use of nutrition support in late stage patients receiving only palliative treatment is seldom indicated, and multiple factors must be taken into account, including the goals of nutritional care and the risks and benefits. Additional factors to consider before initiating nutritional support include patient performance status, ethical considerations, and the anticipated duration of survival (August et al. 2009).

While undernutrition and weight loss are well-recognized in nutritional support of cancer patients, it is equally important for cancer survivors to undertake weight management strategies with significant overweight or obesity. Excess body fat is associated with increased risks of cardiovascular disease, diabetes, and a number of common cancers, including pancreatic cancer, liver cancer, colorectal cancer, postmenopausal breast cancer, endometrial cancer, kidney cancer, and esophageal cancer (Salaun et al. 2017). Weight gain during adulthood can also increase the risk of postmenopausal breast cancer (Salaun et al. 2017, Keum et al. 2015). In addition to increased risk of these primary cancers, data have shown that obesity is associated with an increased risk of breast cancer recurrence (Picon-Ruiz et al. 2017) and may also be associated with increased risk of recurrence in other cancer types (Lin et al. 2018, Cao and Ma 2011).

Along with these concerns, cancer survivors also face a high risk of developing a second primary cancer and other chronic diseases (Ng and Travis 2008). Thus, important overall practices to develop for these survivors include achieving and maintaining a healthy weight, healthy nutrition including colorful fruits and vegetables, and regular physical activity. Ultimately, the goal is to maximize overall health, quality of life, and to reduce the risk of recurrent disease, second primary cancer, and common chronic diseases (Ng and Travis 2008). With these goals in mind, the current American Cancer Society recommendations for cancer survivors include weight management, a diet focused on fruits, vegetables, and whole grains and reduced amounts of fat, red and processed meat, and simple sugars, and limited alcohol consumption for survivors of head and neck cancer (Society 2019).

NUTRITION IN THE CANCER SURVIVOR

Cancer survivors comprise a heterogeneous population of individuals with many different types of cancer at different stages, undergoing different modes and periods of treatment with different period of anticipated survival. Nutritional approaches must be individualized to the unique characteristics of each person. Ideally, there would be specific dietary choices that could be followed to reduce recurrence risk and improve overall survival for each caner type, but due to the complexity of cancer, there is no single overall approach that is ideal.

Determining precise nutrition exposures affecting outcomes such as disease-specific survival, progression-free survival, and recurrence proves difficult, and therefore, current dietary recommendations for survivors are to follow the guidance for prevention of cancer in conjunction with personalized nutritional care from a medical professional. Nutritional treatment following diagnosis and into the long-term survival period should be tailored to the individual based on their type of disease, stage, and time period following treatment (Research 2018).

SPECIFIC NUTRIENTS AND FOOD COMPOUNDS

A number of studies have investigated the role of specific nutrients, foods, or food compounds and their effects in patients with cancer. A majority of these studies have occurred in survivors of breast cancer, with emerging studies for other cancer types. Many of these studies have focused on the effects of prediagnosis food intake on disease development and survival periods, while fewer have analyzed the effects of intake following diagnosis (Schwedhelm et al. 2016). The Women's Intervention Nutrition Study (WINS) randomized controlled trial evaluated the effect of dietary fat reduction on relapse-free survival in postmenopausal women with early stage breast cancer (Chlebowski et al. 2006). Those in the intervention group achieved fat intake reduction from 29.6% to 20.3% of total calories (Hoy et al. 2009). They were also found to have lower total energy intake, higher fiber intake, and had a statistically significant weight reduction of six pounds versus the control group (Hoy et al. 2009). The intervention group had a reduced hazard ratio for relapse events, though the change in weight and nutrient intake apart from fat could have affected the outcome (Hoy et al. 2009).

Soy foods are a complete protein frequently avoided unnecessarily following a diagnosis of breast cancer based on observations in animals (Hilakivi-Clarke, Andrade, and Helferich 2010). In a pooled analysis of cohort studies involving breast cancer survivors from the United States and China, results showed intake of soy food ≥10 mg of soy isoflavones per day following diagnosis was associated with a statistically significant reduced risk of recurrence, in Chinese, US, and non-Asian US survivors (Nechuta et al. 2012).

Dietary fiber consumption and its effects on the breast cancer survivors has been evaluated, with some studies suggesting that higher fiber intake is inversely associated with mortality; however, these findings are not definitive across all studies (Belle et al. 2011, McEligot et al. 2006, De Cicco et al. 2019).

Observational evidence suggests that in prostate cancer survivors, a diet lower in fat and specifically saturated fat may reduce tumor angiogenesis and cancer recurrence (Di Sebastiano and Mourtzakis 2014). Evaluation of a cohort from the Health Professionals Follow-up Study, analyzing pre- and postdiagnosis diet, suggested that intake of fish and tomato sauce after diagnosis is inversely associated with risk of prostate cancer progression (Chan et al. 2006). The association of tomato sauce may be due to its lycopene content and the association of lycopene with inverse risk of certain cancers, including prostate (Giovannucci 1999).

Prospective data in individuals with stage I to III colorectal cancer in the Nurses' Health Study and Health Professionals Follow-up Study showed an association between higher fiber intake following diagnosis and lower disease-specific and overall mortality (Song et al. 2018). In a separate study of individuals with stage III colon cancer enrolled in an adjuvant chemotherapy trial, a diet that included two or more servings of tree nuts per week, compared with no intake of nuts, was associated with significant improvements in recurrence, disease-free survival, and all-cause mortality (Fadelu et al. 2018).

Many other observational studies evaluating the effects of nutrients or foods on recurrence and survival in cancer show conflicting results. While such observational studies can provide new research insights, investigating individual foods or their components does not account for the dynamic interaction between compounds, nutrients, and foods as part of an overall dietary pattern and the interaction with other lifestyle factors, making it difficult to ascertain definitive and comprehensive dietary recommendations for cancer survivors. It is often more practical to consider overall dietary pattern and its important role for the cancer survivor.

ALCOHOL USE IN SURVIVORS

It is established that alcohol intake increases risk of several cancer types, including mouth, pharynx, larynx, esophagus, and pre- and postmenopausal breast cancer. Two or more alcohol drinks per day increases risk of colorectal cancer and three or more alcohol drinks per day increases the risk of stomach and liver cancers (Ratna and Mandrekar 2017). For individuals with head and neck cancer, among several negative prognostic factors is alcohol use, which has been associated with an increased risk of overall mortality specific to cancer of the hypopharynx and larynx (Giraldi et al. 2017). When evaluating alcohol use prior to and following diagnosis in patients with breast cancer, the results have been mixed. Some studies show no association between pre- or postdiagnosis alcohol use and survival, with potential for survival benefit with light consumption of alcohol (Newcomb et al. 2013, Minami et al. 2019). Other studies have shown association with alcohol use and increased risk of breast cancer recurrence in postmenopausal women and those with overweight or obesity (Kwan et al. 2010). When examining multiple types of cancer together and alcohol use pre- and postdiagnosis, alcohol intake was found to increase the risk of cancer recurrence, and this association remained when evaluating postdiagnosis alcohol intake alone (Schwedhelm et al. 2016).

DIETARY PATTERN

The complete pattern of dietary intake involves the dynamic interaction between foods, nutrients, and bioactive compounds. It may be more useful to inform individuals as to the effects of dietary pattern rather than individual nutrients on recurrence and mortality following a cancer diagnosis. For example, changes in dietary fat intake imply changes in carbohydrate intake when protein is held constant. Complex interactions among different food components and other lifestyle factors lead to an understanding of the effects of an overall dietary pattern. There is increased interest in studying dietary pattern effects on cancer survival, rather than simply looking at individual nutrients. While this may be an effective strategy to guide patients on nutrition modifications they can implement, more research is needed.

While some studies have evaluated the effects of foods and dietary pattern on overall mortality in different diseases such as cardiovascular disease (Kahleova, Levin, and Barnard 2018), fewer studies have analyzed the association with cancer recurrence, and furthermore, few have specifically evaluated postdiagnosis changes in dietary pattern (Schwedhelm et al. 2016). Nevertheless, in patients with stage III colon cancer enrolled in an adjuvant therapy trial, dietary patterns were analyzed for their effect on cancer recurrence and mortality in survivors (Meyerhardt et al. 2007). Analysis showed that a Western dietary pattern, defined by intake of refined grains, processed and red meats, desserts, high-fat dairy products, and French fries, was associated with significantly worse disease-free, recurrence-free, and overall survival when comparing the highest and lowest intake of these foods. A prudent dietary pattern, defined by high intake of fruits, vegetables, whole grains, legumes, poultry, and fish, was not significantly associated with disease recurrence or mortality (Meyerhardt et al. 2007). In this same cohort of patients, further analysis assessed whether adherence to the American Cancer Society nutrition and physical activity guidelines affected survival in these patients (Van Blarigan et al. 2018). These guidelines recommend achieving and maintaining healthy body weight, regular physical activity, and a dietary pattern high in vegetables, fruits, whole grains, and limited red and processed meats. The study showed a 42% lower risk of death in highest versus lowest adherence to guidelines; this included a 9% absolute risk reduction of death at 5 years (Van Blarigan et al. 2018).

The Women's Healthy Eating and Living (WHEL) randomized trial evaluated dietary changes of an increase in vegetables, fruits, fiber and reduction in fat, and its effect on new primary breast cancer, recurrence, and all-cause mortality in pre- and postmenopausal survivors of early stage breast cancer (Pierce et al. 2007). After a 7.3-year follow up period, there was no observed reduction in recurrence or mortality between the two groups. Notably, there was no significant weight change observed in the groups. Secondary analysis suggested that in women without hot flashes at baseline, there was an association of these dietary changes with reduced risk of breast cancer events (recurrence, distant metastases, or new primary breast cancer), which could relate to circulating estrogen concentrations (Pierce et al. 2009). A separate examination of adherence with the American Cancer Society nutrition recommendations for cancer prevention in breast cancer survivors did not show an association between fruit, vegetable, or whole grain intake with breast cancer-specific or all-cause mortality (McCullough et al. 2016). However, higher consumption of red and processed meat following diagnosis was independently associated with overall mortality (McCullough et al. 2016).

Additional studies have analyzed the effects of concordance with diet-quality indices, dietary patterns, and beverage consumption on recurrence and overall mortality in survivors including a meta-analysis of cohort studies which included survivors of breast, colorectal, head and neck, and gastroesophageal cancers (Schwedhelm et al. 2016). Different food items and food groups were analyzed, along with diet-quality indices such as the Healthy Eating Index, World Cancer Research Fund/American Institute for Cancer Research dietary adherence score, and Mediterranean diet score. All of these diet indices focus on high intakes of fruits and vegetables, whole grains, legumes, and nuts, along with reduced intake of meat. Data-driven dietary patterns categorized as healthy/prudent and unhealthy/Western were also used. Studies evaluating effects on cancer recurrence were fewer and did not conclude significant associations between specific dietary patterns and recurrence; however, higher diet-quality indices and prudent/healthy dietary patterns showed an inverse association with mortality risk and Western dietary pattern showed positive association with mortality risk (Schwedhelm et al. 2016).

In an analysis focusing on survivors of cancer types that have a 10-year survival >50%, a systematic review of two randomized controlled trials and 36 cohort studies investigated the relationship of pre- and postdiagnosis adherence to dietary patterns and intake from major food groups, with cancer recurrence and mortality (Jochems et al. 2018). Studies evaluated the following cancer types: bowel, breast, prostate, non-Hodgkin's lymphoma, bladder, laryngeal, and prostate. In cancers of the bladder, bowel, larynx, prostate, and non-Hodgkin's lymphoma, there were no definitive associations found between foods from the main food groups or adherence to specific dietary patterns/indices and an effect on mortality in survivors of these cancers, mainly due to a paucity of studies or inconsistency in results. The exception in this study was regarding survivors of breast cancer, in which adherence to dietary indices reflecting a healthy nutrition pattern may be associated with decreased overall mortality, and concordance with a Western dietary pattern following diagnosis was associated with higher risk of overall morality (Jochems et al. 2018).

As is evident, determining the potential effects of dietary exposures on different outcomes in cancer survivors is not straightforward. Cancer survivors as a group includes people in different stages of survivorship where different outcome measures hold greater importance, whether it is quality of life, recovery from treatment side effects, disease-free survival, or presence/absence of other medical conditions. There is consistent evidence that increased body fat and obesity is positively associated with breast cancer mortality, all-cause mortality, and development of second primary breast cancers (Picon-Ruiz et al. 2017). In view of the paucity of data for many types of cancer, it is advisable to implement a dietary pattern that is consistent with the available epidemiological literature on the prevention of cancer, which includes maintaining a healthy weight and eating more whole grains, vegetables, fruits, and legumes, avoiding sugary drinks, and limiting the consumption of red meat, processed meats, processed foods high in fat, sugar, and starches while also limiting the consumption of alcohol (Research 2018).

It is important to keep in mind that no one food item or food group alone will necessarily prolong survival or reduce risk of cancer recurrence, but rather the entirety of a nutritional pattern is most important. Dietary advice must be individualized for each patient, based on their cancer diagnosis, previous treatment, current nutritional status, and current and future goals.

DIETARY SUPPLEMENTS

The use of complementary and alternative medicine including botanicals and dietary supplements has increased over a number of decades among cancer survivors, with estimates that 40%–88% of individuals use supplements following a diagnosis of cancer (Horneber et al. 2012, Qureshi, Zelinski, and Carlson 2018). Dietary supplements encompass vitamins, minerals, amino acids, herbs, and botanicals and include any concentrate, metabolite, constituent extract, or combination of these that supplement other nutrition (Rock et al. 2012). Supplement use is higher among adults ages 65 and over, women, non-Hispanic whites, and those with higher levels of education (Kantor et al. 2016). In the United States, 52% of all adults report supplement use, with 25%–33% reporting use of multivitamin/multimineral supplements (Kantor et al. 2016, Velicer and Ulrich 2008). Among cancer survivors, the use of any vitamin or mineral supplement is higher than the overall population and ranges from 64% to 81% of individuals, with multivitamin use ranging from 26% to 77% (Velicer and Ulrich 2008). Importantly, an estimated 15%–50% of individuals begin use following diagnosis of cancer (Du et al. 2020). Prevalence of vitamin and mineral supplement use varies among different types of cancer, with most usage in breast cancer survivors, followed by survivors of colorectal, lung, and prostate cancer (Marian 2017, Bours et al. 2015).

There are a number of motivations for supplement use following a cancer diagnosis, including attempts to prevent disease recurrence, support concurrent therapy, aid recovery from side effects, strengthen the immune system, reduce symptoms of disease or treatment, help cope with physical and psychological stress, improve quality of life, assure adequate nutrient intake, and optimize general health (Bours et al. 2015). Some patients may initiate use on the advice of their medical provider (Marian 2017), while others initiate and continue use without notifying their medical provider (Velicer and Ulrich 2008). While current guidelines recommend that nutritional needs be met through food sources rather than primarily through dietary supplements, supplement use remains prevalent as added nutrition when the diet fails to provide all essential nutrients needed. It is important to recognize and openly discuss supplement use with patients regarding potential risks and benefits, and in order to provide comprehensive nutritional care to each cancer survivor.

VITAMINS AND MINERALS

Among the most commonly used supplements in cancer survivors are vitamin C, vitamin D, vitamin E, vitamin B12, calcium, fish oils (eicosapentaenoic acid and docosahexaenoic acid), and lutein (Du et al. 2020). Compared to those without cancer, cancer survivors tend to consume lesser amounts of several nutrients from foods, and greater amounts of nutrients from dietary supplements.

For some, this translates into excess nutrient intake above the tolerable upper limits for nutrients such as niacin, calcium, zinc, magnesium, vitamin D, and vitamin B6. These findings underscore the need to determine nutritional status and capacity, and to consistently incorporate nutritional factors into the care of cancer survivors.

Multivitamin/multimineral use is common if there is a general concern for a suboptimal level of nutrition. Several studies have investigated the role for use in cancer survivors. Daily use of multivitamin/multimineral supplements in patients with nonsmall cell lung cancer was found to be associated with prolonged survival and increased quality of life measures compared with nonuse of these supplements (Jatoi et al. 2005). In breast cancer, there have been mixed results when evaluating the potential association of multivitamin use with recurrence and survival, with some studies suggesting reduced mortality and others showing no association (Marian 2017, Kwan et al. 2011, Saquib et al. 2011). Multivitamin use in patients with stage III colon cancer, both during and following adjuvant chemotherapy, was not associated with recurrence-free or overall survival (Ng et al. 2010). In postmenopausal cancer survivors, multivitamin use following diagnosis trended toward increased risk of death, specific to individuals with low diet quality measures or declining health (Inoue-Choi et al. 2014), which suggests that it is most important to evaluate supplement use in the context of overall nutritional status.

VITAMIN D

Vitamin D is one of the most commonly used dietary supplements, and studies have shown that there is an inverse association between circulating levels of 25-hydroxyvitamin D and incidence of many types of cancer (Marian 2017). Meta-analyses have shown that higher serum levels of 25-hydroxyvitamin D are associated with reduced risk of lung cancer (Chen et al. 2015, Zhang et al. 2015). In colorectal cancer, higher levels of serum 25-hydroxyvitamin D are shown to be associated with greater survival in both stages I–III and in metastatic disease (Zgaga et al. 2014, Facciorusso et al. 2016). The impact of supplementation to achieve the increased levels, however, remains unclear (Vernieri et al. 2018). In the evaluation of breast cancer recurrence, analysis of the Pathways Study showed that women with advanced-stage tumors had lower serum 25-hydroxyvitamin D levels, and women in the highest tertile of serum levels had greater overall survival (Yao et al. 2017). Further research is needed to more fully define the role of vitamin D supplementation in breast cancer survivors.

Vitamin D supplementation and its effects on prostate cancer suggest there may be benefit in early-stage, low-risk disease during active surveillance; however, this has not been extensively studied (Marshall et al. 2012). A retrospective study of vitamin D in pancreatic cancer did not find any significant association between baseline serum concentration of 25-hydroxyvitamin D and overall survival or time to progression (McGovern et al. 2016).

Vitamin D insufficiency has been associated with poor prognosis in lymphoid malignancies, and an ongoing study is currently evaluating whether vitamin D replacement in the setting of low vitamin D levels affects prognosis in those with lymphoid malignancies (Sfeir et al. 2017). Observational evidence in esophageal cancer suggests that postsurgical vitamin D supplementation may improve disease-free survival and improve quality of life (Wang et al. 2016).

The role of vitamin D in head and neck cancer is unclear, as studies have shown conflicting results in regards to serum 25-hydroxyvitamin D levels, intake of vitamin D, and its effects on recurrence and mortality (Yokosawa et al. 2018). As a whole, more data are needed to determine if supplementation of vitamin D may have benefit in reduction of cancer recurrence and/or mortality as it relates to specific cancer types. In future research, it will be important to determine the serum levels of 25-hydroxyvitamin D that alter risk of cancer recurrence and mortality, the effects of changes to these levels, and how supplementation may or may not be effective at achieving beneficial outcomes. Based on current guidelines, it is best to recommend that individuals deficient in vitamin D be supplemented to maintain adequate levels.

VITAMIN E

Vitamin E supplementation has been investigated for its effect on both incidence and mortality in lung, prostate, and head and neck cancers. In individuals with head and neck cancer treated with radiation therapy, α-tocopherol in a dose of 400 IU per day during and following radiation was significantly associated with an increased risk of second primary cancer and recurrence during the period of supplementation (Bairati et al. 2006). Other studies have suggested a potential role of vitamin E supplementation to reduce risk of recurrence of noninvasive bladder cancer, where such effects may be more prominent in patients who smoke (Mazdak and Zia 2012). Other studies have focused on the effect of supplemental vitamin E on incident cancer of the lung, prostate, colorectum, and mortality in the general population (Harvie 2014). There are multiple forms of vitamin E in cells including four tocopherols and four tocotrienols. The most common form in the diet is γ-tocopherol, and there is a α-tocopherol transfer protein that is consistent with a special physiological role for this tocopherol, but more research is needed to determine the effects they can have on cancer recurrence and mortality.

BETA-CAROTENE

Beta-carotene supplementation has been investigated regarding its effect on colorectal adenoma recurrence (Baron et al. 2003b). Notably, a randomized trial evaluating supplementation showed that in individuals who did not smoke cigarettes or drink alcohol, beta-carotene supplementation decreased risk of recurrent adenomas, whereas supplementation significantly increased adenoma recurrence risk in individuals who both smoked cigarettes and drank alcohol (Baron et al. 2003a). The majority of other studies of beta-carotene have looked at its role in chemoprevention, particular in lung cancer. Results are conflicting and likely dependent on smoking status and baseline risk of lung cancer.

Selenium has not been extensively studied with regard to its potential effect on cancer recurrence. More frequently, it is investigated for chemoprevention or to alleviate toxicity during chemotherapy treatment (Harvie 2014). There was, however, a randomized trial of selenium supplementation as selenium yeast following resection of stage I nonsmall-cell lung cancer, to evaluate its effect on incidence of second primary tumors (Karp et al. 2013). While deemed safe, supplementation with selenium did not provide benefit in reducing the risk of second primary tumors. The Selenium and Bladder Cancer Trial (SELEBLAT) was a separate randomized trial in Belgium that found selenium supplementation reduced the risk of recurrence of noninvasive urothelial carcinoma (Goossens et al. 2016).

VITAMIN C

Vitamin C is also frequently used by individuals following a cancer diagnosis for its potential antioxidant effects. Cohort studies have suggested vitamin C supplementation may be associated with improved survival in breast cancer patients following treatment; however, it is challenging to determine the precise effect of vitamin C due to its frequent use in combination with other antioxidant vitamins (Poole et al. 2013). A meta-analysis of observational studies found that postdiagnosis vitamin C supplementation and dietary vitamin C intake were associated with a reduced risk of breast cancer-specific and total mortality (Harris, Orsini, and Wolk 2014). In a prospective study of Chinese women, supplemental vitamin C intake for >3 months was associated with reduced risk of recurrence and reduced mortality (Nechuta et al. 2011). Such findings need to be further investigated with larger studies of individuals in different postdiagnosis periods.

SUMMARY AND FUTURE DIRECTIONS

Investigations into the role of nutrition and dietary supplements in cancer survivors are complex, due to the unique clinical status of each individual survivor in terms of stage of disease, treatment, and the presence of coexisting conditions. This heterogeneity makes it difficult to assess the role of single or multiple supplements in the context of research on safety and efficacy. Furthermore, many of the studies of dietary supplements do not necessarily document the presupplementation levels of vitamins or minerals, which is important to determine the potential benefit or harm of added supplements.

In general, cancer survivors should prioritize obtaining their nutrients from foods in a dietary pattern to which supplements could be added while always transparently informing their healthcare providers of the nature and amounts of supplements being consumed. If there is a confirmed biochemical or clinical deficiency of one or multiple vitamins or minerals, or if overall dietary intakes are deficient, then supplementation should be provided to address specific deficiencies and ameliorate malnutrition. Most importantly, medical providers must ask their patients about use of dietary supplements, and must be willing to have transparent discussions about their potential risks and benefits.

The majority of current nutritional recommendations in cancer survivors come from studies on the primary prevention of cancer. Therefore, this advice is not based on the specific nutritional needs during all of the phases of survivorship following initial diagnosis.

The largest body of nutrition research in survivorship has occurred in breast cancer survivors and cannot be generalized to all types of cancer. Overall nutrition, dietary patterns, and supplements play different roles in each cancer type and subtype, including interactions with treatments and other medical conditions and their treatments. Based on the available research, it is most prudent to ensure that individuals diagnosed with cancer maintain a healthy weight without excess body fat. Appropriate weight management will vary based on prediagnosis weight and changes that occur during and following treatment. It is also judicious to prioritize a dietary pattern with more frequent intake of vegetables, fruits, whole grains, and legumes, while limiting a pattern that includes processed foods, red or processed meats, and alcohol. While specific food groups may provide added benefit in certain cancers, a healthy complete pattern of nutrition is most important.

Looking forward, future nutrition research in cancer survivors should define the most appropriate outcome measures in each cancer type, so that nutritional exposures or interventions can be better evaluated. This should include studies of longer duration including different groups of survivors with a variety of types of cancer. In addition, subgroup analysis should be analyzed based on treatment exposures. In view of the heterogeneous nature of cancer as a disease, gathering additional data from all parts of the world, to include individuals not frequently represented in prior nutritional research studies, will serve to better define the important role of nutrition and dietary supplements in cancer survivorship.

REFERENCES

August, D. A., M. B. Huhmann, American Society for Parenteral and Enteral Nutrition (A.S.P.E.N.) Board of Directors. 2009. "A.S.P.E.N. clinical guidelines: nutrition support therapy during adult anticancer treatment and in hematopoietic cell transplantation." *JPEN J Parenter Enteral Nutr* 33 (5):472–500. doi: 10.1177/0148607109341804.

Bairati, I., F. Meyer, E. Jobin, M. Gelinas, A. Fortin, A. Nabid, F. Brochet, and B. Tetu. 2006. "Antioxidant vitamins supplementation and mortality: a randomized trial in head and neck cancer patients." *Int J Cancer* 119 (9):2221–4. doi: 10.1002/ijc.22042.

Baron, J. A., B. F. Cole, L. Mott, R. Haile, M. Grau, T. R. Church, G. J. Beck, and E. R. Greenberg. 2003a. "Neoplastic and antineoplastic effects of beta-carotene on colorectal adenoma recurrence: Results of a randomized trial." *J Nat Cancer Inst* 95 (10):717–22. doi: 10.1093/jnci/95.10.717.

Baron, J. A., B. F. Cole, R. S. Sandler, R. W. Haile, D. Ahnen, R. Bresalier, G. McKeown-Eyssen, R. W. Summers, R. Rothstein, C. A. Burke, D. C. Snover, T. R. Church, J. I. Allen, M. Beach, G. J. Beck, J. H. Bond, T. Byers, E. R. Greenberg, J. S. Mandel, N. Marcon, L. A. Mott, L. Pearson, F. Saibil, and R. U. van Stolk. 2003b. "A randomized trial of aspirin to prevent colorectal adenomas." *N Engl J Med* 348 (10):891–9. doi: 10.1056/NEJMoa021735.

Belle, F. N., E. Kampman, A. McTiernan, L. Bernstein, K. Baumgartner, R. Baumgartner, A. Ambs, R. Ballard-Barbash, and M. L. Neuhouser. 2011. "Dietary fiber, carbohydrates, glycemic index, and glycemic load in relation to breast cancer prognosis in the HEAL cohort." *Cancer Epidemiol Biomarkers Prev* 20 (5):890–9. doi: 10.1158/1055-9965.EPI-10-1278.

Berry, L. L., S. W. Davis, A. Godfrey Flynn, J. Landercasper, and K. A. Deming. 2019. "Is it time to reconsider the term "cancer survivor"?" *J Psychosoc Oncol* 37 (4):413–26. doi: 10.1080/07347332.2018.1522411.

Bours, M. J., S. Beijer, R. M. Winkels, F. J. van Duijnhoven, F. Mols, J. J. Breedveld-Peters, E. Kampman, M. P. Weijenberg, and L. V. van de Poll-Franse. 2015. "Dietary changes and dietary supplement use, and underlying motives for these habits reported by colorectal cancer survivors of the Patient Reported Outcomes Following Initial Treatment and Long-Term Evaluation of Survivorship (PROFILES) registry." *Br J Nutr* 114 (2):286–96. doi: 10.1017/S0007114515001798.

Cao, Y., and J. Ma. 2011. "Body mass index, prostate cancer-specific mortality, and biochemical recurrence: a systematic review and meta-analysis." *Cancer Prev Res (Phila)* 4 (4):486–501. doi: 10.1158/1940-6207. CAPR-10-0229.

Capuano, G., P. C. Gentile, F. Bianciardi, M. Tosti, A. Palladino, and M. Di Palma. 2010. "Prevalence and influence of malnutrition on quality of life and performance status in patients with locally advanced head and neck cancer before treatment." *Support Care Cancer* 18 (4):433–7. doi: 10.1007/s00520-009-0681-8.

Chan, J. M., C. N. Holick, M. F. Leitzmann, E. B. Rimm, W. C. Willett, M. J. Stampfer, and E. L. Giovannucci. 2006. "Diet after diagnosis and the risk of prostate cancer progression, recurrence, and death (United States)." *Cancer Causes Control* 17 (2):199–208. doi: 10.1007/s10552-005-0413-4.

Chen, G. C., Z. L. Zhang, Z. X. Wan, L. Wang, P. Weber, M. Eggersdorfer, L. Q. Qin, and W. G. Zhang. 2015. "Circulating 25-hydroxyvitamin D and risk of lung cancer: a dose-response meta-analysis." *Cancer Causes Control* 26 (12):1719–1728. doi: 10.1007/s10552-015-0665-6.

Chlebowski, R. T., G. L. Blackburn, C. A. Thomson, D. W. Nixon, A. Shapiro, M. K. Hoy, M. T. Goodman, A. E. Giuliano, N. Karanja, P. McAndrew, C. Hudis, J. Butler, D. Merkel, A. Kristal, B. Caan, R. Michaelson, V. Vinciguerra, S. Del Prete, M. Winkler, R. Hall, M. Simon, B. L. Winters, and R. M. Elashoff. 2006. "Dietary fat reduction and breast cancer outcome: interim efficacy results from the Women's Intervention Nutrition Study." *J Natl Cancer Inst* 98 (24):1767–76. doi: 10.1093/jnci/djj494.

De Cicco, P., M. V. Catani, V. Gasperi, M. Sibilano, M. Quaglietta, and I. Savini. 2019. "Nutrition and breast cancer: A literature review on prevention, treatment and recurrence." *Nutrients* 11 (7). doi: 10.3390/nu11071514.

Di Sebastiano, K. M., and M. Mourtzakis. 2014. "The role of dietary fat throughout the prostate cancer trajectory." *Nutrients* 6 (12):6095–109. doi: 10.3390/nu6126095.

Du, M., H. Luo, J. B. Blumberg, G. Rogers, F. Chen, M. Ruan, Z. Shan, E. Biever, and F. F. Zhang. 2020. "Dietary supplement use among adult cancer survivors in the United States." *J Nutr* 150 (6):1499–508. doi: 10.1093/jn/nxaa040.

Facciorusso, A., V. Del Prete, N. Muscatiello, N. Crucinio, and M. Barone. 2016. "Prognostic role of 25-hydroxyvitamin D in patients with liver metastases from colorectal cancer treated with radiofrequency ablation." *J Gastroenterol Hepatol* 31 (8):1483–8. doi: 10.1111/jgh.13326.

Fadelu, T., S. Zhang, D. Niedzwiecki, X. Ye, L. B. Saltz, R. J. Mayer, R. B. Mowat, R. Whittom, A. Hantel, A. B. Benson, D. M. Atienza, M. Messino, H. L. Kindler, A. Venook, S. Ogino, K. Ng, K. Wu, W. Willett, E. Giovannucci, J. Meyerhardt, Y. Bao, and C. S. Fuchs. 2018. "Nut consumption and survival in patients with stage III colon cancer: results from CALGB 89803 (Alliance)." *J Clin Oncol* 36 (11):1112–20. doi: 10.1200/JCO.2017.75.5413.

Giovannucci, E. 1999. "Tomatoes, tomato-based products, lycopene, and cancer: review of the epidemiologic literature." *J Natl Cancer Inst* 91 (4):317–31. doi: 10.1093/jnci/91.4.317.

Giraldi, L., E. Leoncini, R. Pastorino, V. Wunsch-Filho, M. de Carvalho, R. Lopez, G. Cadoni, D. Arzani, L. Petrelli, K. Matsuo, C. Bosetti, C. La Vecchia, W. Garavello, J. Polesel, D. Serraino, L. Simonato, C. Canova, L. Richiardi, P. Boffetta, M. Hashibe, Y. C. A. Lee, and S. Boccia. 2017. "Alcohol and cigarette consumption predict mortality in patients with head and neck cancer: a pooled analysis within the International Head and Neck Cancer Epidemiology (INHANCE) consortium." *Ann Oncol* 28 (11):2843–51. doi: 10.1093/annonc/mdx486.

Goossens, M. E., M. P. Zeegers, H. van Poppel, S. Joniau, K. Ackaert, F. Ameye, I. Billiet, J. Braeckman, A. Breugelmans, J. Darras, K. Dilen, L. Goeman, B. Tombal, S. Van Bruwaene, B. Van Cleyenbreugel, F. Van der Aa, K. Vekemans, and F. Buntinx. 2016. "Phase III randomised chemoprevention study with selenium on the recurrence of non-invasive urothelial carcinoma: the SELEnium and BLAdder cancer Trial." *Eur J Cancer* 69:9–18 doi: 10.1016/j.ejca.2016.09.021.

Guo, Z. Q., J. M. Yu, W. Li, Z. M. Fu, Y. Lin, Y. Y. Shi, W. Hu, Y. Ba, S. Y. Li, Z. N. Li, K. H. Wang, J. Wu, Y. He, J. J. Yang, C. H. Xie, X. X. Song, G. Y. Chen, W. J. Ma, S. X. Luo, Z. H. Chen, M. H. Cong, H. Ma, C. L. Zhou, W. Wang, Q. Luo, Y. M. Shi, Y. M. Qi, H. P. Jiang, W. X. Guan, J. Q. Chen, J. X. Chen, Y. Fang, L. Zhou, Y. D. Feng, R. S. Tan, T. Li, J. W. Ou, Q. C. Zhao, J. X. Wu, L. Deng, X. Lin, L. Q. Yang, M. Yang, C. Wang, C. H. Song, H. X. Xu, H. P. Shi, Status Investigation on the Nutrition, and Group Clinical Outcome of Common Cancers. 2020. "Survey and analysis of the nutritional status in hospitalized patients with malignant gastric tumors and its influence on the quality of life." *Support Care Cancer* 28 (1):373–80. doi: 10.1007/s00520-019-04803-3.

Gupta, D., C. G. Lis, J. Granick, J. F. Grutsch, P. G. Vashi, and C. A. Lammersfeld. 2006. "Malnutrition was associated with poor quality of life in colorectal cancer: a retrospective analysis." *J Clin Epidemiol* 59 (7):704–9. doi: 10.1016/j.jclinepi.2005.08.020.

Harris, H. R., N. Orsini, and A. Wolk. 2014. "Vitamin C and survival among women with breast cancer: a meta-analysis." *Eur J Cancer* 50 (7):1223–31. doi: 10.1016/j.ejca.2014.02.013.

Harvie, M. 2014. "Nutritional supplements and cancer: potential benefits and proven harms." *Am Soc Clin Oncol Educ Book*:e478–86. doi: 10.14694/EdBook_AM.2014.34.e478.

Hilakivi-Clarke, L., J. E. Andrade, and W. Helferich. 2010. "Is soy consumption good or bad for the breast?" *J Nutr* 140 (12):2326S–34S. doi: 10.3945/jn.110.124230.

Horneber, M., G. Bueschel, G. Dennert, D. Less, E. Ritter, and M. Zwahlen. 2012. "How many cancer patients use complementary and alternative medicine: a systematic review and metaanalysis." *Integr Cancer Ther* 11 (3):187–203. doi: 10.1177/1534735411423920.

Hoy, M. K., B. L. Winters, R. T. Chlebowski, C. Papoutsakis, A. Shapiro, M. P. Lubin, C. A. Thomson, M. B. Grosvenor, T. Copeland, E. Falk, K. Day, and G. L. Blackburn. 2009. "Implementing a low-fat eating plan in the Women's Intervention Nutrition Study." *J Am Diet Assoc* 109 (4):688–96. doi: 10.1016/j.jada.2008.12.016.

Inoue-Choi, M., H. Greenlee, S. J. Oppeneer, and K. Robien. 2014. "The association between postdiagnosis dietary supplement use and total mortality differs by diet quality among older female cancer survivors." *Cancer Epidemiol Biomarkers Prev* 23 (5):865–75. doi: 10.1158/1055-9965.Epi-13-1303.

Jatoi, A., B. Williams, F. Nichols, R. Marks, M. C. Aubry, J. Wampfler, E. E. Finke, and P. Yang. 2005. "Is voluntary vitamin and mineral supplementation associated with better outcome in non-small cell lung cancer patients? Results from the Mayo Clinic lung cancer cohort." *Lung Cancer* 49 (1):77–84. doi: 10.1016/j.lungcan.2005.01.004.

Jochems, S. H. J., F. H. M. Van Osch, R. T. Bryan, A. Wesselius, F. J. van Schooten, K. K. Cheng, and M. P. Zeegers. 2018. "Impact of dietary patterns and the main food groups on mortality and recurrence in cancer survivors: a systematic review of current epidemiological literature." *BMJ Open* 8 (2):e014530. doi: 10.1136/bmjopen-2016-014530.

Kahleova, H., S. Levin, and N. D. Barnard. 2018. "Vegetarian dietary patterns and cardiovascular disease." *Prog Cardiovasc Dis* 61 (1):54–61. doi: 10.1016/j.pcad.2018.05.002.

Kantor, E. D., C. D. Rehm, M. Du, E. White, and E. L. Giovannucci. 2016. "Trends in dietary supplement use among US adults from 1999 to 2012." *JAMA* 316 (14):1464–74. doi: 10.1001/jama.2016.14403.

Karp, D. D., S. J. Lee, S. M. Keller, G. S. Wright, S. Aisner, S. A. Belinsky, D. H. Johnson, M. R. Johnston, G. Goodman, G. Clamon, G. Okawara, R. Marks, E. Frechette, W. McCaskill-Stevens, S. M. Lippman, J. Ruckdeschel, and F. R. Khuri. 2013. "Randomized, double-blind, placebo-controlled, phase III chemoprevention trial of selenium supplementation in patients with resected stage I non-small-cell lung cancer: ECOG 5597." *J Clin Oncol* 31 (33):4179–87. doi: 10.1200/JCO.2013.49.2173.

Keum, N., D. C. Greenwood, D. H. Lee, R. Kim, D. Aune, W. Ju, F. B. Hu, and E. L. Giovannucci. 2015. "Adult weight gain and adiposity-related cancers: a dose-response meta-analysis of prospective observational studies." *J Natl Cancer Inst* 107 (2). doi: 10.1093/jnci/djv088.

Kwan, M. L., L. H. Kushi, E. Weltzien, E. K. Tam, A. Castillo, C. Sweeney, and B. J. Caan. 2010. "Alcohol consumption and breast cancer recurrence and survival among women with early-stage breast cancer: the life after cancer epidemiology study." *J Clin Oncol* 28 (29):4410–6. doi: 10.1200/JCO.2010.29.2730.

Kwan, M. L., H. Greenlee, V. S. Lee, A. Castillo, E. P. Gunderson, L. A. Habel, L. H. Kushi, C. Sweeney, E. K. Tam, and B. J. Caan. 2011. "Multivitamin use and breast cancer outcomes in women with early-stage breast cancer: the life after cancer epidemiology study." *Breast Cancer Res Treat* 130 (1):195–205. doi: 10.1007/s10549-011-1557-4.

Lin, Y., Y. Wang, Q. Wu, H. Jin, G. Ma, H. Liu, M. Wang, Z. Zhang, and H. Chu. 2018. "Association between obesity and bladder cancer recurrence: a meta-analysis." *Clin Chim Acta* 480:41–6. doi: 10.1016/j.cca.2018.01.039.

Marian, M. J. 2017. "Dietary supplements commonly used by cancer survivors: Are there any benefits?" *Nutr Clin Pract* 32 (5):607–27. doi: 10.1177/0884533617721687.

Marshall, D. T., S. J. Savage, E. Garrett-Mayer, T. E. Keane, B. W. Hollis, R. L. Horst, L. H. Ambrose, M. S. Kindy, and S. Gattoni-Celli. 2012. "Vitamin D3 supplementation at 4000 international units per day for one year results in a decrease of positive cores at repeat biopsy in subjects with low-risk prostate cancer under active surveillance." *J Clin Endocrinol Metab* 97 (7):2315–24. doi: 10.1210/jc.2012-1451.

Marzorati, C., S. Riva, and G. Pravettoni. 2017. "Who is a cancer survivor? A systematic review of published definitions." *J Cancer Educ* 32 (2):228–37. doi: 10.1007/s13187-016-0997-2.

Mazdak, H., and H. Zia. 2012. "Vitamin e reduces superficial bladder cancer recurrence: a randomized controlled trial." *Int J Prev Med* 3 (2):110–5.

McCullough, M. L., S. M. Gapstur, R. Shah, P. T. Campbell, Y. Wang, C. Doyle, and M. M. Gaudet. 2016. "Pre- and postdiagnostic diet in relation to mortality among breast cancer survivors in the CPS-II Nutrition Cohort." *Cancer Causes Control* 27 (11):1303–14. doi: 10.1007/s10552-016-0802-x.

McEligot, A. J., J. Largent, A. Ziogas, D. Peel, and H. Anton-Culver. 2006. "Dietary fat, fiber, vegetable, and micronutrients are associated with overall survival in postmenopausal women diagnosed with breast cancer." *Nutr Cancer* 55 (2):132–40. doi: 10.1207/s15327914nc5502_3.

McGovern, E. M., M. E. Lewis, M. L. Niesley, N. Huynh, and J. B. Hoag. 2016. "Retrospective analysis of the influence of 25-hydroxyvitamin D on disease progression and survival in pancreatic cancer." *Nutr J* 15:17. doi: 10.1186/s12937-016-0135-3.

Meyerhardt, J. A., D. Niedzwiecki, D. Hollis, L. B. Saltz, F. B. Hu, R. J. Mayer, H. Nelson, R. Whittom, A. Hantel, J. Thomas, and C. S. Fuchs. 2007. "Association of dietary patterns with cancer recurrence and survival in patients with stage III colon cancer." *JAMA* 298 (7):754–64. doi: 10.1001/jama.298.7.754.

Miller, K. D., L. Nogueira, A. B. Mariotto, J. H. Rowland, K. R. Yabroff, C. M. Alfano, A. Jemal, J. L. Kramer, and R. L. Siegel. 2019. "Cancer treatment and survivorship statistics, 2019." *CA Cancer J Clin* 69 (5):363–85. doi: 10.3322/caac.21565.

Minami, Y., S. Kanemura, M. Kawai, Y. Nishino, H. Tada, M. Miyashita, T. Ishida, and Y. Kakugawa. 2019. "Alcohol consumption and survival after breast cancer diagnosis in Japanese women: a prospective patient cohort study." *PLoS One* 14 (11):e0224797. doi: 10.1371/journal.pone.0224797.

Nechuta, S. J., B. J. Caan, W. Y. Chen, S. W. Flatt, W. Lu, R. E. Patterson, E. M. Poole, M. L. Kwan, Z. Chen, E. Weltzien, J. P. Pierce, and X. O. Shu. 2011. "The after breast cancer pooling project: rationale, methodology, and breast cancer survivor characteristics." *Cancer Causes Control* 22 (9):1319–31. doi: 10.1007/s10552-011-9805-9.

Nechuta, S. J., B. J. Caan, W. Y. Chen, W. Lu, Z. Chen, M. L. Kwan, S. W. Flatt, Y. Zheng, W. Zheng, J. P. Pierce, and X. O. Shu. 2012. "Soy food intake after diagnosis of breast cancer and survival: an in-depth analysis of combined evidence from cohort studies of US and Chinese women." *Am J Clin Nutr* 96 (1):123–32. doi: 10.3945/ajcn.112.035972.

Newcomb, P. A., E. Kampman, A. Trentham-Dietz, K. M. Egan, L. J. Titus, J. A. Baron, J. M. Hampton, M. N. Passarelli, and W. C. Willett. 2013. "Alcohol consumption before and after breast cancer diagnosis: associations with survival from breast cancer, cardiovascular disease, and other causes." *J Clin Oncol* 31 (16):1939–46. doi: 10.1200/JCO.2012.46.5765.

Ng, A. K., and L. B. Travis. 2008. "Second primary cancers: an overview." *Hematol Oncol Clin North Am* 22 (2):271–89. doi: 10.1016/j.hoc.2008.01.007.

Ng, K., J. A. Meyerhardt, J. A. Chan, D. Niedzwiecki, D. R. Hollis, L. B. Saltz, R. J. Mayer, A. B. Benson, P. L. Schaefer, R. Whittom, A. Hantel, R. M. Goldberg, and C. S. Fuchs. 2010. "Multivitamin use is not associated with cancer recurrence or survival in patients with stage III colon cancer: Findings from CALGB 89803." *J Clin Oncol* 28 (28):4354–63. doi: 10.1200/Jco.2010.28.0362.

Picon-Ruiz, M., C. Morata-Tarifa, J. J. Valle-Goffin, E. R. Friedman, and J. M. Slingerland. 2017. "Obesity and adverse breast cancer risk and outcome: Mechanistic insights and strategies for intervention." *CA Cancer J Clin* 67 (5):378–97. doi: 10.3322/caac.21405.

Pierce, J. P., L. Natarajan, B. J. Caan, B. A. Parker, E. R. Greenberg, S. W. Flatt, C. L. Rock, S. Kealey, W. K. Al-Delaimy, W. A. Bardwell, R. W. Carlson, J. A. Emond, S. Faerber, E. B. Gold, R. A. Hajek, K. Hollenbach, L. A. Jones, N. Karanja, L. Madlensky, J. Marshall, V. A. Newman, C. Ritenbaugh, C. A. Thomson, L. Wasserman, and M. L. Stefanick. 2007. "Influence of a diet very high in vegetables, fruit, and fiber and low in fat on prognosis following treatment for breast cancer: the Women's Healthy Eating and Living (WHEL) randomized trial." *JAMA* 298 (3):289–98. doi: 10.1001/jama.298.3.289.

Pierce, J. P., L. Natarajan, B. J. Caan, S. W. Flatt, S. Kealey, E. B. Gold, R. A. Hajek, V. A. Newman, C. L. Rock, M. Pu, N. Saquib, M. L. Stefanick, C. A. Thomson, and B. Parker. 2009. "Dietary change and reduced breast cancer events among women without hot flashes after treatment of early-stage breast cancer: subgroup analysis of the Women's Healthy Eating and Living Study." *Am J Clin Nutr* 89 (5):1565S–71S. doi: 10.3945/ajcn.2009.26736F.

Poole, E. M., X. Shu, B. J. Caan, S. W. Flatt, M. D. Holmes, W. Lu, M. L. Kwan, S. J. Nechuta, J. P. Pierce, and W. Y. Chen. 2013. "Postdiagnosis supplement use and breast cancer prognosis in the after breast cancer pooling project." *Breast Cancer Res Treat* 139 (2):529–37. doi: 10.1007/s10549-013-2548-4.

Qureshi, M., E. Zelinski, and L. E. Carlson. 2018. "Cancer and complementary therapies: Current trends in survivors' interest and use." *Integr Cancer Ther* 17 (3):844–53. doi: 10.1177/1534735418762496.

Ratna, A., and P. Mandrekar. 2017. "Alcohol and cancer: Mechanisms and therapies." *Biomolecules* 7 (3). doi: 10.3390/biom7030061.

Ravasco, P., I. Monteiro-Grillo, P. M. Vidal, and M. E. Camilo. 2004. "Cancer: disease and nutrition are key determinants of patients' quality of life." *Support Care Cancer* 12 (4):246–52. doi: 10.1007/s00520-003-0568-z.

Research, World Cancer Research Fund/American Institute for Cancer. 2018. Continuous update project expert report 2018. In Survivors of Breast and Other Cancers.

Rock, C. L., C. Doyle, W. Demark-Wahnefried, J. Meyerhardt, K. S. Courneya, A. L. Schwartz, E. V. Bandera, K. K. Hamilton, B. Grant, M. McCullough, T. Byers, and T. Gansler. 2012. "Nutrition and physical activity guidelines for cancer survivors." *CA Cancer J Clin* 62 (4):243–74. doi: 10.3322/caac.21142.

Rowland, J. H., E. E. Kent, L. P. Forsythe, J. H. Loge, L. Hjorth, A. Glaser, V. Mattioli, and S. D. Fossa. 2013. "Cancer survivorship research in Europe and the United States: where have we been, where are we going, and what can we learn from each other?" *Cancer* 119 (Suppl 11):2094–108 doi: 10.1002/cncr.28060.

Salaun, H., J. Thariat, M. Vignot, Y. Merrouche, and S. Vignot. 2017. "Obesity and cancer." *Bull Cancer* 104 (1):30–41. doi: 10.1016/j.bulcan.2016.11.012.

Saquib, J., C. L. Rock, L. Natarajan, N. Saquib, V. A. Newman, R. E. Patterson, C. A. Thomson, W. K. Al-Delaimy, and J. P. Pierce. 2011. "Dietary intake, supplement use, and survival among women diagnosed with early-stage breast cancer." *Nutr Cancer Int J* 63 (3):327–33. doi: 10.1080/01635581.2011.535957.

Schwedhelm, C., H. Boeing, G. Hoffmann, K. Aleksandrova, and L. Schwingshackl. 2016. "Effect of diet on mortality and cancer recurrence among cancer survivors: a systematic review and meta-analysis of cohort studies." *Nutr Rev* 74 (12):737–48. doi: 10.1093/nutrit/nuw045.

Sfeir, J. G., M. T. Drake, B. R. LaPlant, M. J. Maurer, B. K. Link, T. J. Berndt, T. D. Shanafelt, J. R. Cerhan, T. M. Habermann, A. L. Feldman, and T. Witzig. 2017. "Validation of a vitamin D replacement strategy in vitamin D-insufficient patients with lymphoma or chronic lymphocytic leukemia." *Blood Cancer J* 7 (2):e526. doi: 10.1038/bcj.2017.9.

Society, American Cancer. 2019. "Cancer treatment & survivorship facts & figures 2019–2021." Atlanta: American Cancer Society. https://www.cancer.org/content/dam/cancer-org/research/cancer-facts-and-statistics/cancer-treatment-and-survivorship-facts-and-figures/cancer-treatment-and-survivorship-facts-and-figures-2019-2021.pdf.

Song, M., K. Wu, J. A. Meyerhardt, S. Ogino, M. Wang, C. S. Fuchs, E. L. Giovannucci, and A. T. Chan. 2018. "Fiber intake and survival after colorectal cancer diagnosis." *JAMA Oncol* 4 (1):71–79. doi: 10.1001/jamaoncol.2017.3684.

Van Blarigan, E. L., C. S. Fuchs, D. Niedzwiecki, S. Zhang, L. B. Saltz, R. J. Mayer, R. B. Mowat, R. Whittom, A. Hantel, A. Benson, D. Atienza, M. Messino, H. Kindler, A. Venook, S. Ogino, E. L. Giovannucci, K. Ng, and J. A. Meyerhardt. 2018. "Association of survival with adherence to the American Cancer Society Nutrition and Physical Activity Guidelines for cancer survivors after colon cancer diagnosis: The CALGB 89803/Alliance Trial." *JAMA Oncol* 4 (6):783–90. doi: 10.1001/jamaoncol.2018.0126.

Velicer, C. M., and C. M. Ulrich. 2008. "Vitamin and mineral supplement use among US adults after cancer diagnosis: a systematic review." *J Clin Oncol* 26 (4):665–73. doi: 10.1200/JCO.2007.13.5905.

Vernieri, C., F. Nichetti, A. Raimondi, S. Pusceddu, M. Platania, F. Berrino, and F. de Braud. 2018. "Diet and supplements in cancer prevention and treatment: clinical evidences and future perspectives." *Crit Rev Oncol Hematol* 123:57–73. doi: 10.1016/j.critrevonc.2018.01.002.

Wang, L., C. Wang, J. Wang, X. Huang, and Y. Cheng. 2016. "Longitudinal, observational study on associations between postoperative nutritional vitamin D supplementation and clinical outcomes in esophageal cancer patients undergoing esophagectomy." *Sci Rep* 6:38962. doi: 10.1038/srep38962.

Yao, S., M. L. Kwan, I. J. Ergas, J. M. Roh, T. D. Cheng, C. C. Hong, S. E. McCann, L. Tang, W. Davis, S. Liu, C. P. Quesenberry, Jr., M. M. Lee, C. B. Ambrosone, and L. H. Kushi. 2017. "Association of serum level of Vitamin D at diagnosis with breast cancer survival: a case-cohort analysis in the pathways study." *JAMA Oncol* 3 (3):351–7. doi: 10.1001/jamaoncol.2016.4188.

Yokosawa, E. B., A. E. Arthur, K. M. Rentschler, G. T. Wolf, L. S. Rozek, and A. M. Mondul. 2018. "Vitamin D intake and survival and recurrence in head and neck cancer patients." *Laryngoscope* 128 (11):E371–6. doi: 10.1002/lary.27256.

Zgaga, L., E. Theodoratou, S. M. Farrington, F. V. N. Din, L. Y. Ooi, D. Glodzik, S. Johnston, A. Tenesa, H. Campbell, and M. G. Dunlop. 2014. "Plasma vitamin D concentration influences survival outcome after a diagnosis of colorectal cancer." *J Clin Oncol* 32 (23):2430–U220. doi: 10.1200/Jco.2013.54.5947.

Zhang, L. Q., S. H. Wang, X. Y. Che, and X. H. Li. 2015. "Vitamin D and lung cancer risk: A comprehensive review and meta-analysis." *Cell Physiol Biochem* 36 (1):299–305. doi: 10.1159/000374072.

20 Lifestyle Changes and Behavioral Approaches for the Cancer Survivor

William J. McCarthy
UCLA Fielding School of Public Health

Catherine L. Carpenter
UCLA Center for Human Nutrition
Schools of Nursing, Medicine and Public Health

CONTENTS

HEALTHIER LIFESTYLE CHOICES IMPROVE RECURRENCE-FREE SURVIVAL AND QUALITY OF LIFE

The number of Americans who have lived 5 years or more after their cancer diagnosis is projected to increase 35%, to 14 million (Bluethmann, Mariotto, and Rowland 2016). Moreover, the average age and comorbidity burden of the average cancer survivor are expected to increase such that nearly three quarters (73%) of cancer survivors are expected to be 65 years old or older by 2040 (Bluethmann, Mariotto, and Rowland 2016). Inasmuch as healthy lifestyle behaviors have generally been associated with reduced burden of disease and higher quality of life in healthy adults, it should not surprise observers to find that the same principle applies to cancer survivors as well: healthier lifestyle choices will yield superior medical and quality of life outcomes.

"Quality of life" is defined by the World Health Organization (WHO) as "the individual's perception of their position in life in the context of the culture and value systems in which they live and in relation to their goals" (WHO 1997). Quality of life generally refers to a person's overall subjective well-being. For research on behavior change in cancer survivors, however, there are both general health-related quality of life instruments (e.g., the SF-36) (Ware and Sherbourne 1992) and cancer-specific quality of life instruments (e.g., the FACT-G) (Brucker et al. 2005). The general health-related quality of life instruments typically assess physical, social, emotional, and functional well-being. The cancer-specific measures assess similar constructs but take into account stressors and barriers specific to various cancer sites (e.g., lymphedema in breast cancer, impotence in prostate cancer, etc.). The impact of physical activity and/or healthier eating on either general or cancer-specific quality of life outcomes tends to be similar, so reviews of the behavior change literature tend to conflate the two, a practice that we have adopted in this chapter.

CANCER SURVIVORS ARE MOTIVATED TO MAKE LIFESTYLE CHANGES THAT OPTIMIZE THEIR QUALITY OF LIFE

The active treatment phase for controlling a specific cancer typically disrupts one's daily routines quite noticeably, so much so that many working-age adults temporarily withdraw from the workforce during this phase (L'Hotta et al. 2020, in press). Following the end of the active treatment phase, however, cancer survivors can take advantage of this "teachable moment" to undertake lifestyle changes designed to optimize their quality of life and minimize their future risk of cancer (Demark-Wahnefried et al. 2005). Colorectal cancer survivors assessed 7 years after diagnosis who adhered to four recommended lifestyle practices (healthy weight, healthy eating, recreationally active, and nonsmoking) were found to have higher quality of life than survivors who adhered to only two of these recommended lifestyle practices (Schlesinger et al. 2014). An earlier U.S. study of six cancer survivor groups (breast, prostate, colorectal, bladder, uterine, and skin melanoma) showed a similar quality of life benefit associated with adherence to regular physical activity, eating five fruit and vegetable servings daily and not smoking (Blanchard, Courneya, and Stein 2008).

Cancers include 200-plus distinct types, with different etiologies and different physical sequelae. While the physical treatment of these cancers necessarily differs, the psychosocial sequelae of depression, anxiety, and fatigue are remarkably common across cancer types (Miller et al. 2019). Direct (psychosocial counseling) and indirect (behavior change) approaches to coping with cancer survivorship have been shown to increase appreciably survivors' quality of life and the quality of life of their caregivers. This chapter will focus on the quality of life benefits of inducing cancer survivors to adhere to federal dietary, physical activity, and tobacco use guidelines.

In parallel with healthy adults, most cancer survivors fail to adhere to health behavior guidelines (Arem et al. 2020, Blanchard, Courneya, and Stein 2008). While most (86%) cancer survivors avoid tobacco use, 59.6% drink alcohol at least occasionally, 56.6% fail to engage in sufficient regular physical activity, and 64% are overweight or obese (Arem et al. 2020). From the Health Belief Model (National Cancer Institute (NCI) 2005), one would assume that cancer survivors' direct experience with cancer would make them acutely aware of their vulnerability to cancer and motivate them more strongly to exercise regularly, lose excess weight, limit alcohol intake, and eat more fiber-rich, minimally processed plant foods. There does appear to be a short-term burst of improved adherence to selected health behavior recommendations, but less so long-term (Tollosa et al. 2020, in press). Survivors' lack of motivation to adhere to recommended health behaviors is particularly surprising, given that adherence to lifestyle behavior guidelines is not only associated with reduced cancer recurrence and reduced cancer mortality but is also associated with increased quality of life across several cancer sites (Blanchard, Courneya, and Stein 2008). Alarms that were sounded in the 2000s concerning the lost opportunities for improving cancer survivors' physical and emotional prospects were accompanied by suggestions for more intensive individual-level interventions (Blanchard, Courneya, and Stein 2008). After a dozen years of more sophisticated individual-level interventions yielding similar results, alarms are now accompanied by calls for increased investment in research, advocacy, and policy (Arem et al. 2020).

Simply providing environments and resources supportive of the recommended health behaviors is not enough to elicit increased adherence to those behaviors, however. An example was the impact of colocating an exercise facility within a cancer treatment center (Kennedy et al. 2020, in press). At 1-year follow-up, only 12% of patients regularly coming to the center had ever made use of the exercise facility (Kennedy et al. 2020, in press). Supportive education and community resource navigation need to accompany the environmental supports to optimize survivor use of the enhanced local resources (Kennedy et al. 2020, in press).

The scientific literature is clear that tobacco use is a significant influence on taste, smell, absorption of nutrients in the small intestine, fermentation of indigestible carbohydrate in the colon and on whether gut microbial metabolites prevent or facilitate carcinogenesis. This confounder is addressed briefly before discussing the major focus of this chapter on nutrition-related and physical activity-related behavior change interventions involving cancer survivors.

TOBACCO USE CONFOUNDER NEEDS TO BE TAKEN INTO ACCOUNT IN ORDER TO OPTIMIZE THE QUALITY OF LIFE BENEFITS OF HEALTHY EATING AND REGULAR PHYSICAL ACTIVITY

Regular tobacco users worldwide adhere to predictably less healthy dietary patterns than nonusers (Tang et al. 1997, Dallongeville et al. 1998, Larson et al. 2007, Haibach et al. 2015, Osler et al. 2002, Palaniappan et al. 2001). In fact, a consistent nutritional marker of long-term abstinence is increased fruit and vegetable intake of abstainers compared to continuing smokers (Haibach, Homish, and Giovino 2013, Poisson et al. 2012). These consistent associations between tobacco use status and daily food choice behaviors may be mediated by the negative impact of smoking on gut microbiota functioning (Stewart et al. 2018, Savin et al. 2018, Lee et al. 2018, Biedermann et al. 2013b). Gut dysbiosis, as reflected by diminished microbial diversity, increased inflammation, and increased abundance of pathogenic bacteria, is more commonly observed in current smokers compared to abstainers (Biedermann et al. 2013a). Gut dysbiosis, in turn, is associated with reduced expression of the satiety hormones peptide tyrosine tyrosine (PYY) and glucagon-like peptide-1 (GLP-1) (Yamane and Inagaki 2018). Elevated levels of PYY and GLP-1 are consistently but not always associated with better weight control. Smoking has also been shown in preclinical studies to reduce functional olfactory receptors (Ueha et al. 2016). Epidemiological studies consistently show active smokers to have impaired taste sensitivity (Glennon et al. 2019, Frye, Schwartz, and Doty 1990, Vennemann, Hummel, and Berger 2008). Fortunately, most (but not all) ex-smokers regain the taste sensitivity they had before they became regular smokers. Successful change in daily food choice behaviors and in daily engagement in physical activity is consistently less likely in tobacco users than in nontobacco users as reflected by their increased risk of dropping out-of-behavior change programs (Maugeri et al. 2019, Kelly et al. 2017). Fortunately, there is some evidence of synergistic benefit in conjoining smoking cessation with dietary change (Hyman et al. 2007) and change in physical activity (Marcus et al. 1999), particularly when well-integrated into a week-long residential treatment program (Hodgkin et al. 2013, Hays et al. 2001).

PHYSICAL ACTIVITY INFLUENCE ON EATING BEHAVIOR AND DIGESTION

Recent reviews have concluded that breast cancer survivors who engage in physical activity following their breast cancer diagnosis improve both their survival rates and psychosocial health outcomes (Patel et al. 2019, Friedenreich et al. 2020). Other cancer sites with evidence of survival benefit for survivors engaging in regular physical activity include colorectal and prostate and possibly kidney, bladder, endometrial, esophageal, and lung (Patel et al. 2019, Friedenreich et al. 2020). The biological mechanisms responsible for these effects of postdiagnosis physical activity are unclear but could plausibly be mediated by the impact of physical activity on the gut microbiota in association with a fiber-rich diet (Allen et al. 2018). From its inception (Select Committee on Nutrition and Human Needs-U.S. Senate 1977), the *Dietary Guidelines for Americans* has enjoined Americans to engage regularly in physical activity for the purpose of optimizing nutritional status. Adoption and maintenance of physical activity occurs in parallel with adoption and maintenance of a dietary pattern rich in fruits and vegetables (Lounassalo et al. 2019). The few studies that have examined the impact of physical activity on taste preferences indicate increased sensitivity to low levels of sweetness following aerobic physical activity compared to before the activity (Westerterp-Plantenga et al. 1997, Passe, Horn, and Murray 2000). Emerging findings from studies of the human gut microbiota are demonstrating new ways in which aerobic exercise can amplify the microbial conversion of fiber into short-chain fatty acids, at least in lean adults (Allen et al. 2018). The short-chain fatty acid, butyrate, is particularly important for the prevention of colon cancer (O'Keefe et al. 2015). Exercise may protect against colon cancer in other ways as well, such as by speeding up the transit of residue through the colon (Oettle 1991), thereby reducing epithelial exposure to carcinogens in the residue (Bingham and Cummings 1989).

In addition to recurrence-free survival as a benefit of physical activity postdiagnosis, recent reviews (Forbes et al. 2020) have also focused on near-term physical and psychosocial benefits of engaging cancer survivors in regular physical activity. They have concluded that physical activity postdiagnosis improved near-term quality-of-life-related outcomes including fatigue, general and cancer-specific quality of life, distress, depression, and physical functioning (Forbes et al. 2020).

ADHERENCE TO A MEDITERRANEAN DIETARY PATTERN OR SIMILAR DIETARY PATTERNS IS ASSOCIATED WITH INCREASED QUALITY OF LIFE

Whole food choices and food patterns are now the focus of cancer prevention nutritional guidelines instead of the traditional reductionist focus on calories, macronutrients and micronutrients (Rock et al. 2020, U.S. Department of Agriculture 2020). The commercial weight loss services company,

Weight Watchers International, evolved its nutritional recommendations away from its original focus on restricting daily calorie (Carroll 2019) intake toward a focus on eating "zero points" minimally processed, mostly plant foods (Weight Watchers Research Department 2018). The World Cancer Research Fund (WCRF)'s approach to reviewing the world's literature relating lifespan nutritional variations to cancer outcomes evolved in similar fashion. Whereas the WCRF's first two reviews of the world's literature relating cancer outcomes to nutritional exposures focused on studies associating individual macronutrients and micronutrients on cancer risk, the newest review explicitly embraces an ecological perspective, asserting that optimal prevention of nutrition-related cancers requires choosing a healthy dietary pattern such as the Mediterranean diet (WCRF 2018). A 2020 narrative review of dietary patterns and cancer risk confirmed consistent evidence that healthful dietary patterns (e.g., Mediterranean, "prudent diet", DASH) and unhealthful dietary patterns (e.g., "western") are associated with cancer incidence and mortality involving various cancer sites, including breast, prostate, colorectal, esophageal, lung, and pancreatic (Steck and Murphy 2020).

There are several reasons for the clinical shift from a focus on micro- and macronutrients to a focus on whole foods and dietary patterns. One is the fact that major chemoprevention trials failed to show the hypothesized benefit of increasing intake of isolated nutrients (Omenn et al. 1996, Hennekens et al. 1996, Heinonen et al. 1994). Another is the increasing evidence that nutrients interact with other nutrients (Kubena and McMurray 1996), interactions that historically were ignored in single-nutrient trials. A third and clinically most compelling reason is that patients typically do not eat single nutrients but instead eat whole foods (Jacobs and Tapsell 2007) and tend to follow dietary patterns, such as the western dietary pattern (Slattery et al. 1998), or the Mediterranean dietary pattern (Piazzi et al. 2019).

Researchers are sounding a cautionary note on using calorie restriction as a way to reduce obesity before resection of the tumor. Researchers are reporting that across five human safety studies, use of calorie restriction has been associated with either no change in the Ki67 tumor cell proliferation rate or a significant increase in the Ki67 cell proliferation rate (Demark-Wahnefried et al. 2020). On the basis of these consistently disappointing results, the researchers are saying that it would be prudent to delay involving cancer patients in calorie restriction efforts to reduce excess body weight until after the tumor has been resected (Demark-Wahnefried et al. 2020).

HEALTH ORIENTATION, CLARITY OF HEALTH CHANGE GOAL, AND HEALTH LOCUS OF CONTROL

Depending on the person's health status, health orientation and the nature of the health behavior needing change, different behavior change approaches will apply. Immediately after treatment, the person's typical health orientation is focused on health restoration, bringing back the physiological functioning that existed prediagnosis. For the cancer survivor who has recovered the physical functioning that she had prior to her cancer, her primary health orientation is likely to shift to the health enhancement orientation that most healthy adults pursue during their working age years. The feature that most distinguishes health restoration from health enhancement is the person's prior experience with the target health status. In both cases, she is optimizing her quality of life. In the case of health restoration, however, she is working toward a known health status because she has been there before. She does not have to wonder what achieving that health goal feels like, because she has been there before. She can therefore be more self-reliant as she works toward restoring the physical functioning that she had before. In the case of health enhancement, she suspects from what she has been told or learned that her quality of life will be improved if she tries new health behaviors such as urban gardening or Zumba™ dancing. But because she has not done these before, she will benefit from relying on others to help her master these new skills. The Self Determination Theory (Ryan and Deci 2000) approach to behavior change seeks to support the autonomy and perceived competence of the person making the behavior change. It is well-suited to facilitating a cancer survivor's return to the physical activity and dietary patterns that prevailed before her cancer diagnosis (Milne et al. 2008). For facilitating the adoption and mastery of new skills, Social Learning Theory/Social Cognitive Theory (SCT) may be a better choice because learning new behaviors benefits from progressive goal-setting and trial-and-error learning or by emulating others who are acknowledged masters of the desired new lifestyle behaviors (Bandura 2004). Highlights of these two theoretical approaches are described in more detail below.

FOR LONG-TERM MAINTENANCE OF DESIRED HEALTH BEHAVIORS, COMMUNITY SUPPORT IS KEY

During the active change part of the health behavior change process, the individual typically invests disproportionate time, attention, and energy into making the behavior change process work (Ross et al. 2019). There are opportunity costs, such as the time, attention, and energy that should be invested in one's spouse, one's children, and one's community that will eventually force the person to reduce her day-to-day investment in the health behavior change process and compel her to rely on the desired behaviors having become part of her daily routine. For long-term maintenance of desirable health behaviors, it is increasingly recognized that individual volition and intention are not enough (Rock et al. 2020). Relapse is the rule rather than the exception for individuals trying to lose excess weight or quit smoking on their own, without community support (Brownell et al. 1986). With community support, the probability of long-term maintenance of the desired behavior is enhanced (Kilgore et al. 2014). It is easier to be a nonsmoker in Utah than in Nevada despite their similar geographies because their respective histories of community support for nonsmokers are quite different. Utah community standards have long been influenced by the Church of Latter Day Saints, which forbids tobacco use (Enstrom 1978). Nevada, by contrast, is well-known for its tolerance of socially denigrated behaviors such as gambling, extramarital sex and smoking (Burnham 1992). Research on the impact of the home environment on food choices illustrates the power of one's immediate environment to shape one's daily food choices by finding that even the nonparticipating spouses of participants in weight loss regimens that require a change to the home food environment nonetheless experience changes in daily food choices and accompanying weight loss (Gorin et al. 2013). The accumulating evidence of the power of the social and community environment to shape physical activity and daily food choice behaviors has prompted the American Cancer Society (ACS), the WCRF, and the *Dietary Guidelines for Americans* Advisory Committee to include as an explicit part of their respective lifestyle behavior guidelines the need to create and nurture built and community environments supportive of the recommended lifestyle behaviors (U.S. Department of Agriculture (USDA) and U.S. Department of Health and Human Services 2015, Rock et al. 2020, WCRF 2018). The 2015–2020 Dietary Guidelines for Americans (USDA 2016) even included a description of the Social Ecological Model (Ohri-Vachaspati et al. 2015), to encourage nutrition professionals to incorporate multilevel influences in their nutrition interventions.

COMMON BEHAVIORAL APPROACHES TO MOTIVATING CHANGES IN FOOD CHOICE BEHAVIORS AND MAINTAINING THEM

There is no space here to examine every major theoretical approach to motivating desired behavior change in cancer survivors. Fortunately, the NCI has enumerated and summarized the major features of popular theoretical approaches to health behavior change for the purpose of increasing health-related quality of life and recurrence-free survival (NCI 2005). As health orientations change following treatment for cancer and as old age approaches, what might be the most appropriate approach will necessarily change. Figure 20.1 summarizes the changing applicability of major theoretical approaches (Dohnke, Steinhilber, and Fuchs 2015, NCI 2005, Ohri-Vachaspati et al. 2015, Ewart 1991, Ryan and Deci 2000, Brownell et al. 1986) to desired health behavior change as the ultimate change agent shifts from self to family to community.

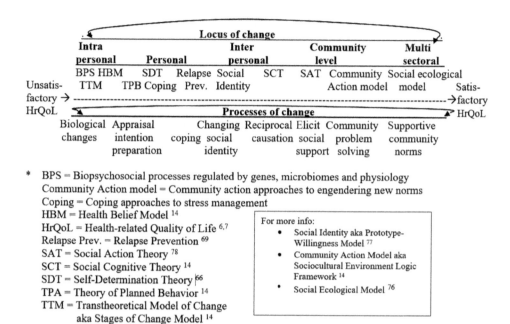

FIGURE 20.1 Traditional lifestyle change models and associated change processes, by theory.

Rigorous research on behavior change interventions ideally tests all major components of the behavioral theories invoked to explain the expected results. The busy clinician, on the other hand, does not have the luxury of evaluating every major component of the behavioral approach(es) that he or she relies on to improve health prospects, nor should she. The typical researcher is focused on predicting behavior change-related outcomes over a small, at most 1-year duration whereas the dedicated clinician should expect to be providing care and optimizing the survivor's health prospects and quality of life over a lifetime. For the individual patient, the behavior change process is a dynamic one (Ross et al. 2019), with different behavior theories optimally deployed at different points during the behavior change trajectory (see box for example).

Example of dynamic nature of behavior change process: Betsy White was diagnosed with stage 2, ER-negative breast cancer at age 55. Her oncologist determined that Betsy had no family history of breast cancer and had no major risk factors, such as obesity, estrogen supplementation, or childlessness. She was sedentary, however, and admitted to being ten pounds overweight. The oncologist asked about her alcohol consumption. Betsy was surprised by the question. "Oh, is alcohol consumption related to breast cancer risk?" she asked. The oncologist noted that the WCRF and the ACS were both recommending avoidance of alcohol for people at risk of breast cancer, based on the best available evidence. Given her now-documented higher risk of a new breast cancer [invoke Health Belief Model], she agreed to stop her regular beer-drinking and wine-drinking. On her oncologist's advice, she enrolled in a CDC-supported Diabetes Prevention Program (DPP) (Ely et al. 2017) to help her control her weight. The progressive goal-setting and self-monitoring [invoke SCT (Bandura 2004)] featured in the DPP helped her lose 9 lbs but she found going to the gym and counting calories tedious, especially when the excess weight started returning. She and her husband, Sam, joined a regional folk-dancing organization that hosted dances in varying regional locales, which kept them engaged in intrinsically enjoyable physical activity [invoke Social Ecological Model (Stokols 1996)] and helped stop the unwanted weight gain.

PREVENTION AND TREATMENT OF OBESITY AS A PRIMARY GOAL FOR HEALTHY CANCER SURVIVORSHIP

The National Comprehensive Cancer Network (National Comprehensive Cancer Network 2020), the WCRF (2018), and the ACS guidelines (Rock et al. 2012) concur that a common determinant of quality of life in cancer survivors is the obesity status of the survivor. There is less agreement, however, on how to optimize survivors' weight control because of the failure of researchers to identify health behavior intervention strategies that result in sustainable long-term weight control (Gimeno, Briere, and Seeley 2020). Based on current empirical evidence, the most effective long-term strategy for reducing and keeping off excess body fat is not behavioral but surgical, namely, bariatric surgery (Gimeno, Briere, and Seeley 2020). Curiously, the effectiveness of bariatric surgery at optimizing satiety and facilitating adherence to healthy eating seems to be more related to the changed architecture of the digestive system than to the constriction in the stomach. It appears that the more rapid gastric emptying and shortened transit time of food through the small intestine results in a higher proportion of carbohydrate-rich foods escaping digestion to become substrate for the microbes in the colon. The consistent result is higher expression of the satiety hormones PYY and GLP-1 with consequent reduction in time being spent feeling hungry. But eating a less processed, more fiber-rich, plant-based diet and exercising regularly can also generate increased expression of these same satiety hormones (Zhao et al. 2018). Researchers are therefore looking to identify the constellation of lifestyle behaviors that can yield metabolic benefits similar to those associated with bariatric surgery (Wang et al. 2019). One behavioral choice that can generate increased generation of the PYY satiety hormone is to eat only foods that are minimally processed (Hall et al. 2019). The degree of food processing, alone, has been shown to influence short-term weight change and markedly change satiety hormone levels (Hall et al. 2019). Ultraprocessed foods include fast food, chips, sugar-sweetened beverages, and pizza (Monteiro et al. 2019). In a cross-over metabolic ward study with meals designed to be matched on calories and macronutrient profile, the same individuals registered significantly lower body weights after 14 days on the unprocessed food diet than they did after 14 days on the ultra-processed food diet (Hall et al. 2019). The investigators noted that the experimental ultra-processed food diet was similar to the study participants' baseline diet (Hall et al. 2019). Epidemiological evidence consistently shows that body weight is elevated in those whose diets consist mostly of ultraprocessed foods relative to those whose diets consist mostly of minimally processed foods (Monteiro et al. 2018, Juul et al. 2018, Costa et al. 2019). Given the importance of obesity as a risk factor for cancer (WCRF 2018), it will surprise no one that there is direct epidemiological evidence that cancer risk is elevated in those consuming mostly ultraprocessed foods relative to those consuming mostly minimally processed foods (Fiolet et al. 2018). A 10% increase in the proportion of ultraprocessed foods in the diet was associated with a >10% increase in risks of cancer in general and breast cancer more specifically (Fiolet et al. 2018). Because of the consensus that obesity increases risk of cancer recurrence for many cancer sites (WCRF 2018), obesity risk reduction is the primary outcome in many of the health behavior intervention trials involving cancer survivors to be discussed below.

SELECTED BEHAVIOR CHANGE THEORIES CHOSEN FOR THEIR FREQUENCY OF INVOCATION IN PUBLICATIONS

Several behavior change theories are invoked often enough in the published literature to warrant highlighting some of their distinctive features, which we do below. In a 2019 review (Grimmett et al. 2019) of 27 randomized controlled physical activity intervention trials involving cancer survivors, the behavior change theories invoked most often were: SCT (12), Transtheoretical Model of Change (TTM) (aka Stages of Change Model) (7), Theory of Planned Behavior (TPB) (4), Self-Determination Theory (1), Cognitive Behavior Therapy (1), Self-regulation Theory (1), Health Action Approach (1), and Social Ecological Model (1). Seven studies invoked no specific behavior change theory and six studies invoked a combination of SCT+TTM. Of 12 studies showing significant between-group effects, only one (8.3%) failed to include an explicit behavior change theory. Of nine studies failing to show significant between group effects but still showing within-group effects, three (33.3%) failed to include an explicit behavior change theory. Of six studies failing to show any significant intervention effects, three (50%) failed to include an explicit behavior change theory. These results confirmed the tentative conclusion of a 2017 review (Bluethmann et al. 2017) that behavior change interventions involving cancer survivors were more likely to be impactful if they incorporated explicit behavior change theory.

SOCIAL COGNITIVE THEORY HIGHLIGHTS

SCT is the behavior change theory most often invoked in dietary change interventions involving primary care patients (de Menezes et al. 2020, Rigby et al. 2020). With roots in behaviorism, SCT's innovations included the insight that people learn from observing others as well as from personal experience (Bandura 2001). Unlike other individual-level behavior change theories (e.g., Health Belief Model (NCI 2005), Theory of Planned Behavior (TPB), NCI 2005), SCT explicitly acknowledges reciprocal determinism, where the client's behavior change can influence her/his social environment and her/his social environment can influence the client's behavior change. SCT is placed in the middle in Figure 20.1 because the locus of change for the SCT is interpersonal, compared to the more individual focus of approaches like the TTM and the TPB. The SCT serves as a bridge, spanning a focus on the individual as the primary determinant of health behavior adherence and a focus on the community/environment as the primary determinant of health behavior adherence. The most dominant individually focused features of SCT include behavior-specific self-efficacy, self-monitoring, progressive goal-setting, and outcome expectancies (Bandura 2001). Behavior-specific self-efficacy, such as exercise self-efficacy or weight loss self-efficacy, is the person's perception that she/he is capable of mastering the exercise goal or weight loss goal not yet achieved but that the person intends to achieve. Progressive goal-setting includes a "goldilocks" rule that overly ambitious goals can be dispiriting whereas unchallenging goals provide no opportunity for growth in mastery (Bandura and Schunk 1981). Ipsative goal-setting, where target individuals set their own challenge goals for behavior change, is an underappreciated approach to personalizing population-level goals while tailoring individual-level goal-setting to conform with the goldilocks rule. For example, more population health benefit may be achieved in helping a community improve its adherence to eating the recommended minimum five serving of fruits and vegetables a day by asking those members currently eating only one serving a day to set a goal of eating two servings a day but concurrently asking members already eating four servings a day to eat five servings a day. The rationale for ipsative goal-setting is that setting the population goal of five-a-day as everyone's immediate personal goal sets up for failure those whose baseline fruit and vegetable consumption is very low. Attempts at overly ambitious behavior change that consistently result in failure tend to diminish self-efficacy; step-by-step goal-setting that sets progressively more challenging goals following the goldilocks rule tends to increase self-efficacy for everyone and ultimately potentiates achievement of the long-term population goal, given enough time (Clark 2016, Fiatarone et al. 1994).

MOTIVATIONAL INTERVIEWING

Motivational interviewing is a minimally directive counseling approach that healthcare providers can use to encourage behavior change in patients (Miller and Rollnick 2013). It is relevant to mention motivational interviewing in the context of SCT inasmuch as enhancing the patient's self-efficacy to undertake behavior change is the ultimate goal of motivational interviewing (Miller and Rollnick 2013). What distinguishes motivational interviewing from traditional counseling is the counselor's nonjudgmental support for however much behavior change the client is ready for. In this regard, motivational interviewing resembles SCT's ipsative goal-setting, where the client's current level of motivation dictates the ambitiousness of the desired behavior change.

In SCT, there are several sources of information that inform the client's perception of self-efficacy, including enactive mastery (trial-and-error learning), vicarious learning (watching others attempt to adhere to the desired behavior), and symbolic learning (learning through reading, listening to lectures, interrogating experts) (Bandura 2001). Of these, enactive mastery has the most impact on the client's perceptions of self-efficacy (Bandura 2001). Motivational interviewing is a counseling approach that compels the client to generate his/her own behavior change prescription; the counselor is only a cheerleader (Miller and Rollnick 2013). If and when the client follows through on the self-prescription, the boost in self-efficacy will be attributable to enactive mastery, not to vicarious or symbolic learning, the usual modes of learning in traditional health education. Motivational interviewing and other methods for boosting client self-efficacy have been used successfully to motivate increased physical activity in long-term cancer survivors (Pinto et al. 2013, Bennett et al. 2007).

TRANSTHEORETICAL MODEL OF CHANGE (AKA STAGES OF CHANGE MODEL) HIGHLIGHTS

The second behavioral theory/model most frequently invoked in behavior change programs involving cancer survivors (Bluethmann et al. 2017, Grimmett et al. 2019) is the TTM, often referred to as the Stages of Change Model (Prochaska, Diclemente, and Norcross 1992, NCI 2005). In Figure 20.1, the TTM is grouped with other intrapersonal approaches to behavior change because most of its stages of change are distinguished by different thoughts within the person. TTM posits that behavior change typically involves a dynamic, cyclical process marked by stages of varying commitment to the desired behavior change. The stages begin with the precontemplation stage, where the person in need of a specific behavior change (e.g., need to lose excess weight) is not at the stage of even contemplating making any changes to her/his daily lifestyle choices. The contemplation, preparation, and action stages are self-explanatory. The maintenance stage has been somewhat problematic inasmuch as no deliberate cognitions concerning stage status are necessary to define it, hence the tautological definition: maintenance is when the desired behavior is being maintained. The five-stage TTM original formulation was revised to include relapse as an additional stage, reflecting the reality that unexpected challenges can derail clients' behavior change intentions. Part of TTM's appeal to behavior change intervention designers is that it distinguished between clients ready and motivated to engage in behavior change and clients with seemingly no appetite for behavior change. Previous behavior change approaches had implicitly assumed that everybody targeted for health behavior change would be responsive to the behavior change intervention. Numerous TTM-inspired interventions created different intervention messages, tailored to the TTM stage of each client. In theory, this tailoring of the intervention prescription should yield overall more impact across a diversity of clients than if one used a one-size-fits-all intervention approach for all clients. In practice, this expectation of increased aggregate impact often did not pan out. Part of the problem with TTM is that full implementation of all of its features is not practical so the model never gets a fair test (Hutchison, Breckon, and Johnston 2009). Another problem is that the implicit TTM assumption that a well-planned (well-contemplated) behavior change will yield more impact than a spontaneous behavior change not preceded by contemplation and preparation may be incorrect. Retrospective data collected from UK adults with a history of smoking showed that unplanned, spontaneous quit attempts were 2.5 times as likely to yield continued abstinence 6 months later than planned attempts to quit (West and Sohal 2006). Finally, administrators of limited public health resources may be tempted to use the TTM to triage potential targets of behavior change interventions who are in the precontemplation stage and target expenditure of those resources to those prepared to undertake the desired behavior change. Contrary to TTM assumptions, some researchers have found the so-called precontemplators just as likely to achieve desired behavior changes (e.g., eat more fruits and vegetables) as those at baseline who were in the contemplation or even preparation stage (Resnicow, McCarty, and Baranowski 2003, Cahill, Lancaster, and Green 2010). The demographic characteristics of adults who are disproportionately found in the precontemplation stage of adhering to federally recommended lifestyle behaviors typically include barriers (e.g., obesity) and lack of resources (e.g., income, education) that would hinder personal health enhancement efforts (Kearney et al. 1999, de Vet et al. 2005). In other words, those with the greatest barriers and fewest resources to undertake the desired behavior change would be the ones most likely to report being in the precontemplation stage (Emmons et al. 1994) and thus the ones that public health administrators would be least likely to invest limited public health resources in, which would exacerbate health disparities rather than reduce them.

TPB HIGHLIGHTS

In Figure 20.1, the TPB is placed next to intrapersonal approaches because it assumes that behavioral intention (an intrapersonal phenomenon) is the most important determinant of whether a client will make efforts to adopt a new health behavior (NCI 2005). What sets it apart from other theories that consider attitudes and beliefs to be important determinants of behavior change is that the TPB includes a moderator of behavioral intention that other behavior change theories do not, namely, normative beliefs. For this theory, normative beliefs refer to the beliefs of people important to the client that support or oppose the desired behavior change. It is because of its normative beliefs component that the TPB is placed in Figure 20.1 next to approaches characterized by explicit recognition of the importance of social influences, like the SCT. In tobacco control research, normative beliefs have consistently been shown to be important determinants of smoking behavior and explain significant variance in intervention outcomes (Andrews, Hampson, and Barckley 2008). The attitudes of family members and friends, for instance, influence one's daily food choices (Gorin et al. 2011).

SELF-DETERMINATION THEORY HIGHLIGHTS

When people engage in desired health behaviors spontaneously, without being induced to do so by money, encouragement of a personal trainer or because it is a condition of employment (e.g., military), they are said to be intrinsically motivated. The goal of Self-Determination Theory (Ryan and Deci 2000) is to cultivate in clients intrinsic motivation to eat more healthfully, exercise 5 days a week, etc. It has been long observed in behavior change research that clients adopt and maintain the desired health behavior as long as their behavior is being monitored by a coach or counselor but as soon as the external monitoring ends (Hall and Kahan 2018) as happens with many structured behavior change intervention programs that end, the client's continued maintenance of the desirable health behavior drops off markedly (Frensham et al. 2014). The clients who continue adhering to the recommended behavior even after the external monitoring has ended are those who are intrinsically motivated. The keys to cultivating intrinsic motivation in a client to maintain a desired health behavior are the client's perceive autonomy in practicing the desired behavior, the client's competence in practicing the desired behavior, and the client's autonomy support, the social, and physical supports that make it possible for the client to practice the desired behavior autonomously (Deci and Ryan 2008).

SOCIAL ECOLOGICAL MODEL HIGHLIGHTS

Features of the Social Ecological Model are highlighted here in part because none of the other theories or models listed in Figure 20.1 focus explicitly on environmental influences, with a partial exception for the Social Cognitive Model. The Social Ecological Model had its roots in Bronfenbrenner's Ecological Framework for Human Development (Bronfenbrenner 1977). This framework assumed that in order to understand human development, the entire ecological system in which growth occurs needs to be taken into account. This ecological system includes genes, the human microbiota, physiological functioning, family dynamics, and community-level influences. The social determinants of health would fall under the purview of the Social Ecological Model and have been shown to be major predictors of daily food choices (de Mello et al. 2020) and long-term health prospects (Chetty et al. 2016). The Social Ecological Model is important because, with respect to encouraging healthier eating practices, clinicians have been remiss in not paying more attention to the role of the patient's home and community food environments for influencing their patients' daily food choices. Ridding the home environment of sugary drinks and savory snacks and assiduously maintaining a countertop bowl filled with fresh fruit have been shown to improve household residents' weight control prospects (Gorin et al. 2013). Minimizing the time that family members are exposed to food commercials while eating dinner by moving the family TV set out of the family dining area or by keeping it off during meal times is associated with healthier food choices and reduced risk of obesity (Robinson 1999). Living in a home environment supportive of healthier food choices reduces the need for external incentives to motivate healthier food choices (Parks et al. 2018).

EVALUATING BEHAVIOR CHANGE TECHNIQUES REGARDLESS OF BEHAVIOR CHANGE THEORY

Researchers have begun evaluating the full range of behavior change techniques used in past behavior change interventions but doing so now without explicitly embedding them in the behavior change theory(ies) that they might be associated with. A taxonomy of 93 behavior change techniques has been extracted from the full range of established behavior change theories (Michie et al. 2013). A 2019 meta-analysis (Sheeran et al. 2019) of randomized controlled trials promoting physical activity among cancer survivors identified several behavior change techniques across the reviewed interventions that were associated with increased or decreased intervention effect size. One consistent finding was that greater contact time during supervised exercise programs was associated with optimal intervention effect (Sheeran et al. 2019). For unsupervised (i.e., self-help) programs, establishing specific outcome expectations and targeting overweight or sedentary clients were associated with increased effect sizes. For unsupervised programs, providing detailed workbooks or highlighting barriers to watch out for were surprisingly counterproductive, yielding lower effect sizes than evident in participants assigned to the control condition. The authors inferred that highlighting barriers to watch out for had the inadvertent effect of reducing clients' self-efficacy, thereby reducing their motivation to exercise (Sheeran et al. 2019). For evaluation purposes, being able to screen published health behavior change studies for the full range of behavior change techniques provides insights into specific techniques that may be uncommonly effective in motivating desirable behavior change. For the purpose of designing effective behavior change interventions, however, invoking integrated behavioral theories with established track records for effectiveness appears to be a more prudent choice than selecting behavior change techniques haphazardly (Bluethmann et al. 2017).

BEHAVIOR CHANGE RESEARCH, STRATIFIED BY CANCER SITE

Below, we highlight major health behavior change studies designed to help cancer patients/survivors improve their health prospects and optimize their quality of life. We have stratified these studies by cancer site, beginning with breast cancer, the cancer site that has garnered the most attention from behavior change researchers.

More behavior change research has involved breast cancer survivorship than any other cancer. One reflection of this fact is the number of hits obtained in typing "behavior change", "nutrition",/"diet",/"physical activity"/"exercise", and "[cancer name]" in searches of the ISI Web of Knowledge database on July 21, 2020 (See Table 20.1). Depending on the search terms for diet and

TABLE 20.1

Number of Hits When Searching ISI Database for Behavior Change Involving Various Cancer Sites

Cancer	Hits—Nutrition	%	Hits—Diet	%	Hits—Physical Activity	%	Hits—Exercise	%
Breast cancer	177	55.5%	433	54.9%	652	64.2%	464	66.3%
Colorectal cancer	71	22.3%	226	28.6%	250	24.6%	147	21.0%
Lung cancer	33	10.3%	64	8.1%	75	7.4%	57	8.1%
Head and neck cancers	21	6.6%	21	2.7%	7	0.7%	13	1.9%
Liver cancer	15	4.7%	32	4.1%	13	1.3%	10	1.4%
Melanoma	2	0.6%	13	1.6%	18	1.8%	9	1.3%
Totals	319		789		1015		700	

Source: ISI Webofknowledge.com database. Search terms included: "behavior change", "nutrition"/"diet"/"physical activity"/"exercise", and "[cancer name]". Date of search: July 21, 2020.

physical activity, breast cancer accounts for 55%–66% of all the behavior change research involving cancer patients/survivors. Colorectal cancer comes next, with 21%–29% of studies, lung cancer accounts for 7%–10% of studies, head and neck cancers account for 1%–7% of studies, liver cancer accounts for 1%–5% of studies, and melanoma accounts for 1%–2% of studies.

BEHAVIOR CHANGE RESEARCH SPECIFIC TO BREAST CANCER SURVIVORSHIP

U.S. breast cancer projected incidence is 30% of all cancers, easily topping the second most incident cancer in women, namely, cancer of the lung and bronchus (12%). These two cancer sites reverse their order, however, when it comes to mortality from the cancer (22% for lung and bronchus; 15% for breast cancer). The 10-year relative survival of women diagnosed with invasive breast cancer is 84% (ACS 2020). Among other implications is that half of the women diagnosed with breast cancer will survive the diagnosis long enough to die from some other cause of death, typically heart disease, stroke or nonbreast cancer (Afifi et al. 2020). The high proportion of survivors and the lengthy periods of breast cancer survivorship help to explain why there has been so much more behavior change research involving breast cancer survivors compared to survivors of other cancers.

FOCUS ON DIETARY CHANGE APPROACH TO INCREASING RECURRENCE-FREE SURVIVAL AND QUALITY OF LIFE IN BREAST CANCER SURVIVORS

Table 20.1 indicates that diet-alone interventions involving breast cancer patients and survivors are ~40% less common than physical-alone interventions. This difference may probably be in part because of the relative dearth of objective measures of dietary change compared to the objective measures of change in physical activity (e.g., accelerometry measures, aerobic fitness, 6-minute walk test). Also notable to consider is the etiologically relevant time period of dietary consumption. Cancer development takes decades and a central question in nutritional epidemiologic studies is when during the developmental time period is dietary consumption most important in relationship to cancer risk. The two most popular methods of assessment are the 24-hour diet recall, which assesses recent dietary intake, and the semi-quantitative food frequency questionnaire, which measures usual dietary consumption, typically over the last year. The gold standard for dietary assessment is the multipass 24-hour recall, which requires a well-trained nutritionist and a study participant with good recall of all dietary ingredients consumed in the last 24 hours

(Conway et al. 2003). Other dietary assessment instruments included semiquantitative food frequency questionnaires, which rely on the study participant's memory for typical foods consumed over the last 12 months, and a Mediterranean diet adherence questionnaire (Ruiz-Vozmediano et al. 2020). All these instruments depend on study participant self-report and are therefore subject to social desirability-related and memory-related biases. Compounding the imprecision of dietary assessment is the lack of consensus concerning how best to design cancer-preventive dietary interventions. In pursuit of scientific replicability, early dietary-focused cancer prevention efforts consisted of "chemoprevention" trials, where the dietary intervention consisted of single-nutrient pills or placebo pills. These chemoprevention trials fell into disfavor after some notable failures, where the ostensibly protective nutrient turned out to increase risk instead of decrease risk when taken in superphysiological doses (Omenn et al. 1996, Heinonen et al. 1994). In the aughts, the focus of cancer preventive dietary interventions were constraints on the daily intake of calories (Greenlee et al. 2013), macronutrients, or high-glycemic foods (Belle et al. 2011). More recently, the focus has shifted to dietary patterns such as the Mediterranean diet (Zuniga et al. 2019) but there are many different versions of the Mediterranean diet, making comparisons across studies problematic. The search for a consensus, replicable dietary pattern well-designed to help breast cancer survivors optimize recurrence-free survival and quality of life continues.

The results of a randomized controlled trial indicated that a reduction in low-fat dietary intake can increase relapse-free survival of breast cancer patients receiving conventional cancer treatment (Chlebowski et al. 2006) but inconsistent results from other low-fat dietary intake trials reduce confidence in this particular dietary approach to reducing mortality from breast cancer. There is more consensus that dietary pattern interventions (Barchitta et al. 2020), particularly if accompanied by physical activity intervention (Ruiz-Vozmediano et al. 2020), result in increased quality of life (e.g., increased physical functioning, increased role functioning, reduced depressive symptoms) (Ruiz-Vozmediano et al. 2020).

Insights from the recent surge in studies of the human gut microbiota (Proctor et al. 2019) shed new light on the results of two major diet intervention trials intended to reduce breast cancer recurrence in breast cancer survivors. The first was the Women's Intervention Nutrition Study (WINS) trial (Chlebowski et al. 2006), in which 2,437 women with resected, early-stage breast cancer receiving conventional cancer management were randomized. The control arm received minimal nutrition counseling. The intervention arm received intensive training in how to adhere to a low-fat eating plan. The stated goal of the intervention arm was to get participants to reduce their daily fat intake to 15% of total calories but the statistical power of the study was premised on intervention participants achieving 20% of total calories from dietary fat. More specifically, participants on the low-fat eating plan were expected to (1) reduce consumption of oils, high-fat spreads, high-fat salad dressings, and high-fat sauces; (2) choose low-fat dairy products; (3) choose low-fat fish, poultry without skin, lean cuts of meat; (4) eat more fruits, vegetables, legumes, and whole grains; and (5) replace high-fat desserts, snacks, and beverages with low-fat substitutes (Winters et al. 2004). Behavioral strategies were informed by SCT (Bandura 2004) and included self-monitoring (fat gram counting and recording), progressive goal setting, dietitian modeling of desirable behaviors, eliciting social support from family members and friends, and relapse prevention strategies for how to get back on track when participants strayed from acceptable adherence to their fat goal prescription. Individual fat gram goals were based on baseline energy intake and were designed to help the participant maintain her body weight. No counseling on weight reduction was provided. The low-fat eating plan was initiated during eight 1-hour biweekly individual, in-person counseling sessions. Subsequent dietitian contacts (visits or calls) occurred every 3 months, with available, optional monthly dietary group sessions for those wanting additional dietitian counseling. Women in the dietary intervention group were instructed to keep a written record of their daily fat gram intake. Participants in the control condition had one baseline dietitian visit and contacts with a dietitian every 3 months. They received written information concerning general dietary guidelines but were otherwise counseled only on nutritional adequacy for vitamin and mineral intake.

Several things, in hindsight, were missing in this intervention that current research on the human gut microbiota would suggest would have been good to include. One is distinguishing between proinflammatory and anti-inflammatory fats. Implicitly, the WINS special intervention did encourage disproportionate reduction of proinflammatory saturated fats by urging participants to limit their intake of high-fat animal foods such as high-fat dairy and meat (Turner-McGrievy et al. 2015) but the intervention might have done better by also encouraging participants to replace meat with fish rich in omega-3 fatty acids (Rosell et al. 2006) and replace corn oil with canola oil (Alfenas and Mattes 2003). The second is highlighting the satiety-signaling and glucose management benefits of plant foods rich in fiber (Zhao et al. 2018). The third is stressing the synergistic benefit of accompanying the dietary change with increased adherence to regular physical activity (Johns et al. 2014). While fiber intake is key to maintaining healthy levels of short-chain fatty acids in the colon (O'Keefe 2019), regular aerobic physical activity can independently boost short chain fatty acids (Allen et al. 2018), which, in turn, can help prevent unwanted weight gain and reduce systemic inflammation (McNabney and Henagan 2017). Regular physical activity also facilitates adherence to recommended dietary changes (Maugeri et al. 2019), possibly because of its effect on reducing depressive symptoms via the gut-brain axis (Gubert et al. 2020). This combination of increased gut homeostasis, reduced inflammation, and improved glucose control facilitates adherence to the recommended behavior changes by providing the participant with palpable evidence of physical and psychological benefit (Klem et al. 2000).

Despite these deficiencies, the participants in the low-fat diet intervention did experience significant reduction in dietary fat intake and significantly increased relapse-free survival relative to controls (Chlebowski et al. 2006). This effect was particularly strong in women with hormone receptor-negative cancer. The authors noted that a predominant influence of the dietary intervention on hormone receptor-negative women would imply that factors other than estrogen mediated the effect of dietary change on their likelihood of relapse-free survival. The candidate alternative mediators that they suggested might be part of the causal pathway explaining their results included reduced insulin levels (Borugian et al. 2004, Goodwin et al. 2002), reduced insulin resistance (Pollak et al. 2006) or reduced inflammation (Barnard et al. 2006, Clifton et al. 2005), all of which would have been more powerfully addressed had insights from the study of the human gut microbiota mentioned above been incorporated into the dietary intervention.

The second major intervention trial was the Women's Healthy Eating and Living (WHEL) randomized controlled trial (Pierce et al. 2007). A computer-assisted protocol based on SCT had three phases of decreasing intensity. During the first phase (3–8 calls in 4–6 weeks), counselors focused on building self-efficacy to implement the study nutritional targets, which consisted of daily intake of 5 vegetable servings plus 16 ounces of vegetable juice, 3 fruit servings, 30 g of fiber, and 15%–20% of energy intake from fat. Phase 2 (through 5 months) focused on self-monitoring and dealt with barriers to adherence. Phase 3 (through study completion) focused on retaining motivation for the study dietary pattern and preventing setbacks. The daily vegetable juice intake goal was explained as a way of maximizing vegetable nutrients without excessive bulk (Pierce et al. 2004). A major goal of this intervention was to boost levels of plasma carotenoids in special intervention participants measured at 12 and 36 months follow-up. The biggest problem for this intervention was its contravention of the WCRF recommendation that adults limit their juice intake in favor of consuming whole fruits and vegetables (WCRF 2018, p. 33). Juices typically have only a fraction of the fiber found in equicaloric quantities of the whole fruit or vegetable from which they were derived, thereby reducing the satiety-signaling and glucose management benefits of plant foods rich in fiber (Zhao et al. 2018). The special nutrition intervention did explicitly encourage increased consumption of fiber-rich foods but the 3-g, 14.7% increase in fiber intake observed at 72 months follow-up relative to baseline may have been too little to affect the gut microbiota (Pierce et al. 2004). The complete absence of intervention messaging concerning the benefits of regular physical activity is another obvious lacuna, given the direct and indirect contribution of regular physical activity to enhanced gut homeostasis (Allen et al. 2018) and enhanced quality of life (Xu et al. 2018).

As intended, the WHEL intervention successfully boosted intensive intervention participants' serum carotenoid levels, validating self-reports of increased fruit and vegetable intake (Pierce et al. 2007). Unlike the WINS trial, however, the WHEL intervention failed to reduce the number of invasive breast cancer events relative to the control condition over 7.3 years of follow-up. Curiously, the mean weight of the participants in the intensive nutrition intervention increased 0.6 kg over the course of the trial compared to an increase of 0.4 kg for the participants in the control condition. This finding is curious because most intensive nutrition interventions featuring increased fruit and vegetable intake (and lower fat intake) have yielded significant weight loss compared to controls (Howard et al. 2006, Ello-Martin, Roe, and Rolls 2004, Ledikwe et al. 2007). It is worth noting that none of these other trials promoted daily consumption of juices.

Most breast cancer survivors complain of profound fatigue after cancer treatment has ended (Puigpinos-Riera et al. 2020). Both physical activity interventions (Parra et al. 2020, Alizadeh et al. 2019) and dietary pattern interventions (Zick et al. 2017) have been shown to decrease risk of cancer-related fatigue by reducing elevated low-grade inflammation.

FOCUS ON PHYSICAL ACTIVITY CHANGE APPROACH TO INCREASING RECURRENCE-FREE SURVIVAL AND QUALITY OF LIFE IN BREAST CANCER SURVIVORS

As evident from the relative number of hits in Table 20.1 that were elicited from bibliographic searches of the ISI webofknowledge.com data base, there is ~50% more scientific literature addressing the impact of physical activity interventions than diet-related interventions on cancer survivor recurrence-free survival and quality of life. If we subtract the 336 hits for multimodal interventions that included both diet and physical activity interventions, then the number of physical activity-only interventions is closer to 80% more numerous than diet-only interventions. The relatively greater popularity of physical activity-only interventions may be attributable to the greater availability of objective measures of physical activity and physical fitness than is true of diet or body nutrient concentration. Probably the most common measure of increased physical activity capacity used in these studies was the 6-minute walk distance test, which is an inexpensive, reliable, safe way to assess physical activity capacity of older patients (Wesolowski, Orlowski, and Kram 2020). Accelerometers, typically worn around the waist, have facilitated objective assessment of minutes of moderate and vigorous physical activity (Adlard et al. 2019). Physical activity trackers, often built into watches worn on the wrist, have proven useful in providing survivors with objective information about their daily level of physical activity (Lynch et al. 2019).

A 2018 Cochrane review (Lahart et al. 2018) of published trials concluded that the available evidence is not yet sufficient to say with confidence that getting breast cancer survivors to adopt increased physical activity will decrease mortality or increase relapse-free survival. The authors of this review were more confident in concluding that getting breast cancer survivors to increase their daily physical activity (mostly walking or resistance training) appreciably increased their quality of life, their cardiorespiratory fitness, and emotional health relative to controls (Lahart et al. 2018).

A 2019 review (Abdin et al. 2019) was prefaced by a statement that the scientific consensus had determined that engaging in physical activity following a diagnosis in breast cancer patients improves both survival rates and psychosocial health outcomes. Going beyond these "settled" questions, the questions these investigators wanted their review to answer were: (1) Which exercise modes were most helpful? (2) Are group exercise classes more effective than individual efforts at sustaining the desired exercise levels long-term? This review identified 17 randomized, controlled physical activity intervention trials involving women diagnosed with breast cancer. The authors concluded that type of exercise mode (aerobic, resistance, walking) seemed not to matter-all were associated with better post-treatment functioning (physical function, 12-minute walk test, quality of life, positive mood, pain, endocrine symptoms) at least short-term, than controls (Abdin et al. 2019). Six of the trials featured resistance training. All featured some form of aerobic exercise or walking interventions. Only five trials provided group-based exercise intervention. Five of the twelve individual-focused trials reported long-term maintenance of the observed beneficial short-term effects, as did only one of the five group-based trials. The varied outcomes across trials made it impossible to compare the relative effectiveness of individual-focused versus group-based trials. No detrimental effects of the physical activity interventions were apparent in any of the trials (Abdin et al. 2019).

Prescription of aromatase inhibitors is now standard of care for postmenopausal women with hormone receptor-positive breast cancer (Burstein et al. 2019), because it has been shown to be effective in reducing recurrence (Dowsett et al. 2015). Unfortunately, aromatase inhibitor treatment is associated with a high incidence of aromatase inhibitor-induced musculoskeletal symptoms (Roberts et al. 2017b), often described as pain and soreness in the joints, musculoskeletal pain, and joint stiffness. These symptoms reduce compliance with aromatase inhibitors, potentially compromising breast cancer outcomes. Exercise has been investigated for the prevention and treatment of these joint and musculoskeletal symptoms but no consistent benefits have been observed so far, including on stiffness, grip strength, overall health-related quality of life, or cancer-related quality of life (Roberts et al. 2020).

A 15-year follow-up of an observational cohort study of 153 breast cancer survivors and 4,778 same-age Australian women without breast cancer (Tollosa et al. 2020, in press) observed no difference in adherence to a range of recommended health behaviors between the two groups prior to diagnosis. After diagnosis, the breast cancer survivors significantly increased their adherence to recommended participation in regular physical activity and recommended daily fruit intake, but reduced their adherence to recommended body weight level in the first few years postdiagnosis (Tollosa et al. 2020, in press). The proportion of nonalcohol drinkers and nonsmokers increased slightly over the survivorship period. Dietary data collected periodically using a semiquantitative food frequency questionnaire showed increased consumption of nonstarchy vegetables and increased total calories but otherwise no significant difference in consumption of other dietary constituents relative to nonbreast cancer survivors, including no difference in consumption of saturated fat, dietary fiber, or alcohol (Tollosa et al. 2020, in press). The recommended level of alcohol consumption is zero for breast cancer survivors (Rock et al. 2012), but only 14%–16% of participants during the near-term and long-term survivorship periods adhered to this recommendation, similar to adherence levels reported for breast cancer survivors in the US 2–4 years postdiagnosis (Lin et al. 2019). The authors noted that most of the unwanted weight gain occurred in the period immediately following diagnosis (Tollosa et al. 2020, in press). They inferred that the unwanted weight gain was related to the women's breast cancer treatment (Tollosa et al. 2020, in press). The consistently low level of adherence to recommended daily dietary fiber intake and to recommended limits on saturated fat intake may have contributed to inadequate levels of the satiety hormone GLP-1 (Bodnaruc et al. 2016). Adequate levels of GLP-1 satiety-signaling could have protected the women from excessive consumption of daily calories (Flint et al. 1998).

From the foregoing, we conclude that breast cancer survivors need to improve their daily health behaviors in order to optimize their health prospects and quality of life. Behavior change theory-driven approaches that take into account the survivor's health status and social supports can facilitate adoption and maintenance of desirable health behaviors and that doing so increases recurrence-free survival and quality of life. There is growing support for multimodal (e.g., dietary change + increased physical activity + stress management) interventions yielding greater impact than interventions focused on improving a single health behavior. With respect to dietary interventions, the healthy dietary pattern approach (e.g., Mediterranean diet) appears to be more effective than macronutrient or micronutrient approaches in improving survivors' physical health prospects and quality of life. We conjecture that the gut microbiota is likely to be the site for the biological integration of the physiological impact of these health behavior changes, as reflected by reduced low-grade systemic inflammation and increased abundance of short-chain fatty acid-generating commensal gut bacteria.

BEHAVIOR CHANGE RESEARCH SPECIFIC TO
COLORECTAL CANCER SURVIVORSHIP

A 2019 update of a review of the role of dietary patterns in colorectal cancer incidence concluded that healthy dietary patterns, as assessed by the Healthy Eating Index, a Mediterranean diet index, or Dietary Inflammatory Index, were generally associated with reduced risk of colorectal cancer (Fernandez-Villa et al. 2020). Unfortunately, adherence to healthy dietary patterns by U.S. colorectal cancer survivors tends to be low (Van Blarigan et al. 2018, Guinter et al. 2018). Seeking to remedy this poor dietary adherence to healthy eating, a 2020 pilot study showed promising results for the use of automated text messages to inform and motivate the survivors to make healthier daily food choices (Van Blarigan et al. 2020). The intervention design benefited from the researchers invoking the TPB and SCT by addressing outcome expectations, self-efficacy, goal setting, self-monitoring, and social support (Stacey et al. 2015, Pinto and Floyd 2008).

A 2005 randomized, controlled nutrition intervention (Ravasco et al. 2005a) involved 111 colorectal cancer patients receiving radiotherapy. Three-month follow-up results showed that intensive dietary counseling was associated with lower radiotherapy toxicity, that is, lower rates of anorexia, nausea, vomiting, and diarrhea compared to the usual care control condition, as well as higher quality of life. At the subsequent 7-year follow-up (Ravasco, Monteiro-Grillo, and Camila 2012), late radiotherapy toxicity was lower and quality of life was higher in the group that received the intensive nutritional counseling compared to the controls (Ravasco, Monteiro-Grillo, and Camila 2012).

In its 2018 review of the literature associating daily food choices and physical activity levels to cancer outcomes, the WCRF concluded that evidence is convincing that physical activity prevents colon cancer (WCRF 2018). Evidence is more limited that physical activity prevents recurrence in colon cancer survivors (Cormie et al. 2017).

A 2020 physical activity-focused Cochrane review (McGettigan et al. 2020) identified 16 randomized, controlled physical activity intervention trials involving 992 participants who were diagnosed with nonadvanced colorectal cancer, staged as T1–4 N0–2 M0, treated surgically or with neoadjuvant and/or adjuvant therapy (i.e., chemotherapy, radiotherapy, or chemoradiotherapy). Ten studies included participants who had finished active treatment, two studies included participants who were receiving active treatment, two studies included both those receiving and finished active treatment. Treatment status was unclear in the four remaining studies. Three studies opted for supervised interventions, five for home-based self-directed interventions, and seven studies opted for a combination of supervised and self-directed programs. The most common intervention duration was 12 weeks (7 studies). The type of physical activity included walking, cycling, resistance exercise, yoga, and core stabilization exercise. Results showed positive effects of physical activity intervention on aerobic fitness, cancer-related fatigue, and health-related quality of life at immediate-term but not medium-term follow-up (McGettigan et al. 2020). Where reported, adverse events were generally minor.

Historically, the health behavior change efforts involving people diagnosed with colorectal cancer were applied only post-treatment. In recent years, however, researchers have wanted to see if engaging colorectal cancer patients in behavior change interventions before surgery could yield health benefits similar to or better than those generated post-treatment. They called this "prehabilitation" (Meneses-Echavez et al. 2020). Because early exercise-only prehabilitation interventions yielded mixed results (Carli et al. 2010, Moran et al. 2016), more recent efforts have been multimodal. A 2019 multimodal 4-week pilot prehabilitation intervention involving 50 colorectal cancer patients featured (1) protein supplementation; (2) supervised vigorous aerobic and resistance exercise; (3) individual psychological counseling to reduce anxiety; and (4) smoking cessation for those who smoked (van Rooijen et al. 2019). In this nonrandomized, controlled trial, 86% of the participants in the multimodal intervention group recovered baseline functional capacity compared to only 40% of the participants in the usual care group. A 2018 systematic review identified five randomized controlled trials and four cohort studies involving colorectal cancer patients that concluded that nutritional prehabilitation alone or combined with exercise decreased hospital length of stay by 2 days after undergoing colorectal surgery (Gillis et al. 2018).

Based on the results of preclinical studies, the emerging scientific consensus is that the salubrious effects of regular physical activity and healthy dietary patterns on reducing colon cancer risk are probably mediated by their influences on the composition of each person's gut microbiota (Piazzi et al. 2019, Song and Chan 2019).

BEHAVIOR CHANGE RESEARCH SPECIFIC TO LUNG CANCER SURVIVORSHIP

Whereas unwanted weight gain is the fear most commonly seen in persons with breast cancer (Stan, Loprinzi, and Ruddy 2013), the opposite (i.e., unwanted weight loss) is true for persons with lung cancer (Naito 2019). Cachexia is arguably the most important nutrition-related challenge associated with lung cancer survivorship (Laviano et al. 2020). The root cause of cachexia is unknown but nutrition interventions may provide at least partial remedies (Naito 2019).

A 2019 physical activity-focused Cochrane review (Cavalheri et al. 2019) reported the results of eight randomized controlled trials involving a total of 450 lung cancer survivors exposed to physical activity interventions within a month of lung resection. Six studies examined the effects of combined aerobic and resistance training; one examined the effects of combined aerobic and inspiratory muscle training; and one examined the effects of combined aerobic, resistance, inspiratory muscle training, and balance training (Cavalheri et al. 2019). The length of the exercise programs ranged from 4 to 20 weeks, with exercises performed twice to 5 days a week. The authors concluded with moderate to high confidence that lung cancer survivors exposed to the exercise trainings enjoyed significantly increased exercise capacity (Cavalheri et al. 2019). They concluded with moderate confidence that lung cancer survivors exposed to the exercise interventions did not experience increased risk of injury, excess weight loss, or other exercise-related challenge to their physical health. They concluded with a low-level confidence that lung cancer survivors exposed to the exercise intervention enjoyed increased quality of life compared to controls (Cavalheri et al. 2019).

For persons with advanced lung cancer, exercise capacity is critical in a patient's ability to participate in life's activities. A second 2019 physical activity-focused Cochrane review (Peddle-McIntyre et al. 2019) reported the results of six randomized controlled trials involving a total of 221 participants with advanced lung cancer. Despite the comorbidities associated with advanced lung cancer, the results overlapped with the results of the previously discussed 2019 Cochrane review (Cavalheri et al. 2019). Despite metastatic disease, lung cancer survivors induced to exercise regularly were more physically fit and enjoyed a higher quality of life than lung cancer survivors not encouraged to exercise (Peddle-McIntyre et al. 2019).

BEHAVIOR CHANGE RESEARCH SPECIFIC TO PROSTATE CANCER SURVIVORSHIP

An observational study involving prostate cancer survivors found an inverse relationship between adherence to WCRF lifestyle recommendations and prostate cancer aggressiveness, with 13% risk reduction benefit for every 1-point increase in the total adherence score (Arab et al. 2013). A 2020 review of barriers and facilitators to physical activity in men with prostate cancer concluded that heterogeneity and unsystematic reporting of quantitative study methods prohibited a quantitative data synthesis but that both quantitative and qualitative evaluation of the literature consistently identified incontinence as a specific barrier to exercise among prostate cancer survivors treated surgically (Fox et al. 2020, in press).

In terms of possible nutrition interventions to reduce the negative side effects of androgen deprivation therapy, a 2019 review of 16 relevant studies concluded that the critical mass of evidence needed for nutritional guidelines has not yet been achieved but said that additional trials of nutrition interventions were warranted (Barnes et al. 2019).

BEHAVIOR CHANGE RESEARCH SPECIFIC TO MELANOMA CANCER SURVIVORSHIP

A 2019 review (Patel et al. 2019) noted that risk of melanoma was found to increase with physical activity in contrast to most other epithelial cancers, where risk decreased with increasing levels of physical activity. The authors attributed the increased risk of melanoma associated with exercise to the increased exposure to radiation from the sun that commonly accompanies increased exercise (Patel et al. 2019). If the excess solar radiation hazard is avoided, then increased physical activity for melanoma patients should yield physical and psychosocial benefits previously observed in survivors of other cancers, such as reduction in treatment-related fatigue (Hyatt et al. 2020, Cormie et al. 2017).

BEHAVIOR CHANGE RESEARCH SPECIFIC TO HEAD AND NECK CANCER SURVIVORSHIP

Unlike other cancer sites, where nutrition interventions are seen as adjunctive, for head and neck cancer survivors, learning to eat healthfully is central to achieving an acceptable quality of life. Eating problems and other late effects can be long-lasting if not treated (Kristensen et al. 2020). These problems include dysphagia (swallowing difficulties), xerostomia (dry mouth), dysgeusia (taste disturbances), and trismus (reduced mouth opening) (Crowder et al. 2019).

One much-cited randomized, controlled nutrition intervention involving 75 head and neck patients referred for radiotherapy was published in 2005 (Ravasco et al. 2005b). Results showed that 90% of patients who received intensive nutrition counseling reported reduced side effects of radiotherapy toxicity at 3 months follow-up compared to 51% of patients in usual care (Ravasco et al. 2005b). Patients receiving the intensive nutritional counseling also reported either maintaining or increasing their quality of life in contrast to patients in the usual care condition, who reported either just maintaining or seeing their quality of life actually decreasing (Ravasco et al. 2005b).

BEHAVIOR CHANGE RESEARCH SPECIFIC TO SURVIVING DIAGNOSES INVOLVING MULTIPLE CANCER SITES

Some intervention research has targeted survivors of different cancer sites concurrently.

For example, a 2020 report of an Australian study of a postrehabilitation physical activity maintenance intervention enrolled all cancer survivors regardless of cancer site who had successfully completed a 12-week medical center sponsored exercise-based oncology rehabilitation program. The oncology rehabilitation program consisted of twice weekly, supervised exercise sessions and encouragement to engage in at least 30 minutes of physical activity on most days. Fifty-seven percent of the 66 participants were breast cancer survivors. The remaining participants included survivors of cervical, endometrial, lung, leukemia, lymphoma, urinary, melanoma, rectal, oral, ovarian, and prostate cancers. The participants were randomized either to a Fitbit-only control condition for 8 weeks or to a Fitbit+health coach+25 text messages intervention. The health coach called the intervention participants three times over the 8 weeks to remind them of the health and emotional benefits of physical activity, to identify and problem-solve barriers to adhering to the 30 minutes/day exercise prescription and to help them to assess and revise their physical activity goals. At the end of 8 weeks, research accelerometry data showed that the coach- and text-message-supported participants had continued to adhere fully to the 30 minutes/day exercise prescription for 8 of the 8 weeks whereas the Fitbit-only group no longer adhered fully to the 30 minutes/day exercise prescription on any of the 8 weeks of the physical activity maintenance follow-up period. There were no indications that results differed by cancer diagnosis. Results showed that maintenance of a desired health behavior that was initially adopted with intensive support from an oncology rehabilitation program benefited from continued coaching support at a less intensive and more intermittent level following graduation from the more structured, more intensive rehabilitation program. With respect to Figure 20.1, this represents a transition in the locus of behavior change from the interpersonal (coach to client) to the social ecological (text messages programmed to encourage the client).

Guidelines for management of the profound fatigue that often accompanies treatment for cancer have identified psychosocial interventions as effective for alleviating fatigue in survivors of various cancers (Bower et al. 2014). The American Society of Clinical Oncology (ASCO) guidelines, for example, provided detailed guidance and encouragement to engage unspecified cancer survivors in physical activity as a way to alleviate post-treatment fatigue. Their recommendations included:

- Initiating/maintaining adequate levels of physical activity can reduce cancer-related fatigue in post-treatment survivors.
- Actively encourage all patients to engage in a moderate level of physical activity after cancer treatment (e.g., 150 minutes of moderate aerobic exercise [such as fast walking, cycling, or swimming] per week with an additional two to three strength training [such as weight lifting] sessions per week, unless contraindicated.
- Walking programs are generally safe for most cancer survivors; the American College of Sports Medicine recommends that cancer survivors can begin this type of program after consulting with their doctors, but without any formal exercise testing (such as a stress test).
- Survivors at higher risk of injury (e.g., those living with neuropathy, cardiomyopathy, or other long-term effects of therapy other than comorbidities) should be referred to a physical therapist or exercise specialist. Breast cancer survivors with lymphedema should also consider meeting with an exercise specialist before initiating upper body strength-training exercise.

The ASCO guidelines were not comparably specific about how nutrition interventions could help alleviate fatigue in cancer survivors other than to recommend that oncologists screen for and manage "nutritional issues" or "nutritional deficits" (Bower et al. 2014). This was surprising inasmuch as inflammation has been identified as a key contributor to post-treatment fatigue (Bower and Lamkin 2013) has been identified as one mechanism by which regular physical activity reduces post-treatment fatigue (Alizadeh et al. 2019), and is widely regarded as importantly determined by daily food choices (Correa and Rogero 2019, Zhang, Wang, and Zhang 2018, Akbaraly et al. 2015, Alfano et al. 2012).

ONLINE BEHAVIOR CHANGE PROGRAMS FOR CANCER SURVIVORS

The external monitoring provided by a primary care provider, oncologist, or lifestyle coach that helps motivate patients/clients to adhere to better eating and physical activity practices is labor-intensive and expensive to maintain (Vandelanotte et al. 2016). An increasing number of mobile health solutions (mhealth) are being developed to provide some of the same benefits normally associated with extensive external monitoring by a care provider at a fraction of the cost (Vandelanotte et al. 2016). But how effective are these mhealth solutions when applied to cancer survivors? A 2017 meta-analysis identified 15 internet-based programs that delivered a physical activity and/or diet intervention tailored for cancer survivors (Roberts et al. 2017a). A consistent positive effect was found for increasing physical activity and reducing body mass index, but findings were mixed or inconclusive for cancer treatment–related symptoms, health-related quality of life, self-efficacy, and dietary change. For those who make full use of the mhealth program, there is usually some benefit but the number who make full use of an mhealth program after logging onto it at least once is typically small (e.g., 23%) (Gianfredi et al. 2020). These weaknesses notwithstanding, the field of mhealth will keep expanding mhealth resources for cancer survivors because of the drive to provide greater access to lifestyle coaching resources to more patients/clients at lower cost (Vandelanotte et al. 2016).

STRUCTURAL BARRIERS TO HEALTHCARE PROVIDERS PROMOTING HEALTHIER BEHAVIORS TO CANCER SURVIVORS

Structural barriers to healthcare providers promoting physical activity to cancer survivors include lack of time, lack of provider knowledge about the health benefits of physical activity, provider attitude that physical activity promotion was not a legitimate part of their professional role, insufficiently engaged patients (Spellman, Craike, and Livingston 2014) and safety concerns (Nadler et al. 2017).

SUMMARY

The evidence to date supports the conclusion that cancer survivors are deriving significant, if small, recurrence-free survival and quality of life benefits from the health behavior promotion efforts that they have participated in. Some of the lessons learned in promoting healthier ways of living in breast cancer survivors should be applicable to survivors of other cancer diagnoses, given common features of recovery from cytotoxic and radiographic cancer treatment across cancer diagnoses.

There has been a convergence of lifestyle recommendations by the major voluntary health organizations: American Heart Association, ACS, and American Diabetes Association (Kushi et al. 2012). Hence, some of the lessons learned about lifestyle behavior change strategies designed to reduce risk of heart disease or type 2 diabetes may also apply to cancer survivors. A 2020 review of cardiac rehabilitation interventions that included cancer survivors identified nine studies that included a total of 662 cancer survivors (Cuthbertson et al. 2020, in press). This scoping review concluded that of cancer survivors participating in cardiac rehabilitation, 60% of enrolled cancer survivors completed the rehabilitation programs and enjoyed some of the same physical and psychosocial benefits that other cancer survivors have experienced in cancer-specific lifestyle behavior change programs (Cuthbertson et al. 2020, in press).

RECOMMENDATIONS TO ACCELERATE PROGRESS IN OPTIMIZING CANCER SURVIVOR QUALITY OF LIFE THROUGH MOTIVATING THEM TO ENGAGE IN HEALTHFUL LIFESTYLE CHANGE

In clinical behavior change intervention research, include explicitly theory-based behavior change elements so that results can be more informative about putative causal processes.

For busy clinicians, invoke different behavior change theories (see Figure 20.1) depending on the cancer survivor's progress in achieving an acceptable quality of life with family and community supports recognized as necessary for the long-term sustainability of the desired behaviors.

The new insights afforded by the advent of high-throughput gene sequencing have illuminated alternative causal pathways involving metabolic functioning that differ from hypothesized causal pathways previously assumed to explain the phenomenon of unwanted weight gain. Future research on behavior change approaches to reducing unwanted weight gain in cancer survivors would benefit from capitalizing on these insights. More specifically, behavior change researchers should focus on increasing cancer survivors' exposure to prebiotic and anti-inflammatory features of common dietary patterns such as the Mediterranean or DASH dietary patterns.

The increasing recognition of the role of inflammation in promoting carcinogenesis should motivate researchers to incorporate greater frequency and possibly intensity of physical activity in health promotion efforts. The consistent anti-inflammatory effect of regular physical activity may synergistically magnify the anti-inflammatory effects of healthier daily food choices.

Similar reasoning justifies including smoking cessation efforts for those cancer survivors who continue to smoke. In other words, physical activity promotion and smoking cessation are essential for the cancer survivor to derive maximum health benefit from her efforts to improve her daily food choices.

Clinicians should feel free to refer cancer survivors to community health promotion programs (e.g., YMCA DPP), if their current health status permits. Programs designed to improve the physical health and emotional well-being of healthy community members are good bets for improving the physical health and emotional well-being of cancer survivors as well.

In short, there is much that cancer survivors can do using accessible community resources at their disposal to improve their physical health prospects and optimize their overall quality of life. There is much that their healthcare providers, caretakers, and interested community members can do to optimize cancer survivors' use of community resources to enhance their physical health and quality of life.

REFERENCES

Abdin, S., J. F. Lavallee, J. Faulkner, and M. Husted. 2019. "A systematic review of the effectiveness of physical activity interventions in adults with breast cancer by physical activity type and mode of participation." *Psycho-Oncology* 28 (7):1381–1393. doi: 10.1002/pon.5101.

Adlard, K. N., D. G. Jenkins, C. E. Salisbury, K. A. Bolam, S. R. Gomersall, J. F. Aitken, S. K. Chambers, J. C. Dunn, K. S. Courneya, and T. L. Skinner. 2019. "Peer support for the maintenance of physical activity and health in cancer survivors: The PEER trial - a study protocol of a randomised controlled trial." *BMC Cancer* 19:15. doi: 10.1186/s12885-019-5853-4.

Afifi, A. M., A. M. Saad, M. J. Al-Husseini, A. O. Elmehrath, D. W. Northfelt, and M. B. Sonbol. 2020. "Causes of death after breast cancer diagnosis: A US population-based analysis." *Cancer* 126 (7):1559–1567. doi: 10.1002/cncr.32648.

Akbaraly, T. N., M. J. Shipley, J. E. Ferrie, M. Virtanen, G. Lowe, M. Hamer, and M. Kivimaki. 2015. "Long-term adherence to healthy dietary guidelines and chronic inflammation in the prospective Whitehall II study." *American Journal of Medicine* 128 (2):152–U162. doi: 10.1016/j.amjmed.2014.10.002.

Alfano, C. M., I. Imayama, M. L. Neuhouser, J. K. Kiecolt-Glaser, A. W. Smith, A. Meeske, A. McTiernan, L. Bernstein, K. B. Baumgartner, C. M. Ulrich, and R. Ballard-Barbash. 2012. "Fatigue, inflammation, and omega-3 and omega-6 fatty acid intake among breast cancer survivors." *Journal of Clinical Oncology* 30 (12):1280–1287. doi: 10.1200/jco.2011.36.4109.

Alfenas, R. C. G., and R. D. Mattes. 2003. "Effect of fat sources on satiety." *Obesity Research* 11 (2):183–187. doi: 10.1038/oby.2003.29.

Alizadeh, A. M., A. Isanejad, S. Sadighi, M. Mardani, B. Kalaghchi, and Z. M. Hassan. 2019. "High-intensity interval training can modulate the systemic inflammation and HSP70 in the breast cancer: A randomized control trial." *Journal of Cancer Research and Clinical Oncology* 145 (10):2583–2593. doi: 10.1007/s00432-019-02996-y.

Allen, J. M., L. J. Mailing, G. M. Niemiro, R. Moore, M. D. Cook, B. A. White, H. D. Holscher, and J. A. Woods. 2018. "Exercise alters gut microbiota composition and function in lean and obese humans." *Medicine & Science in Sports & Exercise* 50 (4):747–757. doi: 10.1249/mss.0000000000001495.

American Cancer Society (ACS). 2020. *Cancer Facts and Figures 2020.* Atlanta, GA: American Cancer Society. https://www.cancer.org/content/dam/cancer-org/research/cancer-facts-and-statistics/annual-cancer-facts-and-figures/2020/cancer-facts-and-figures-2020.pdf (accessed July 3, 2020).

Andrews, J. A., S. Hampson, and M. Barckley. 2008. "The effect of subjective normative social images of smokers on children's intentions to smoke." *Nicotine & Tobacco Research* 10 (4):589–597. doi: 10.1080/14622200801975819.

Arab, L., J. Su, S. E. Steck, A. Ang, E. T. H. Fontham, J. T. Bensen, and J. L. Mohler. 2013. "Adherence to World Cancer Research Fund/American Institute for Cancer Research Lifestyle Recommendations Reduces Prostate Cancer Aggressiveness Among African and Caucasian Americans." *Nutrition and Cancer: An International Journal* 65 (5):633–643. doi: 10.1080/01635581.2013.789540.

Arem, H., S. K. Mama, X. J. Duan, J. H. Rowland, K. M. Bellizzi, and D. K. Ehlers. 2020. "Prevalence of healthy behaviors among cancer survivors in the United States: How far have we come?" *Cancer Epidemiology Biomarkers & Prevention* 29 (6):1179–1187. doi: 10.1158/1055-9965.epi-19-1318.

Bandura, A. 2001. "Social cognitive theory: An agentic perspective." *Annual Review of Psychology* 52:1–26. doi: 10.1146/annurev.psych.52.1.1.

Bandura, A. 2004. "Health promotion by social cognitive means." *Health Education & Behavior* 31 (2):143–164.

Bandura, A., and D. H. Schunk. 1981. "Cultivating competence, self-efficacy, and intrinsic interest through proximal self-motivation." *Journal of Personality and Social Psychology* 41 (3):586–598.

Barchitta, M., A. Maugeri, R. M. San Lio, A. Quattrocchi, F. Degrassi, F. Catalano, G. Basile, and A. Agodi. 2020. "The effects of diet and dietary interventions on the quality of life among breast cancer survivors: A cross-sectional analysis and a systematic review of experimental studies." *Cancers* 12 (2):15. doi: 10.3390/cancers12020322.

Barnard, R. J., J. H. Gonzalez, M. E. Liva, and T. H. Ngo. 2006. "Effects of a low-fat, high-fiber diet and exercise program on breast cancer risk factors in vivo and tumor cell growth and apoptosis in vitro." *Nutrition and Cancer: An International Journal* 55 (1):28–34. doi: 10.1207/s15327914nc5501_4.

Barnes, K. A., L. E. Ball, D. A. Galvao, R. U. Newton, and S. K. Chambers. 2019. "Nutrition care guidelines for men with prostate cancer undergoing androgen deprivation therapy: Do we have enough evidence?" *Prostate Cancer and Prostatic Diseases* 22 (2):221–234. doi: 10.1038/s41391-018-0099-9.

Belle, F. N., E. Kampman, A. McTiernan, L. Bernstein, K. Baumgartner, R. Baumgartner, A. Ambs, R. Ballard-Barbash, and M. L. Neuhouser. 2011. "Dietary fiber, carbohydrates, glycemic index, and glycemic load in relation to breast cancer prognosis in the HEAL cohort." *Cancer Epidemiology Biomarkers & Prevention* 20 (5):890–899. doi: 10.1158/1055-9965.epi-10-1278.

Bennett, J. A., K. S. Lyons, K. Winters-Stone, L. M. Nail, and J. Scherer. 2007. "Motivational interviewing to increase physical activity in long-term cancer survivors: A randomized controlled trial." *Nursing Research* 56 (1):18–27. doi: 10.1097/00006199-200701000-00003.

Biedermann, L., J. Zeitz, J. Mwinyi, E. Sutter-Minder, A. Rehman, S. J. Ott, C. Steurer-Stey, A. Frei, P. Frei, M. Scharl, M. J. Loessner, S. R. Vavricka, M. Fried, S. Schreiber, M. Schuppler, and G. Rogler. 2013a. "Smoking cessation induces profound changes in the composition of the intestinal microbiota in humans." *PLos One* 8 (3):8. doi: 10.1371/journal.pone.0059260.

Bingham, S. A., and J. H. Cummings. 1989. "Effect of exercise and physical fitness on large intestinal function." *Gastroenterology* 97 (6):1389–1399. doi: 10.1016/0016-5085(89)90381-8.

Blanchard, C. M., K. S. Courneya, and K. Stein. 2008. "Cancer survivors' adherence to lifestyle behavior recommendations and associations with health-related quality of life: Results from the American Cancer Society's SCS-II." *Journal of Clinical Oncology* 26 (13):2198–2204. doi: 10.1200/jco.2007.14.6217.

Bluethmann, S. M., A. B. Mariotto, and J. H. Rowland. 2016. "Anticipating the "Silver Tsunami": Prevalence trajectories and comorbidity burden among older cancer survivors in the United States." *Cancer Epidemiology Biomarkers & Prevention* 25 (7):1029–1036. doi: 10.1158/1055-9965.epi-16-0133.

Bluethmann, S. M., L. K. Bartholomew, C. C. Murphy, and S. W. Vernon. 2017. "Use of theory in behavior change interventions: An analysis of programs to increase physical activity in posttreatment breast cancer survivors." *Health Education & Behavior* 44 (2):245–253. doi: 10.1177/1090198116647712.

Bodnaruc, A. M., D. Prud'homme, R. Blanchet, and I. Giroux. 2016. "Nutritional modulation of endogenous glucagon-like peptide-1 secretion: A review." *Nutrition & Metabolism* 13:16. doi: 10.1186/s12986-016-0153-3.

Borugian, M. J., S. B. Sheps, C. Kim-Sing, C. Van Patten, J. D. Potter, B. Dunn, R. P. Gallagher, and T. G. Hislop. 2004. "Insulin, macronutrient intake, and physical activity: Are potential indicators of insulin resistance associated with mortality from breast cancer?" *Cancer Epidemiology Biomarkers & Prevention* 13 (7):1163–1172.

Bower, J. E., and D. M. Lamkin. 2013. "Inflammation and cancer-related fatigue: Mechanisms, contributing factors, and treatment implications." *Brain Behavior and Immunity* 30:S48–S57. doi: 10.1016/j.bbi.2012.06.011.

Bower, J. E., K. Bak, A. Berger, W. Breitbart, C. P. Escalante, P. A. Ganz, H. H. Schnipper, C. Lacchetti, J. A. Ligibel, G. H. Lyman, M. S. Ogaily, W. F. Pirl, and P. B. Jacobsen. 2014. "Screening, assessment, and management of fatigue in adult survivors of cancer: An American Society of Clinical Oncology clinical practice guideline adaptation." *Journal of Clinical Oncology* 32 (17):1840–U127. doi: 10.1200/jco.2013.53.4495.

Bronfenbrenner, U. 1977. "Toward an experimental ecology of human development." *American Psychologist* 32 (7):513–531. doi: 10.1037/0003-066x.32.7.513.

Brownell, K. D., G. A. Marlatt, E. Lichtenstein, and G. T. Wilson. 1986. "Understanding and preventing relapse." *American Psychologist* 41 (7):765–782. doi: 10.1037//0003-066x.41.7.765.

Brucker, P. S., K. Yost, J. Cashy, K. Webster, and D. Cella. 2005. "General population and cancer patient norms for the functional assessment of cancer therapy-general (FACT-G)." *Evaluation & the Health Professions* 28 (2):192–211. doi: 10.1177/0163278705275341.

Burnham, J. C., ed. 1992. *Bad Habits: Drinking, Smoking, Taking Drugs, Gambling, Sexual Misbehavior and Swearing in American History.* New York: NYU Press.

Burstein, H. J., C. Lacchetti, H. Anderson, T. A. Buchholz, N. E. Davidson, K. A. Gelmon, S. H. Giordano, C. A. Hudis, A. J. Solky, V. Stearns, E. P. Winer, and J. J. Griggs. 2019. "Adjuvant endocrine therapy for women with hormone receptor-positive breast cancer: ASCO clinical practice guideline focused update." *Journal of Clinical Oncology* 37 (5):423–438. doi: 10.1200/jco.18.01160.

Cahill, K., T. Lancaster, and N. Green. 2010. "Stage-based interventions for smoking cessation." *Cochrane Database of Systematic Reviews* (11):105. doi: 10.1002/14651858.CD004492.pub4.

Carli, F., P. Charlebois, B. Stein, L. Feldman, G. Zavorsky, D. J. Kim, S. Scott, and N. E. Mayo. 2010. "Randomized clinical trial of prehabilitation in colorectal surgery." *British Journal of Surgery* 97 (8):1187–1197. doi: 10.1002/bjs.7102.

Carroll, C. 2019. "What is weight watchers?" verywellfit.com, accessed July 14. https://www.verywellfit.com/weight-watchers-overview-4691074?print.

Cavalheri, V., C. Burtin, V. R. Formico, M. L. Nonoyama, S. Jenkins, M. A. Spruit, and K. Hill. 2019. "Exercise training undertaken by people within 12 months of lung resection for non-small cell lung cancer." *Cochrane Database of Systematic Reviews* (6):62. doi: 10.1002/14651858.CD009955.pub3.

Chetty, R., M. Stepner, S. Abraham, S. Lin, B. Scuderi, N. Turner, A. Bergeron, and D. Cutler. 2016. "The association between income and life expectancy in the United States, 2001–2014." *JAMA-Journal of the American Medical Association* 315 (16):1750–1766. doi: 10.1001/jama.2016.4226.

Chlebowski, R. T., G. L. Blackburn, C. A. Thomson, D. W. Nixon, A. Shapiro, M. K. Hoy, M. T. Goodman, A. E. Giuliano, N. Karanja, P. McAndrew, C. Hudis, J. Butler, D. Merkel, A. Kristal, B. Caan, R. Michaelson, V. Vinciguerra, S. Del Prete, M. Winkler, R. Hall, M. Simon, B. L. Winters, and R. M. Elashoff. 2006. "Dietary fat reduction and breast cancer outcome: Interim efficacy results from the women's intervention nutrition study." *Journal of the National Cancer Institute* 98 (24):1767–1776. doi: 10.1093/jnci/djj494.

Clark, J. E. 2016. "The impact of duration on effectiveness of exercise, the implication for periodization of training and goal setting for individuals who are overfat, a meta-analysis." *Biology of Sport* 33 (4):309–333. doi: 10.5604/20831862.1212974.

Clifton, P. M., J. B. Keogh, P. R. Foster, and M. Noakes. 2005. "Effect of weight loss on inflammatory and endothelial markers and FMD using two low-fat diets." *International Journal of Obesity* 29 (12):1445–1451. doi: 10.1038/sj.ijo.0803039.

Conway, J. M., L. A. Ingwersen, B. T. Vinyard, and A. J. Moshfegh. 2003. "Effectiveness of the US department of agriculture 5-step multiple-pass method in assessing food intake in obese and nonobese women." *American Journal of Clinical Nutrition* 77 (5):1171–1178.

Cormie, P., E. M. Zopf, X. C. Zhang, and K. H. Schmitz. 2017. "The impact of exercise on cancer mortality, recurrence, and treatment-related adverse effects." *Epidemiologic Reviews* 39 (1):71–92. doi: 10.1093/epirev/mxx007.

Correa, T. A. F., and M. M. Rogero. 2019. "Polyphenols regulating microRNAs and inflammation biomarkers in obesity." *Nutrition* 59:150–157 doi: 10.1016/j.nut.2018.08.010.

Costa, C. S., F. Rauber, P. S. Leffa, C. N. Sangalli, P. D. B. Campagnolo, and M. R. Vitolo. 2019. "Ultra-processed food consumption and its effects on anthropometric and glucose profile: A longitudinal study during childhood." *Nutrition Metabolism and Cardiovascular Diseases* 29 (2):177–184. doi: 10.1016/j.numecd.2018.11.003.

Crowder, S. L., K. G. Douglas, A. D. Fruge, W. R. Carroll, S. A. Spencer, J. L. Locher, W. Demark-Wahnefried, L. Q. Rogers, and A. E. Arthur. 2019. "Head and neck cancer survivors' preferences for and evaluations of a post-treatment dietary intervention." *Nutrition Journal* 18 (1):8. doi: 10.1186/s12937-019-0479-6.

Cuthbertson, C. C., E. E. Pearce, C. G. Valle, and K. R. Evenson. 2020. "Cardiac rehabilitation programs for cancer survivors: A scoping review." *Current Epidemiology Reports*:15, in press. doi: 10.1007/s40471-020-00235-4.

Dallongeville, J., N. Marecaux, J. C. Fruchart, and P. Amouyel. 1998. "Cigarette smoking is associated with unhealthy patterns of nutrient intake: A meta-analysis." *Journal of Nutrition* 128 (9):1450–1457.

de Mello, A. V., J. L. Pereira, A. C. B. Leme, M. Goldbaum, C. L. G. Cesar, and R. M. Fisberg. 2020. "Social determinants, lifestyle and diet quality: A population-based study from the 2015 Health Survey of Sao Paulo, Brazil." *Public Health Nutrition* 23 (10):1766–1777. doi: 10.1017/s1368980019003483.

de Menezes, M. C., C. K. Duarte, D. V. D. Costa, M. S. Lopes, P. P. de Freitas, S. F. Campos, and A. C. S. Lopes. 2020. "A systematic review of effects, potentialities, and limitations of nutritional interventions aimed at managing obesity in primary and secondary health care." *Nutrition* 75–76:13. doi: 10.1016/j.nut.2020.110784.

de Vet, E., J. De Nooijer, N. K. De Vries, and J. Brug. 2005. "Stages of change in fruit intake: A longitudinal examination of stability, stage transitions and transition profiles." *Psychology & Health* 20 (4):415–428.

Deci, E. L., and R. M. Ryan. 2008. "Self-determination theory: A macrotheory of human motivation, development, and health." *Canadian Psychology-Psychologie Canadienne* 49 (3):182–185. doi: 10.1037/a0012801.

Demark-Wahnefried, W., N. M. Aziz, J. H. Rowland, and B. M. Pinto. 2005. "Riding the crest of the teachable moment: Promoting long-term health after the diagnosis of cancer." *Journal of Clinical Oncology* 23 (24):5814–5830. doi: 10.1200/jco.2005.01.230.

Demark-Wahnefried, W., L. Q. Rogers, J. T. Gibson, S. Harada, A. D. Frug, R. A. Oster, W. E. Grizzle, L. A. Norian, E. S. Yang, D. Della Manna, L. W. Jones, M. Azrad, and H. Krontiras. 2020. "Randomized trial of weight loss in primary breast cancer: Impact on body composition, circulating biomarkers and tumor characteristics." *International Journal of Cancer* 146 (10):2784–2796. doi: 10.1002/ijc.32637.

Dohnke, B., A. Steinhilber, and T. Fuchs. 2015. "Adolescents' eating behaviour in general and in the peer context: Testing the prototype-willingness model." *Psychology & Health* 30 (4):381–399. doi: 10.1080/08870446.2014.974604.

Dowsett, M., J. F. Forbes, R. Bradley, J. Ingle, T. Aihara, J. Bliss, F. Boccardo, A. Coates, R. C. Coombes, J. Cuzick, P. Dubsky, M. Gnant, M. Kaufmann, L. Kilburn, F. Perrone, D. Rea, B. Thurlimann, C. van de Velde, H. Pan, R. Peto, C. Davies, R. Gray, M. Baum, A. Buzdar, J. Cuzick, M. Dowsett, J. F. Forbes, I. Sestak, C. Markopoulos, P. Dubsky, C. Fesl, M. Gnant, R. Jakesz, A. Coates, M. Colleoni, J. F. Forbes, R. Gelber, M. Regan, M. Kaufmann, G. von Minckwitz, J. Bliss, A. Coates, R. C. Coombes, J. F. Forbes, L. Kilburn, C. Snowdon, F. Boccardo, F. Perrone, P. Goss, J. Ingle, K. Pritchard, S. Anderson, J. Costantino, E. Mamounas, T. Aihara, Y. Ohashi, T. Watanabe, E. Bastiaannet, C. van de Velde, D. Rea, and Trialists Early Breast Canc. 2015. "Aromatase inhibitors versus tamoxifen in early breast cancer: Patient-level meta-analysis of the randomised trials." *Lancet* 386 (10001):1341–1352. doi: 10.1016/s0140-6736(15)61074-1.

Ello-Martin, J., L. Roe, and B. Rolls. 2004. "A diet reduced in energy density results in greater weight loss than a diet reduced in fat." *Obesity Research* 12:A23.

Ely, E. K., S. M. Gruss, E. T. Luman, E. W. Gregg, M. K. Ali, K. Nhim, D. B. Rolka, and A. L. Albright. 2017. "A national effort to prevent type 2 diabetes: Participant-level evaluation of CDC's national diabetes prevention program." *Diabetes Care* 40 (10):1331–1341. doi: 10.2337/dc16-2099.

Emmons, K. M., B. H. Marcus, L. Linnan, J. S. Rossi, and D. B. Abrams. 1994. "Mechanisms in multiple risk factor interventions-smoking, physical activity, and dietary fat intake among manufacturing workers." *Preventive Medicine* 23 (4):481–489. doi: 10.1006/pmed.1994.1066.

Enstrom, J. E. 1978. "Cancer and total mortality among active Mormons." *Cancer* 42 (4):1943–1951. doi: 10.1002/1097-0142(197810)42:4<1943::aid-cncr2820420437>3.0.co;2-l.

Ewart, C. K. 1991. "Social action theory for a public health psychology." *American Psychologist* 46 (9):931–946. doi: 10.1037//0003-066x.46.9.931.

Fernandez-Villa, T., L. Alvarez-Alvarez, M. Rubin-Garcia, M. Obon-Santacana, and V. Moreno. 2020. "The role of dietary patterns in colorectal cancer: A 2019 update." *Expert Review of Gastroenterology & Hepatology* 14 (4):281–290. doi: 10.1080/17474124.2020.1736043.

Fiatarone, M. A., E. F. Oneill, N. D. Ryan, K. M. Clements, G. R. Solares, M. E. Nelson, S. B. Roberts, J. J. Kehayias, L. A. Lipsitz, and W. J. Evans. 1994. "Exercise training and nutritional supplementation for physical frailty in very elderly people." *New England Journal of Medicine* 330 (25):1769–1775.

Fiolet, T., B. Srour, L. Sellem, E. Kesse-Guyo, B. Alles, C. Mejean, M. Deschasaux, P. Fassier, P. Latino-Martel, M. Beslay, S. Hercberg, C. Lavalette, C. A. Monteiro, C. Julia, and M. Touvier. 2018. "Consumption of ultra-processed foods and cancer risk: Results from NutriNet-Sante prospective cohort." *BMJ-British Medical Journal* 360:11. doi: 10.1136/bmj.k322.

Flint, A., A. Raben, A. Astrup, and J. J. Holst. 1998. "Glucagon-like peptide 1 promotes satiety and suppresses energy intake in humans." *Journal of Clinical Investigation* 101 (3):515–520. doi: 10.1172/jci990.

Forbes, C. C., F. Swan, S. L. Greenley, M. Lind, and M. J. Johnson. 2020. "Physical activity and nutrition interventions for older adults with cancer: A systematic review." *Journal of Cancer Survivorship*:23, in press. doi: 10.1007/s11764-020-00883-x.

Fox, L., T. Wiseman, D. Cahill, K. Beyer, N. Peat, E. Rammant, and M. Van Hemelrijck. 2020. "Barriers and facilitators to physical activity in men with prostate cancer: A qualitative and quantitative systematic review." *Psycho-Oncology*:16, in press. doi: 10.1002/pon.5240.

Frensham, L. J., D. M. Zarnowiecki, G. Parfitt, R. M. Stanley, and J. Dollman. 2014. "Steps toward improving diet and exercise for cancer survivors (STRIDE): A quasi-randomised controlled trial protocol." *BMC Cancer* 14:7. doi: 10.1186/1471-2407-14-428.

Friedenreich, C. M., C. R. Stone, W. Y. Cheung, and S. C. Hayes. 2020. "Physical activity and mortality in cancer survivors: A systematic review and meta-analysis." *JNCI Cancer Spectrum* 4 (1):pkz080. doi: 10.1093/jncics/pkz080.

Frye, R. E., B. S. Schwartz, and R. L. Doty. 1990. "Dose-related effects of cigarette smoking on olfactory function." *JAMA-Journal of the American Medical Association* 263 (9):1233–1236. doi: 10.1001/jama.263.9.1233.

Gianfredi, V., D. Nucci, M. Balzarini, M. Acito, M. Moretti, A. Villarini, and M. Villarini. 2020. "E-coaching: The DianaWeb study to prevent breast cancer recurrences." *Clinica Terapeutica* 171 (1):E59–E65. doi: 10.7417/ct.2020.2190.

Gillis, C., K. Buhler, L. Bresee, F. Carli, L. Gramlich, N. Culos-Reed, T. T. Sajobi, and T. R. Fenton. 2018. "Effects of nutritional prehabilitation, with and without exercise, on outcomes of patients who undergo colorectal surgery: A systematic review and meta-analysis." *Gastroenterology* 155 (2):391–410. doi: 10.1053/j.gastro.2018.05.012.

Gimeno, R. E., D. A. Briere, and R. J. Seeley. 2020. "Leveraging the gut to treat metabolic disease." *Cell Metabolism* 31 (4):679–698. doi: 10.1016/j.cmet.2020.02.014.

Glennon, S. G., T. Huedo-Medina, S. Rawal, H. J. Hoffman, M. D. Litt, and V. B. Duffy. 2019. "Chronic cigarette smoking associates directly and indirectly with self-reported olfactory alterations: Analysis of the 2011–2014 National Health and Nutrition Examination survey." *Nicotine & Tobacco Research* 21 (6):818–827. doi: 10.1093/ntr/ntx242.

Goodwin, P. J., M. Ennis, K. I. Pritchard, M. E. Trudeau, J. Koo, Y. Madarnas, W. Hartwick, B. Hoffman, and N. Hood. 2002. "Fasting insulin and outcome in early-stage breast cancer: Results of a prospective cohort study." *Journal of Clinical Oncology* 20 (1):42–51. doi: 10.1200/jco.20.1.42.

Gorin, A. A., S. Phelan, H. Raynor, and R. R. Wing. 2011. "Home food and exercise environments of normal-weight and overweight adults." *American Journal of Health Behavior* 35 (5):618–626.

Gorin, A. A., H. A. Raynor, J. Fava, K. Maguire, E. Robichaud, J. Trautvetter, M. Crane, and R. R. Wing. 2013. "Randomized controlled trial of a comprehensive home environment-focused weight-loss program for adults." *Health Psychology* 32 (2):128–137. doi: 10.1037/a0026959.

Greenlee, H. A., K. D. Crew, J. M. Mata, P. S. McKinley, A. G. Rundle, W. F. Zhang, Y. Y. Liao, W. Y. Tsai, and D. L. Hershman. 2013. "A pilot randomized controlled trial of a commercial diet and exercise weight loss program in minority breast cancer survivors." *Obesity* 21 (1):65–76. doi: 10.1002/oby.20245.

Grimmett, C., T. Corbett, J. Brunet, J. Shepherd, B. M. Pinto, C. R. May, and C. Foster. 2019. "Systematic review and meta-analysis of maintenance of physical activity behaviour change in cancer survivors." *International Journal of Behavioral Nutrition and Physical Activity* 16:20. doi: 10.1186/s12966-019-0787-4.

Gubert, C., G. Kong, T. Renoir, and A. J. Hannan. 2020. "Exercise, diet and stress as modulators of gut microbiota: Implications for neurodegenerative diseases." *Neurobiology of Disease* 134:16. doi: 10.1016/j.nbd.2019.104621.

Guinter, M. A., M. L. McCullough, S. M. Gapstur, and P. T. Campbell. 2018. "Associations of pre- and post-diagnosis diet quality with risk of mortality among men and women with colorectal cancer." *Journal of Clinical Oncology* 36 (34):3404. doi: 10.1200/jco.18.00714.

Haibach, J. P., G. G. Homish, and G. A. Giovino. 2013. "A longitudinal evaluation of fruit and vegetable consumption and cigarette smoking." *Nicotine & Tobacco Research* 15 (2):355–363. doi: 10.1093/ntr/nts130.

Haibach, J. P., G. G. Homish, R. L. Collins, C. B. Ambrosone, and G. A. Giovino. 2015. "An evaluation of fruit and vegetable consumption and cigarette smoking among youth." *Nicotine & Tobacco Research* 17 (6):719–726. doi: 10.1093/ntr/ntu215.

Hall, K. D., and S. Kahan. 2018. "Maintenance of lost weight and long-term management of obesity." *Medical Clinics of North America* 102 (1):183–197. doi: 10.1016/j.mcna.2017.08.012.

Hall, K. D., A. Ayuketah, R. Brychta, H. Y. Cai, T. Cassimatis, K. Y. Chen, S. T. Chung, E. Costa, A. Courville, V. Darcey, L. A. Fletcher, C. G. Forde, A. M. Gharib, J. Guo, R. Howard, P. V. Joseph, S. McGehee, R. Ouwerkerk, K. Raisinger, I. Rozga, M. Stagliano, M. Walter, P. J. Walter, S. Yang, and M. G. Zhou. 2019. "Ultra-processed diets cause excess calorie intake and weight gain: An inpatient randomized controlled trial of Ad libitum food intake." *Cell Metabolism* 30 (1):67–77. doi: 10.1016/j.cmet.2019.05.008.

Hays, J. T., T. D. Wolter, K. M. Eberman, I. T. Croghan, K. P. Offord, and R. D. Hurt. 2001. "Residential (inpatient) treatment compared with outpatient treatment for nicotine dependence." *Mayo Clinic Proceedings* 76 (2):124–133.

Heinonen, O. P., J. K. Huttunen, D. Albanes, J. Haapakoski, J. Palmgren, P. Pietinen, J. Pikkarainen, M. Rautalahti, J. Virtamo, B. K. Edwards, P. Greenwald, A. M. Hartman, P. R. Taylor, J. Haukka, P. Jarvinen, N. Malila, S. Rapola, P. Jokinen, J. Karjalainen, J. Lauronen, J. Mutikainen, M. Sarjakoski, A. Suorsa, M. Tiainen, M. Verkasalo, M. Barrett, G. Alfthan, C. Ehnholm, C. G. Gref, J. Sundvall, E. Haapa, M. L. Ovaskainen, M. Palvaalhola, E. Roos, E. Pukkala, L. Teppo, H. Frick, A. Pasternack, B. W. Brown, D. L. Demets, K. Kokkola, E. Tala, E. Aalto, V. Maenpaa, L. Tienhaara, M. Jarvinen, I. Kuuliala, L. Linko, E. Mikkola, J. Nyrhinen, A. Ronkanen, A. Vuorela, S. Koskinen, P. Lohela, T. Viljanen, K. Godenhjelm, T. Kallio, M. Kaskinen, M. Havu, P. Kirves, K. Taubert, H. Alkio, R. Koskinen, K. Laine, K. Makitalo, S. Rastas, P. Tani, M. Niemisto, T. L. Sellergren, C. Aikas, P. S. Pekkanen, R. Tarvala, K. Alanko, K. Makipaja, S. Vaara, H. Siuko, V. Tuominen, L. Alaketola, A. Haapanen, M. Haveri, L. Keskinisula, E. Kokko, M. Koskenkari, P. Linden, A. Nurmenniemi, R. Raninen, T. Raudaskoski, S. K. Toivakka, H. Vierola, S. Kyronpalokauppinen, E. Schoultz, M. Jaakkola, E. Lehtinen, K. Rautaseppa, M. Saarikoski, K. Liippo, K. Reunanen, E. R. Salomaa, D. Ettinger, P. Hietanen, H. Maenpaa, L. Teerenhovi, G. Prout, E. Taskinen, F. Askin, Y. Erozan, S. Nordling, M. Virolainen, L. Koss, P. Sipponen, K. Lewin, K. Franssila, P. Karkkainen, M. Heinonen, L. Hyvonen, P. Koivistoinen, V. Ollilainen, V. Piironen, P. Varo, W. Bilhuber, R. Salkeld, W. Schalch, and R. Speiser. 1994. "Effect of vitamin E and beta carotene on the incidence of lung cancer and other cancers in male smokers." *New England Journal of Medicine* 330 (15):1029–1035.

Hennekens, C. H., J. E. Buring, J. E. Manson, M. Stampfer, B. Rosner, N. R. Cook, C. Belanger, F. LaMotte, J. M. Gaziano, P. M. Ridker, W. Willett, and R. Peto. 1996. "Lack of effect of long-term supplementation with beta carotene on the incidence of malignant neoplasms and cardiovascular disease." *New England Journal of Medicine* 334 (18):1145–1149. doi: 10.1056/nejm199605023341801.

Hodgkin, J. E., D. P. L. Sachs, G. E. Swan, L. M. Jack, B. L. Titus, S. J. S. Waldron, B. L. Sachs, and J. Brigham. 2013. "Outcomes from a patient-centered residential treatment plan for tobacco dependence." *Mayo Clinic Proceedings* 88 (9):970–976. doi: 10.1016/j.mayocp.2013.05.027.

Howard, B. V., J. E. Manson, M. L. Stefanick, S. A. Beresford, G. Frank, B. T. Jones, R. J. Rodabough, L. Snetselaar, C. Thomson, L. Tinker, M. Vitolins, and R. Prentice. 2006. "Low-fat dietary pattern and weight change over 7 years: The women's health initiative dietary modification trial." *JAMA-Journal of the American Medical Association* 295 (1):39–49. doi: 10.1001/jama.295.1.39.

Hutchison, A. J., J. D. Breckon, and L. H. Johnston. 2009. "Physical activity behavior change interventions based on the transtheoretical model: A systematic review." *Health Education & Behavior* 36 (5):829–845. doi: 10.1177/1090198108318491.

Hyatt, A., K. Gough, A. Murnane, G. Au-Yeung, T. Dawson, E. Pearson, H. Dhillon, S. Sandhu, N. Williams, E. Paton, A. Billett, A. Traill, H. Andersen, V. Beedle, and D. Milne. 2020. "i-Move, a personalised exercise intervention for patients with advanced melanoma receiving immunotherapy: A randomised feasibility trial protocol." *BMJ Open* 10 (2):9. doi: 10.1136/bmjopen-2019-036059.

Hyman, D. J., V. N. Pavlik, W. C. Taylor, K. Goodrick, and L. Moye. 2007. "Simultaneous vs sequential counseling for multiple behavior change." *Archives of Internal Medicine* 167 (11):1152–1158.

Jacobs, D. R., and L. C. Tapsell. 2007. "Food, not nutrients, is the fundamental unit in nutrition." *Nutrition Reviews* 65 (10):439–450. doi: 10.1301/nr.2007.oct.439-450.

Johns, D. J., J. Hartmann-Boyce, S. A. Jebb, P. Aveyard, and Group Behavioural Weight Management Review. 2014. "Diet or exercise interventions vs combined behavioral weight management programs: A systematic review and meta-analysis of direct comparisons." *Journal of the Academy of Nutrition and Dietetics* 114 (10):1557–1568. doi: 10.1016/j.jand.2014.07.005.

Juul, F., E. Martinez-Steele, N. Parekh, C. A. Monteiro, and V. W. Chang. 2018. "Ultra-processed food consumption and excess weight among US adults." *British Journal of Nutrition* 120 (1):90–100. doi: 10.1017/s0007114518001046.

Kearney, J. M., C. de Graaf, S. Damkjaer, and L. M. Engstrom. 1999. "Stages of change towards physical activity in a nationally representative sample in the European Union." *Public Health Nutrition* 2 (1A):115–124. doi: 10.1017/s1368980099000166.

Kelly, M. C., G. C. Rae, D. Walker, S. Partington, C. J. Dodd-Reynolds, and N. Caplan. 2017. "Retrospective cohort study of the South Tyneside exercise referral scheme 2009–14: Predictors of dropout and barriers to adherence." *Journal of Public Health* 39 (4):E257–E264. doi: 10.1093/pubmed/fdw122.

Kennedy, M. A., S. Bayes, D. A. Galvao, F. Singh, N. A. Spry, M. Davis, R. Chee, Y. Zissiadis, N. H. Hart, D. R. Taaffe, and R. U. Newton. 2020. "If you build it, will they come? Evaluation of a co-located exercise clinic and cancer treatment centre using the RE-AIM framework." *European Journal of Cancer Care*:12, in press. doi: 10.1111/ecc.13251.

Kilgore, E. A., J. Mandel-Ricci, M. Johns, M. H. Coady, S. B. Perl, A. Goodman, and S. M. Kansagra. 2014. "Making it harder to smoke and easier to quit: The effect of 10 years of tobacco control in New York City." *American Journal of Public Health* 104 (6):E5–E8. doi: 10.2105/ajph.2014.301940.

Klem, M. L., R. R. Wing, C. C. H. Chang, W. Lang, M. T. McGuire, H. J. Sugerman, S. L. Hutchison, A. L. Makovich, and J. O. Hill. 2000. "A case-control study of successful maintenance of a substantial weight loss: Individuals who lost weight through surgery versus those who lost weight through non-surgical means." *International Journal of Obesity* 24 (5):573–579.

Kristensen, M. B., I. Wessel, A. M. Beck, K. B. Dieperink, T. B. Mikkelsen, J. J. K. Moller, and A. D. Zwisler. 2020. "Rationale and design of a randomised controlled trial investigating the effect of multidisciplinary nutritional rehabilitation for patients treated for head and neck cancer (the NUTRI-HAB trial)." *Nutrition Journal* 19 (1):15. doi: 10.1186/s12937-020-00539-7.

Kubena, K. S., and D. N. McMurray. 1996. "Nutrition and the immune system: A review of nutrient-nutrient interactions." *Journal of the American Dietetic Association* 96 (11):1156–1164. doi: 10.1016/s0002-8223(96)00297-0.

Kushi, L. H., C. Doyle, M. McCullough, C. L. Rock, W. Demark-Wahnefried, E. V. Bandera, S. Gapstur, A. V. Patel, K. Andrews, T. Gansler, and The ACS 2010 Nutrition and Physical Activity Guidelines Advisory Committee. 2012. "American cancer society guidelines on nutrition and physical activity for cancer prevention." *CA: A Cancer Journal for Clinicians* 62:30–67.

L'Hotta, A. J., T. E. Varughese, K. D. Lyons, L. Simon, and A. A. King. 2020. "Assessments used to measure participation in life activities in individuals with cancer: A scoping review." *Supportive Care in Cancer*:12, in press. doi: 10.1007/s00520-020-05441-w.

Lahart, I. M., G. S. Metsios, A. M. Nevill, and A. R. Carmichael. 2018. "Physical activity for women with breast cancer after adjuvant therapy." *Cochrane Database of Systematic Reviews* (1):937. doi: 10.1002/14651858.CD011292.pub2.

Larson, N. I., M. Story, C. L. Perry, D. Neumark-Sztainer, and P. J. Hannan. 2007. "Are diet and physical activity patterns related to cigarette smoking in adolescents? Findings from project EAT." *Preventing Chronic Disease* 4 (3):A51.

Laviano, A., P. C. Calder, Amwj Schols, F. Lonnqvist, M. Bech, and M. Muscaritoli. 2020. "Safety and tolerability of targeted medical nutrition for cachexia in non-small-cell lung cancer: A randomized, double-blind, controlled pilot trial." *Nutrition and Cancer: An International Journal* 72 (3):12. doi: 10.1080/01635581.2019.1634746.

Ledikwe, J. H., B. J. Rolls, H. Smiciklas-Wright, D. C. Mitchell, J. D. Ard, C. Champagne, N. Karanja, P. H. Lin, V. J. Stevens, and L. J. Appel. 2007. "Reductions in dietary energy density are associated with weight loss in overweight and obese participants in the PREMIER trial." *American Journal of Clinical Nutrition* 85 (5):1212–1221.

Lee, S. H., Y. Yun, S. J. Kim, E. J. Lee, Y. Chang, S. Ryu, H. Shin, H. L. Kim, H. N. Kim, and J. H. Lee. 2018. "Association between cigarette smoking status and composition of gut microbiota: Population-based cross-sectional study." *Journal of Clinical Medicine* 7 (9):13. doi: 10.3390/jcm7090282.

Lin, H. Y., P. Fisher, D. Harris, and T. S. Tseng. 2019. "Alcohol intake patterns for cancer and non-cancer individuals: A population study." *Translational Cancer Research* 8:S334–S345. doi: 10.21037/tcr.2019.06.31.

Lounassalo, I., M. Hirvensalo, A. Kankaanpaa, A. Tolvanen, S. Palomaki, K. Salin, M. Fogelholm, X. L. Yang, K. Pahkala, S. Rovio, N. Hutri-Kahonen, O. Raitakari, and T. H. Tammelin. 2019. "Associations of leisure-time physical activity trajectories with fruit and vegetable consumption from childhood to adulthood: The cardiovascular risk in young finns study." *International Journal of Environmental Research and Public Health* 16 (22):17. doi: 10.3390/ijerph16224437.

Lynch, B. M., N. H. Nguyen, M. M. Moore, M. M. Reeves, D. E. Rosenberg, T. Boyle, J. K. Vallance, S. Milton, C. M. Friedenreich, and D. R. English. 2019. "A randomized controlled trial of a wearable technology-based intervention for increasing moderate to vigorous physical activity and reducing sedentary behavior in breast cancer survivors: The ACTIVATE trial." *Cancer* 125 (16):2846–2855. doi: 10.1002/cncr.32143.

Marcus, B. H., A. E. Albrecht, T. K. King, A. F. Parisi, B. M. Pinto, M. Roberts, R. S. Niaura, and D. B. Abrams. 1999. "The efficacy of exercise as an aid for smoking cessation in women: A randomized controlled trial." *Archives of Internal Medicine* 159 (11):1229–1234. doi: 10.1001/archinte.159.11.1229.

Maugeri, A., M. Barchitta, V. Fiore, G. Rosta, G. Favara, C. La Mastra, M. C. La Rosa, R. M. San Lio, and A. Agodi. 2019. "Determinants of adherence to the mediterranean diet: Findings from a cross-sectional study in women from southern Italy." *International Journal of Environmental Research and Public Health* 16 (16):14. doi: 10.3390/ijerph16162963.

McGettigan, M., C. R. Cardwell, M. M. Cantwell, and M. A. Tully. 2020. "Physical activity interventions for disease-related physical and mental health during and following treatment in people with non-advanced colorectal cancer." *Cochrane Database of Systematic Reviews* (5):133. doi: 10.1002/14651858. CD012864.pub2.

McNabney, S. M., and T. M. Henagan. 2017. "Short chain fatty acids in the colon and peripheral tissues: A focus on butyrate, colon cancer, obesity and insulin resistance." *Nutrients* 9 (12):28. doi: 10.3390/nu9121348.

Meneses-Echavez, J. F., A. F. Loaiza-Betancur, V. Diaz-Lopez, and A. M. Echavarria-Rodriguez. 2020. "Prehabilitation programs for cancer patients: A systematic review of randomized controlled trials (protocol)." *Systematic Reviews* 9 (1):5. doi: 10.1186/s13643-020-1282-3.

Michie, S., M. Richardson, M. Johnston, C. Abraham, J. Francis, W. Hardeman, M. P. Eccles, J. Cane, and C. E. Wood. 2013. "The behavior change technique taxonomy (v1) of 93 hierarchically clustered techniques: Building an international consensus for the reporting of behavior change interventions." *Annals of Behavioral Medicine* 46 (1):81–95. doi: 10.1007/s12160-013-9486-6.

Miller, W., and S. Rollnick. 2013. *Motivational Interviewing: Preparing People for Change*, 3rd Edition. New York: Guilford Press.

Miller, K. D., L. Nogueira, A. B. Mariotto, J. H. Rowland, K. R. Yabroff, C. M. Alfano, A. Jemal, J. L. Kramer, and R. L. Siegel. 2019. "Cancer treatment and survivorship statistics, 2019." *CA: A Cancer Journal for Clinicians* 69 (5):363–385. doi: 10.3322/caac.21565.

Milne, H. M., K. E. Wallman, A. Guilfoyle, S. Gordon, and K. S. Courneya. 2008. "Self-determination theory and physical activity among breast cancer survivors." *Journal of Sport & Exercise Psychology* 30 (1):23–38. doi: 10.1123/jsep.30.1.23.

Monteiro, C. A., J.-C. Moubarac, R. B. Levy, D. S. Canella, M. L. da Costa Louzada, and G. Cannon. 2018. "Household availability of ultra-processed foods and obesity in nineteen European countries." *Public Health Nutrition* 21 (1):18–26. doi: 10.1017/s1368980017001379.

Monteiro, C. A., G. Cannon, R. B. Levy, J. C. Moubarac, M. L. C. Louzada, F. Rauber, N. Khandpur, G. Cediel, D. Neri, E. Martinez-Steele, L. G. Baraldi, and P. C. Jaime. 2019. "Ultra-processed foods: What they are and how to identify them." *Public Health Nutrition* 22 (5):936–941. doi: 10.1017/s1368980018003762.

Moran, J., E. Guinan, P. McCormick, J. Larkin, D. Mockler, J. Hussey, J. Moriarty, and F. Wilson. 2016. "The ability of prehabilitation to influence postoperative outcome after intra-abdominal operation: A systematic review and meta-analysis." *Surgery* 160 (5):1189–1201. doi: 10.1016/j.surg.2016.05.014.

Nadler, M., D. Bainbridge, J. Tomasone, O. Cheifetz, R. A. Juergens, and J. Sussman. 2017. "Oncology care provider perspectives on exercise promotion in people with cancer: An examination of knowledge, practices, barriers, and facilitators." *Supportive Care in Cancer* 25 (7):2297–2304. doi: 10.1007/s00520-017-3640-9.

Naito, T. 2019. "Emerging treatment options for cancer-associated cachexia: A literature review." *Therapeutics and Clinical Risk Management* 15:1253–1266. doi: 10.2147/tcrm.s196802.

National Cancer Institute (NCI). 2005. *Theory at a Glance*, 2nd Edition. National Cancer Institute. http://www.cancer.gov/cancertopics/cancerlibrary/theory.pdf (accessed May 11, 2014).

National Comprehensive Cancer Network. 2020. *Nutrition for Cancer Survivors*. National Comprehensive Cancer Network. https://www.nccn.org/patients/resources/life_after_cancer/nutrition.aspx (accessed June 15, 2020).

O'Keefe, S. J. 2019. "The association between dietary fibre deficiency and high-income lifestyle-associated diseases: Burkitt's hypothesis revisited." *Lancet Gastroenterology & Hepatology* 4 (12):984–996. doi: 10.1016/s2468-1253(19)30257-2.

O'Keefe, S. J., J. V. Li, L. Lahti, J. Ou, F. Carbonero, K. Mohammed, J. M. Posma, J. Kinross, E. Wahl, E. Ruder, K. I. Vipperla, V. Naidoo, L. Mtshali, S. Tims, P. G. B. Puylaert, J. P. DeLany, A. Krasinskas, A. C. Benefiel, H. O. Kaseb, K. Newton, J. K. Nicholson, and W. M. de Vos. 2015. "Fat, fibre and cancer risk in African Americans and rural Africans." *Nature Communications* 6:6342.

Oettle, G. J. 1991. "Effect of moderate exercise on bowel habit." *Gut* 32 (8):941–944. doi: 10.1136/gut.32.8.941.

Ohri-Vachaspati, P., D. Delia, R. S. DeWeese, N. C. Crespo, M. Todd, and M. J. Yedidia. 2015. "The relative contribution of layers of the social ecological model to childhood obesity." *Public Health Nutrition* 18 (11):2055–2066. doi: 10.1017/s1368980014002365.

Omenn, G. S., G. E. Goodman, M. D. Thornquist, J. Balmes, M. R. Cullen, A. Glass, J. P. Keogh, F. L. Meyskens, B. Valanis, J. H. Williams, S. Barnhart, and S. Hammar. 1996. "Effects of a combination of beta carotene and vitamin A on lung cancer and cardiovascular disease." *New England Journal of Medicine* 334 (18):1150–1155. doi: 10.1056/nejm199605023341802.

Osler, M., A. Tjonneland, M. Suntum, B. L. Thomsen, C. Stripp, M. Gronbaek, and K. Overvad. 2002. "Does the association between smoking status and selected healthy foods depend on gender? A population-based study of 54 417 middle-aged Danes." *European Journal of Clinical Nutrition* 56 (1):57–63. doi: 10.1038/sj.ejcn.1601280.

Palaniappan, U., L. J. Starkey, J. O'Loughlin, and K. Gray-Donald. 2001. "Fruit and vegetable consumption is lower and saturated fat intake is higher among Canadians reporting smoking." *Journal of Nutrition* 131 (7):1952–1958.

Parks, C. A., C. Blaser, T. M. Smith, E. E. Calloway, A. Y. Oh, L. A. Dwyer, B. M. Liu, L. C. Nebeling, and A. L. Yaroch. 2018. "Correlates of fruit and vegetable intake among parents and adolescents: Findings from the Family Life, Activity, Sun, Health, and Eating (FLASHE) study." *Public Health Nutrition* 21 (11):2079–2087. doi: 10.1017/s1368980018000770.

Parra, M. T., N. Esmeaeli, J. Kohn, B. L. Henry, S. Klagholz, S. Jain, C. Pruitt, D. Vicario, W. Jonas, and P. J. Mills. 2020. "Greater well-being in more physically active cancer patients who are enrolled in supportive care services." *Integrative Cancer Therapies* 19:17. doi: 10.1177/1534735420921439.

Passe, D. H., M. Horn, and R. Murray. 2000. "Impact of beverage acceptability on fluid intake during exercise." *Appetite* 35 (3):219–229.

Patel, A. V., C. M. Friedenreich, S. C. Moore, S. C. Hayes, J. K. Silver, K. L. Campbell, K. Winters-Stone, L. H. Gerber, S. M. George, J. E. Fulton, C. Denlinger, G. S. Morris, T. Hue, K. H. Schmitz, and C. E. Matthews. 2019. "American college of sports medicine roundtable report on physical activity, sedentary behavior, and cancer prevention and control." *Medicine and Science in Sports and Exercise* 51 (11):2391–2402. doi: 10.1249/mss.0000000000002117.

Peddle-McIntyre, C. J., F. Singh, R. Thomas, R. U. Newton, D. A. Galvao, and V. Cavalheri. 2019. "Exercise training for advanced lung cancer." *Cochrane Database of Systematic Reviews* (2):59. doi: 10.1002/14651858.CD012685.pub2.

Piazzi, G., A. Prossomariti, M. Baldassarre, C. Montagna, P. Vitaglione, V. Fogliano, E. Biagi, M. Candela, P. Brigidi, T. Balbi, A. Munarini, A. Belluzzi, M. Pariali, F. Bazzoli, and L. Ricciardiello. 2019. "A mediterranean diet mix has chemopreventive effects in a murine model of colorectal cancer modulating apoptosis and the gut microbiota." *Frontiers in Oncology* 9:11. doi: 10.3389/fonc.2019.00140.

Pierce, J. P., V. A. Newman, S. W. Flatt, S. Faerber, C. L. Rock, L. Natarajan, B. J. Caan, E. B. Gold, K. A. Hollenbach, L. Wasserman, L. Jones, C. Ritenbaugh, M. L. Stefanick, C. A. Thomson, S. Kealey, and Whel Study Group. 2004. "Telephone counseling intervention increases intakes of micronutrient-and phytochemical-rich vegetables, fruit and fiber in breast cancer survivors." *Journal of Nutrition* 134 (2):452–458.

Pierce, J. P., L. Natarajan, B. J. Caan, B. A. Parker, E. R. Greenberg, S. W. Flatt, C. L. Rock, S. Kealey, W. K. Al-Delaimy, W. A. Bardwell, R. W. Carlson, J. A. Emond, S. Faerber, E. B. Gold, R. A. Hajek, K. Hollenbach, L. A. Jones, N. Karanja, L. Madlensky, J. Marshall, V. A. Newman, C. Ritenbaugh, C. A. Thomson, L. Wasserman, and M. L. Stefanick. 2007. "Influence of a diet very high in vegetables, fruit, and fiber and low in fat on prognosis following treatment for breast cancer: The Women's Healthy Eating and Living (WHEL) randomized trial." *JAMA-Journal of the American Medical Association* 298 (3):289–298. doi: 10.1001/jama.298.3.289.

Pinto, B. M., and A. Floyd. 2008. "Theories underlying health promotion interventions among cancer survivors." *Seminars in Oncology Nursing* 24 (3):153–163. doi: 10.1016/j.soncn.2008.05.003.

Pinto, B. M., G. D. Papandonatos, M. G. Goldstein, B. H. Marcus, and N. Farrell. 2013. "Home-based physical activity intervention for colorectal cancer survivors." *Psycho-Oncology* 22 (1):54–64. doi: 10.1002/pon.2047.

Poisson, T., J. Dallongeville, A. Evans, P. Ducimetierre, P. Amouyel, J. Yarnell, A. Bingham, F. Kee, and L. Dauchet. 2012. "Fruit and vegetable intake and smoking cessation." *European Journal of Clinical Nutrition* 66 (11):1247–1253. doi: 10.1038/ejcn.2012.70.

Pollak, M. N., J. W. Chapman, L. Shepherd, D. Meng, P. Richardson, C. Wilson, B. Orme, and K. I. Pritchard. 2006. "Insulin resistance, estimated by serum C-peptide level, is associated with reduced event-free survival for postmenopausal women in NCICCTG MA.14 adjuvant breast cancer trial." *Journal of Clinical Oncology* 24 (18):9S.

Prochaska, J. O., C. C. Diclemente, and J. C. Norcross. 1992. "In search of how people change: Applications to addictive behaviors." *American Psychologist* 47 (9):1102–1114. doi: 10.1037/0003-066x.47.9.1102.

Proctor, L., J. LoTempio, A. Marquitz, P. Daschner, D. Xi, R. Flores, L. Brown, R. Ranallo, P. Maruvada, K. Regan, R. D. Lunsford, M. Reddy, L. Caler, and NIH Human Microbiome Portfolio Ana. 2019. "A review of 10 years of human microbiome research activities at the US National Institutes of Health, Fiscal Years 2007–2016." *Microbiome* 7:19. doi: 10.1186/s40168-019-0620-y.

Puigpinos-Riera, R., G. Serral, M. Sala, X. Bargallo, M. J. Quintana, M. Espinosa, R. Manzanera, M. Domenech, F. Macia, J. Grau, and E. Vidal. 2020. "Cancer-related fatigue and its determinants in a cohort of women with breast cancer: The DAMA cohort." *Supportive Care in Cancer*:9. doi: 10.1007/s00520-020-05337-9.

Ravasco, P., I. Monteiro-Grillo, and M. Camila. 2012. "Individualized nutrition intervention is of major benefit to colorectal cancer patients: Long-term follow-up of a randomized controlled trial of nutritional therapy." *American Journal of Clinical Nutrition* 96 (6):1346–1353. doi: 10.3945/ajcn.111.018838.

Ravasco, P., I. Monteiro-Grillo, P. M. Vidal, and M. E. Camilo. 2005a. "Dietary counseling improves patient outcomes: A prospective, randomized, controlled trial in colorectal cancer patients undergoing radiotherapy." *Journal of Clinical Oncology* 23 (7):1431–1438. doi: 10.1200/jco.2005.02.054.

Ravasco, P., I. Monteiro-Grillo, P. M. Vidal, and M. E. Camilo. 2005b. "Impact of nutrition on outcome: A prospective randomized controlled trial in patients with head and neck cancer undergoing radiotherapy." *Nutrition and Patient Outcomes* 27 (8):659–668. doi: 10.1002/hed.20221.

Resnicow, K., F. McCarty, and T. Baranowski. 2003. "Are precontemplators less likely to change their dietary behavior? A prospective analysis." *Health Education Research* 18 (6):693–705. doi: 10.1093/her/cyf052.

Rigby, R. R., L. J. Mitchell, K. Hamilton, and L. T. Williams. 2020. "The use of behavior change theories in dietetics practice in primary health care: A systematic review of randomized controlled trials." *Journal of the Academy of Nutrition and Dietetics* 120 (7):1172–1197.

Roberts, A. L., A. Fisher, L. Smith, M. Heinrich, and H. W. W. Potts. 2017a. "Digital health behaviour change interventions targeting physical activity and diet in cancer survivors: A systematic review and meta-analysis." *Journal of Cancer Survivorship* 11 (6):704–719. doi: 10.1007/s11764-017-0632-1.

Roberts, K., K. Rickett, R. Greer, and N. Woodward. 2017b. "Management of aromatase inhibitor induced musculoskeletal symptoms in postmenopausal early Breast cancer: A systematic review and meta-analysis." *Critical Reviews in Oncology Hematology* 111:66–80. doi: 10.1016/j.critrevonc.2017.01.010.

Roberts, K. E., K. Rickett, S. Feng, D. Vagenas, and N. E. Woodward. 2020. "Exercise therapies for preventing or treating aromatase inhibitor-induced musculoskeletal symptoms in early breast cancer." *Cochrane Database of Systematic Reviews* 1:57. doi: 10.1002/14651858.CD012988.pub2.

Robinson, T. N. 1999. "Reducing children's television viewing to prevent obesity: A randomized controlled trial." *JAMA-Journal of the American Medical Association* 282 (16):1561–1567. doi: 10.1001/jama.282.16.1561.

Rock, C. L., C. Doyle, W. Demark-Wahnefried, J. Meyerhardt, K. S. Courneya, A. L. Schwartz, E. V. Bandera, K. K. Hamilton, B. Grant, M. McCullough, T. Byers, and T. Gansler. 2012. "Nutrition and physical activity guidelines for cancer survivors." *CA: A Cancer Journal for Clinicians* 62 (4):243–274. doi: 10.3322/caac.21142.

Rock, C. L., C. Thomson, T. Gansler, S. M. Gapstur, M. L. McCullough, A. V. Patel, K. S. Andrews, E. V. Bandera, C. K. Spees, K. Robien, S. Hartman, K. Sullivan, B. L. Grant, K. K. Hamilton, L. H. Kushi, B. J. Caan, D. Kibbe, J. D. Black, T. L. Wiedt, C. McMahon, K. Sloan, and C. Doyle. 2020. "American Cancer Society guideline for diet and physical activity for cancer prevention." *CA: A Cancer Journal for Clinicians*. doi: 10.3322/caac.21591.

Rosell, M., P. Appleby, E. Spencer, and T. Key. 2006. "Weight gain over 5 years in 21 966 meat-eating, fish-eating, vegetarian, and vegan men and women in EPIC-Oxford." *International Journal of Obesity* 30 (9):1389–1396.

Ross, K. M., P. H. Qiu, L. You, and R. R. Wing. 2019. "Week-to-week predictors of weight loss and regain." *Health Psychology* 38 (12):1150–1158. doi: 10.1037/hea0000798.

Ruiz-Vozmediano, J., S. Lohnchen, L. Jurado, R. Recio, A. Rodriguez-Carrillo, M. Lopez, V. Mustieles, M. Exposito, M. Arroyo-Morales, and M. F. Fernandez. 2020. "Influence of a multidisciplinary program of diet, exercise, and mindfulness on the quality of life of stage IIA-IIB breast cancer survivors." *Integrative Cancer Therapies* 19:11. doi: 10.1177/1534735420924757.

Ryan, R. M., and E. L. Deci. 2000. "Self-determination theory and the facilitation of intrinsic motivation, social development, and well-being." *American Psychologist* 55 (1):68–78. doi: 10.1037//0003-066x.55.1.68.

Savin, Z., S. Kivity, H. Yonath, and S. Yehuda. 2018. "Smoking and the intestinal microbiome." *Archives of Microbiology* 200 (5):677–684. doi: 10.1007/s00203-018-1506-2.

Schlesinger, S., J. Walter, J. Hampe, W. von Schonfels, S. Hinz, T. Kuchler, G. Jacobs, C. Schafmayer, and U. Nothlings. 2014. "Lifestyle factors and health-related quality of life in colorectal cancer survivors." *Cancer Causes & Control* 25 (1):99–110. doi: 10.1007/s10552-013-0313-y.

Select Committee on Nutrition and Human Needs-U.S. Senate. 1977. *Dietary Goals for the United States*, 2nd Edition. Washington DC: U.S. Printing Office. file:///D:/Gigo/McGovern%20Senate%20Select%20Committee%20on%20Nutrition.Dietary%20Goals%20for%20the%20US.1977.pdf (accessed July 4, 2020).

Sheeran, P., C. Abraham, K. Jones, M. E. Villegas, A. Avishai, Y. R. Symes, H. Ellinger, E. Miles, K. M. Gates, C. E. Wright, K. M. Ribisl, and D. K. Mayer. 2019. "Promoting physical activity among cancer survivors: Meta-analysis and meta-CART analysis of randomized controlled trials." *Health Psychology* 38 (6):467–482. doi: 10.1037/hea0000712.

Slattery, M. L., K. M. Boucher, B. J. Caan, J. D. Potter, and K. N. Ma. 1998. "Eating patterns and risk of colon cancer." *American Journal of Epidemiology* 148 (1):4–16.

Song, M., and A. T. Chan. 2019. "Environmental factors, gut microbiota, and colorectal cancer prevention." *Clinical Gastroenterology and Hepatology* 17 (2):275–289. doi: 10.1016/j.cgh.2018.07.012.

Spellman, C., M. Craike, and P. M. Livingston. 2014. "Knowledge, attitudes and practices of clinicians in promoting physical activity to prostate cancer survivors." *Health Education Journal* 73 (5):566–575. doi: 10.1177/0017896913508395.

Stacey, F. G., E. L. James, K. Chapman, K. S. Courneya, and D. R. Lubans. 2015. "A systematic review and meta-analysis of social cognitive theory-based physical activity and/or nutrition behavior change interventions for cancer survivors." *Journal of Cancer Survivorship* 9 (2):305–338. doi: 10.1007/s11764-014-0413-z.

Stan, D., C. L. Loprinzi, and K. J. Ruddy. 2013. "Breast cancer survivorship issues." *Hematology-Oncology Clinics of North America* 27 (4):805–827. doi: 10.1016/j.hoc.2013.05.005.

Steck, S. E., and E. A. Murphy. 2020. "Dietary patterns and cancer risk." *Nature Reviews Cancer* 20 (2):125–138. doi: 10.1038/s41568-019-0227-4.

Stewart, C. J., T. A. Auchtung, N. J. Ajami, K. Velasquez, D. P. Smith, R. De La Garza, R. Salas, and J. F. Petrosino. 2018. "Effects of tobacco smoke and electronic cigarette vapor exposure on the oral and gut microbiota in humans: A pilot study." *PeerJ* 6:16. doi: 10.7717/peerj.4693.

Stokols, D. 1996. "Translating social ecological theory into guidelines for community health promotion." *American Journal of Health Promotion* 10 (4):282–298.

Tang, J. L., J. Muir, T. Lancaster, L. Jones, and G. Fowler. 1997. "Health profiles of current and former smokers and lifelong abstainers." *Journal of the Royal College of Physicians of London* 31 (3):304–309.

Tollosa, D. N., E. Holliday, A. Hure, M. Tavener, and E. L. James. 2020. "A 15-year follow-up study on long-term adherence to health behaviour recommendations in women diagnosed with breast cancer." *Breast Cancer Research and Treatment*:12, in press. doi: 10.1007/s10549-020-05704-4.

Turner-McGrievy, G. M., M. D. Wirth, N. Shivappa, E. E. Wingard, R. Fayad, S. Wilcox, E. A. Frongillo, and J. R. Hebert. 2015. "Randomization to plant-based dietary approaches leads to larger short-term improvements in dietary inflammatory index scores and macronutrient intake compared with diets that contain meat." *Nutrition Research* 35 (2):97–106. doi: 10.1016/j.nutres.2014.11.007.

U.S. Department of Agriculture (USDA). 2016. *Dietary Guidelines for Americans 2015–2020*, 8th Edition. Rockville, MD: U.S. Department of Health and Human Services, accessed January 7. http://health.gov/dietaryguidelines/2015/guidelines/.

U.S. Department of Agriculture. 2020. *History of Dietary Guidelines for Americans*. Rockville, MD: U.S. Department of Agriculture. https://www.dietaryguidelines.gov/about-dietary-guidelines/history-dietary-guidelines (accessed July 04, 2020).

U.S. Department of Agriculture (USDA) & U.S. Department of Health and Human Services. 2015. *Scientific Report of the 2015 Dietary Guidelines Advisory Committee*. Rockville, MD: U.S. Department of Agriculture, accessed March 17. http://www.health.gov/dietaryguidelines/2015-scientific-report/.

Ueha, R., S. Ueha, K. Kondo, T. Sakamoto, S. Kikuta, K. Kanaya, H. Nishijima, K. Matsushima, and T. Yamasoba. 2016. "Damage to olfactory progenitor cells is involved in cigarette smoke-induced olfactory dysfunction in mice." *American Journal of Pathology* 186 (3):579–586. doi: 10.1016/j.ajpath.2015.11.009.

Van Blarigan, E. L., C. S. Fuchs, D. Niedzwiecki, S. Zhang, L. B. Saltz, R. J. Mayer, R. B. Mowat, R. Whittom, A. Hantel, A. Benson, D. Atienza, M. Messino, H. Kindler, A. Venook, S. Ogino, E. L. Giovannucci, K. Ng, and J. A. Meyerhardt. 2018. "Association of survival with adherence to the American cancer society nutrition and physical activity guidelines for cancer survivors after colon cancer diagnosis the CALGB 89803/alliance trial." *JAMA Oncology* 4 (6):783–790. doi: 10.1001/jamaoncol.2018.0126.

Van Blarigan, E. L., S. A. Kenfield, J. M. Chan, K. Van Loon, A. Paciorek, L. Zhang, H. Chan, M. B. Savoie, A. G. Bocobo, V. N. Liu, L. X. Wong, A. Laffan, C. E. Atreya, C. Miaskowski, Y. Fukuoka, J. A. Meyerhardt, and A. P. Venook. 2020. "Feasibility and acceptability of a web-based dietary intervention with text messages for colorectal cancer: A randomized pilot trial." *Cancer Epidemiology Biomarkers & Prevention* 29 (4):752–760. doi: 10.1158/1055-9965.epi-19-0840.

van Rooijen, S. J., C. J. L. Molenaar, G. Schep, R. van Lieshout, S. Beijer, R. Dubbers, N. Rademakers, N. E. Papen-Botterhuis, S. van Kempen, F. Carli, R. M. H. Roumen, and G. D. Slooter. 2019. "Making patients fit for surgery introducing a four pillar multimodal prehabilitation program in colorectal cancer." *American Journal of Physical Medicine & Rehabilitation* 98 (10):888–896. doi: 10.1097/phm.0000000000001221.

Vandelanotte, C., A. M. Muller, C. E. Short, M. Hingle, N. Nathan, S. L. Williams, M. L. Lopez, S. Parekh, and C. A. Maher. 2016. "Past, present, and future of ehealth and mhealth research to improve physical activity and dietary behaviors." *Journal of Nutrition Education and Behavior* 48 (3):219–228. doi: 10.1016/j.jneb.2015.12.006.

Vennemann, M. M., T. Hummel, and K. Berger. 2008. "The association between smoking and smell and taste impairment in the general population." *Journal of Neurology* 255 (8):1121–1126. doi: 10.1007/s00415-008-0807-9.

Wang, Y. M., X. M. Guo, X. Lu, S. Mattar, and G. Kassab. 2019. "Mechanisms of weight loss after sleeve gastrectomy and adjustable gastric banding: Far more than just restriction." *Obesity* 27 (11):1776–1783. doi: 10.1002/oby.22623.

Ware, J. E., and C. D. Sherbourne. 1992. "The MOS 36-item short form health survey (SF-36). 1. Conceptual framework and item selection." *Medical Care* 30 (6):473–483. doi: 10.1097/00005650-199206000-00002.

Weight Watchers Research Department. 2018. "The four pillars: Food: How weight watchers fits in with many different eating preferences and styles." Weight Watchers International, accessed May 14. https://www.weightwatchers.com/util/art/index_art.aspx?tabnum=1&art_id=20751&sc=807.

Wesolowski, S., T. M. Orlowski, and M. Kram. 2020. "The 6-min walk test in the functional evaluation of patients with lung cancer qualified for lobectomy." *Interactive Cardiovascular and Thoracic Surgery* 30 (4):559–564. doi: 10.1093/icvts/ivz313.

West, R., and T. Sohal. 2006. ""Catastrophic" pathways to smoking cessation: Findings from national survey." *British Medical Journal* 332 (7539):458–460. doi: 10.1136/bmj.38723.573866.AE.

Westerterp-Plantenga, M. S., C. R. T. Verwegen, M. J. W. Ijedema, N. E. G. Wijckmans, and W. H. M. Saris. 1997. "Acute effects of exercise or sauna on appetite in obese and nonobese men." *Physiology & Behavior* 62 (6):1345–1354.

Winters, B. L., D. C. Mitchell, H. Smiciklas-Wright, M. B. Grosvenor, W. Q. Liu, and G. L. Blackburn. 2004. "Dietary patterns in women treated for breast cancer who successfully reduce fat intake: The Women's Intervention Nutrition Study (WINS)." *Journal of the American Dietetic Association* 104 (4):551–559. doi: 10.1016/j.jada.2004.01.012.

World Cancer Research Fund (WCRF). 2018. *Diet, Nutrition, Physical Activity and Cancer: A Global Perspective.* Continuous Update Project Expert Report 2018. London: World Cancer Research Foundation - American Institute of Cancer Research. www.dietandcancerreport.org (accessed June 4, 2018).

World Health Organization (WHO). 1997. *WHOQOL: Measuring Quality of Life.* Geneva: World Health Organization. https://www.who.int/healthinfo/survey/whoqol-qualityoflife/en/ (accessed July 28, 2020).

Xu, F. R., S. A. Cohen, I. E. Lofgren, G. W. Greene, M. J. Delmonico, and M. L. Greaney. 2018. "Relationship between diet quality, physical activity and health-related quality of life in older adults: Findings from 2007–2014 National Health and Nutrition Examination Survey." *Journal of Nutrition Health & Aging* 22 (9):1072–1079. doi: 10.1007/s12603-018-1050-4.

Yamane, S., and N. Inagaki. 2018. "Regulation of glucagon-like peptide-1 sensitivity by gut microbiota dysbiosis." *Journal of Diabetes Investigation* 9 (2):262–264. doi: 10.1111/jdi.12762.

Zhang, C. X., W. J. Wang, and D. F. Zhang. 2018. "Association between dietary inflammation index and the risk of colorectal cancer: A meta-analysis." *Nutrition and Cancer: An International Journal* 70 (1):14–22. doi: 10.1080/01635581.2017.1374418.

Zhao, L. P., F. Zhang, X. Y. Ding, G. J. Wu, Y. Y. Lam, X. J. Wang, H. Q. Fu, X. H. Xue, C. H. Lu, J. L. Ma, L. H. Yu, C. M. Xu, Z. Y. Ren, Y. Xu, S. M. Xu, H. L. Shen, X. L. Zhu, Y. Shi, Q. Y. Shen, W. P. Dong, R. Liu, Y. X. Ling, Y. Zeng, X. P. Wang, Q. P. Zhang, J. Wang, L. H. Wang, Y. Q. Wu, B. H. Zeng, H. Wei, M. H. Zhang, Y. D. Peng, and C. H. Zhang. 2018. "Gut bacteria selectively promoted by dietary fibers alleviate type 2 diabetes." *Science* 359 (6380):1151–1156. doi: 10.1126/science.aao5774.

Zick, S. M., J. Colacino, M. Cornellier, T. Khabir, K. Surnow, and Z. Djuric. 2017. "Fatigue reduction diet in breast cancer survivors: A pilot randomized clinical trial." *Breast Cancer Research and Treatment* 161 (2):299–310. doi: 10.1007/s10549-016-4070-y.

Zuniga, K. E., D. L. Parma, E. Munoz, M. Spaniol, M. Wargovich, and A. G. Ramirez. 2019. "Dietary intervention among breast cancer survivors increased adherence to a mediterranean-style, anti-inflammatory dietary pattern: The Rx for better breast health randomized controlled trial." *Breast Cancer Research and Treatment* 173 (1):145–154. doi: 10.1007/s10549-018-4982-9.

21 Environmental Factors in Cancer Risk

Lishi Xie and Gail S. Prins
University of Illinois at Chicago

CONTENTS

INTRODUCTION

"God does not play dice with the universe" is one of Albert Einstein's most famous quotes, which represents human nature's search for causes behind catastrophic events, including cancer, to rule out mere "chance" or "bad luck". Recently, modelling studies by Tomasetti and Vogelstein (Tomasetti and Vogelstein 2015, Tomasetti et al. 2017) suggested that two-thirds of all cancer burdens may be explained by "bad luck": the random mistakes made during normal DNA replication in normal, noncancerous stem cells. As expected, this provocative conclusion gained extensive media attention and rekindled old debates on the role of environmental factors in cancer risk among researchers in the public health field.

The debates usually start with a basic question: do factors other than mere "bad luck" of DNA replication, especially environmental factors, make significant contributions to the lifetime cancer risk? Through decades of study involving multiple disciplines, we have achieved significant progress in our understanding of cancer etiology as well as in prevention, early detection, and treatment (Chabner and Roberts 2005, Verellen et al. 2007, Vineis and Wild 2014, Yang 2015), leading to a decline of cancer mortality in the industrialized world. Meanwhile, the incidence of certain cancer types continues to increase worldwide due, in part, to longer lifespans and changing patterns of cancer risk factors (Fitzmaurice et al. 2018). For example, growing evidence demonstrates an impact of the obesity epidemic on cancers, increasing the risk of at least 13 different types of cancer (Steele et al. 2017, Avgerinos et al. 2019). Furthermore, significant disparities in age-adjusted cancer incidence rates have been observed across different regions of the world (Hemminki et al. 2014), in certain racial/ethnic groups (Ashktorab et al. 2017), and even between twins with identical genetic backgrounds (Lichtenstein et al. 2000). Collectively, the cancerous process is a result of disturbed cell function, which involves contributions from replication, hereditary, and environmental factors as well as from the interactions of those factors.

The next question posed is what is considered as environmental factors. Cell division and organ development are finely regulated processes. The dysregulation of the molecular mechanisms involved in these processes may cause cancer, which is a consequence of a series of intrinsic and/ or extrinsic events both inside and outside the body. In this context, scientists consider everything outside the body that interacts with humans as the environmental factors, which excludes replication and hereditary factors. Inside the body, cellular DNA damage can be triggered by spontaneous hydrolysis, reactive oxygen species, aberrant metabolism, or other perturbations that cause DNA damage. Environmental factors from outside the body can damage the DNA directly, such as ultraviolet (UV) exposure induced DNA damage in skin (Sample and He 2018), or indirectly through altering cellular metabolism or affecting the ability of cells to interact with the microenvironment (Carbone et al. 2020). It has been challenging to identify certain environmental factors as carcinogens due, in part, to the typically long interval between carcinogen exposure and cancer diagnosis; thus there remains a large knowledge gap of these factors despite extensive study over decades (Wu et al. 2018, Carbone et al. 2020).

One of the most important questions related to public health is whether cancers are preventable. At its core, cancer results from cells that are dividing with intrinsic random mistakes causing mutations. Although mutations are the engine for evolution, they can also destroy the cooperative processes of cells, leading to uncontrolled replication. However, it is critical to realize that nonintrinsic factors can increase the risk of developing cancer, and as such, there remains considerable room for the intervention of nonintrinsic factors to reduce overall cancer rates. For example, nonsmokers have a lifetime risk of lung cancer of 0.2%–1%, while whether a smoker develops lung cancer or not, an event that has a probability of 10%–25%, depends on other factors including their gender and degree of smoking (Wu et al. 2018). In fact, smoking reduction by 50% significantly reduces the risk of lung cancer among individuals who smoke 15 or more cigarettes per day (Godtfredsen et al. 2005). Furthermore, cancer risk factors often do not act independently and the most likely scenario is that they cooperatively contribute to cancer development. Thus cancer risk can be modified through prevention or intervention strategies targeting interactions of intrinsic and nonintrinsic factors. Anti-inflammatory agents such as aspirin and other nonsteroidal anti-inflammatory drugs have demonstrated the preventive effects on colorectal cancer in individuals with Hereditary Nonpolyposis Colorectal Cancer Syndrome who carry germline mutations in DNA repair genes, which increase DNA mutation rate from intrinsic replication errors (Bibbins-Domingo 2016, Todoric et al. 2016). Indeed, the result of another modeling study provides evidence that intrinsic risk factors by themselves, without interactions with other factors, contribute less than 10%–30% of lifetime risk in most common cancer types (Wu et al. 2016). Cancer risk is thus heavily influenced by extrinsic factors, including environmental factors, which lead to the conclusion that most cancers are preventable. Addressing the question of how to reduce cancer risks will rely on a better understanding of cancer etiology and effective strategies for cancer prevention, research, and public health.

In this chapter, we will review the current understanding of environmental factors in cancer risk from a biological perspective, trying to answer the question of how environmental factors affect the initiation and progression of cancer at various levels ranging from molecular, cellular to organismic. While all environmental factors that contribute to cancer risks cannot be covered in one chapter, we hope this discussion will provide insights into the design of novel and effective strategies for cancer prevention and therapy in the light of nutritional oncology.

ENVIRONMENTAL FACTORS AND GENETIC ALTERATIONS

Cancer is primarily a genetic disease caused by the clonal evolution of tumor cell populations through cycles of mutation and selection that eventually result in a metastatic tumor (Nowell 1976). Indeed, it is the enormous capacity to generate heterogeneity via mutations that renders cancer the ability to survive treatment as well as to escape natural defenses, such as the immune system (Zhang and Vijg 2018, Marusyk et al. 2020).

DNA, as the carrier of the genetic information for almost all life forms on earth, was generally assumed to be a very stable molecule (Watson and Crick 1953). However, it has become clear that DNA is highly vulnerable, under physiological conditions, to damage varying from hydrolysis and alkylation to oxidation (Lindahl 1993). It is a highly conserved system of genome maintenance mechanisms that renders the apparent stability of DNA in the genome and eliminates many thousands of chemical lesions generated each day in a typical cell (Lindahl 1993, Hoeijmakers 2001). In the history of life, genes encoding the DNA damage repair system were likely among the first genetic traits selected for a survival advantage to the protocells using DNA instead of the even more vulnerable RNA (de Duve 2005). Indeed, deficiencies inherited or acquired in genome maintenance systems significantly contribute to the onset of cancer (Hoeijmakers 2001).

DNA mutation is different from DNA damage. The term "DNA damage" refers to physical changes of the DNA structure such as breaks, cross-links, and modified bases. DNA mutations are alterations in the genetic information encoded by the combination of DNA base pairs, varying from the very large chromosomal aberrations and copy number variations to smaller deletions and insertions. Therefore, while DNA damage can be repaired, DNA mutations cannot be recognized by the DNA repair system and can be removed only through the death of the cell or the entire organism carrying the mutations (Zhang and Vijg 2018). As a result of errors during DNA damage repair, replication, and mitosis, DNA mutations, at least in the germline, generate genetic variation in organisms and drive evolution together with natural selection in the population which is inherent to life and necessary for its continuation as a species. Meanwhile, for individuals, one end product of mutations, usually in somatic cells, is cancer.

For multicellular organisms, mutations in the germ cells and that of the somatic cells are distinct; they follow different natural selection rules. Germline mutations occur in gametes and are passed onto offspring where every cell in the new entire organism will be affected. Somatic mutations only occur in a single body cell and are inherited only in daughter cells of division. Thus only tissues derived from mutated cells are affected. The human germline mutation rate, determined by DNA sequencing of somatic tissue from parents and children, is around $1.0-1.2 \times 10^{-8}$ per nucleotide per generation, corresponding to about 60 new germline mutations per generation (Conrad et al. 2011, Kong et al. 2012). In each newborn, only <10% of these germline mutations are considered weakly deleterious due to purifying selection (Kong et al. 2012). For somatic mutations, the pressure of natural selection in most adult tissues is minimal. Hence, the somatic mutations provide the majority of the genetic heterogeneity required for the evolution of normal cells to cancer cells. The Cancer Gene Census database contains genes recurrently mutated in cancer, of which ~90% are derived from somatic mutations and ~20% from germline mutations that predispose to cancer (family cancer) (Forbes et al. 2015). As an example of Darwinian evolution, cancer has been linked with somatic mutation.

Recent advances in high-throughput sequencing have made it possible to determine the somatic mutations in individual tumors (Avgerinos et al. 2019) and findings indicate that environmental factors are extensively involved in the somatic mutational process of cancer. In fact, the causal relationship between mutations and cancer was strongly supported by the discovery that many carcinogenic chemicals are also mutagenic (Loeb and Harris 2008). Environmental factors can damage the DNA directly, including chemicals, UV light, and ionizing radiation; or indirectly through interaction with endogenous factors, such as reactive species and aldehydes. It is worth mentioning that recent studies reveal that even normal sun-exposed skin demonstrated a high burden of somatic mutations similar to that seen in many cancers with strong positive selection for multiple cancer genes (Martincorena et al. 2015). This study provides fundamental insights into the role of environmental factors in the initiation of cancer.

Environmental factors can also introduce DNA mutations by affecting the genome maintenance systems such as loss of DNA repair pathways or chromosome integrity checkpoints (Alexandrov et al. 2013) leading to dramatically increased mutation rates. E-cigarette smoke (ECS) is promoted as noncarcinogenic and a revolutionary cure for tobacco smokers by delivering nicotine directly through aerosols without burning tobacco. However, studies reveal that ECS induces DNA damage in various tissues of mice and reduces DNA-repair functions in the lungs leading to enhanced mutations and malignant transformation of cultured human lung cells (Lee et al. 2018).

In addition, as a biological environmental factor, viruses can cause DNA mutations in the host genome by insertions of DNA fragments (Martincorena and Campbell 2015). A recent study using next-generation sequencing (NGS) to detect viral sequences in human genome revealed that nearly all tumor and normal tissues examined contained viral sequences. This study further confirmed reported associations of Hepatitis B and C virus (HBV, HCV) with liver cancer, and human papillomaviruses (HPV) with cervical cancer, and head and neck cancer (Cantalupo et al. 2018).

Environmental factors can further affect cancer risk through gene–environment interactions. The Lynch syndrome (LS) is the most common autosomal tumor predisposition syndrome, which is caused by germline mutations of DNA mismatch repair genes. LS patients have increased cancer risk due to high mutation rates (Jiricny and Nyström-Lahti 2000). However, families with LS in Asia have a higher incidence of stomach cancer than families in Western countries, indicating that gene–environment interactions determine the final cancer risk (Wei et al. 2010, Park et al. 2016).

ENVIRONMENTAL FACTORS AND EPIGENETIC ALTERATIONS

Epigenetic alterations play profound and ubiquitous roles in cancer which is typically considered a genetic disease. Through epigenetic mechanisms, a vast repertoire of gene expression patterns, responsible for hundreds of cell types and adaptations to different developmental and environmental conditions, are generated for the whole organism from a single genome without changing its genetic information. The human genome contains 6 million bases of DNA which are wrapped about 30 million nucleosomes, forming a macromolecular complex named chromatin. The chromatin is the essential platform through which transcription factors, signaling pathways, and other cues alter gene activity and cellular responses (Margueron and Reinberg 2010). Aberrations in chromatin are associated with a wide range of common diseases, including cancer (Flavahan et al. 2017). A large-scale cancer genome sequencing analysis revealed that roughly half of the human cancers harbor mutations in chromatin proteins (You and Jones 2012, Shen and Laird 2013).

Environmental factors along with genetic and metabolic factors can also affect cancer risk through epigenetic alterations. In fact, only 2% of the genome encodes proteins, the remaining 98% comprises regulatory elements that orchestrate context-specific gene activity (Flavahan, Gaskell et al. 2017). Proximal and distal regulatory factors (promoters and enhancers, respectively) control gene expression in response to developmental or environmental cues. As mentioned above, the genome is wrapped on nucleosomes and further packaged into chromatin. Active genes are accessible to transcription factors and transcriptional machinery, while inactive genes are sequestered within compact and inaccessible structures that prevent their aberrant activation (Margueron and Reinberg 2010, Allis and Jenuwein 2016). Environmental factors that affect the state of chromatin by increasing resistance may result in a restrictive state that prevents normal biological programs, such as differentiation. Those that decrease chromatin resistance may result in a permissive state called epigenetic plasticity. It is proposed that plasticity allows premalignant or malignant cells to stochastically activate genes and gives rise to adaptive clonal evolution necessary for cancer progression. Further, acquired epigenetic alterations are inherited through mitosis including DNA methylation, genomic imprinting, specific histone modifications, and noncoding RNAs (Mazzio and Soliman 2012, Flavahan et al. 2017).

It is believed that the most critical impact of the environmental factors on the resulting phenotype occurs when exposure occurs at the earlier stage of development. In fact, long-term phenotypic changes are largely initiated when the organism is introduced to the external world following the in utero/perinatal periods (Martínez-Frías 2010). In animal studies, early-life exposures to estradiol benzoate and bisphenol A (BPA) have been linked to increased prostate cancer risk through multiple epigenetic mechanisms, including genomic DNA methylation (Cheong et al. 2016), histone modifications (Prins et al. 2018), and alterations in noncoding RNA (Ho et al. 2015). Epigenetic alterations due to early-life environmental exposures may result in a permissive state of chromatin, elevating the basal and inductive expression of environmental factor reprogrammed genes into adulthood (Wang et al. 2016). Importantly, the epigenetic alterations induced by environmental factors may act like a driver mutation. Bronchial epithelial cells chronically exposed to cigarette smoke displayed epigenetic alterations leading to activation of KRAS, WNT, and epidermal growth factor receptor signaling (Vaz et al. 2017). Furthermore, the epigenetic alterations can become transgenerational, lasting for three to four generations even though the initiating stimuli are long discontinued (Titus-Ernstoff et al. 2008, Skinner and Guerrero-Bosagna 2009).

ENVIRONMENTAL FACTORS AND PROTEIN HOMEOSTASIS

As a major risk factor for cancer development, organismal aging is associated with the gradual accumulation of damaged biomolecules due to a time-dependent decline in physiological organ function. Proteins carry out the majority of cellular functions, thus proteome quality control is critical for normal cellular function. Two main degradation machineries, namely, the ubiquitin-proteasome system (UPS) and autophagy-lysosome pathways (ALP), are key components of the proteostasis network by which cells regulate essential biological processes such as the cell cycle, DNA damage repair, and cell death. Alteration of specific proteostasis factors is associated with cancer progression (Carvalho et al. 2016, Wedel et al. 2018).

The UPS is composed of ubiquitin-activating, conjugating, and ligating enzymes and the proteasome where cells degrade short-lived, poly-ubiquitinated normal or damaged proteins or polypeptides. Cytosolic or estrogen receptor-bound proteasomes play a central role in quality control of protein synthesis, by which nonfunctional newly synthesized polypeptides are targeted. Nuclear proteasomes are involved in DNA damage response, while outer mitochondrial membrane located proteasomes are responsible for mitochondrial quality control (Wedel et al. 2018). Environmental factors can affect the proteasome activity or the key events of the UPS. For example, UV radiation decreases proteasome activity through the induction of cellular oxidative stress due to protein oxidation (Bulteau et al. 2002). In the case of HPV infection-related cervical cancer, E3 ubiquitin ligase activity of HPV E6 protein targets p53, a well-known tumor suppression gene, for proteasomal degradation (Vlachostergios et al. 2009).

The other main cellular degradation and recycling pathway in eukaryotic cells is ALP. Macroautophagy (hereafter referred to as autophagy) encloses cellular material in double-membrane vesicles termed autophagosome, and their subsequent fusion with lysosomes allows for their degradation (Kimmelman and White 2017). ALP has been shown to be essential for multiple aspects of cancer development, including cell metabolism, protein and organelle turnover, and cell survival. On the one hand, ALP constrains tumor initiation through maintaining cellular and genomic integrity. On the other hand, ALP helps established tumor maintenance, allowing tumors to survive environmental stress (Santana-Codina et al. 2017). A number of environmental chemicals such as pesticides and metals have been shown to interfere with APL processes at various molecular levels (Pesonen and Vähäkangas 2019). Recently, inorganic arsenic was shown to inhibit lysosome acidification leading to impaired ALP and subsequent transformation of prostate stem-progenitor cells (Xie et al. 2020). In another example, UV-radiation targets the autophagy gene Atg7 in the epidermis, contributing to skin carcinogenesis (Qiang et al. 2017).

ENVIRONMENTAL FACTORS AND STEM CELLS

Stem cells are unspecialized cells that duplicate through cell division, termed self-renewal, and differentiate to committed progenitor lineages and eventually, fully differentiated cells. Embryonic stem cells are pluripotent cells that give rise to the whole organism, whereas organ-specific stem cells are responsible for the generation of the tissue during development, life-long tissue maintenance, and injury repair (Brazhnik et al. 2020).

Given the pivotal role of stem cells in maintaining the integrity of multicellular organisms throughout the lifespan, it is not surprising to find that stem cells adopt multiple mechanisms to prevent malignant transformation. For example, single-cell sequencing has revealed that considerably lower mutation frequencies are observed in liver stem cells (Brazhnik et al. 2020). Both normal and cancer stem cells (CSCs) have a superior capacity of DNA damage repair and CSCs are particularly tolerant to DNA damage during progression or therapy (Vitale et al. 2017). Other mechanisms applied to maintain stem cell homeostasis include asymmetric division, enhanced autophagy, lower numbers of mitochondria, and cell cycle quiescence (Revuelta and Matheu 2017, Vitale et al. 2017, Venkei and Yamashita 2018, Zhang et al. 2018).

In the past decades, significant progress has been made to identify the cells of origin in cancers. Accumulating evidence suggests that adult stem cells (ASCs) or early-stage progenitors can also be responsible for cancer development. First, ASCs are long-lived and gradually accumulate genetic mutations leading to various age-related diseases, including cancer. Mutations accumulate steadily over time in ASCs from various tissues, at a rate of ~40 novel mutations per year (Blokzijl et al. 2016). Second, ASCs are multipotent which could explain the cellular heterogeneity found within most tumors and the cell state transitions necessary for successful metastasis of aggressive cancers (Lambert et al. 2017). Third, ASCs have significant self-renewal capability, which could be critical for tumor expansion (White and Lowry 2015). Indeed, experimental evidence from lineage tracing implicates that ASCs may be a cell origin of various solid tumors (Blanpain 2013).

CSCs are defined by their ability to propagate tumors when serially transplanted (Reya et al. 2001). Although CSCs have similar properties and gene expression patterns to ASCs, it remains unclear where there is a causal relationship between them. It is postulated that CSCs may stem from oncogenic transformed normal ASCs or from differentiated cells that acquire the properties of stem cells through genetic or epigenetic alterations. CSCs play a critical role in cancer progression by actively remodeling their microenvironment to establish a sustainable niche (Prager et al. 2019). More importantly, stem-cell pathways promote plasticity in tumor cells, fueling their therapy-resistance and metastatic competence in aggressive cancers (Soundararajan et al. 2018).

Environmental factors can affect cancer risk through altering the function and homeostasis of stem cells. It is well known that high-caloric diets and obesity are associated with increased cancer risk. Studies using mice and intestinal organoid cultures demonstrated that a long-term high-fat diet (HFD) increased the number and function of intestinal ASCs; enforced activation of HFD induced the peroxisome proliferator-activated receptor delta (PPARd) pathway and led to tumor formation after loss of tumor suppressor (Beyaz et al. 2016). In a carcinogen-induced breast cancer mouse model, exposure to HFD in utero doubled mammary cancer risk along with an increased size of the mammary ASC population (Lambertz et al. 2017).

ENDOCRINE DISRUPTING CHEMICALS AND CANCER RISK

The high incidence of breast and prostate cancer in industrialized countries suggests a significant environmental component in their etiology. As these and others are hormone-dependent cancers, endocrine disrupting chemicals (EDCs) are of particular concern. The Endocrine Society defines EDCs as "an exogenous compound or mixture of chemicals that can interfere with any aspect of hormone action" (Zoeller et al. 2012). Exposure to EDCs may occur during various activities of daily life due to the ubiquitous existence of synthesized chemicals in water, soil, and air, which includes chemicals in plastic products, metal food cans, detergents, flame retardants, food, toys, and pesticides. It is estimated that ~1,000 manufactured chemicals have endocrine-disrupting properties among thousands evaluated to date. Since EDCs alter normal hormone functions, studies show that they may pose a greater risk during prenatal and early postnatal development (Yilmaz et al. 2020).

EDCs may increase cancer risk through various mechanisms. EDCs may target the stem cells, which is a compelling cancer target in organisms during development and cancer progression (Kopras et al. 2014). As the fate of the stem cells is regulated by environmental cues, exposure to EDCs can alter the properties of both embryonic and ASCs at multiple levels, depending on the developmental stage (Annab et al. 2012). BPA is a well-characterized xenoestrogen, which activates estrogen receptor signaling in exposed organisms. Prostate stem-progenitors express a high level of estrogen receptors through which BPA epigenetically reprograms their fate during early-life exposure, ultimately leading to higher prostate cancer risk in adulthood (Hu et al. 2012, Prins et al. 2018). Likewise, BPA increases mammary tumor incidence and drives carcinomas in rodent models, also through epigenetic and structural alterations (Dhimolea et al. 2014, Seachrist et al. 2016, Montévil et al. 2020). EDCs can also promote cancer progression. Phthalates are a group of EDCs associated with increased breast cancer risk (López-Carrillo et al. 2010). Though activation of estrogen receptor and histone deacetylase 6, phthalates promote a metastatic phenotype, such as epithelial-mesenchymal transition (EMT), cell migration, and cell invasion in breast stem cells (Hsieh et al. 2012).

Some EDCs, such as tributyltin and phthalates which activate PPARd, exert obesogenic effects that result in alternated energy homeostasis (Egusquiza and Blumberg 2020). As such, these chemicals can drive metabolic syndrome and promote obesity which is positively associated with elevated cancer incidence (Salamanca-Fernández et al. 2020). It is noteworthy that many EDCs are lipophilic and bioaccumulate in body fat over the years. Thus, the association between obesity and cancer may also due to prolonged exposure to EDCs (Yilmaz et al. 2020). Furthermore, studies indicate that EDCs affect the immune system function, resulting in hyperimmunity or immune suppression (Bansal et al. 2018), and EDCs may alter immune responses to infections and tumor cells and thereby increase cancer risk.

AIR POLLUTION AND CANCER RISK

With the fast economic growth and urbanization in the past decades, exposure to ambient air pollution has become a significant contributor to the cancer burden. Although the relative risk of developing cancer from air pollution is generally small, the attributable risk is high due to the high numbers of exposed people. Air pollution is well-known to be associated with respiratory and cardiovascular diseases, but cancer is also an important outcome. Lung cancer has the most robust association with prolonged exposure to air pollution (Fajersztajn et al. 2013). A recent large prospective study found that air pollution was also significantly associated with kidney, bladder, and colorectal cancers among 29 anatomic sites (Turner et al. 2017). Moreover, a growing body of evidence links air pollution with increased cancer risk in other tissues, such as breast (Crouse et al. 2010, Chen and Bina 2012), ovarian (García-Pérez et al. 2015, Wang et al. 2019), prostate (Cohen et al. 2018, Shekarrizfard et al. 2018, Wang et al. 2019), and hematopoietic tissues (Whitworth et al. 2008, Weng et al. 2009, Wang et al. 2019).

Outdoor air pollution is a mixture of multiple pollutants originating from natural or anthropogenic sources, including transportation, power generation, industrial activity, biomass burning, domestic heating, and cooking (Loomis et al. 2013). Diverse indexes have been applied to measure air pollution, such as NO_2, SO_2, O_3, and particulate matter (PM). PM is a mixture of air pollution sources that are present in the air rather than a single pollutant, and PM is classified according to their size, which ranges from 0.005 to 100 μm in diameter (Fajersztajn et al. 2013). PM2.5 is a fine PM with a median aerodynamic diameter of <2.5 μm, which is increasingly used as an indicator pollutant, with annual average concentrations ranging from 10 to more than 100 μg/m³ globally (Loomis et al. 2013). The smaller sized PM has more potential to penetrate deep into the respiratory tract. In fact, there is a higher association of lung cancer risk with air pollution expressed in terms of PM2.5 (Fajersztajn et al. 2013). The composition of PM includes various classes of organic and inorganic chemicals, such as heavy and transition metals, hydrocarbons, ions, and microorganisms.

Diesel emissions, a substantial component of urban particles, were considered to be class I carcinogens by the International Agency of Research on Cancer (Benbrahim-Tallaa et al. 2012).

Studies of cohorts occupationally exposed to air pollution, such as traffic police, drivers, and street vendors, have shown increased chromosome aberrations in lymphocytes (de Marini 2013). Air pollution is also associated with altered expression of genes involved in genome maintenance, inflammation, immune, and oxidative stress responses; epigenetic alteration such as DNA methylation (Loomis et al. 2013). Furthermore, genetic alterations and DNA damage were also observed in mammals, birds, and plants exposed to outdoor air pollution (Somers 2011).

OPPORTUNITIES FOR CANCER PREVENTION

Since the British surgeon Percivall Pott observed that scrotal cancer was a common disease among chimney sweeps in 1775 (Brown and Thornton 1957), multiple approaches have been applied over many decades to understand environmental factors and cancer risk. Nonetheless, it remains a challenge to establish causal relationships due to the typical long interval between carcinogen exposures and cancer diagnosis.

During this temporal gap, usually decades, intrinsic, heritable, and environmental factors cooperatively affect the integrity of multicellular organisms, and cancer is one of the end products of this process. Retrospective case–control studies have been used to generate numerous hypotheses about the role of environmental factors in cancer risk. A historical study involving 40,000 British people conducted by Doll and Hill (1950) discovered that tobacco smoking was strongly over-represented in lung cancer cases compared with matched controls (Doll and Hill 1950). The positive association between lung cancer and smoking was further confirmed 4 years later in a prospective cohort study of more than 30,000 British physicians (Doll and Hill 1954). In a follow-up study of 34,439 male British doctors 50 year later, while cigarette smoking from early adult life was found to triple age-specific mortality rates due to multiple diseases including cancer, cessation at age 50 halved the risk, and cessation at age 30 avoided almost all of it (Doll et al. 2004). In the studies over more than half a century, enormous progress has been achieved in our understanding of the mechanisms of smoking-induced changes at multiple levels, including genetic and epigenetic alterations (Vaz et al. 2017). The story of smoking and lung cancer also provides a valuable angle for cancer prevention and intervention by modifying other environmental factors.

The rapid development of NGS technology has revolutionized the knowledge of somatic mutations in cancer. The findings from large-scale tumor sequencing provide not only new insight into the role of intrinsic vs nonintrinsic cancer risk factors but also link specific mutation signatures to specific factors. More than 30 unique mutation signatures were revealed in various cancers, of which 10 can be partially linked to known mutagens (Alexandrov et al. 2013). Two signatures strongly correlated with age in most cancer types and thus are most likely to be intrinsic factors since DNA mutations introduced by DNA replication would accumulate in a monotonic fashion over time. In contrast, all known carcinogen-specific signatures are uncorrelated with age and demonstrate a tumor-specific pattern. Therefore, the other unknown signatures may also result from certain unknown carcinogens (Wu et al. 2018). Based on the distribution of the mutation signatures, it was posited that no more than 10%–30% of all cancer incidence is a result of intrinsic risk alone (Wu et al. 2016), which is the "bad luck" part of cancer risk.

Inheritable and environmental factors comprise the nonintrinsic part of cancer risk factors, which are the cornerstone of cancer prevention and intervention. Inheritable factors, such as aging and genetic susceptibility, are unchangeable per se. However, in view of gene-environment interactions (G×E interactions), they are partially modifiable. For example, individuals with germline mutations of TP53, a well-known tumor suppression gene, have increased oxidative metabolism. In a mouse model of TP53 mutation, decreasing oxidative stress by inhibition of mitochondrial respiration using metformin prevented cancer onset (Wang et al. 2017). Thus a better understanding of the etiology of cancer as well as principles of life sciences will certainly benefit the goal of cancer prevention and intervention.

Environmental factors are exogenous risk factors, including radiation, carcinogens, infectious agents, diet, and lifestyles. A recent NGS study revealed a strong mutation signature for UV light which has long been known to induce somatic mutations in the skin (Alexandrov et al. 2013). This finding provides a proof of principle for identifying the effect of mutagens without knowing their origin and highlights its potential to reveal individual exposure history to carcinogens. For example, exposure to aristolochic acid, which has been linked with urothelial carcinoma of the upper urinary tract, shows a highly specific signature (Hoang et al. 2013). In human-induced pluripotent stem cells, a recent study examined the mutational signatures of 79 known or suspected environmental carcinogens. Forty-one demonstrated distinct mutational signatures, in which some were similar to signatures found in human tumors (Kucab et al. 2019). The findings of this study provided a valuable signature map for further exploration of environmental factors in cancer etiology and underscore the vulnerability of stem cell DNA to environmental factors. With the advance of approaches to characterize carcinogens, more modifiable environmental factors are expected to be uncovered. Nonetheless, some factors are not readily modifiable, such as radon exposure, a known factor for lung cancer for the entire population, second only to smoking (Wu et al. 2018).

The misinterpretation of two-thirds of the cancer burden as "bad luck" is detrimental to cancer prevention. It underestimates the impact of prevention on reducing the cancer burden in public health and may impede progress in identifying modifiable factors for cancer prevention. It is generally believed that at least three hits are necessary for solid tumors to develop and fewer for blood tumors (Wu et al. 2018). Thus, cancer may still be preventable even if "bad luck" occurs. Indeed, Cancer Research UK estimated that 42% of cancer cases are preventable (https://www.cancerresearchuk.org/health-professional/cancer-statistics/risk/preventable-cancers) while in the US, the Centers for Disease Control and Prevention estimated that 21% of annual cancer deaths could be prevented (https://www.cdc.gov/media/releases/2014/p0501-preventable-deaths.html). After aristolochic acid was identified as a strong carcinogen-inducing DNA mutation, the Taiwanese government imposed a ban on aristolochic acid-containing Chinese herbal products. In an interrupted time-series analysis, the incidence rate of urological cancers was decreased considerably after 2008 and 2011 (Jhuang et al. 2019). This finding underlines the impact of modifiable environmental factors in cancer prevention.

Awareness is an essential part of cancer prevention. In fact, increasing public awareness is one of the goals of this book. The examples of smoking and aristolochic acid demonstrated the importance of both studies to establish the causal relationship between specific carcinogen exposures and specific cancer diagnoses and the effective strategies in cancer prevention. Carcinogen awareness at the scientific level requires extensive studies by researchers from multiple disciplines including epidemiologists, physicians, and scientists. However, public awareness of carcinogens is also an essential component for effectively reducing the cancer burden of public health and this requires creative and effective strategies to deliver the knowledge from the biomedical science field to the public. For example, inorganic arsenic is a well-known carcinogen for bladder, skin, and prostate cancers and chronic exposure to well water arsenic remains a major rural health challenge in Bangladesh and other countries worldwide. Findings from a recent study in Bangladesh demonstrated that school-based intervention can effectively reduce arsenic exposure by motivating teachers, children, and parents (Khan et al. 2015) as well as governmental regulators.

CONCLUSIONS

Cancer is primarily a genetic disease, and intrinsic, hereditary, and environmental factors affect its initiation and progression, as summarized in Figure 21.1. DNA is the most shared carrier of genetic information for carbon-based life forms on earth and is highly vulnerable under physiological conditions.

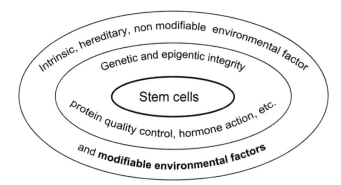

FIGURE 21.1   This diagram illustrates the types of cancer risk factors and the aspects of the organism they affect.

It is the genome maintenance system that renders DNA stability of the genome and eliminates the many thousands of chemical lesions from daily life. Somatic DNA mutations largely contribute to the risk of all cancers and environmental factors may induce somatic mutations directly or indirectly through interaction with intrinsic and hereditary factors. Environmental factors are also associated with cancer risk through interfering with epigenetic mechanisms, protein quality maintenance systems, and hormone actions. Many identified carcinogens are EDCs and increase cancer risk either directly or indirectly through interference with aspects of hormone action. Stem cells are a compelling target of cancer progression and are affected by environmental factors leading to a disturbed balance of self-renewal and differentiation.

Significant progress has been achieved over the past few decades to understand environmental factors and cancer risk. The multiple-hit model of cancer etiology serves as the cornerstone of cancer prevention. The proportion of currently preventable cancers is mostly a subset of cancers with known nonintrinsic risk factors, including environmental factors (Wu et al. 2018). From our perspective, critical challenges going forward in understanding the causal association between environmental factors and cancer risk include a better understanding of cancer etiology and novel approaches to identity environmental carcinogens through NGS and stem cell studies, which may overcome the difficulty of the typically long interval between exposure and cancer diagnosis.

REFERENCES

Alexandrov, L. B., S. Nik-Zainal, D. C. Wedge, S. A. J. R. Aparicio, S. Behjati, A. V. Biankin, G. R. Bignell, N. Bolli, A. Borg, A.-L. Børresen-Dale, S. Boyault, B. Burkhardt, A. P. Butler, C. Caldas, H. R. Davies, C. Desmedt, R. Eils, J. E. Eyfjörd, J. A. Foekens, M. Greaves, F. Hosoda, B. Hutter, T. Ilicic, S. Imbeaud, M. Imielinski, N. Jäger, D. T. W. Jones, D. Jones, S. Knappskog, M. Kool, S. R. Lakhani, C. López-Otín, S. Martin, N. C. Munshi, H. Nakamura, P. A. Northcott, M. Pajic, E. Papaemmanuil, A. Paradiso, J. V. Pearson, X. S. Puente, K. Raine, M. Ramakrishna, A. L. Richardson, J. Richter, P. Rosenstiel, M. Schlesner, T. N. Schumacher, P. N. Span, J. W. Teague, Y. Totoki, A. N. J. Tutt, R. Valdés-Mas, M. M. van Buuren, L. van't Veer, A. Vincent-Salomon, N. Waddell, L. R. Yates, J. Zucman-Rossi, P. Andrew Futreal, U. McDermott, P. Lichter, M. Meyerson, S. M. Grimmond, R. Siebert, E. Campo, T. Shibata, S. M. Pfister, P. J. Campbell, M. R. Stratton, Australian Pancreatic Cancer Genome Initiative, Inflammatory Breast Cancer International Consortium, IMS Global Learning Consortium and ICGC PedBrain (2013). "Signatures of mutational processes in human cancer." *Nature* **500**(7463): 415–421.

Allis, C. D. and T. Jenuwein (2016). "The molecular hallmarks of epigenetic control." *Nat Rev Genet* **17**(8): 487–500.

Annab, L. A., C. D. Bortner, M. I. Sifre, J. M. Collins, R. R. Shah, D. Dixon, H. Karimi Kinyamu and T. K. Archer (2012). "Differential responses to retinoic acid and endocrine disruptor compounds of subpopulations within human embryonic stem cell lines." *Differentiation* **84**(4): 330–343.

Ashktorab, H., S. S. Kupfer, H. Brim and J. M. Carethers (2017). "Racial disparity in gastrointestinal cancer risk." *Gastroenterology* **153**(4): 910–923.

Avgerinos, K. I., N. Spyrou, C. S. Mantzoros and M. Dalamaga (2019). "Obesity and cancer risk: Emerging biological mechanisms and perspectives." *Metabolism* **92**: 121–135.

Bansal, A., J. Henao-Mejia and R. A. Simmons (2018). "Immune system: an emerging player in mediating effects of endocrine disruptors on metabolic health." *Endocrinology* **159**(1): 32–45.

Benbrahim-Tallaa, L., R. A. Baan, Y. Grosse, B. Lauby-Secretan, F. El Ghissassi, V. Bouvard, N. Guha, D. Loomis and K. Straif (2012). "Carcinogenicity of diesel-engine and gasoline-engine exhausts and some nitroarenes." *Lancet Oncol* **13**(7): 663–664.

Beyaz, S., M. D. Mana, J. Roper, D. Kedrin, A. Saadatpour, S.-J. Hong, K. E. Bauer-Rowe, M. E. Xifaras, A. Akkad, E. Arias, L. Pinello, Y. Katz, S. Shinagare, M. Abu-Remaileh, M. M. Mihaylova, D. W. Lamming, R. Dogum, G. Guo, G. W. Bell, M. Selig, G. P. Nielsen, N. Gupta, C. R. Ferrone, V. Deshpande, G.-C. Yuan, S. H. Orkin, D. M. Sabatini and Ö. H. Yilmaz (2016). "High-fat diet enhances stemness and tumorigenicity of intestinal progenitors." *Nature* **531**(7592): 53–58.

Bibbins-Domingo, K. (2016). "Aspirin use for the primary prevention of cardiovascular disease and colorectal cancer: U.S. preventive services task force recommendation statement." *Ann Intern Med* **164**(12): 836–845.

Blanpain, C. (2013). "Tracing the cellular origin of cancer." *Nature Cell Biology* **15**(2): 126–134.

Blokzijl, F., J. de Ligt, M. Jager, V. Sasselli, S. Roerink, N. Sasaki, M. Huch, S. Boymans, E. Kuijk, P. Prins, I. J. Nijman, I. Martincorena, M. Mokry, C. L. Wiegerinck, S. Middendorp, T. Sato, G. Schwank, E. E. Nieuwenhuis, M. M. Verstegen, L. J. van der Laan, J. de Jonge, I. J. JN, R. G. Vries, M. van de Wetering, M. R. Stratton, H. Clevers, E. Cuppen and R. van Boxtel (2016). "Tissue-specific mutation accumulation in human adult stem cells during life." *Nature* **538**(7624): 260–264.

Brazhnik, K., S. Sun, O. Alani, M. Kinkhabwala, A. W. Wolkoff, A. Y. Maslov, X. Dong and J. Vijg (2020). "Single-cell analysis reveals different age-related somatic mutation profiles between stem and differentiated cells in human liver." *Sci Adv* **6**(5): eaax2659.

Brown, J. R. and J. L. Thornton (1957). "Percivall Pott (1714-1788) and chimney sweepers' cancer of the scrotum." *Br J Ind Med* **14**(1): 68–70.

Bulteau, A. L., M. Moreau, C. Nizard and B. Friguet (2002). "Impairment of proteasome function upon UVA- and UVB-irradiation of human keratinocytes." *Free Radic Biol Med* **32**(11): 1157–1170.

Cantalupo, P. G., J. P. Katz and J. M. Pipas (2018). "Viral sequences in human cancer." *Virology* **513**: 208–216.

Carbone, M., S. T. Arron, B. Beutler, A. Bononi, W. Cavenee, J. E. Cleaver, C. M. Croce, A. D'Andrea, W. D. Foulkes, G. Gaudino, J. L. Groden, E. P. Henske, I. D. Hickson, P. M. Hwang, R. D. Kolodner, T. W. Mak, D. Malkin, R. J. Monnat, Jr., F. Novelli, H. I. Pass, J. H. Petrini, L. S. Schmidt and H. Yang (2020). "Tumour predisposition and cancer syndromes as models to study gene-environment interactions." *Nat Rev Cancer* **20**(9): 533–549.

Carvalho, A. S., M. S. Rodríguez and R. Matthiesen (2016). "Review and literature mining on proteostasis factors and cancer." *Methods Mol Biol* **1449**: 71–84.

Chabner, B. A. and T. G. Roberts, Jr. (2005). "Timeline: Chemotherapy and the war on cancer." *Nat Rev Cancer* **5**(1): 65–72.

Chen, F. and W. F. Bina (2012). "Correlation of white female breast cancer incidence trends with nitrogen dioxide emission levels and motor vehicle density patterns." *Breast Cancer Res Treat* **132**(1): 327–333.

Cheong, A., X. Zhang, Y. Y. Cheung, W. Y. Tang, J. Chen, S. H. Ye, M. Medvedovic, Y. K. Leung, G. S. Prins and S. M. Ho (2016). "DNA methylome changes by estradiol benzoate and bisphenol A links early-life environmental exposures to prostate cancer risk." *Epigenetics* **11**(9): 674–689.

Cohen, G., I. Levy, Yuval, J. D. Kark, N. Levin, G. Witberg, Z. Iakobishvili, T. Bental, D. M. Broday, D. M. Steinberg, R. Kornowski and Y. Gerber (2018). "Chronic exposure to traffic-related air pollution and cancer incidence among 10,000 patients undergoing percutaneous coronary interventions: A historical prospective study." *Eur J Prev Cardiol* **25**(6): 659–670.

Conrad, D. F., J. E. Keebler, M. A. DePristo, S. J. Lindsay, Y. Zhang, F. Casals, Y. Idaghdour, C. L. Hartl, C. Torroja, K. V. Garimella, M. Zilversmit, R. Cartwright, G. A. Rouleau, M. Daly, E. A. Stone, M. E. Hurles and P. Awadalla (2011). "Variation in genome-wide mutation rates within and between human families." *Nat Genet* **43**(7): 712–714.

Crouse, D. L., M. S. Goldberg, N. A. Ross, H. Chen and F. Labrèche (2010). "Postmenopausal breast cancer is associated with exposure to traffic-related air pollution in Montreal, Canada: A case-control study." *Environ Health Perspect* **118**(11): 1578–1583.

de Duve, C. (2005). "The onset of selection." *Nature* **433**(7026): 581–582.

de Marini, D. M. (2013). "Genotoxicity biomarkers associated with exposure to traffic and near-road atmospheres: a review." *Mutagenesis* **28**(5): 485–505.

Dhimolea, E., P. R. Wadia, T. J. Murray, M. L. Settles, J. D. Treitman, C. Sonnenschein, T. Shioda and A. M. Soto (2014). "Prenatal exposure to BPA alters the epigenome of the rat mammary gland and increases the propensity to neoplastic development." *PLoS One* **9**(7): e99800.

Doll, R. and A. B. Hill (1950). "Smoking and carcinoma of the lung; preliminary report." *Br Med J* **2**(4682): 739–748.

Doll, R. and A. B. Hill (1954). "The mortality of doctors in relation to their smoking habits: A preliminary report. 1954." *BMJ* **328**(7455): 1529–1533.

Doll, R., R. Peto, J. Boreham and I. Sutherland (2004). "Mortality in relation to smoking: 50 years' observations on male British doctors." *BMJ* **328**(7455): 1519.

Egusquiza, R. J. and B. Blumberg (2020). "Environmental obesogens and their impact on susceptibility to obesity: New mechanisms and chemicals." *Endocrinology* **161**(3): 1–14.

Fajersztajn, L., M. Veras, L. V. Barrozo and P. Saldiva (2013). "Air pollution: A potentially modifiable risk factor for lung cancer." *Nat Rev Cancer* **13**(9): 674–678.

Fitzmaurice, C., et al. (2018). "Global, regional, and national cancer incidence, mortality, years of life lost, years lived with disability, and disability-adjusted life-years for 29 cancer groups, 1990 to 2016: A systematic analysis for the global burden of disease study global burden of disease cancer collaboration." *JAMA Oncology* **4**(11): 1553–1568.

Flavahan, W. A., E. Gaskell and B. E. Bernstein (2017). "Epigenetic plasticity and the hallmarks of cancer." *Science* **357**(6348): eaal2380.

Forbes, S. A., D. Beare, P. Gunasekaran, K. Leung, N. Bindal, H. Boutselakis, M. Ding, S. Bamford, C. Cole, S. Ward, C. Y. Kok, M. Jia, T. De, J. W. Teague, M. R. Stratton, U. McDermott and P. J. Campbell (2015). "COSMIC: Exploring the world's knowledge of somatic mutations in human cancer." *Nucleic Acids Res* **43**(Database issue): D805–D811.

García-Pérez, J., V. Lope, G. López-Abente, M. González-Sánchez and P. Fernández-Navarro (2015). "Ovarian cancer mortality and industrial pollution." *Environ Pollut* **205**: 103–110.

Godtfredsen, N. S., E. Prescott and M. Osler (2005). "Effect of smoking reduction on lung cancer risk." *JAMA* **294**(12): 1505–1510.

Hemminki, K., A. Försti, M. Khyatti, W. A. Anwar and M. Mousavi (2014). "Cancer in immigrants as a pointer to the causes of cancer." *Eur J Public Health* **24**(Suppl 1): 64–71.

Ho, S. M., A. Cheong, H. M. Lam, W. Y. Hu, G. B. Shi, X. Zhu, J. Chen, X. Zhang, M. Medvedovic, Y. K. Leung and G. S. Prins (2015). "Exposure of human prostaspheres to bisphenol a epigenetically regulates SNORD family noncoding RNAs via histone modification." *Endocrinology* **156**(11): 3984–3995.

Hoang, M. L., C. H. Chen, V. S. Sidorenko, J. He, K. G. Dickman, B. H. Yun, M. Moriya, N. Niknafs, C. Douville, R. Karchin, R. J. Turesky, Y. S. Pu, B. Vogelstein, N. Papadopoulos, A. P. Grollman, K. W. Kinzler and T. A. Rosenquist (2013). "Mutational signature of aristolochic acid exposure as revealed by whole-exome sequencing." *Sci Transl Med* **5**(197): 197ra102.

Hoeijmakers, J. H. (2001). "Genome maintenance mechanisms for preventing cancer." *Nature* **411**(6835): 366–374.

Hsieh, T. H., C. F. Tsai, C. Y. Hsu, P. L. Kuo, J. N. Lee, C. Y. Chai, M. F. Hou, C. C. Chang, C. Y. Long, Y. C. Ko and E. M. Tsai (2012). "Phthalates stimulate the epithelial to mesenchymal transition through an HDAC6-dependent mechanism in human breast epithelial stem cells." *Toxicol Sci* **128**(2): 365–376.

Hu, W. Y., G. B. Shi, D. P. Hu, J. L. Nelles and G. S. Prins (2012). "Actions of estrogens and endocrine disrupting chemicals on human prostate stem/progenitor cells and prostate cancer risk." *Mol Cell Endocrinol* **354**(1–2): 63–73.

Jhuang, J. R., C. J. Chiang, S. Y. Su, Y. W. Yang and W. C. Lee (2019). "Reduction in the incidence of urological cancers after the ban on chinese herbal products containing aristolochic acid: An interrupted time-series analysis." *Sci Rep* **9**(1): 19860.

Jiricny, J. and M. Nyström-Lahti (2000). "Mismatch repair defects in cancer." *Curr Opin Genet Dev* **10**(2): 157–161.

Khan, K., E. Ahmed, P. Factor-Litvak, X. Liu, A. B. Siddique, G. A. Wasserman, V. Slavkovich, D. Levy, J. L. Mey, A. van Geen and J. H. Graziano (2015). "Evaluation of an elementary school-based educational intervention for reducing arsenic exposure in Bangladesh." *Environ Health Perspect* **123**(12): 1331–1336.

Kimmelman, A. C. and E. White (2017). "Autophagy and tumor metabolism." *Cell Metab* **25**(5): 1037–1043.

Kong, A., M. L. Frigge, G. Masson, S. Besenbacher, P. Sulem, G. Magnusson, S. A. Gudjonsson, A. Sigurdsson, A. Jonasdottir, A. Jonasdottir, W. S. Wong, G. Sigurdsson, G. B. Walters, S. Steinberg, H. Helgason, G. Thorleifsson, D. F. Gudbjartsson, A. Helgason, O. T. Magnusson, U. Thorsteinsdottir and K. Stefansson (2012). "Rate of de novo mutations and the importance of father's age to disease risk." *Nature* **488**(7412): 471–475.

Kopras, E., V. Potluri, M. L. Bermudez, K. Williams, S. Belcher and S. Kasper (2014). "Actions of endocrine-disrupting chemicals on stem/progenitor cells during development and disease." *Endocr Relat Cancer* **21**(2): T1–T12.

Kucab, J. E., X. Zou, S. Morganella, M. Joel, A. S. Nanda, E. Nagy, C. Gomez, A. Degasperi, R. Harris, S. P. Jackson, V. M. Arlt, D. H. Phillips and S. Nik-Zainal (2019). "A compendium of mutational signatures of environmental agents." *Cell* **177**(4): 821–836.e816.

Lambert, A. W., D. R. Pattabiraman and R. A. Weinberg (2017). "Emerging biological principles of metastasis." *Cell* **168**(4): 670–691.

Lambertz, I. U., L. Luo, T. R. Berton, S. L. Schwartz, S. D. Hursting, C. J. Conti and R. Fuchs-Young (2017). "Early exposure to a high fat/high sugar diet increases the mammary stem cell compartment and mammary tumor risk in female mice." *Cancer Prev Res (Phila)* **10**(10): 553–562.

Lee, H. W., S. H. Park, M. W. Weng, H. T. Wang, W. C. Huang, H. Lepor, X. R. Wu, L. C. Chen and M. S. Tang (2018). "E-cigarette smoke damages DNA and reduces repair activity in mouse lung, heart, and bladder as well as in human lung and bladder cells." *Proc Natl Acad Sci U S A* **115**(7): E1560–E1569.

Lichtenstein, P., N. V. Holm, P. K. Verkasalo, A. Iliadou, J. Kaprio, M. Koskenvuo, E. Pukkala, A. Skytthe and K. Hemminki (2000). "Environmental and heritable factors in the causation of cancer: Analyses of cohorts of twins from Sweden, Denmark, and Finland." *N Engl J Med* **343**(2): 78–85.

Lindahl, T. (1993). "Instability and decay of the primary structure of DNA." *Nature* **362**(6422): 709–715.

Loeb, L. A. and C. C. Harris (2008). "Advances in chemical carcinogenesis: A historical review and prospective." *Cancer Res* **68**(17): 6863–6872.

Loomis, D., Y. Grosse, B. Lauby-Secretan, F. El Ghissassi, V. Bouvard, L. Benbrahim-Tallaa, N. Guha, R. Baan, H. Mattock and K. Straif (2013). "The carcinogenicity of outdoor air pollution." *Lancet Oncol* **14**(13): 1262–1263.

López-Carrillo, L., R. U. Hernández-Ramírez, A. M. Calafat, L. Torres-Sánchez, M. Galván-Portillo, L. L. Needham, R. Ruiz-Ramos and M. E. Cebrián (2010). "Exposure to phthalates and breast cancer risk in Northern Mexico." *Environ Health Perspect* **118**(4): 539–544.

Margueron, R. and D. Reinberg (2010). "Chromatin structure and the inheritance of epigenetic information." *Nat Rev Genet* **11**(4): 285–296.

Martincorena, I. and P. J. Campbell (2015). "Somatic mutation in cancer and normal cells." *Science* **349**(6255): 1483–1489.

Martincorena, I., A. Roshan, M. Gerstung, P. Ellis, P. Van Loo, S. McLaren, D. C. Wedge, A. Fullam, L. B. Alexandrov, J. M. Tubio, L. Stebbings, A. Menzies, S. Widaa, M. R. Stratton, P. H. Jones and P. J. Campbell (2015). "High burden and pervasive positive selection of somatic mutations in normal human skin." *Science* **348**(6237): 880–886.

Martínez-Frías, M. L. (2010). "Can our understanding of epigenetics assist with primary prevention of congenital defects?" *J Med Genet* **47**(2): 73–80.

Marusyk, A., M. Janiszewska and K. Polyak (2020). "Intratumor heterogeneity: The Rosetta stone of therapy resistance." *Cancer Cell* **37**(4): 471–484.

Mazzio, E. A. and K. F. Soliman (2012). "Basic concepts of epigenetics: Impact of environmental signals on gene expression." *Epigenetics* **7**(2): 119–130.

Montévil, M., N. Acevedo, C. M. Schaeberle, M. Bharadwaj, S. E. Fenton and A. M. Soto (2020). "A combined morphometric and statistical approach to assess nonmonotonicity in the developing mammary gland of rats in the CLARITY-BPA study." *Environ Health Perspect* **128**(5): 57001.

Nowell, P. C. (1976). "The clonal evolution of tumor cell populations." *Science* **194**(4260): 23–28.

Park, H. M., H. Woo, S. J. Jung, K. W. Jung, H. R. Shin and A. Shin (2016). "Colorectal cancer incidence in 5 Asian countries by subsite: An analysis of cancer incidence in five continents (1998-2007)." *Cancer Epidemiol* **45**: 65–70.

Pesonen, M. and K. Vähäkangas (2019). "Autophagy in exposure to environmental chemicals." *Toxicol Lett* **305**: 1–9.

Prager, B. C., Q. Xie, S. Bao and J. N. Rich (2019). "Cancer stem cells: The architects of the tumor ecosystem." *Cell Stem Cell* **24**(1): 41–53.

Prins, G. S., W. Y. Hu, L. Xie, G. B. Shi, D. P. Hu, L. Birch and M. C. Bosland (2018). "Evaluation of Bisphenol A (BPA) exposures on prostate stem cell homeostasis and prostate cancer risk in the NCTR-Sprague-Dawley Rat: An NIEHS/FDA CLARITY-BPA consortium study." *Environ Health Perspect* **126**(11): 117001.

Qiang, L., A. Sample, C. R. Shea, K. Soltani, K. F. Macleod and Y. Y. He (2017). "Autophagy gene ATG7 regulates ultraviolet radiation-induced inflammation and skin tumorigenesis." *Autophagy* **13**(12): 2086–2103.

Revuelta, M. and A. Matheu (2017). "Autophagy in stem cell aging." *Aging Cell* **16**(5): 912–915.

Reya, T., S. J. Morrison, M. F. Clarke and I. L. Weissman (2001). "Stem cells, cancer, and cancer stem cells." *Nature* **414**(6859): 105–111.

Salamanca-Fernández, E., L. M. Iribarne-Durán, M. Rodríguez-Barranco, F. Vela-Soria, N. Olea, M. J. Sánchez-Pérez and J. P. Arrebola (2020). "Historical exposure to non-persistent environmental pollutants and risk of type 2 diabetes in a Spanish sub-cohort from the European prospective investigation into cancer and nutrition study." *Environ Res* **185**: 109383.

Sample, A. and Y. Y. He (2018). "Mechanisms and prevention of UV-induced melanoma." *Photodermatol Photoimmunol Photomed* **34**(1): 13–24.

Santana-Codina, N., J. D. Mancias and A. C. Kimmelman (2017). "The role of autophagy in cancer." *Annu Rev Cancer Biol* **1**: 19–39.

Seachrist, D. D., K. W. Bonk, S. M. Ho, G. S. Prins, A. M. Soto and R. A. Keri (2016). "A review of the carcinogenic potential of bisphenol A." *Reprod Toxicol* **59**: 167–182.

Shekarrizfard, M., M.-F. Valois, S. Weichenthal, M. S. Goldberg, M. Fallah-Shorshani, L. D. Cavellin, D. Crouse, M.-E. Parent and M. Hatzopoulou (2018). "Investigating the effects of multiple exposure measures to traffic-related air pollution on the risk of breast and prostate cancer." *J Transport Health* **11**: 34–46.

Shen, H. and P. W. Laird (2013). "Interplay between the cancer genome and epigenome." *Cell* **153**(1): 38–55.

Skinner, M. K. and C. Guerrero-Bosagna (2009). "Environmental signals and transgenerational epigenetics." *Epigenomics* **1**(1): 111–117.

Somers, C. M. (2011). "Ambient air pollution exposure and damage to male gametes: Human studies and in situ 'sentinel' animal experiments." *Syst Biol Reprod Med* **57**(1–2): 63–71.

Soundararajan, R., A. N. Paranjape, S. Maity, A. Aparicio and S. A. Mani (2018). "EMT, stemness and tumor plasticity in aggressive variant neuroendocrine prostate cancers." *Biochim Biophys Acta Rev Cancer* **1870**(2): 229–238.

Steele, C. B., C. C. Thomas, S. J. Henley, G. M. Massetti, D. A. Galuska, T. Agurs-Collins, M. Puckett and L. C. Richardson (2017). "Vital signs: Trends in incidence of cancers associated with overweight and obesity: United States, 2005-2014." *MMWR Morb Mortal Wkly Rep* **66**(39): 1052–1058.

Titus-Ernstoff, L., R. Troisi, E. E. Hatch, M. Hyer, L. A. Wise, J. R. Palmer, R. Kaufman, E. Adam, K. Noller, A. L. Herbst, W. Strohsnitter, B. F. Cole, P. Hartge and R. N. Hoover (2008). "Offspring of women exposed in utero to diethylstilbestrol (DES): A preliminary report of benign and malignant pathology in the third generation." *Epidemiology* **19**(2): 251–257.

Todoric, J., L. Antonucci and M. Karin (2016). "Targeting inflammation in cancer prevention and therapy." *Cancer Prev Res (Phila)* **9**(12): 895–905.

Tomasetti, C. and B. Vogelstein (2015). "Variation in cancer risk among tissues can be explained by the number of stem cell divisions." *Science* **347**(6217): 78–81.

Tomasetti, C., L. Li and B. Vogelstein (2017). "Stem cell divisions, somatic mutations, cancer etiology, and cancer prevention." *Science* **355**(6331): 1330–1334.

Turner, M. C., D. Krewski, W. R. Diver, C. A. Pope, R. T. Burnett, M. Jerrett, J. D. Marshall and S. M. Gapstur (2017). "Ambient air pollution and cancer mortality in the cancer prevention study II." *Environ Health Perspect* **125**(8): 087013.

Vaz, M., S. Y. Hwang, I. Kagiampakis, J. Phallen, A. Patil, H. M. O'Hagan, L. Murphy, C. A. Zahnow, E. Gabrielson, V. E. Velculescu, H. P. Easwaran and S. B. Baylin (2017). "Chronic cigarette smoke-induced epigenomic changes precede sensitization of bronchial epithelial cells to single-step transformation by KRAS mutations." *Cancer Cell* **32**(3): 360–376.e366.

Venkei, Z. G. and Y. M. Yamashita (2018). "Emerging mechanisms of asymmetric stem cell division." *J Cell Biol* **217**(11): 3785–3795.

Verellen, D., M. De Ridder, N. Linthout, K. Tournel, G. Soete and G. Storme (2007). "Innovations in image-guided radiotherapy." *Nat Rev Cancer* **7**(12): 949–960.

Vineis, P. and C. P. Wild (2014). "Global cancer patterns: Causes and prevention." *Lancet* **383**(9916): 549–557.

Vitale, I., G. Manic, R. De Maria, G. Kroemer and L. Galluzzi (2017). "DNA damage in stem cells." *Mol Cell* **66**(3): 306–319.

Vlachostergios, P. J., A. Patrikidou, D. D. Daliani and C. N. Papandreou (2009). "The ubiquitin-proteasome system in cancer, a major player in DNA repair. Part 1: Post-translational regulation." *J Cell Mol Med* **13**(9b): 3006–3018.

Wang, Q., L. S. Trevino, R. L. Wong, M. Medvedovic, J. Chen, S. M. Ho, J. Shen, C. E. Foulds, C. Coarfa, B. W. O'Malley, A. Shilatifard and C. L. Walker (2016). "Reprogramming of the epigenome by MLL1 links early-life environmental exposures to prostate cancer risk." *Mol Endocrinol* **30**(8): 856–871.

Wang, P. Y., J. Li, F. L. Walcott, J. G. Kang, M. F. Starost, S. L. Talagala, J. Zhuang, J. H. Park, R. D. Huffstutler, C. M. Bryla, P. L. Mai, M. Pollak, C. M. Annunziata, S. A. Savage, A. T. Fojo and P. M. Hwang (2017). "Inhibiting mitochondrial respiration prevents cancer in a mouse model of Li-Fraumeni syndrome." *J Clin Invest* **127**(1): 132–136.

Wang, H., Z. Gao, J. Ren, Y. Liu, L. T. Chang, K. Cheung, Y. Feng and Y. Li (2019). "An urban-rural and sex differences in cancer incidence and mortality and the relationship with PM(2.5) exposure: An ecological study in the southeastern side of Hu line." *Chemosphere* **216**: 766–773.

Watson, J. D. and F. H. Crick (1953). "Molecular structure of nucleic acids; a structure for deoxyribose nucleic acid." *Nature* **171**(4356): 737–738.

Wedel, S., M. Manola, M. Cavinato, I. P. Trougakos and P. Jansen-Dürr (2018). "Targeting protein quality control mechanisms by natural products to promote healthy ageing." *Molecules* **23**(5):1219.

Wei, W., L. Liu, J. Chen, K. Jin, F. Jiang, F. Liu, R. Fan, Z. Cheng, M. Shen, C. Xue, S. Cai, Y. Xu and P. Nan (2010). "Racial differences in MLH1 and MSH2 mutation: An analysis of yellow race and white race based on the InSiGHT database." *J Bioinform Comput Biol* **8** (Suppl 1): 111–125.

Weng, H. H., S. S. Tsai, H. F. Chiu, T. N. Wu and C. Y. Yang (2009). "Childhood leukemia and traffic air pollution in Taiwan: Petrol station density as an indicator." *J Toxicol Environ Health A* **72**(2): 83–87.

White, A. C. and W. E. Lowry (2015). "Refining the role for adult stem cells as cancer cells of origin." *Trends Cell Biol* **25**(1): 11–20.

Whitworth, K. W., E. Symanski and A. L. Coker (2008). "Childhood lymphohematopoietic cancer incidence and hazardous air pollutants in southeast Texas, 1995-2004." *Environ Health Perspect* **116**(11): 1576–1580.

Wu, S., S. Powers, W. Zhu and Y. A. Hannun (2016). "Substantial contribution of extrinsic risk factors to cancer development." *Nature* **529**(7584): 43–47.

Wu, S., W. Zhu, P. Thompson and Y. A. Hannun (2018). "Evaluating intrinsic and non-intrinsic cancer risk factors." *Nat Commun* **9**(1): 3490.

Xie, L., W. Y. Hu, D. P. Hu, G. Shi, Y. Li, J. Yang and G. S. Prins (2020). "Effects of inorganic arsenic on human prostate stem-progenitor cell transformation, autophagic flux blockade, and NRF2 pathway activation." *Environ Health Perspect* **128**(6): 67008.

Yang, Y. (2015). "Cancer immunotherapy: Harnessing the immune system to battle cancer." *J Clin Invest* **125**(9): 3335–3337.

Yilmaz, B., H. Terekeci, S. Sandal and F. Kelestimur (2020). "Endocrine disrupting chemicals: Exposure, effects on human health, mechanism of action, models for testing and strategies for prevention." *Rev Endocr Metab Disord* **21**(1): 127–147.

You, J. S. and P. A. Jones (2012). "Cancer genetics and epigenetics: Two sides of the same coin?" *Cancer Cell* **22**(1): 9–20.

Zhang, L. and J. Vijg (2018). "Somatic mutagenesis in mammals and its implications for human disease and aging." *Annu Rev Genet* **52**: 397–419.

Zhang, H., K. J. Menzies and J. Auwerx (2018). "The role of mitochondria in stem cell fate and aging." *Development* **145**(8): dev143420.

Zoeller, R. T., T. R. Brown, L. L. Doan, A. C. Gore, N. E. Skakkebaek, A. M. Soto, T. J. Woodruff and F. S. Vom Saal (2012). "Endocrine-disrupting chemicals and public health protection: A statement of principles from the endocrine society." *Endocrinology* **153**(9): 4097–4110.

22 Minority Health Disparities in Nutrition and Cancer

Keith C. Norris
David Geffen School of Medicine at UCLA

Bettina M. Beech
University of Houston College of Medicine

David Heber
UCLA Center for Human Nutrition

CONTENTS

INTRODUCTION

While overall cancer incidence and mortality for many forms of cancer have decreased in the United States, certain groups continue to be at increased risk of developing or dying from particular cancers. African Americans have higher death rates than all other groups for many, although not all, cancer types. African American women are much more likely than White women to die of breast cancer (Yedjou et al. 2019). African American women are nearly twice as likely as White women to be diagnosed with triple-negative breast cancer, which is more aggressive and harder to treat than other subtypes of breast cancer (Sharma 2016). African Americans are more than twice as likely as Whites to die of prostate cancer (McAllister 2019) and nearly twice as likely to die of stomach cancer (Klapheke, Carvajal-Carmona, and Cress 2019). Colorectal cancer incidence is higher in African Americans than in Whites despite an overall decreased in incidence among African Americans (Rogers et al. 2019). There are large differences among racial/ethnic groups in colorectal cancer screening rates, with Spanish-speaking Hispanics less likely to be screened than Whites or English-speaking Hispanics (Valdovinos et al. 2016, Wittich et al. 2019). Related biological and factors in the organizational framework of healthcare are associated with minority health disparities including many cancer disparities secondary to poverty, poor nutrition, obesity, and lack of quality medical care. Addressing these various factors is not simple, but requires a coordinated response by public health officials and political leaders (Alvidrez et al. 2019). Food insecurity is more common in minority populations and can lead to decreased intakes of protein, fruits, and vegetables being replaced by high fat and high sugar foods, which may play a factor in the increased incidence of obesity observed in minority populations contributing to an increased risk of many common forms of cancer (Johnson et al. 2018).

ORGANIZATIONAL FRAMEWORK

The overall health of communities including cancer-related risk factors is affected by the organizational framework of healthcare including social and economic factors, income, economic stability, education, built environment, and healthcare resources (Asare, Flannery, and Kamen 2017). Minority communities have a history of discrimination by the majority-dominated society which can lead to difficulty engaging with healthcare systems that have historically exploited minority communities (Mays, Cochran, and Barnes 2007). Lack of trust among minority populations has reduced their participation in research studies and clinical trials limiting access to some forms of therapy. Minority mistrust is based in part on historical precedents of discrimination, as well as unethical research experiments, such as the Tuskegee Syphilis Study (Alsan and Wanamaker 2018, Jaiswal and Halkitis 2019) that has resulted in reduced participation in clinical trials that may contribute to persistent health disparities in cancer prevention and treatment (Klabunde et al. 1999).

There are multiple factors that contribute to minority health disparities in nutrition and cancer: (1) Disparities in socioeconomic status including lower income, lower employment, higher expenses, and increased debt can have a negative impact on an individual's ability to access healthcare. In addition, poor living conditions can increase environmental and nutritional cancer risk factors (Stepanikova and Oates 2017). (2) Disparities in education can lead to low health literacy. As a result, individuals' ability to access, understand, and act on complex health information, communicate with health team members, and fully engage in healthcare decision making can impair cancer detection, prevention, and care (Purnell et al. 2016). (3) Disparities in the built environment and neighborhoods include the availability of transportation, safe and modem housing, safe walking paths and sidewalks, and other infrastructure elements. Lack of accessible and affordable transportation to doctors' appointments can restrict access to healthcare (Sarpel et al. 2018). (4) Disparities in the availability of health coverage and specialist healthcare providers, the quality of care and the cultural competency of healthcare providers across healthcare settings can also compromise an individual's cancer care (Baldwin et al. 2017). (5) Disparities in the psychosocial aspects of a community including social integration, community engagement, trust, and social support can affect the community response to prevention and detection efforts as well as the tendency to seek medical care early in the course of cancer (Harrison et al. 2019).

NUTRITION

Disparities in food access have been well-documented in minority communities across the United States (Bower et al. 2014, Larson, Story, and Nelson 2009). Low-income and minority communities tend to have more small convenience stores and liquor stores than predominantly White middle income communities. These stores sell mostly high-fat/high-sugar and energy-dense foods with little fresh produce or nutrient-dense foods (Cavanaugh et al. 2013, Zenk et al. 2006). There are also fewer supermarkets, which typically would carry a greater variety of nutritious food including colorful fruits and vegetables at lower prices than small convenience stores (Cannuscio et al. 2013). Low-income African American and Hispanic communities have the fewest supermarkets (Powell et al. 2007). These disparities in food access often described as "food deserts" contribute to an environment where healthy foods are both inaccessible and unaffordable for minority residents.

Healthy food access is associated with better population health (Thornton et al. 2016). Lower risks of heart disease and diabetes have been attributed to community level access to healthy food (Christine et al. 2015, Wing et al. 2016). Greater exposure to unhealthy foods is also associated with increased rates of overweight and obesity which can increase cancer risk (Feng et al. 2018).

Improving access to and consumption of healthy, safe, and affordable food and at the same time reducing access to and consumption of calorie-dense, nutrient-poor foods is a strategy that could reduce minority health disparities in cancer risk.

Low-income neighborhoods also have more pharmacies compared to those with lesser levels of poverty (Amstislavski et al. 2012). Snack foods are found for sale in almost all neighborhood pharmacies and community clinics were found to have substantially more packaged snacks, candy and sugar-sweetened beverages than commercial or hospital-based pharmacies (Whitehouse et al. 2012). Candy, sweetened beverages, salty snacks, and baked sweets were found in one survey near cash registers in 96% of pharmacies in this country (Farley et al. 2010).

Analyses of the availability of healthy food items were conducted among corner/small grocery stores, gas-marts, pharmacies, and dollar stores in 119 locations in Minneapolis and St. Paul, Minnesota, which were not participating in the Special Supplemental Nutrition Program for Women, Infants, and Children. Data from store inventories were used to examine the availability of 12 healthy food types used to develop an overall healthy food supply score. Interviews with 71 store managers assessed stocking practices and profitability (Caspi et al. 2016). Only corner/small grocery stores commonly sold fresh vegetables (63% vs. 8% of gas-marts, 0% of dollar stores, and 23% of pharmacies). More than half of managers stocking produce relied on cash-and-carry practices to stock fresh fruit (53%) and vegetables (55%), instead of direct store delivery. The store managers judged that healthy foods had average but not high profitability. So the least healthy snack foods and beverages were the most profitable items in these small stores.

The combination of increased access to both convenience stores and pharmacies observed in the lowest income census tracts may further expose low-income residents to abundant energy-dense, nutrient-poor foods (Ohri-Vachaspati et al. 2019).

OBESITY

The prevalence of obesity is significantly higher in ethnic minority, low-income, and lower socio-economic populations (Kumanyika 2019). Adverse social circumstances are caused by a deeper problem of systemic social dynamics that reduce opportunities for advancement (Bailey et al. 2017). Social inequities and reduced opportunity lead to a greater likelihood of living in poor-quality housing and in socially disadvantaged neighborhoods where there are limited options for healthy eating and physical activity as already reviewed above (Lovasi et al. 2009).

The age-adjusted prevalence of obesity in 2015–2016 demonstrated key differences in obesity among non-Hispanic Black men and women, and Hispanic men and women as well as non-Hispanic Asian men and women (Hales et al. 2017). Hispanic (47.0%) and non-Hispanic Black (46.8%) adults had a significantly higher prevalence of obesity than non-Hispanic White adults (37.9%). Among women, the prevalence of obesity was 38.0% in non-Hispanic White, 54.8% in non-Hispanic Black, 14.8% in non-Hispanic Asian, and 50.6% in Hispanic women. The prevalence of obesity in men was lower in non-Hispanic Asian adults (10.1%) compared with non-Hispanic White (37.9%), non-Hispanic Black (36.9%), and Hispanic (43.1%) men (see Figure 22.1).

Overweight and obesity are associated with increased death rates for all cancers combined and for cancers at multiple specific sites (Calle et al. 2003). It has been almost 20 years since the largest population study of obesity and cancer was completed and published in the New England Journal of Medicine. The study followed some 900,000 individuals over 21 years and found that in men and women, increased body-mass index was significantly associated with higher rates of death due to cancer of the esophagus, colon and rectum, liver, gallbladder, pancreas, and kidney. In addition, increased death rates due to non-Hodgkin's lymphoma and multiple myeloma were observed. There were significant trends for increased risk of higher body-mass-index values for death from cancers of the stomach and prostate in men and for death from cancers of the breast, uterus, cervix, and ovary in women. Based on these observations it was estimated that overweight and obesity in the United States could account for 14% of all deaths from cancer in men and 20% of those in women.

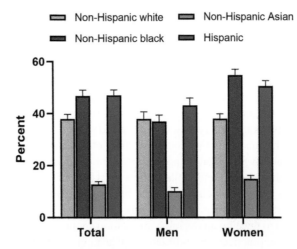

FIGURE 22.1 Age-adjusted prevalence of obesity among adults aged 20 and over, by sex and race and Hispanic origin: United States, 2015–2016 (Craig M. Hales 2017). Orange color: Significantly different from non-Hispanic Asian persons. Grey color: Significantly different from non-Hispanic white persons. Green color: Significantly different from Hispanic persons. Blue color: Significantly different from women of same race and Hispanic origin.

Therefore, the increased rates of obesity observed in minorities are a significant factor in minority health disparities linking nutrition and cancer.

OXIDATIVE STRESS

Racial disparities in cancer morbidity and mortality may be due in part to biological processes and these processes may interact with social and psychological factors to contribute to the observed disparities. Oxidative stress is central to initiation and progression of common forms of cancer. Oxidative stress contributes to the initiation of carcinogenesis and the promotion of tumor progression through increasing cell proliferation, chronic inflammation, DNA damage, and genomic instability. These processes are also associated with increased visceral abdominal fat in overweight and obese individuals. Therefore, oxidative stress and immune function are influenced by host factors that may explain minority health disparities in cancer. These host factors such as dietary behaviors, physical activity, and discrimination-based psychosocial stresses may result in biological effects independent of race (Bailey et al. 2017). African Americans demonstrated significantly greater levels of oxidative stress compared to Caucasian Americans after controlling for differences in inflammation and risk factors for cardiovascular disease (Morris et al. 2012). Stress secondary to racial discrimination has been associated with oxidative stress among African Americans as shown by greater red blood cell oxidative stress in a community-based study (Szanton et al. 2012). These observations suggest that racial disparities in cancer may be in part due to differences in oxidative stress as a result of psychosocial and behavioral stressors leading ultimately to biological processes that mediate minority health disparities in nutrition and cancer.

GENOMICS

Breast cancer is the most common form of cancer affecting women of all racial/ethnic groups in the United States. Protein expression of estrogen receptors (ER), progesterone receptors (PR), and human epidermal growth factor 2 (HER2) detected by standard immunohistochemical methods has been used to identify the gene expression subtypes in patient specimens. Triple negative (TN) breast cancer (ER–, PR–, HER2–) overlaps with basal cancer, ER-positive cancers closely define luminal cancers, and the ER-negative, PR-negative, and HER+ cancers approximate the HER2-expressing subtype. The incidence of basal-like breast cancer or TN breast cancer in Black women especially at younger ages is twice the incidence observed in White women (Yedjou et al. 2019). Compared to other subtypes of breast cancer, these are high-grade tumors which are also an aggressive subtype of breast cancer.

There are a number of possible biological properties of TN breast tumors related to the disparity between Black women and White women that could influence breast cancer treatment outcomes between the two ethnic groups. TN tumors have marked genomic instability with the highest average frequency of genome-wide copy number alterations (both increases and decreases in copy number) compared to the other breast cancer subtypes (Loo et al. 2011). These tumors commonly express high-molecular-weight basal cytokeratins (cytokeratin 5/6, cytokeratin 14, and cytokeratin 17), epidermal growth factor receptor, vimentin, p-cadherin, αB-crystallin, fascin, and caveolins 1 and 2 (Reis-Filho and Tutt 2008). There is research proceeding to further understand the heterogeneity observed in TN breast cancers in an attempt to define potential targeted treatments.

African American men are at higher risk for developing prostate cancer and experience higher death rates as compared to other ethnic groups. African American men have 1.7 times higher incidence, and 2.4 times higher mortality rate than Caucasian men (DeSantis et al. 2016). Prostate cancer demonstrates genetic susceptibility markers identified from family-based studies, candidate gene association studies, and genome-wide association studies. Replication of susceptibility loci across race, ethnicity, and geography has been very limited due to the low numbers of African American men included in large-scale genomic studies.

Even after adjusting for the effects of socioeconomic factors, significant minority disparities in the incidence and mortality rates of common forms of cancer remain, suggesting other social determinants and/or a contribution from molecular and genetic factors which may interact with environmental and lifestyle factors. An observed higher prevalence of well-known oncogenic mutations in just four genes; BRAF, NRAS, HRAS, and LKB1 mutations were detected in 90% (47 of 52 patients) of East Asian nonsmoking females with lung adenocarcinomas. Careful genomic testing and targeted therapies in these patients could lead to better overall survival (Sun et al. 2010).

To address the lack of minority representation in genetic research and cancer trials, the National Institutes of Health developed Policy and Guidelines on Inclusion of Women and Minority as Subjects in Clinical Research (Knerr, Wayman, and Bonham 2011). Hopefully, this will lead to large cohort studies using next generation sequencing to identify more targets of therapy especially useful in reducing minority health disparities in cancer prevention and treatment.

CANCER INCIDENCE

African Americans have the highest death rate and shortest survival of any racial or ethnic group for most cancers. There are many complex reasons for these minority health disparities reflecting social and economic disparities to a greater extent than biological differences. As documented by the American Cancer Society, 26% of Blacks compared with 10% of non-Hispanic Whites were living below the federal poverty level in 2014 (DeSantis et al. 2016). Minorities as outlined above have fewer opportunities for physical activity and less access to fresh fruits and vegetables both of which are associated with reduced cancer risks. At the same time, the incidence of obesity is greater in minorities and obesity is associated with a number of common forms of cancer.

Prostate cancer is expected to be the most commonly diagnosed cancer in Africa American men, and breast cancer is expected to be the most commonly diagnosed cancer in African American women as last estimated in 2016 (DeSantis et al. 2016). Lung cancer and colorectal cancer follow as the second and third most common forms of cancer in Africa-American men and Black women. In sum, the four most common forms of cancer account for more than half of all cancer cases.

The incidence of cancer increased in African Americans from the 1970s to the early 1990s. From 2003 to 2012, incidence rates decreased by 2% per year in Black males but remained stable in females, similar to the pattern in non-Hispanic Caucasians. The declines in cancer cases among men were largely explained by reduced incidences of lung cancer and prostate cancer.

Hispanics represent the largest ethnic minority group in the United States and accounted for 17.4% of the American population in 2014 (Siegel et al. 2015). The majority of Hispanics are of Mexican origin (64.3%), followed by Puerto Rican (9.5%), Salvadoran (3.7%), Cuban (3.7%), and Dominican (3.1%). Interestingly, Hispanics have a 20% lower overall incidence of cancers and 30% lower death rates compared with non-Hispanic Caucasians, despite having a higher incidence of obesity and diabetes than the non-Hispanic Caucasian population (Health United States 2018, 2019). Even with a lower cancer death rate than other populations, cancer is the leading cause of death (Heron 2019) among American Hispanics. There is some variation among Hispanics with Mexican Hispanics having the lowest cancer rates except for cancers secondary to infections. The challenge for reducing cancer risk in Hispanic populations includes increasing the acceptance and utilization of preventive screening and targeted interventions to reduce obesity, tobacco use, and alcohol consumption.

In a recent study in San Francisco, US-born Asian American women had a lower risk of breast cancer than American women (Morey et al. 2019). It has been established by many studies that breast cancer incidence rates are four to seven times greater in the United States than in China or Japan. When Asian women migrate to the United States, their breast cancer risk rises over several generations. Asian immigrants who had lived in California for a decade or more had an 80% increased risk of breast cancer compared to more recent immigrants. These observations are consistent with the concept that Western diet, lifestyles, and environmental exposures increase breast cancer risk in women of Asian origin.

Ongoing surveillance of cancer rates in minority populations is critical to the evolution of methods of addressing minority health disparities in nutrition and cancer.

HEALTH WORKERS

Community health workers who are trained and culturally sensitive can link patients and healthcare providers in order to reduce healthcare disparities (Albarran, Heilemann, and Koniak-Griffin 2014). Patient navigators, community health workers, outreach workers, promotoras, lay health educators, health advocates, peer counselors, or in some cases medical assistants can all serve this key role in reducing minority disparities (Hurtado et al. 2014). Unlike physicians and nurses, community health navigators do not provide any healthcare services directly, but rather offer culturally specific educational and support services to patients that can aid communication between patients and physicians and guide patients in overcoming barriers to obtaining appropriate cancer screening and care. As the cost of cancer diagnosis and treatment continues to rise, many patients are faced with significant financial burdens. Community healthcare workers can guide patients through many aspects of care and are often considerate of the financial distresses caused by a cancer diagnosis. These healthcare workers can also establish support groups for cancer patients which can provide further help with adopting diet and lifestyle changes that could impact cancer prevention and treatment concerns.

CONCLUSION

Numerous scientific advances in cancer diagnosis and treatment have improved outcomes in the overall population, but racial and ethnic minorities, underprivileged, and lower socioeconomic populations continue to have increased incidences and poorer cancer outcomes resulting in minority health disparities in nutrition and cancer (Polite et al. 2017). Collaborative approaches involving public health experts, oncology researchers, and nutrition scientists have the opportunity to address minority health disparities in nutrition and cancer. Improving community conditions could make a difference in improving health outcomes (Yelton et al. 2020). Building healthy communities requires involving community stakeholders and local resources such as schools, hospitals, recreational facilities, retail outlets, and housing. Healthier communities with health-promoting environments such as parks, safe walking spaces, maintained homes, full-service food stores, and environmental protection are likely to result in reduced cancer risk among minority populations (Alcaraz et al. 2020, Williams, Mohammed, and Shields 2016). Policy initiatives in a community setting include improved economic opportunity, higher quality schools, local businesses offering healthier foods, more open green space, and effective community policing (Alcaraz et al. 2020). Cancer and nutrition-coordinated healthcare that addresses the behaviors that increase cancer risk and emphasize adherence to screening and treatment as well as addressing the cultural aspects of cancer prevention and treatment in minority populations.

REFERENCES

Alcaraz, K. I., T. L. Wiedt, E. C. Daniels, K. R. Yabroff, C. E. Guerra, and R. C. Wender. 2020. "Understanding and addressing social determinants to advance cancer health equity in the United States: A blueprint for practice, research, and policy." *CA Cancer J Clin* 70 (1):31–46. doi: 10.3322/caac.21586.

Alsan, M., and M. Wanamaker. 2018. "Tuskegee and the health of black men." *Q J Econ* 133 (1):407–455. doi: 10.1093/qje/qjx029.

Alvidrez, J., D. Castille, M. Laude-Sharp, A. Rosario, and D. Tabor. 2019. "The national institute on minority health and health disparities research framework." *Am J Public Health* 109 (S1):S16–S20. doi: 10.2105/AJPH.2018.304883.

Amstislavski, P., A. Matthews, S. Sheffield, A. R. Maroko, and J. Weedon. 2012. "Medication deserts: Survey of neighborhood disparities in availability of prescription medications." *Int J Health Geogr* 11:48. doi: 10.1186/1476-072X-11-48.

Asare, M., M. Flannery, and C. Kamen. 2017. "Social determinants of health: A framework for studying cancer health disparities and minority participation in research." *Oncol Nurs Forum* 44 (1):20–23. doi: 10.1188/17.ONF.20-23.

Bailey, Z. D., N. Krieger, M. Agenor, J. Graves, N. Linos, and M. T. Bassett. 2017. "Structural racism and health inequities in the USA: Evidence and interventions." *Lancet* 389 (10077):1453–1463. doi: 10.1016/S0140-6736(17)30569-X.

Baldwin, M. R., J. L. Sell, N. Heyden, A. Javaid, D. A. Berlin, W. C. Gonzalez, P. B. Bach, M. S. Maurer, G. S. Lovasi, and D. J. Lederer. 2017. "Race, ethnicity, health insurance, and mortality in older survivors of critical illness." *Crit Care Med* 45 (6):e583–e591. doi: 10.1097/CCM.0000000000002313.

Bower, K. M., R. J. Thorpe, Jr., C. Rohde, and D. J. Gaskin. 2014. "The intersection of neighborhood racial segregation, poverty, and urbanicity and its impact on food store availability in the United States." *Prev Med* 58:33–9 doi: 10.1016/j.ypmed.2013.10.010.

Calle, E. E., C. Rodriguez, K. Walker-Thurmond, and M. J. Thun. 2003. "Overweight, obesity, and mortality from cancer in a prospectively studied cohort of U.S. adults." *N Engl J Med* 348 (17):1625–38. doi: 10.1056/NEJMoa021423.

Cannuscio, C. C., K. Tappe, A. Hillier, A. Buttenheim, A. Karpyn, and K. Glanz. 2013. "Urban food environments and residents' shopping behaviors." *Am J Prev Med* 45 (5):606–14. doi: 10.1016/j.amepre.2013.06.021.

Caspi, C. E., J. E. Pelletier, L. Harnack, D. J. Erickson, and M. N. Laska. 2016. "Differences in healthy food supply and stocking practices between small grocery stores, gas-marts, pharmacies and dollar stores." *Public Health Nutr* 19 (3):540–7. doi: 10.1017/S1368980015002724.

Cavanaugh, E., G. Mallya, C. Brensinger, A. Tierney, and K. Glanz. 2013. "Nutrition environments in corner stores in Philadelphia." *Prev Med* 56 (2):149–51. doi: 10.1016/j.ypmed.2012.12.007.

Christine, P. J., A. H. Auchincloss, A. G. Bertoni, M. R. Carnethon, B. N. Sanchez, K. Moore, S. D. Adar, T. B. Horwich, K. E. Watson, and A. V. Diez Roux. 2015. "Longitudinal associations between neighborhood physical and social environments and incident type 2 diabetes mellitus: The multi-ethnic study of atherosclerosis (MESA)." *JAMA Int Med* 175 (8):1311–20. doi: 10.1001/jamainternmed.2015.2691.

DeSantis, C. E., R. L. Siegel, A. G. Sauer, K. D. Miller, S. A. Fedewa, K. I. Alcaraz, and A. Jemal. 2016. "Cancer statistics for African Americans, 2016: Progress and opportunities in reducing racial disparities." *CA Cancer J Clin* 66 (4):290–308. doi: 10.3322/caac.21340.

Farley, T. A., E. T. Baker, L. Futrell, and J. C. Rice. 2010. "The ubiquity of energy-dense snack foods: A national multicity study." *Am J Public Health* 100 (2):306–11. doi: 10.2105/AJPH.2009.178681.

Feng, X., T. Astell-Burt, H. Badland, S. Mavoa, and B. Giles-Corti. 2018. "Modest ratios of fast food outlets to supermarkets and green grocers are associated with higher body mass index: Longitudinal analysis of a sample of 15,229 Australians aged 45 years and older in the Australian National Liveability Study." *Health Place* 49:101–110 doi: 10.1016/j.healthplace.2017.10.004.

Hales, C. M., M. D. Carroll, C. D. Fryar, and C. L. Ogden. 2017. "Prevalence of obesity among adults and youth: United States, 2015–2016." *NCHS Data Brief* no. 288:1–8.

Harrison, R., M. Walton, A. Chauhan, E. Manias, U. Chitkara, M. Latanik, and D. Leone. 2019. "What is the role of cultural competence in ethnic minority consumer engagement? An analysis in community healthcare." *Int J Equity Health* 18 (1):191. doi: 10.1186/s12939-019-1104-1.

Health United States 2018. 2019. National Center for Health Statistics. Hyattsville, MD.

Heron, M. 2019. *Deaths: Leading Causes for 2017*, National Vital Statistics Reports. Hyattsville, MD: National Center for Health Statistics.

Jaiswal, J., and P. N. Halkitis. 2019. "Towards a more inclusive and dynamic understanding of medical mistrust informed by science." *Behav Med* 45 (2):79–85. doi: 10.1080/08964289.2019.1619511.

Johnson, C. M., J. R. Sharkey, M. J. Lackey, L. S. Adair, A. E. Aiello, S. K. Bowen, W. Fang, V. L. Flax, and A. S. Ammerman. 2018. "Relationship of food insecurity to women's dietary outcomes: A systematic review." *Nutr Rev* 76 (12):910–928. doi: 10.1093/nutrit/nuy042.

Klabunde, C. N., B. C. Springer, B. Butler, M. S. White, and J. Atkins. 1999. "Factors influencing enrollment in clinical trials for cancer treatment." *South Med J* 92 (12):1189–93. doi: 10.1097/00007611-199912000-00011.

Klapheke, A. K., L. G. Carvajal-Carmona, and R. D. Cress. 2019. "Racial/ethnic differences in survival among gastric cancer patients in California." *Cancer Causes Control* 30 (7):687–696. doi: 10.1007/s10552-019-01184-0.

Knerr, S., D. Wayman, and V. L. Bonham. 2011. "Inclusion of racial and ethnic minorities in genetic research: Advance the spirit by changing the rules?" *J Law Med Ethics* 39 (3):502–12. doi: 10.1111/j.1748-720X.2011.00617.x.

Kumanyika, S. K. 2019. "A framework for increasing equity impact in obesity prevention." *Am J Public Health* 109 (10):1350–7. doi: 10.2105/AJPH.2019.305221.

Larson, N. I., M. T. Story, and M. C. Nelson. 2009. "Neighborhood environments: Disparities in access to healthy foods in the U.S." *Am J Prev Med* 36 (1):74–81. doi: 10.1016/j.amepre.2008.09.025.

Loo, L. W., Y. Wang, E. M. Flynn, M. J. Lund, E. J. Bowles, D. S. Buist, J. M. Liff, E. W. Flagg, R. J. Coates, J. W. Eley, L. Hsu, and P. L. Porter. 2011. "Genome-wide copy number alterations in subtypes of invasive breast cancers in young white and African American women." *Breast Cancer Res Treat* 127 (1):297–308. doi: 10.1007/s10549-010-1297-x.

Lovasi, G. S., M. A. Hutson, M. Guerra, and K. M. Neckerman. 2009. "Built environments and obesity in disadvantaged populations." *Epidemiol Rev* 31:7–20 doi: 10.1093/epirev/mxp005.

Mays, V. M., S. D. Cochran, and N. W. Barnes. 2007. "Race, race-based discrimination, and health outcomes among African Americans." *Annu Rev Psychol* 58:201–25 doi: 10.1146/annurev.psych.57.102904.190212.

McAllister, B. J. 2019. "The association between ethnic background and prostate cancer." *Br J Nurs* 28 (18):S4–S10. doi: 10.12968/bjon.2019.28.18.S4.

Morris, A. A., L. Zhao, R. S. Patel, D. P. Jones, Y. Ahmed, N. Stoyanova, G. H. Gibbons, V. Vaccarino, R. Din-Dzietham, and A. A. Quyyumi. 2012. "Differences in systemic oxidative stress based on race and the metabolic syndrome: The Morehouse and Emory Team up to Eliminate Health Disparities (META-Health) study." *Metab Syndr Relat Disord* 10 (4):252–9. doi: 10.1089/met.2011.0117.

Ohri-Vachaspati, P., R. S. DeWeese, F. Acciai, D. DeLia, D. Tulloch, D. Tong, C. Lorts, and M. Yedidia. 2019. "Healthy food access in low-income high-minority communities: A longitudinal assessment-2009–2017." *Int J Environ Res Public Health* 16 (13). doi: 10.3390/ijerph16132354.

Polite, B. N., L. L. Adams-Campbell, O. W. Brawley, N. Bickell, J. M. Carethers, C. R. Flowers, M. Foti, S. L. Gomez, J. J. Griggs, C. S. Lathan, C. I. Li, J. L. Lichtenfeld, W. McCaskill-Stevens, and E. D. Paskett. 2017. "Charting the future of cancer health disparities research: A position statement from the American Association for Cancer research, the American Cancer Society, the American Society of Clinical Oncology, and the National Cancer Institute." *J Clin Oncol* 35 (26):3075–82. doi: 10.1200/JCO.2017.73.6546.

Powell, L. M., S. Slater, D. Mirtcheva, Y. Bao, and F. J. Chaloupka. 2007. "Food store availability and neighborhood characteristics in the United States." *Prev Med* 44 (3):189–95. doi: 10.1016/j.ypmed.2006.08.008.

Purnell, T. S., E. A. Calhoun, S. H. Golden, J. R. Halladay, J. L. Krok-Schoen, B. M. Appelhans, and L. A. Cooper. 2016. "Achieving health equity: Closing the gaps in health care disparities, interventions, and research." *Health Aff (Millwood)* 35 (8):1410–5. doi: 10.1377/hlthaff.2016.0158.

Reis-Filho, J. S., and A. N. Tutt. 2008. "Triple negative tumours: A critical review." *Histopathology* 52 (1):108–18. doi: 10.1111/j.1365-2559.2007.02889.x.

Rogers, C. R., K. Okuyemi, E. D. Paskett, R. J. Thorpe, Jr., T. N. Rogers, M. Hung, S. Zickmund, C. Riley, and M. D. Fetters. 2019. "Study protocol for developing #CuttingCRC: A barbershop-based trial on masculinity barriers to care and colorectal cancer screening uptake among African-American men using an exploratory sequential mixed-methods design." *BMJ Open* 9 (7):e030000. doi: 10.1136/bmjopen-2019-030000.

Sarpel, U., X. Huang, C. Austin, and F. Gany. 2018. "Barriers to care in chinese immigrants with hepatocellular carcinoma: A focus group study in New York City." *J Community Health* 43 (6):1161–71. doi: 10.1007/s10900-018-0536-7.

Sharma, P. 2016. "Biology and management of patients with triple-negative breast cancer." *Oncologist* 21 (9):1050–62. doi: 10.1634/theoncologist.2016-0067.

Stepanikova, I., and G. R. Oates. 2017. "Perceived discrimination and privilege in health care: The role of socioeconomic status and race." *Am J Prev Med* 52 (1S1):S86–S94. doi: 10.1016/j.amepre.2016.09.024.

Sun, Y., Y. Ren, Z. Fang, C. Li, R. Fang, B. Gao, X. Han, W. Tian, W. Pao, H. Chen, and H. Ji. 2010. "Lung adenocarcinoma from East Asian never-smokers is a disease largely defined by targetable oncogenic mutant kinases." *J Clin Oncol* 28 (30):4616–20. doi: 10.1200/JCO.2010.29.6038.

Szanton, S. L., J. M. Rifkind, J. G. Mohanty, E. R. Miller, 3rd, R. J. Thorpe, E. Nagababu, E. S. Epel, A. B. Zonderman, and M. K. Evans. 2012. "Racial discrimination is associated with a measure of red blood cell oxidative stress: A potential pathway for racial health disparities." *Int J Behav Med* 19 (4):489–95. doi: 10.1007/s12529-011-9188-z.

Thornton, R. L., C. M. Glover, C. W. Cene, D. C. Glik, J. A. Henderson, and D. R. Williams. 2016. "Evaluating strategies for reducing health disparities by addressing the social determinants of health." *Health Aff (Millwood)* 35 (8):1416–23. doi: 10.1377/hlthaff.2015.1357.

Valdovinos, C., F. J. Penedo, C. R. Isasi, M. Jung, R. C. Kaplan, R. E. Giacinto, P. Gonzalez, V. L. Malcarne, K. Perreira, H. Salgado, M. A. Simon, L. M. Wruck, and H. A. Greenlee. 2016. "Perceived discrimination and cancer screening behaviors in US Hispanics: The Hispanic Community Health Study/Study of Latinos Sociocultural Ancillary Study." *Cancer Causes Control* 27 (1):27–37. doi: 10.1007/s10552-015-0679-0.

Whitehouse, A., A. Simon, S. A. French, and J. Wolfson. 2012. "Availability of snacks, candy and beverages in hospital, community clinic and commercial pharmacies." *Public Health Nutr* 15 (6):1117–23. doi: 10.1017/S1368980011003600.

Williams, D. R., S. A. Mohammed, and A. E. Shields. 2016. "Understanding and effectively addressing breast cancer in African American women: Unpacking the social context." *Cancer* 122 (14):2138–49. doi: 10.1002/cncr.29935.

Wing, J. J., E. August, S. D. Adar, A. L. Dannenberg, A. Hajat, B. N. Sanchez, J. H. Stein, M. C. Tattersall, and A. V. Diez Roux. 2016. "Change in neighborhood characteristics and change in coronary artery calcium: A longitudinal investigation in the MESA (multi-ethnic study of atherosclerosis) cohort." *Circulation* 134 (7):504–13. doi: 10.1161/CIRCULATIONAHA.115.020534.

Wittich, A. R., L. A. Shay, B. Flores, E. M. De La Rosa, T. Mackay, and M. A. Valerio. 2019. "Colorectal cancer screening: Understanding the health literacy needs of hispanic rural residents." *AIMS Public Health* 6 (2):107–120. doi: 10.3934/publichealth.2019.2.107.

Yedjou, C. G., J. N. Sims, L. Miele, F. Noubissi, L. Lowe, D. D. Fonseca, R. A. Alo, M. Payton, and P. B. Tchounwou. 2019. "Health and racial disparity in breast cancer." *Adv Exp Med Biol* 1152:31–49 doi: 10.1007/978-3-030-20301-6_3.

Yelton, B., H. M. Brandt, S. A. Adams, J. R. Ureda, J. R. Lead, D. Fedrick, K. Lewis, S. Kulkarni, and D. B. Friedman. 2020. ""Talk about cancer and build healthy communities": How visuals are starting the conversation about breast cancer within African-American communities." *Int Q Community Health Educ.* doi: 10.1177/0272684X20942076.

Zenk, S. N., A. J. Schulz, B. A. Israel, S. A. James, S. Bao, and M. L. Wilson. 2006. "Fruit and vegetable access differs by community racial composition and socioeconomic position in Detroit, Michigan." *Ethn Dis* 16 (1):275–80.

23 The Critical Questions on Nutrition and Cancer That Remain

David Heber and Zhaoping Li
UCLA Center for Human Nutrition

CONTENTS

INTRODUCTION

The dual and co-existing nutrition science and genetic oncology revolutions including the discovery of the microbiome, diet, and nutrient interactions at the genetic, epigenetic, endocrine, and metabolic levels have created new challenges and opportunities for researchers, clinicians, and other healthcare providers to contribute to the fusion of these separate fields in new research initiatives. Ultimately, the translation of insights gleaned from basic and epidemiological research on nutrition and cancer into real benefits for people requires clinical investigation.

Clinical investigations of many of the most interesting hypotheses raised by epidemiological and basic research with regard to nutrition and cancer have been hampered by many factors characteristic of nutritional intervention studies in general. These challenges include lack of adherence to diet and difficulties in monitoring dietary intake and physical activities in free-living populations.

Added to these complexities in nutrition and cancer intervention studies is the heterogeneous nature of the cancer biology making generalization difficult. Better biomarkers of cancer that can be used earlier in the course of cancer and metastasis such as cell-free DNA will aid in research on nutrition and cancer, but improved methods of monitoring dietary intake, body composition, and physical activity are also critical to future progress. The lack of ethnic and racial diversity in many cancer studies also limits the generalizability of research findings to the growing immigrant and minority communities as well as for those living in the developing world.

Nutrients modulate gene expression and changes in gene expression affect nutrition and metabolism. Complex interactions at a genetic and epigenetic level which can be heritable and modified by nutrients, diet, and lifestyle can affect the risk for developing many age-related chronic diseases including cancer. Some studies have related the metabolic abnormalities characteristic of the global epidemics of type 2 diabetes and obesity to increased risks of cancer demonstrating the potential impact of widespread changes in nutrition through public health and agriculture and food production in cancer prevention (Gallagher and LeRoith 2015).

Nutrients have been shown to affect DNA methylation, histone modifications, and gene silencing in association with an increased or decreased risk for cancer (Sapienza and Issa 2016). Evidence from population studies clearly indicates that dietary patterns, foods, and nutrients are associated with anticancer effects including reduced tumor progression (Steck and Murphy 2020). Basic research has demonstrated the important role of angiogenesis and modifications of the tumor microenvironment including effects on immune cells (Ramjiawan, Griffioen, and Duda 2017). Immunotherapy and the discovery of the role of the gut microflora in modulating immune function have provided new opportunities for nutrition in cancer prevention and treatment research (Gopalakrishnan et al. 2018). Precision Oncology has revolutionized cancer diagnosis and treatment (Saadeh, Bright, and Rustem 2019) in parallel to increased research in Personalized Nutrition demonstrating the individual variability in postprandial glucose responses to the same food or nutrient (Zeevi et al. 2015). While nutritional intakes from foods cannot be adequately controlled through simple public health advice, the role of nutrients in the biology of tumor growth and progression has led to more research aimed at developing novel dietary supplements and botanicals as adjuncts to cancer prevention and treatment (Vernieri et al. 2018).

It is clear that nutrition and cancer research has moved a long way from its initial focus on nutritional deficiencies associated with cancer cachexia to considerations at the heart of public health nutrition research. However, the challenges around cancer cachexia remain to be solved. In Public Health Nutrition, similarly, the challenge remains of translating information on nutrition and cancer into simple and accessible policy advice and programs that can aid in the prevention and treatment of common forms of cancer (Di Sebastiano et al. 2019).

A new generation of clinical studies can combine Precision Oncology and Personalized Nutrition in order to develop the insights needed to engage nutrition as a tool to be used not only in cancer prevention but hopefully also in cancer treatment and relapse prevention. This chapter will review the most promising areas of future research to address the critical questions that remain in nutrition and cancer.

OBESITY AND INFLAMMATION

Obesity is often referred to as the elephant in the room, meaning that we know obesity exists within the population of cancer patients and is associated with the cause and in some cases the outcome of common forms of cancer, but it remains unrecognized and inconsistently approached in research and practice. Cancer patients are generally lumped together in research on treatment options with the exception of dose adjustments for body size and some recognition that achieving a healthy body weight may be helpful in cancer survivors especially in breast cancer and prostate cancer (Park et al. 2014, Avgerinos et al. 2019, Kolb, Sutterwala, and Zhang 2016).

What remains to be done is to examine the effects of obesity and excess adiposity on the course of disease and the effects of weight management on response to cancer therapy and cancer prevention interventions. Given the common and growing incidence of obesity in the United States and globally, the metabolic effects of excess body fat and inflammation secondary to excess fat in the abdomen and other ectopic sites including breast fat and periprostatic fat may affect carcinogenesis, tumor progression, and cancer recurrence.

Inflammation associated with excess obesity especially in abdominal fat can affect immune function systemically by infiltrating adipose tissue (Han and Levings 2013). Macrophages enter white adipose tissue under conditions of excess abdominal fat and stimulate the release of inflammatory cytokines locally and systemically (Weisberg et al. 2003). Fat cells are endocrine cells and immune cells in their function (Sun, Kusminski, and Scherer 2011). They release chemokines, including CCL2, CCL3, and RANTES/CCL5 that attract macrophages as part of the innate immune response. As adipocytes grow rapidly in abdominal fat and other depots, they can outgrow the blood supplied by angiogenesis leading to fat cell death and the release of free fatty acids and other cell debris providing an enhanced signal to recruit macrophages to digest and remove dead adipocytes and further stimulating local and systemic inflammation.

Adipocytes in the microenvironment of cancer cells can contribute to tumor cell growth and metastasis. Studies in breast tumors have demonstrated that adipocytes at the junction of stroma and tumor cells convert to a phenotype resembling fibroblasts that can promote tumor invasion locally through release of protease enzymes and proinflammatory cytokines (Yang et al. 2015, Bochet et al. 2013). As a result, dense stroma filled with collagen forms a stiff extracellular matrix. The attraction, migration, and invasion of ovarian cancer cells to the omentum where ovarian cancer cells most commonly metastasize is promoted by omental fat cell secretion of cytokines including interleukin (IL)-6 and IL-8 (Nieman et al. 2011). The free fatty acids released from omental fat cells through lipolysis are potential energy source for ovarian metastatic tumor cells. Periprostatic fat cells release the chemokine CCL7, which diffuses from this local fat depot to the peripheral zone of the prostate gland where it stimulates the migration of CCR3 expressing prostate cancer cells leading to local spread of prostate cancer (Laurent et al. 2016) in common with other tumors the stromal vascular fraction which makes up the bulk of the prostate gland contributes to tumor growth. These stromal cells include stem cells derived from adipocytes, preadipocytes, lymphocytes, macrophages, fibroblasts, and vascular endothelial cells. The interactions of these various cell types with tumor cells are potentially important ways that obesity and inflammation can promote tumor growth, invasion, and metastasis and deserve much more research to examine how these processes interact with targeted therapies in the era of precision oncology.

NUTRITION AND IMMUNOTHERAPY

In addition to the advances in the genomic understanding of cancer, the discovery of immunotherapy has provided a new branch to Precision Oncology recognized by the award of the Nobel Prize in 2018 (Teillaud 2019). Immunotherapy unmasks even metastatic tumors to the immune system by blocking proteins generated by tumors. Immunotherapy can be used as either a first line or second line therapy (Li et al. 2018). When successful, this therapy leads to long-term effects compared to standard chemotherapy approaches. It has been observed that only a portion of cancers respond to this treatment (Shergold, Millar, and Nibbs 2019), providing the challenge to understand whether nutrition can improve the effectiveness of immunotherapy through effects on the gut microbiome.

Changes in the gut microbiome have been associated with responses to immunotherapy in melanoma patients and confirmed in animal model studies (Gopalakrishnan et al. 2018). In 2015 demonstrating that the composition of the gut microbiota could influence the response to immune checkpoint inhibitors including both cytotoxic T lymphocyte antigen-4 (CTLA-4) and programmed death receptor-1 (PD-1) (Vetizou et al. 2015, Sivan et al. 2015).

Following CTLA-4 blockade in mice, changes can be found in the gut microbiome in mice in association with reduced efficacy of immunotherapy. In germ-free mice or mice treated with broad-spectrum antibiotics the efficacy of immunotherapy is also significantly reduced. Probiotics can restore responses to immunotherapy in these mice and were shown to be involved in the anticancer effects of cyclophosphamide chemotherapy in mice. In patients, fecal microbiome transplants with samples rich in Bacteroides species were shown to result in improved responses to immunotherapy (Viaud et al. 2013, Vetizou et al. 2015).

Studies examining the effects of gut bacteria in response to PD-1 blockade found significant differences in response to immunotherapy in mice with different gut microbiomes. Probiotics given to mice with unfavorable gut microbiomes containing Bifidobacterium restored responses to PDL1-blockade. In these studies, there was stimulation of dendritic cell maturation and increased tumor-directed CD8+ T-cell lymphocyte activity (Sivan et al. 2015).

The critical question which remains is to examine how nutrients, supplements, and dietary patterns can affect and modulate responses to immunotherapy through effects on the gut-associated lymphoid tissue immune cells in direct communication with dietary constituents. Proinflammatory and anti-inflammatory effects of foods and dietary patterns have been demonstrated (Soldati et al. 2018). There is much to learn about optimal strategies to modulate the gut microbiome in order to enhance responses to cancer immunotherapy and to strengthen immune function during cancer treatment. There are many ways to change the microbiome including prebiotics, probiotics, and synbiotics that need to be tested carefully in the context of clinical trials. These studies also have the potential to develop new regimens before during and after cancer diagnosis and treatment to enhance immune surveillance of cancer.

CACHEXIA

Cancer cachexia is the advanced stage of malnutrition and energy imbalance in cancer patients characterized by a failure to gain weight despite the administration of apparently adequate calories or even aggressive nutrition via total parenteral nutrition (Evans et al. 1985). It has been estimated that the cachexia is the primary cause of death in 20% of cancer patients (Fearon, Arends, and Baracos 2013). Systemic inflammation, body weight loss, atrophy of adipose tissue and loss of skeletal muscle, and loss of immune function ultimately cause death. There are only a limited number of interventions which can be used to address this primary cause of death in many cancer patients, and a key remaining issue is the development of therapies that address energy imbalance and the relative roles of adipose tissue and muscle that lead to the development and progression of cancer cachexia.

Prior to muscle wasting in cancer cachexia, white adipose tissue converts to brown fat which may help to explain the energy imbalance in cancer cachexia. This so-called browning is associated with a phenotypic change that can be observed as an increased number of mitochondria within the brown fat cell and increased gene expression of uncoupling protein 1 (UCP1), which results in increased thermogenesis rather than adenosine triphosphate (ATP) synthesis. These metabolic changes in fat cells lead to increased lipid mobilization and energy imbalance in mice before there is muscle wasting. In animal studies, the inflammatory cytokine IL-6 increases UCP1 expression in white adipose tissue and treatments that reduce inflammation or beta-adrenergic blockade reduce white adipose tissue browning and reduce the degree of cachexia in mice. UCP1 staining is also observed in white adipose tissue from patients with cancer cachexia (Petruzzelli and Wagner 2016).

In mice with Lewis lung cancer implants, a reduced ATP synthesis rate can be demonstrated in muscle and has been implicated in the molecular mechanisms underlying muscle wasting in cancer cachexia. Whole genome studies in mice demonstrate atypical gene expression of regulatory genes for muscle including peroxisomal proliferator-activated receptor gamma coactivator 1 beta which is involved in mitochondrial biogenesis and the gene for mitochondrial uncoupling protein 3 (UCP3) (Constantinou et al. 2011). Cancer patients without cachexia or any limitation in activities of daily living demonstrate decreases in muscle efficiency during exercise such as knee extension which does not appear to be explained by muscle loss (Dalise et al. 2020). However, these conclusions need to be re-examined using newer methods of assessing muscle mass specifically (Evans et al. 2019). To what extent rehabilitative exercises begun at the time of diagnosis of cancer may be able to modify mitochondrial metabolism as was shown for the changes in muscle function occurring with aging and sedentary lifestyle is a remaining question to be examined (Naseeb and Volpe 2017). Assessment of skeletal muscle mass using the D3-Creatine dilution method in prospective cohort studies may reveal the course of sarcopenia and the potential benefits of treatments designed to reduce the rate of muscle loss in cancer patients before and during cancer malnutrition and cachexia (Evans et al. 2019).

Reduced ATP synthesis is linked to mitochondrial dysfunction, ultimately leading to skeletal muscle wasting and skeletal muscle dysfunction in cancer patients. A number of intracellular signals involved in protein turnover and wasting have been identified including those for inflammatory cytokines released by tumor cells or immune cells in the microenvironment including adjacent adipose tissue. Proinflammatory cytokines including tumor necrosis factor (TNF)α and IL-1 activate the nuclear factor-κB and p38 MAPK pathways resulting in an increased expression of the key E3 ligases and muscle atrophy F-box protein which mediate structural muscle protein breakdown and inhibition of protein synthesis (Glass 2010).

These questions around the changes in fat cells and muscle cells in cancer patients as cachexia is addressed or develops unchecked is an important area for future research that can support the development of novel therapeutics and nutritional strategies to combat cachexia. To date, despite existing studies and some clinical trials, effective methods to prevent and treat cancer cachexia are still lacking and remain an unanswered question in nutrition and cancer research.

CANCER METABOLISM AND AUTOPHAGY

Nutrition affects carcinogenesis beginning at the cellular level and extending throughout the body's homeostatic organ and tissue systems through the effects of diet and lifestyle. At the cellular level, the genetic changes that occur in cancer cells transform normal metabolic pathways in ways that benefit the growth of cancer cells and also utilize substrates in perturbed normal metabolic pathways in ways that promote tumor growth (Boroughs and DeBerardinis 2015). Autophagy in cells is a normal homeostatic mechanism that prevents accumulation of damaged proteins and organelles including mitochondria. In this way, autophagy limits oxidative stress and chronic tissue damage. By reducing oncogenic signaling through reactive oxygen species, normal autophagy acts to limit cancer initiation generally. The stimulation of homeostatic autophagy may be a useful strategy in cancer prevention. On the other hand cancers are demonstrated to induce autophagy for survival by recycling substrates to maintain mitochondrial energy production for the specialized metabolic needs of cancer cells for growth. Autophagy inhibition could be beneficial in some cases for cancer therapy. The investigation of the regulation of autophagy at a molecular level is extensive, but the extent to which inhibition of autophagy or stimulation of autophagy can be used in humans remains an open question (White, Mehnert, and Chan 2015).

Oncologists have largely overlooked tumor metabolism as a potential therapeutic target as a result of the view that cancer affects the genome primarily and that nutritional and metabolic changes were secondary. Metabolism was put aside as molecular approaches targeted the driver mutations in cancer cells. The Warburg effect in cancer cells links anaerobic glucose metabolism to cancer cell growth but within a tumor there is heterogeneity of both aerobic and anaerobic metabolism related to the oxygen tension in tumor tissues (Liberti and Locasale 2016). Changes in glutamine catabolism also interact with glucose metabolism and glutaminase inhibitors have been examined for their potential use in therapy (Vander Heiden and DeBerardinis 2017). There are also changes within cancer cells in de novo synthesis and catabolism of fatty acids providing further targets for therapy (Munir et al. 2019). All of these changes are demonstrable in basic studies but have not been translated into clinical trials that integrate nutrition into cancer therapy.

There are several examples of recently discovered small molecules that target cellular proteins controlling cancer cell metabolism including cyclin-dependent kinase 4 and 6, poly(adenosine diphosphate-ribose) polymerase, and phosphoinositide 3-kinase in breast cancer among others (Phan, Yeung, and Lee 2014, Nur Husna et al. 2018). The remaining question is whether these and future metabolic inhibitors of cancer cell growth based on genetic profiling and precision oncology can yield less toxic and more cancer-specific treatments for cancer.

EPIGENETICS

Research for a connection between diet and human cancer has led to the realization that altering diet can alter the epigenetic state of cancer-associated genes (Nebbioso et al. 2018). DNA methylation, chromatin remodeling, histone modification, and noncoding RNA are all implicated in cancer prevention and treatment. It has been demonstrated in animal studies that epigenetic alterations have the potential to increase or decrease cancer risk. However, the conclusion that diet is linked directly to epigenetic alterations and that these epigenetic alterations directly increase or decrease the risk of human cancer is a critical question that remains in nutrition and cancer research.

Nutrition can alter gene expression as well as the susceptibility to age-related chronic diseases, including common forms of cancer, through changes in the epigenome through mechanisms that include DNA dietary intakes, and microbiota exhibit daily and seasonal variations which can affect gene expression as metabolic pathways shift to meet changing demands (Riscuta et al. 2018). DNA methylation has been linked to both aging and cancer (Pal and Tyler 2016, Sapienza and Issa 2016). The effects of nutrients on the epigenetics of cancer have the potential to lead to the development of dietary supplements that can be used in conjunction with established cancer therapies or in cancer prevention. Clinical studies are critical to translate findings from animal studies in order to evaluate the efficacy and safety of dietary compounds, and to establish the most efficient strategies for implementation.

ANGIOGENESIS

The tumor microenvironment consists of not only tumor cells but also various cellular components including endothelial cells, pericytes, fibroblasts, inflammatory cells, and red blood cells (Kim and Bae 2016). Cancer cells often produce signaling molecules to manipulate host cells in the local microenvironment to facilitate their detachment, invasion, and metastasis. Direct stimulation of angiogenesis by the vascular endothelial growth factor signal pathway can promote both tumor growth and metastasis (Melincovici et al. 2018). The complex tumor microenvironment and the influence of nutrition have never been fully investigated and remain an important area for basic and clinical investigation.

BOTANICALS

The identification and characterization of plant-based botanical dietary supplements have progressed significantly. Methods including plant genetics and metabolomics can monitor the impact of changes in cultivation practices on the phytochemical contents and physiological effects of botanical dietary supplements. The therapeutic and preventive anticancer effects of botanicals are demonstrated by the observation that about a third of all drugs approved for cancer treatment including paclitaxel and vincristine are based on compounds found in plants (Benatrehina et al. 2018). The synergy of multiple phytochemicals in botanicals on endpoints including tumor cell proliferation and apoptosis has been demonstrated repeatedly. This synergy which is little investigation in classical pharmacotherapy provides a potential pathway to increased efficacy with reduced toxicity. The exploration and characterization of botanicals may lead not only to new drugs but also to botanical dietary supplements based on food extracts that concentrate beneficial compounds. Many fruits and vegetables have been bred and domesticated to eliminate the bitter polyphenols found in the original plants of ancient times. In more recent times, many varieties of fruits and vegetables are grown under conditions where production of antioxidant phytochemicals is not monitored or valued. Phytochemicals found in botanical are known to have useful properties including inhibition of angiogenesis, oxidant stress, and inflammation. Many botanicals are well tolerated and are inactivated by metabolic pathways and in the liver, kidney, and microbiome which limit toxicity. Unfortunately, regulatory authorities have taken a dim view of botanicals emphasizing toxicity and lack of regulation (Brown 2017). The appropriate regulation of good manufacturing practices and postmarketing surveillance for safety combined with new initiatives in clinical research could make use of botanical dietary supplement part of cancer prevention, cancer treatment, and prevention of relapse strategies in the future.

BIG DATA

Big data that combine genomic data with nutrition information in conjunction with treatment and outcome data across multiple studies have the potential to transform our understanding of how precision oncology and precision nutrition may interact. Data sharing is critical in advancing this agenda. The NCI Blue Ribbon Panel report from the Cancer Moonshot Initiative (2016) was advocated in response to the call for broader data sharing on cancer genomics. In response, several other big-data initiatives including the National Institute of Health (NIH) Genomic Data Commons, the American Association for Cancer Research (AACR) Project GENIE, and the Global Alliance for Genomics and Health have been established in order to centralize and standardize genomic data on cancer and accelerate progress toward identifying improved therapeutic strategies (Siu et al. 2016, Jensen et al. 2017, AACR Project GENIE Consortium 2017). A critical question remaining for nutrition and cancer research is how to integrate with these big data efforts in a meaningful way that leads to new insights into nutrition and cancer.

The current evidence linking diet, exercise, and physical activity to cancer in humans has largely relied on self-reported questionnaire data. Studies on adiposity and cancer risk rely on weight and height to estimate body mass index. New validated measures of body shape using 3D cameras have the potential to add precision data on body shape including 14 circumferences and estimated body composition using noninvasive infrared radiation (Ng et al. 2019). To refine current concepts researchers have started incorporating other emerging technologies for measuring diet and physical activity in human populations including the use of wearable devices that monitor movement. Using Global Positioning System (GPS) satellite data, it is possible to follow the movements of individuals in the environment although this has raised issues of individual freedom and privacy (Scully et al. 2017). Monitoring food intake has been more challenging despite attempts to use food photography to estimate portion size (Most et al. 2018).

Blood glucose levels can now be monitored continuously over 14 days as individuals consume a diet of foods that can be recorded (Bailey et al. 2015). There is already a great deal of evidence that individuals react differently in terms of postprandial blood glucose increases after eating the same food (Bailey et al. 2015). This new technology could be applied to specific foods and dietary patterns and supplemented with monitoring of hormone levels that regulate metabolism in cancer patients.

Significant technological advances have been made in machine-learning technologies, graphics processing, cloud computing, and data storage (DeGregory et al. 2018). These big data computing advances may make it feasible to begin to explore trends and patterns of the effects of nutrition on early-stage cancers in numbers never imagined before. A critical remaining question in nutrition and cancer research is how to combine multiple, independent data collections from social media, online search and food shopping histories, exercise and physical movement data, and clinical, pathological, and molecular clinical cancer data through artificial intelligence and predictive algorithms to integrate and analyze the interactions of nutrition and cancer in prevention, treatment, and prevention of relapse.

PUBLIC POLICY

Although much has been done to develop national guidelines on nutrition and cancer there is still much that needs to be done to translate these guidelines into actions by the public that reduce cancer risk (Di Sebastiano et al. 2019). There has been consistent messaging around healthy eating for decades including summaries of the evidence supporting the role of diet and nutrition in cancer prevention. However, this advice is unfortunately seen as inconsistent by both healthcare providers and the public (Niederdeppe and Levy 2007). In addition, many in the public have the fatalistic view that nothing can be done to prevent cancer. These beliefs are more prevalent among minorities who suffer other health disparities. While issuing guidelines appears to be highly ineffective in changing behavior, changes in economic and farm policy and food production can increase nutritional habits that are recognized as leading to reductions in cancer risk. Effective behavioral strategies to motivate change need to be employed rather than simply providing information and education. Solutions to minority health disparities in nutrition and cancer remain unsolved.

CONCLUSION

This book has been written at an exciting time in the science of nutrition and in the understanding of carcinogenesis. The advances in genomic technology have advanced a new understanding of the biology of cancer. At the same time, the discovery of the microbiome and its association with immune function has opened new vistas for research in nutrition and cancer. Basic scientists and clinical investigators have the opportunity to translate advances from the bench to the bedside if the typical issues in nutrition research can be overcome. Artificial intelligence applied to big data sets holds out the promise of developing overarching principles and information from the complexities of diet, nutrition, physical activity, and lifestyle. The challenge of integrating information from different fields each with their own jargon that is constantly evolving requires more than ever a dedication to lifelong learning by researchers and clinicians working in cancer prevention, cancer treatment, and the prevention of recurrence.

REFERENCES

AACR Project GENIE Consortium. 2017. "AACR Project GENIE: Powering precision medicine through an international consortium." *Cancer Discov* 7 (8):818–31. doi: 10.1158/2159-8290.CD-17-0151.

Avgerinos, K. I., N. Spyrou, C. S. Mantzoros, and M. Dalamaga. 2019. "Obesity and cancer risk: Emerging biological mechanisms and perspectives." *Metabolism* 92:121–35. doi: 10.1016/j.metabol.2018.11.001.

Bailey, T., B. W. Bode, M. P. Christiansen, L. J. Klaff, and S. Alva. 2015. "The performance and usability of a factory-calibrated flash glucose monitoring system." *Diabetes Technol Ther* 17 (11):787–94. doi: 10.1089/dia.2014.0378.

Benatrehina, P. A., L. Pan, C. B. Naman, J. Li, and A. D. Kinghorn. 2018. "Usage, biological activity, and safety of selected botanical dietary supplements consumed in the United States." *J Tradit Complement Med* 8 (2):267–77. doi: 10.1016/j.jtcme.2018.01.006.

Bochet, L., C. Lehuede, S. Dauvillier, Y. Y. Wang, B. Dirat, V. Laurent, C. Dray, R. Guiet, I. Maridonneau-Parini, S. Le Gonidec, B. Couderc, G. Escourrou, P. Valet, and C. Muller. 2013. "Adipocyte-derived fibroblasts promote tumor progression and contribute to the desmoplastic reaction in breast cancer." *Cancer Res* 73 (18):5657–68. doi: 10.1158/0008-5472.CAN-13-0530.

Boroughs, L. K., and R. J. DeBerardinis. 2015. "Metabolic pathways promoting cancer cell survival and growth." *Nat Cell Biol* 17 (4):351–9. doi: 10.1038/ncb3124.

Brown, A. C. 2017. "An overview of herb and dietary supplement efficacy, safety and government regulations in the United States with suggested improvements. Part 1 of 5 series." *Food Chem Toxicol* 107 (Pt A):449–71. doi: 10.1016/j.fct.2016.11.001.

Constantinou, C., C. C. Fontes de Oliveira, D. Mintzopoulos, S. Busquets, J. He, M. Kesarwani, M. Mindrinos, L. G. Rahme, J. M. Argiles, and A. A. Tzika. 2011. "Nuclear magnetic resonance in conjunction with functional genomics suggests mitochondrial dysfunction in a murine model of cancer cachexia." *Int J Mol Med* 27 (1):15–24. doi: 10.3892/ijmm.2010.557.

Dalise, S., P. Tropea, L. Galli, A. Sbrana, and C. Chisari. 2020. "Muscle function impairment in cancer patients in pre-cachexia stage." *Eur J Transl Myol* 30 (2):8931. doi: 10.4081/ejtm.2019.8931.

DeGregory, K. W., P. Kuiper, T. DeSilvio, J. D. Pleuss, R. Miller, J. W. Roginski, C. B. Fisher, D. Harness, S. Viswanath, S. B. Heymsfield, I. Dungan, and D. M. Thomas. 2018. "A review of machine learning in obesity." *Obes Rev* 19 (5):668–85. doi: 10.1111/obr.12667.

Di Sebastiano, K. M., G. Murthy, K. L. Campbell, S. Desroches, and R. A. Murphy. 2019. "Nutrition and cancer prevention: Why is the evidence lost in translation?" *Adv Nutr* 10 (3):410–8. doi: 10.1093/advances/nmy089.

Evans, W. K., R. Makuch, G. H. Clamon, R. Feld, R. S. Weiner, E. Moran, R. Blum, F. A. Shepherd, K. N. Jeejeebhoy, and W. D. DeWys. 1985. "Limited impact of total parenteral nutrition on nutritional status during treatment for small cell lung cancer." *Cancer Res* 45 (7):3347–53.

Evans, W. J., M. Hellerstein, E. Orwoll, S. Cummings, and P. M. Cawthon. 2019. "D3-creatine dilution and the importance of accuracy in the assessment of skeletal muscle mass." *J Cachexia Sarcopenia Muscle* 10 (1):14–21. doi: 10.1002/jcsm.12390.

Fearon, K., J. Arends, and V. Baracos. 2013. "Understanding the mechanisms and treatment options in cancer cachexia." *Nat Rev Clin Oncol* 10 (2):90–9. doi: 10.1038/nrclinonc.2012.209.

Gallagher, E. J., and D. LeRoith. 2015. "Obesity and diabetes: The increased risk of cancer and cancer-related mortality." *Physiol Rev* 95 (3):727–48. doi: 10.1152/physrev.00030.2014.

Glass, D. J. 2010. "Signaling pathways perturbing muscle mass." *Curr Opin Clin Nutr Metab Care* 13 (3):225–9. doi: 10.1097/mco.0b013e32833862df.

Gopalakrishnan, V., B. A. Helmink, C. N. Spencer, A. Reuben, and J. A. Wargo. 2018. "The influence of the gut microbiome on cancer, immunity, and cancer immunotherapy." *Cancer Cell* 33 (4):570–80. doi: 10.1016/j.ccell.2018.03.015.

Han, J. M., and M. K. Levings. 2013. "Immune regulation in obesity-associated adipose inflammation." *J Immunol* 191 (2):527–32. doi: 10.4049/jimmunol.1301035.

Jensen, M. A., V. Ferretti, R. L. Grossman, and L. M. Staudt. 2017. "The NCI genomic data commons as an engine for precision medicine." *Blood* 130 (4):453–9. doi: 10.1182/blood-2017-03-735654.

Kim, J., and J. S. Bae. 2016. "Tumor-associated macrophages and neutrophils in tumor microenvironment." *Mediators Inflamm* 2016:6058147. doi: 10.1155/2016/6058147.

Kolb, R., F. S. Sutterwala, and W. Zhang. 2016. "Obesity and cancer: Inflammation bridges the two." *Curr Opin Pharmacol* 29:77–89. doi: 10.1016/j.coph.2016.07.005.

Laurent, V., A. Guerard, C. Mazerolles, S. Le Gonidec, A. Toulet, L. Nieto, F. Zaidi, B. Majed, D. Garandeau, Y. Socrier, M. Golzio, T. Cadoudal, K. Chaoui, C. Dray, B. Monsarrat, O. Schiltz, Y. Y. Wang, B. Couderc, P. Valet, B. Malavaud, and C. Muller. 2016. "Periprostatic adipocytes act as a driving force for prostate cancer progression in obesity." *Nat Commun* 7:10230. doi: 10.1038/ncomms10230.

Li, Z., W. Song, M. Rubinstein, and D. Liu. 2018. "Recent updates in cancer immunotherapy: A comprehensive review and perspective of the 2018 China Cancer Immunotherapy Workshop in Beijing." *J Hematol Oncol* 11 (1):142. doi: 10.1186/s13045-018-0684-3.

Liberti, M. V., and J. W. Locasale. 2016. "The Warburg effect: How does it benefit cancer cells?" *Trends Biochem Sci* 41 (3):211–8. doi: 10.1016/j.tibs.2015.12.001.

Melincovici, C. S., A. B. Bosca, S. Susman, M. Marginean, C. Mihu, M. Istrate, I. M. Moldovan, A. L. Roman, and C. M. Mihu. 2018. "Vascular endothelial growth factor (VEGF): Key factor in normal and pathological angiogenesis." *Rom J Morphol Embryol* 59 (2):455–67.

Most, J., P. M. Vallo, A. D. Altazan, L. A. Gilmore, E. F. Sutton, L. E. Cain, J. H. Burton, C. K. Martin, and L. M. Redman. 2018. "Food photography is not an accurate measure of energy intake in obese, pregnant women." *J Nutr* 148 (4):658–63. doi: 10.1093/jn/nxy009.

Munir, R., J. Lisec, J. V. Swinnen, and N. Zaidi. 2019. "Lipid metabolism in cancer cells under metabolic stress." *Br J Cancer* 120 (12):1090–8. doi: 10.1038/s41416-019-0451-4.

Naseeb, M. A., and S. L. Volpe. 2017. "Protein and exercise in the prevention of sarcopenia and aging." *Nutr Res* 40:1–20. doi: 10.1016/j.nutres.2017.01.001.

Nebbioso, A., F. P. Tambaro, C. Dell'Aversana, and L. Altucci. 2018. "Cancer epigenetics: Moving forward." *PLoS Genet* 14 (6):e1007362. doi: 10.1371/journal.pgen.1007362.

Ng, B. K., M. J. Sommer, M. C. Wong, I. Pagano, Y. Nie, B. Fan, S. Kennedy, B. Bourgeois, N. Kelly, Y. E. Liu, P. Hwaung, A. K. Garber, D. Chow, C. Vaisse, B. Curless, S. B. Heymsfield, and J. A. Shepherd. 2019. "Detailed 3-dimensional body shape features predict body composition, blood metabolites, and functional strength: the Shape Up! studies." *Am J Clin Nutr* 110 (6):1316–26. doi: 10.1093/ajcn/nqz218.

Niederdeppe, J., and A. G. Levy. 2007. "Fatalistic beliefs about cancer prevention and three prevention behaviors." *Cancer Epidemiol Biomarkers Prev* 16 (5):998–1003. doi: 10.1158/1055-9965.EPI-06-0608.

Nieman, K. M., H. A. Kenny, C. V. Penicka, A. Ladanyi, R. Buell-Gutbrod, M. R. Zillhardt, I. L. Romero, M. S. Carey, G. B. Mills, G. S. Hotamisligil, S. D. Yamada, M. E. Peter, K. Gwin, and E. Lengyel. 2011. "Adipocytes promote ovarian cancer metastasis and provide energy for rapid tumor growth." *Nat Med* 17 (11):1498–503. doi: 10.1038/nm.2492.

Nur Husna, S. M., H. T. Tan, R. Mohamud, A. Dyhl-Polk, and K. K. Wong. 2018. "Inhibitors targeting CDK4/6, PARP and PI3K in breast cancer: A review." *Ther Adv Med Oncol* 10. doi: 10.1177/1758835918808509.

Pal, S., and J. K. Tyler. 2016. "Epigenetics and aging." *Sci Adv* 2 (7):e1600584. doi: 10.1126/sciadv.1600584.

Park, J., T. S. Morley, M. Kim, D. J. Clegg, and P. E. Scherer. 2014. "Obesity and cancer--mechanisms underlying tumour progression and recurrence." *Nat Rev Endocrinol* 10 (8):455–65. doi: 10.1038/nrendo.2014.94.

Petruzzelli, M., and E. F. Wagner. 2016. "Mechanisms of metabolic dysfunction in cancer-associated cachexia." *Genes Dev* 30 (5):489–501. doi: 10.1101/gad.276733.115.

Phan, L. M., S. C. Yeung, and M. H. Lee. 2014. "Cancer metabolic reprogramming: Importance, main features, and potentials for precise targeted anti-cancer therapies." *Cancer Biol Med* 11 (1):1–19. doi: 10.7497/j.issn.2095-3941.2014.01.001.

Ramjiawan, R. R., A. W. Griffioen, and D. G. Duda. 2017. "Anti-angiogenesis for cancer revisited: Is there a role for combinations with immunotherapy?" *Angiogenesis* 20 (2):185–204. doi: 10.1007/s10456-017-9552-y.

Riscuta, G., D. Xi, D. Pierre-Victor, P. Starke-Reed, J. Khalsa, and L. Duffy. 2018. "Diet, microbiome, and epigenetics in the era of precision medicine." *Methods Mol Biol* 1856:141–56. doi: 10.1007/978-1-4939-8751-1_8.

Saadeh, C., D. Bright, and D. Rustem. 2019. "Precision medicine in oncology pharmacy practice." *Acta Med Acad* 48 (1):90–104. doi: 10.5644/ama2006-124.246.

Sapienza, C., and J. P. Issa. 2016. "Diet, nutrition, and cancer epigenetics." *Annu Rev Nutr* 36:665–81. doi: 10.1146/annurev-nutr-121415-112634.

Scully, J. Y., A. Vernez Moudon, P. M. Hurvitz, A. Aggarwal, and A. Drewnowski. 2017. "GPS or travel diary: Comparing spatial and temporal characteristics of visits to fast food restaurants and supermarkets." *PLoS One* 12 (4):e0174859. doi: 10.1371/journal.pone.0174859.

Shergold, A. L., R. Millar, and R. J. B. Nibbs. 2019. "Understanding and overcoming the resistance of cancer to PD-1/PD-L1 blockade." *Pharmacol Res* 145:104258. doi: 10.1016/j.phrs.2019.104258.

Siu, L. L., M. Lawler, D. Haussler, B. M. Knoppers, J. Lewin, D. J. Vis, R. G. Liao, F. Andre, I. Banks, J. C. Barrett, C. Caldas, A. A. Camargo, R. C. Fitzgerald, M. Mao, J. E. Mattison, W. Pao, W. R. Sellers, P. Sullivan, B. T. Teh, R. L. Ward, J. C. ZenKlusen, C. L. Sawyers, and E. E. Voest. 2016. "Facilitating a culture of responsible and effective sharing of cancer genome data." *Nat Med* 22 (5):464–71. doi: 10.1038/nm.4089.

Sivan, A., L. Corrales, N. Hubert, J. B. Williams, K. Aquino-Michaels, Z. M. Earley, F. W. Benyamin, Y. M. Lei, B. Jabri, M. L. Alegre, E. B. Chang, and T. F. Gajewski. 2015. "Commensal bifidobacterium promotes antitumor immunity and facilitates anti-PD-L1 efficacy." *Science* 350 (6264):1084–9. doi: 10.1126/science.aac4255.

Soldati, L., L. Di Renzo, E. Jirillo, P. A. Ascierto, F. M. Marincola, and A. De Lorenzo. 2018. "The influence of diet on anti-cancer immune responsiveness." *J Transl Med* 16 (1):75. doi: 10.1186/s12967-018-1448-0.

Steck, S. E., and E. A. Murphy. 2020. "Dietary patterns and cancer risk." *Nat Rev Cancer* 20 (2):125–38. doi: 10.1038/s41568-019-0227-4.

Sun, K., C. M. Kusminski, and P. E. Scherer. 2011. "Adipose tissue remodeling and obesity." *J Clin Invest* 121 (6):2094–101. doi: 10.1172/JCI45887.

Teillaud, J. L. 2019. "Cancer immunotherapy crowned with Nobel prize in physiology or medicine awarded to James Allison and Tasuku Honjo." *Med Sci (Paris)* 35 (4):365–6. doi: 10.1051/medsci/2019073.

Vander Heiden, M. G., and R. J. DeBerardinis. 2017. "Understanding the intersections between metabolism and cancer biology." *Cell* 168 (4):657–69. doi: 10.1016/j.cell.2016.12.039.

Vernieri, C., F. Nichetti, A. Raimondi, S. Pusceddu, M. Platania, F. Berrino, and F. de Braud. 2018. "Diet and supplements in cancer prevention and treatment: Clinical evidences and future perspectives." *Crit Rev Oncol Hematol* 123:57–73. doi: 10.1016/j.critrevonc.2018.01.002.

Vetizou, M., J. M. Pitt, R. Daillere, P. Lepage, N. Waldschmitt, C. Flament, S. Rusakiewicz, B. Routy, M. P. Roberti, C. P. Duong, V. Poirier-Colame, A. Roux, S. Becharef, S. Formenti, E. Golden, S. Cording, G. Eberl, A. Schlitzer, F. Ginhoux, S. Mani, T. Yamazaki, N. Jacquelot, D. P. Enot, M. Berard, J. Nigou, P. Opolon, A. Eggermont, P. L. Woerther, E. Chachaty, N. Chaput, C. Robert, C. Mateus, G. Kroemer, D. Raoult, I. G. Boneca, F. Carbonnel, M. Chamaillard, and L. Zitvogel. 2015. "Anticancer immunotherapy by CTLA-4 blockade relies on the gut microbiota." *Science* 350 (6264):1079–84. doi: 10.1126/science.aad1329.

Viaud, S., F. Saccheri, G. Mignot, T. Yamazaki, R. Daillere, D. Hannani, D. P. Enot, C. Pfirschke, C. Engblom, M. J. Pittet, A. Schlitzer, F. Ginhoux, L. Apetoh, E. Chachaty, P. L. Woerther, G. Eberl, M. Berard, C. Ecobichon, D. Clermont, C. Bizet, V. Gaboriau-Routhiau, N. Cerf-Bensussan, P. Opolon, N. Yessaad, E. Vivier, B. Ryffel, C. O. Elson, J. Dore, G. Kroemer, P. Lepage, I. G. Boneca, F. Ghiringhelli, and L. Zitvogel. 2013. "The intestinal microbiota modulates the anticancer immune effects of cyclophosphamide." *Science* 342 (6161):971–6. doi: 10.1126/science.1240537.

Weisberg, S. P., D. McCann, M. Desai, M. Rosenbaum, R. L. Leibel, and A. W. Ferrante, Jr. 2003. "Obesity is associated with macrophage accumulation in adipose tissue." *J Clin Invest* 112 (12):1796–808. doi: 10.1172/JCI19246.

White, E., J. M. Mehnert, and C. S. Chan. 2015. "Autophagy, metabolism, and cancer." *Clin Cancer Res* 21 (22):5037–46. doi: 10.1158/1078-0432.CCR-15-0490.

Yang, L., E. S. Calay, J. Fan, A. Arduini, R. C. Kunz, S. P. Gygi, A. Yalcin, S. Fu, and G. S. Hotamisligil. 2015. "METABOLISM: S-Nitrosylation links obesity-associated inflammation to endoplasmic reticulum dysfunction." *Science* 349 (6247):500–6. doi: 10.1126/science.aaa0079.

Zeevi, D., T. Korem, N. Zmora, D. Israeli, D. Rothschild, A. Weinberger, O. Ben-Yacov, D. Lador, T. Avnit-Sagi, M. Lotan-Pompan, J. Suez, J. A. Mahdi, E. Matot, G. Malka, N. Kosower, M. Rein, G. Zilberman-Schapira, L. Dohnalova, M. Pevsner-Fischer, R. Bikovsky, Z. Halpern, E. Elinav, and E. Segal. 2015. "Personalized nutrition by prediction of glycemic responses." *Cell* 163 (5):1079–94. doi: 10.1016/j.cell.2015.11.001.

Index

Note: **Bold** page numbers refer to tables and *italic* page numbers refer to figures.